PEDIATRIC EMERGENCY MEDICINE

PEDIATRIC EMERGENCY MEDICINE

Senior Editor

Frank E. Ehrlich, MD
Head of the Department of Emergency/Trauma Service
The Buffalo General Hospital
Buffalo, New York

Co-Editors

Fred J. Heldrich, MD
Chairman of the Department of Pediatrics
St. Agnes Hospital
and
Associate Professor of Pediatrics
The Johns Hopkins School of Medicine
Baltimore, Maryland

J.J. Tepas III, MD
Associate Professor of Pediatric Surgery
University of Florida
Jacksonville, Florida

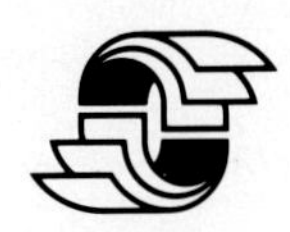

AN ASPEN PUBLICATION®
Aspen Publishers, Inc.
Rockville, Maryland
Royal Tunbridge Wells
1987

Library of Congress Cataloging-in-Publication Data

Pediatric emergency medicine.

"An Aspen publication."
Includes bibliographies and index.
1. Pediatric emergencies. I. Ehrlich, Frank E., 1939- . II. Heldrich, Fred J. III. Tepas, J.J.
[DNLM: 1. Emergencies — in infancy & childhood — handbooks. 2. Emergency Medicine — in infancy & childhood — handbooks. WS 39 P3713]
RJ370.P45 1987 618.92'025 86-22347
ISBN: 0-87189-298-7

The authors have made every effort to ensure the accuracy of the information herein. However, appropriate information sources should be consulted, especially for new or unfamiliar procedures. It is the responsibility of every practitioner to evaluate the appropriateness of a particular opinion in the context of actual clinical situations and with due considerations to new developments. Authors, editors, and the publisher cannot be held responsible for any typographical or other errors found in this book.

Editorial Services: Ruth Bloom

Library of Congress Catalog Card Number: 86-22347
ISBN: 0-87189-298-7

Printed in the United States of America

1 2 3 4 5

Table of Contents

PART IV DISORDERS OF THE CENTRAL NERVOUS SYSTEM

PART V GASTROENTEROLOGIC DISORDERS

Contributors

Robert J. Ancona, MD
Chief, Department of Pediatrics
Union Memorial Hospital
Baltimore, MD
Assistant Professor of Pediatrics
University of Maryland School of Medicine
Baltimore, MD
Assistant Professor of Pediatrics
Johns Hopkins University School of Medicine
Baltimore, MD

Michael B. Andorsky, MD
Assistant Professor of Pediatrics
Johns Hopkins University School of Medicine
Baltimore, MD

Richard J. Andrassy, MD
Division of Pediatric Surgery
University of Texas Health Science Center
Houston, TX

Robert M. Arensman, MD
Chief of Pediatric Surgery
Oschner Clinic
New Orleans, LA

Pat L. Aulicino, MD
Associate Professor of Orthopedic Surgery
Eastern Virginia Medical School
Norfolk, Virginia
Hand Surgery Associates
Chesapeake, Virginia

William Carl Bailey, MD
Director, Burn Center
Department of General Pediatric Surgery
The Children's Hospital
Denver, CO

Nancy K. Barnett, MD
Assistant Professor of Pediatrics and Dermatology
Johns Hopkins University School of Medicine
Baltimore, MD

Mark F. Bellinger, MD
Chief, Pediatric Urology
Children's Hospital of Pittsburgh
Associate Professor of Surgery
University of Pittsburgh Medical School
Pittsburgh, Pennsylvania

Catherine DeAngelis, MD, MPH
Deputy Director
Department of Pediatrics
Johns Hopkins Medical Institutions
Baltimore, MD

Bernard J. D'Souza, MD
Associate Professor of Pediatrics
Chief, Division of Pediatric Neurology
Duke University Medical Center
Durham, NC

Theodore E. DuPuy, MD
Clinical Professor of Orthopedics
Eastern Virginia Medical School
Norfolk, Virginia
Hand Surgery Associates
Chesapeake, VA

Frank E. Ehrlich, MD
Head of the Department of Emergency/Trauma Service
The Buffalo General Hospital
Buffalo, New York

Kenneth W. Falterman, MD
Chief, Division of Pediatric Surgery
Associate Professor of Surgery and Pediatrics
Louisiana State University Medical Center, New Orleans
Staff Surgeon
Ochsner Clinic
New Orleans, Louisiana

B. Gregory Fernandopulle, MD
Director, Division of Child and Adolescent Psychiatry
St. Agnes Hospital
Baltimore, MD

Francis T. Ferry, MD
Underwood-Memorial Hospital
Thomas Jefferson University
Family Practice Residency Program
Woodbury, NJ

Arnold D. Gale, MD
Assistant Professor
Department of Neurology
Department of Child Health and Development
George Washington University School of Medicine and Health Sciences
Children's Hospital National Medical Center
Washington, DC

Howard E. Gendelman, MD
Clinical and Research Fellow
Departments of Medicine and Neurology
Johns Hopkins University School of Medicine
Baltimore, MD

E. Stevers Golladay, MD
Professor of Surgery and Pediatrics
Chief, Pediatric Surgery
Arkansas Children's Hospital
Little Rock, AK

Jay L. Grosfeld, MD
James Whitcombe Riley Hospital for Children
Indiana University Medical Center
Indianapolis, Indiana

Jean-Jacques Gunning, MD
Captain, Medical Corps
United States Navy (Retired)
Medical Director
St. Agnes Hospital
Baltimore, MD
Instructor, Department of Internal Medicine
University of Maryland School of Medicine
Baltimore, MD

Harold E. Harrison, MD
Professor Emeritus of Pediatrics
Johns Hopkins University School of Medicine
Baltimore, MD

Dennis L. Headings, MD
Assistant Professor of Pediatrics
Johns Hopkins University School of Medicine
Baltimore, MD

Fred J. Heldrich, MD
Chairman, Department of Pediatrics
St. Agnes Hospital
Associate Professor of Pediatrics
The Johns Hopkins University School of Medicine
Baltimore, Maryland

William Herndon, MD
Associate Professor of Orthopedics
University of Oklahoma School of Medicine
Department of Orthopedic Surgery
Children's Memorial Hospital
Oklahoma City, OK

Dennis J. Hoelzer, MD
Assistant Professor, Pediatric Surgery
University of Oklahoma
College of Medicine
Oklahoma City, OK

Antoinette F. Hood, MD
Associate Professor of Dermatology
Johns Hopkins University School of Medicine
Baltimore, MD

Dennis L. Hoover, MD
Director, Pediatric Urology
Associate Professor of Surgery
University of South Florida
College of South Florida
College of Medicine
Tampa, FL

Thomas H. Howard, MD
Assistant Professor of Pediatrics
Childrens Hospital of Alabama
University of Alabama
Birmingham, AL

Raymond S. Kandt, MD
Assistant Professor
Division of Pediatric Neurology
Department of Pediatrics
Duke University Medical Center
Durham, NC

Richard A. Kaplan, MD
Clinical Fellow
Children's Hospital of Philadelphia
Research Fellow
Department of Physics and Biochemistry
University of Pennsylvania
Philadelphia, PA

Michael S. Kappy, MD, PhD
Program Director
Children's Health Center
St. Joseph's Hospital and Medical Center
Phoenix, AZ

Charles R. Medani, MD
Assistant Professor of Pediatrics
University of Maryland School of Medicine
Baltimore, MD

William H. Meyer, MD
Assistant Professor of Pediatrics
University of Virginia School of Medicine
Charlottesville, VA

William C. Mobley, MD
Department of Neurology
University of California, San Francisco
San Francisco, CA

Randall W. Powell, MD
Associate Professor of Surgery
Department of Pediatrics
University of South Alabama
Mobile, AL

Arnold M. Salzberg, MD
Professor of Surgery
Medical College of Virginia
Richmond, Virginia

Dennis W. Shermeta, MD
Professor of Surgery and Surgeon-in-Chief
Wyler Children's Hospital
University of Chicago
Chicago, IL

Charles I. Shubin, MD
Assistant Professor of Pediatrics
Johns Hopkins University School of Medicine
Baltimore, MD

Edward M. Sills, MD
Associate Professor of Pediatrics
Johns Hopkins University School of Medicine
Baltimore, MD

Perry W. Stafford, MD
Chief Resident, Pediatric Surgery
Children's Hospital
Columbus, OH

Dennis C. Stokes, MD
Assistant Professor of Pediatrics
Johns Hopkins University School of Medicine
Baltimore, MD

Bruce D. Taylor, MD
Director of Anesthesia and Attending Physician
Pediatric Intensive Care Unit
Cook-Fort Worth Children's Medical Center
Fort Worth, Texas

J. J. Tepas III, MD
Associate Professor of Pediatric Surgery
University of Florida
Jacksonville, Florida

Charles Turner, MD
Assistant Professor of Surgery
Division of Pediatric Surgery
Bowman Gray School of Medicine
Wake Forest University
Winston-Salem, NC

Dennis W. Vane, MD
James Whitcombe Riley Hospital for Children
Indiana University Medical Center
Indianapolis, Indiana

John D. Ward, MD
Department of Neurosurgery
Medical College of Virginia
Virginia Commonwealth University
Richmond, VA

Thomas R. Weber, MD
Cardinal-Glennon Children's Hospital
St. Louis, MS

Thomas V. Whalen, CDR, MC, USN
Division of Pediatric Surgery
Naval Hospital
Portsmouth, Virginia

William Ernest Winter, MD
Assistant Professor of Pathology and Pediatrics
University of Florida College of Medicine
Gainesville, FL

Stephen A. Wolf, MD
Associate Professor of Surgery
Division of Pediatric Surgery
Marshall University School of Medicine
Huntington, West Virginia

Robert A. Wood, MD
Fellow, Pediatric Allergy and Immunology
Johns Hopkins University School of Medicine
Baltimore, Maryland

Jerry S. Wolinsky, MD
Professor, Department of Neurology
University of Texas Health Sciences Center
Houston, Texas

Andrew M. Yeager, MD
Assistant Professor of Oncology and Pediatrics
Johns Hopkins University School of Medicine
Baltimore, Maryland

Kenneth G. Zahka, MD
Assistant Professor of Pediatrics
Division of Pediatric Cardiology
Johns Hopkins University School of Medicine
Baltimore, Maryland

Moritz M. Ziegler, MD
Children's Hospital
Philadelphia, PA

Foreword

Infants, children, and youths, the special focus of this book, constitute one third of the population of this country. Although they fall prey to unique diseases, most of their disorders are recognizable to physicians who deal primarily with adults. Unfortunately, the different substrate upon which the disease acts often precludes identical action and requires alteration in information and thinking. In pediatric, surgical, and general emergency units, this need for pediatric orientation is compounded by a virtual epidemic of young patients requesting care for acute and chronic medical illnesses and major and minor surgical complaints.

Physicians and parents know that infants and children never become ill at convenient times. Pain always worsens at night and accidents never happen during office hours. Add to these factors the restricted ability of working parents to make morning and afternoon appointments, and the increased pediatric patient traffic in emergency departments is more than partially explained.

The situation is perhaps even worse for rural or inner city children who have no regular source of medical care. They have used, and will continue to use, the emergency department as a physician substitute. Commonly, their needs are less urgent from the physician's perspective than from the perspective of parent and child.

Finally, the advanced technology of the modern hospital, as well as improvements in communication and transportation, has made the emergency department the logical place for the care of a select group of children with pressing medical problems, such as serious trauma, significant drug overdose, status epilepticus and asthmaticus, child abuse, psychiatric and gynecologic emergencies, aspirated foreign bodies, burns, or bite wounds. No office can or should be organized to care for these complex and expensive problems.

All these areas and concerns mandate the printing of and are well addressed in *Pediatric Emergency Medicine*. This book was written for the emergency department physician, the generalist who sees infants and children, and the pediatrician working in an emergency environment. This will be apparent to child health care providers when faced with the unexpected in the hospital, office, or on the phone. Decision-making information must be committed to memory or quickly available to appropriately treat, stabilize, and refer the patient while supporting the parents.

The authors deserve some scrutiny. They are not older clinicians who have shed the subject matter of this book for more esoteric and elective diseases and operations. By and large, these contributors are in, or have recently come from, busy emergency departments and the information in this volume is first hand.

The content of the various chapters is extensive in scope. The geographic position of the emergency facility and its physicians is not isolated from the whole. The contributors have made detailed remarks concerning the diagnosis and management of the spectrum of disorders seen in emergency departments and have extended this discussion into the hospital course and management of patients, so that integration has been accomplished. The emergency department and its personnel and equipment are seen as a vital part of the entire health management organization. It becomes, then, more rational and satisfying for physicians in this symphony to recognize their irreplaceable roles in the total process.

Written by pediatricians, pediatric surgeons, and other specialists, this book serves as a meeting ground for many disciplines and provides a sense of common language, administrative cooperation, and cohesive consultation when facing a common goal: the health of the pediatric patient.

Joseph Zanga, M.D.
Associate Professor of Pediatrics
Director, Child and Adolescent Emergency Unit
Medical College of Virginia

Arnold M. Salzberg, M.D.
Professor of Surgery
Chairman, Division of Pediatric Surgery
Medical College of Virginia

Preface

Emergency medicine is now a recognized medical specialty. Since 1979 significant progress has been made in developing the foundations for this new discipline. There is one component of this framework that remains somewhat elusive for practicing emergency medicine physicians in their quest for training and continuing medical education, namely, pediatric emergency medicine.

The majority of patients who visit a general hospital emergency department are adults. It is estimated that in a non-children's hospital emergency department, less than 15% of the patients are in the pediatric age group. Furthermore, the majority of those children are brought in for a minor illness or injury. It is therefore difficult for a practicing emergency medicine physician to maintain the knowledge base and skill level required to manage the child with more than a simple laceration or urinary tract infection.

When the senior editor first began practicing emergency medicine, it was apparent that emergency medicine physicians needed education in the management of pediatric emergencies and information that could be used in the practical setting of their own emergency department. From this point came the beginnings for this book. It was the senior editor's intent to develop a textbook with surgical chapters and pediatric nonsurgical chapters so that the information presented would represent current knowledge at the time of publication. The associate editors then developed the chapters and sections in accord with this premise. The authors of each chapter were specifically requested to write their chapter with an orientation to the practicing emergency medicine physician and not a pediatrician working in a children's hospital emergency department. We believe this requirement has been met.

It was then decided to divide the book into systems so as to make it a more usable reference on the library shelf of a busy community hospital emergency department. Furthermore, by setting up the book in this manner, that is having a chapter on pediatric surgical musculoskeletal problems written by a pediatric surgeon immediately adjacent to a chapter on pediatric nonsurgical musculoskeletal problems written by a pediatrician, the reader can gain an overview of all musculoskeletal problems. In the emergency setting the format allows reference material for any given diagnosis to be more easily found.

We would like to thank all of the chapter authors for their extensive work in writing their chapters and revising them when requested. Their willingness to continue with this effort and to make it as up-to-date as publication constraints would allow speaks highly for their dedication and willingness to participate in the continuing education of emergency medicine physicians.

No preface would be complete without an appropriate thank you to our secretaries Jan Amigh,

Sharon Tringali, Linda Laughton, and Barbara Burns, for their unending support in the retyping and rewriting of this book. Our thanks also go to Anne Patterson of Aspen Publishers, whose monumental efforts to keep us on track have helped to bring you this text.

Finally, to our wives and children, a most sincere and loving thank you for understanding the hours spent without us and for always being there when we needed the support to continue.

It is our sincere hope that through our efforts and the efforts of everyone connected with this book the children of our world will lead a healthier and happier life. To those same children we say thank you for the joy and happiness you bring our world.

Frank Ehrlich, M.D.
Fred J. Heldrich, M.D.
J. J. Tepas III, M.D.

Part I

Cardiopulmonary Resuscitation

Fred J. Heldrich
Robert A. Wood

1 Cardiopulmonary Resuscitation

Cardiopulmonary resuscitation is an emergency procedure used to restore circulation and respiratory effort when one or both of these functions have failed. For optimum effectiveness of the resuscitative effort, it is necessary to accomplish the following:

1. Rapidly recognize failure of effective circulation and/or respiration.
2. Establish an airway and effective ventilation.
3. Establish an effective circulation.
4. Recognize specific reasons for cardiopulmonary failure that require special management.

Speed and organization are essential to a successful resuscitative effort. Thus preliminary planning greatly increases the effectiveness of the therapy. This includes being familiar with the principles and techniques of resuscitation and having equipment and medications immediately available. Such equipment and medication should be stored in a "crash cart" located in the treatment area. The crash cart should contain supplies and equipment for a variety of pediatric emergencies, not only cardiopulmonary resuscitation (Exhibit 1-1). The contents of the crash cart should be checked at least daily to ensure that required material is always available and functioning. There is no substitute for adequate preparation. Equally important is the prompt response of competent personnel. For optimal organization and procedural efficiency, one of the team members should direct the resuscitative effort to synchronize the work of each individual and assess the effectiveness of the resuscitation as it proceeds.

In children the primary event in cardiopulmonary arrest is usually respiratory failure. The hypoxia that develops then leads to acidosis and subsequent cardiac failure. Less often, cardiac failure is the initial event. Frequently, by the time the patient is seen, both cardiac and pulmonary failure are present.

Cardiac failure results in cessation of blood flow to the brain. Pupillary dilation begins within 45 seconds of failure of cerebral perfusion and is complete within just less than 2 minutes. The general rule is that irreversible brain damage occurs after 4 minutes of circulatory failure, although preexisting hypoxia may shorten the interval. Hypothermia, if present, can play a protective role, allowing the brain to withstand the anoxic insult for periods slightly longer than 4 minutes.[1]

Although the immediate problem of cardiopulmonary arrest must be dealt with urgently, the underlying cause for the arrest also must be identified and may require special consideration.[2] Conditions usually associated with an emergency setting are summarized in Exhibit 1-2.

To prevent death and reduce the incidence of sequelae, the diagnosis of cardiopulmonary arrest must be made promptly. The signs and symptoms of

EXHIBIT 1-1 Equipment and Material on "Crash Cart"*

Top of Cart
- Suction machine with nonconductive connecting tubing
- Face masks: 1 adult, 1 small adult, 1 infant, 1 newborn
- Oxygen connecting tubing and nasal cannula tubing
- Suction catheters: nos. 8, 10, 14 (2 each)

Drawer 1
- Laryngoscope handle
- Laryngoscope blades: nos. 1, 2, 3; 1 straight and 1 curved of each
- Oropharyngeal airways: nos. 1, 2, 3, 5 (1 each)
- Endotracheal tubes (mm): 2.5, 3.5, 4.5, 5.0, 6.0, 7.0, 8.0, 9.0, 10.0
- Nasogastric tubes: nos. 8, 12
- 1 Yankauer suction handle
- 1 stylette
- 1 tubing clamp
- 1 Salem sump tube no. 16
- 1 20-mL eccentric tip disposable syringe, no. 5694
- 1 5/8-inch, 25-gauge disposable needle
- 6 4 × 4-inch sterile sponges
- 4 packets sterile surgical lubricant
- 1 35-mL disposable catheter tip syringe
- 1 1-inch roll adhesive tape

Drawer 2
- Sponges—Tape
  - 6 4 × 3-inch Curity cover sterile sponges
  - 20 alcohol prep sponges
  - 1 2-inch roll poly-vent adhesive tape
- Syringes
  - 4 35-mL Luer-Lok tip
  - 1 60-mL Luer-Lok tip
  - 1 20-mL Luer-Lok tip
  - 4 arterial blood gas syringe packages
  - 10 3-mL with 1½-inch, 22-gauge needles
  - 10 10-mL with 1½-inch, 20-gauge needles
  - 10 1-mL tuberculin syringes
  - 3 disposable stopcocks
  - 1 male deadhead
- Needles
  - 5 18 gauge, 3½-inch length
  - 8 (each) 16, 19, 20, 22, 25 gauge, each 1½-inch length
  - 2 (each) butterfly needles: 21, 23, 25 gauge
  - 2 (each) Quick-cath: 22, 20, 18 gauge
  - 1 1-oz bottle povidone-iodine solution
  - 2 povidone-iodine ointment packages

Drawer 3

Drugs

No. of Units	Unit Size	Drug	Strength
1	20-mL vial	Atropine	0.4 mg/mL
3	10-mL ampule	Calcium chloride	100 mg/mL
3	10-mL ampule	Calcium gluconate	100 mg/mL
1	50-mL vial	Dextrose 25%	250 mg/mL
2	2-mL ampule	Diazepam	5 mg/mL
2	5-mL vial	Dopamine	40 mg/mL
3	1-mL ampule	Epinephrine 1 : 1000	1 mg/mL
6	10-mL syringe	Epinephrine 1 : 10,000	0.1 mg/mL
2	4-mL ampule	Furosemide	10 mg/mL
1	10-mL ampule	Heparin	1000 U/mL
2	5-mL ampule	Isoproterenol	0.2 mg/mL
2	5-mL syringe	Lidocaine 2%	20 mg/mL
2	25-mL vial	Lidocaine 4%	40 mg/mL
1	50-mL vial	Mannitol 25%	250 mg/mL
1	10-mL vial	Quinidine	80 mg/mL
4	10-mL syringe	Sodium bicarbonate 8.4%	1 mEq/mL
8	50-mL syringe	Sodium bicarbonate 7.5%	0.9 mEq/mL

Clipboard with flow sheet for recording RESUS procedure

Exhibit 1-1 continued

Drawer 4
- IV equipment
  - 1 pediatric venesection tray
  - 2 22-gauge Intracath, 8 inches, with 19-gauge needle
  - 2 19-gauge Intracath, 8 inches, with 17-gauge needle
  - 2 16-gauge Intracath, 8 inches, with 14-gauge needle
  - 2 150-mL burettes with minidrip with "Y" connectors
  - 5 IV solution administration sets with "Y" connectors
  - 1 blood administration set
  - 2 150-mL in-line burettes
  - 2 tourniquets
- Fluids
  - 3 500 mL 5% dextrose in water (D5W)
  - 3 500 mL D5/0.45% NaCl
  - 2 500 mL D5/0.2% NaCl
- Other equipment
  - 2 pairs each sterile gloves: sizes 7½ and 8½
  - 1 plastic bag (trash)
  - 1 cardboard needle-and-syringe box (trash)

* Contents of the pediatric crash carts in use at St. Agnes Hospital on the Pediatric-Adolescent Unit and Emergency Room.

EXHIBIT 1-2 Conditions Associated with Cardiopulmonary Arrest

- Respiratory
  - Foreign body aspiration
  - Laryngotracheobronchitis
  - Epiglottitis
  - Asthma
  - Pneumonia
  - Angioedema
  - Near drowning
  - Smoke inhalation
- Cardiovascular
  - Myocarditis
  - Arrhythmia
  - Congenital heart disease
  - Hypovolemia—dehydration
- Trauma
  - Blood loss
  - Head injury
  - Chest injury
  - Electrocution
- Central Nervous System
  - Seizures
  - Encephalitis
  - Mass lesions
  - Polyneuritis (Guillain-Barré syndrome)
- Drug Overdose
- Sudden Infant Death Syndrome—"Near Miss"
- Child Abuse

arrest or impending arrest are quite clear and easily recognized:

- loss of consciousness
- gasping or cessation of breathing
- cyanosis
- absent pulse or severe bradycardia
- no heart sounds
- pupillary dilatation

Should any doubt exist concerning the diagnosis, assume that the patient has gone into arrest, implement the resuscitative effort immediately,[1] and simultaneously summon the appropriate personnel by calling "Resus" or some similar identifying signal. Each institution should have its own code to summon personnel to the area where the resuscitation is being carried out.

Note the precise time the resuscitation begins, and record all the therapeutic maneuvers undertaken, as well as the patient's response. This information will be useful in determining ongoing therapy and in evaluating the effectiveness of the resuscitative effort during the procedure.

STEP I. RESPIRATORY SUPPORT

Establishing the Airway

1. Clear the oropharynx with a suction catheter or bulb syringe. A finger can be used to clear material from the oropharynx, but this should not be done blindly for fear of forcing debris down the trachea.[3,4]
2. Position the patient's neck to maximize the upper airway. To best accomplish this, place several fingers or a hand under the patient's neck and lift it slightly while tilting the head back, or lift the mandible while tilting the head back. In infants, slightly elevate the head before slightly extending the neck or lifting the mandible. If a neck injury is suspected, take care to maintain neck stability to prevent further injury.

3. As soon as the airway is open, determine if there is a flow of air by placing an ear over the patient's nose and mouth to hear or feel the flow of air, while observing for a rise and fall of the chest and abdomen. If there is no flow, initiate respiration.

Initiating Respiration

1. Place your mouth over the mouth and nose of young children and infants. For older patients, pinch the nose closed and place your mouth over the mouth of the patient.
2. Deliver four quick breaths and look for chest motion. For infants, 24 breaths per minute (1 every 2.5 seconds); for young children, 20 breaths per minute (1 every 3 seconds); and for older children, 15 breaths per minute (1 every 4 seconds) are the desired respiratory rates.[4] Exhaled air provides an oxygen concentration of 16%[2] and will sustain an arterial oxygen pressure of approximately 60 mm Hg.
3. Use a resuscitation bag and mask with 100% oxygen if they are available. If the patient is unconscious, insert an oropharyngeal airway to depress the tongue and maintain a patent airway. However, in a conscious patient the oropharyngeal airway can induce vomiting.[2]
4. If spontaneous respirations are initiated by the aforementioned procedures, then supplemental oxygen can be supplied by face mask or nasal cannula.

Endotracheal Intubation

Endotracheal tubes provide a most effective means of ventilation and should be used to ventilate patients in whom bag and mask methods have failed, in unconscious patients, or in those who need continued ventilatory assistance. Determine the approximate size of the endotracheal tube (internal diameter) by the following formula:[4]

$$\text{Endotracheal tube size (mm)} = \frac{\text{age in years} + 16}{4}.$$

When the patient's age can only be approximated, use the following guide:[2]

Age	Size (mm ± 0.5)
18 mo	4
5 yr	5
8 yr	6
16 yr	7

Use uncuffed tubes in infants and young children.

When attempting endotracheal tube intubation use mouth-to-mouth or bag-and-mask ventilation at intervals of no more than every 15 seconds until the intubation has been accomplished. Do not allow ventilation to be interrupted for more than 30 seconds.[2] Secure the endotracheal tube carefully by sutures placed through the wall of the endotracheal tube and then through plaster placed on the patient's upper lip, or by adhesive tape.

Once the endotracheal tube has been inserted, auscultate the lungs to determine the bilateral entry of air. Further check the position of the endotracheal tube by roentgenography as soon as possible if ventilator assistance must be continued.

STEP II. CIRCULATORY SUPPORT

Rapid determination of the presence or absence of a pulse is critical to survival. If the pulse cannot be determined with certainty, start external cardiac massage in addition to pulmonary resuscitation.

External Cardiac Massage

Apply pressure to the sternum and depress it 2 cm in the infant to as much as 5 cm in the older child.[1] This pressure ejects blood from the heart and enables adequate perfusion; the elastic recoil of the chest when pressure is removed allows refilling of the heart. Rhythmic compression of the sternum can reestablish circulation. Sternal compression can be applied with the fingers or encircling thumbs for infants, the heel of the hand for young children, and the heel of one hand with the other on top (two hands) for older children and adolescents. The location for applying sternal pressure is the midsternal area for the infant and young child, and the lower third of the sternum above the xiphoid in the older child. Apply the force in the midline of the sternum, perpendicular to the sternum to avoid rib fractures, laceration of the lungs, or trauma to abdominal viscera.

Synchronize sternal compression with ventilation at a ratio of 5:1 when two persons are providing the resuscitative effort. If it is a one-person resuscitation, then the compression-to-ventilation ratio should be 15:2. However, in very young infants, a ratio of 5:1 should be maintained, even if there is only one resuscitator. The sternal compression rate should be 60 to 80/min for older children and adolescents but should increase to 80 to 100/min for younger children and 100 to 120/min for infants; the youngest patient requires the most rapid rate.[4]

The patient should be lying on a firm surface such as the cardiac board. Start electrocardiographic monitoring immediately since this becomes the means for determining the need for medications or defibrillation.

STEP III. DRUGS

While the resuscitation is proceeding, establish an intravenous line. Perform a cut-down if a good-sized vessel is not immediately available. A work sheet for the drugs most commonly needed and their dosage schedules are outlined in Table 1-1.

Epinephrine

Epinephrine, one of the cardinal drugs, is indicated for asystole or ventricular fibrillation. It acts on the myocardium to improve contractility and elevate perfusion pressure by its vasoconstrictive effect. It also has the capacity to increase cardiac muscle tone and thereby convert fine fibrillary contractions to coarse fibrillary contractions. These coarse fibrillations are more easily corrected by countershock. A 1:10,000 dilution (.1 mg/mL) is used and the dose is .01 mg/kg of body weight, with a maximum dose of 0.5 mg. This dose can be repeated every 5 to 10 minutes. The route of administration can be intravenous, intracardiac, or by instillation in the endotracheal tube.

Sodium Bicarbonate

Severe metabolic acidosis reduces the effectiveness of epinephrine, and its correction should be attempted. The acidosis that accompanies cardiopulmonary arrest is both respiratory and metabolic. Ventilation is critical to the correction of the respiratory component, while sodium bicarbonate, 1 mEq/kg IV, should be given for correction of the metabolic component. Subsequent doses should be given in response to pH determination. The depressant effects of acidosis include

- decreased diastolic depolarization
- reduction of spontaneous myocardial activity
- decreased electrical threshold to ventricular fibrillation
- decreased ventricular contractile force
- decreased cardiac sensitivity to catecholamines

The degree of acidosis required to produce these effects in pediatric patients is not accurately known but probably is at a pH less than 7.1.

TABLE 1-1 Pediatric Drug Work Sheet

			Patient Weight ______ kg	
Drug	Concentration/mL	Dose/kg	mL × wt	= Final Dose
Epinephrine (1:10,000)	.1 mg	.01 mg (max = .5 mg)	.1 ×	= ml epinephrine (max = 5 mL)
$NaHCO_3$	1 mEq	1 mEq	1 ×	= ml $NaHCO_3$
Atropine	.1 mg	.01 mg–.03 mg (max = .5 mg)	.1 ×	= ml atropine (max = 5 mL)
Ca Chloride 10%	100 mg	10 mg–25 mg (max = 1 g)	.1 ×	= ml CaCl (max = 10 mL)
Ca Gluconate 10%	100 mg	100 mg (max = 2 g)	.1 ×	= ml CaGL (max = 20 mL)
Naloxone	.4 mg	.01 mg	.025 ×	= mL Naloxone

Drug	Concentration/mL	Dose/kg/h	Solutions for IV infusion	Rate
Lidocaine 2%	20 mg/mL	1.2–3 mg	1 mg/kg as bolus, then 6 mL in 100 mL D5W = 1.2 mg/mL	1–2.5 mL/kg/h
Dopamine	40 mg	120–600 μg	1.5 mL in 100 mL D5W = 600 μg/mL	.2–1 mL/kg/h
Isoproterenol	.2 mg	6–120 μg	5 mL in 100 mL D5W = 100 μg/ml	.6–12 mL/kg/h
Defibrillation	2 watts/sec/kg			

Calcium

For asystole or wide QRS complexes, calcium is indicated. Ventricular excitability and conduction velocities are enhanced and myocardial contractility is increased by an infusion of calcium. Calcium chloride is the drug of choice because of its greater calcium ion concentration per volume; 10 to 25 mg/kg (maximum dose, 1 g) is given IV. This should be administered slowly to prevent bradycardia or, in digitalized patients, a dysrhythmia. Calcium chloride should not be given in a solution containing sodium bicarbonate because calcium will precipitate to form insoluble calcium carbonate.

Atropine

Atropine is used in the presence of atrioventricular block or sinus bradycardia. This parasympatholytic drug reduces vagal tone and increases sinoauricular node firing and atrioventricular node conduction. A dose of 0.1 mg/kg (with a minimum of 0.1 mg and a maximum of 2 mg), either IV or via endotracheal tube, is given and can be repeated in 20 minutes. In insufficient doses a paroxysmal bradycardia can occur.

Lidocaine

Lidocaine is indicated for ventricular fibrillation, ventricular irritability, ventricular tachycardia, and premature ventricular contractions. It reduces cardiac automaticity, increases the cardiac threshold to fibrillation, and diminishes reentrant tachycardia. Initially, a bolus of 1 mg/kg IV is given, followed by IV infusion at 20 μg/kg/min (1.2 mg/kg/h). The dose can be increased to 50 μg/kg/min (3 mg/kg/h). Since lidocaine is metabolized by the liver, hepatic disease can lead to excessive blood levels and signs of toxicity including lethargy, nausea, altered sensorium, coma, or seizures.

Dopamine

Hypotension that is not secondary to hypovolemia is managed by an intravenous infusion of dopamine or isoproterenol. The action of dopamine, which has both an α- and β-adrenergic effect, is dependent on the rate of infusion. At a rate of 1 to 7 μg/kg/min, dilation of renal, mesenteric, coronary, and cerebral vessels occurs. Inotropic and chronotropic effects lead to increased stroke volume and cardiac output at a rate of infusion between 7 and 20 μg/kg/min. At a rate greater than 20 μg/kg/min, there is peripheral vasoconstriction and reduction in renal blood flow. The rate of infusion is adjusted in accordance with patient response, but it is usually between 2 and 20 μg/kg/min (120 to 1200 μg/kg/h).

Isoproterenol

Isoproterenol is a β-adrenergic stimulant. It affects the heart by increasing heart rate, improving myocardial contractility and tone, and increasing cardiac output. Oxygen consumption by the myocardium is increased. It also produces peripheral arterial vasodilatation, and the risk of hypotension is great if the patient is hypovolemic. Isoproterenol is primarily used for status asthmaticus with impending respiratory failure, but it also can be used for patients in cardiogenic shock who are unresponsive to dopamine. When used for status asthmaticus, the dose begins with 0.02 μg/kg/min, rapidly increasing to 0.1 μg/kg/min if necessary. The dose should not exceed 0.5 μg/kg/min. If used for shock refractory to dopamine, the starting dose is 0.1 μg/kg/min, the rate increasing as needed. Higher doses may be required, up to 1.5 μg/kg/min, but the risks of tachycardia and arrhythmias demand careful observation.

Nitroprusside

Should the course of arrest be related to a hypertensive crisis, then nitroprusside, an agent that reduces blood pressure by its direct dilating effect on blood vessels, should be given. It is infused at a rate of 0.5 to 8.0 μg/kg/min (usually 3 μg/kg/min), with titration by continuous monitoring of blood pressure. Its effect is terminated as soon as infusion is discontinued.

Bretylium

Bretylium is available for refractory ventricular fibrillation and tachycardia. It is useful when lidocaine has failed. First administered IV as a 5 mg/kg bolus, it can be increased by 5 mg/kg to a maximum of 30 mg/kg. Doses can be repeated every 15 to 30 minutes.

Naloxone Hydrochloride

When cardiopulmonary arrest occurs secondary to narcotic depression, the specific antidote is naloxone hydrochloride. No adverse effect can occur from a single dose, making it a safe drug to use when the clinical diagnosis of narcotic depression is made. Given IV at a dose of 0.01 mg/kg, it can produce prompt improvement, but repeated doses may be required at 5- to 10-minute intervals.

Defibrillation

With evidence of ventricular fibrillation, defibrillation may be warranted. If complexes are seen on the electrocardiographic tracing, but there is no palpable pulse, calcium may be required. The use of epinephrine and bolus doses of lidocaine may have terminated the ventricular fibrillation; if not, then electric shock should be used.[1]

1. Cover the paddles with electrode paste and place one over the cardiac apex, the other at the sternal notch.
2. Disconnect all electrical equipment.
3. Have all personnel stand away from the patient.
4. Deliver the electric shock.
5. If unsuccessful, double the wattage and repeat.
6. Repeat drugs, if necessary.

STEP IV. FOLLOW-UP

Following resuscitation, the patient requires intensive monitoring of respiration, cardiovascular status, and fluid intake and output (urine flow). Other important considerations are abnormal neurologic signs, which can result from cerebral anoxia and require specific therapy; glucose homeostasis; temperature control; and prevention or treatment of infection.[1,5]

STEP V. TERMINATION OF THE RESUSCITATIVE EFFORT

Deciding when to terminate resuscitative efforts is difficult, but after an unsuccessful attempt has been made for 1 hour, indications for discontinuing resuscitation can be identified:[2,5]

1. no spontaneous respiration, verified by discontinuing the ventilator for 3 minutes if the carbon dioxide pressure is normal at the time
2. no ventricular electrical activity
3. fixed, dilated pupils
4. absent corneal reflexes
5. positive doll's eyes sign
6. unresponsive to all stimuli
7. no drug depression or hypothermia (temperature below 32.2° C)

The resiliency of the pediatric patient and/or the associated presence of hypothermia are reasons for continuing resuscitative efforts for long periods.

References

1. Anthony CL Jr, Crawford EW, Morgan BC: Management of cardiac and respiratory arrest in children. A survey of major principles of therapy. *Clin Pediatr* 1969;8:647–654.
2. Smith RM: Respiratory arrest and its sequelae, in Smith CA (ed): *The Critically Ill Child: Diagnosis and Management.* Philadelphia, WB Saunders Co, 1972, pp 124–138.
3. Standards and guidelines for cardiopulmonary resuscitation (CPR) and emergency cardiac care (ECC). *JAMA* 1980;244:453–509.
4. Orlowski JP: Cardiopulmonary resuscitation in children. *Pediatr Clin North Am* 1980;27:495–512.
5. Levin DL, Morris FC, Moore GC: Intensive care, in Shirkey HC (ed): *Pediatric Therapy,* ed 6. St Louis, CV Mosby Co, 1980, pp 167–210.

Robert M. Arensman
Kenneth W. Falterman

2

Initial Care of the Injured Child: The First 30 Minutes

The initial care of the injured child begins long before a patient ever arrives in an emergency department. Essentially, that care begins when pediatric health providers ask who the injured child is, how many such injured children are likely to be seen, what the nature of their injuries is, and what facilities and supplies are needed for their immediate care and evaluation. Fortunately, the answers to these questions are available from recent trauma reviews;[1,2] the medical statistics of the U.S. Department of Health, Education and Welfare;[3] and the experience of centers that have established well-supplied and -staffed pediatric emergency facilities.

BACKGROUND

Who and How Many

Of the 19 million children per year who are injured severely enough to seek medical care or to restrict usual activity, more than 100,000[4] are permanently disabled and 15,000[5,6] die. Death by accident is the leading cause of mortality for those from 1 year of age to early adulthood.[7–10] Males outnumber females two to one in all age categories.

Types of Injuries

Lacerations repeatedly head the list as the most common injury of childhood; these are followed by contusions and abrasions, fractures and dislocations, ingestions, and bites.[11] In fatal injuries the mechanisms of trauma are quite different, and motor vehicle accidents account for almost half of all pediatric deaths in patients under 14 years of age (20% of motor vehicle fatalities are victims younger than 18 years of age).[5] Drownings, burns, ingestions, and falls follow in order. Tragically, over 600 children die each year from firearm injuries.[12]

Facilities and Supplies

The considerations of an emergency treatment facility are similar, whether it treats adults or children. However, because the provision of supplies is remarkably different, one can easily recognize an emergency department seriously committed to the treatment of pediatric injury.

Regardless of patient age, the facility should have

1. easy accessibility for both ambulatory and transported victims
2. sufficient space to handle the expected number of patients
3. good lighting
4. availability of oxygen, suction, and compressed air
5. facilities for on-site x-ray studies
6. rapid access to laboratory service.

In addition, a full-time, experienced, and fully trained nursing staff dedicated to delivering trauma care is essential.[13,14]

It is really in the area of supplies and equipment that an emergency department demonstrates its readiness and ability to care for the injured child. There is little chance of successful evaluation and resuscitation if time is wasted finding materials of appropriate sizes after a victim arrives. Consequently, every emergency department that anticipates receiving children should establish a coded cart containing the appropriate supplies. In our own institution such carts have been established using a Sears Craftsman tool case (Figures 2-1 to 2-5). This large and mobile storage cabinet is readily available and easily accommodates all the materials needed for a standard pediatric emergency. Within the eight drawers a selection of intravenous fluids (5% dextrose in water [D5W], lactated Ringer's solution, D5/0.2% NaCl, and /0.45% NaCl) are stored with appropriate intravenous needles, catheters, and

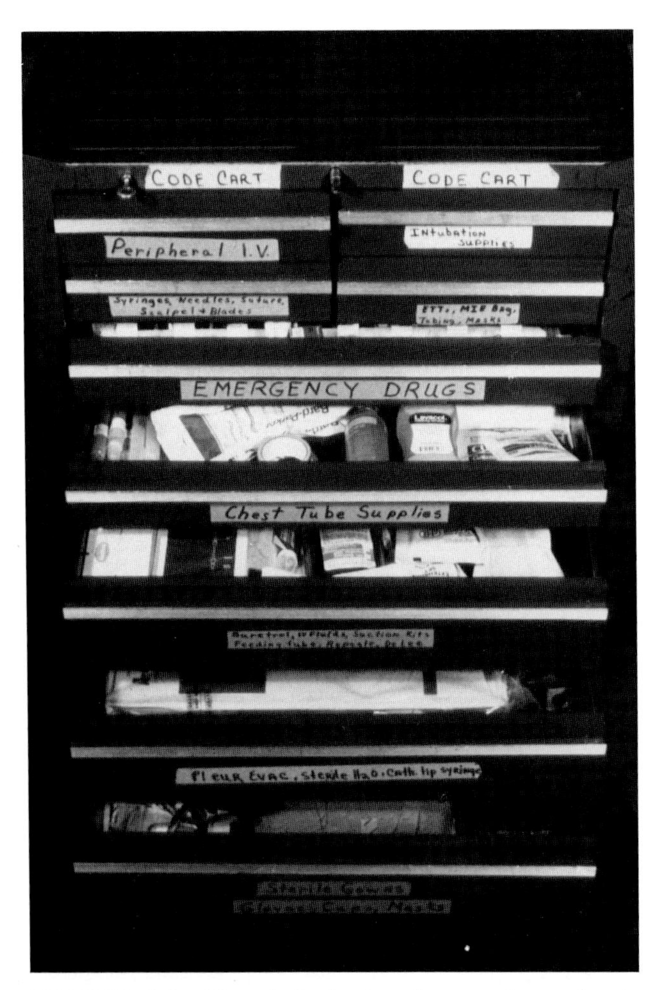

FIGURE 2-1 Closed, locked code cart for pediatric trauma victims.

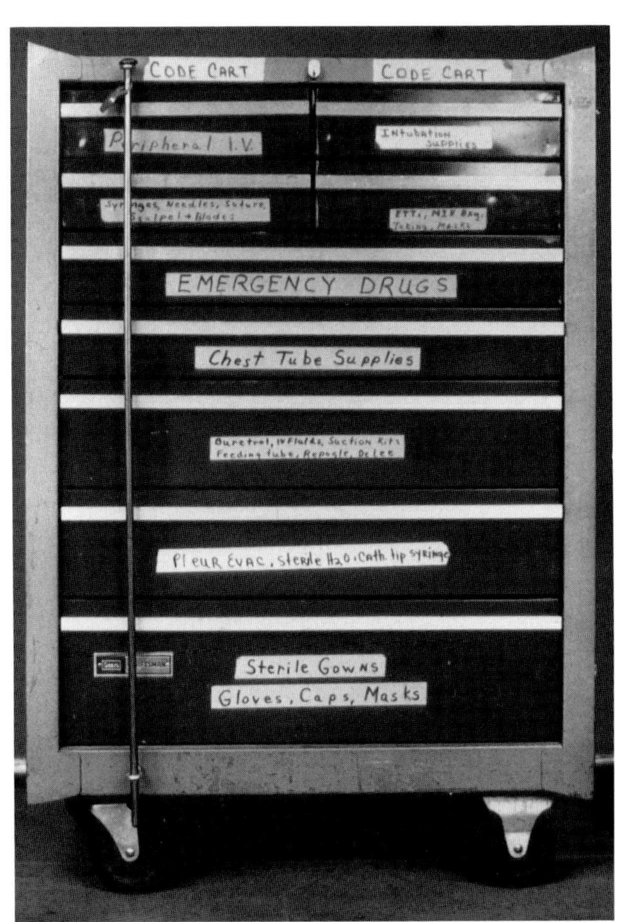

FIGURE 2-2 Distribution of equipment allows for rapid access to immediately lifesaving supplies.

burettes. Respiratory equipment consists of endotracheal tubes from 2.5 to 8.0 mm with laryngoscopes, an assortment of blades, 2 Ambu bags, and various sized face masks. Several sterile instrument trays are stored with appropriate pediatric instruments and drapes. One drawer is devoted to drugs in dosages appropriate for children. In addition, books are now readily available that provide pediatric dosages and dosages calculated by body weight, and these are attached to the cart. Suctioning equipment and catheters are attached to the top of the cabinet for emergency use.

INITIAL EVALUATION

If one has defined *who* constitutes the injured child, and if one has provided appropriate space and supplies for pediatric care, then a plan can be established to care for these very special patients. Initially, this involves a triage approach to determine

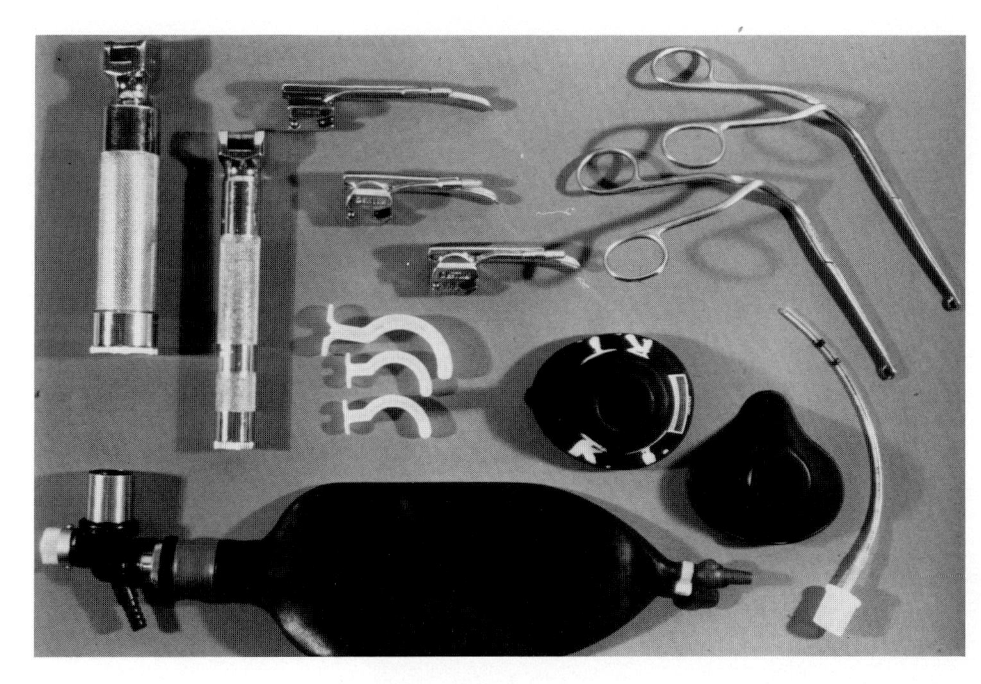

FIGURE 2-3 First concern: airway management supplies.

seriousness of injury.[15–17] In the event that the injury falls into one of the more common and less serious categories (e.g., minor lacerations, contusions, abrasions), the initial evaluation involves taking a history, recording vital signs, and assessing the completeness of immunizations. The specific injury then can be addressed and appropriately handled. If triage establishes the presence of a life-threatening injury, the child should be moved immediately to the emergency critical care room where priorities are assessed and therapy is instituted (Figure 2-6).

Respiration

Since life depends upon successful oxygenation and cardiac action, a rapid assessment of those functions is the first priority. If apnea is present, a check for foreign matter in the oral cavity followed by extension of the lower jaw—maintaining at all times

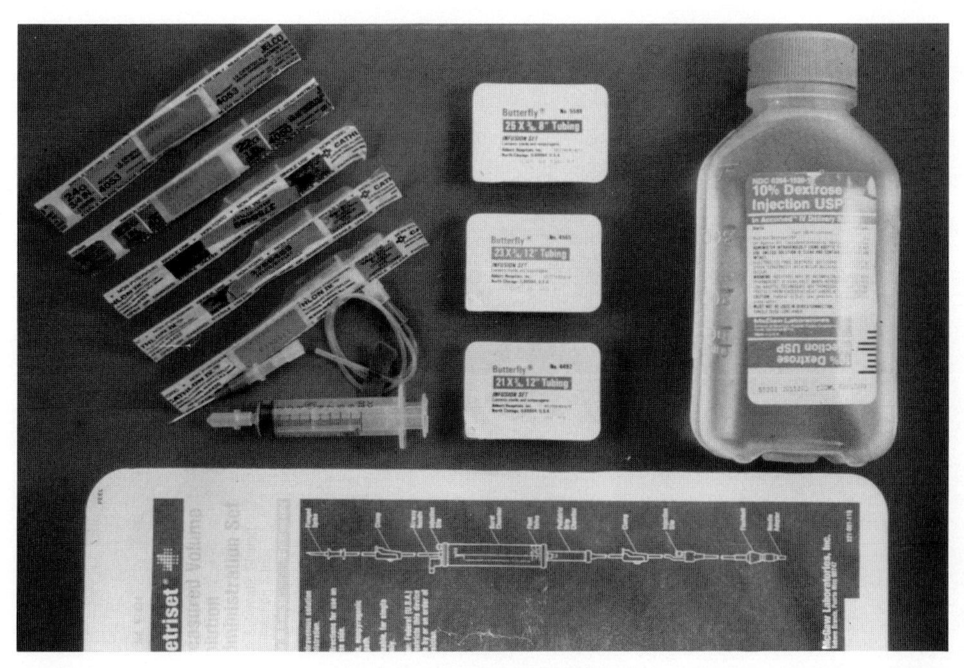

FIGURE 2-4 Second concern: intravenous access supplies.

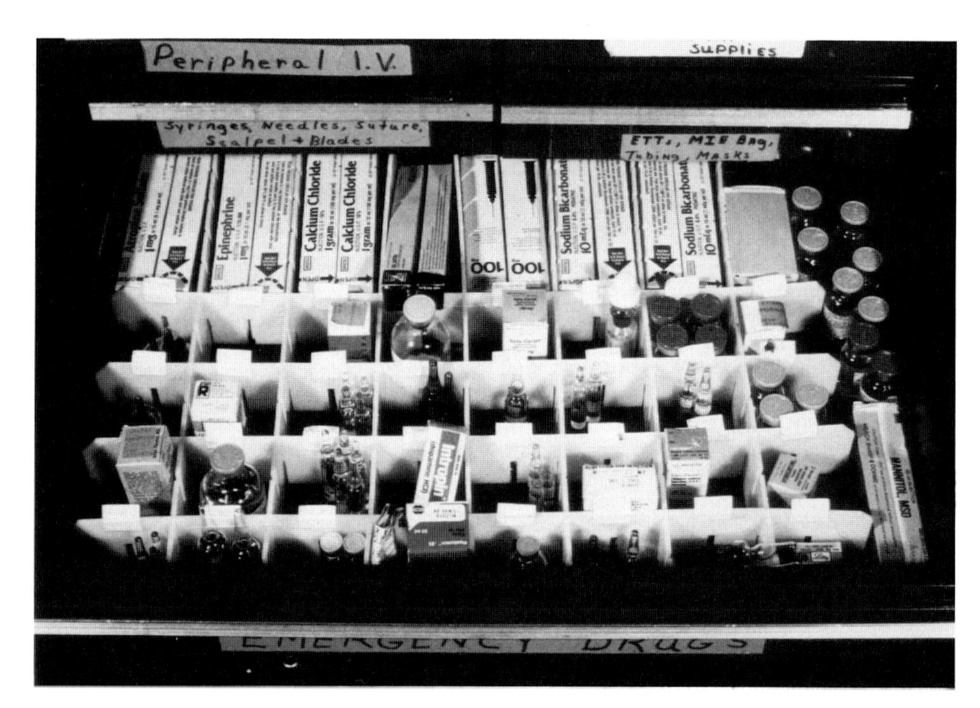

FIGURE 2-5 Third concern: drug drawer.

cervical in-line traction—is the appropriate first maneuver to clear the mouth or to relieve obstruction secondary to the tongue in an unconscious child. If obstruction persists, suctioning of blood or foreign matter in the hypopharynx may be indicated. If the airway is clear, respiration can be maintained with mask and bag; however, the unreliability of this method plus the uncontrolled insufflation of air into the stomach favors early intubation to secure respiration in the apneic trauma victim.

Cardiac Action

The seriousness of the injury or external blood loss can result in loss of cardiac action. Simple palpation of carotid or femoral pulses proves the presence of cardiac action and gives a rough estimate of the adequacy of cardiac output. Blood pressure readings and placement of electrocardiographic leads more fully document cardiac activity; however, if the child is pulseless, one should not wait for these

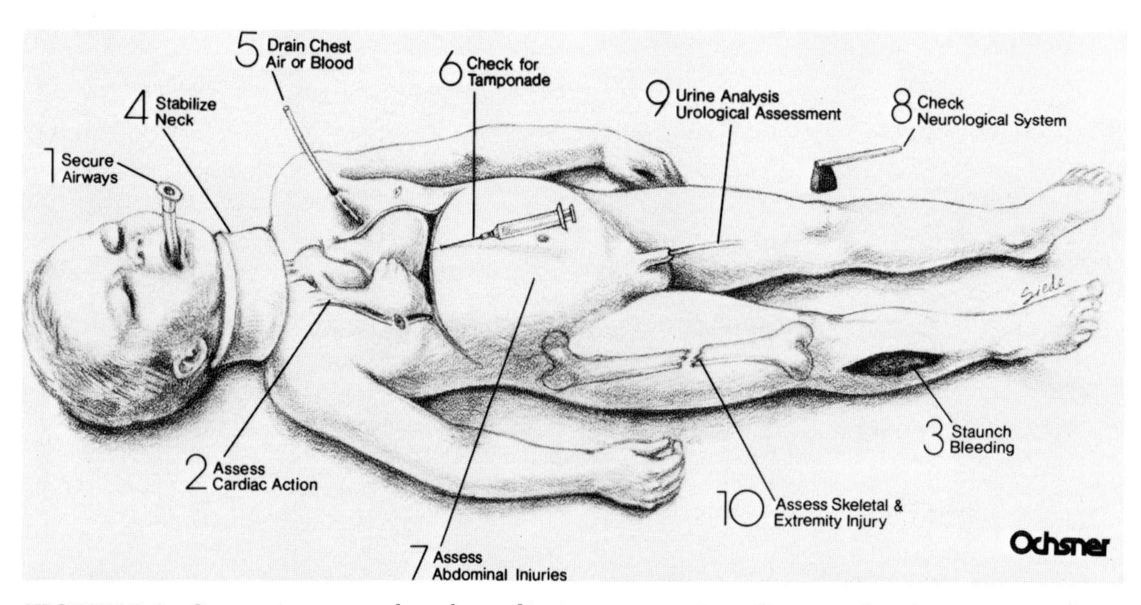

FIGURE 2-6 Composite approach to the pediatric trauma patient. (Reprinted with permission from Arensman RM, Falterman KW: *Postgraduate Medicine* 1984;75(1):257–265.

measurements. External cardiac massage should be started. For infants this is done by pushing the lower sternum downward with two fingers at a rate of 100/min.[18] For the older child the heel of the hand can be used as in adults, attempting to achieve a rate of 80/min.[18] For all ages the presence and fullness of peripheral pulses indicate the degree of success.

Hemostasis

The next priority is hemostasis. External exsanguinating hemorrhage is usually quite visible and should be quickly controlled. Simple direct pressure on the wound or to the proximal feeding artery generally achieves control. Although a tourniquet is rarely required, a child occasionally reaches the emergency department with a tourniquet in place. Inspection of the wound and placement of a hemostat across the injured vessel allow removal of the device; however, one must remember that major nerves often accompany arteries and should be identified to prevent injury.

SECONDARY EVALUATION

After securing the airway, assessing circulatory adequacy, and establishing hemostasis, the physician can initiate the secondary evaluation. Since this evaluation must cover the remainder of the entire body, a systematic but prioritized search should ensue.[19] This allows one to be thorough and yet assess the possibilities in descending order of seriousness.

Cervical Injury

The possibility of cervical injury is generally anticipated by members of the emergency transport team. In the event of severe head injury or unconsciousness, a patient usually is cervically immobilized and moved on a back board. If this has not been done, the head and neck should be immobilized immediately. Once the cervical area is secured, cervical x-ray films should be taken to confirm injury or rule out danger.

Chest Injury

Attention next should turn to the possibility of chest injury. Sucking chest wounds from penetrating trauma can be satisfactorily controlled with an occlusive dressing. A patient with a flail segment usually requires immediate intubation and assisted respiration.[20] More difficult to diagnose is tension pneumothorax, which leads to mediastinal shift and loss of cardiac venous return. Occasionally, a hemothorax produces the same problem. Loss of respiratory sounds may suggest the correct diagnosis, and if time permits, a chest film will confirm it. However, needle aspiration both confirms the diagnosis and serves as initial therapy until a tube thoracostomy is performed.[21–23]

Another intrathoracic injury often associated with penetrating wounds is cardiac tamponade, which demands immediate recognition and treatment to prevent disaster. Physical signs are often subtle: a weak pulse, distant heart sounds, and distended neck veins. A chest film and an electrocardiogram can confirm this diagnosis; needle aspiration from the subxiphoid position is both diagnostic and therapeutic.

Abdominal Injury

Because the abdominal cavity is the other large space in which hidden hemorrhage can occur, with severe consequences to the traumatized child, a search for injury in this area should be the next step. In the conscious child the presence of tenderness is a reliable guide to injury, although the severity can vary from minimal to life threatening. Progressive distension, recorded over a period of observation, is another reliable indicator of intra-abdominal injury. Both signs suggest the need for further diagnostic tests. Plain x-ray films in children can be the source of considerable information. Sonography and radionucleotide studies require more time but are now widely used to document hepatic and splenic lacerations and intra-abdominal hematomas. Abdominal taps and lavage appear to be as reliable in children as in adults,[24] but they are not greatly recommended by pediatric surgeons. Serial abdominal examinations are often difficult to perform after lavage because of tenderness from the catheter insertion. Moreover, since the nonoperative approach to ruptured spleens is widely accepted and practiced,[25,26] the information gained by lavage is no longer as critical as it once was.

Penetrating wounds are still widely regarded as an indication for abdominal exploration. However, in recent years some centers have reported observation of stab victims who show no signs of severe intra-abdominal injury,[27–29] especially if a sinogram suggests no celomic penetration. In any event, a penetrating wound warrants immediate surgical consultation, and a decision can be made according to the experience and practice of the pediatric surgical service.

Finally, one must remember that children are particularly prone to develop gastric dilation.[17] If this is severe enough, it can impede venous return and cause emesis and aspiration. Thus early placement of a nasogastric tube is advised for any child with substantial trauma.

Neurologic Injury

Neurologic evaluation is the next priority. The examination should first consider cerebral function and then proceed to evaluate the cranial nerves and the peripheral neurologic system. Accurate assessment of the level of consciousness is followed by ocular evaluation for papilledema or lateralizing extraocular muscle paresis. Examination for extremity paralysis, long tract signs, and sensory deficits completes the evaluation. Cranial x-ray films to rule out unrecognized skull fracture(s) are taken when time permits or condition warrants.

Genitourinary Injury

The genitourinary system usually has low priority in a trauma assessment. It is frequently involved in trauma but seldom represents life-threatening injury. On the initial examination one should check for blood at the urethral orifice. Such a finding suggests a urethral tear and possibly transection. Catheterization in such a situation is difficult and often dangerous. Urologic consultation should be considered prior to instrumentation. Otherwise, urinalysis is a quick, simple test for trauma. Even minor blunt trauma in children can lead to hematuria. An intravenous pyelogram can be obtained simply by infusion of meglumine diatrizoate at 2 mL/kg. In the event of renal nonvisualization, an arteriogram should be performed promptly so that renal artery transection can be documented. Renal artery reconstruction must be done before irreversible renal ischemia occurs.

Extremity Injury

Finally, extremity trauma should be assessed. Actually, evaluation of the other systems may have already revealed any significant injury. These injuries are most likely fractures or vascular-neurologic damage. Although deformity, tenderness, and swelling are the typical signs of fracture, x-ray films are necessary to reveal or confirm the occasional occult fracture.

Peripheral vascular injury is often subtle and initially missed. An absent or substantially decreased pulse is often the only early sign. Pallor and coolness are additional signs but often are hard to assess in a child who is in shock. Any time a difference in pulse quality is even suspected, Doppler evaluation and comparison to the contralateral pulse should be carried out.

STABILIZATION AND TRANSPORTATION

In an age of rapid air evacuation and specialty care units, traumatized children can often be moved to a center with a pediatric intensive care unit or a pediatric trauma unit.[30,31] Obviously, stabilization, as outlined in the preceding section, must be achieved first. Then the emergency physician must evaluate the chance of a successful transport. Unfortunately, some children who arrive at the emergency department are so severely injured that no action can sustain life. An injudicious decision to hastily transport such a patient only increases parental anguish in the event death occurs en route.

Once the patient is stabilized and triage assessment suggests that the patient might survive movement, the physician must consider the method of transport. Under the best circumstances the nearest pediatric intensive care unit will have both a transport team to accompany the injured child and an existing system of transport. In less than optimal situations, the referring physician must arrange air or surface transport and must determine the personnel needed to accompany the patient. Generally, such a system cannot be arranged after the injured child arrives. Therefore, if a hospital is not prepared to admit an injured child, then a well-planned and -equipped transport mechanism should exist as part of the overall emergency design.

The four major considerations in pediatric transport are

1. availability of appropriate supplies
2. availability of appropriate personnel[30]
3. mode of transport
4. special requirements of children.

Supplies are similar to those outlined previously but are reduced in quantity. In our unit all supplies are stored in two portable cases that move with the team. These are sufficiently complete to effect stabilization at a referring institution and to allow for almost any emergency that might arise in transport.

Appropriate personnel would include

- transport physicians to accompany all severely injured children

- mobile pediatric intensive care nurses
- mobile pediatric respiratory therapists, if needed
- clerical and administrative personnel to staff the dispatch area 24 hours each day.

In our particular instance all of these functions are handled through the present staff of the pediatric intensive care unit.

Modes of transport are, of course, surface or air, and in some localities air transport may be by helicopter or fixed-wing aircraft. The transportation chosen obviously varies according to each individual's locality and depends on such factors as weather conditions, terrain, and the availability of helicopters or fixed-wing aircraft. Our experience has shown that surface transport is the most expeditious method for victims within 50 miles of our intensive care unit. Beyond this distance, all of our experience has been by air transport, which has been most satisfactory but occasionally impractical because of weather conditions.

Finally, one must anticipate special requirements associated with children. Foremost among these is thermal control, especially for the smaller child. Because the large surface-area-to-mass ratio leads to rapid heat loss, even in transport, constant attention to temperature control is necessary.

CONCLUSION

In conclusion, one fifth of America's trauma victims are members of the pediatric age group. This segment of our injured population often has tremendous physiologic and psychologic reserves. Children survive and overcome many of the worst injuries provided they receive the same level of initial care and evaluation that would be given an injured adult. Anticipation and preparation for these pediatric trauma victims can and do increase their chances of survival.

References

1. Gratz RR: Accidental injury in childhood: a literature review on pediatric trauma. *J Trauma* 1979;19:551–555.
2. Velcek FT, Weiss A, DiMaio D, et al: Traumatic death in urban children. *Ped Surg* 1977;12:375–384.
3. Garfinkle J, Chabot JJ, Pratt MW: *Infant, Maternal and Childhood Mortality in the US*, US Department of Health, Education, and Welfare publication No. (HSA) 75-5013. Rockville, MD, Health Services Administration, 1968–1973.
4. Haller JA: Problems in children's trauma. *J Trauma* 1970;10:269–271.
5. White House Conference on Children: *Profiles on Children*. Washington, DC, Government Printing Office, 1970.
6. Randolph JG: Children as accident victims, in Randolph JG, Ravich M, Welch K, et al (eds): *The Injured Child: Surgical Management*. Chicago, Year Book Medical Publishers Inc, 1979, pp 1–5.
7. Haggerty R: Childhood accidents, in Green M, Haggerty R (eds): *Ambulatory Pediatrics*. Philadelphia, WB Saunders Co, 1968, pp 813–817.
8. Chisolm JJ: Accidents and poisoning, in Cooke RE (ed): *The Biologic Basis of Pediatric Practice*. New York, McGraw-Hill Book Co, 1968, pp 1591–1608.
9. Haddon W, Suchman EA, Klein D (eds): *Accident Research: Methods and Approaches*. New York, Harper and Row Publishers, 1964.
10. Haller JA: Newer concepts in emergency care for children with major injuries. *Md State Med J* 1973;22:65–68.
11. Izant RJ, Hubay CA: The annual injury of 15,000,000 children: A limited study of childhood accidental injury and death. *J Trauma* 1966;6:65–74.
12. Childhood homicide—United States. *MMWR* 1982;31:292–293.
13. Cowley RA, Scanlan E: University trauma center: Operation, design and staffing. *Am Surg* 1979;45: 79–85.
14. Halpern R, Meyers A, Alpert J: Utilization of pediatric emergency services: A critical review. *Pediatr Clin North Am* 1979;26:747–757.
15. Morse TS: Step by step with an injured child. *Emergency Medicine* 1974; 6 (May):121–133.
16. Feins NR: Multiple trauma. *Pediatr Clin North Am* 1979;26:759–771.
17. Morse TS: Evaluation and initial management, in Touloukian RJ (ed): *Pediatric Trauma*. New York, Wiley Medical Publications, 1978, chap 2.
18. McIntyre KM (chairman): 1979 National Conference on Cardiopulmonary Resuscitation and Emergency Cardiac Care. Standards and Guidelines for Cardiopulmonary Resuscitation (CPR) and Emergency Cardiac Care (ECC). *JAMA* 1980;244:453–509.
19. Steichen FN: Emergency management of the severely injured child, in Randolf J, Ravich M, Welch K, et al (eds): *The Injured Child: Surgical Management*. Chicago, Year Book Medical Publishers Inc, 1979, pp 7–28.
20. Cullen P: Treatment of flail chest: Use of intermittent mandatory ventilation and positive end-expiratory pressure. *Arch Surg* 1975;110:1099–1103.
21. Sturm JP, Points BJ, Perry JF: Hemopneumothorax following blunt trauma of the thorax. *Surg Gynecol Obstet* 1975;141:539–540.
22. Welch KJ: Abdominal and thoracic injuries, in Mustard WT, Ravitch MM, Snyder WH (eds): *Pediatric Surgery*, ed 2. Chicago, Year Book Medical Publishers Inc, 1969, pp 708–731.
23. Ballinger WF, Rutherford RB, Zuidema JD (eds): *The Management of Trauma*. Philadelphia, WB Saunders Co, 1973.

24. Powell RW, Smith DE, Zarins CK, et al: Peritoneal lavage in children with blunt abdominal trauma. *J Pediatr Surg* 1976;11:973–977.
25. Upadhyaya P, Simpson JS: Splenic trauma in children. *Surg Gynecol Obstet* 1968;126:781–790.
26. Douglas GJ, Simpson JS: The conservative management of splenic trauma. *J Pediatr Surg* 1971;6:565–570.
27. Jordan GL Jr: Conservatism in the management of abdominal trauma. *Am J Surg* 1973;126:581–582.
28. Nance FC, Wennar MH, Johnson LW, et al: Surgical judgment and management of penetrating wounds of the abdomen: Experience with 2,212 patients. *Ann Surg* 1974;179:639–646.
29. Thavendran A: Selective surgery for abdominal stab wounds. *Br J Surg* 1975;62:750–752.
30. Dobrin RS, Block B, Gilman JI, et al: The development of a pediatric emergency transport system. *Pediatr Clin North Am* 1980;27:633–646.
31. Duke JH, Clarke WP: A university staffed, private hospital-based air transport service. *Arch Surg* 1981;116:702–706.

Part II

Common Pediatric Emergencies

Frank E. Ehrlich

3

Common Pediatric Emergencies

The majority of general hospital emergency departments primarily treat adults. When small children appear in one of these emergency departments, they usually create anxiety among the emergency personnel. It is therefore imperative that the staff prepare themselves for the arrival of these patients. It is likely that no patient is easier to treat in the emergency department, since there is generally no secondary gain involved. A child who appears sick is in fact a sick child. A playful, romping child has, more than likely, no significant acute illness.

"Children are not small adults." This statement is something that health professionals must be reminded of regularly. Pediatric patients have their own pathophysiology, which emergency physicians should become familiar with.

INITIAL ASSESSMENT

Any emergency department situation involving pediatric patients involves a triangular relationship bringing into play the patient, the patient's parents or guardian, and the emergency department personnel. If this is managed thoughtfully, many problems in the initial assessment can be resolved.

The first corner of the triangle and the most important is the patient. Emergency department personnel realize that invariably they are dealing with a frightened patient. Hospitals and people in white uniforms often evoke memories of previous traumatic experiences. Even a child who has never been in an emergency department can sense the similarity to a physician's office. It is therefore imperative that every effort be made to make the hospital experience as atraumatic as possible. It should be remembered that a child who has a bad experience today may be an unmanageable patient in the future.

Separating children from parents to facilitate diagnostic procedures, often enhances their fear. A thoughtful and understanding staff can do much to alleviate this problem. On the other hand, efforts directed at convincing a small child to voluntarily submit to a painful procedure are largely wasted time and energy. The effort to convince a 4-year-old to hold still for blood drawing may be productive, but if the child does not cooperate readily, the child should be properly restrained and the blood drawn. It is much better to do what is necessary in an understanding yet firm manner than to battle a screaming, frightened, unrestrained child.

Another important aspect of pediatric patients is that they live in a world of simple truths—to deceive, lie, or create distrust destroys all hope of dealing with them. Children should be given all the necessary information in terms they can deal with. As an example, telling a child that the needle used for drawing blood will not hurt or that an injection will not hurt creates distrust for any future efforts. A

Note: This chapter has been excerpted from Ehrlich, F.E., "Common Pediatric Emergencies," in Kravis, T.C. and Warner, C.G. (Eds.), *Emergency Medicine: A Comprehensive Review*. Rockville, MD: Aspen Publishers, Inc. © 1983.

gentle, firm, honest, and reassuring approach with the child over 3 years of age often enables the physician to perform a complete initial assessment with minimal difficulty. Explaining procedures in detail to the patient under the age of 3 is usually a waste of time. It is better to tell the child what is going to happen, restrain the child properly, and then carry out the necessary procedures.

At the second corner of the triangle are the parents of the patient. It is absolutely essential for emergency personnel to remember that they are dealing not only with a patient but the parents of that patient as well. For most parents, their child's illness is a frightening experience. They feel helpless and may even sense failure over the situation. They may feel guilty because the child is ill or injured and wonder if it was something they could have prevented. All of this leads to an anxiety-laden experience. Their behavior may be totally different from when the illness involves one of them. Understanding this situation will lead to a better experience for all concerned.

Parents should be completely informed of the physician's impressions of the cause of the problem and what studies and treatment are planned. Just as no secrets should be kept from the patient, none should be kept from the parents either. A helpful and thoughtful word from the physicians and nurses will do much to alleviate anxiety.

The mother appearing in the emergency department at three o'clock in the morning with a child whose temperature is 101°F (38°C) and who has a runny nose, is herself in need of help. The child probably has nothing more than an upper respiratory infection, but the mother is telling the staff, "I am insecure and do not really understand what to do for my child." She is indirectly asking for help. The child will be helped as much by educating the mother as by a prescription for a decongestant.

The final corner in the triangle is the emergency department personnel. The arrival of a pediatric patient can create significant anxiety for the staff. First, personnel are often afraid of dealing with such small patients. They are unable to understand the child's pathophysiology, uneasy performing the necessary diagnostic procedures, and often uncertain as to the appropriate therapy. Finally, they are afraid of similar problems with their own children. It is imperative that emergency personnel deal with their anxieties in a constructive way and not allow them to interfere with relationships with parents and patients.

The staff must serve as the conductor, orchestrating the relationships surrounding a pediatric patient. It is interesting to talk with children and parents who have been treated in the emergency department of a pediatric hospital. In these institutions the staff are readily familiar with pediatric patients and have voluntarily chosen to work with them. The anxiety level among this staff is usually much lower. The experience in these emergency departments, for child and parent alike, is better when compared with that in a general hospital emergency department. Obviously, effort must be put forth to offset this problem.

History

Another point to remember is that for the vast majority of children the medical history comes primarily from the parents. Nevertheless, when taking a history always have the child in the room with the parents; talking with the parents away from the child usually arouses distrust on the part of the child. In addition, it is sometimes beneficial to ask questions directly of the child but in the presence of the parents. The child who understands the question will give a reliable answer. This same technique is helpful in completing the physical examination since the presence of a parent will help to alleviate fear and distrust.

The details of history-taking are quite similar to the adult patient. The one point that should be emphasized for the pediatric group is the time factor. In a small child, such as a 6-month-old infant, tremendous devastation can occur in a short period of time. Twenty-four hours of diarrhea in a 6-month-old can produce far more significant fluid loss than 24 hours of diarrhea in a 20-year-old.

Physical Examination

As for the physical examination the basic premise is that nothing should be done to frighten or startle the child and initiate fear and crying. Instruments should be room temperature; nothing is more frightening to a small infant or child than to have a cold instrument placed on the chest or abdomen. Likewise, the examiner's hands should be warm. Along these same lines it is imperative that the examiner have available pediatric-size instruments. This includes otoscope attachments, a pediatric stethoscope so that pulmonary and heart sounds can be adequately localized, and needles and syringes for drawing blood samples.

It is important that the blood pressure cuff be of the appropriate size. The correct size cuff covers approximately two-thirds of the upper arm. If the cuff is narrower, readings will be erroneously high and if the cuff is wider, erroneously low.

During this stage of the initial assessment the parent may hold the child. In particular, examination of the chest is aided by the parent's holding the child to the chest with the child's back turned to the examiner. The object, once again, is to maintain the child's sense of security. If for some reason the parents must leave the room, it is advisable to explain to the child why they are leaving and what will happen while the parents are away. It is often helpful to allow the child the opportunity of playing with some of the instruments and exploring them prior to using them on the patient.

It is important to realize that the sequence of the adult physical examination, which usually begins at the head and proceeds to the toes, is not appropriate for small children. It is easier for everyone if those areas which are most apt to produce crying are examined at the very end. Therefore a good beginning is listening to the chest, a procedure which is the least invasive and least obnoxious to the child and enables the child to stay in the parent's arms and be most secure. Then proceed to auscultation of the heart and anterior chest.

Then if the abdomen is not involved with the problem, examine that area, perhaps tickling the child and beginning some sort of play relationship.

In general, examining the ears, throat, and nose produces the child's most vivid response. Distracting the child by pretending to produce things from the child's ears may make it possible to carry out this part of the assessment without difficulty. However, if the child has an earache on one side, then that will certainly be the last area to examine. If the problem is external otitis, expect minimal cooperation from the child. When the physician examines the throat and ears of small children an assistant should restrain the child in order to make the procedure as atraumatic and rapid as possible.

It is important when examining a sick child to be as patient as possible. Haste will only result in pain, needless trauma, and fear. In turn this will result in the least amount of cooperation and produce a sequence that benefits no one.

Restraining the Child

A child can be restrained in three ways. The simplest method is to ask a staff assistant to hold the child in the proper position. Parents often shrink from using the force required to restrain their children. During the initial assessment, the parent may be allowed to hold the child's feet since this maintains contact between them. Another form of restraint entails the use of a commercially available device that consists of a board and Velcro straps. These are, in general, quite effective. They are especially useful when dealing with patients with lacerations. The third type of restraint involves "mummifying" the child in a bed sheet. This is probably the most inexpensive effective way to immobilize a small child for examination of the areas around the upper extremities and head.

PROBLEMS IN THE FIRST YEAR OF LIFE

Infants in this age group are probably the most frightening patients to the staff of a general hospital emergency department. At the same time they are often the easiest to diagnose and treat. The majority of patients in this age group are brought to the emergency department for some form of infection. The presenting complaint is usually fever, a frightening experience for most parents when it involves their own children. Usually, they make some effort to control the fever and when that fails they bring the child immediately to the emergency department. If the child has additional symptoms such as diarrhea or vomiting or is tugging at an ear, then the diagnosis is simplified.

On the other hand, many children are brought to the emergency department with a complaint of fever and no localizing signs or symptoms. The physician must then do a thorough head-to-toe examination looking for the cause. Otitis media, urinary tract infections, and pharyngitis are often hidden causes for fever. If a cause is found treatment is rendered accordingly. If no cause is found then the laboratory should be used for assistance. A complete blood cell count (CBC), urinalysis, and chest roentgenogram should be done. Throat and blood cultures are done as indicated, as is a cerebrospinal fluid (CSF) evaluation.

The appropriate dosage for aspirin and acetaminophen products is based on the weight of the patient. The dose for aspirin used as an antipyretic is 30 to 60 mg/kg/day. This is given orally and divided into doses every four hours. Another good general rule to teach parents is to administer 1¼ grains of aspirin for every year of life. Since most of the pediatric aspirin tablet preparations come as 1¼ grain tablets, this is a simple system to use. The American Academy of Pediatrics recommends avoiding the use of aspirin in young children with flu or chicken pox, because of the risk of Reye's syndrome. The dose for acetaminophen, for infants under 1 year of age is 60 mg orally every four hours; for children under 3 years of age 120 mg every 4 hours orally; and for children over 3 years of age 120 to 240 mg every three or four hours orally. Parents should be advised that for children who are vomiting, both medications are available in suppository form. The dosage for aspirin and acetaminophen administered rectally is the same as the dosage orally. It is often helpful in the management of high fevers to use both medications, alternating them at two-hour intervals.

Fever in the first 3 months of life is a serious symptom and any temperature over 101°F (38°C) most likely warrants hospital admission and a com plete work-up in terms of diagnostic studies, including lumbar puncture, cultures, chest roentgenogram, CBC, and urinalysis.

Respiratory Infections

In the case of a child under 1 year of age with an upper respiratory infection, management should include humidification and increased fluid intake and should not include the use of antibiotics, decongestants, or antihistamines. (See Chapter 7).

Urinary Tract Infections

Urinary tract infections in children in this age-group are difficult to diagnose because of the lack of symptoms. Sterile urine for culture must be collected in order to make the diagnosis. Various commercial kits are available for strapping the child in order to collect a sample. If these do not work then a suprapubic tap is indicated. Once the diagnosis of a urinary tract infection is established, appropriate antibiotic therapy should be instituted and a diagnostic work-up of the urinary tract should be initiated by referral to a urologist. (See Chapter 21.)

Gastrointestinal (GI) Infections

Another form of infection common in this age-group involves the GI tract. Therapy entails replacement of fluid loss. An important consideration is that for the outpatient management of children with GI infections and fluid loss, the oral replacement fluid should be a simple electrolyte solution. The child should be fed small amounts of these liquids at frequent intervals and no attempt made to give large bolus volumes. Agents such as Kaopectate and Lomotil should be avoided in the management of diarrhea since they may prolong the problem. If any of these problems persists to such a degree that adequate oral intake cannot be given and the child seems to be worsening clinically, hospital admission for IV fluid replacement and a culture work-up is required. (See Chapter 14.)

Surgical Conditions

A few surgical conditions that occur in the first year of life can present as problems to the emergency department. Chronologically, the first of these is pyloric stenosis. This usually presents in a patient between 2 and 6 weeks of age. The infant is brought to the emergency department because of persistent projectile vomiting. The vomiting is usually worse later in the day than in the morning. The characteristic history and the palpable mass in the child's right upper quadrant lead to the definitive diagnosis. The treatment is, of course, surgery.

Another surgical problem is intussusception. These children are usually between 6 months and 1 year of age, and more often male than female. The patient usually presents with intermittent crampy abdominal pain. Often the parents describe the child as having "fits"—drawing up the legs and crying in apparent pain. There may be bloody diarrhea and emesis, depending on the degree of intestinal obstruction. Physical examination usually reveals a tender abdomen and on occasion a palpable mass on the right side of the abdomen. This can be a difficult diagnosis to make and requires a high index of suspicion. The treatment is to obtain the diagnostic (and often therapeutic) barium enema after a surgical consultation.

Inguinal hernias can present as a problem in this age-group. They are usually frightening to the parents and get far more attention than they deserve. If the hernia can be reduced, then the parents should be reassured and referred to their pediatrician for eventual surgical consultation. Efforts to reduce the hernia can be made but an overzealous effort to squeeze the hernia contents back into the abdominal cavity should be avoided. If the hernia cannot be reduced easily, then immediate surgical consultation is required. (See Chapter 21.)

SEIZURES

Febrile seizures are common in the pediatric population, and are associated with some form of febrile illness such as viral gastroenteritis or roseola. They usually occur between 6 months and 5 years of age. They are of short duration lasting generally less than ten minutes.

The important steps in management involve immediate supportive treatment. This consists of airway maintenance, oxygen, and initiating an IV line. Anticonvulsants are used when indicated, the most appropriate being diazepam. It can be given in a dose of 0.5 mg/kg up to a maximum dose of 5 mg in small children. The intramuscular (IM) route is by no means as effective as the rectal or IV route. If diazepam is given IV it should be administered slowly. Since it may be difficult to establish an IV in a small child, rectal administration of the standard IV diazepam preparation in the same dosage, via a small rubber catheter is recommended. The dosage should be titrated carefully, since respiratory depression may occur with an overdose.

Once the seizure has been controlled then the fever should be evaluated and the child treated with appropriate medications. The central nervous system should be evaluated as a possible source of the convulsion. Whether these children should be placed on daily prophylactic therapy, whether they should be given prophylactic phenobarbital during febrile episodes, or whether they should be managed with neither is controversial. A careful review of the literature suggests that doing nothing is most likely the best management. (See Chapter 11.)

COMMON VIRAL INFECTIONS

It is imperative for the emergency physician in a general hospital to be adept at recognizing certain of the viral infections common to the pediatric population. These include rubeola, rubella, roseola, erythema infectiosum, varicella, and mumps. (See Chapter 36.)

Rubeola

Rubeola, or measles, has an incubation period of 10 to 12 days. The prodromal phase is characterized by a low-grade to moderate fever, a mild cough, and the general symptoms of an upper respiratory infection. This in turn is followed by the appearance of Koplik's spots which are pathognomonic of measles. These spots are grayish punctate lesions on the buccal mucosa opposite the lower molars. Next the rash of measles begins to appear, first as macules along the neck and face area. Then it becomes more maculopapular as the rash spreads over the upper body and arms, then to the torso and abdomen, and eventually the feet. The rash may take two to three days to reach the distal lower extremity. The rash may be confluent. Pruritus is unusual. Isolation should be continued for approximately one week after the rash starts. The rapid decline in the number of cases of measles throughout the United States only underscores the need for greater awareness on the part of the emergency physician as to the diagnosis.

Rubella

Rubella, or German measles, has an incubation period of two to three weeks. The prodromal period consists of mild catarrhal symptoms and often goes unnoticed. The characteristic physical finding in rubella is the posterior or retroauricular lymphadenopathy. These nodes are often quite large and tender. Few alternative diagnoses cause this finding in this age population. The rash of rubella varies from discrete maculopapular lesions to flushing with confluence of the maculopapular lesions particularly over the face. The rash usually lasts about three days. The photophobia (light sensitivity) present with measles is not present in German measles. Fever is usually low-grade, and pruritus is not generally a problem.

Roseola

Roseola, or exanthem subitum, is characterized by the sudden onset of four to five days of high-grade fever, often as high as 103° to 105°F (39° to 40°C). Febrile seizures are not uncommon when the fever is this high. There may be minimal symptoms of an upper respiratory infection. The most outstanding characteristic of roseola is the complete absence of any physical findings to explain the fever. This clinical characteristic is often used to support the diagnosis. The disease occurs most commonly in infants and young children. The fever usually falls precipitously around the fourth day and at about the same time a macular or maculopapular eruption appears over the trunk and then spreads to the arms, neck, and finally the face and legs. The rash usually lasts only 24 hours and then fades.

Erythema Infectiosum

Fifth disease, or erythema infectiosum, is characterized by a rash which seems to appear in two separate stages. The rash may be preceded by very nonspecific signs and symptoms of an upper respiratory infection, including sore throat and coryza. The first stage of the disease is characterized by erythematous, coalescent, maculopapular lesions overlying the cheeks—the so-called "slapped cheeks." The rest of the face is usually spared. The lesions resemble, at least superficially, early erysipelas. The facial rash generally lasts one to four days.

The second-stage rash, which begins about one day after the first, consists of an erythematous maculopapular eruption on the extensor surfaces of the arms, hands, and then shortly thereafter the thighs and buttocks. The trunk is usually spared. The rash spreads to the flexor surface of the arms as the extensor surface lesions begin to clear. The rash may take from one to two weeks to fade completely with the entire course of the disease lasting up to 24 days. A peculiar characteristic of the rash of fifth disease is its marked variation in intensity from moment to moment. There is often mild pruritus. These patients are usually afebrile particularly in the latter stages of the disease.

Varicella

Varicella, or chickenpox, has an incubation period of two to three weeks. The prodromal symptoms consist of a mild fever with malaise. Following this, the specific rash of chickenpox appears. It begins as small red papules that shortly thereafter develop into clear vesicles overlying an erythematous base. Subsequently the vesicle content becomes cloudy. The vesicles are broken easily and are coated with an eschar. Vesicle eruption continues for between two and five days. They spread from the trunk to the face and scalp, sparing the extremities. Pruritus is a predominant symptom of varicella. The fever may range from low-grade to as high as 105°F (40°C).

Mumps

Mumps has an incubation period of two to three weeks. Prodromal symptoms are rare but, if present, usually consist of mild myalgia in the neck area. The onset of the illness is characterized by pain and then swelling in the area of one or both parotid glands. These symptoms persist for one to three days and then over the ensuing week gradually subside. Bilateral swelling is much more common than unilateral. High fever is a rare complication of mumps. On occasion, the submandibular gland may be swollen as well or may even be the only gland involved with mumps.

ACUTE ABDOMEN

One of the most common problems for which children are brought to an emergency department is abdominal pain. It is absolutely essential that an emergency medicine physician be adept at discerning the nonsurgically from the surgically treatable causes. The emergency physician must be able to decide that a child most likely has appendicitis and will require surgery or has a viral mesenteric adenitis and can go home. (See Chapters 14 and 15.)

Appendicitis

The story of epigastric pain followed by nausea, anorexia, vomiting, malaise, and subsequent migration of the pain to the right lower quadrant is classical for appendicitis. The diagnosis of appendicitis in a child should be based on clinical findings and not laboratory tests. The physician must take a careful history of the nature, onset, and progression of the pain, and must elicit a history of the child's overall behavior during the time of the illness. A child who has been playing and jovial throughout the illness is much less likely to have appendicitis than one who has been lying around watching television or playing quietly in bed or on the couch. The critical part of this diagnosis is a careful abdominal examination and eliciting peritoneal signs along with localized right lower quadrant abdominal tenderness.

The standard technique for producing rebound tenderness is to push into the abdominal cavity and then sharply release the abdominal wall. This should *never* be done as part of the examination of children. It produces a pain over which the child has no control. It will assuredly destroy the examiner's rapport with the child. A far better technique for discovering the same information is to use the cough rebound sign. If in fact the peritoneum is irritated, the child will limit the excursion of the cough and protect the abdomen.

At this point the diagnosis of acute appendicitis should be entertained and, whether or not the white blood cell count (WBC) is elevated, surgical consultation should be requested. Many children have had a gangrenous appendix removed while their WBC count was normal, and many children with a WBC count of 20,000 to 25,000 have been operated upon only to find a normal appendix. Although the majority of patients with acute appendicitis have a mildly to moderately elevated WBC count, emergency department physicians cannot allow themselves the luxury of using it as a basis for diagnosis. They should base their impressions on the physical examination and history, particularly if they intend to avoid the catastrophe of sending a patient out of the emergency department with acute appendicitis.

Once the diagnosis of acute appendicitis has been clinically ruled out, the child often can be managed as an outpatient. One exception involves the abdominal pain of sickle cell disease.

It is imperative that a child sent home with abdominal pain and instructions for outpatient management have a follow-up visit arranged for the next day.

COMMON PEDIATRIC TRAUMAS

A child can be traumatized in any area and the ability to manage these injuries is required of all emergency department physicians. This section covers some of the common forms of trauma. The battered child, pediatric orthopedic injuries, drowning, burns, or injuries to the genitourinary tract are discussed in other chapters.

Foreign Bodies

A common problem for which children are brought to the emergency department involves the ingestion of a foreign body. If the foreign body is in the tracheobronchial tree, immediate surgical consultation is required. This should be done only after the child's airway has been evaluated and secured. (See Chapter 9.)

If the foreign body has been swallowed and is in the stomach then therapy will depend on the nature of the object. If it is a blunt object such as a coin, no further attention is necessary. These patients can be followed once a week with routine roentgenograms so as to follow the course of the foreign body. In addition, the parents should be instructed to check the bowel movements for the foreign body. If the child has swallowed a pointed or sharp object, the type and location of the object will determine the management.

Esophageal foreign bodies need immediate attention. In the child under the age of 4, coins can be removed from the esophagus without the use of the esophagoscope. This can be done with a Foley catheter. The technique involves placement of the Foley catheter in the esophagus. Inflation of the Foley balloon is done under the fluoroscope with radiopaque dye so that it is exactly the same size as the coin. This prevents any damage to the esophagus by the balloon. The child is then tipped head down and the Foley catheter withdrawn. The coin will fall out onto the table. The child is then observed overnight on a liquid diet and sent home after a repeat chest roentgenogram. (See Chapter 20.)

Foreign bodies in the ears and nose can pose a difficult problem. Many foreign bodies lodged in the nose can be extracted with fine forceps. If this does not work, then a small Foley catheter can usually be passed beyond the object, the balloon inflated, and the object and catheter withdrawn simultaneously.

Foreign bodies in the ear can be difficult to remove, and most of them should be referred directly to an otolaryngologist. They require a great deal of expertise in working through an otoscope with a head mirror, light, and delicate instruments. If the ear canal is irritated and bleeding initiated, the task of the otolaryngologist will only be more difficult and general anesthesia and an operating room may be needed.

Another site for foreign body presentation is the vagina. Little girls whom you suspect of having vaginal foreign bodies should be examined with thought and patience and only in the presence of their mothers and a nurse. A good deal of explanation will be necessary, as well as reassurance and a gentle manner. The correct size instruments are an absolute prerequisite. (See Chapter 23.)

Lacerations

Lacerations around the head, eyes, ears, nose, and face are common in this age-group. The management of these injuries is the same for children as for adults. (See Chapter 29.)

One injury more common in children than adults involves lacerations of the tongue. This can be a difficult injury to treat, particularly at three in the morning with minimal assistance. Suturing such a laceration should be done only after conservative means to control the bleeding fail. Also, the minimum number of assistants is two and appropriate lighting and equipment must be available. The mouth should be held open, with the tongue outside the oral cavity, my means of some form of mouth gag or an assistant. This requires fine absorbable suture material as well as a great deal of suction and patience. Anything less is doomed to failure. If repair cannot be accomplished in the emergency department, the patient should be managed by the appropriate specialist and will more than likely require general anesthesia and an operating room.

Electric Burns

Another common injury involves burns around the mouth from contact with electrical current. Such injuries usually occur because the child bit into a plug or electrical cord and sustained an injury, most often in the corner of the mouth. This injury may look like a superficial burn initially and be covered with an eschar. The eschar in turn will slough around the fifth to the seventh day at which time significant bleeding may occur. All of these children should be admitted to the hospital if any tissue loss has taken place. They can be treated conservatively and appropriate surgical consultations obtained as needed. (See Chapter 30.)

MAJOR TRAUMA

The management of a child with major multisystem trauma resembles that of an adult with similar trauma. Attention to the ABCs of trauma resuscitation are paramount. The possibility of a fracture of the cervical spine must constantly be emphasized. The ability to gain airway control in a child with head and neck trauma requires a skilled intubationist or a skilled surgeon to perform a tracheostomy or cricothyroidotomy. A tracheostomy in a traumatized 3-year-old child, in the best of hands, is a difficult procedure. Cricothyroidotomy, while difficult, is certainly easier than a tracheostomy and should be a skill in which the emergency physician maintains some degree of expertise.

Access to the circulation of a child via the various large peripheral veins is another skill required of an emergency physician. Venous cutdown at the saphenous vein in the ankle or groin or the basilic or cephalic veins in the upper extremity, and the percutaneous techniques of external jugular or subclavian puncture are procedures that may need to be performed rapidly in a small child.

The necessary steps for evaluation of injuries to the chest, abdomen, and head are similar in children and adults. One major difference is that peritoneal lavage should be a routine part of the management of the pediatric patient with an abdominal injury. Since the history is often difficult to obtain and may be of doubtful validity, peritoneal lavage provides a basis, but not a definitive one, for the initial diagnosis. That is, a positive lavage has meaning while a negative lavage does not. The administration of fluids and maintenance of adequate urine output, with appropriate monitoring of either wedge pressure or central venous pressure, are mandatory for the pediatric patient.

The basic format for trauma management outlined in the Advanced Trauma Life Support course of the American College of Surgeons should be familiar to every emergency department physician managing a traumatized pediatric patient. (See Chapters 17 and 25.)

BIBLIOGRAPHY

Gellis SS, Kagan M: *Current Pediatric Trauma*, ed 11. Philadelphia, WB Saunders, 1984.

Irving G: Pediatric emergencies, in Schwartz GR (ed): *Principles and Practice in Emergency Medicine*, Philadelphia, WB Saunders, 1978.

Smith C: *The Critically Ill Child*, ed 2. Philadelphia, WB Saunders, 1977.

Vaughan VC, McKay RJ, Behran RE: *Nelson Text Book of Pediatrics*, ed 11. Philadelphia, WB Saunders, 1979.

American College of Emergency Physicians: *The Study Guide in Emergency Medicine*. November 1980.

Fred J. Heldrich

4 Anaphylaxis

Anaphylaxis is a sudden allergic reaction, ranging from life threatening to mild, that follows exposure to a stimulus to which the patient is allergic. Symptoms can occur after initial exposure or exposure to a stimulus to which the patient has been previously sensitized. The list of potential stimuli includes antibiotics, biologicals, other pharmaceuticals, insect stings, and foods. Severity of the reaction is usually greatest when the interval between exposure to the stimulus and onset of symptoms is shortest.

Usually beginning with a generalized erythema, symptoms can rapidly increase and include a sense of apprehension, itching, and hives. Edema of the larynx is first manifested by coughing, followed by dyspnea, wheezing, and inspiratory stridor leading to hypoxia and cyanosis. Gastrointestinal symptoms of nausea and vomiting can also occur. Cardiovascular collapse may follow. Symptoms may not progress to such an extreme but could be limited to generalized urticaria or perhaps moderate wheezing. Early intervention is imperative and has two stages: emergency and continuing.

EMERGENCY THERAPY

The following are used in the emergency treatment of anaphylaxis:

1. Aqueous epinephrine, 1 : 1000 (1 mg/mL): administer 0.01 mL/kg (maximum, 0.5 mL) SC. Give a similar dose simultaneously at the site of the bite or injection, but in the latter case, only if the initial dose was given subcutaneously. For *shock*, administer a 1 : 10,000 (0.1 mg/mL) dilution of aqueous epinephrine, 1 to 2 mL IV.
2. Tourniquet: apply proximal to the site of the bite or injection.
3. Oxygen: administer via mask to prevent hypoxemia.
4. Diphenhydramine (Benadryl) for urticaria: administer 2 mg/kg IV, then 5 mg/kg/24 h orally for several days.

CONTINUING THERAPY

Any of the following may be necessary, depending on the initial response to treatment:

1. Intravenous fluids: use normal saline, lactated Ringer's solution, or 5% serum albumin to correct hypovolemia and maintain blood pressure.
2. Vasopressor—metaraminol bitartrate (Aramine): add 0.4 mg/kg to intravenous fluids and titrate the flow rate to stabilize blood pressure or dopamine at an infusion rate of 7 to 20 μg/kg/min may be given.
3. Bronchodilator—aminophylline: dilute 6 mg/kg in two equal volumes of saline and administer IV over 10 to 15 minutes. If necessary, follow with

continuous aminophylline drip at a rate of 1 mg/kg/h.
4. Adrenocorticosteroids: Although of little value in managing the acute stage, these can be used as supplemental therapy for several days.

COMPLICATIONS

Airway obstruction, metabolic acidosis, hypoxic seizures, and cardiac arrhythmias require further specific care and hospitalization. Hospitalization is also indicated for those patients who do not respond promptly to emergency measures discussed here. Relapses are not uncommon after an initial clinical response to treatment.

Upon discharge, patients should be supplied with a kit containing epinephrine for immediate use should it be necessary. Desensitization is a useful protective measure for anaphylaxis secondary to stings of bees, wasps, yellow jackets, and hornets (see Chapter 33).

Bibliography

Smith CA (ed): *The Critically Ill Child: Diagnosis and Management*. Philadelphia, WB Saunders Co, 1972.
Vaughn VA III, McKay RJ, Behrman RE, et al (eds): *Nelson Textbook of Pediatrics*, ed 11. Philadelphia, WB Saunders Co, 1978.

Charles S. Turner

5 Anesthetic Management

Anesthetic care of an injured child in the emergency department is a challenge for the physician. First of all, the psychologic situation must be managed.[1] Fear of pain or possible separation from parents and especially fear of the unknown are the major reactions of the injured child. Parental anxiety, which is easily sensed by the child, can heighten the child's fear. Add to this the possibility of a cold and impersonal environment and an almost impossible situation is produced.

The physician who takes care of the child must feel confident. This confidence is sensed easily by both the child and the parents. Taking time to talk calmly with the parents while obtaining a history of the accident and past medical history allows the parents to relax. This relaxation and rapport with the parents help the child realize that the physician is not only caring but also nonthreatening.

Even more important, the physician must take time to develop a friendship with the patient. Questions about the child's age, siblings, friends, pets, school, and the like, show a sincere interest in the child beyond the injury and help allay anxiety and fear. Offering an object to play with, such as a stethoscope or reflex hammer, provides a distraction while talking with the child and the parents. The child also is less apt to be frightened when these instruments are needed diagnostically.

Once the child is acclimated to the environment of the emergency department and has confidence in the physician, a careful examination can be carried out. The injury amenable to repair in the emergency department and therefore requiring some anesthetic is usually a soft tissue injury.[1] Examination of the wound can be facilitated by sedation, but this also can interfere with an accurate assessment of nerve and tendon injuries. With care and good rapport, the physician can evaluate most injuries and determine the need for general anesthesia in the operating room. If the injury is to be handled in the emergency department then the issue of sedation, anesthesia, and restraints must be addressed.

SEDATION

For the child under 6 years of age, sedation can be very helpful. In the very young child, adequate examination of the injury often requires sedation as well as a local anesthetic.[1,2] Then it can be determined whether the child needs general anesthesia for more extensive repair. In this regard, it is crucial to inform the operating room anesthesiologist of the medications given in the emergency department to ensure a smooth transition to general anesthesia if necessary.

Sedation alone is not satisfactory for minor procedures performed in the emergency department, and therefore an analgesic should be provided as well. Likewise, an analgesic alone does not provide the

TABLE 5-1 Sedation of Infants and Children

Meperidine (Demerol)	1.0 mg/kg
Chlorpromazine (Thorazine)	0.5 mg/kg
Promethazine (Phenergan)	0.5 mg/kg
Morphine sulfate	0.2 mg/kg
Hydroxyzine (Vistaril)	1.0 mg/kg
Secobarbital (Seconal)	3.0 mg/kg

Source: From Seashore JH: Soft tissue injuries, in Touloukian RJ (ed): *Pediatric Trauma,* p 220. Copyright © 1978 John Wiley & Sons, Inc. Reprinted by permission of John Wiley & Sons, Inc.

relief from fear and anxiety that a sedative does. Indeed, an analgesic alone (e.g., meperidine) can accentuate a child's hyperactive state. There are several combinations of drugs that can be used to provide not only systemic analgesia but also amnesia and sedation (Table 5-1).[3] It is very important to weigh the child and calculate accurate doses rather than approximating the weight and thus the dose.

RESTRAINTS

Some sort of physical restraint is necessary for children under 2 years of age.[1] A child this age is unable to understand and cooperate. Even with sedation, restraints are needed to keep the child still during the procedure. Restraining some preschoolers may relieve their anxiety about moving when they should not. In the child from 2 to 4 years of age, the use of restraints must be individualized. Whether restraints are used in the older child depends on the type of injury to be repaired and the response of the child to sedation but mostly on the amount of time and effort the physician takes in comforting the child. It is worth taking a few extra minutes to explain what is wrong and what needs to be done in order to gain the child's confidence and cooperation. Restraints used in a child 4 years of age or older can be a sign of the physician's failure to fulfill the obligation of total care of the patient. It serves no purpose to terrify further a child already terrified by injury and fear.

Once rapport is established, children realize that there may be discomfort but that nothing will be forced upon them. They can handle discomfort if they are honestly informed and given time to adjust. In this regard, it is important not to hide equipment from children. Likewise, a child's face and eyes should not be covered with drapes if at all possible. Secretiveness builds mistrust and covering the face enhances an already terrifying situation. "No surprises" is the most comforting phrase a child can hear during a procedure.

During the procedure, it is important to communicate constantly with the child. This not only allows the child time to adjust and to understand what is being done but also serves as a distraction. Questions again about schooling, friends, pets, etc., can help focus attention away from the procedure. Once the child is calmed with a "lytic cocktail" and gentle restraints, the area to be repaired must be anesthetized. In the pediatric emergency department, the regional anesthetic techniques include[3]

- topical anesthesia/ethyl chloride spray
- infiltration: injecting anesthetic into the tissue to be incised or debrided (Figures 5-1 and 5-2)
- field block: injecting anesthetic into the tissue on the periphery of the area to be repaired (Figures 5-3 and 5-4)

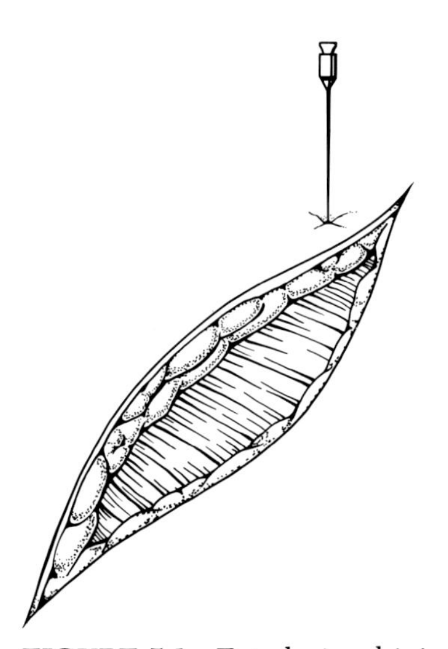

FIGURE 5-1 Extralesional injection.

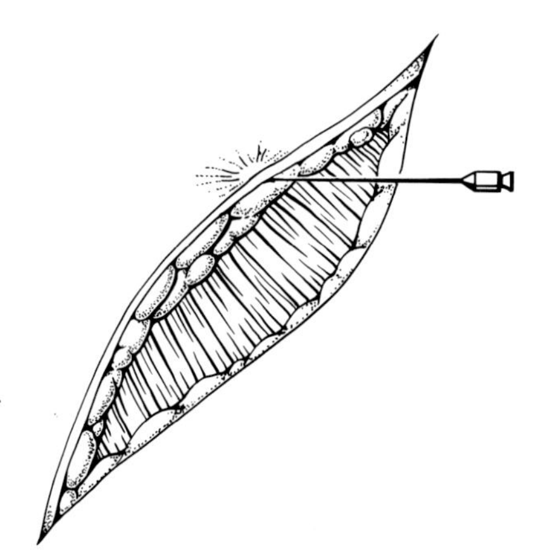

FIGURE 5-2 Intralesional injection. Injecting through the edge of the wound does not increase the chance of infection and is less painful.

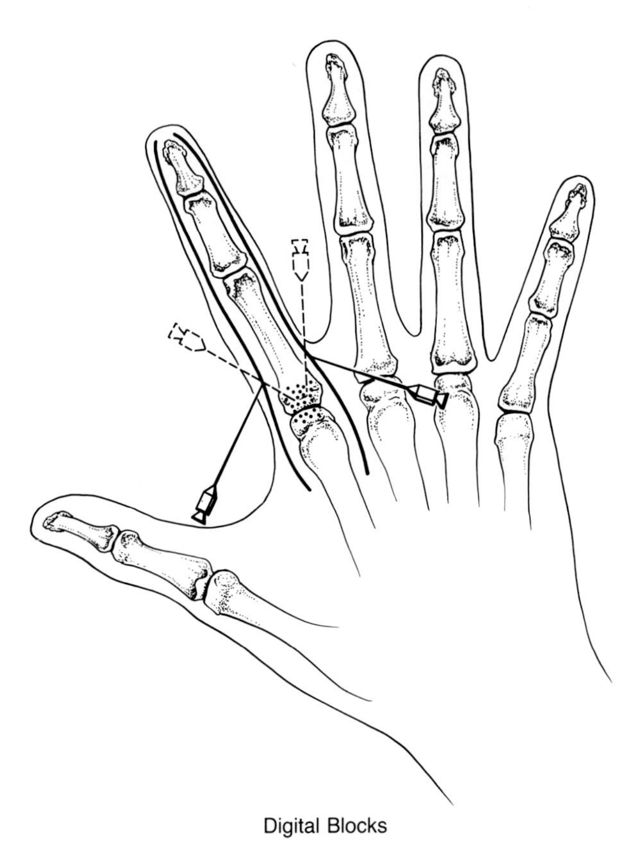

FIGURE 5-3 Digital blocks. Use 1% lidocaine; never use epinephrine in the anesthetic. Cleanse the dorsal surface and palpate the distal metatarsal head. Make a skin wheal with a 25- or 26-gauge needle at the lateral border of the head. Slowly advance the needle to the side of the head and inject the anesthetic. Keeping the needle under the skin, pull back and advance the needle to the other side of the metatarsal head and make a wheal in the dermis. Then insert the needle in the other side of the head and inject the anesthetic.

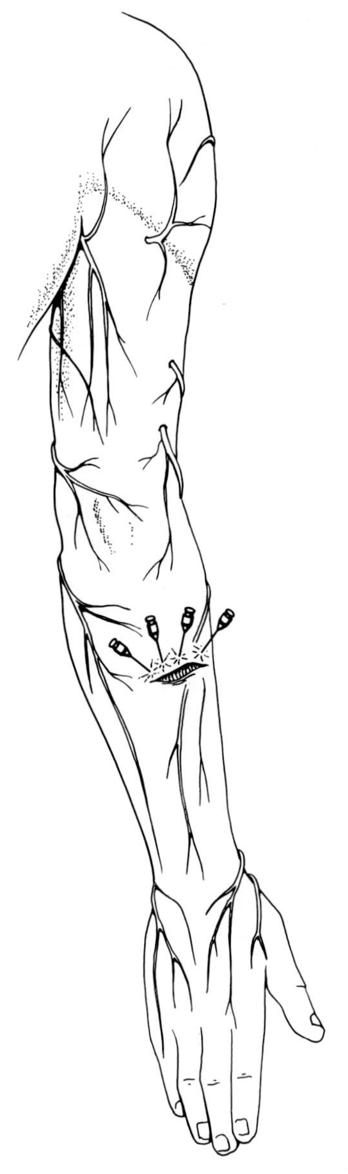

FIGURE 5-4 Field blocks.

Generally, for infiltrative anesthesia 0.5% to 1.0% lidocaine is used; for field block, 1%; and for a truncal block, if attempted, 1.5% or 2.0%.

When selecting the type and route of anesthetic, the smallest effective amount of the least toxic substance in the safest possible manner should be used (Table 5-2). Severe side effects are possible with any of the local anesthetics,[4] and these must be recognized early and treated rapidly. Resuscitative equipment and medications must be readily available, and the physician in charge must be familiar with their use.

Many factors affect the toxicity of local anesthetics.[2,4] The rapidity of attaining a high plasma level depends on the total dose of the agent and the speed with which the dose is injected. Injection into a highly vascularized area or into a vessel itself increases the risk of a high blood level and subsequent toxic reactions. Hyperpyrexia increases absorption whereas debility, shock, and anemia decrease the metabolic clearance of the anesthetic. Liver disease and severe anemia also diminish the level of plasma pseudocholinesterase, and therefore detoxification of ester-type drugs is retarded. Renal disease with failure to eliminate the breakdown products of anesthetics will prolong their action. Vasoconstrictors, such as epinephrine, can not only decrease the absorption and therefore the blood

TABLE 5-2 Guideline for Doses of Local Anesthetics

	Concentration (%)		
Anesthetic	Infiltration	Nerve Block	Maximum Dose (mg/kg body wt)
Procaine hydrochloride (Novocain)	0.5–1.0	1–1.5	15
Chloroprocaine hydrochloride (Nesacaine)	0.5–1.0	1–1.5	20
Lidocaine (Xylocaine)	0.25–0.5 (infants) 0.5–1.0 (children)	1.0	7
Tetracaine hydrochloride (Pontocaine)		0.1–0.15	2

Source: Adapted with permission from Eather KF: Regional anesthesia for infants and children. *Int Anesthesiol Clin* 1975;13(3):30.

level of the anesthetic but also be very hazardous. A local anesthetic containing epinephrine should never be used on the fingers, toes, nose, ear lobes, or penis because it may cause ischemic gangrene.

Throughout subsequent chapters a variety of techniques for providing local anesthesia are discussed along with the injuries to which they are applicable. In each case the principles mentioned here should be applied. Good rapport and effective therapy invariably yield a rapid recovery.

References

1. Seashore JH: Soft tissue injuries, in Touloukian RJ (ed): *Pediatric Trauma*. New York, John Wiley & Sons Inc, 1978, pp 219–237.
2. Collins VJ (ed): *Principles of Anesthesiology*, ed 2. Philadelphia, Lea & Febiger, 1976, chaps 45 and 48.
3. Eather KF: Regional anesthesia for infants and children. *Int Anesthesiol Clin* 1975;13:19–48.
4. Owens WD (ed): Anesthetic side effects and complications: Seeking, finding, and treating. *Int Anesthesiol Clin* 1980;18:1–23.

Harold E. Harrison

6 Parenteral Fluid Therapy

WATER REQUIREMENTS OF CHILDREN

Parenteral fluid therapy is most frequently used to meet the water needs of patients who are unable to take oral fluids.[1] A wide range of conditions are involved:

- severe infections, particularly with disturbances of consciousness, such as meningitis or encephalitis
- poisonings
- burns*
- head injuries
- postoperative states
- disorders of the gastrointestinal tract

Since physicians caring for children deal with subjects varying from newborns weighing 3 kg or less to adolescents of perhaps 60 kg, some method is needed to estimate the maintenance water requirements of children of varying age and size who have additional needs arising from various disease states. Although these estimates are only rough approximations, the order of magnitude of water need should be understood: overloading the sick infant or child with fluids can be harmful, and yet an adequate intake for physiologic requirements is essential. It is not surprising, therefore, that considerable attention has been given to various methods for computing the water requirements of the sick infant and child.

Maintenance water needs are not directly proportional to weight over the entire range of age and weight from infancy to adolescence. It has been suggested that surface area be used as a basis for estimating maintenance water needs, and this has been accepted by many workers interested in the problem.[2] We are in agreement with Darrow[3] and others who have suggested that maintenance water requirements can best be related to total kilocalories metabolized. Since basal energy metabolism is approximately proportional to surface area, these two methods of calculation give similar results under basal conditions.[2] However, total energy metabolism in the restless or febrile child can be much greater than basal values, so that even rough estimates of calories metabolized, under varying conditions, would appear to offer the most useful basis for calculating minimal water needs.

Table 6-1 indicates the average weight, surface area, and the basal kilocalorie expenditure per 24 hours for children from the first week of life through adolescence. The minimal water needs under basal conditions are also given on the basis of 1 mL/kcal metabolized.[2] This minimal basal water requirement includes the insensible water loss (i.e., the water evaporated through lungs and skin in the ab-

* Because the treatment of burns is discussed in Chapter 31, it is not included here.

TABLE 6-1 Basal Water Requirements in Relation to Age, Weight, Surface Area, and Basal Caloric Requirements

Age	Weight		Surface Area (m^2)	Basal	Minimal Basal Water Requirement		
	lb	kg		Metabolism (kcal/24 h)*	mL/24 h	mL/m^2	mL/kg
1 wk	7.5	3.3	0.20	200	200	1000	60
2 mo	11.0	5.0	0.25	270	270	1080	54
6 mo	17.5	8.0	0.35	400	400	1140	50
12 mo	22.0	10.0	0.45	500	500	1110	50
3 yr	33.0	15.0	0.60	700	700	1170	47
5 yr	44.0	20.0	0.80	900	900	1120	45
8 yr	66.0	30.0	1.05	1100	1100	1050	37
15 yr	132.0	60.0	1.70	1600	1600	940	27

* Water requirement = 1 mL/kcal.

sence of visible sweating), water loss in the stool, and also the urine water needed for solute excretion. The insensible water loss is directly proportional to energy metabolism and is about 0.4 mL/kcal. The urine water need is related to solute excretion, but under fasting conditions, which prevail in the situations in which parenteral fluids are given, the solute load is a function of tissue breakdown and therefore varies with energy metabolism. Stool loss approximates 0.1 mL/kcal, and urine loss, 0.5 mL/kcal. Water requirements thus can be calculated in terms of energy metabolism; when the preceding values are summed, the minimal need for replacement of evaporative water loss, stool water, and urine water is about 1 mL/kcal.[2] Since the energy output of the restless or active child exceeds basal level, the basal calories should be multiplied by 1.5 to provide for the needs of the nonfebrile but restless or active patient. If fever and restlessness are present, the energy output can be twice the basal values. For example, the minimal fasting water requirement for a febrile, restless 1-year-old child weighing 10 kg would be 1000 mL/d.[2] Thus an extra 500 mL or 50 mL/kg would be provided to cover the extra water losses through skin or lungs if profuse sweating or hyperpnea was present. Water intake greater than basal need also can be ordered to provide more calories as glucose without the need to give markedly hypertonic solutions.

The electrolyte needs of the fasting child maintained on parenteral fluids usually can be met by providing 2 to 3 mEq each of sodium, chloride, and potassium per 100 kcal metabolized.[2] A solution containing 30 mEq of sodium per liter and 20 mEq of potassium per liter provides for this requirement. Such solutions are available commercially or can be prepared by (1) using 0.2% NaCl in 5% dextrose in water (D5W) and adding 20 mEq of potassium acetate per liter, or (2) diluting with water either lactated Ringer's solution (Hartmann) or physiologic saline and adding 1.5 g (20 mEq) potassium chloride per liter. When given in appropriate quantities, these solutions provide for water and electrolyte needs during fasting periods of several days' duration and also supply sufficient glucose to prevent glycogen depletion and ketosis.

DEPLETION OF EXTRACELLULAR VOLUME

The most frequent major problem in water and electrolyte balance demanding emergency attention is depletion of extracellular fluid volume to such a degree that plasma volume is reduced. This decrease in circulating blood volume leads to constriction of peripheral arterioles and reduction of visceral and renal blood flow to maintain blood pressure and brain perfusion. The reduction of renal perfusion further distorts extracellular concentration of solutes, particularly increasing acidosis, because of failing renal hydrogen ion secretion and organic acid excretion. The poor perfusion of skeletal muscle results in accumulation of lactic acid, compounding the severity of metabolic acidosis.[4]

Extracellular fluid volume depletion results from loss of sodium salts and water. A major cause of such loss is failure to reabsorb gastrointestinal secretions, which in essence are specialized extracellular fluids. These fluids can be lost because of vomiting and diarrhea, intestinal obstruction with accumulation of fluid in the intestinal lumen, or continued fluid aspiration resulting from ileus or mechanical obstruction. Another mechanism of sodium salt and water loss is excessive renal excretion of sodium, which can occur in diabetes mellitus because of glycosuria-induced osmotic diuresis plus the loss of sodium to balance the excessive excretion of the

TABLE 6-2 Dehydration and Estimated Loss of Total Body Water

Dehydration	Clinical State	Estimated Loss of Total Body Water (%) Infant	Child (>10 yr)
Mild	History of abnormal fluid loss Sticky mucous membranes	5	3
Moderate	Dry mucous membranes Poor skin turgor Tearing reduced Oliguric Sunken eyes Lethargy Depressed fontanelle	10	6
Severe	Pallor Tenting of skin Hyperpnea Anuric Hypotension Weak, rapid pulse	15	9

organic anions in urine, β-hydroxybutyric acid and acetoacetic acid. Renal sodium loss in urine also occurs in adrenal insufficiency with hypoaldosteronism. An unusual site of sodium loss is the skin in cystic fibrosis patients who sweat profusely, since the sweat in this disorder has a high sodium content.

Recognition of extracellular volume depletion depends on changes resulting from loss of both interstitial fluid and plasma volume (Table 6-2). The signs of the former are

1. changes in skin turgor, with loss of elasticity
2. reduction of retro-orbital tissue fluid, with sinking of the eyeballs into the orbits
3. loss of intraocular fluid, with soft eyeballs
4. reduction of cerebrospinal fluid volume, manifested by sunken fontanelle in the infant with open fontanelle

The reduction of intravascular fluid volume is recognized initially by the compensatory responses:

1. tachycardia
2. peripheral arteriolar constriction with cold, cyanotic hands and feet
3. reduced blood pressure and shock

Changes in consciousness occur when circulatory insufficiency is so marked that brain perfusion is reduced or when acidosis is severe, with reduction of blood pH below 7.0. The neurologic manifestations of hypernatremic dehydration, which do not

TABLE 6-3 Distribution of Body Water as a Percentage of Body Weight

Age Group	Distribution (% of Body Weight) Intracellular	Extracellular: Interstitial	Extracellular: Intravascular	Total
Infant	45	25	5	75
Child	45	20	5	70
Adult	40	15	5	60

depend primarily on circulatory insufficiency, are discussed in a later section.

The extracellular fluid volume in the infant under 6 months of age, excluding the first 2 weeks of life, approximates 30% of body weight. In the older infant and young child up to 2 to 3 years of age, this value is 25% of body weight. For the older child the value of 20% of body weight can be used (Table 6-3).[1] The signs of severe extracellular fluid volume depletion, with manifest reduction of plasma volume, indicate a loss of approximately one third of the original extracellular fluid volume, ranging from 10% of body weight in the young infant to 7% of body weight in the older child. The actual loss of body weight in patients with loss of gastrointestinal secretions or diabetic ketoacidosis can exceed this because of reduction of intracellular fluid as well as tissue solids. The sodium deficit, assuming isonatremic dehydration and a sodium concentration in extracellular fluid of 140 mEq/L, approximates 10 mEq/kg in the older child and can be as high as 14 mEq/kg in the young infant. Since the concentration of chloride in extracellular fluid is 80% of that of sodium, the chloride deficits are 8 to 11 mEq/kg.

Treatment

The treatment of extracellular fluid depletion can be divided into three phases: emergency, replacement, and maintenance (Exhibit 6-1). The initial

EXHIBIT 6-1 Management of Dehydration

Initial Assessment
- Evaluate the degree of dehydration.
- Order appropriate laboratory studies.

Emergency Management
- See Table 6-4.

Immediate Management
- Replace the deficit (see Table 6-5).

Continuing Management
- Replace remaining specific electrolyte deficits as calculated.
- Replace continuing abnormal losses.
- Provide basic daily requirements.
- Provide additional nutritional needs.

TABLE 6-4 Emergency Management of Severe Dehydration

Fluid*	Amount	Time	Comment
Lactated Ringer's solution with 5% dextrose; or saline-bicarbonate solution†	20 mL/kg of either; can be repeated	Administer over 30–60 min; can be repeated	Observe the patient for clinical response. Replace the deficit as soon as the patient's condition indicates.

* May be preceded by plasma or 5% serum albumin (shock).
† Saline-bicarbonate solution: 750 mL 0.85% NaCl in D5W, 225 mL D5W, and 25 mL 8.4% $NaHCO_3$.

emergency treatment (Table 6-4) is aimed at rapid expansion of intravascular volume to improve renal and muscular perfusion. Infusion of plasma or 5% albumin solution, 20 mL/kg, could be used for this purpose but is required only in patients who are in severe circulatory collapse. In the child dehydrated from loss of gastrointestinal secretions and depleted of glycogen because of starvation, the rapid infusion of lactated Ringer's solution with 5% dextrose or of a saline-bicarbonate solution (see Table 6-4), at a dose of 20 mL/kg, can produce striking improvement by supplying metabolic substrate as well as expansion of plasma volume. The 20 mL/kg dose of these solutions given initially provides 3 mEq of sodium per kilogram.[5] In patients with profoundly compromised peripheral perfusion, the use of the solution containing bicarbonate, rather than lactate, may be preferred. Administration of a sodium chloride solution alone, while increasing volume, dilutes the extracellular bicarbonate concentration until the extra chloride is excreted in the urine. The concentration of dissolved CO_2 is not proportionately diluted, since carbon dioxide partial pressure (P_{CO_2}) depends upon respiratory control. The reduced bicarbonate concentration without change in P_{CO_2} decreases extracellular pH. If the patient is already markedly acidotic, this further decrease in pH can compromise cardiac and brain metabolism.

After the emergency treatment, the replacement of deficit (Table 6-5) can be provided over the next

TABLE 6-5 Replacement Management of Dehydration

Type of Dehydration	Fluid	Amount	Time
Hypertonic ($Na^+ > 150$ mEq)	0.2% NaCl in D5W with 20 mEq of K acetate per liter*	Calculated basic daily requirement for 48 h plus calculated deficit	Administer at a constant rate of flow over 48 h
Isotonic ($Na^+ = 130–150$ mEq)	0.45% NaCl in D5W with 20 mEq of K acetate per liter to replace deficit, plus 0.2% NaCl in D5W with 20 mEq of K acetate per liter to provide basic daily requirement	Calculated deficit† plus calculated basic daily requirement	Give half the total in the first 8 h; give second half over the next 16 h
Hypotonic ($Na^+ < 130$ mEq)			
Sodium loss	0.9% NaCl in D5W with 20 mEq of K acetate per liter to replace deficit until Na^+ reaches 130 mEq, then 0.45% NaCl in D5W with 20 mEq of K acetate per liter to replace remaining deficit plus 0.2% NaCl in D5W with 20 mEq of K acetate per liter to provide basic daily requirement	Calculated deficit plus calculated basic daily requirement	Give half the total in the first 8 h; give second half over the next 16 h

* K acetate to be added after urine flow is established.
† Amount of crystalloid given in emergency management to be substracted from deficit volume required.

12 hours by a solution of 0.45% saline in D5W at a rate of 8 to 10 mL/kg/h. This contains 75 mEq of sodium per liter so that during the 12 hours of treatment, an additional 7.5 to 9.0 mEq of sodium per kilogram is given, supplementing the emergency dose of 3 mEq/kg. This solution also provides the water for urine output and evaporative water losses through skin and lungs. A solution with a more favorable ratio of sodium to chloride, such as equal parts lactated Ringer's solution and D5W or D10W, may be preferable, but it is difficult to show clear superiority over saline in clinical experience.

Potassium replacement is begun when acidosis is corrected and urine output is adequate (≥1 mL/kg/h).[5] Potassium losses occur in gastrointestinal secretions of patients with diarrhea and vomiting or intestinal obstruction, or in the urine of patients in diabetic ketoacidosis, which depletes intracellular potassium. During the acute stage of dehydration, the serum potassium concentration may be normal or even elevated, despite depletion of body potassium because of renal dysfunction and acidosis. The latter state causes potassium to leak out of the cells. When extracellular fluid volume and renal function are restored and acidosis is corrected, serum potassium concentrations drop as potassium is taken up by cells. Hypokalemia is associated with loss of smooth muscle tone, skeletal muscle weakness, and myocardial function disturbances, which are reflected in the electrocardiogram. Potassium salts can be added to the intravenous fluid regimen in the form of potassium chloride or potassium acetate at a concentration of 20 to 40 mEq/L in the final infusion solution. The lower concentration is preferred; the higher one is used only if serum potassium concentrations persist at levels below 3 mEq/L. In patients with diabetic ketoacidosis, serum phosphate concentrations decrease after insulin treatment as glucose enters the cells and glycogen is stored. Potassium phosphate can be used during this state, and a combination of potassium chloride and potassium phosphate, each supplying 10 mEq/L, has been found to be safe. Higher concentrations of potassium phosphate can reduce calcium ion concentration and produce tetany.

After the initial 12-hour replacement phase, the required maintenance therapy can be instituted with solutions providing 25 to 40 mEq of sodium per liter (0.2% saline = 34 mEq/L) and 20 mEq of potassium per liter plus glucose, given at a rate of 4 to 5 mL/kg/h. During the first 24 hours, therefore, the total fluid intake is 40 mL/kg during the first hour of emergency treatment, 95 to 120 mL/kg over the next 12 hours, and about 40 to 50 mL/kg during the final portion of the initial 24-hour regimen. The total fluid administered during the 24-hour period is 175 to 210 mL/kg, replacing the extracellular fluid deficit of 70 to 100 mL/kg and supplying extra water for urine excretion, evaporative water loss, and continued losses of gastrointestinal secretions in the case of vomiting and diarrhea. In patients with intestinal obstruction and continuous nasogastric aspiration of gastrointestinal fluids, such fluids should be measured and the treatment should be modified to replace the continued losses as well as the original deficit.

The regimens discussed can be modified as long as the major principles are adhered to: emergency increase of plasma volume and rapid restoration of deficits of sodium salts and water, with extra water and electrolytes for maintenance requirements and ongoing losses (Table 6-6). After initial correction specific deficits that remain can be calculated (Exhibit 6-2); normal values of plasma electrolyte concentrations must be used (Table 6-7). A variety of electrolyte solutions of known composition are available for use (Table 6-8).

TABLE 6-6 Electrolyte Composition of Abnormal Fluid Loss

Fluid Loss	Electrolyte (estimated mEq/L)		
	Na^+	K^+	Cl^-
Vomiting			
Gastric	20–80	5–20	100–150
Small intestine	100–140	5–15	90–130
Diarrhea	10–90	10–80	10–110

EXHIBIT 6-2 Formula for Correction of Specific Electrolyte Deficits

1. Desired value (mEq/L) − actual value (mEq/L) = deficit (mEq/L).
2. Deficit (mEq/L) × body weight (kg) × distribution factor* = mEq required.

* Distribution factors: bicarbonate, 0.5; chloride, 0.2; sodium, 0.7.

TABLE 6-7 Normal Concentrations of Plasma Electrolytes

Cations	mEq/L	Anions	mEq/L
Na^+	140	Cl^-	102
K^+	4	HCO_3^-	24
Ca^{++}	5	SO_4^{--}	1
Mg^{++}	2	HPO_4^-	2
		Organic acids	6
		Proteins	16
Total	151	Total	151

TABLE 6-8 Composition of Frequently Used Parenteral Fluids

Liquid	CHO	Prot.*	kcal/L	Na	K	Cl	HCO_3†	Ca	p+
	(g/100 mL)			(mEq/L‡)					(mg/dL)
D_5W	5		170						
$D_{10}W$	10		340						
Normal saline (0.9% NaCl)				154		154			
½ Normal saline (0.45% NaCl)	5			77		77			
D_5 + 0.2% NaCl			170	34		34			
3% Saline				513		513			
8.4% Sodium bicarbonate (1 mEq/mL)				1000			1000		
Ringer's	0–10		0–340	147	4	155.5		4.5	
Ringer's lactate	0–10		0–340	130	4	109	28	3	
Amino acid 8.5% (Travasol)		8.5	340	3		34	52		
Plasmanate		5	200	110	2	50	29		
Albumin 25% (salt poor)		25	1000	100–160	1	120			
Intralipid (Cutter)§	2.25		1100	2.5	0.5	4.0			0.8

* Protein or amino acid equivalent.
† Bicarbonate or equivalent (citrate, acetate, lactate).
‡ Approximate values: actual values may vary somewhat in various localities, depending on electrolyte composition of water supply used to reconstitute solution.
§ Values are approximate—may vary from lot to lot.
Source: Reproduced with permission from Johns Hopkins Hospital: THE HARRIET LANE HANDBOOK, 9th edition, edited by J. A. Biller and A. M. Yeager. Copyright © 1981 by Year Book Medical Publishers, Inc., Chicago.

HYPOCHLOREMIA AND METABOLIC ALKALOSIS

Dehydration resulting from losses of gastric secretions differs from the previously discussed states in that the chloride deficit exceeds that of sodium, so that the loss of extracellular fluid volume is associated with hypochloremia and metabolic alkalosis.[5] Replacement therapy requires larger amounts of chloride than in other forms of extracellular fluid deficit. If the dehydration is severe, the estimated water deficit is about 100 mL/kg. If this volume plus the maintenance requirement of 80 to 100 mL/kg is replaced by a solution supplying 75 mEq of sodium per liter and 75 mEq of chloride per liter, a total of 15 mEq of sodium and of chloride per kilogram will be given in the first 24 hours. This is an excessive amount of sodium, but the surplus is lost through the excretion of an alkaline urine, whereas the needed chloride is retained. Therefore, a solution of equal parts of 0.85% saline and glucose in water is the solution of choice, given in a volume corresponding to the deficit plus the maintenance requirement. Whole blood transfusions, 20 mL/kg, are given preoperatively to infants who have been severely malnourished or dehydrated. Deficiencies of potassium can be great in the infant whose course has been prolonged and who has shown a marked metabolic alkalosis. An indication of such severe potassium deficiency is persistent hypochloremia despite treatment with large amounts of sodium chloride. Under these circumstances parenteral potassium is given preoperatively, after circulation and urine output have been improved by the initial therapy with saline and glucose in water. A solution of 0.3% potassium chloride in glucose can be added to the parenteral fluids; 75 mL of this solution per kilogram supplies 3 mEq of potassium per kilogram and can be given over a 6- to 8-hour period. Correction of the potassium deficit and metabolic alkalosis in such cases should be done before operation.

HYPERNATREMIA

Loss of water from the body without proportionate loss of sodium results in increased concentration of sodium in extracellular fluid, known as hypernatremic dehydration.[6] Hypernatremia also can result from excess salt loading; in this instance there is no water deficit but an absolute sodium excess. The major physiologic effect of hypernatremia is loss of intracellular water since there is osmotic equilibrium between cells and extracellular fluid, although the cell cation is predominantly potassium rather than sodium, as in extracellular fluid. Cell dehydration, particularly dehydration of nerve cells, causes physiologic dysfunction. The major manifestations of hypernatremia are disorders of brain function, i.e., disturbances of consciousness and, in the more severe states, convulsive seizures. Since water is withdrawn from the cells, extracellular volume depletion is minimized, and the clinical manifestations of reduced intravascular volume are not ordinarily seen.

Hypernatremic dehydration can occur as a result of diarrhea, particularly in young infants. The profuse watery stools can contain low concentrations of sodium and high concentrations of potassium, resulting from sodium-potassium exchange in the colon. The water loss in stools can be intensified by malabsorption of ingested carbohydrates, particularly lactose or other disaccharides or oligosaccharides, because of the osmotic effect of the unabsorbed sugars and the products of their fermentation by bacteria.[6] Another cause of hypernatremic dehydration is diabetes insipidus, whether due to lack of antidiuretic hormone (ADH) or of the nephrogenic variety. In infants osmotic diuresis from excessively high protein intake via improper feeding mixtures can cause severe hypernatremia. Mistaken addition of excessive salt, either to infant feeding preparations or to homemade oral electrolyte mixtures used for treatment of diarrhea, can result in salt poisoning with hypernatremia.

Treatment

The major guiding principle in the treatment of hypernatremic dehydration is gradual restoration of normal extracellular sodium concentration and osmolality. Too rapid dilution of the hyperosmolar extracellular fluid results in excessive uptake of water by the cerebrospinal fluid and brain cells, resulting in brain edema and convulsive seizures. This is the result of slow equilibration of sodium between cerebrospinal fluid and the plasma, and of metabolite production in the brain cells, which increases intracellular osmotic pressure in response to the hyperosmolality of extracellular fluid. The normal state must be approached gradually to allow physiologic and metabolic equilibrium to occur. A rule of thumb is to give fluids at a rate that will restore serum sodium concentrations to the normal range in about 48 hours.[6] The fluid deficit in hypernatremic dehydration is approximately 50 mL/kg if serum sodium is 150 mEq/L, 90 mL/kg if serum sodium is 160 mEq/L, and 140 mL/kg with a serum sodium of 170 mEq/L. The solutions to be given intravenously should contain sodium at a concentration of 25 to 35 mEq/L to avoid reducing the extracellular sodium concentration too rapidly and also because some degree of sodium deficit may be present despite hypernatremia, especially in infants who have developed hypernatremia because of diarrhea. A 0.2% solution of sodium chloride in D5W or lactated Ringer's solution diluted with D5W are convenient solutions. The infusion is given at a constant rate calculated to restore the water deficit in 48 hours and to provide the additional maintenance water needed for urine and evaporative water loss. In the case of hypernatremia due to nephrogenic diabetes insipidus, the expected urine output is at least five times that calculated for the normal infant, so the maintenance water requirement will be 3 mL/kcal rather than 1 mL/kcal. The safest procedure for this disorder is to measure urine output and use this as a guide to the rate of fluid administration. Potassium deficit is an important complication of hypernatremic dehydration, particularly that associated with diarrhea. Addition of a potassium salt, in a final concentration of 20 to 40 mEq/L in the intravenous solution, should be made with the same precautions as in the treatment of extracellular depletion.

HYPONATREMIA

With Appropriate ADH Secretion

The normal stimuli for secretion of ADH are increased osmolality of extracellular fluid, usually because of increased sodium concentration, and decreased intravascular volume. Hyponatremia with appropriate ADH secretion can occur when sodium loss from the body is replaced with dextrose in water or oral water without adequate sodium salts so that extracellular sodium is diluted by water retention. The reduced osmolality of extracellular fluid results in water uptake by the cells, and thus extracellular volume is greatly depleted. Patients with this condition show all the manifestations of extracellular volume depletion, including circulatory insufficiency and failure of renal function. Serum urea nitrogen and creatinine concentrations are increased. In addition, patients may show the neurologic symptoms of water intoxication because of water uptake by brain cells and cerebrospinal fluid.

Treatment should be rapid replacement of sodium. Although hypertonic sodium chloride solutions (3% sodium chloride) have been used by some, an isotonic sodium chloride solution can be used in the treatment and may be safer in that sodium overloading with too rapid increase of plasma volume could result from excessive administration of hypertonic saline.[2]

With Inappropriate ADH Secretion

Inappropriate ADH secretion, i.e., continued secretion of ADH despite dilution of extracellular fluid osmolality and expansion of body water, is an expected finding in patients with intracranial infections such as meningitis or encephalitis and after head trauma with brain edema. It also may be seen in severe infections without intracranial extension. These patients exhibit hyponatremia if given the usual amounts of water.

It is important to differentiate this state from hyponatremic dehydration with appropriate ADH secretion because the total body water content of subjects with inappropriate ADH is increased, and if given large amounts of sodium salts, they can develop intravascular fluid overload with brain and pulmonary edema, complicating already serious problems. The diagnosis is made on clinical grounds and by examination of renal function. Because there is no depletion of extracellular fluid volume, plasma volume is not reduced and renal perfusion is normal. Although urine output is reduced because of highly concentrated urine, serum urea nitrogen and creatinine are not elevated but may be low because of dilution of total body water. The major clinical manifestations, in addition to those of the illness or injury predisposing to inappropriate ADH secretion, are those of water intoxication if excessive fluids are given, i.e., brain edema and convulsions.

The appropriate treatment is water restriction to prevent excessive water retention. The amount of water given is only that necessary to provide for minimal output of urine plus evaporative water losses. If water intoxication is already manifest, rapid removal of water via the urine should be started. This can be done by osmotic diuresis, i.e., IV injection of a 20% mannitol solution, 5 mL/kg, which causes diuresis with less loss of sodium than of water. This treatment can be repeated after 6 hours if water removal is not adequate after the initial injection. An alternative method of diuresis is injection of furosemide, 1 mg/kg, with replacement of urine sodium by a volume of isotonic sodium chloride solution equivalent to urine output.[2]

OTHER ELECTROLYTE ABNORMALITIES

Excess Hydrogen Ions

Reference already has been made to increased hydrogen ion concentration (reduction of pH) caused by loss of bicarbonate, either in intestinal fluids or by replacement with organic acids. If renal function is adequate, the excess H^+ is removed in the urine by H^+-Na^+ exchange and by trapping of NH_3 in the tubular contents to form NH_4^+ so that Na^+ is conserved and HCO_3^- is regenerated. For this reason replacement of extracellular fluid volume with a sodium chloride solution can correct acidosis. However, such replacement temporarily lowers the bicarbonate concentration by dilution, as stated earlier. If acidosis is severe (blood pH ≤ 7.0), some bicarbonate should be given to prevent further reduction. It is possible to estimate the amount of bicarbonate necessary to raise serum bicarbonate to 12 mEq/L by the following formula:

$$\text{mEq NaHCO}_3 = (12 - \text{serum HCO}_3^- \text{ [mEq/L]}) \times 0.5 \text{ body weight (kg)}.$$

In the initial dehydration treatment, if a solution containing 50 mEq of $NaHCO_3^-$ per liter is given in a volume of 20 mL/kg, the extracellular bicarbonate should be raised 2 mEq/L. If renal function is restored after this initial infusion, further replacement of sodium can be continued with 0.85% saline. If there are doubts about renal function, solutions supplying an excess of sodium over chloride, such as saline-bicarbonate or lactated Ringer's solutions, should be used to replace the deficit of sodium salts.

Hypocalcemia

Hypocalcemia can be seen as a complication of severe infections and in hypernatremic dehydration. The mechanism is not completely understood, but potassium and magnesium deficiency due to starvation and excessive losses of these ions in gastrointestinal secretions or urine may be important factors in the failure of calcium homeostasis. Serum calcium concentrations should be monitored under these conditions, and if levels are below 8 mg/dL, a 10% calcium gluconate solution, 2 to 6 mL/kg, can be added to the intravenous solution for a total dose of 18 to 54 mg/kg/24 h, depending upon the degree of hypocalcemia. (See also Chapter 35.)

Hypomagnesemia

Magnesium deficiency can result from the loss of this ion in gastrointestinal secretions and also from urinary loss in patients receiving aminoglycoside antibiotics. These antibiotics are nephrotoxic, and one of the early manifestations of renal tubule injury is wasting of potassium and magnesium in the urine. Magnesium deficiency prevents normal parathyroid hormone secretion and function, resulting in hypocalcemia. Hyperexcitability of the nervous system is both a direct effect of reduced magnesium concentration and a result of the secondary hypocalcemia. Magnesium can be replaced by 50% $MgSO_4 \cdot 7H_2O$, either 0.2 mL/kg IM or added to the volume of continuous intravenous solution given over a period of 4 hours. This dose provides 0.9 mEq of magnesium per kilogram and can be repeated at 4- to 6-hour intervals until the serum magnesium concentration is restored to normal. If the patient is anuric, the serum magnesium concentration must be monitored closely to prevent hypermagnesemia.

Hypermagnesemia

Hypermagnesemia, serum magnesium concentrations greater than 5 mEq/L, causes depression of central nervous system activity. The earliest manifestation is depression of spinal reflexes, which should be recognized as a premonitory sign that can be followed by depression of medullary centers and respiratory arrest. This entity can occur in infants delivered of mothers who have been given magnesium sulfate intravenously for control of eclampsia. Treatment consists of 10% calcium gluconate, 2 mL/kg IV; the infusion rate should be monitored to avoid too rapid elevation of serum Ca^{++}, which slows the heart rate and can cause cardiac arrest.

Hypophosphatemia

Depression of serum phosphate concentrations is seen in acute infections associated with low phosphate intake and increased cell metabolic activity. Infants who are starved because of vomiting and diarrhea and given intravenous glucose can develop marked hypophosphatemia. Similarly, hypophosphatemia is commonly seen in patients with diabetic ketoacidosis after institution of insulin treatment and redeposition of glycogen in liver and muscle tissue. There is uncertainty about the need to treat acute hypophosphatemia, but potassium phosphate can be given for this purpose, as described in the management of hypophosphatemia with diabetic ketoacidosis in this section.

Hyperphosphatemia

Hyperphosphatemia occurs when there is rapid cell destruction and impaired kidney function. This combination is seen in children with acute leukemia after institution of antileukemic treatment with rapid cytolysis of leukocytes. Prevention of renal shutdown by inducing diuresis before and during treatment and prevention of hyperuricemia by administering allopurinol reduce the likelihood of this complication. Hyperphosphatemia reduces the concentrations of Ca^{++} and Mg^{+} in extracellular fluid, and cautious replacement of these ions is required.[2]

References

1. Heird WC, Winters RW: Total parenteral nutrition—the state of the art. *J Pediatr* 1975;86:2–16.
2. Finberg L, Kravath RE, Fleischman AR: *Water and Mineral Metabolism in Pediatrics: Physiology, Pathophysiology, and Treatment.* Philadelphia, WB Saunders Co, 1982.
3. Darrow DC: Body-fluid physiology: relation of tissue composition to problems of water and electrolyte balance. *New Eng J Med* 1945;233:91–97.
4. Reactor FC Jr (ed): Symposium on acid-base homeostasis. *Kidney Int* 1972;1:273–379.
5. Sperotto G, Carrazza FR, Marcondes E: Treatment of diarrheal dehydration. *Am J Clin Nutr* 1977;30:1447–1456.
6. Harrison HE, Finberg L: Hypernatremic dehydration. *Pediatr Clin North Am* 1964;11:955–961.

Part III

Respiratory Disorders

Dennis C. Stokes

7 Respiratory Disorders

Disorders of the respiratory system are the most common and dramatic pediatric emergencies. This chapter focuses first on the initial assessment of pediatric patients with common respiratory emergencies and acute problems, and second on management of specific disorders frequently encountered in the emergency department or clinic. Children with chronic respiratory disorders, such as asthma, also make up a large segment of pediatric patients seen for emergency care, and the practitioner must know how to recognize these disorders and their complications and arrange for long-term follow-up care.

SIGNS AND SYMPTOMS

Acute Respiratory Distress

Respiratory distress is a general term that covers several abnormalities of breathing, including tachypnea, dyspnea, cyanosis, and retractions. Obviously, respiratory *distress* should not be confused with respiratory failure—many children with very labored breathing are not in respiratory failure whereas others with severe respiratory failure, such as that associated with neuromuscular disorders or respiratory muscle exhaustion, may have little or no apparent increased respiratory effort. Respiratory failure exists when the compensatory mechanisms of the respiratory system are inadequate to maintain gas exchange, resulting in significant hypoxemia and/or hypercapnea (carbon dioxide partial pressure [P_{CO_2}] > 55 mmHg).

Tachypnea refers to increased rate of breathing over the age-specific normal values. Hyperpnea suggests increased depth of breathing and can be difficult to assess adequately by clinical exam. Many factors other than lung disease can affect both the depth and frequency of the respiratory rate (Exhibit 7-1). Dyspnea refers to a subjective feeling (symptom) of increased effort in breathing, and therefore it is less often applicable to young patients, although the observation of increased work of breathing (e.g., retractions, flaring of the nasal alae) is also commonly termed dyspnea. Common causes of acute dyspnea in pediatric patients include pneumonia, asthma, congestive heart failure, foreign bodies, and acute pneumothorax. Dyspnea only with exercise is an important symptom that occurs in several situations, including congestive heart failure and exercise-induced asthma.

Retractions of different parts of the thorax are often striking in infants and young children with airway diseases because of the highly compliant chest wall. Marked retractions of the intercostal spaces, lower sternum, and subcostal areas are seen in many types of obstructive airway diseases. Use of the accessory muscles of respiration, including the scalene and sternocleidomastoid muscles, corre-

Exhibit 7-1 Nonpulmonary Causes of Tachypnea or Hyperpnea

Respiratory compensation for acidosis (e.g., renal failure, diabetic ketoacidosis)
Meningitis
Increased intracranial pressure
Fever
Anxiety
Abdominal pain
Ingestion of salicylates, amphetamines
Carbon monoxide poisoning

lates well with the severity of airway obstruction in asthma and other disorders of increased ventilatory effort.

Wheezing

The wheeze is a continuous, high-pitched, musical sound that does not normally occur in the lung. It is generally, but not exclusively, expiratory and results from vibration of larger airway walls during narrowing. The rhonchus is a lower pitched, continuous "snoring" sound that is usually associated with excessive secretions in the lower respiratory tract and often accompanies wheezing. Although wheezing primarily originates from larger intrathoracic airways and is therefore prominent in a disorder like asthma, it also occurs with bronchiolitis, which produces obstruction mainly in small airways (subsegmental). Parents often associate wheezing with upper airway noise during breathing, particularly in infants with nasal congestion or laryngomalacia. The differential diagnosis of wheezing is extensive (Table 7-1). Diagnostic points that are particularly useful include the age and suddenness of onset, associated physical findings, and historical aspects, such as a family history of asthma and cystic fibrosis (CF) or a history of foreign body ingestion. Wheezing in the infant is often related to acute viral infection with bronchiolitis. Asymmetrical wheezing is often a clue to the presence of a foreign body but also can be seen in other disorders, such as asthma or CF, when mucous obstruction leads to irregular aeration. Congestive heart failure is associated with wheezing in infancy; thus the presence of murmurs, hepatomegaly, a third heart sound, or edema can be important associated physical findings.

The evaluation of wheezing may be as simple as a trial of bronchodilators, provided other major disorders such as a foreign body or CF have been excluded, because asthma is the most common cause of wheezing. Response to bronchodilators (usually subcutaneous epinephrine or terbutaline) has been used frequently to distinguish asthma from bronchiolitis in wheezy infants. However, response to bronchodilators is very poor in most patients under 18 months of age, even those later shown to have asthma, so this is an unreliable differential test. Studies to consider in patients who wheeze are shown in Table 7-2.

TABLE 7-1 Causes of Wheezing

Age Group	Common	Uncommon
Infant	Upper airway congestion Bronchiolitis Asthma	Congenital lesions Congestive heart failure Cystic fibrosis Foreign body Vascular ring Immotile cilia syndrome Immunodeficiency disorders Gastroesophageal reflux
Toddler	Asthma Foreign body Pneumonia Cystic fibrosis	Include above
Child	Asthma Pneumonia Foreign body	Include above
Adolescent	Asthma	Include above Mediastinal mass Collagen vascular diseases

Cough

Cough is a common pediatric symptom that is normally the result of acute viral respiratory tract infections. A cough persisting for more than 3 weeks without an obvious cause is considered chronic and generally indicates an underlying disorder (Exhibit 7-2). There are several reports of chronic cough, particularly nocturnal cough, as a frequent symptom of asthma (or hyperreactive airways disease), both in children and adults. This observation has therapeutic importance since bronchodilators may be effective in treating cough in

TABLE 7-2 Evaluation of Patients with Wheezing

Initial	Later
Chest x-ray film	Computed tomography scan
Complete blood count, differential	Bronchoscopy
Electrocardiogram	Esophageal manometry
Airway films	Esophageal pH determinations
Sweat test	Esophagoscopy
Immunoglobulins	
Immunoglobulin E	
Barium cine-esophagram	
Pulmonary function tests	

Exhibit 7-2 Causes of a Chronic or Persistent Cough

Infectious organisms
- *Bordatella pertussis*
- *Mycoplasma*
- *M. tuberculosis*
- *Chlamydia*

Chronic lung disorders
- Asthma
- CF
- Bronchiectasis (± sinusitis, situs inversus)

Foreign body
Chronic aspiration syndromes, e.g., tracheoesophageal fistula, gastroesophageal reflux
Postnasal drip
Smoking
Nervous or psychogenic cough

this group of patients. Cough plays an important role in pulmonary defense; thus cough suppressants have little use in pediatric patients and are generally ineffective in any case. Expectorants, such as guaifenesin, or iodides are also ineffective, and chronic use of the latter can result in goiter.

Stridor

Stridor refers to respiratory distress secondary to upper airway obstruction, generally associated with inspiration. Careful examination of the child with stridor usually indicates the site of obstruction. Severe inspiratory stridor occurs in extrathoracic obstruction, because of the lower intratracheal pressures on inspiration, which favor airway narrowing. In contrast, intrathoracic obstruction is typically worse on expiration as the trachea and intrathoracic airways narrow because of increasing positive pleural pressure. The most important causes of stridor are those associated with the croup syndromes. Congenital airway lesions causing stridor often are accompanied by a respiratory infection. The clue to the existence of a congenital lesion may be the presence of associated findings such as a cutaneous or mucous membrane hemangioma or a history of unusually severe, prolonged, or recurrent stridor. Radiologic techniques are particularly useful in the patient with stridor, providing excellent visualization of the upper airway. If there remains any doubt as to the presence of a lesion, careful laryngoscopy by an experienced observer is indicated, even if radiographic studies are normal.

Cyanosis

Cyanosis is unusual as an isolated sign, although it can be seen in many clinical settings associated with congenital heart disease or respiratory distress. Cyanosis should be sought only in central tissues such as the tongue and face. Peripheral cyanosis can result from poor tissue perfusion (shock), from hypothermia, or as normal physiologic response in infants. It is important to recognize that the absence of cyanosis is an unreliable sign that oxygenation is adequate; arterial blood gas measurements are the only reliable indicators of ventilation and oxygenation. Cyanosis is a particularly unreliable clinical sign in the presence of anemia or low cardiac output states such as shock. Other disorders can mimic the appearance of cyanosis, including skin staining from clothing dyes, methemoglobinemia (ingestions, congenital hemoglobinopathy), and polycythemia.

Exhibit 7-3 Causes of Chest Pain in Pediatric and Adolescent Patients

Pneumonia
Pleurisy
Costochondritis
Bronchitis
Muscle strain
Trauma
Spontaneous pneumothorax or pneumomediastinum
Subclinical asthma
Pericarditis
Esophagitis
Early herpes zoster infection
Referred pain
- Fitz-Hugh-Curtis syndrome
- Cholecystitis

Cardiac conditions
- Severe aortic stenosis
- Arrhythmias

Idiopathic

Chest Pain

Chest pain is a frequent complaint in the older pediatric age group, although serious causes are less common than in the adult age group (Exhibit 7-3). A careful history, physical examination, chest radiograph, and electrocardiogram usually separate out those patients who need more extensive evaluations.

PHYSICAL EXAMINATION

The rapidity of the physical examination of the respiratory tract obviously depends upon the acuteness of the condition. Basically, a few simple questions should be asked first (Table 7-3) before pro-

TABLE 7-3 Assessment of Acute Respiratory Distress

Question	Assessment	Action
1. Is ventilation currently adequate?	Examination Arterial blood gases	If *no*, prepare for intubation, assisted ventilation. (See Chapter 1, "Cardiopulmonary Resuscitation.")
2. Is respiratory arrest likely in near future?	Evidence of fatigue, such as paradoxical respiratory motion Changes in consciousness, somnolence, agitation	Intubation and assisted ventilation
3. Is there upper or lower airway obstruction?	Upper: inspiratory stridor, hoarseness, "croup" Lower: expiratory obstruction > inspiratory, adventitial lung sounds (wheeze, rhonchi)	Define specific cause
4. Is acute bacterial supraglottitis or severe tracheitis possible?	Abrupt onset of upper airway obstruction, fever, toxicity, positive radiograph for "thumb" sign of epiglottis swelling	To operating room for intubation and examination
5. How long have symptoms been present?	History	
6. Is there a history of asthma, foreign body aspiration, trauma, smoke inhalation, ingestion, etc.?	History	Appropriate therapy

ceeding to other aspects of the examination. Although the adequacy of gas exchange is difficult to judge from physical examination alone, the most important physical signs and symptoms of hypoxemia or hypercapnea include cyanosis (hypoxemia), tachycardia (both), agitation (hypoxemia), and somnolence (both). The respiratory rate and use of accessory muscles of respiration are also important findings to note at the beginning of the evaluation.

DIAGNOSTIC PROCEDURES

Arterial Blood Gas Measurements

An arterial blood gas sample is essential to establish the adequacy of gas exchange. As noted, physical signs are notoriously unreliable in assessing patients with respiratory failure. Arterial samples should be collected in heparinized glass syringes, stored in ice, and immediately processed for accurate determination. The most common errors in performing blood gas studies are (1) addition to too much anticoagulant solution, resulting primarily in errors in P_{CO_2} (oxygen partial pressure $[P_{O_2}] = 150$ mmHg, $P_{CO_2} = 0$ mmHg); (2) introduction of air bubbles; and (3) delay in processing. The results from an individual study are often less important than trends in several studies. For example, early in an asthma attack, there is usually hypoxemia with a low P_{CO_2}. As the attack worsens, a rise in P_{CO_2} to the normal range can indicate a worsening clinical course.

The normal values for blood gases are shown in Table 7-4. Note that the normal arterial P_{O_2} (Pa_{O_2}) depends upon age and that the normal Pa_{O_2} values for infants are lower than those for older children and adults.

TABLE 7-4 Normal Blood Gas Values (Room Air)

Age Group	pH	Pa_{CO_2} (mmHg)	Pa_{O_2} (mmHg)	HCO_3^- (mEq/L)
Newborn	7.26–7.29	34–45	40–70	24–26
Infant	7.38–7.41	34–35	70–80	24–26
Child	7.38–7.41	34–35	>80	24–26
Adult	7.35–7.45	34–45	>80	24–26

Pulmonary Function Testing

Routine equipment for measurement of simple pulmonary functions should be available in every emergency facility. Portable spirometers and simple peak-flow measuring devices provide objective bedside evaluation that can supplement the physical examination. The most common of these devices in use is the Wright peak-flow meter, which measures peak flow over a very short portion of expiration. These measurements are particularly valuable in the outpatient asthmatic because serial peak-flow rates can be used to assess response to bronchodilator therapy. Simple pulmonary function tests also can be used to evaluate symptoms such as dyspnea and chronic cough. An obstructive pattern, recorded by bedside spirometry, that improves with bronchodilators can be useful in diagnosing unrecognized asthma.

Radiologic Techniques

Chest Radiograph

The importance of an adequate quality chest radiograph cannot be overemphasized since pediatric patients are often overtreated for pneumonia on the basis of poor films or movement artifacts. A lateral radiograph is also important, particularly with left lower lobe processes, which are hidden by the cardiac shadows on the plain posteroanterior film. Access to previous chest radiographs is critical in the interpretation of recurrent or persistent infiltrates; if possible, prior radiographs should be obtained for every child with pneumonia seen in the emergency department.

Upper Airway Films

Excellent resolution of the structure of the upper airway can be achieved using high-kilovoltage techniques.

Fluoroscopy

Fluoroscopy of the upper airway often can define airway lesions and the level of stridor or obstruction. Fluoroscopy of the diaphragm can be useful in patients with respiratory distress when unilateral diaphragm paralysis is suspected. Unilateral air trapping as a result of foreign bodies can often be appreciated on fluoroscopy in children too young for radiographs on inspiration and expiration.

Computed Axial Tomography of the Chest

Although hardly a routine outpatient procedure, the computed tomography scan, if available, can be very useful in evaluating complex bronchial anatomy, unusual intrathoracic lesions, or mediastinal masses.

Barium Cine-Esophagram

This technique is used primarily for additional diagnostic evaluation of patients with recurrent pneumonias (tracheoesophageal fistula, gastroesophageal reflux) or stridor (vascular ring).

Examination of Sputum

Direct examination of sputum is a frequently overlooked diagnostic test in pediatric patients. Although younger children generally swallow their secretions, many older children can produce sputum with encouragement. Careful examination of wet preparations and Gram's and Wright's stains of sputum can demonstrate polymorphonuclear leukocytes and bacterial pathogens in pneumonia, and eosinophils and bronchiolar casts (Curschmann's spirals) in asthma (Table 7-5). The patient with CF typically produces thick, greenish yellow, and highly tenacious mucus. The major difficulty in most patients is obtaining adequate sputum for examination. Occasionally, direct tracheal suctioning or transtracheal aspiration in older children and adolescents is indicated to obtain sputum for culture and examination in patients with significant lower respiratory tract infections.

Obtaining Material for Culture and Immunologic Studies

In addition to expectorated sputum and tracheal aspiration, there are other methods for obtaining material from the lower respiratory tract. Direct lung aspiration can be performed in selected patients with complicated pneumonia and has a very low rate of complications. Bronchoscopy can be used to obtain uncontaminated cultures of the lower respiratory tract by utilizing catheters, which reduce contamination with upper airway flora.

Thoracentesis

Diagnostic thoracentesis is indicated in any child with an unexplained pleural effusion to obtain fluid for culture and to rule out the presence of empyema. Pleural fluid should be tested for pH, specific gravity, protein content, glucose, and lactate dehydrogenase (LDH); examined cytologically for malignant cells; and cultured for anaerobic, aerobic, and acid-fast organisms (Table 7-6).

TABLE 7-5 Examination of Sputum

Method	Finding	Probable Cause
Wet preparations and Wright's stain	Eosinophils, bronchiolar casts	Asthma
	Polymorphonuclear leukocytes	Infection
Gram's stain	Gram-positive diplococci	Pneumococcal pneumonia
KOH preparation	Hyphae	Fungal infection or colonization
Acid-fast stain	Acid-fast organism	Tuberculosis
	Partially acid-fast organisms	Nocardiosis

TABLE 7-6 Pleural Fluid Examination*

Finding	Conclusion
Protein < 3 g/dL	Transudate: congestive heart failure, hypoproteinemia, liver cirrhosis
Protein > 3 g/dL (pleural fluid protein : serum protein > 0.5)	Exudate : infection, inflammatory or malignant process
LDH : serum LDH > 0.6	Exudate
pH < 7.20	Pneumonia likely to require drainage
Glucose reduced	Infection
Triglyceride ≈ 400 mg/dL	Chylothorax
Smear and cultures positive	Infecting organism
Cytology positive	Malignancy

* Cell count and differential of limited usefulness.

Laryngoscopy and Bronchoscopy

Indirect laryngoscopy often can be performed in cooperative children if the physician is patient. Direct laryngoscopy can be useful in patients with unexplained stridor, and the new, small fiberoptic laryngoscopes will undoubtedly be helpful in the outpatient setting for this purpose. Examination of the upper airway in children is best performed by an observer familiar with the normal anatomic features at different ages, one proficient in examining the upper airway in order to avoid missing potentially treatable lesions such as hemangiomas. Patients with suspected epiglottitis should *not* be examined in the emergency department but be moved to the operating room, where intubation or tracheostomy can be performed safely, if indicated.

Bronchoscopy with the newer pediatric flexible bronchoscopes can also be useful in evaluation of the upper and lower airway. In addition, difficult tracheal intubations are possible under direct visualization with a flexible bronchoscope placed through the endotracheal tube.

THERAPEUTIC PROCEDURES

Chest Physiotherapy

Frequently, patients with asthma or pneumonia receive chest physiotherapy from the emergency department nursing staff. There is little evidence to suggest that such measures are beneficial to most patients; in fact, younger patients with significant respiratory distress may tolerate these procedures poorly. However, some patients with significant mucous obstruction benefit noticeably from chest physiotherapy, and children with persistent atelectasis often benefit from a program of chest physiotherapy to aid bronchial drainage.

Inhalation Therapy

Many drugs are given effectively by the aerosol route, including bronchodilators, such as metaproterenol or isoetharine. Aerosol racemic epinephrine also has been used for improvement of nonbacterial croup. Medications given by intermittent positive-pressure breathing are no more effective than those given by simple aerosol and have a greater risk of pneumothorax.

Intubation

The techniques for emergency intubation are described in Chapter 1 and should be familiar to every physician working in an emergency care setting. Although nasotracheal intubation offers the advantage of a more secure placement, it is technically more difficult, and, in an emergency, placement of an oral tracheal tube is usually preferable. The most frequent error in intubation is attempting to hyperextend the entire head and neck, rather than lifting up on the mandible to bring the glottis into view. The next most common errors are failure to prepare suctioning equipment and failure to establish ventilation by use of a bag and face mask before attempting endotracheal intubation. Difficult intubations are encountered in patients with facial, cervical spine, or upper airway anomalies. If an emergency airway cannot be obtained by intubation, there are other alternatives in an emergency. A cricothyrotomy can be made, using a special large-bore needle. Alternatively, in a life-threatening situation an emergency tracheotomy must be performed (see Chapter 8).

Chest Tube Drainage of the Pleural Space

Closed chest tube drainage is indicated in patients with empyema (particularly *Staphylococcus aureus*) and pneumothorax. Simple needle aspiration is usually sufficient for diagnostic purposes when effusions are not purulent.

DISORDERS OF THE UPPER RESPIRATORY TRACT

Rhinitis

Nasal discharges can be clear and watery, mucoid, or mucopurulent. The major causes of acute rhinitis are viral acute upper respiratory tract infections (URIs; i.e., the common cold), including those caused by rhinoviruses. Allergic rhinitis is distinguished by a seasonal history of symptoms and the presence of eosinophils in nasal smears, whereas perennial allergic rhinitis can occur without a seasonal history. Vasomotor rhinitis is more common in adults and older children, who have watery rhinorrhea and nasal obstruction. Although the cause of most acute rhinitis is viral, occasionally a persistent mucopurulent discharge from the nose will culture a pure growth of an organism such as the pneumococcus. Purulent discharges, particularly if chronic, foul-smelling, or unilateral, should prompt a careful examination for a nasal foreign body (e.g., wadded paper, coins, crayons).

Acute viral rhinitis is self-limited, and therapy is aimed at alleviation of symptoms. Infants and young children are provided relief from nasal congestion by the use of buffered saline nose drops or sprays. Decongestants can produce agitation and irritability in infants and young children and should be avoided. Antihistamines are used for patients with allergic rhinitis. Antibiotic treatment should be reserved for patients with purulent rhinitis, and the choice of antibiotics is determined by the results from culturing the nasal discharge.

Epistaxis

Epistaxis or nosebleeds are common childhood complaints. They usually are associated with a URI in an individual with fragile superficial surface vessels (Kesselbach's plexus). Other contributing factors include trauma; drying of the nasal mucosa during cold, dry winters; or chronic inflammatory conditions such as allergic rhinitis. Rarely, epistaxis is associated with systemic illnesses such as thrombocytopenia, clotting disorders, or hypertension. Trauma—picking the nose—can lead to nocturnal epistaxis.

In addition to careful examination of the nares, turbinates, and posterior pharynx to localize the site of bleeding, evaluation also should include a hematocrit, smear for platelet estimation, and blood pressure measurement. Most epistaxis responds to simple pressure or pressure with ice. Vasoconstriction with a topical solution of epinephrine or, more rarely, nasal packs may be necessary if bleeding persists. Repeated bleeding from an obvious site can be treated by cauterization with silver nitrate. Saline nose drops, increased room humidification, or petroleum jelly applied to the anterior nares can also be recommended.

Polyps

Nasal polyps usually create no symptoms but frequently accompany chronic allergic rhinitis and CF. They are diagnosed by finding a glistening gray mass in the turbinates. Because of the importance of excluding CF, a sweat test for CF should be done in any patient with nasal polyps. Treatment is surgical although antihistamines may be helpful in those with an allergic basis.

Pharyngitis

Sore throat is a common complaint in the emergency care clinic. Although acute viral infections and group A β-hemolytic streptococcus are common causes of pharyngitis, other causes include postnasal drip, tumors, thyromegaly, and gastroesophageal reflux.

After examination, most sore throats require only symptomatic treatment. When there is fever, an exudative tonsillitis, and cervical lymphadenopathy, the exudate should be cultured to exclude streptococcal pharyngitis and the need for oral penicillin therapy. If there is a high likelihood of streptococcal disease by clinical assessment, then a 10-day course of penicillin should be started even before culture results are available. A follow-up throat culture and examination should be arranged for all patients with streptococcal pharyngitis to document elimination of the organism.

Sinusitis

Sinusitis is uncommon in children because of the normal delay in sinus development, but when it occurs, it is often difficult to diagnose in young children. Ethmoidal sinuses are present at birth, maxillary sinuses develop during the first year, and frontal sinuses only appear after 6 years of age. Symptoms of sinusitis can be nonspecific, such as fever, chronic purulent nasal discharge, or chronic cough. Older children more commonly exhibit classic symptoms of sinusitis such as headache, facial pain, or swelling. Methods for diagnosing sinusitis include transillumination of the sinuses, sinus radiographs, and needle aspiration of the sinuses. Most acute sinus infections are caused by nontypable *Haemophilus influenzae* and *Streptococcus pneumoniae*. Ethmoid sinusitis is often associated with erosion into the periorbital space, resulting in acute orbital cellulitis. Other serious complications of sinus infection include subdural empyemas, meningitis, and dural sinus thrombosis.

Treatment of sinusitis includes appropriate antibiotic therapy such as ampicillin, based on the usual pathogens just mentioned (or guided by cultures from sinus aspiration), and irrigation and drainage in selected cases. Patients with chronic sinus disease associated with bronchitis or other chronic respiratory symptoms should be evaluated for causes of chronic sinopulmonary disease such as immunodeficiency syndromes, CF, or immotile cilia syndrome.

Upper Respiratory Tract Infections

URTIs result from a variety of viral agents, primarily the rhinoviruses. Symptomatic treatment for the common cold is generally ineffective, although subjective improvement can occur with antihistamines or decongestants. In the emergency department the complaint of a "cold" is often an irritation to the busy staff. Such a seemingly trivial complaint should be evaluated carefully, however. Is this a new mother who needs further support in the care of her child? Is there something different about this "cold," such as increased lethargy or poor feeding, that brings in the parents of a young infant and that may indicate a more serious disorder such as sepsis? Another common complaint is that a child "keeps a cold." Often factors can be identified that account for "keeping a cold"—an older sibling just starting school and exposed to frequent viral infections, an allergic family background—but each patient with this complaint should be carefully evaluated.

Adenoiditis

Many clinicians observe patients with purulent nasopharyngeal secretions who appear to have primary involvement of adenoidal tissue. Infants and young children can experience malaise, anorexia, irritability, and low-grade fever. The choice of antibiotics should be based on the results of nasopharyngeal culture. Patients with recurrent infection may benefit from adenoidectomy. Chronic adenoidal and tonsillar hypertrophy results in recurrent otitis media, mouth breathing, and, occasionally, severe obstructive sleep apnea.

Otitis Externa

Otitis externa generally results when the protective waxy layers of the external auditory canal are removed or damaged by trauma or frequent immersion. The canal is generally filled with exudate and exquisitely tender so that complete examination of the middle ear is impossible. Pain when the pinna is moved is usually diagnostic of otitis externa.

Causative organisms include common "waterbugs" such as *Pseudomonas*, and treatment consists of irrigations with dilute acetic acid solutions (2%) or half-strength Burrow's solution. Staphylococcal infections frequently produce furuncles in the canal and require systemic penicillinase-resistant penicillins as well as local therapy. A cotton wick saturated with an antibiotic-corticosteroid preparation is effective. If there is fever or a history of middle ear disease suggesting that the otitis externa may be due to perforation of the tympanic membrane secondary to acute otitis media, then oral antibiotic therapy is also indicated. Frequent swimmers may benefit from prophylactic treatment with dilute acetic acid in the external auditory canals or by wearing ear plugs.

Otitis Media

The usual symptoms of otitis media include pain, manifested by an earache in older children or crying, irritability, and fever in infants. Erythema of the tympanic membrane is an early sign, followed by loss of landmarks, bulging of the drum as fluid accumulates behind it, and loss of mobility.

Acute otitis media results from a variety of bacterial and viral agents but is generally treated with antibiotics since clinical judgments as to a viral cause are unreliable. Several antibiotics are suitable for treatment of otitis media, based on the organisms that are typically cultured from middle ear fluid. These organisms include *S. pneumoniae* and *H. influenzae* (in children under 5 years of age). Ampicillin, penicillin, and sulfisoxazole or erythromycin-sulfisoxazole combinations are suitable initial choices in younger patients; in older patients penicillin or erythromycin is sufficient therapy. Regardless of antibiotic choice, careful follow-up should be arranged at 2 days and 10 to 14 days to exclude antibiotic failure or persistent middle ear effusions. Should an initial course of treatment with these antibiotics fail, then an additional 10-day course of a trimethoprim-sulfisoxazole combination, ampicillin-clavuanate combination, or cefaclor can be tried.

Otitis media in neonates or very young infants is more likely the result of Gram-negative organisms resistant to the usual oral antibiotics. For this reason these infants are usually admitted for parenteral antibiotic therapy. A tympanocentesis may be performed as a guide to antibiotic selection. Although this is generally safe in experienced hands, complications such as bleeding and middle ear damage can occur. Tympanocentesis preferably should be done through an operating microscope.

Patients with a history of recurrent acute otitis media or chronic otitis media with effusion require particularly careful follow-up. Factors predisposing to chronic disease include allergy, immunodeficiency disorders (hypogammaglobulinemia, immunoglobulin A (IgA) deficiency), adenoidal hypertrophy, immotile cilia syndrome, and facial disorders such as cleft palate and achondroplasia.

Acute Upper Airway Obstruction: Croup Syndromes

Viral Laryngotracheobronchitis

Viral laryngotracheobronchitis or croup is an acute respiratory tract infection caused by a variety of viral agents including parainfluenza virus, influenza virus, and adenovirus. Croup characteristically is a winter disease, with 80% of cases occurring between October and April. There is often a community outbreak of the viral agents responsible. Approximately two thirds of cases are under 3 years of age, with males predominating. Beginning with a nonspecific URTI, the patient develops hoarseness, a "croupy" cough, and finally stridorous breathing and a variable degree of sternal, subcostal, and supraclavicular retraction. Fever, if present, is low grade and patients usually are not in a toxic state. Typically, symptoms are worse in the middle of the night. Assessment of croup depends upon careful history (noting findings such as preceding URTI, history of recurrent croup, evidence of fatigue and decreased appetite, and prolonged course with patient fatigue) and physical examination. Soft tissue radiographs of the neck may show subglottic narrowing of the airway.

Management of viral croup includes a high-humidity environment at home, if possible. Patients showing evidence of fatigue, moderate respiratory distress, or dehydration should be admitted for intravenous hydration, high-humidity environment, and close observation. An objective scoring system (Table 7-7) is useful for following the course of these patients when hospitalization is necessary. Symptoms usually persist for several days. Supplemental oxygen therapy may be necessary. Racemic epinephrine by nebulizer (2.25% solution diluted in saline, 0.05 mL/kg/dose) generally produces a transient improvement in stridor; but because of the short duration of its effect, this treatment only should be given to patients who are admitted to the hospital. Neither antibiotics nor corticosteroids have proven effectiveness in altering the course of viral croup. If there is evidence of acute respiratory failure, then intubation or tracheostomy is necessary. Fortunately, 10% or less of croup patients require an artificial airway.

Epiglottitis or Supraglottitis

Epiglottitis or supraglottitis is a true respiratory emergency. Epiglottitis is caused primarily by *H. influenzae* type b, although a few other types of bacterial infections may involve the same area. The disease appears most commonly in the 2- to 6-year-old age group but also can occur in older children and adults. The typical history differs from that of viral laryngotracheobronchitis in that the onset is acute, with high fever, toxic effects, and rapid progression to severe obstruction. There is often severe dysphagia to the extent that drooling occurs. The patient typically assumes a position sitting forward, appears anxious, and is in severe distress. Careful examination of the oropharynx can reveal a swollen, red epiglottis at the base of the tongue. Since any manipulation of the airway can precipitate complete obstruction, a carefully planned approach should be followed. The patient is kept in a sitting position and given humidified air or O_2. As soon as possible the patient should be transferred to the operating room for direct laryngoscopy under general anesthesia. Generally, nasotracheal intubation is now the preferred procedure for management of

TABLE 7-7 Upper Airway Obstruction (Croup) Score

Sign	Score		
	0	1	2
Stridor	None	Inspiratory	Inspiratory and expiratory
Cough	None	Hoarse cry	Bark
Retractions and nasal flaring	None	Flaring and suprasternal retractions	Also subcostal and intercostal retractions
Cyanosis	None	In air	In 40% O_2
Inspiratory breath	Normal	Harsh with wheezing or rhonchi	Delayed

epiglottitis. A nasotracheal tube several sizes smaller than the patient's age would indicate can be used. In institutions where nasotracheal intubation cannot be safely maintained, a tracheostomy is the procedure of choice.

After cultures of the blood and epiglottis, therapy with intravenous ampicillin and chloramphenicol, or chloramphenicol alone, is begun to cover ampicillin-resistant *H. influenzae.* After fever and other manifestations of acute infection have resolved (24 to 48 hours), extubation can be attempted in the operating room.

Although lateral x-rays of the neck may reveal the swollen epiglottis, they are unnecessary in patients suspected of having acute epiglottitis since direct visualization is mandatory and provides absolute proof of the swollen, inflamed epiglottis. Transport of a patient to the radiology department for x-ray studies increases the danger of acute decompensation and can delay the definitive diagnostic and therapeutic procedure—direct visualization. In patients in whom the primary clinical diagnosis is laryngotracheobronchitis, a negative lateral neck x-ray may be of some value in confirming the diagnosis.

Every emergency care facility should have a protocol for managing this disorder.

Bacterial Tracheitis

Bacterial tracheitis is also a severe disorder causing acute upper airway obstruction. In this disorder, however, the epiglottis is normal, and, clinically, these patients frequently appear to have laryngotracheobronchitis but fail to respond to therapy and get progressively worse. The site of severe inflammation is the subglottic region. Fever, toxic effects, and a course progressing to respiratory arrest are seen in this entity. Airway films may show severe narrowing of the trachea. Examination and culture under anesthesia, with placement of an endotracheal tube, are recommended management for this disorder. Systemic antibiotic therapy, including coverage for *S. aureus,* is also begun.

Comparisons of the major clinical features of viral laryngotracheobronchitis, epiglottitis, and bacterial tracheitis are shown in Table 7-8.

Acute Spasmodic Croup

This form of croup is characterized by a sudden onset of inspiratory stridor, usually occurring in the night. Children between the ages of 1 and 3 years are most commonly affected. Typically, the child who has been well during the day, except perhaps for a mild URI, awakens soon after going to bed in severe respiratory distress with a barking cough, extreme anxiety, and noticeable inspiratory stridor. Cyanosis can be present, but there is no fever. The attack is self-limited and may cease after placing the child in a warm, humid environment; after vomiting; or, frequently, en route to the hospital. Some hoarseness can persist and a recurrence of symptoms the next evening can be anticipated. Patients typically have recurrent attacks for the first several years of life. The cause is unknown, but hypersensitivity and emotional factors are felt to play a role.

Other causes of upper airway obstruction include tumors, subglottic stenosis, angioneurotic edema, and foreign bodies.

DISORDERS OF THE LOWER RESPIRATORY TRACT

Bronchiolitis

Wheezing and rales in infants are often related to acute viral infections associated with bronchiolitis. Bronchiolitis is primarily a winter, epidemic illness of infants between 2 and 6 months of age, caused by several different viral agents, including respiratory syncytial virus (RSV), parainfluenza virus, and adenovirus. The principal effects are inflammation,

TABLE 7-8 Viral Laryngotracheobronchitis (Croup), Bacterial Epiglottitis (Supraglottitis), and Bacterial Tracheitis

	Viral Croup	Epiglottitis	Tracheitis
Frequency	80% cases	20% cases	?
Cause	Parainfluenza virus 1, 2, 3 (50%); adenovirus; echovirus	*H. influenzae* type b	*S. aureus*, pneumococcus; others?
Age group (yr)	0–3 (61%) 3–6 (32%) 6 (3%)	0–3 (27%) 3–6 (70%) 6 (1%)	Variable
Season	Oct–Apr, but can occur year round	Oct–April	Any
Onset	Preceding URI, cough, coryza	Rapid	Rapid
Laboratory findings	No leukocytosis	Leukocytosis, positive cultures of blood and epiglottis	Leukocytosis, positive tracheal cultures
Radiologic findings	Croup or "steeple" sign of subglottic edema	"Thumb" sign of swollen epiglottis	Subglottic narrowing with normal epiglottis; tracheal membranes
Therapy	Close observation; follow-up moist, cool air; tracheal or NT* intubation for severe cases; racemic epinephrine in hospitalized patients	NT intubation, IV chloramphenicol	NT intubation, methicillin and chloramphenicol

* Nasotracheal.

edema, and obstruction of the small airways by inflammatory exudate and mucus. Generally, it is a limited illness and begins with a nonspecific URTI and cough. Infants often look well despite tachypnea and audible wheezing, and they usually have minimal fever; thus the presence of high fever should alert one to the presence of a bacterial complication such as otitis or pneumonia. Rapid respirations (over 60/min), somnolence or irritability, or a prolonged course with evidence of fatigue should prompt hospital admission and observation.

Since infants with bronchiolitis frequently are hyperinflated, with downward displacement of the diaphragm, the liver may appear enlarged, suggesting congestive heart failure. Another frequently confusing diagnosis is asthma—so-called "wheezy bronchitis" in the British literature—in the younger infant up to age 18 months. Distinguishing clinical features include

- the typical younger age of the infant with bronchiolitis
- the absence of recurrent disease (although occasional infants will have two or three bouts of virus-associated bronchiolitis)
- the presence of a winter epidemic of RSV, and the absence of a family history of asthma (Table 7-9)

While several studies indicate that most "wheezing" infants under 18 months of age respond poorly to bronchodilators, the interpretation of clinical response to a single subcutaneous epinephrine dose can be helpful.

Therapy for bronchiolitis is guided by first identifying those at risk for respiratory failure. This is best accomplished by measuring arterial blood

TABLE 7-9 Bronchiolitis versus Asthma: "Wheezy Bronchitis"

Characteristic	Asthma	Bronchiolitis
Family history of asthma or atopic disease	Frequent	Less frequent
Recurrent attacks	Frequent	Occasional
Associated with respiratory infection (i.e., URI symptoms)	Frequent	Frequent
Elevated IgE	Common	Common
Eosinophilia	Common	Less common
Response to bronchodilators	Favorable	Uncommon

gases and resting respiratory rate. Patients with significant hypoxia should be admitted and given oxygen, humidification, and careful observation. Mildly affected infants can be observed at home provided they continue good fluid intake, with no worsening of their symptoms. Unfortunately, sudden deaths are associated with RSV infections, but at present there is no reliable guide to judge those at risk for this complication.

Bronchitis

Acute bronchitis often accompanies viral infections of the respiratory tract and is the usual cause for cough. It is doubtful whether children ever develop the equivalent of chronic bronchitis in adults, with chronic cough and sputum production, and usually causes other than bronchitis can be found in the child who "keeps a cough." These include asthma, immunodeficiency, and CF. Acute viral bronchitis generally does not require antibiotic therapy.

Pneumonia

Pneumonia is recognized clinically by the presence of fever, tachypnea, and auscultatory findings of rales and consolidation with decreased breath sounds. Patients with pneumonia frequently have had a preceding URI for several days, followed by a sudden rise in temperature, increase in respiratory rate, and, in older children, a cough. In the infant or young child, the sudden onset of fever can lead to convulsions. Infants are restless and irritable; older children may complain of chest pain, particularly if the pneumonia is caused by pneumococcus. Respiratory distress increases, with grunting, flaring of nasal alae, and retractions. Fever, tachypnea, and reduced fluid intake lead to dehydration.

Chest radiographs confirm the diagnosis by demonstrating areas of infiltration or consolidation. Pleural reaction and pleural effusions may be present.

The bacterial organisms responsible for pneumonia in children include *S. aureus, H. influenzae* (in children under 7 years of age), and *S. pneumoniae*. These organisms and their appropriate antibiotic treatments are summarized in Table 7-10). Viral agents include RSV, parainfluenza virus, influenza virus, and adenovirus. *Mycoplasma* is a cause of atypical pneumonia, usually in older pediatric patients, but also causes other types of airway disease—bronchiolitis, otitis—in younger patients.

Staphylococcal pneumonia is often a rapidly progressive process, so the initial chest radiograph may reveal little. Infants with pneumonia who are in a toxic state or have evidence of pneumatocele formation should be hospitalized, treated, and observed carefully for complications of staphylococcal pneumonia (pyopneumothoraces, empyema). The presence of fluid on the chest radiograph, particularly in a child under 2 years of age, can indicate *H. influenzae* or staphylococcal pneumonia and requires inpatient management. Appropriate cultures of the fluid obtained by thoracentesis can show the etiologic agent. Other indications for hospitalization of children with pneumonia are listed in Exhibit 7-4.

Seizures and meningismus demand the exclusion of meningitis. Abdominal pain accompanied by ileus can suggest serious abdominal emergency in patients with pneumonia of the lower lobes.

In uncomplicated pneumonia a follow-up radiograph 6 to 8 weeks after treatment is useful in ruling out chronic or persistent lung changes. Radiographs should not be repeated too early or too frequently, provided the child is improving satisfactorily. The evaluation of children with recurrent pneumonias or persistent pulmonary infiltrates is covered later in this chapter.

TABLE 7-10 Causes and Treatment of Childhood Pneumonia

Organism	Antibiotic Dose
S. pneumoniae	Penicillin V: 50,000 U/kg/d IV or PO, divided q6h
H. influenzae	Ampicillin: 200–400 mg/kg/d IV IV, divided q6h
	Choramphenicol: 50–100 mg/kg/d IV, divided q6h; monitor levels in infants and young children
S. aureus	Methicillin: 100–400 mg/kg/d IV, divided q4–6h
Klebsiella pneumoniae	Gentamicin: 5–7.5 mg/kg/d IV, divided q8h
Mycoplasma pneumoniae	Erythromycin: 50–100 mg/kg/d PO, divided q6–8h; or 15–20 mg/kg/d IV, divided q4–6h

Exhibit 7-4 Indications for Admission of Children with Pneumonia

Infants less than 8 weeks of age
Toxic effects
  Temperature > 40°C
  White blood cell count > 25,000/μL
Hypoxemia in room air
Hypercapnea
Evidence of fatigue
Medication noncompliance
Presence of pleural effusion

Emphysema and Hyperinflation

Emphysema is a term that is properly applied to situations in which there is actual destruction and enlargement of air spaces; it is rare in pediatric patients. Hyperlucency on chest radiographs, with or without hyperinflation, is more common.

Localized emphysema can cause hyperinflation with mediastinal shift. Congenital lobar emphysema is one cause of respiratory distress in infants. Generalized emphysema usually occurs secondary to an underlying disease that destroys lung parenchyma, such as cystic fibrosis or α-1-antitrypsin deficiency.

Treatment of the underlying disease plus supportive care is indicated for generalized disease. Unilateral interstitial emphysema has responded to selective intubation of the uninvolved lung. Surgical resection of the affected lobe may be required in congenital lobar emphysema.

Partial obstruction of a large radicle of the tracheobronchial tree is a major cause of lobar hyperinflation. Aspiration of a foreign object, a mucous plug, and extrinsic pressure on a bronchus by an enlarged lymph node or tumor are examples of lesions that can lead to this entity. Asthma and reactive airway disease are leading causes of generalized hyperinflation. Treatment is dictated by the cause: removal of foreign material, relief of extrinsic pressure by antibiotics or chemotherapy, and relief of bronchospasm by the use of brochodilators.

Atelectasis

Atelectasis accompanies obstruction of a large airway when collateral ventilation is insufficient to aerate the lung beyond the obstruction. Because of the small size of pediatric airways, relatively poor collateral ventilation, and low elastic lung recoil, there is a great tendency for atelectasis in the major obstructive airway diseases of childhood, such as asthma or CF.

Atelectasis in asthma frequently resolves spontaneously or with appropriate bronchodilator therapy. Radiographs may reveal a mass producing external pressure on the bronchus. Bronchoscopy to rule out a foreign body is often indicated in patients with persistent atelectasis. Right middle lobe atelectasis is particularly difficult to resolve, especially if associated with repeated infection in that area.

Pneumothorax and Pneumomediastinum

Spontaneous pneumothoraces generally occur in adolescent males (often with a family history) and can recur. Symptoms include acute dyspnea and chest pain and are related to rupture of small subpleural, usually apical, blebs. Asthmatic patients occasionally develop pneumothorax or pneumomediastinum during acute asthma attacks. In addition to the classic physical findings of air dissection into the mediastinum (Hamman's crunch—a click heard in synchrony with the heart beat—or crepitus caused by subcutaneous air), there may be a history of sudden chest pain or refractory wheezing. CF is also complicated by the development of pneumothoraces. These tend to occur with advanced disease and to be recurrent. Other causes of pneumothoraces include diffuse lung disorders, such as histiocytosis, and trauma (either penetrating or blunt). The latter is particularly likely to be associated with hemopneumothorax (see Chapter 8).

Tension pneumothorax occurs when air accumulates in the pleural space under pressure and can be recognized by flattening of the diaphragm, marked shift of the mediastinum away from the pneumothorax, and severe cardiopulmonary distress.

Needle aspiration (for small accumulations) or closed chest tube drainage may be necessary with pneumothoraces. Occasionally, pleural sclerosing therapy with tetracycline or by surgery is required for recurrent spontaneous pneumothoraces.

Pleural Effusions

Fluid in the pleural space can be produced by a variety of mechanisms. In pediatric patients the most common cause of fluid is infection. Evaluation of pleural fluid obtained at thoracentesis is aimed at excluding infection and differentiating it from other causes (see Table 7-6). The results of pleural fluid cultures determine antibiotic therapy.

Empyema

Empyema refers to the presence of infected material within the pleural space. Although *S. aureus* was the major cause of empyema in previous years, other organisms such as *H. influenzae* and pneumococcus are more commonly associated with empyema now. Viral and *Mycoplasma* infections are also occasionally associated with the presence of pleural effusions. Tuberculous effusions are generally difficult to culture for *M. tuberculosis*, although a pleural biopsy may grow the organism or demonstrate it with acid-fast staining. Appropriate antibiotic therapy is the treatment of choice, but surgical drainage may be necessary in some instances.

Pleurisy

Pleurisy is inflammation of the parietal or visceral pleura and is usually associated with viral infections or infection in the adjacent pulmonary or diaphragmatic areas. Pleural involvement is also associated with a variety of systemic disorders including malignancies, pulmonary infarction (e.g., sickle cell disease), and connective tissue disorders.

Symptoms of pleuritic involvement are nonspecific in the younger child—tachypnea and shallow breathing—whereas older children may complain of dyspnea, pain on inspiration, or cough. Pleural friction rubs may be audible on auscultation. With increased duration of irritation, pleural fluid accumulates.

Therapy of pleurisy depends upon the underlying condition. Anesthesia of the pleural surface by local intercostal nerve block can be useful Local heat and analgesics also help alleviate pain.

Acute Asthma

Asthma is defined as airway obstruction of the large and small lower airways that is reversible, either with time or with therapy. The patient with typical acute asthma has difficulty breathing (primarily due to expiratory obstruction), cough, a hyperinflated chest, and wheezing. Asthma is associated with a number of precipitating factors, including infection, allergy, emotion, and exercise. Although it is usually easy to recognize typical acute asthma, it is important also to recognize that many asthmatics have atypical presentation, with chronic cough, recurrent pulmonary infiltrates (primarily atelectasis), and exercise dyspnea—all of which respond to appropriate bronchodilator therapy.

The etiology of asthma is unknown, but it affects up to 10% of the general population and accounts for a large percentage of emergency department visits by children, second only to trauma in many areas. Although much of childhood asthma has an allergic basis, respiratory infections (usually viral) play a major role in exacerbating symptoms in most childhood asthmatics. IgE-mediated antibody interaction with sensitized airway mast cells, with release of bronchoconstricting mediators, is also a possible major mechanism in asthma.

The muscular tone of the airways is under control of both adrenergic and cholinergic systems. The drugs used in asthma are aimed at increasing activity of β-receptors by direct stimulation (epinephrine, isoproterenol) and by blocking breakdown of cyclic adenosine 3′, 5′-monophosphate, the active metabolite responsible for smooth muscle relaxation (theophylline). The pathophysiology of asthma is not related only to smooth muscle constriction. There is also prominent mucous hypersecretion, inflammation, and edema during the acute asthma attack, all of which contribute to airway obstruction and are major factors in severe, fatal asthma.

The differential diagnosis of wheezing is extensive (Table 7-1), so it cannot be assumed that all wheezing is asthma. The evaluation of the first-time asthmatic should include a careful history of possible precipitating factors and family history. A careful physical examination and chest radiograph can exclude most other chronic lung disorders such as CF. Patients with asthma generally do not show clubbing, although occasionally growth is poor in inadequately controlled asthma.

Treatment of the acute asthma attack is aimed at (1) reversing the acute symptomatology and (2) preventing recurrent symptoms. Although the standard emergency department treatment in this country has been subcutaneous epinephrine, selective β_2 agents, including aerosols, are generally replacing subcutaneous epinephrine in most circumstances (Exhibit 7-5). Another major advance in emergency care is the rapid determination of theophylline levels, allowing patients to achieve and maintain therapeutic levels of medication.

Complications of acute asthma include respiratory failure, pneumomediastinum, pneumothoraces, and acute cor pulmonale. Because the cardiopulmonary mechanics of the acute asthma attack favor accumulation of interstitial fluid (high negative intrathoracic pressures), minimal fluids should

Exhibit 7-5 Drug Management of Acute Asthma

Administer one of the following:

Epinephrine (1 : 1000 solution)
0.01 mL/kg (maximum single dose, 0./3 mL) SC every 15–20 min for three doses

or

Terbutaline, 0.05 mg/kg SC every 20 min for three doses

or

Isoetharine, 0.5 mL/2.5 mL normal saline per nebulizer over 20 min; repeat in 1–4 h

or

Metaproterenol, 1–2 puffs by metered dose inhaler (650 μg per puff), or 0.2–0.3 mL/2.5 mL normal saline per nebulizer over 20 min: repeat in 1–4 h

Immediately obtain theophylline level in patients receiving oral preparations containing theophylline.

Administer aminophylline (5–8 mg/kg) IV over 20–30 min, followed by a continuous infusion of 0.9 mg/kg/h. Check levels. Reduce dose by half in patients receiving oral theophylline if level is not known.

be given to replace losses (e.g., from vomiting) and meet maintenance requirements.

Severe Acute Asthma This is a major medical emergency that must be treated aggressively. These patients may have a relatively brief history of symptoms but have the physical findings of severe airway obstruction: hyperinflation, minimal air movement (and consequently minimal wheezing), pulsus paradoxus, and accessory muscle use. As noted in the section on physical examination, changes in consciousness are often ominous signs of hypoxemia or hypercapnea. Patients with severe acute asthma should be placed in a quiet, neutral environment and be given supplemental oxygen immediately during the initial assessment. A rapid-acting bronchodilator, epinephrine or terbutaline, by subcutaneous route is probably preferable to aerosol medications for initial therapy in severe asthma. An intravenous line should be set up to begin hydration and provide a route for additional drug therapy, including aminophylline. There is controversy over the role of corticosteroids in the management of acute severe asthma, but patients who have required long-term steroid therapy should receive additional therapy early in the course of a severe attack because of the delay in onset of steroid action.

Status Asthmaticus This condition is defined as asthma refractory to usual outpatient management. It is important to recognize when a patient is likely to fail outpatient therapy so that admission can be quickly arranged (Exhibit 7-6).

Foreign Body Aspiration

Foreign body aspiration should be suspected in any pediatric patient with an acute onset of wheezing or stridor and in patients with chronic or recurrent localized pulmonary infiltrates. Hofznecht's sign—unilateral hyperlucency—can be a useful radiologic clue to the presence of a foreign body. Inspiratory-expiratory films (or decubitus films in younger patients) and fluoroscopy are useful in demonstrating air trapping when a foreign body is suspected. Treatment for aspirated foreign bodies is removal by rigid bronchoscopy in most instances. Chest physical therapy when a foreign body is present carries the risk of dislodging it into a central airway or the larynx, resulting in acute respiratory arrest. (For a more detailed discussion, see Chapter 20.)

Exhibit 7-6 Risk Factors in Status Asthmaticus That Require Hospitalization and Prolonged Therapy

Prior history of hospitalization or respiratory failure
Asthma requiring multiple drug therapy for control
Chronic or intermittent corticosteroid use
History of poor asthma control for several days or weeks: repeated visits to the emergency department, frequent use of inhaler, etc.
Evidence of fatigue
Poor initial response to emergency treatment
Significant gas exchange abnormalities: hypoxemia, hypercapnea
Evidence of concurrent infection

Smoke Inhalation

Accidental fires are a major cause of deaths in children and as many die from smoke inhalation as from thermal injury. Smoke contains a variety of substances toxic to the respiratory tract, and the high respiratory rates of children as well as the small size of their airways contribute to the severity of lung injury with smoke inhalation. Carbon monoxide poisoning often accompanies smoke inhalation, and CO levels should be measured in every child trapped in a fire. Smoke-related injury should be suspected in any child taken from a burning building, even if thermal burns are not obvious. Thermal injury primarily occurs to the upper airway and trachea because heated air is rapidly cooled to body temperature as it is inspired. Such thermal injury poses a significant risk of acute airway obstruction, so that an immediate tracheostomy may be necessary to establish an airway.

Chemical injuries related to toxic products from smoke are a major cause of delayed lung injury. These products, such as hydrogen chloride and aldehydes, are toxic to pulmonary parenchymal cells. Within 24 hours of injury, ciliated bronchial type I alveolar cells and the alveolar-capillary membrane are injured, leading to bronchiolitis, edema, and atelectasis. Superinfection also can occur during this injury phase. The primary physiologic disorder with this type of injury is hypoxemia.

The treatment of smoke inhalation includes intubation and ventilation if there is evidence of respiratory insufficiency, difficulty in handling secretions, laryngeal edema, or severe burns of the face. After the patient is stabilized, arterial blood gas levels should be obtained, and oxygen and fluid therapy should be administered as needed. Examination of the upper airway and trachea by flexible fiberoptic bronchoscopy can be used to gauge the extent of airway injury. Often acute respiratory injury complicates the resuscitation therapy for surface thermal burns, since too vigorous fluid administration in the face of alveolar injury results in pulmonary edema.

Carbon Monoxide Poisoning

Poisoning from carbon monoxide is a risk of closed-space fires such as those from faulty space heaters. CO has a high affinity for hemoglobin and myoglobin, resulting in a leftward shift of the oxyhemoglobin dissociation curve (increased affinity), leading to decreased tissue O_2 delivery. CO also inhibits respiration at the cellular level by competing with molecular O_2. Clinical examination to determine CO poisoning is unreliable, particularly in children, in whom impaired psychomotor functioning—the earliest sign of significant CO levels—is often difficult to judge in an emergency situation. There is no cyanosis and PaO_2 and saturation are normal. Therefore, direct measurement of carboxyhemoglobin levels is essential. CO levels less than 20% are associated with headaches and decreased higher cerebral functions. With levels from 20% to 40%—moderate toxicity—there is irritability, diminished visual acuity, nausea, and impaired mental abilities. Levels from 40% to 60% result in confusion, hallucinations, and coma. If CO poisoning is strongly suspected, the patient should be placed in 100% oxygen until the CO level is known. If the level is greater than 25% or there is strong reason to suspect high levels, hyperbaric oxygen is indicated. If there is anemia, transfusion or even a partial exchange transfusion should be done to improve O_2 delivery.

Aspiration Syndromes, Including Hydrocarbon Pneumonitis

The lungs of the child are at major risk for injury by aspiration, including aspiration of meconium at birth, refluxed gastric contents, and ingested foreign substances such as hydrocarbons. This section focuses primarily on hydrocarbon pneumonitis because it is a major respiratory emergency and is the second most common form of childhood poisoning (after salicylates).

Although both the central nervous system and viscera are affected in hydrocarbon ingestion, death usually results from pulmonary involvement. Commonly ingested hydrocarbons include furniture polish, lighter fluid, gasoline, and kerosene. Because the solutions are generally quite irritating to the oral mucosa, the volumes ingested are often small. Most patients with significant ingestion show pulmonary symptoms within the first 24 hours, but physical and radiographic findings may be minimal within the first few hours after ingestion. The type of product ingested affects the incidence and severity of pulmonary complications: generally the more volatile hydrocarbons are more likely to result in injury.

The management of hydrocarbon ingestion includes (1) hospitalization, (2) supportive fluids and O_2 therapy, and (3) mechanical ventilation and continuous positive pressure to maintain oxygenation, if necessary. Careful gastric lavage does not appear to affect outcome, but vomiting (either spontaneous or provoked by lavage) is likely to increase complications. Use of corticosteroids is controversial but is probably of little use in most circumstances. Follow-up studies of pulmonary function suggest that residual abnormalities are common after hydrocarbon ingestion.

Near-Drowning

Near-drowning can occur with or without aspiration of water because reflex laryngospasm may protect the lungs during immersion (Figure 7-1). Thus the damage that ensues is due either to hypoxia alone or hypoxia plus aspiration. The pattern of fluid and electrolyte alterations depends upon whether drowning occurs in fresh or salt water (Table 7-11), and the prognosis is better when the immersion occurs in cold water. Aspiration of contaminated water can lead to secondary problems such as bacterial pneumonitis.

The outcome of near-drowning probably depends more on what happens during initial resuscitation than upon subsequent treatment. Immediate establishment of an airway, initiation of ventilation (by mouth-to-mouth or mechanical ventilators), and

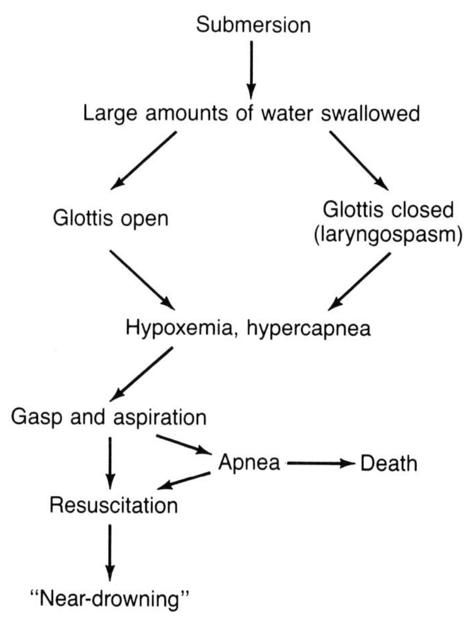

FIGURE 7-1 Pathophysiology of near-drowning.

TABLE 7-11 Respiratory, Fluid, and Electrolyte Alterations in Fresh and Salt Water Near-Drowning

Fresh Water	Salt Water
ARDS:* altered surfactant	ARDS: fluid-filled alveoli
Hypoxemia	Hypoxemia
Hyperkalemia	Hypovolemia (rare)
Hyponatremia (mild)	
Hemodilution (rare)	
Hypervolemia (rare)	
Late: pneumonia, secondary lung injury, aspiration syndromes, neurologic sequelae	

* Acute respiratory distress syndrome.

closed-chest massage to establish circulation are critical to a good outcome. Subsequent pathophysiology of drowning is related primarily to respiratory complications, since the metabolic, cardiovascular, and renal complications are rarely severe.

At admission to the hospital, if a pulse has not yet been established, immediate tracheal epinephrine should be administered while an electrocardiographic tracing is obtained to indicate ventricular fibrillation or asystole. After restoration of circulation and ventilation, initial laboratory studies should be obtained, including hematocrit, electrolyte levels, type and crossmatch for transfusion, and arterial blood gas measurements. Hypoxemia is the major disturbance in blood gas status, often accompanied by a persistent metabolic and/or respiratory acidosis. Although the initial hypoxemia is related to asphyxia, other mechanisms become important, depending on whether salt or fresh water has been aspirated. With salt water, fluid is drawn into the alveolus, resulting in pulmonary edema, loss of compliance, and loss of effective surface for gas exchange. With fresh water, surface tension properties within the alveolus are altered, resulting in reduced compliance and atelectasis.

Significant life-threatening alterations in either hematocrit or electrolyte values are rare with either type of drowning. If serious hemolysis occurs with fresh water drowning (related to both hypotonicity and hypoxemia), then a partial exchange transfusion should be started. With salt water, shifts of plasma volume from the intravascular space into the lungs occur, resulting in hemoconcentration and hypotension.

In addition to supplemental oxygen and correction of acidosis and metabolic problems, the major aspect of treatment for near-drowning is ventilation with positive-end expiratory pressure to maintain adequate oxygenation (although only oxygen may be necessary initially). Patients should be followed for 24 to 48 hours to rule out progressive respiratory distress. If the initial radiograph is completely negative, this indicates a good pulmonary prognosis.

Although the emphasis here has been on the pulmonary complications of near-drowning the fact is that pulmonary injury is rarely the cause of death in drowning victims. More recently, therapy has focused on cerebral injury following the asphyxia of drowning and how improvements in control of cerebral edema and blood flow alterations may improve neurologic outcome in these patients. Cerebral resuscitation is covered more completely in Chapter 12.

Cystic Fibrosis

CF is an autosomal recessive genetic disorder characterized by chronic obstructive pulmonary disease, pancreatic insufficiency, and elevations of sweat electrolytes (sodium and chloride). Pulmonary manifestations include a persistent moist cough, wheezing, and recurrent bouts of pneumonia. Nasal polyps and sinusitis are evidence of upper respiratory tract involvement. The gastrointestinal manifestation is frequent, loose, and foul-smelling stools. Failure to thrive secondary to malabsorption and recurrent bouts of pneumonia with ultimate progression to respiratory failure are the rule. CF patients are frequent visitors to the emergency department because of the acute respiratory and gastrointestinal complications that occur in this disorder (Exhibit 7-7). Occasionally, the diagnosis of CF has not been made at the time the patient is admitted with one of these complications.

Exhibit 7-7 Acute Complications of CF That May Require Emergency Care

Pulmonary
- Hemoptysis, occasionally massive
- Pneumothorax, pneumomediastinum
- Acute exacerbations of obstructive pulmonary disease: respiratory failure
- Lobar atelectasis (mucous plugging)
- Cor pulmonale, with clinical manifestations of heart failure: edema, hepatomegaly

Gastrointestinal
- Meconium ileus equivalent (intestinal obstruction): intussusception, abdominal masses
- Rectal prolapse
- Acute pancreatitis
- Esophageal bleeding (secondary to cirrhosis, varices)
- Edema and hypoproteinemia (infants)

Metabolic
- Hyponatremic dehydration and shock
- Diabetes mellitus (rarely ketoacidosis)

Other
- Bleeding diathesis (vitamin K deficiency)
- Hypertrophic osteoarthropathy (pain in the extremities)

Recurrent Pneumonia

When a patient with pneumonia is seen in an emergency care setting, one should always ask about previous lower respiratory tract infections. Patients with two or more pneumonias, separated by at least 6 to 8 weeks and by radiologic evidence of clearing, are said to have recurrent pneumonia and should have further diagnostic studies. The first priority always is to obtain and review all old radiographs. Second, a follow-up radiograph should be obtained in all such patients after a suitable interval of appropriate antibiotic therapy (6 to 8 weeks). Appropriate evaluation for a patient with recurrent pneumonia is shown in Exhibit 7-8.

Chronic Obstructive Pulmonary Disease

The pediatric equivalent of the adult with chronic obstructive lung disease is now common in many emergency departments. Patients who are survivors of prematurity, severe hyaline membrane disease, and oxygen toxicity can have significant chronic obstructive lung disease. Many still require supplemental oxygen at home and are more likely to develop severe complications such as wheezing, recurrent pneumonias, atelectasis, and apneas.

Exhibit 7-8 Evaluation of Recurrent Pneumonia

Initial
- Careful history: family, birth and neonatal period, travel, environmental exposures, dates and details of all previous significant infections, growth and development, feeding problems, gastrointestinal symptoms, etc.
- Physical examination: resting respiratory rate, clubbing, cyanosis, pulmonary and chest wall examination, neurologic evaluation, etc.
- Review all available chest radiographs, in order.
- Laboratory tests:
  - Complete blood count, with white blood-cell count and differential, to detect anemia, leukocytosis, neutropenia, lymphopenia, eosinophilia
  - Sputum examination and culture
  - Quantitative pilocarpine iontophoresis ("sweat test")
  - Quantitative immunoglobulines, including IgE

Subsequent (as indicated)
- Sinus films
- Arterial blood gas measurements
- Pulmonary function studies
- Complement levels
- Functional antibody levels to detect diphtheria, tetanus
- Skin tests (T-cell function) to detect *Candida*, mumps, *Trichophyton* α-1-Antitrypsin level
- Skin testing for hypersensitivity
- Barium esophagram
- Nasal cilia biopsy for ultrastructure

"Near-Miss" Sudden Infant Death Syndrome (SIDS) and Apnea of Various Causes

The near-miss SIDS patient is defined as a previously healthy infant under 1 year of age (usually 2 weeks to 6 months) who is found with absent or shallow respirations, cyanosis, or cardiac arrest without an apparent medical cause such a pneumonia, sepsis, or meningitis. These events are usually associated with sleep or feeding. Such infants may be successfully resuscitated by parents or paramedics and then brought to the emergency department, where physical examination is often normal except for lethargy. Laboratory evaluation may show leukocytosis and elevated values in liver function tests, both consistent with anoxia and catecholamine release. A chest radiograph may show evidence of aspiration.

Subsequent management of these infants is a difficult problem. Although it is accepted that many of these infants are at risk for SIDS, defining this risk is very difficult: the criteria vary with different centers and can include being a sibling of a SIDS victim. Such children usually are admitted to the hospital for a period of observation and monitoring. Many facilities now also provide "apnea" screening programs including monitoring of a sleep electroencephalogram, respiration, and transcutaneous oxygen and CO_2 levels, as well as 24-hour esophageal pH levels, if indicated. Control of breathing and other automatic functions appear to be abnormal in some of these infants; thus detailed studies of response to hypercapnea and hypoxia can be useful.

Screening studies using a portable electrocardiograph and respiratory monitors can also be done at home to provide evidence of cardiac irregularities and abnormal breathing patterns. Infants at risk for SIDS are discharged home from the hospital with an apnea and an electrocardiographic monitor until the parents and physician are comfortable that risk is minimal for significant apneic events.

Obstructive sleep apnea is another disorder that may be seen in the emergency department. Common causes in pediatric patients include enlarged tonsils and adenoids and genetic syndromes such as Pierre Robin anomaly or Down's syndrome. Patients often have associated problems such as difficulties in school (secondary to disturbed sleep patterns or chronic hypoxia), nocturnal enuresis, unexplained cor pulmonale, and failure to thrive. Careful observation during sleep—for chest and abdominal motion without obvious movement of air—is often quite useful, but if symptoms are significant, referral to a regional sleep center should be made for a more detailed sleep study.

Bibliography

General

Hughes WT, Buescher ES (eds): *Pediatric Procedures.* Philadelphia, WB Saunders Co, 1980.

Kendig EL, Chernick V (eds): *Disorders of the Respiratory Tract in Children.* Philadelphia, WB Saunders Co, 1977.

Levison H (ed): *Pediatric Clinics of North America.* Philadelphia, WB Saunders Co, 1979, vol 26, no. 3: *The Chest.*

Shapiro BA, Harrison RA, Walton JR (eds): *Clinical Application of Blood Gases.* Chicago, Year Book Medical Publishers, 1982.

West JB (ed): *Pulmonary Pathophysiology: The Essentials.* Baltimore, Williams & Wilkins Co, 1977.

Common Signs and Symptoms

Eigen H: The clinical evaluation of chronic cough. *Pediatr Clin North Am* 1982;29:67.

Irwin RS, Rosen MJ, Braman SS: Cough: A comprehensive review. *Arch Intern Med* 1977;137:1186.

Mellis CM: Evaluation and treatment of chronic cough in children. *Pediatr Clin North Am* 1979;26:553.

Tom LWC, Weisman RA, Handler SD: Hemoptysis in children. *Ann Otol Rhinol Laryngol* 1980;89:419.

Yudkin S: Six children with coughs: The second diagnosis. *Lancet* 1961;2:561.

Evaluation

Downes JJ, et al: Arterial blood gases and acid-base disorders in infants and children with status asthmaticus. *Pediatrics* 1968;42:238.

Joseph PM, et al: Upper airway obstruction in infants and small children. *Radiology* 1976;121:143.

McFadden ER, Kiesen R, deGroot W: Acute bronchial asthma: Relations between clinical and physiologic manifestations. *N Engl J Med* 1973;288:221.

Pharyngitis

Schwartz RH, Wientzin RL, Grundfast KM: Sore throat in adolescents. *Pediatr Infect Dis* 1982;1:443.

Sinusitis

Wald ER, et al: Acute maxillary sinusitis in children. *N Engl J Med* 1981;304:749.

Wald ER, et al: Sinusitis and its complications in the pediatric patient. *Pediatr Clin North Am* 1981;28:777.

Otitis Media

Berman S, Balkany T, Simmons M: Otitis media in infants less than 12 weeks of age: Differing bacteriology among inpatients and outpatients. *J Pediatr* 1978;93:453.

Klein JO, Bluestone CD: Acute otitis media. *Pediatr Infect Dis* 1982;1:66.

Croup Syndromes

Barker GA: Current management of croup and epiglottitis. *Pediatr Clin North Am* 1979;26:565.

Bass JW, Bruhn FW, Merritt WT: Corticosteroids and racemic epinephrine with IPPB in the treatment of croup. *J Pediatr* 1980;96:173.

Fried MP: Controversies in the management of supraglottitis and croup. *Pediatr Clin North Am* 1979;26:931.

Liston SL, Gehrz RC, Jarvis CW: Bacterial tracheitis. *Arch Otolaryngol* 1981;107:561.

McCook TA, Felman AH: Retropharyngeal masses in infants and young children. *Am J Dis Child* 1979;133:41.

Newth C, et al: The respiratory status of children with croup. *J Pediatr* 1972;81:1068.

Oliphant M, Grossman H: Acute upper airway obstruction: Clinico-radiologic approach. *Pediatr Ann* 1975;5:650.

Bronchiolitis

Lenney W, Milner AD: Alpha and beta adrenergic stimulants in bronchiolitis and wheezy bronchitis in children under 18 months of age. *Arch Dis Child* 1978;53:707.

Reynolds EOR: Arterial blood gas tensions in acute disease of the lower respiratory tract in infancy. *Br Med J* 1963;2:1192.

Workshop on bronchiolitis. *Pediatr Res* 1977;11:209.

Bronchitis

Taussig LM, Smith SM, Blumenfield R: Chronic bronchitis in childhood: What is it? *Pediatrics* 1981;66:1.

Pneumonia

Honig P, Pasquariello P, Stool S: *H. influenzae* pneumonia in infants and children. *J Pediatr* 1973;83:215.

Jay S, Johanson W, Pierce A: The radiographic resolution of *Streptococcus pneumoniae* pneumonia. *N Engl J Med* 1975;293:798.

Mimica I, et al: Lung puncture in the etiologic diagnosis of pneumonia. *Am J Dis Child* 1971;122:278.

Seto D, Heller R: Acute respiratory infections. *Pediatr Clin N Am* 1974;21:683.

Emphysema

Dickman GL, Short BL, Krauss DR: Selective bronchial intubation in the management of unilateral pulmonary interstitial emphysema. *Am J Dis Child* 1977;131:365.

Pneumothorax

Bierman C: Pneumomediastinum and pneumothorax complicating asthma in children. *Am J Dis Child* 1967;114:42.

Pleural Effusions, Empyema, and Pleurisy

Finland M, Barnes MW: Changing ecology of acute bacterial empyema: Occurrence and mortality at Boston City Hospital during 12 selected years from 1935–1972. *J Infect Dis* 1978;137:274.

Light RW, MacGregor M, Luchsinger PC, et al: Pleural effusions: The diagnostic separation of transudates and exudates. *Ann Intern Med* 1972;77:507.

Pagtakhan RC, Chernick V: Pleurisy and empyema. Liquid and air in the pleural space, in Kendig EL, Chernick V (eds): *Disorders of the Respiratory Tract in Children.* Philadelphia, WB Saunders, 1977, pp 475–487, 602–607.

Asthma

Becker AB, Nelson NA, Simmons FER: Inhaled sabutamol (albuterol) vs injected epinephrine in the treatment of acute asthma in children. *J Pediatr* 1983;102:465.

Cloutier MM, Loughlin GM: Chronic cough in children: Manifestations of airway hyperreactivity. *Pediatrics* 1981;67:6.

Fischl MA, Pitchenik A, Gardner LB: An index predicting relapse and need for hospitalization in patients with acute bronchial asthma. *N Engl J Med* 1981;305:783.

Franklin W: Asthma in the emergency room: Assessment and treatment. *N Engl J Med* 1981;305:826.

Gluck JC, Busto R, Marks M: Pulsus paradoxus in childhood asthma: Its prognostic value. *Ann Allergy* 1977;38:405.

Kattan M, Gurwitz D, Levison H: Corticosteroids in status asthmaticus. *J Pediatr* 1980;96:596.

Kravis L: The complications of acute asthma in children. *Clin Pediatr* 1973;12:538.

Lee HS, Evans HE: Albuterol by aerosol and orally administered theophylline in asthmatic children. *J Pediatr* 1982;101:632.

Leffert F: The management of acute severe asthma. *J Pediatr* 1980;96:1.

Lenny W, Milner AD: At what age do bronchodilators work? *Arch Dis Child* 1978;53:532.

Lulla S, Newcomb RW: Emergency management of asthma in children. *J Pediatr* 1980;97:346.

Management of asthma. *Pediatrics* 1981;68:874.

McFadden ER: Exertional dyspnea and cough as preludes to acute attacks of bronchial asthma. *N Engl J Med* 1975;292:555.

McFadden ER Jr, Lyons HA: Arterial-blood gas tension in asthma. *N Engl J Med* 1968;278:1027.

Richards W: Differential diagnosis of childhood asthma. *Curr Probl Pediatr* 1974;4:1.

Schwartz AL, et al: Management of acute asthma in childhood: A randomized evaluation of β-adrenergic agents. *Am J Dis Child* 1980;134:474.

Stalcup SA, Mellins RB: Mechanical forces producing pulmonary edema in acute asthma. *N Engl J Med* 1977;297:592.

Weinberger M, Hendeles L, Ahrens R: Clinical pharmacology of drugs used for asthma. *Pediatr Clin North Am* 1981;28:47.

Foreign Body Aspiration

Kim I, et al: Foreign body in the airway. *Laryngoscope* 1973;83:347.

Smoke Inhalation

Charnock EL, Meehan JJ: Postburn respiratory injuries in children. *Pediatr Clin North Am* 1980;27:661.

Mellins RB, Park S: Respiratory complications of smoke inhalation in victims of fires. *J Pediatr* 1975;87:1.

O'Neill JA: Evaluation and treatment of the burned child. *Pediatr Clin North Am* 1975;22:407.

Aspiration Syndromes

Eade NR, Taussig LM, Marks MI: Hydrocarbon pneumonitis. *Pediatrics* 1974;54:351.

Wolfsdorf J: Kerosene intoxication: An experimental approach to the etiology of CNS manifestations in primates. *J Pediatr* 1976;88:1037.

Wynne JW, Modell JH: Respiratory aspiration of stomach contents. *Ann Intern Med* 1977;87:466.

Near-Drowning

Fandel I, BanCaleri E: Near-drowning in children: Clinical aspects. *Pediatrics* 1976;58:573.

Giammona S: Drowning: Pathophysiology and management. *Curr Probl Pediatr* 1971;1:1

Modell JH, Graves SA, Ketover A: Clinical course of 91 consecutive near-drowning victims. *Chest* 1976; 70:231.

Cystic Fibrosis

General

Gurwitz D, et al: Perspectives in cystic fibrosis. *Pediatr Clin North Am* 1979;26:603.

Rosenstein BJ, Langbaum TS, Metz ST: Cystic fibrosis: Diagnostic consideration. *Johns Hopkins Med J* 1982;150:113.

Wood RE, Boat T, Doershuk C: State of the art: Cystic fibrosis. *Am Rev Respir Dis* 1976;113:833.

Hemoptysis

Fellows KE, et al: Bronchial artery embolization in cystic fibrosis: Technique and long term results. *J Pediatr* 1979;95:959.

Remy J, et al: Treatment of hemoptysis by embolization of bronchial arteries. *Radiology* 1977;122:33.

Pneumothorax

Boat JF, et al: Pneumothorax in cystic fibrosis. *JAMA* 1969;209:1498.

McLaughlin FJ, Matthews WJ, Strieder DJ, et al: Pneumothorax in cystic fibrosis: Management and outcome. *J Pediatr* 1982;100:863.

Stowe SM, et al: Open thoracotomy for pneumothorax in CF. *Am Rev Respir Dis* 1975;111:611.

Respiratory Failure

Davis P, diSant Agnese P: Assisted ventilation for patients with cystic fibrosis. *JAMA* 1978;239:1851.

Recurrent Pneumonia

Davis PB, et al: Familial bronchiectasis. *J Pediatr* 1983;102:177.

Huang NN: Evaluation of recurrent respiratory tract infections. *Pediatr Ann* 1977;6:27.

Seto D: Recurrent pneumonia in children. *Drug Therapy (Hosp)*, January 1977, p 54.

Chronic Lung Disorders

Smyth JA, et al: Pulmonary function and bronchial hyperreactivity in long-term survivors of bronchopulmonary dysplasia. *Pediatrics* 1981;68:336.

Near-Miss SIDS

Beckwith JB: The sudden infant death syndrome. *Curr Probl Pediatr* 1973;3:1.

Gould JB: Management of the near-miss infant: A personal perspective. *Pediatr Clin North Am* 1979;26:857.

Kelly D, Shannon D, O'Connell K: Care of infants with near-miss sudden infant death syndrome. *Pediatrics* 1978;61:511.

Acute Respiratory Failure

Downes JJ, et al: Acute respiratory failure in infants and children. *Pediatr Clin North Am* 1972;19:423.

Holbrook PR, et al: Adult respiratory distress syndrome in children. *Pediatr Clin North Am* 1980;27:677.

Newth CJL: Recognition and management of respiratory failure. *Pediatr Clin North Am* 1979;26:617.

Lungs in Trauma

Haller JA, Shermeta DW: Major thoracic trauma in children. *Pediatr Clin North Am* 1975;341.

Milley JR, Nugent SK, Rogers MC: Neurogenic pulmonary edema in childhood. *J Pediatr* 1979;94:706.

Pfenninger J, et al: Adult respiratory distress syndrome in children. *J Pediatr* 1982;101:352.

Tuberculosis

Glassroth J, Robins AG, Snider DE: Tuberculosis in the 1980's. *N Engl J Med* 1980;26:1441.

Guidelines for the investigation and management of tuberculosis contacts. *Am Rev Respir Dis* 1976;114:459.

E. Stevers Golladay

8 Thoracic Injuries

Chest trauma is seen less frequently in children than in adults.[1] Until the adolescent years most thoracic injuries in the childhood age group are secondary to blunt trauma. During the teenage years intentional penetrating injuries (i.e., stab and gunshot wounds) are more prevalent. However, throughout the childhood age group, penetrating injuries usually occur from accidental impalement or from fractured or displaced ribs. With blunt injuries of similar force, a relatively higher mortality is found in children than in adults since the force of injury is inadequately dissipated by the pliable chest wall. The mortality of isolated chest injuries averages 8% but doubles with involvement of one other organ system and quadruples with three or more organ systems involved.

INITIAL ASSESSMENT AND STABILIZATION

The approach to the accident victim is initially tailored by the mechanism of injury.[1,2] A child who falls from a chair fits into an entirely different category than one struck by a truck. Preexisting conditions, including the use of medication or a history of allergy, must be noted during the initial analysis. A willingness to alter the diagnosis or treatment plan after completion of that analysis is essential if the clinical situation changes or the diagnoses reached do not correlate with the physical, laboratory, or roentgenographic findings. Any child who has a history suggestive of injury or has signs or symptoms of thoracic trauma requires complete investigation because even seemingly trivial episodes can cause devastating damage.

Inadequate respiration, circulation, or mentation demand a rapid management sequence. First, airway patency must be assured. A large obstruction, such as a foreign body or clot, must be removed immediately. After it is determined that the cervical spine is not fractured, the neck can be placed in slight extension, which prevents pharyngeal occlusion in the small child. The posterior pharynx of the infant buckles because the occiput is relatively large in comparison to the neck and shoulders. Examination for dislocation of odontic devices or loss of teeth and for tracheobronchial or pulmonary trauma can give clues to the cause of respiratory distress.

Endotracheal intubation may be required to establish and maintain adequate ventilation. To aid intubation in patients with fractures of the face, cervical spine, or trachea, a fiberoptic bronchoscope can be passed through an endotracheal tube and both advanced until the vocal cords are visualized. Transtracheal ventilation can be used as an emergency means temporarily to stabilize the critically ill patient. Cricothyroidotomy can be rapidly accomplished in the emergency department.[3]

In evaluating clinical and laboratory parameters as to the necessity for intubation, no single value is nearly as helpful as serial measurements. Factors used to assess the need for ventilation are listed by availability and reproducibility:

1. a minute ventilation of greater than 150% of the norm for the child's age;
2. evidence of impending cardiorespiratory arrest;
3. Pa_{O_2} less than 60 mmHg forced inspiratory oxygen (FI_{O_2}) greater than 50%;
4. Pa_{CO_2} greater than 55 torr;
5. tidal volume less than 4 mL/kg;
6. maximum inspiratory pressure less than 20 cm negative water pressure;
7. vital capacity less than 10 mL/kg;
8. forced expiratory volume less than 10.

The reverse of these measurements on minimal ventilator settings can be used as indications for extubation. The following initial ventilator settings are usually adequate to maintain ventilation:

- continous positive airway pressure, 3 cm
- peak inspiratory pressure, 20 cm
- FI_{O_2}, 40%
- intermittent mandatory ventilation, 30

If ventilation is adequate but hypotension or poor perfusion is present, extrathoracic causes must be considered.[2,4] A rapid infusion of lactated Ringer's solution, 20 to 30 mL/kg, to restore right atrial filling pressure should be given by peripheral vein prior to any extensive diagnostic maneuvers. Hypotension in the child usually indicates at least a 30% blood volume loss. Preexisting cardiac illness is unusual, but a cardiac, cerebral, or pulmonary contusion can dictate the need for fluid restriction and accurate fluid replacement. However, placement of a percutaneous subclavian catheter for assessment of a central venous pressure has no place in the management of a hypotensive, frightened, and struggling child. Volume repletion must first be accomplished. Iatrogenic injuries to the brachial plexus, lung, or subclavian artery, as well as the difficulty in placing the catheter in a collapsed subclavian vein, establish the saphenous or external jugular veins as the proper conduits for initial administration of fluid. The external jugular vein usually can be used to thread a catheter to a central position. Gentle pressure over the liver allows better definition of the external jugular vein. Frequently, percutaneous puncture is then possible, but cutdowns are easily and readily accomplished by seeking the vein at the midpoint between the mastoid and clavicle on the posterior border of the sternocleidomastoid muscle. If the external jugular catheter cannot be threaded to a central position, and central venous pressure measurements are necessary, an internal jugular or subclavian vein placement can be done under controlled conditions after partial volume replacement. Using this method reduces the probability that difficulties such as subclavian artery puncture or pneumothorax may result.

Arterial gas measurements should be obtained early in the management of thoracic trauma. If the arterial pH is less than 7.20 because of a metabolic cause, one should give 2 mEq of sodium bicarbonate per kilogram. Blood gases may indicate the need for intubation or supplemental oxygen.

Inspection, Palpation, Percussion, and Auscultation

Quick inspection of the undressed child allows easy recognition of several signs:

- labored respirations
- chest wall instability
- splinting or asymmetry
- alar flaring
- subcostal or suprasternal retractions
- cyanosis (not apparent with low hemoglobin levels)
- pallor
- diaphoresis
- distended neck veins
- the gray color of poor perfusion and ventilation

Careful palpation assesses

- tracheal position
- pulse volumes of both upper and lower extremities (with special attention to the possibility of the paradoxical pulse of cardiac tamponade)
- point tenderness of the clavicles, ribs, thoracic spine, or sternum
- crepitus, indicating the air in the subcutaneous tissues

Entrance and exit wounds should be noted. Petechiae suggestive of traumatic asphyxia and ecchymoses overlying the chest can herald significant intrathoracic injuries.

Percussion can assess the heart's position and the possibility of cardiomegaly. It also may detect the hyperresonance of pneumothorax or the dullness of hemothorax. Auscultation for quality of heart sounds, murmurs, xiphisternal crunch (Hamman's sign of mediastinal air), and quality of breath sounds concludes initial assessment.

The agitation and distress secondary to borderline hypovolemia or hypoxemia can exacerbate or simulate pain, but sedation for pain can cause hypotension and inadequate ventilation. Sedation with diazepam or pentobarbital, however, is occasionally useful when treating a stable but anxious child. Phenothiazines should be avoided because of their adverse effect on blood pressure regulation. Narcotics must not be used because children with thoracic injuries often have associated head or abdominal injuries. Pupillary response as well as reactivity to pain and tenderness is altered with narcotic analgesia. A brief period spent in acquiring rapport with a parent and child is more worthwhile than medications. The replacement of fluid loss and an increase in the inspired oxygen concentration or assisted ventilation are used to combat the hypovolemia or hypoxemia before consideration is given to sedation.

Gastric decompression should be an early and essential part of the management of blunt thoracic injury in the child. The blunt trauma victim is aerophagic and has gastric atony. This combination produces (1) diaphragmatic elevation in a diaphragmatic breather, (2) vomiting with the potential hazard of aspiration, and (3) marked distortion of physical findings by the distended and painful stomach.

Laboratory Tests and Monitoring

When there are significant injuries, laboratory tests must include hematocrit, hemoglobin level, a type and crossmatch, and arterial gas measurements. The severely injured patient also may require

- electrolyte measurements
- assessment of urine volumes
- central venous pressure readings
- wedge pressure measurements
- electrocardiographic monitoring
- ear oximetry
- percutaneous oxygen readings
- PT, PTT and platelet count

Twelve-lead electrocardiograms are indicated in all patients with fractures of the first three ribs, sternal fractures, precordial injury, or any other significant chest trauma.

Roentgenograms

Chest films should be obtained as a second priority after cervical spine films when these examinations are dictated by the clinical situation. Portable films may be necessary for an initial assessment. Before transportation to the radiology department, the child must be stabilized. A seriously injured victim should be attended by a physician during any radiologic evaluation. Chest roentgenograms are preferably obtained in the upright posteroanterior and lateral positions. Entrance and exit wounds of penetrating injuries should be marked.

Chest films should be systematically inspected for fractures of the chest cage; shift, widening, or emphysema of the mediastinum; abnormalities of the heart shadow or diaphragm; and abnormal densities or lucencies in the lung fields. An esophagram with water-soluble contrast is indicated when esophageal perforation is suspected because of proximity to the injury, mediastinal emphysema, or presence of esophageal contents in thoracostomy tube drainage. Aortography is performed for a widened mediastinum or other signs of aortic rupture.

Tracheostomy

Unless the circumstances are extraordinary, a tracheostomy should be performed in the operating room under general anesthesia. After the neck is placed in a moderately extended position, a transverse neck incision is made a finger's breadth above the suprasternal notch. The strap muscles are separated and the pretracheal fascia are incised. Then a vertical incision is made through tracheal rings 2, 3, and 4. A stay suture is placed in the third cartilage on either side of the tracheal incision and taped to the chest to allow easy reinsertion should accidental extubation occur. A plastic or Silastic tracheostomy tube of appropriate size is inserted. The skin is not closed. (See Figure 8-1.)

Thoracotomy in the Emergency Department

Indications for immediate thoracotomy occur in less than 10% of trauma victims.[2–4] These indications can be divided into those for emergency department thoracotomy and those for rapid transport to the operating room. Emergency department thoracotomy should be performed for

1. penetrating thoracic injury with uncontrolled hemorrhage or impending cardiac arrest,
2. a suspected blunt or penetrating major vessel injury with intrapleural exsanguination,
3. cardiac arrest in a patient with a flail chest,
4. failure of external cardiac compression or defibrillation secondary to chest wall abnormality or nontraumatic cardiac problem,
5. penetrating abdominal wound with emergency department cardiac arrest.

The need for rapid transport to the operating room may be indicated by

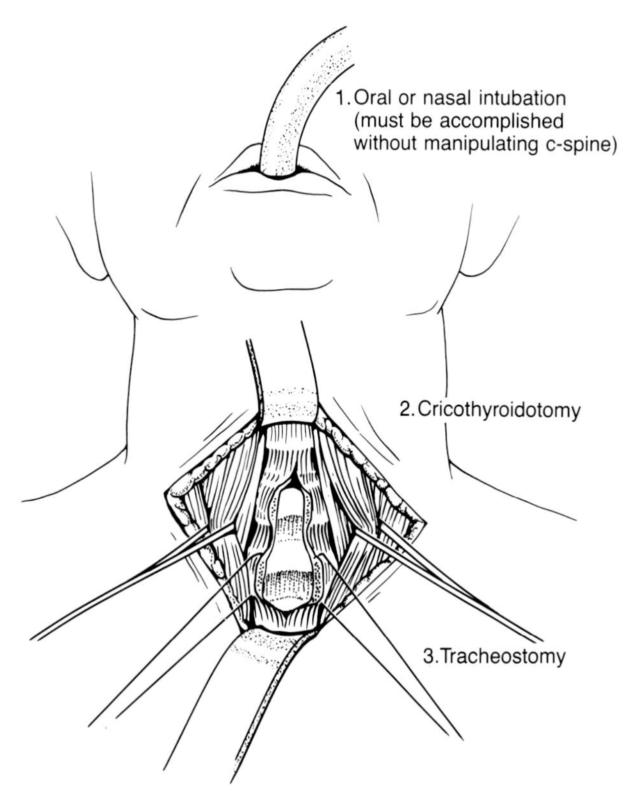

FIGURE 8-1 Oral intubation and surgical exposure for tracheostomy. Note tracheal stay sutures.

1. chest tube losses of blood greater than 10 mL/kg/h, greater than 20 mL/kg/3 hr, or a cumulative total of greater than 40 mL/kg;
2. cardiac tamponade;
3. penetrating cardiac injury and arrest;
4. widened mediastinum with a left hemothorax;
5. confirmed aortic disruption;
6. a ruptured esophagus;
7. an open pneumothorax with a major chest wall defect;
8. a major bronchial injury;
9. gross contamination with a large foreign body;
10. diaphragmatic hernia;
11. a clotted hemothorax with a mediastinal shift.

Precise establishment of the bleeding rate is not possible. Therefore, the decision for a thoracotomy should be based on the rate of bleeding, patency of the evacuation tubes, availability of blood for transfusion, and the patient's response to resuscitative measures.

After rapid skin decontamination, emergency department thoracotomy is performed through a fourth or fifth intercostal space incision from the anterior axillary line to the sternum on the side involved, as determined by physical examination or x-ray film, or on the left side if the laterality is not obvious (Figure 8-2). Care must be taken to avoid the internal mammary artery on the medial margin of the incision and the intercostal vessels on the superior margin of the intercostal space. A clamp is placed on the descending thoracic aorta, taking care not to clamp the esophagus.[3] This maneuver increases perfusion of the cranium and heart. If the pericardium is bulging, the pericardial sac should be opened anterior to the phrenic nerve. The heart is then elevated into the left side of the chest. Bleeding is controlled with finger pressure or insertion of a balloon catheter. Repair is accomplished with pledgeted, nonabsorbable, horizontal mattress sutures. If the wound is on the right or posterior aspect of the heart, extension into the right side of the chest should be made to gain better access to the wound. Pulmonary lacerations are managed by clamping the pulmonary hilus with a large vascular clamp.

Tube Thoracostomy

For tube thoracostomy (Figure 8-3) the skin is antiseptically prepared and the proposed incision site is

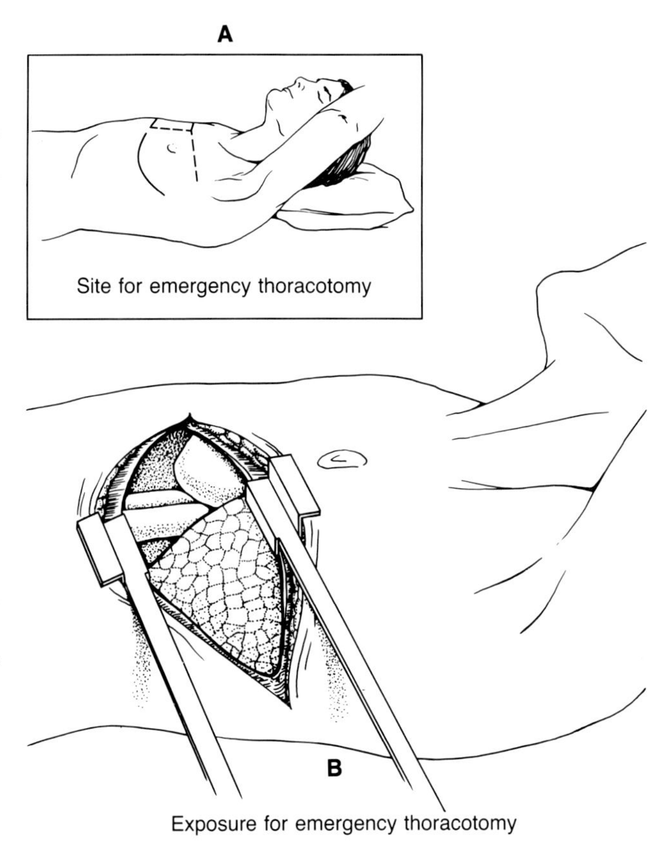

FIGURE 8-2 Site (A) and exposure (B) for emergency thoracotomy.

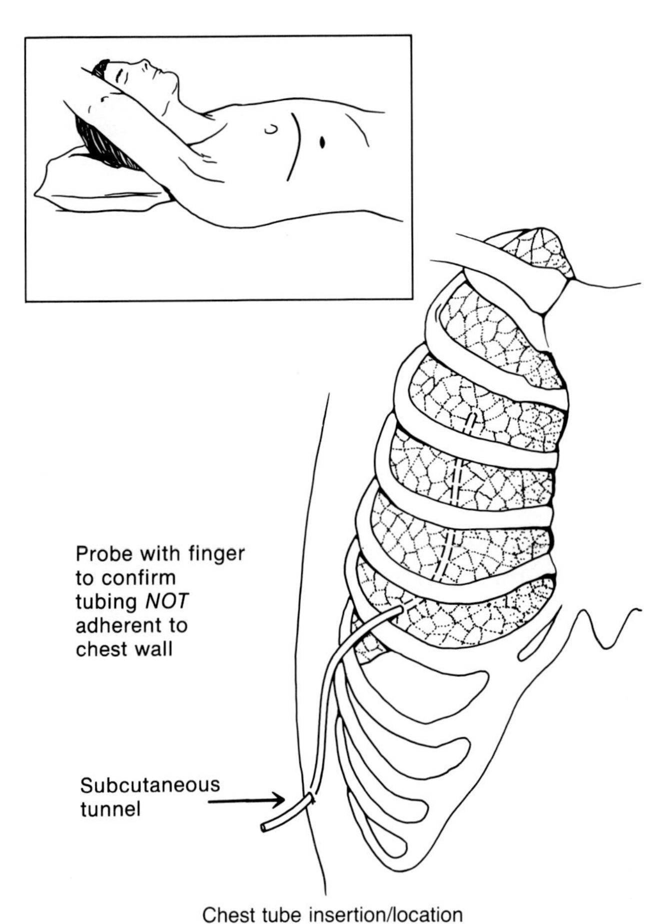

FIGURE 8-3 Placement of tube thoracostomy.

infiltrated with local anesthesia. The tube size selected should be approximately the same width as the interspace through which it is placed (e.g., if the interspace is 7 mm, use a 21 French tube; 8 mm, a 24-gauge French tube). The skin incision should be made in the anterior axillary line overlying the seventh rib. Dissection with a hemostat is done to provide an entrance into the chest in the mid to posterior axillary line in the fifth or sixth intercostal space. The tube is grasped in a hemostat and emplaced into the pleural cavity, with care to avoid the intercostal vessels beneath the ribs. With a small child the hole on the sentinel line should be placed just inside the pleural cavity, and the tip of the tube should be located in the posterior third intercostal space. The tube length from the tip of the sentinel hole may need shortening in an infant. The tube should be secured with two heavy nonabsorbable sutures to prevent inadvertent dislodgment. Heimlich or flutter valves can be useful until an underwater seal or suction (at a 5 to 15 cm water pressure) is instituted. After placement, films are essential to verify positioning and adequacy of hemopneumothorax drainage and to visualize previously indistinct areas of the chest.

Pericardiocentesis

The child with hypotension and potential cardiac injury should undergo pericardiocentesis (Figure 8-4). Ideally this should be performed in the operating room, with preparation for a major thoracotomy. After skin preparation the needle is inserted in the left xiphocostal angle with the tip of the needle directed toward the left shoulder. The procedure is performed with a long large-bore needle connected to a 20-mL syringe with a three-way stopcock. A chest lead is attached to the pericardial needle. The needle is advanced with frequent aspirations until a pop is felt as the pericardium is penetrated. A current of injury will show on the electrocardiogram if the epicardium is contacted. If blood can be withdrawn quite freely and it clots, the needle may be in a heart chamber. Careful attention should be paid to the electrocardiogram as the needle is slowly withdrawn. When one is sure the needle tip is in the pericardial space, blood is withdrawn until it is no longer possible to do so. If no blood is aspirated, insertion of a stylette or injection of saline will assure a patent needle. If signs and symptoms of tam-

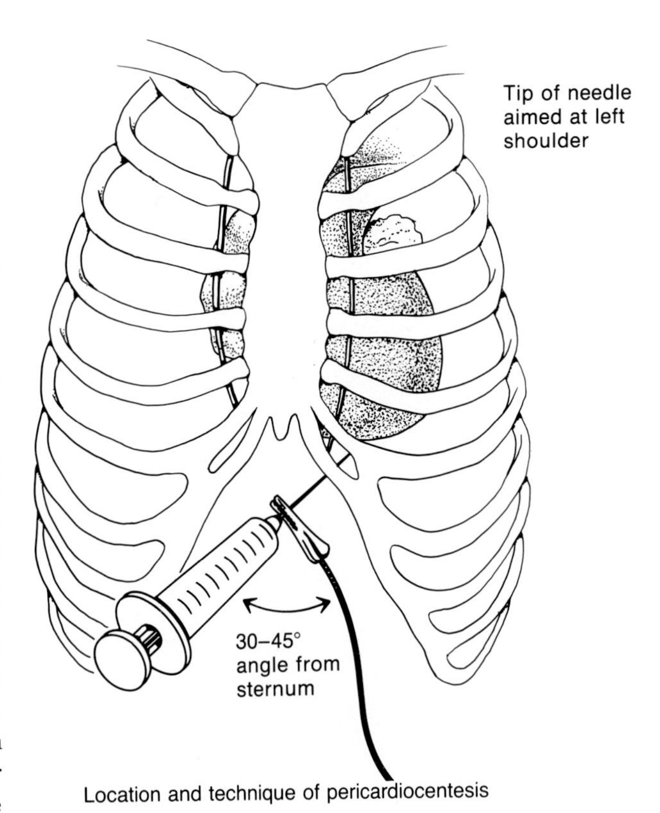

FIGURE 8-4 Technique for pericardiocentesis.

ponade persist, a subxiphoid pericardiotomy is necessary since one fourth of patients with acute cardiac tamponade have a negative pericardiocentesis. An over-the-needle plastic cannula is useful in continued decompression after emergency pericardiocentesis.

SPECIFIC INJURIES

Management of specific injuries is detailed in the remainder of the chapter. These discussions are presented in a sequence based on the area involved, relative frequency, and life-threatening potential, in accordance with advanced trauma life-support standards. They are intended to help the emergency physician recognize and stabilize these injuries.

Tension Pneumothorax

Tension pneumothorax creates a critical emergency in which an air leak accumulates without a means of escape and collects to compress both ipsilateral and contralateral lungs through a shift of the flexible mediastinum. The superior vena cava and inferior vena cava are distorted, thus reducing venous return and consequently cardiac output. The usual causes are tracheal, bronchial, or esophageal perforations; chest injuries with oblique tracts; or an oblique pulmonary parenchymal laceration. Relatively common causes after institution of therapy include high-pressure positive ventilation and tight skin closure around a tracheostomy site. The clinical signs of pneumothorax are

- tachypnea
- dyspnea
- cyanosis
- bulging of the involved hemithorax
- distension of neck veins
- hyperresonance
- decreased breath sounds over the involved hemithorax
- marked tracheal shift to the contralateral side

Immediate percutaneous needle puncture of the involved hemithorax followed by rapid insertion of a tube thoracostomy is the appropriate management sequence.

Open Pneumothorax

The diagnosis of a sucking chest wound should be obvious on inspection.[2,4] The wound is covered by the cleanest means rapidly available, as effective ventilation is impossible with an open pneumothorax. A dressing consisting of multiple layers of petrolatum-impregnated gauze extending at least 5 cm beyond the wound edges and taped securely on three edges makes the chest airtight again and provides a flutter-type valve. A tube thoracostomy is placed through a separate incision to vent the pleural space. Chest films are obtained to ascertain the presence of other injuries or intrathoracic foreign bodies. Large or grossly contaminated wounds should be debrided. Maintenance of adequate ventilation sometimes requires intubation and assisted ventilation.

Hemothorax

Blood in the chest cavity can result from blunt or penetrating injuries.[3,5] Recognition of the possibility of associated abdominal injury with penetrating injury at the nipple level or below is essential. Internal mammary, intercostal, pulmonary, cardiac, or great vessel lacerations can be responsible for hemothorax. Large volumes of blood do not usually result from pulmonary injury since the lung is a low-pressure system and contraction of the elastic lung and the action of vasoactive substances cause quick cessation of flow. Symptoms occur from large-volume blood loss with attendent hypotension or from bilateral pulmonary compression causing hypoxemia. Forty percent of the blood volume can be lost into either pleural cavity. Dyspnea, hypotension, decreased breath sounds, dullness to percussion, and tracheal shift to the contralateral side are the most frequent indications of hemothorax. The lost blood usually remains fluid because of defibrination. A pneumothorax is also present in most traumatic hemothoraces. Upright films show collections of blood in the costophrenic, cardiophrenic, and subpulmonic areas. There may be a wide separation of the gastric air bubble from the inferior margin of the lung. Supine films show a differential radiolucency of the two lung fields.

After institution of volume replacement, tube thoracostomy should be performed. The tube expands the collapsed lung, reduces the risk of fibrothorax, and provides a guide to continuing blood loss. A large loss of blood via chest tube loss may indicate the need for emergency department thoracostomy. If the blood is not evacuated by tube thoracostomy, the clotted hemothorax is best treated by early removal of the fibrin and blood via thoracostomy. Traumatic hemothorax has a 2% incidence of empyema. The mortality of isolated hemothorax is small for a penetrating injury but approaches 70%

with combined blunt trauma to the head, abdomen, and chest.

Flail Chest

The paradoxical inward motion during inspiration secondary to multiple rib fractures is pathognomonic of flail chest. Uneven motion of the chest wall should be sought on physical examination. Initially the injury may be so well splinted that this paradoxical motion does not become apparent until the patient tires. Flail chest is more likely with fractures of the sternum and is less likely with posterior injuries because of the stabilizing effect of the local musculature. Although chest films may show multiple rib fractures, this does not constitute flail chest. Likewise, a child can have costochondral separation as a part of the flail segment and this not be visualized on chest film. Close analysis for evidence of pulmonary contusion is essential in those patients suspected of having flail chest.[4]

The injured side should be placed in a dependent position to provide some stabilization while the need for mechanical ventilation is determined. The initial difficulty is that the pressure gradient is dissipated, so air exchange is hampered. Subsequently, pulmonary contusion is the source of impaired oxygen exchange. Although internal pneumatic stabilization with positive-pressure ventilation is often necessary, an alternate treatment method has been suggested:

1. fluid restriction,
2. diuresis,
3. tracheobronchial therapy that includes coughing and deep breathing,
4. supplemental oxygen to maintain a Pa_{O_2} greater than 80 mmHg,
5. control of chest wall pain.

Bronchodilators and antibiotics can be added. Use of corticosteroids is controversial but may ameliorate the clinical course when given in large doses for the first 48 hours.

Close, continuous monitoring allows early recognition of increased tachypnea, restlessness, anxiety, and Pa_{CO_2}; decreased tidal volume; or a Pa_{O_2} below 60 mmHg despite an FI_{O_2} greater than 40%. Adverse alteration in these or the other parameters detailed under ventilation needs (see "Initial Assessment and Stabilization") should alert one to the need for mechanical assistance. Experiments have shown that early application of constant positive airway pressure reduces mortality and should be provided in this circumstance. Decreased cardiac output can indicate associated myocardial contusion. In patients who have flail chest and shock, the mortality approaches 95%. The higher mortality appears to be in those children with more than seven rib segments or with more than two associated injuries.

Hemopericardium

Hemopericardium can result from injuries to epicardial, myocardial, or pericardial vessels; from chamber rupture; or from intrapericardial rupture of great vessels or laceration of coronary vessels.[5] The symptoms include

- decreased blood pressure
- vasoconstriction
- distended neck veins
- distant heart sounds
- narrow pulse pressure
- pulsus paradoxus
- Kussmaul's sign (increased neck vein distention during inspiration)
- a flat parasternal percussion sound

The diagnosis of pericardial tamponade (Figure 8-5) is more difficult to establish in the child than in the adult because the respiratory rate makes pulsus paradoxus difficult to measure. A smaller volume of pericardial blood can cause trouble in the child, particularly since there is a lesser margin of safety between perfusion pressure and normal blood pressure. In addition, associated injuries and hypovolemia can prevent venous distension. The electrocardiogram may show low-voltage or peaked T waves late in the course of the injury. Chest films show increased cardiac shadow or an increased space between the epicardial fat line and the pericardium.

Initial management of hemopericardium with signs of tamponade includes (1) increasing the filling pressure until a central venous pressure of over 15 cm of water results; (2) an infusion of isoproterenol to increase the heart rate and decrease the end-systolic and diastolic volumes, and (3) pericardiocentesis, as previously described. Thoracotomy should soon follow pericardiocentesis. Should rapid deterioration occur, emergency department thoracotomy is necessary.

Penetrating Cardiac Injuries

Infants are the most likely to be injured from accidental penetration of the chest wall by pins or needles. Older children may have an esophageal foreign body penetrate the heart. The varied activities of adolescence are responsible for the preteen and teen injuries.

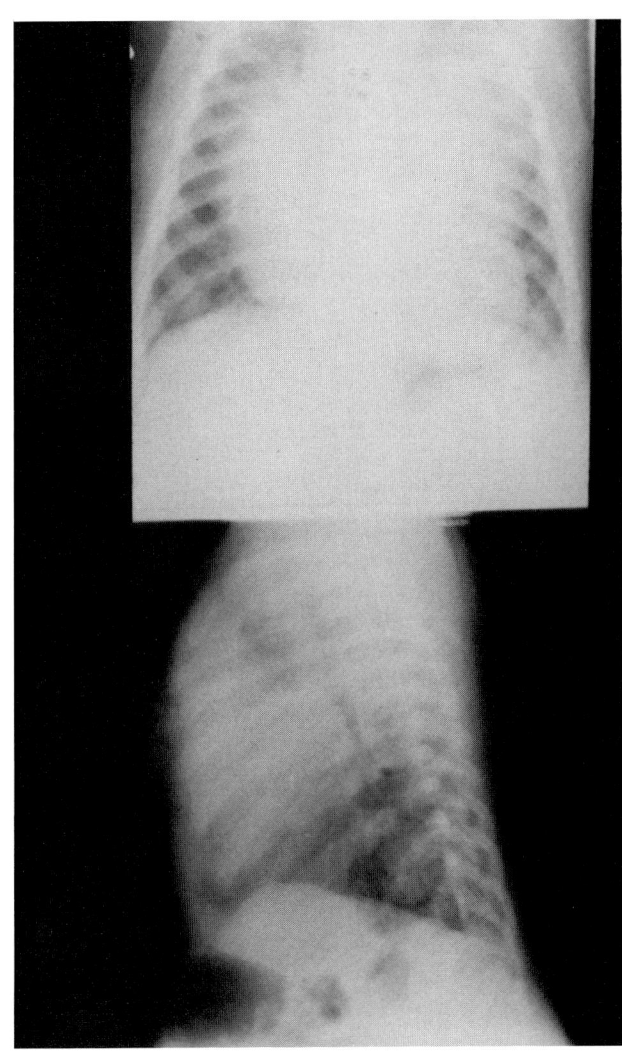

FIGURE 8-5 Pericardial tamponade.

Needle puncture can go undetected initially and be manifest much later as chest pain or irritability. Other symptoms of needle puncture are those of pericardial effusion and tamponade and fever of unknown origin. Chest roentgenograms of acute injury may demonstrate a foreign body in or near the heart, hemothorax, pneumothorax, pneumopericardium, or widened mediastinum (the thymus can imitate this sign in the younger child). The cardiac silhouette usually remains normal. The possibility of embolization to a peripheral location must be considered if there is a penetrating foreign body that has not been detected on the chest film. Stab wounds in the ventricle can seal, but the blast injury of a gunshot wound usually destroys enough cardiac muscle to cause rapid death. Treatment of penetrating cardiac injuries should be the same as for hemopericardium.

Pulmonary Contusion

Pulmonary contusion is the most common serious chest lesion resulting from trauma in children. The damage can be quite localized and have little importance or be widely disseminated. The lungs react to any injury by a graded physiologic response, which varies from minimal interstitial edema to rapid intra-alveolar extravasation of blood and fluid. Impaired cough (as in flail chest), central nervous system depression, or an elevated diaphragm compounds any pulmonary injury. Signs and symptoms such as dyspnea, wheezes, crackles, dullness over the area, hemoptysis, and hypoxemia may not be present initially. The chest film may initially be normal but then progress to soft peribronchial and perivascular infiltration and then to complete consolidation (Figure 8-6). Immediate assessment of arterial gases allows early recognition of a significant pulmonary contusion. Special attention should be paid to children with the following conditions because they are associated with significant contusion:

- impaired consciousness
- multiple rib fractures
- flail chest
- abdominal injury resulting in ileus or operation or the need for operation
- large-volume resuscitation
- multiple soft tissue contusions
- multiple skeletal injuries
- renal failure
- progressive deterioration

Management of the pulmonary contusion should be the same as detailed in the section on flail chest.

Aortic Rupture

Although aortic rupture is a common cause of death in adults after traffic accidents, it rarely occurs in children. It can happen because of blunt force to the chest, vertical deceleration as in a fall, or horizontal deceleration as occurs in auto-pedestrian accidents. The most common site of rupture in decelerating injuries is just distal to the left subclavian artery. In falls from heights, the ascending aorta is involved. In ascending aorta injuries 80% of the victims have severe associated injuries and the combination is usually fatal. The hemopericardium that is common in ascending aortic injury also contributes significantly to the high mortality. Temporary survival occurs in patients in whom the adventitia remains intact.

The patient may have massive hemothorax, hy-

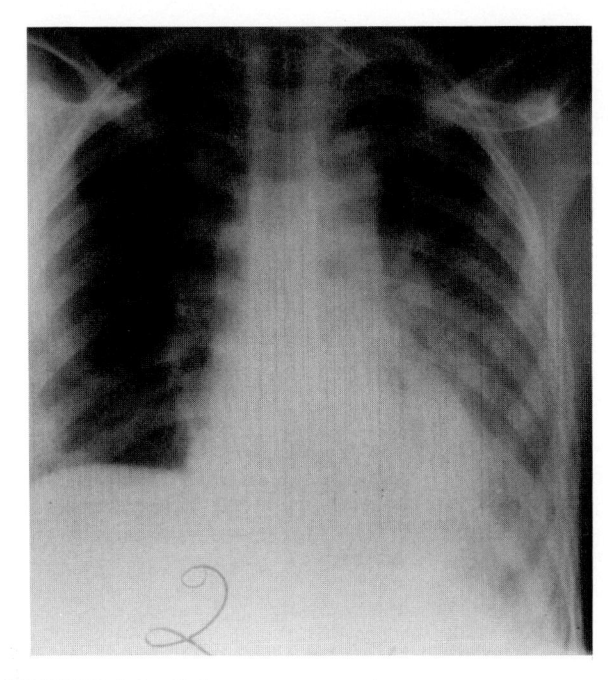

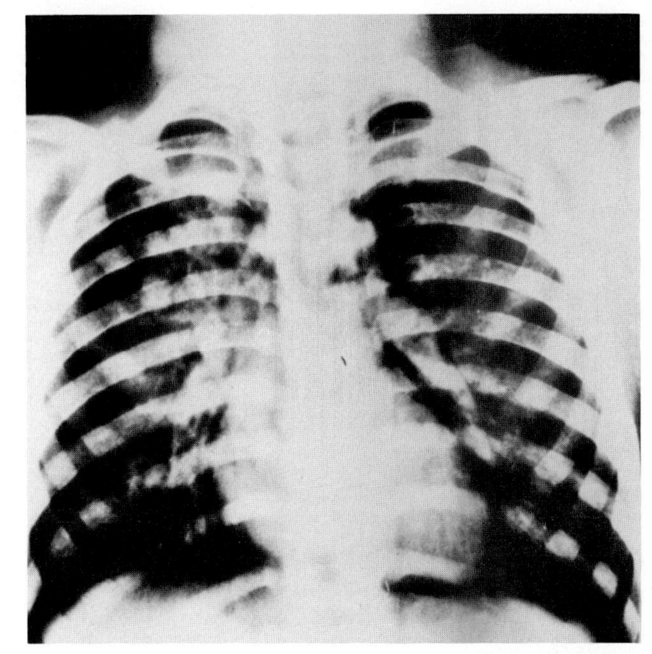

FIGURE 8-6 Pulmonary contusion.

potension, or extensive chest wall contusion; occasionally, a sharp systolic murmur is present. Paraplegia exists secondary to intercostal or spinal artery compression. Additional findings include decreased femoral pulses, dysphagia secondary to esophageal compression, presence of blood in the supraclavicular area, and hypertension in the upper extremities. Associated lesions can mask any of these signs or symptoms. If the patient exhibits upper extremity hypertension, hypotensive treatment should be considered. Trimethephan (Arfonad) in a 5% dextrose drip is infused at 0.1 mg/kg/min to maintain normotension, as assessed by arterial monitoring.

Chest roentgenograms can show the following:

- a widened mediastinum
- inferior displacement of the left mainstem bronchus
- deviation of the trachea to the right
- left pleural fluid or cap
- haziness of the aortic knob
- a full retrosternum
- fractures of the first three ribs
- deviation of the nasogastric tube to the left

Misinterpretation of these findings is common in these critically ill patients and thus film should be carefully reviewed in those patients with severe horizontal or vertical deceleration injuries. The plain film findings must then be confirmed with aortography (Figure 8-7). In more stable patients aor-

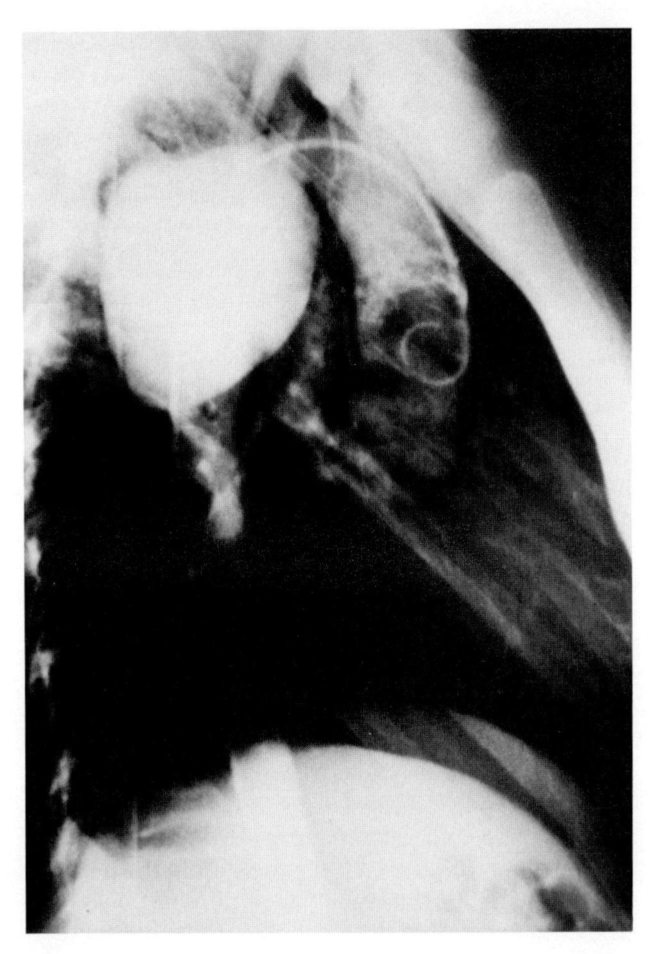

FIGURE 8-7 Aortographic demonstration of aortic rupture.

tography should be done by conventional femoral approach unless there is a large differential blood pressure between the upper and lower extremities. Then the brachial route is preferable.

If an accident victim has bleeding into the left side of the chest, a left anterolateral thoracotomy should be performed and the bleeding should be controlled by pressure. To complete the operation a cardiopulmonary bypass or a heparinized shunt is often required. Recently, direct suture under clamp control and induced hypotension have been used. An interposition graft may be needed. Late rupture of the aneurysm can occur if it is unrepaired.

Bronchopulmonary Laceration

After extensive chest trauma a laceration of the lung can produce a hemopneumothorax with a continuing air leak.[2,4,5] Immediate management is that for hemothorax or pneumothorax, but persistent hemorrhage or massive air leak may require thoracotomy.

Pulmonary hematomas result from extravasation of blood into the pulmonary parenchyma. Hematomas appear on chest films as radiodensities with fluffy outlines, which, over a period of several days, become indistinguishable from coin lesions of other origins. These hematomas may be from 2 to 5 cm in diameter and are usually located in the posterior lower lobes. Resolution occurs most often in less than a month. If resolution has not occurred in 3 to 4 weeks, a biopsy may be necessary to distinguish this lesion from a pulmonary lesion of nontraumatic origin.

Esophageal Injuries

The cervical esophagus can be injured by a garrote mechanism. Penetrating injuries are produced by stab or gunshot wounds. If the path of the trauma is near the esophagus and there is dysphagia or crepitus, this area should be promptly investigated. Verification is sometimes possible by an esophagram with water-soluble contrast. Transgression of the mucosal barrier of the cervical esophagus mandates exploration and drainage.

Intrathoracic penetrating injuries of the esophagus can occur at any level.[5] Substernal pain, often disproportionate to the injury; fever; subcutaneous emphysema; mediastinal crunch; pleural effusion; or saliva appearing in chest tube drainage are signs of mediastinal perforation. Chest tube drainage can be evaluated for amylase content if the appearance is that of saliva. A bedside diagnosis can be established by a methylene blue swallow, which then appears in the thoracostomy tube.

Chest films show pleural fluid, pneumothorax, or pneumomediastinum (Figure 8-8). Immediate treatment consists of fluid administration, antibiotics, and drainage. Definitive care includes a two-layer closure with gastric, pleural, pericardial, or muscle flap coverage.

Blunt esophageal rupture can occur from severe epigastric trauma. Perforation of the distal third of the esophagus results in spillage of gastric and esophageal contents into the right chest. This diagnosis should be considered in the child with persistent pneumothorax after blunt thoracoabdominal trauma. The character of the drainage may enhance suspicion and amylase content can distinguish the esophagus as the cause. The management of blunt perforation is much the same as that of a penetrating injury, but exclusion procedures are more often necessary.

Tracheoesophageal Fistula

Tracheobronchial rupture occurring simultaneously with esophageal injury can cause tracheoesophageal fistula. The initial signs are those of localized tracheal or esophageal leak: fever and mediastinitis. Three to four days after injury, a paroxysmal cough may be precipitated by feeding or swallowing. This cough should prompt an esophageal swallow with

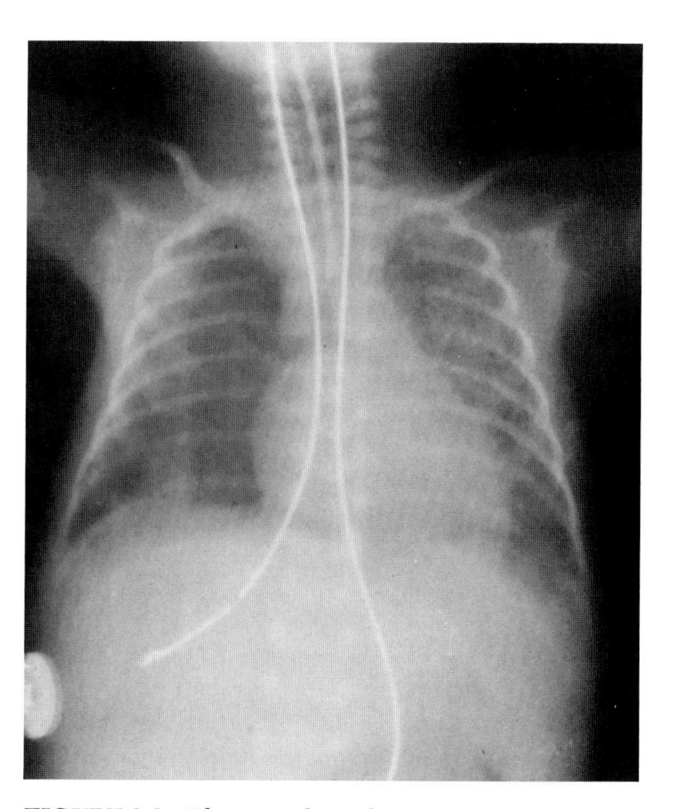

FIGURE 8-8 Blunt esophageal rupture and pneumomediastinum.

metrizamide. Delayed rupture after esophageal exclusion results in long-term survival of 75% of accident victims with posttraumatic tracheoesophageal fistulas.

Injuries to the Pharynx, Larynx, and Intrathoracic Trachea

Trauma to the pharynx, larynx, and trachea usually is iatrogenic in children below 18 months of age; in older children it results from various childhood activities and battering.[3] Eighty percent of the injuries involve the trachea.[3] The cervical trachea is injured three times as often as the intrathoracic trachea. Sudden compression of the chest can cause a traction split of the trachea or crush the bronchus against the spine.

Thirty-five to forty percent of tracheobronchial ruptures have no notable initial findings. The following findings can indicate a tracheal tear:

- atelectasis
- hemoptysis
- subcutaneous or mediastinal emphysema
- dyspnea
- a large-volume air leak
- tension pneumothorax

Tension pneumothorax is especially suspect since the tear often occurs some distance from the pleural entrance. Therefore, tension pneumothorax mandates bronchoscopy, as do hemoptysis and mediastinal emphysema.

Chest films may show lateral displacement of the collapsed lung—the opposite of the normal configuration for a pneumothorax. There may be a bayonet deformity of the air column, a fine air collection paralleling the bronchus, and mediastinal emphysema; in half of reported cases, one of the first three ribs is broken.

Early detection and repair of bronchial injuries is essential since suppuration beyond a point of stenosis commonly results. Immediate treatment requires intercostal tube placement. The preferred definitive treatment is primary suture of the laceration. The overall mortality for this injury is 30% but is only 10% in those who reach the hospital.

Diaphragmatic Injuries

Rupture of the diaphragm occurs from upper abdominal pressure as a result of a high fall or an automobile accident.[6] The incidence appears to be 4% to 5% in severe multiple injuries. Penetration of the diaphragm can occur with a stab or gunshot wound to the chest below the fourth intercostal space. The small hole from a penetrating injury is more likely to cause chronic symptoms or be delayed in recognition than would a larger tear resulting from blunt trauma.

The left side is most often involved with blunt injuries. There is usually a large, ragged linear tear of the central diaphragm in a coronal plane. As a result of the peritoneal-pleural pressure gradient, abdominal contents—stomach, omentum, spleen, and colon—then herniate into the chest. If herniation is acute, dyspnea and pain in the left side of the chest may be present, as well as dullness to percussion, decreased breath sounds, bowel sounds in the chest, a mediastinal shift, and a scaphoid abdomen. Symptoms increase as air collects in the bowel, after which the pathophysiology is similar to tension pneumothorax. An acute diaphragmatic injury from blunt trauma has a 90% association with intra-abdominal injuries; fracture of the lumbar spine is not uncommon. The diaphragmatic injury may not be associated with hemoperitoneum and can be masked by associated injuries. Occasionally, peritoneal lavage fluid is recovered in the chest tube, but lavage per se is inadequate in diagnosing acute diaphragmatic rupture.

The chest film (Figure 8-9) shows herniated viscera, although a loculated pneumothorax, elevation

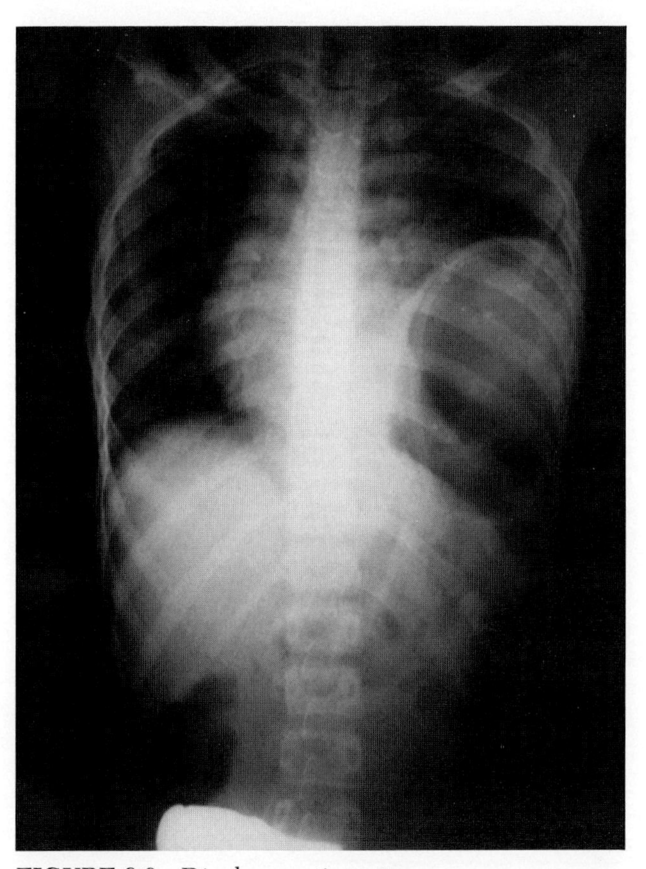

FIGURE 8-9 Diaphragmatic rupture.

of the diaphragm, and cystic pulmonary lesions are entities commonly confused with a diaphragmatic hernia.[7] It should be emphasized that distinction from pneumothorax is usually possible by recognizing the convex shadow of the upper border of the stomach in the chest. Simple passage of a nasogastric tube is frequently useful in diagnosis and is essential in initial management to vent swallowed air. Positive-contrast peritoneography may accurately delineate a diaphragmatic defect. Bowel contrast studies can be helpful in difficult cases.

The victim with a diaphragmatic hernia should have immediate repair through an abdominal approach. One third of traumatic diaphragmatic hernias are recognized late, so a careful history for recent trauma must be part of the initial examination of any child with chest pain or dyspnea. Chronic diaphragmatic hernias are better repaired via a thoracic approach.

Myocardial Contusion and Concussion

Myocardial concussion is brought about by a sharp precordial force, with immediate but transient nonspecific changes in the ST segment. Myocardial contusion is the result of a violent force causing lasting, localized ST-T segment changes and an elevated MB-creatine phosphokinase isoenzyme fraction.[8] When carefully sought, myocardial contusion or concussion is found in approximately 25% of severe chest injuries.

The child with myocardial contusion may have greatly decreased cardiac output and thus impaired resuscitation.[9,10] The signs and symptoms most suggestive of myocardial contusion are tachycardia and precordial pain identical to that of myocardial infarction. There may also be

- bruising of the precordium
- dyspnea
- diaphoresis
- an increase in the venous pressure
- a decrease in blood pressure
- a pericardial rub
- a characteristic tick-tick quality to the heart sounds

There is usually a loss of consciousness at the time of injury, but the other signs and symptoms may not appear for several days. There is an average of 3.5 associated injuries, and the symptoms from these injuries can mask those of myocardial contusion.[9]

Any suspicion of myocardial contusion warrants a 12-lead electrocardiogram, which most characteristically reveals flattened or inverted T waves, flattening of the QRS complex, ventricular premature beats, and ventricular tachycardia; there may also be heart block, atrial fibrillation, or atrial flutter.[8–10] Chest film findings that warrant suspicion include fractures of the sternum or first rib. The cardiac silhouette is rarely enlarged. Because of the possible existence of cardiac contusion with major thoracic injury, serial electrocardiographic evaluation of every such patient is essential. Although electrocardiographic changes following trauma in a child are suggestive of myocardial contusion, there are many other causes for electrical abnormalities, including aberrant coronary arteries and head trauma. Creatine phosphokinase isoenzymes may confirm the diagnosis.

Immediate referral is a must whenever an electrocardiographic abnormality is noted in an injured child. Interim management includes oxygen administration, electrocardiographic monitoring, and treatment of arrhythmias and congestive heart failure. Recovery without residual effects is the most common course.

Septal and Valve Injuries

Although rare, atrial and ventricular septal defects and injuries to the papillary muscles, chordae tendineae, and cardiac valves can occur after both blunt and penetrating cardiac trauma. In children they most often occur in association with myocardial contusion. Recognition of a heart murmur after trauma should prompt further assessment by echocardiography or cardiac catheterization. A ventricular septal defect may spontaneously close, but congestive heart failure can precipitate operative closure earlier than the optimal 2 months. Atrial septal defects require more urgent repair.

Valvular injuries usually require rapid repair by valve replacement, but delay for healing of associated injuries is desirable. Aneurysms of the ventricle can occur later after a blunt or penetrating myocardial injury.

Pneumothorax

Isolated pneumothorax usually results from a stab wound. Decreased breath sounds, respiratory distress, hyperresonance to percussion, and tracheal shifts are signs of pneumothorax. Expiratory films can allow recognition of even a minor collection of air. The noncooperative child can be x-rayed in both right and left decubitus positions to enhance recognition on chest films. The presence of subcutaneous emphysema or a rib fracture, on either physical or radiologic examination, should enhance suspicion. A factitious pneumothorax from folds of skin or clothing is recognizable because the line is nonparallel to the chest or extends beyond the pulmonary boundary. If there is a massive contusion or there are previous adhesions present, the lung may not collapse significantly, but the mediastinum will shift. Proper recognition is essential prior to ventilator use because positive-pressure ventilation will convert a simple pneumothorax to a tension pneumothorax.

For more traumatic pneumothoraces a chest tube should be placed, utilizing the previously described technique. Indications for tube placement include

- moderate-to-large pneumothorax
- respiratory symptoms
- increasing size of the pneumothorax on serial examinations
- assisted ventilation or general anesthesia
- associated hemothorax
- bilateral pneumothorax
- tension pneumothorax

Persistent air leak after tube thoracostomy usually indicates a large bronchopleural fistula, pulmonary penetration by the tube, esophageal rupture or penetration, or a leak around the chest tube, either at the entrance site or at one of the connectors.

Traumatic Asphyxia

Traumatic asphyxia occurs as a result of chest compression during maintenance of a closed glottis.[11] The resultant transmitted pressure causes a sudden, sharp rise in the supraclavicular venular and capillary pressures. The predominant clinical feature is craniocervical cyanosis in a supraclavicular pattern. A V-shaped distribution of discoloration is common in the posterior intrascapular area. Petechiae can occur over the same distribution as the cyanosis. Frequently occurring signs and symptoms include

- subconjunctival hemorrhage
- blurred vision
- mental dullness
- hyperpyrexia
- hemoptysis
- pulmonary contusion
- epistaxis
- hematemesis

Peripheral or spinal paralysis happens rarely. Associated injuries are unusual, but cardiac injuries should be considered. An attendant pulmonary contusion is usually responsible for the most frequent and severe morbidity. Skin changes resolve in about 10 days and conjunctival changes in about 30 days, but optic atrophy can occur later. Recovery without sequelae occurs in more than 90% of cases.[11]

Rib Fractures

Fractures of the ribs do not occur frequently until adult life because of the elasticity of the rib cage during childhood. Rib fractures in a child are usually the result of sharply applied local force. In infancy battering is often implicated. Injury to the first three ribs implies a severe force because of the protection provided by the heavy musculature of the upper thorax, and it is frequently associated with bronchial, cardiac, or aortic rupture. Fractured lower ribs suggest an underlying abdominal visceral injury. Rib fracture is diagnosed when localized pain is aggravated by deep breathing, cough, or positional change. Respiratory excursion may be noticeably restricted.

Roentgenograms of the chest are superior to physical examination in the detection of rib fractures in protected locales (Figure 8-10). Intercostal nerve block should be utilized if pain is not controlled by moderate analgesics. A small volume of bupivacaine (0.25%) is injected posterior to the injury at the lower margins of the two ribs above and below the injured area.

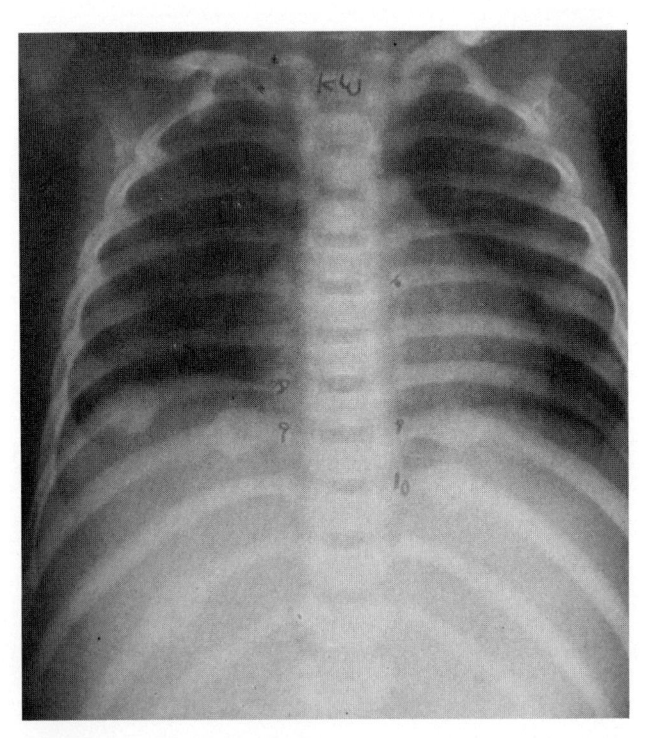

FIGURE 8-10 Chest film showing multiple healing rib fractures.

Subcutaneous Emphysema

Interstitial air occurs as a result of a major break in the pleura, disruption of mediastinal air from rupture of the bronchus or esophagus, or, rarely, from a direct connection with a subcutaneous wound. Treatment is directed toward the underlying cause rather than the emphysema. Indeed, regression of the boundary can indicate that treatment of the responsible injury has been effective. Oxygen washout, needle aspiration, venting of skin incisions, and cervical mediastinotomy have all been used to treat subcutaneous emphysema but are only rarely necessary.

Traumatic Intercostal Hernia

Severe localized disruption of the intercostal muscles has been reported in children. These bulges expand on expiration and disappear on inspiration, and dyspnea can result. Spontaneous closure does occur; therefore, delay to await that closure appears indicated if symptoms are minimal. Simple closure of the defect by utilizing surrounding structures is most often effective if operative therapy is needed.

Sternal Fractures

Because the child's sternum is largely cartilaginous and the usual mechanism for sternal injury is compression by a steering wheel, sternal fracture is quite unusual in the childhood age group. Localized tenderness is usually hidden by other injuries. Associated injuries take precedence in the management sequence since a 25% to 30% mortality results from associated injuries to the aorta or the cranium. There is no specific treatment necessary unless there is marked displacement of the heart, false motion, or severe depression of the chest wall. Reduction should not ordinarily take place for weeks to allow complete management of associated injuries. An electrocardiogram should always be obtained to assess the possibility of myocardial contusion. When surgical repair is indicated, open reduction and fixation with heavy wire sutures is a useful method.

Traumatic Lung Cysts

Acute cystic lesions of the lung resulting from trauma are found mostly in children. They can cause hemoptysis, chest pain, fever, and leukocytosis or create no symptoms at all. Although a hematoma may obscure the cyst initially, the chest film ultimately shows a single cyst or multiple cysts resembling abscess formation in the area of trauma or sometimes in a contrecoup distribution. Further therapy is not needed, and the lesions disappear in a few weeks to a few months.

Posttraumatic Pericarditis

Posttraumatic pericarditis causes severe chest pain exacerbated by inspiration, the supine position, or by swallowing. There may be fever and pericardial or pleural friction rubs. Electrocardiograms may show ST-T interval changes. A large effusion can produce muffled heart sounds, venous distension, hypotension, and paradoxical pulse. Chest films show enlargement of the cardiac shadow. An echocardiogram can confirm the diagnosis. If signs of tamponade are present, pericardiocentesis should be performed.

Chylothorax

Penetrating and blunt injuries of the thorax can cause chylothorax. Symptoms do not usually appear until 2 to 3 days after injury. When oral feedings are begun, the volume in the thoracic duct increases and loss of fluid into the chest with associated hypotension and dyspnea are then the symptoms. Aspiration of a milky fluid, rich in protein and lymphocytes, confirms the diagnosis. Intrathoracic sequestration of a large volume of chyle can produce lymphocytopenia and hypoproteinemia. Chest films are pathognomonic and should prompt appropriate referral. Nonoperative management is often successful.

References

1. Feliciano DV, Mattox KL: Indications, technique and pitfalls of emergency thoracotomy. *Surgical Rounds* 1981;4:32–40
2. Haller JA, Shermeta DW: Acute thoracic injuries in children. *Pediatr Ann* 1976;5:71–79.
3. Holinger PH, Schild JA: Pharyngeal, laryngeal and tracheal injuries in the pediatric age group. *Ann Otol Rhinol Laryngol* 1972;81:538–545.
4. Kirsh MM, Pellegrini RV, Sloan HE: Treatment of blunt chest trauma. *Surgery* 1972;4:51–90.
5. Reynolds J, Davis JT: Injuries of the chest wall, pleura, pericardium, lungs, bronchi and esophagus. *Radiol Clin North Am* 1966;4:383–401.
6. McCune R, Roda CP, Ackert C: Rupture of the diaphragm caused by blunt trauma. *J Trauma* 1976;16:531–537.

7. Sorsdahl OA, Powell JW: Cavitary pulmonary lesions following nonpenetrating chest trauma in children. *Am J Roentgenol* 1965;95:118–124.
8. Michelson WB: CPK-MB isoenzyme determinations: Diagnostic and prognostic value in evaluation of blunt chest trauma. *Ann Emerg Med* 1980; 9:562.
9. Saunders CR, Doty DB: Myocardial contusion. *Surg Gynecol Obstet* 1977;144:595–603.
10. Liedtke AJ, DeMuth WE Jr: Nonpenetrating cardiac injuries: A collective review. *Am Heart J* 1973;86:687–697.
11. Fred HL, Chadler F: Traumatic asphyxia. *Am J Med* 1960;29:508.

Randall W. Powell

9 Foreign Bodies in the Respiratory Tract

In 1976 the U.S. Public Health Service[1] reported 3033 deaths due to inhalation or ingestion of food or other objects leading to obstruction or suffocation, with 625 deaths occurring in the age group up to 19 years. Four hundred fifty-five children were less than 5 years of age. Inhalation of foreign bodies is the leading cause of accidental deaths at home in children less than 6 years of age.[2] Jackson[2] described a 50% mortality from foreign bodies in the tracheobronchial tree in childhood prior to the advent of bronchoscopic removal. The mortality rate now is approximately 1%,[2] and in several large series it has been reported at 0%.[3,4]

In addition to the significant mortality caused by foreign body inhalation, morbidity also can be high. The incidence of major neurologic deficits due to hypoxia is unknown but may be significant. The number and variety of foreign bodies that can be aspirated by children is restricted only by the limits of the child's active, exploring mind; the ability to reach an object; and the natural tendency to explore new objects by the sense of taste. The problem is compounded by the frequent carelessness of parents in allowing small objects or unsuitable foods to be accessible to the young child. Aspiration of foreign bodies is usually preventable, and preventive measures should be emphasized to parents whenever possible.

HISTORY

In 1952 Clerf[5] published a brief history of the medical aspects of foreign body inhalation and ingestion, some details of which are discussed here. Muys in 1690 in his *Practical Surgery* reported the case of a 7-year-old dying from suffocation 3 weeks after aspirating a bean. In 1759 Louis reported 28 collected cases in a paper entitled "Memoir on Bronchotomy." The first large collection of cases, entitled "Treatise on Foreign Bodies in the Air Passages," was published in 1854 by Gross; this work included many of the now well-known physical signs and symptoms. Gross also described the typical "cafe coronary" and ended with these words: "Many a coroner's inquest has been held upon the bodies of the victims of such accidents, and a verdict rendered that they died by the visitation of God, when the actual cause of death lay quietly and unobserved at the door of the windpipe of the deceased."

According to Clerf[5] foreign bodies were initially managed by medical means, including measures to expel the foreign body (emetics and sternutatories) and to prevent the effects induced by the foreign body (bleeding, expectorants, purgatives, and counterirrigation). Gross condemned inversion of the patient or backslapping because of possibly causing complete laryngeal obstruction. In 1650 Bonetus recommended bronchotomy for a boy who had inhaled a bone, but the medical attendent overruled this. The first recorded case of surgical removal was by Verduc in 1717 and involved a tracheal incision to remove a fragment of bone. In 1882 Weist reported a study of 1000 patients with foreign bodies: of 937 cases 599 did not undergo bronchotomy and 399 did; the mortality rates were 23.2% and 27.42%, respectively.

Clerf[5] also discussed the development of esophagoscopy and bronchoscopy. The former was inspired by sword swallowers; the latter, by the success of tracheal intubation. These developments were heralded by Hippocrates' suggestion that tracheal intubation be done when suffocation was imminent. Kirstein performed the first direct laryngoscopy in April 1895 and later that year passed a tube into a bronchus. Two years later Killian removed a fragment of bone from the bronchus of a 63-year-old man. Collidge in 1898 performed the first successful bronchoscopy in the United States in Boston when he removed a foreign body from the right main stem bronchus of a 23-year-old man. In 1902 Einhorn introduced the distally illuminated tube. The credit for refining the instruments and techniques used for extraction of foreign bodies in the respiratory and gastrointestinal tracts must go to Chevalier Jackson, whose many papers and books on the topic remain the basis for evaluation and management of these problems today.

CLINICAL FEATURES

The typical patient with an aspirated foreign body has a history of a severe episode of coughing or choking. The parent may provide clues as to the type of foreign body involved, e.g., the child was eating peanuts or playing with a small toy. The initial episode often is followed by a relatively asymptomatic period unless the object causes significant obstruction of the upper airway. In the latter instance there are the usual signs of severe respiratory distress: cyanosis, retractions caused by accessory muscles, and stridor. The initial episode also can include gagging, aphonia, dysphonia, wheezing, dyspnea, vomiting, and pain (Figure 9-1). If the child was not observed during aspiration, a history of chronic cough and wheezing, unresolved pneumonia, or "bronchitis" may be obtained.[6] A small number of patients have no symptoms, and their foreign body is noted on a radiograph obtained for other reasons such as trauma to the neck or chest.

Children seen for aspiration most commonly fall

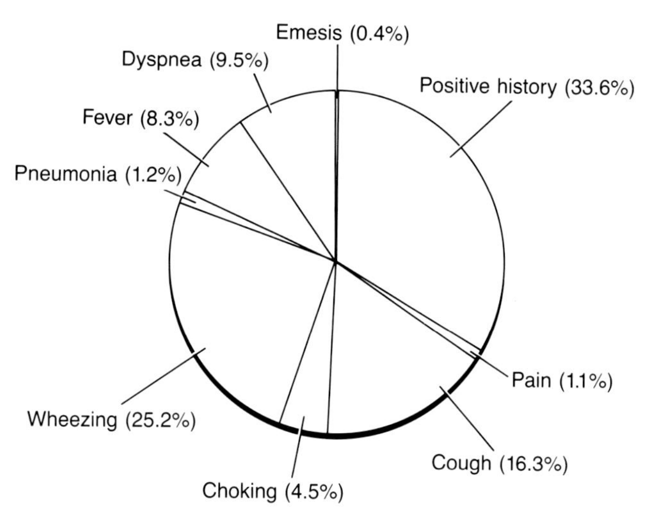

FIGURE 9-1 Symptoms of foreign body aspiration (n = 710 patients). (Data from Refs. 4 and 7–9.)

in the age range from 6 months to 4 years (Figure 9-2). Foreign body aspiration under the age of 6 months is rare because the infant has not reached the exploratory stage. The older child may be reluctant to give a history of aspiration in fear of punishment for wrong-doing.[6]

The type of foreign body aspirated varies widely. In the United States the object most commonly aspirated by a child is a peanut (Figure 9-3). Often the child is too young to be eating such an object and is unable to properly chew the material because of an absence of molar teeth for grinding. A fall or startle (often while watching television) results in a sudden inspiration during which the peanut is aspirated. In addition to its effect as a foreign body, the peanut, being usually salted and oily, chemically irritates the bronchus ("vegetable bronchitis").[2,7]

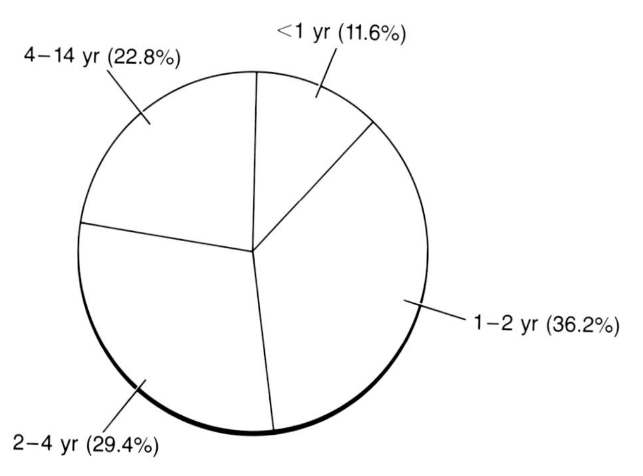

FIGURE 9-2 Age distribution for foreign body aspiration. (Data from Refs. 2, 6, 9, and 10.)

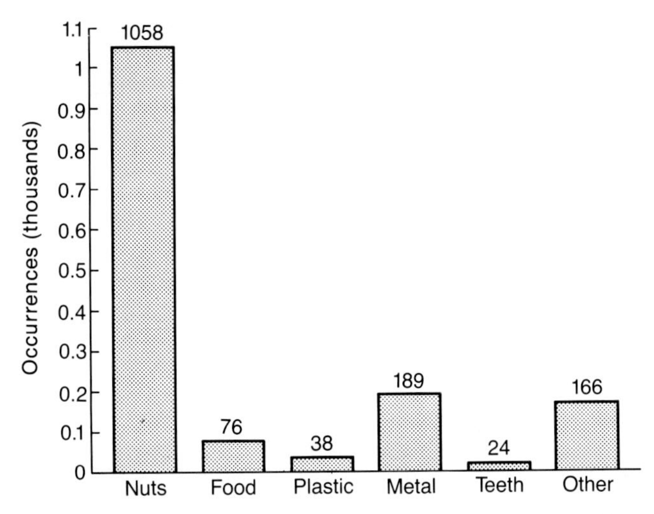

FIGURE 9-3 Types of material aspirated (n = 710). (Data from Refs. 2, 3, 6, 9, and 10.)

This marked inflammatory response and the tendency for the peanut to fragment when grasped with forceps make peanut removal a formidable task. In reports from Middle Eastern countries,[2,9] melon seeds represent the most common material aspirated since they are plentiful and often prepared for eating.

Food particles are frequent offenders, with partially chewed carrots, bits of bacon, and beans representing the most frequent offenders.[3] Dried beans represent a particular hazard since they tend to swell as they absorb bronchial secretions and thus obstruct a larger portion of the airway.[3] After hard candy is aspirated, it dissolves into a thick, viscous material that can cause patchy atelectasis.[3] Due to the hyperosmolar solution from the sugar, marked edema of the airway mucosa occurs, requiring close observation and even ventilator support for up to 48 hours.[11] Aspirated chewing gum also represents a distinct challenge because during removal it sticks to the forceps, bronchoscope, suction apparatus, and airway wall.[3]

Among the nonfood foreign bodies, plastic objects, mainly toys or parts of toys, are appearing more frequently because of the increased use of plastic. Metal objects are probably the easiest to diagnose and locate because they are radiopaque and usually easily visualized on radiographs. Many metallic objects possess sharp points and are more likely to perforate the airway or cause bleeding.

Another foreign body easily seen on x-ray films but frequently missed is a tooth.[12] The usual clinical setting occurs in a child with multiple traumatic injuries: while the more serious injuries are attended to, the absent tooth is overlooked. A quick examination of the mouth and appropriate radiographs should eliminate this type of foreign body as a late complication.[12]

A distinguishing feature of foreign body aspiration in children is the site of lodgment. In adults the right main stem bronchus represents the most frequent site whereas in children the right and left bronchus are involved nearly equally, and in some series the left bronchus is more often involved (Figure 9-4). The reasons for this include a less acute take-off of the left main stem bronchus in children and the fact that the child is often lying down when the object is aspirated.[13]

The physical signs and radiographic findings depend on the different effects that a foreign body causes. There are four types of bronchial obstruction that can occur:[2]

1. Check-valve mechanism: air is inhaled but not expelled, leading to emphysema.
2. Stop-valve mechanism: no inhaled air is allowed to pass, resulting in distal atelectasis.
3. Ball-valve mechanism: the foreign body dislodges during expiration and reimpacts on inspiration, leading to early atelectasis.
4. Bypass-valve mechanism: inflow and outflow are partially obstructed, leading to decreased aeration and opacity on the affected side.

Physical findings also differ in relation to the level of obstruction. Laryngeal obstruction results in severe respiratory distress with extensive cervical, sternal, and intercostal retractions and little to no air exchange audible to auscultation. Stridor may or may not be present depending on the volume of air the child is able to move. The child may not be

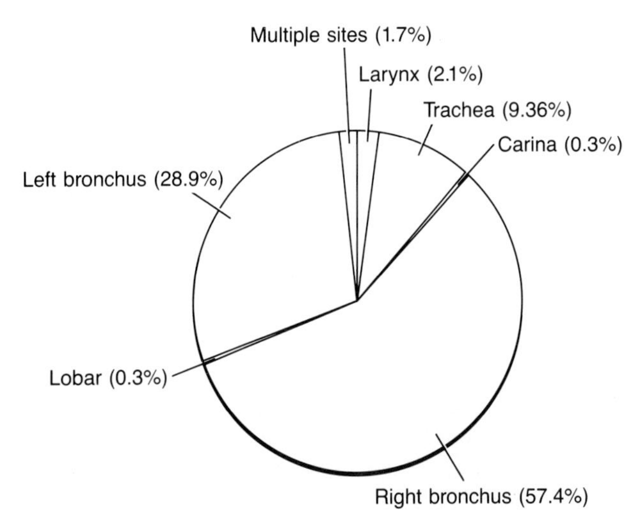

FIGURE 9-4 Location of aspirated material (n = 1516). (Data from Refs. 2, 4, 7–10, 13, and 14.)

able to vocalize or cry. This represents the least common occurrence and requires the most urgent management to prevent brain anoxia and death.

A foreign body in the trachea causes bilateral wheezing and retractions if the obstruction to airflow is significant. If the foreign body moves in the trachea with ventilation, a thud or snap at the end of expiration may be heard. This represents the object striking the cords.[5] In this instance bilateral wheezing also may be heard. An older child may describe a tickling sensation in the trachea, also a result of this movement.[5]

When the foreign body obstructs one of the major bronchi, tachypnea with mild retractions can occur, but the chest wall on the affected side will not move as well as the ventilated side if the obstruction is complete. Depending on the degree of obstruction, the breath sounds may be absent or diminished and a unilateral wheeze may be heard. Obstructions of more distal bronchi usually result in little respiratory distress, and physical findings may be limited to a unilateral wheeze.

If the aspiration has been chronic, there can be signs of pneumonia, including dullness to percussion, rhonchi and rales, and abnormal tubular breath sounds. Yet in some patients the physical examination is entirely normal.

The most common physical findings include decreased air entry, wheezing or rhonchi, and stridor (Figure 9-5). Fever is often seen with vegetable objects and in chronic cases.[13] When there is sudden onset of wheezing in a previous healthy child and a unilateral wheeze on auscultation, a foreign body should be considered the cause.[4]

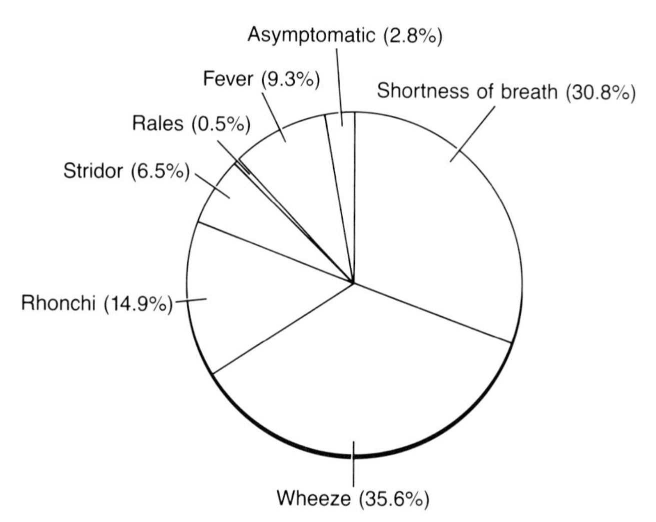

FIGURE 9-5 Physical examination findings. (Data from Refs. 4, 7, 8, and 14.)

DIAGNOSIS

Radiographic studies are the mainstay in diagnosing foreign body aspiration. For a complete examination, posteroanterior and lateral views of the chest, including the neck and upper abdomen, should be obtained. Deep inspiratory and complete expiratory (at the end of a cry in the uncooperative child or young infant) views complete the examination. The most common radiographic findings are emphysema, atelectasis, pneumonia, and a radiopaque foreign body (Figure 9-6). Other findings include narrowing of air passages, lung abscess, bronchiectasis, pneumothorax, pneumomediastinum, mediastinal shift,[2] and pneumopericardium.[15] Figures 9-7 through 9-10 illustrate common radiographic findings.

If the plain chest radiographs fail to visualize the usual abnormal findings, fluoroscopy may reveal subtle changes. During rapid breathing, induced at times by crying, the fluoroscope may show the mediastinum shifting toward the side of a partially obstructing bronchial foreign body on inspiration. In the presence of a tracheal foreign body, paradoxical movement of the mediastinum often occurs.[16] With partial tracheal obstruction the negative intrapleural pressure increases during inspiration, and the mediastinum enlarges because of the increased pool of blood in the venous structures. During expiration a more positive intrapleural pressure is blocked, and the mediastinum is squeezed and appears small. This is the reverse of the normal sequence.[16]

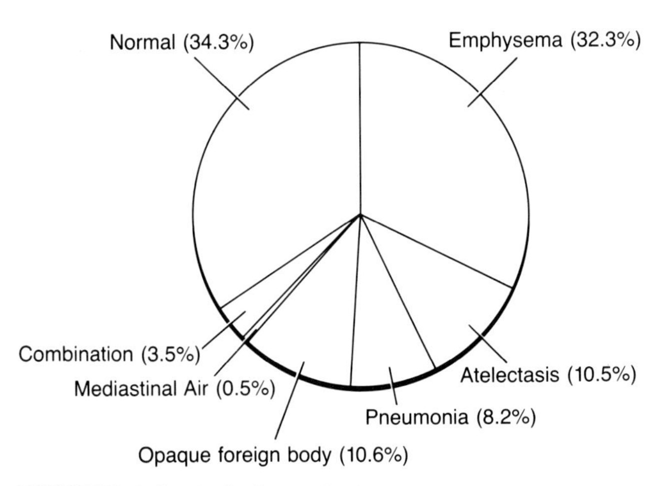

FIGURE 9-6 Radiologic findings. (Data from Refs. 4 and 7–9.)

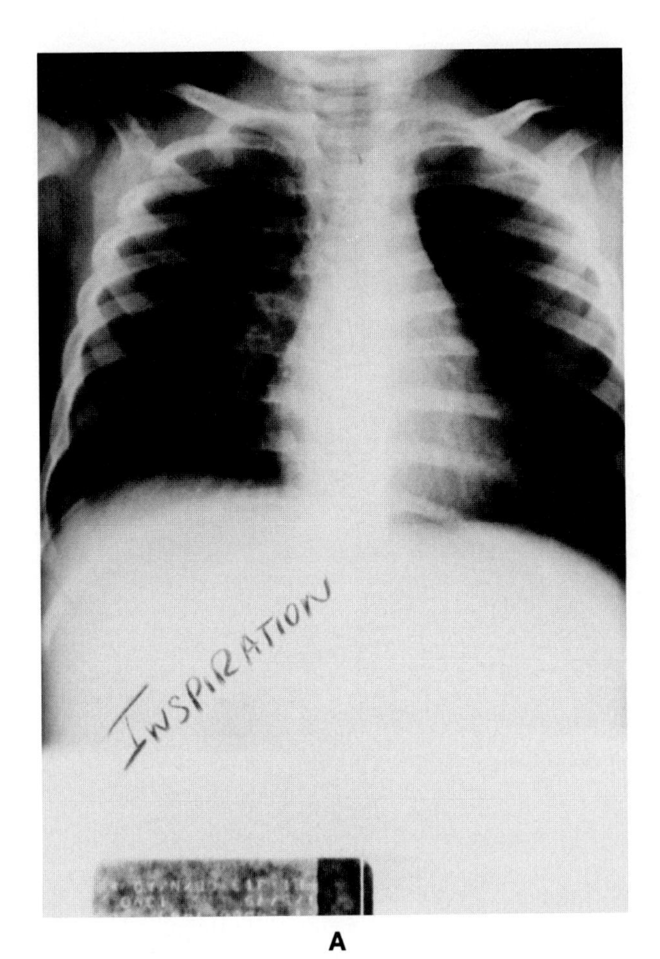

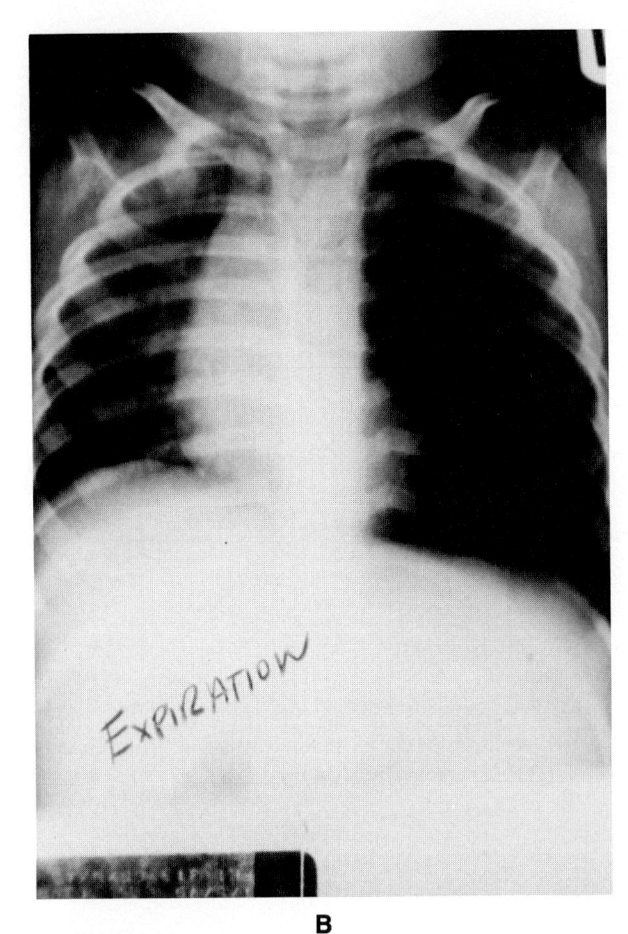

A B

FIGURE 9-7A, B, C Inspiratory, expiratory, and forced expiratory films reveal the emphysema caused by a vegetable foreign body in the left main stem bronchus in a 13-month-old male. A: Inspiration; B: Expiration; C: Forced expiration.

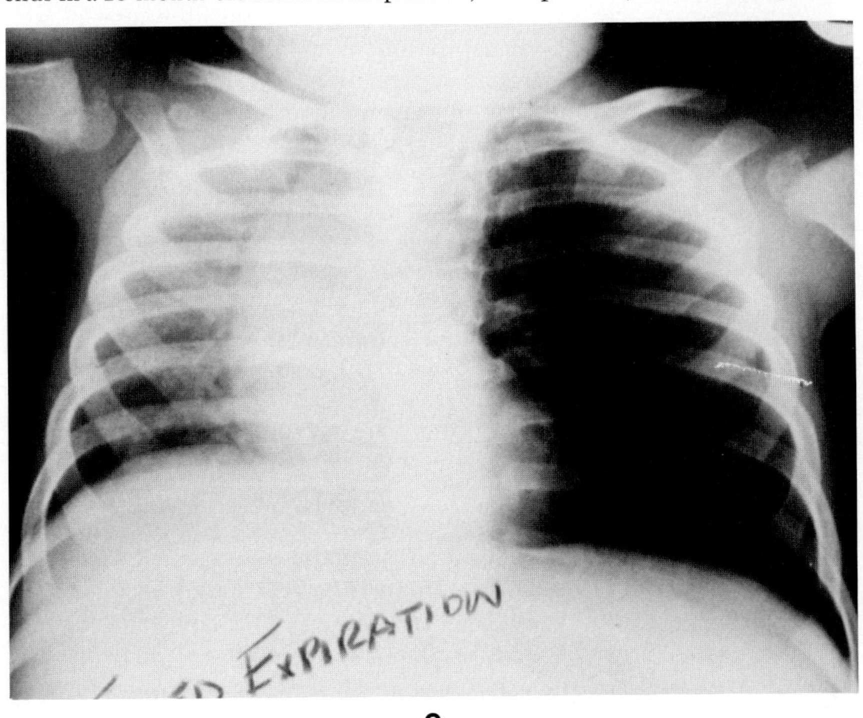

C

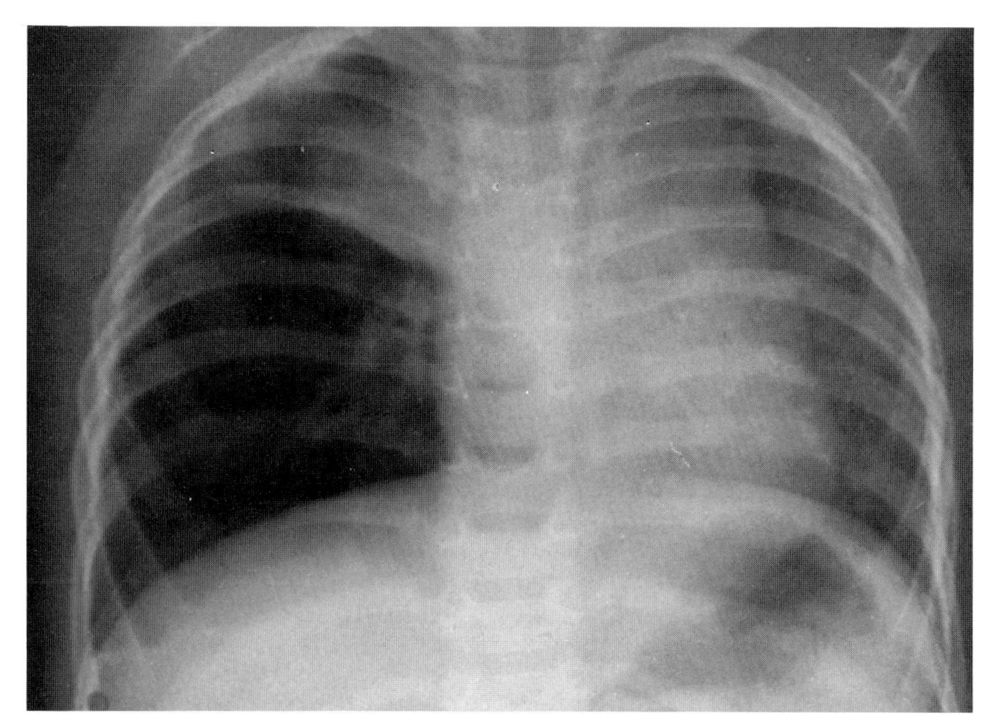

FIGURE 9-8 Expiratory film of child reveals increased emphysema of the right lower lobe with mediastinal shift.

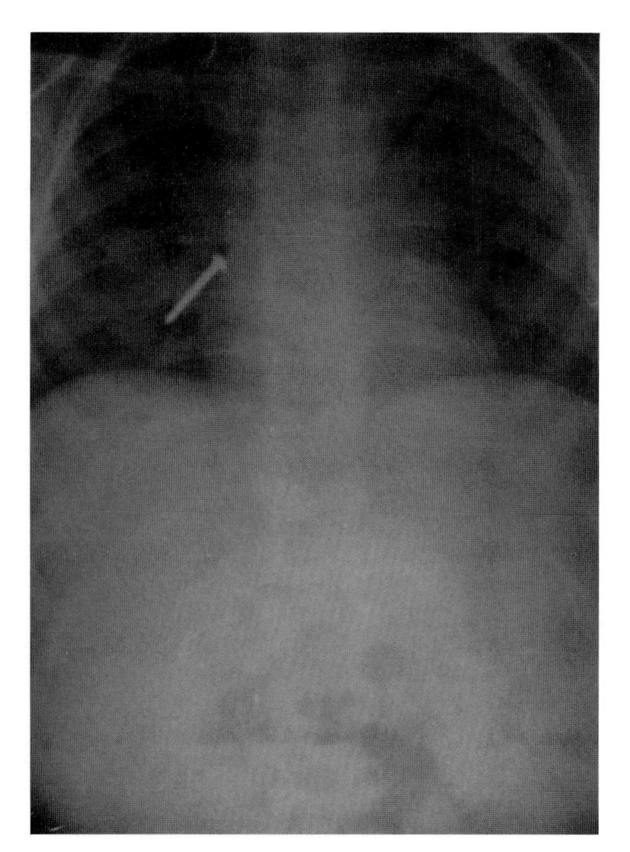

FIGURE 9-9 This three-year-old had a history of the sudden onset coughing and the chest radiograph revealed the radiopaque foreign body in the right lower lobe bronchus.

MANAGEMENT

The major step in management is the definite diagnosis or a strong suspicion—from the history, physical examination, or radiographic findings—of foreign body aspiration. Common pitfalls include the absence of a positive history, a normal chest radiograph, incomplete radiographic studies, failure to consider the diagnosis, and inexperienced consultants.[17] A delay in diagnosis can result in pneumonia, foreign body erosion through the trachea or bronchus, lung abscess, hemoptysis, bronchiectasis, and increased difficulty in removing the foreign body by bronchoscopy, thereby necessitating thoracotomy.[18] One would do well to remember Chevalier Jackson's famous quote, "All that wheezes is not asthma," when dealing with a small child who has bronchopulmonary symptoms but no history of aspiration. In the reverse situation this also applies: in the child with a positive history of foreign body aspiration and normal physical and radiographic findings, a diagnostic-therapeutic bronchoscopy to definitely determine the presence or absence of a foreign body is indicated.[18] The risk of bronchoscopy in the hands of an experienced pediatric endoscopist is quite small compared to the possible deleterious effects of a delay in removing a foreign body from the respiratory tract.

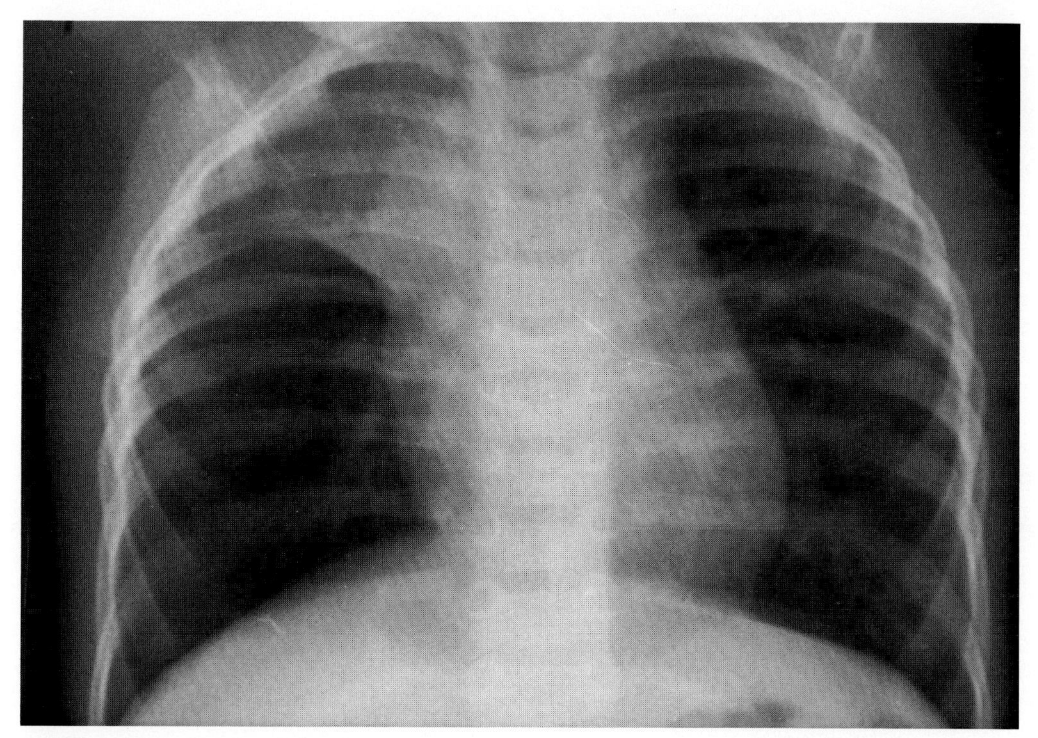

FIGURE 9-10 In this three-year-old male, a neglected or unrecognized right main stem foreign body resulted in a right lung pneumonia and empyema. He died during extraction of the foreign body when an abscess cavity ruptured into the bronchus and flooded the left lung.

Emergency department management of the infant or child with foreign body aspiration varies depending on the site of obstruction and degree of symptoms. In rare situations immediate intervention in the emergency department is necessary. The patient with acute obstruction of the larynx who is unable to ventilate requires immediate action to relieve the obstruction. The successful use of the Heimlich maneuver can be lifesaving. If measures to relieve the obstruction fail, access to the airway is obtained by large-bore needle puncture of the trachea in infants and of the cricothyroid membrane in older children. Cricothyroidostomy in children is not recommended because of the potential for severe complications.[17] If the obstruction appears to be at the laryngeal or tracheal level and the child is able to ventilate, efforts in the emergency department to expel the foreign body can result in acute obstruction. This type of patient is best managed in the operating room by experienced pediatric endoscopists and pediatric anesthesiologists.

Nonobstructing foreign bodies of the trachea and nearly all bronchial foreign bodies in children require no short-term intervention in the emergency department. Appropriate diagnostic studies and consultation should be arranged. If personnel experienced in the endoscopic and anesthetic management of pediatric patients are not available, transfer to an institution where such expertise is available is definitely in the best interest of the patient.

Laryngoscopic or bronchoscopic removal of foreign bodies remains the standard treatment of choice.[2,3,17] With refinements in technique and instrumentation pioneered by Jackson,[3,19] excellent success rates in removal and low mortality have been reported in large series of patients.[2–4,8,10] Even better results can be expected with the advances in fiberoptic lighting and the new Hopkins lens system. A detailed description of bronchoscopic techniques is beyond the scope of this chapter, but appropriate references can be utilized for more detailed information on foreign body removal.[9,10,17,19]

Alternative techniques for the management of foreign body aspiration in children include inhalation therapy with postural drainage[14,20,21] and foreign body extraction utilizing the flexible bronchoscope.[22] In 1972 Burrington and Cotton[21] compared a series of 75 patients undergoing bronchoscopic removal of a foreign body and 28 patients undergoing inhalation therapy with a bronchodilator followed by postural drainage. Twenty-four of the 28 patients coughed out the foreign body within 2 days of treatment. They recommend a 24-hour trial of inhalation and postural drainage prior to bronchoscopy. Two patients experienced cardiac arrest while undergoing treatment when the foreign body became dislodged from one bronchus and obstructed the other bronchus, leading to severe hypoxia and arrest.[20] In another evaluation of this technique, Law and Kosloske[14] reported success in 12 of 49 patients (25%); the other 37 required bronchoscopies, 5 of which were endoscopic failures. They recommend inhalation-postural drainage on an inpatient basis, preferably in an intensive care unit because of the reports of cardiac arrest. Bronchoscopy should be done after 24 hours of unsuccessful treatment.[14] Immediate bronchoscopy remains the primary treatment of choice for significant respiratory distress or long-standing aspirations.[14]

In a series of 300 patients, Cunanan[22] reported successful foreign body extraction with the flexible bronchoscope in 130 patients, ranging in age from 10 to 15 years. One hundred twenty-one patients required only local anesthesia. The flexible bronchoscope has limited application to the pediatric patient because of the small diameter of the trachea and inability to ventilate the child properly during the extraction procedure.[17]

In summary, often the most difficult aspect of the management of children with foreign body aspiration is the diagnosis. A high index of suspicion is necessary when a history of aspiration is not present. The reverse situation, in which the history is positive but the physical and radiographic findings are normal, requires either further evaluation or consultation with those more experienced in the management of this problem. Failure to diagnose foreign body aspiration can result in significant life-threatening complications including pneumonia, airway obstruction, hemoptysis, migration of the foreign body outside the bronchial tree, bronchiectasis, and inability to remove the foreign body by bronchoscopy.

References

1. *Vital Statistics of the United States. Vol 2: Mortality, Part A.* U.S. Department of Health and Human Services, Public Health Service, 1976, pp 1–245.
2. Aytac A, Yurdakul Y, Ikizler C, et al: Inhalation of foreign bodies in children: Report of 500 cases. *J Thorac Cardiovasc Surg* 1977;74:145–151.
3. Holinger PH, Holinger ID: Use of the open tube bronchoscope in the extraction of foreign bodies. *Chest* 1978;73:721–724.
4. Rothmann BF, Boeckman CR: Foreign bodies in the larynx and tracheobronchial tree in children: A review of 225 cases. *Ann Otol Rhinol Laryngol* 1980;89:434–436.
5. Clerf LH: Historical aspects of foreign bodies in the air and food passages. *Ann Otol Rhinol Laryngol* 1952;61:5–17.
6. Benjamin B, Vandeleur T: Inhaled foreign bodies in children. *Med J Aust* 1974;1:355–358.
7. Keith FM, Charrette EJP, Lunn RB, et al: Inhalation of foreign bodies by children: A continuing challenge in management. *Can Med Assoc J* 1980;122:52–57.
8. Kim IG, Brummitt WM, Humphry A, et al: Foreign body in the airway: A review of 202 cases. *Laryngoscope* 1973;83:347–354.
9. Abdulmajid OA, Ebeid AM, Motaweh MM, et al: Aspirated foreign body in the tracheobronchial tree: Report of 250 cases. *Thorax* 1976;31:635–640.
10. Cohen SR, Lewis GB Jr, Herbert WI, et al: Foreign bodies in the airway: Five-year retrospective study with special relevance to management. *Ann Otol Rhinol Laryngol* 1980;89:437–442.
11. Meanns AF, England RM: Dissolving foreign bodies in the trachea and bronchus. *Thorax* 1975;30:461–463.
12. Pochaczevsky R, Leonidas JC, Feldman F, et al: Aspirated and ingested teeth in children. *Clin Radiol* 1973;24:349–353.
13. Daniilidis J, Symeonidis B, Triaridis K, et al: Foreign body in the airway: A review of 90 cases. *Arch Otolarnyngol* 1977;103:570–573.
14. Law D, Kosloske AM: Management of tracheobronchial foreign bodies in children: A reevaluation of postural drainage and bronchoscopy. *Pediatrics* 1976;58:362–367.
15. Tjhen KY, Schmaltz AA, Ibrahim Z, et al: *Pediatr Radiol* 1978;7:121–123.
16. Grünebaum M, Adler S, Varsano I: The paradoxical movement of the mediastinum: A diagnostic sign of foreign body aspiration during childhood. *Pediatr Radiol* 1979;8:213–218.
17. Cohen SR: Unusual presentations and problems created by mismanagement of foreign bodies in the aerodigestive tract of the pediatric patient. *Ann Otol Rhinol Laryngol* 1981;90:316–322.
18. Fearon B: Inhalation of foreign bodies by children. *Can Med Assoc J* 1980;122:8–9.
19. Jackson C, Jackson CI: *Diseases of the Air and Food Passages of Foreign Body Origin.* Philadelphia, WB Saunders Co, 1936.
20. Cotton EK, Abrams G, Vanhoutte J, et al: Removal of aspirated foreign bodies by inhalation and postural drainage: A survey of 24 cases. *Clin Pediatr (Phila)* 1973;12:270–276.
21. Burrington JD, Cotton EK: Removal of foreign bodies from the tracheo-bronchial tree. *J Pediatr Surg* 1972;7:119–122.
22. Cunanan OS: The flexible fiberoptic bronchoscope in foreign body removal: Experience in 300 cases. *Chest* 1978;73:725–726.

Kenneth G. Zahka

10 Cardiovascular Disorders

The orderly assessment, beginning with the history and physical examination, of the child suspected of having heart disease often provides an accurate cardiovascular diagnosis. When it is supplemented by the electrocardiogram, echocardiogram, chest x-ray film, and other noninvasive studies, an accurate diagnosis and initial management plan can be developed for nearly all children with heart disease.

Occasionally, children with previously undiagnosed congenital heart disease or acute primary heart disease appear at the emergency department. More often, however, children with previously diagnosed congenital heart disease come to the emergency department because of other illnesses that either affect their cardiac status or are complications of the primary cardiac lesion. Basic to solving these problems is an understanding of the primary entity. This chapter discusses the differential diagnosis of the most common of these entities on the basis of their signs and symptoms. Management, secondary problems, and complications are included.

EVALUATION

History

The familial, gestational, and perinatal history may help identify those children at increased risk of congenital heart disease. The presence of congenital heart disease in a first-degree relative increases the risk of heart disease in the children from subsequent pregnancies fivefold to 3% to 4%. Maternal drug ingestion (particularly alcohol and phenytoin), diabetes, or viral infections from a rubella virus and possibly coxsackievirus are recognized risk factors.[1] Children with certain genetic syndromes or other multisystem problems are more likely to have congenital heart disease than the general population. The diagnosis of a particular syndrome often suggests a frequently accompanying heart defect (Table 10-1).[2]

A useful indication of the impact of a defect on a child is an estimation of exercise tolerance. For an older child this would be the ability to keep up with peers while playing or, for the more severely limited, dyspnea upon walking or climbing stairs. In infants the feeding history in terms of the daily volume of formula, as well as breathlessness or sweating during feeding, is a useful sign of "exercise" tolerance.

A history of frequent cough or pneumonia is often found in children with congestive heart failure. Chest pain, although usually noncardiac in origin, can result from mitral valve prolapse or from myocardial ischemia in a child with severe aortic stenosis. Palpitations can be a symptom of a dysrhythmia in children without underlying heart disease or in those with structural heart disease, especially after surgery.

TABLE 10-1 Cardiac Defects Associated with Genetic Syndromes

Syndrome	Cardiac Defect
Holt-Oram	ASD*
Hurler's	Mitral and aortic thickening
Marfan's	Aortic aneurysms, AR, MR
Neurofibromatosis	PS, pheochromocytoma
Noonan's	PS, ASD, IHSS
Trisomy 13	VSD, PDA, DXC
Trisomy 18	VSD, PDA, PS
Trisomy 21 (Down's)	VSD, ECD, TOF
Tuberous sclerosis	Myocardial rhabdomyoma
Turner's	COA, AS, ASD

* Abbreviations: ASD, atrial septal defect; AR, aortic regurgitation; MR, mitral regurgitation; PS, pulmonary stenosis; IHSS, idiopathic hypertrophic subaortic stenosis; VSD, ventricular septal defect; PDA, patent ductus arteriosus; DXC, dextrocardia; ECD, endocardial cushion defect; TOF, tetralogy of Fallot; COA, coarctation of the aorta; AS, aortic stenosis.

Physical Examination

Vital Signs

Vital signs must be interpreted in view of the child's age and activity. Moderate tachycardia may occur with fever or be a sign of congestive heart failure and not indicate an intrinsic dysrhythmia. Tachypnea is often a sign of pulmonary congestion in children with large left-to-right shunts or obstruction in the left side of the heart, especially in the absence of an intercurrent pneumonia. In the child with an acute change who has been otherwise stable, a fever can indicate an infection that has placed a further load on an already compromised cardiovascular system.

Blood Pressure

The technique for measuring blood pressure must be tailored to the size of the child. Systolic blood pressure in infants under 6 months of age is best measured with a Doppler system or an automated sphygmomanometer. In older children standard auscultation techniques are possible and permit measurement of both systolic and diastolic pressure. The cuff size is particularly important in younger children, and usually the largest cuff to fit comfortably between the shoulder and elbow should be used. The length of the cuff bladder should be sufficient to encircle nearly the entire circumference of the arm. The cuff should be snugly applied, inflated rapidly, and deflated at 2 to 5 mmHg/s.

Height and Weight

The height and weight are most useful when followed serially. A cardiovascular cause of failure to thrive should be considered in a child who is below the fifth percentile for age or is failing to maintain a given percentile. Sharp fluctuations in weight are due to changes in water balance and can be followed to assess the response to treatment of congestive heart failure.

Cyanosis

The presence of central cyanosis indicates an abnormally low oxygen saturation in the blood. The degree of cyanosis is a function of both the arterial oxygen saturation and the hematocrit. Cyanosis generally becomes evident when there is 3 to 5 g of unsaturated hemoglobin per deciliter of blood.[3] Peripheral cyanosis in the absence of central cyanosis usually indicates an impaired peripheral circulation and in many infants is a normal response to a cold environment. Clubbing is commonly the result of chronic hypoxia.

Precordial Activity

The precordial activity is helpful in assessing the physiologic impact of a cardiac defect. An active left ventricular impulse suggests a volume overload of the left ventricle, as can be seen in left-to-right shunts (patent ductus arteriosus, ventricular septal defect) and regurgitant lesions (aortic or mitral regurgitation) or with severe anemia. A sustained impulse may be found in a child with aortic stenosis. A parasternal right ventricular heave might accompany either right ventricular volume overload (atrial septal defect, pulmonary regurgitation) or pressure overload (pulmonary stenosis, pulmonary hypertension).

Heart Sounds

The first heart sound is generally single and best heard at the apex, but it can be narrowly split in normal children. It is more widely split in children with right bundle-branch block following open heart surgery.

The nature of the second heart sound is valuable in the diagnosis of congenital heart disease. The normal second heart sound is single during expiration and split during inspiration. The splitting may be more prominent in the supine position. A single second heart sound is always abnormal after the first few days of life and indicates pulmonary hypertension, an abnormal position of the great arteries, or severe pulmonary stenosis or atresia. Conversely, it can be widely split with some variation in pulmonic stenosis or right bundle-branch block. Wide, fixed splitting of the second heart sound suggests an atrial septal defect.

A third heart sound is occasionally heard in normal children, although it can indicate increased rapid ventricular filling in early diastole, especially when heard as a gallop rhythm. A fourth heart sound suggests a noncompliant, hypertrophied left ventricle.

An early systolic click can be of pulmonic or aortic origin. Pulmonic clicks vary in intensity with position and respiration and are generally best heard at the left sternal border in the supine patient during expiration. They usually are present in valvular pulmonic stenosis; however, they can be an isolated finding in a child with idiopathic dilatation of the pulmonary artery or a bicuspid pulmonic valve. An aortic click does not vary with respiration or position and is also best heard at the left sternal border. It may be heard in a child with a bicuspid aortic valve or, when accompanied by a murmur, in valvular aortic stenosis. The apical midsystolic click of mitral valve prolapse is accentuated by maneuvers that tend to decrease the left ventricular systolic volume, such as sitting, standing, or during a Valsalva maneuver. Conversely, the click comes later in systole with squatting or leg raising, which increases systolic volume.

Heart Murmurs

Heart murmurs are characterized by their loudness (Table 10-2), quality, type, site of maximum intensity, and radiation. Functional murmurs generally are not louder than grade 2. The intensity of a murmur in a child with structural heart disease is not always an accurate guide to its severity.

The quality of the murmur can suggest its cause. A vibratory murmur has a low, uniform frequency; is associated with relatively nonturbulent blood flow; and is often functional in nature. A harsh murmur suggests more turbulent flow and can result from a stenotic lesion or a ventricular septal defect. A higher pitched, blowing murmur may be heard with semilunar or atrioventricular (AV) valve regurgitation. A honking murmur is typical of mitral regurgitation secondary to mitral valve prolapse. A rumbling murmur is of very low frequency and is often heard in mitral or tricuspid stenosis.

TABLE 10-2 Murmur Intensity Grades

Grade	Description
1	Requires concentration or quiet room
2	Easily heard when stethoscope first placed on chest
3	Loud murmur without a thrill
4	Murmur accompanied by thrill
5	Heard with only the edge of the stethoscope on the chest
6	Heard with the stethoscope off the chest

An ejection murmur is a crescendo-decrescendo murmur that begins after the first heart sound, ends before the second heart sound, and is associated with flow through the semilunar valves and great arteries. A holosystolic murmur is even in intensity throughout systole, beginning with the first heart sound and ending with the second heart sound. It is found in children with a ventricular septal defect or AV valve regurgitation. A decrescendo early systolic murmur begins with the first heart sound and ends before the second heart sound and may be associated with a small ventricular septal defect. The mid- or late systolic murmur of mitral prolapse begins after a systolic click and can extend to the second heart sound. A continuous murmur peaks at and extends through the second heart sound but does not necessarily continue through all of diastole. Although a continuous murmur is typically heard in a child with a patent ductus arteriosus, it also can arise from any systemic-to-pulmonary communication or arteriovenous fistula.

Early diastolic murmurs usually are due to either aortic or pulmonary valve regurgitation. Aortic regurgitation results in a decrescendo murmur, whereas pulmonary regurgitation with low systolic pulmonary artery pressure produces a crescendo-decrescendo murmur. Middiastolic murmurs can result from actual stenosis of the tricuspid or mitral valve or from defects that cause an abnormally large flow of blood to pass through a normal valve.

Peripheral Pulses

Peripheral pulses of poor quality and amplitude are an indication of either poor cardiac output or left ventricular outflow tract obstruction. Bounding pulses are found in any defect with diastolic runoff, such as patent ductus arteriosus or aortic regurgitation. A discrepancy in amplitude and timing between the pulses in the upper and lower extremities is diagnostic of a coarctation of the aorta distal to the left subclavian artery.

Other Signs

Hepatomegaly, especially when followed serially, is a useful sign of systemic venous congestion. Pulmonary rales, rhonchi, and wheezing are found in some children with congestive heart failure due to left-to-right shunts or with left ventricular outflow tract obstruction.

Laboratory Studies

Electrocardiogram

The electrocardiogram provides an assessment of cardiac rhythm, conduction, and chamber hypertro-

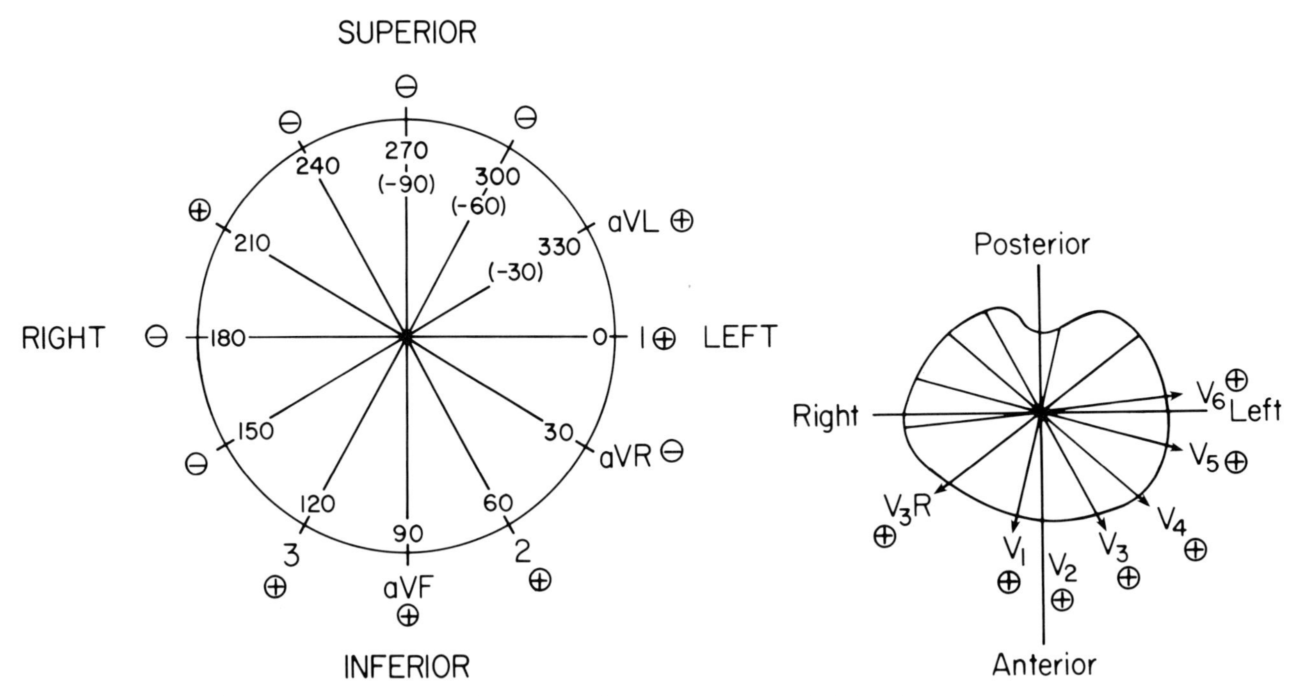

FIGURE 10-1 The frontal plane axis (*left*) and the horizontal plane axis (*right*).

phy. Normal values for many features of the electrocardiogram change with age, and therefore interpretation must be made with a knowledge of the child's age. Most studies are recorded at a paper speed of 25 mm/s and a sensitivity of 1 mV/cm. Alteration of these settings also must be noted to permit accurate interpretation. The standard limb and augmented leads (I, II, III, aV_R, aV_L, aV_F) evaluate the frontal plane (superior-inferior, right-left), while the chest leads record the horizontal plane (antero-posterior, right-left) of the heart (Figure 10-1). Standard nomenclature labels atrial depolarization as the P wave, ventricular depolarization as the QRS complex, and ventricular repolarization as the T wave. The initial negative component of the QRS complex, if present, is a Q wave, the following positive deflection is the R wave, and the next negative deflection is the S wave. Any subsequent positive or negative components are, respectively, R′ and S′ waves. The PR interval is the time from the earliest onset of the P wave in any lead to the first deflection of the QRS complex. This usually occurs in lead II. The QRS duration is the time from the onset of the Q or R wave to the end of the QRS complex. Similarly, the QT interval is from the onset of the QRS complex to the end of the T wave. The QT interval is corrected for heart rate by dividing by the square root of RR interval (the time elapsing between two consecutive QRS complexes). The normal value is less than 0.425 s (Figure 10-2).

The heart rate is determined by a number of methods including measuring the average RR interval and dividing it into 60 or by counting the number of beats over 6 seconds and multiplying by 10. The mean electrical axis in the frontal plane is calculated using the diagram in Figure 10-1 (*left*). Leads I and aV_F define in which quadrant the axis lies (0° to 90°: I positive, aV_F positive; 90° to 180°: I negative, aV_F positive; 180° to 270°: I negative, aV_F

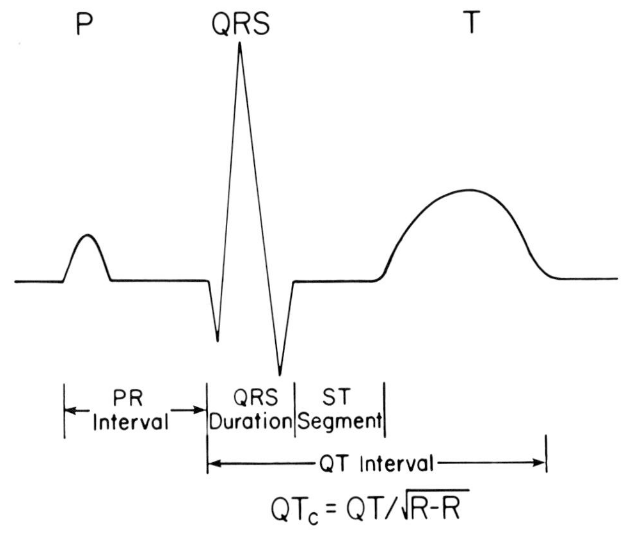

FIGURE 10-2 Standard nomenclature of the electrocardiogram including P wave, QRS complex, and T wave.

negative; 270° to 360°: I positive, aV_F negative). In a similar fashion the remaining four leads permit determining the axis to the nearest 30°. To further define the axis, the two leads adjacent to the 30° segment are examined. If the major deflection is of equal size in both leads, then the axis lies directly between the two leads. If the amplitude of one lead is greater than the other, then the axis is closer to that lead. In the event one of the leads is isoelectric (i.e., equally positive and negative), then the axis is directly perpendicular to that lead. Right axis deviation is an axis greater than normal for age and left axis deviation less than normal.

The normal values for heart rate, PR interval, and QRS duration vary with age (Table 10-3). Abnormally short or long intervals usually indicate a disorder of conduction. ST-T segment abnormalities, in addition to those seen with ventricular hypertrophy, are present in many children with myocardial, metabolic, or central nervous system derangement (Table 10-4). Suggested criteria for the diagnosis of atrial and ventricular hypertrophy are outlined in Table 10-5. With increasing age the contribution of the right ventricular forces to the precordial leads decreases (Table 10-6). In contrast, criteria for atrial hypertrophy vary little with age.

Chest Roentgenogram

Frontal and lateral chest x-ray films are usually readily available and can give a rapid assessment of overall heart size, pulmonary vascularity, position of the aortic arch and state of the lung fields. Further determination of specific chamber enlargement can be difficult in children and is more accurately assessed by echocardiography.

Prominence of the pulmonary vasculature is due either to excessive arterial flow in defects that result in left-to-right shunts or to venous congestion in children with obstruction at any level of the left side of the heart. Arterial enlargement is suggested by well-defined vessels that are enlarged when compared to the adjoining bronchus. Pulmonary venous congestion results in enlarged and hazy vasculature.

The aortic arch normally is to the left of the trachea, causing the trachea to buckle to the right. A right aortic arch is seen most frequently in tetralogy of Fallot, truncus arteriosus, and transposition of the great arteries with ventricular septal defect and pulmonic stenosis; it results in buckling of the trachea to the left. In addition, the trachea may be at the left edge of the mediastinum, indicating that the aorta must be to the right of the trachea.

TABLE 10-3 Normal Electrocardiographic Data

Age	Heart Rate (beats/min)	PR Interval(s)	QRS Axis (degrees)
0–24 h	119 (94–145)	0.10 (0.07–0.12)	135 (60–180)
1–7 d	133 (100–175)	0.09 (0.07–0.12)	125 (80–160)
8–30 d	163 (115–190)	0.09 (0.07–0.11)	110 (60–160)
1–3 mo	154 (124–190)	0.10 (0.07–0.13)	80 (40–120)
3–6 mo	140 (111–179)	0.10 (0.07–0.13)	65 (20–80)
6–12 mo	140 (112–177)	0.10 (0.08–0.13)	65 (0–100)
1–3 yr	126 (98–163)	0.11 (0.08–0.15)	55 (20–100)
3–5 yr	98 (65–132)	0.12 (0.09–0.15)	60 (40–80)
5–8 yr	96 (70–115)	0.13 (0.10–0.16)	65 (40–100)
8–12 yr	79 (55–107)	0.14 (0.10–0.17)	65 (20–80)
12–16 yr	75 (55–102)	0.14 (0.11–0.16)	65 (20–80)

Source: Adapted with permission from Moss AJ, Adams FH, Emmanouilides GE (eds): *Heart Disease in Infants, Children and Adolescents*, ed 2. Baltimore, The Williams & Wilkins Co, 1977, pp 32, 40. Copyright 1977, The Williams & Wilkins Co.

TABLE 10-4 Electrocardiographic Changes Induced by Electrolytes and Drugs

Condition or Drug	Electrocardiographic Findings
Hyperkalemia	Peaked T waves (mild), wide QRS complex (severe)
Hypokalemia	Flat T waves, prominent U waves
Hypercalcemia	Shortened QTc, ventricular dysrhythmias
Hypocalcemia	Prolonged QTc
Hypomagnesemia	Prolonged QTc
Digitalis	Prolonged PR, ST-segment changes (effect); bradycardia, AV block, atrial and ventricular dysrhythmias (toxicity)
Quinidine	Prolonged PR, QRS-interval duration, and QTc

TABLE 10-5 Electrocardiographic Diagnosis of Hypertrophy

Type	Electrocardiographic Findings
Right atrial	Peaked P waves (greater than 3 mm), especially in leads II and V_1
Left atrial	Notched, broad (greater than 0.08 s) P waves or deep terminal inversion of the P wave in lead V_1
Right ventricular	RV_1* or SV_6 greater than 95th percentile for age Upright TV_1 after 4 days R : S ratio in V_1 = 2 after 6 months qR in V_{3R}/V_1
Left ventricular	SV_1, SV_2, RV_6 greater than 95th percentile for age R : S ratio in V_1 < 0.1 after 6 months Q wave greater than 4 mm in V_5 or V_6
Biventricular	Criteria for both right and left ventricular hypertrophy

Source: Adapted with permission from Moss AJ, Adams FH, Emmanouilides GE (eds): *Heart Disease in Infants, Children and Adolescents*, ed 2. Baltimore, The Williams & Wilkins Co, 1977, p 60. Copyright 1977, The Williams & Wilkins Co.

* Abbreviations: RV_1, R wave in V_1; SV_6, S wave in V_6; TV_1, T wave in V_1; etc.

TABLE 10-6 Normal Electrocardiographic Data

Age	RV_1	SV_1	RV_2	SV_2	RV_6	SV_6
30 h	11.9 (4.3–21)*	9.7 (1.1–19.1)			5.4 (1.5–11.3)	5.6 (1.0–13.8)
1 mo	11.1 (3.3–18.7)	6.1 (0.0–15.0)			10.8 (1.0–16.2)	4.8 (0.0–9.5)
2–3 mo	11.2 (4.5–18.0)	7.5 (0.5–17.1)			12.8 (5.4–20.8)	4.2 (0.1–9.1)
4–5 mo	11.2 (4.5–17.4)	8.6 (1.0–16.8)			13.9 (4.4–22.4)	3.5 (0.0–8.0)
6–8 mo	11.4 (3.2–21.2)	10.7 (1.5–25.7)			13.0 (6.0–22.0)	2.5 (0.2–4.4)
9 mo–2 yr	9.7 (2.5–15.6)	8.5 (2.0–17.2)	15.3 (3.0–15.3)	14.2 (5.0–25.5)	12.1 (5.7–20.0)	2.3 (0.3–5.2)
2–5 yr	7.5 (2.1–13.9)	10.9 (2.1–21.6)	12.5 (4.2–20.8)	17.3 (5.4–29.7)	14.4 (6.4–22.1)	1.5 (0.0–3.7)
6–13 yr	5.3 (1.1–10.7)	12.6 (3.8–22.3)	9.7 (3.7–15.9)	9.5 (8.6–29.8)	15.7 (7.7–23.3)	1.4 (0.0–4.1)
13–19 yr	3.0 (1.0–8.0)	12.0 (4.7–20.2)	7.0 (3.0–15.2)	17.0 (6.7–30.0)	12.8 (7.0–20.0)	1.0 (0.0–3.0)

Source: Adapted with permission from Moss AJ, Adams FH, Emmanouilides GE (eds): *Heart Disease in Infants, Children and Adolescents*, ed 2. Baltimore, The Williams & Wilkins Co, 1977, pp 2–40 Copyright 1977, The Williams and Wilkins Co.
* All values shown are in mm.

Pneumonia is seen as a complication of congenital heart disease, and the chest film is useful in its localization. Atelectasis of the lower lobe of the left lung because of an enlarged left atrium and compression of the bronchus may be first diagnosed on the chest film.

Blood Tests

Measuring arterial blood gases in blood samples taken while the child is breathing room air provides not only a determination of the baseline oxygen saturation and P_{O_2} but also an assessment of the child's acid-base status. Hypoxia on room air can result from intracardiac shunting of blood or pulmonary dysfunction. Determining arterial blood gases from samples of blood taken while the child breathes 100% oxygen helps differentiate these two conditions. Children with intracardiac right-to-left shunting generally do not raise their P_{O_2} above 100 mmHg on 100% oxygen. If pulmonary dysfunction is present, high inspired oxygen concentration may alleviate the hypoxia and the P_{O_2} will rise above 100 mmHg.

The venous hematocrit increases in children with chronic cyanosis and thus can indicate the degree of hypoxia. It also identifies those children with severe polycythemia (hematocrit greater than 65%) who may be at risk for cerebrovascular accidents.

Other Tests

Several other tests, including two-dimensional and Doppler echocardiography, Doppler monitoring, 24-hour ambulatory electrocardiographic monitoring, and exercise stress testing have become important and very powerful tools for the assessment of management of children with heart disease. Two-dimensional echocardiography permits noninvasive imaging of cardiac anatomy and function. Doppler monitoring is used to quantify valvular stenosis, valvular regurgitation, and cardiac output. Although these studies have dramatically improved the ease and accuracy of diagnosing children with heart disease, they are most often performed after referral to the pediatric cardiologist and thus are not discussed in detail in this chapter. The reader is referred to any of several excellent reviews and texts on these subjects.[4–6]

DIFFERENTIAL DIAGNOSIS

Functional Murmurs

Functional, "innocent", murmurs occur in a large proportion of children. They are vibratory ejection murmurs that are best heard along the left sternal border. The precordium, heart sounds, and pulses are normal. The electrocardiogram, echocardiogram, and chest film, if done, are normal. The murmur results from the ejection of blood from the right or left ventricle into its respective great artery and may be more prominent at times when the cardiac output is increased, such as with fever or anemia.

Peripheral pulmonic stenosis is a functional murmur heard in many premature babies and infants. It is thought to result from the acute angulation of the branch pulmonary arteries in young children, resulting in mildly turbulent blood flow in the pulmonary arterial branches. However, it is also a vibratory ejection murmur that is uniformly heard over the entire chest. As the child grows and the pulmonary arteries become less angulated, the murmur diminishes in intensity.

A venous hum is a rumbling sound best heard at the upper sternal borders during diastole with the child in the sitting position facing forward. It represents flow through the systemic veins and can usually be obliterated by the supine position, compression of the jugular veins, or turning the head to the side.

Cranial and carotid bruits can be heard in normal children, although they should raise the possibility of left ventricular outflow tract obstruction or increased cardiac output, such as with an arteriovenous malformation.

Cyanotic Congenital Heart Disease

The differential diagnosis of the cyanotic child is extensive, and a variety of cardiac and noncardiac etiologies should be carefully considered during the initial evaluation (Exhibit 10-1).

Tetralogy of Fallot

Tetralogy of Fallot is a relatively common congenital heart lesion, representing approximately 9% of all defects.[7] The basic anatomic abnormality is a large ventricular septal defect with moderate-to-severe right ventricular outflow tract obstruction at either the pulmonary infundibular, valve, or artery level. In the most severe case, there may be total atresia of the pulmonary valve or outflow tract. The other classic features are severe right ventricular hypertrophy and the aorta overriding the ventricular septum.

Signs and Symptoms Children with tetralogy of Fallot may come to medical attention any time in the first year of life. At several hours of age, a newborn with tetralogy of Fallot and pulmonary atresia may exhibit intense cyanosis following spontaneous ductal closure. In contrast, a child with moderate obstruction or a large patent ductus arteriosus may be diagnosed at an older age with minimal cyanosis and a murmur as the signs.

Symptoms are usually limited to those resulting from hypoxia, such as squatting and cyanotic spells. Spells, paroxysms of hyperpnea associated with intense cyanosis, occur at any time in infancy and may be followed by limpness and occasionally loss of consciousness or seizures. They often occur upon awakening from sleep and can be precipitated by crying or feeding. The spells usually end spontaneously with full recovery, but thus can also result in stroke or death. Squatting is frequently noted in older children as they begin to ambulate and is a means of improving arterial oxygen during exercise.[8]

The physical findings of children with tetralogy of Fallot include a right ventricular heave and a single second heart sound. A harsh systolic ejection murmur resulting from the pulmonic stenosis is heard along the left sternal border; its intensity is inversely proportional to the severity of the obstruction. A separate, often continuous murmur of a pat-

Exhibit 10-1 Differential Diagnosis of Cyanosis in Infancy and Childhood

Congenital Heart Disease with Intracardiac Shunting
- Predominantly atrial level shunt
  - Ebstein's anomaly
  - Pulmonic stenosis or atresia with intact ventricular septum
  - Total anomalous pulmonary venous return
  - Tricuspid atresia
  - Tricuspid regurgitation
- Predominantly ventricular level shunt
  - Double outlet right ventricle
  - Double outlet right ventricle with pulmonary stenosis
  - Single ventricle with or without pulmonic stenosis
  - Tetralogy of Fallot
  - Tetralogy of Fallot with pulmonary atresia
  - Truncus arteriosus
- Transposition of the great arteries
  - Intact ventricular septum
  - Ventricular septal defect
  - Ventricular septal defect with pulmonic stenosis

Intrapulmonary Shunting Due to Congestive Heart Failure
- Structural heart disease
  - Anomalous left coronary artery from pulmonary artery
  - AV canal
  - Coarctation of the aorta/aortic arch interruption
  - Critical aortic stenosis
  - Hypoplastic left heart/mitral atresia
  - Systemic arteriovenous fistula
  - Ventricular septal defect/patent ductus/aortic-pulmonary window
- Myocardial dysfunction
  - Complete heart block
  - Myocarditis/endocardial fibroelastosis
  - Supraventricular tachycardia
  - Ventricular tachycardia

Structural Abnormality with intrapulmonary Shunt
- Pulmonary arteriovenous malformation

Nonstructural Heart Disease with Atrial or Great Vessel Shunt
- Persistence of the transitional circulation

Primary Lung Disease
- Hyaline membrane disease
- Meconium aspiration
- Pneumonia
- Pulmonary hemorrhage
- Pulmonary hypoplasia/agenesis

Mechanical Interference with Lung Function
- Choanal atresia
- Diaphragmatic hernia
- Lobar emphysema
- Mucous plugs/atelectasis
- Pneumothorax

Central Nervous System Disease
- Intracranial hemorrhage
- Seizure disorders

Methemoglobinemia

Hypoglycemia

Polycythemia

Sepsis/Shock

Respiratory Depression Secondary to Drugs

ent ductus arteriosus or systemic-to-pulmonary collaterals may be audible over the anterior chest or back. The peripheral pulses are normal and the liver is not enlarged.

The electrocardiogram shows right axis deviation and right ventricular hypertrophy. Left ventricular hypertrophy may be found in children with a large associated patent ductus arteriosus. The chest film usually demonstrates a "boot-shaped" heart and diminished pulmonary arterial vascularity. A right aortic arch is present in approximately 25% of children with tetralogy of Fallot. The two-dimensional echocardiogram documents the ventricular septal defect and the degree of pulmonary stenosis and pulmonary arterial hypoplasia. The Pa_{O_2} or venous hematocrit depends on the amount of pulmonary blood flow through the pulmonary outflow tract or from the aorta via the ductus arteriosus or collaterals. Cardiac catheterization is indicated prior to surgery to demonstrate the right ventricular outflow tract and pulmonary artery anatomy as well as to delineate other sources of pulmonary blood flow and the coronary artery anatomy.

Management Specific therapy must be tailored to the severity of the child's defect. Profoundly hypoxic newborns usually show improvement in their Pa_{O_2} in response to prostaglandin E_1 administration to dilate the ductus arteriosus.[9] These infants can then undergo a palliative systemic-to-pulmonary shunt to establish a reliable source of pulmonary blood flow. The most common shunts in current use are the Blalock-Taussig anastomosis between the subclavian artery and the pulmonary artery, and a Gore-Tex interposition graft between the aorta and pulmonary artery.

After the newborn period most children can be offered total correction—i.e., ventricular septal defect closure and relief of the pulmonary stenosis—at any time in the first year of life. The timing of the operation is usually dictated by the progression of cyanosis or the occurrence of cyanotic spells. Mild pulmonary regurgitation or stenosis is not unusual following correction and is usually well tolerated. Late postoperative complications are infrequent but include right ventricular dysfunction and ventricular dysrhythmias. Children with unrelieved pulmonary stenosis or severe pulmonary artery hypoplasia are particularly prone to serious dysrhythmias, and reports of sudden death in these patients make the diagnosis and control of these dysrhythmias important.

Transposition of the Great Arteries

Transposition of the great arteries is the most common heart defect appearing in the first week of life and comprises 10% of all congenital heart defects.[7] The aorta arises from the right ventricle and the pulmonary artery from the left ventricle. Poorly oxygenated systemic venous blood is ejected into the aorta and fully oxygenated pulmonary venous blood recirculates into the pulmonary artery. Ventricular septal defect, patent ductus arteriosus, pulmonic stenosis, and coarctation can be present as associated defects. Survival depends on mixing of the systemic and pulmonary circulations at either the atrial level or, if a ventricular septal defect is present, the ventricular level. Untreated, the mortality is 50% by 1 month of age.[10]

Signs and Symptoms The majority of children with transposition of the great arteries are cyanotic during the first week of life. If there is an associated ventricular septal defect, the cyanosis may be less marked, and they may be diagnosed in the first several months of life with a murmur and signs of congestive heart failure.

Since the right ventricle pumps blood into the aorta, the right ventricular pressure is high and a right ventricular heave is present. The second heart sound is loud and single because of the anterior placement of the aorta. A harsh murmur, if heard, is usually from an associated ventricular septal defect or pulmonic stenosis.

The electrocardiogram shows right axis deviation and right ventricular hypertrophy. The chest film typically demonstrates a narrow mediastinum and an egg-shaped heart. The two-dimensional echocardiogram confirms the origin of the great arteries and images any septal defects.[11] The Pa_{O_2} is usually less than 40 mmHg and does not rise above 75 mmHg on 100% oxygen.

Management Balloon septostomy[12] (Rashkind procedure) is indicated at the time of clinical and echocardiographic diagnosis to improve intracardiac mixing by enlarging the patent foramen ovale. Atrial baffling (Mustard or Senning procedure) to direct the pulmonary venous blood through the tricuspid valve and the systemic venous blood through the mitral valve can be offered to any child with transposition of the great arteries and an intact ventricular septum in the first 6 months of life, including the newborn period. Atrial dysrhythmias, including sick sinus syndrome, atrial flutter, and supraventricular tachycardia, are common following atrial surgery for transposition of the great arteries. Other long-term complications are unusual and include right ventricular failure, tricuspid regurgitation, and pulmonary or systemic venous obstruction. The *arterial* switch operation (Jatene) is, in many centers, currently reserved for those children with transposition of the great arteries and ventricular septal defect. The initial results of this operation are promising; however, potential long-term complications include obstruction of the aorta, pulmonary artery, or coronary arteries at the suture lines, or aortic regurgitation resulting from distortion of the aortic anulus.

Tricuspid Atresia

Tricuspid atresia represents approximately 3% of all heart defects.[7] In addition to tricuspid atresia, a ventricular septal defect and some degree of right ventricular and pulmonary arterial hypoplasia are usually present. The entire systemic venous return must cross the atrial septum through a persistently patent foramen ovale or an atrial septal defect. It mixes with the pulmonary venous return in the left atrium, which results in arterial desaturation. The pulmonary blood flow must arise from the left ventricle through a ventricular septal defect or a patent ductus arteriosus. The degree of cyanosis is proportional to the relative volume of pulmonary blood flow as compared to systemic blood flow. Those children with associated pulmonary atresia are totally dependent on ductal blood flow.

Signs and Symptoms Findings include an increased left ventricular impulse, a single or widely split second heart sound with a diminished pulmonary component, and a harsh systolic ejection murmur at the left sternal border. The liver may be enlarged and pulsatile if the atrial defect is restrictive.

The electrocardiogram, even in the newborn, is distinctive and reveals left axis deviation, right atrial hypertrophy, and left ventricular hypertrophy. The pulmonary vascular prominence on the chest film is inversely proportional to the degree of right ventricular hypoplasia. The two-dimensional echocardiogram documents the size of the atrial and ventricular defects as well as the degree of right ventricular and pulmonary arterial hypoplasia, and shows a smooth wall in the usual position of the tricuspid valve. The Pa_{O_2} is a function of the pulmonary blood flow, but it is generally between 30 and 45 mmHg. The unusual child with a relatively normal right ventricle and a large ventricular septal defect will have a higher P_{O_2} and may increase it to over 100 mmHg on supplemental oxygen. Cardiac catheterization is useful to document the adequacy and sources of pulmonary blood flow and the atrial pressures.

Management Prostaglandin E_1 may be needed to stabilize the newborn with severely limited pulmonary blood flow after spontaneous closure of the ductus arteriosus. Balloon septostomy is indicated at the time of diagnostic catheterization to enlarge the atrial septal defect and thus permit unrestricted blood flow from the right to the left atrium.[12] Palliative systemic-to-pulmonary shunts are often required for cyanosis in newborns or infants. For those children with large ventricular septal defects and pulmonary hypertension, pulmonary artery banding is necessary to decrease pulmonary blood flow and pressure.

The major long-term surgical goal in children with tricuspid atresia is to separate the systemic and pulmonary venous returns. This is currently accomplished by direct anastomosis of the right atrium to the pulmonary artery, with closure of the atrial septal defect, pulmonary valve, and any systemic-to-pulmonary shunts (Fontan procedure). After the Fontan procedure the systemic venous return enters the lung directly without the additional force of the right ventricle; thus systemic venous congestion with pleural effusion or ascites is occasionally encountered. Other long-term problems include dysrhythmias and mild exercise intolerance.

Total Anomalous Pulmonary Venous Return

Total anomalous pulmonary venous return is an unusual malformation in which the pulmonary veins enter the superior vena cava, right atrium, or inferior vena cava instead of the left atrium.[13] This results in complete mixing of the pulmonary and systemic venous return and thus cyanosis. An atrial septal defect must be present to permit blood to enter the left atrium and supply the systemic circulation. The large left-to-right shunt at the venous level results in increased pulmonary blood flow. Pulmonary venous obstruction may be present, especially when the anomalous connection is to the inferior vena cava below the diaphragm.

Signs and Symptoms In the absence of pulmonary venous obstruction, children with total anomalous pulmonary venous return can be remarkably asymptomatic during the first weeks of life. Since there is complete mixing and the pulmonary blood flow is increased, cyanosis is mild. As the pulmonary vascular resistance falls, pulmonary blood flow increases, leading to congestive heart failure. In children with pulmonary venous obstruction, symptoms of pulmonary edema are evident in the first days of life.

The precordium is very active with a right ventricular heave. The second heart sound is widely split, with an accentuated pulmonic component, or single if pulmonary hypertension is present. A systolic ejection murmur results from the increased blood flow across the pulmonary valve and arteries. The liver is usually enlarged and the pulses are normal.

Right axis deviation and right ventricular hypertrophy, often with a qR pattern in V_1, are found on the electrocardiogram. The chest film shows right ventricular enlargement and increased pulmonary vascularity. When the anomalous drainage is to the superior vena cava, the dilated veins above the cardiac silhouette give the appearance of a "snowman" on the chest film. If the pulmonary venous return is obstructed, the heart is usually small and pulmonary edema is present. The two-dimensional echocardiogram shows the atrial septal defect and a dilated right ventricle, and may delineate the anomalous insertion of the pulmonary veins. Since the pulmonary blood flow is increased, the P_{O_2} on room air may be 50 to 60 mmHg and often increases to 100 to 150 mmHg on 100% oxygen. Cardiac catheterization and angiography demonstrate the pulmonary venous anatomy and permit measurement of pulmonary artery pressure.

Management Current management of total anomalous pulmonary venous return is to offer total correction—i.e., anastomosis of the common pulmonary vein to the left atrium and ligation of the anomalous venous connection—to infants at the time of diagnosis. Infants with pulmonary venous obstruction must undergo repair on an emergency basis. Long-term complications are rare but include obstruction of the pulmonary venous-left atrial anastomosis.

Truncus Arteriosus

Truncus arteriosus represents approximately 1% of all congenital heart defects.[7] The pulmonary artery and aorta share a common origin from a single, large semilunar valve. The valve is almost always abnormal and can be stenotic or permit regurgitation. There is a large associated ventricular septal defect. Unless pulmonary arterial branch stenosis is present, there is pulmonary hypertension and increased pulmonary blood flow.[14]

Signs and Symptoms In the first 2 months of life, children with truncus arteriosus usually exhibit congestive heart failure and mild cyanosis. Other findings include failure to thrive, tachypnea, and a diffusely active precordium. The first heart sound may be followed by a click, especially if the truncal valve is stenotic, and the second heart sound is usually single. A harsh systolic ejection murmur is present along the left sternal border, and if truncal valve regurgitation exists, a blowing diastolic murmur is heard along the lower left sternal border. The liver is usually enlarged and the pulses are bounding.

The electrocardiogram usually indicates both right and left ventricular hypertrophy, and the chest film shows cardiomegaly, increased pulmonary blood flow, and, in 25% of children with this defect, a right aortic arch. The two-dimensional echocardiogram defines the truncal anatomy and the ventricular septal defect. Cardiac catheterization is indicated to precisely define the truncal anatomy and to measure the pulmonary artery pressure.

Management Total correction of truncus arteriosus consists of closure of the ventricular septal defect, separation of the pulmonary arteries from the truncus, and establishment of right ventricular-to-pulmonary artery continuity by an extracardiac conduit. This is usually required between the ages of 2 and 6 months to treat the severe congestive heart failure accompanying the cyanosis in this defect. The extracardiac conduit frequently becomes obstructed or is outgrown within 5 years and must be replaced.

Acyanotic Congenital Heart Disease

The acyanotic child with heart disease can be identified by a murmur, high blood pressure, or the incidental finding of cardiomegaly on a chest film. Others may have signs and symptoms of congestive heart failure, a clinical syndrome characterized by tachypnea, precordial hyperactivity, hepatomegaly, cardiomegaly, poor feeding, and failure to thrive (Exhibit 10-2).

Ventricular Septal Defect

An isolated ventricular septal defect is one of the most common congenital heart lesions, comprising about 15% to 20% of all congenital heart defects.[7] The membranous septum, that area just below the crista supraventricularis on the superior aspect of the septum, is the most frequent site for the defect. Less frequently, the lesion occurs inferiorly in the muscular septum. In approximately 5% of children, the ventricular septal defect is located above the crista supraventricularis, just below the pulmonary valve. Finally, a defect adjacent to the tricuspid and mitral valves occurs as part of the spectrum of endocardial cushion defects. The defects range in size from a pinhole to 1.5 cm in diameter.

The opening in the ventricular septum permits blood to shunt from the left ventricle into the pulmonary artery. When a large, nonrestrictive defect is present, the right and left ventricular pressures

Exhibit 10-2 Differential Diagnosis of Heart Failure in Infancy and Childhood

- Congenital Cardiovascular Malformations
  - Large left-to-right shunts
    - Aortic-pulmonary window
    - Arteriovenous fistula
    - AV canal
    - Patent ductus arteriosus
    - Total anomalous pulmonary venous return
    - Transposition with ventricular septal defect
    - Tricuspid atresia with ventricular septal defect and normal pulmonary artery development
    - Truncus arteriosus
    - Ventricular septal defect
  - Obstructive lesions
    - Aortic stenosis
    - Coarctation of the aorta
    - Hypoplastic left heart syndrome
    - Interruption of the aortic arch
    - Mitral stenosis
    - Pulmonic stenosis
  - Regurgitant lesions
    - Absent pulmonic valve
    - Aortic regurgitation
    - Mitral regurgitation
- Myocardial Diseases
  - Anomalous origin of the left coronary artery from the pulmonary artery
  - Endocardial fibroelastosis
  - Mucocutaneous lymph node syndrome
  - Myocarditis (viral)
  - Neonatal transient myocardial ischemia
- Dysrhythmias
  - Atrial flutter
  - Complete heart block
  - Supraventricular tachycardia
  - Ventricular tachycardia
- Miscellaneous
  - Anemia
  - Atrial myxoma
  - Cor pulmonale
  - Polycythemia
  - Renal insufficiency
  - Upper airway obstruction

are equal, and the degree of shunting is determined by the relative pulmonary and systemic vascular resistances. As the pulmonary vascular resistance falls postnatally, the pulmonary blood flow (normal systemic venous return plus left-to-right shunt) increases and can reach five to six times the systemic blood flow. In a smaller restrictive defect, the right ventricular pressure remains less than the left, and the degree of shunting depends on both the pulmonary vascular resistance and the resistance offered by the defect itself.

Signs and Symptoms The severity of the symptoms and the abnormal physical findings usually parallels the amount of shunting. As the pulmonary vascular resistance falls after birth, left-to-right shunting begins and the typical findings become evident.

In the first 2 months of life, a child with a large ventricular septal defect usually exhibits tachypnea. The precordium is active with an apical impulse, the first heart sound is normal, and the second heart sound is single or narrowly split, with increased intensity of the pulmonic component because of pulmonary hypertension. A third heart sound is present, and there is a harsh holosystolic murmur that radiates widely and is best heard at the lower left sternal border. A rumbling middiastolic murmur may be present in children with pulmonary blood flow that is more than twice the systemic blood flow. The pulses are normal and the liver may be enlarged.

In a child with a small defect, the only abnormal physical finding is a harsh holosystolic or early systolic murmur that varies little with respiration or position. Those children with intermediate size defects have abnormalities in their exam usually in proportion to the degree of left-to-right shunting.

The electrocardiogram shows left ventricular hypertrophy, and, when pulmonary hypertension is present, right axis deviation and right ventricular hypertrophy. The chest film demonstrates cardiomegaly and pulmonary vascular prominence. The degree of left atrial and left ventricular enlargement on the echocardiogram is proportional to the amount of left-to-right shunting. The two-dimensional echocardiogram often images the actual defect (Figure 10-3). Cardiac catheterization is indicated in children with congestive heart failure to document the pulmonary artery pressure and pulmonary-to-systemic flow ratio.

Management Nearly 50% of ventricular septal defects, including some large defects, undergo complete spontaneous closure or a decrease in size, with improvement in symptoms or signs. The natural history of a persistent large defect with pulmonary hypertension is well established.[15,16] Pulmonary vascular resistance gradually increases because of muscular hypertrophy and fibrosis of the pulmonary arterioles, producing the Eisenmenger syndrome. While the increased pulmonary vascular resistance initially improves the congestive heart failure, it eventually results in right-to-left shunting and cyanosis. The pulmonary vascular disease is irreversible and surgical closure of the defect is no longer possible. Thus it is critical to recognize those children who are clinically improved but nevertheless continue to have signs or noninvasive evidence of pulmonary hypertension, in order to intervene

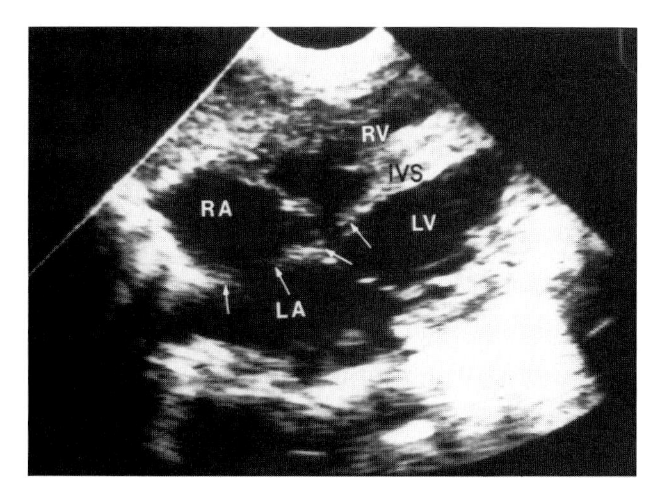

FIGURE 10-3 A two-dimensional echocardiogram, four-chamber view in an infant demonstrates a large atrial septal defect (*arrows*) and ventricular septal defect (*arrows*) in the membranous interventricular septum (IVS). A large pulmonary vein enters the left atrium (LA) near the atrial defect. The tricuspid and mitral valves are closed, separating the right atrium (RA) and right ventricle (RV), and left atrium and left ventricle (LV), respectively.

surgically before the pulmonary vascular disease becomes irreversible. Bacterial endocarditis is an infrequent but important complication, and antibiotic prophylaxis is indicated for dental and certain surgical procedures.

Surgical closure is indicated in infancy for those children who fail to thrive despite digoxin or diuretic therapy for congestive heart failure or who have pulmonary hypertension. The results of operation are frequently dramatic, with a significant increase in growth velocity and normalization of heart size and pulmonary artery pressure. In the asymptomatic child surgical closure is usually undertaken at the age of 4 years if the pulmonary blood flow is twice the normal amount. Small residual defects are occasionally encountered, and right bundle-branch block is common following repair; both cause no difficulty. Serious complications such as complete heart block or a large residual defect are rare.

Patent Ductus Arteriosus

Patent ductus arteriosus is a common defect, both as an isolated finding and in association with other congenital heart defects. Normally, the ductus arteriosus is functionally closed by the end of the first week of life. If it remains patent, it permits blood to shunt left to right, from the aorta to the pulmonary artery. The degree of shunting and thus of left ventricular volume overload is determined by the size of the ductus arteriosus and the relative pulmonary and systemic vascular resistances.

Signs and Symptoms The usual feature is a continuous "machinery"-type murmur at the upper left sternal border. If the ductus is large, the apical impulse is active, the second heart sound is accentuated, and the pulses are bounding. A small lesion has normal findings with the exception of the murmur.

The abnormalities found on the noninvasive studies usually parallel the degree of shunting. With a large shunt the pulmonary vascularity is prominent on chest film and left ventricular hypertrophy is present on the electrocardiogram. The left atrium and ventricle are dilated and the patent ductus is visualized on the echocardiogram. Doppler echocardiography shows continuous flow in the pulmonary artery. Cardiac catheterization is usually not necessary to confirm the diagnosis.

Management Although medical management may ameliorate the symptoms of congestive heart failure in a child with a large shunt, prompt surgical ligation is safe and effective at any age in the symptomatic child. For the asymptomatic child elective ligation after 6 to 12 months of age is usually undertaken to decrease the risk of infective endocarditis.[17]

Atrial Septal Defect

An isolated defect in the middle (secundum) portion of the atrial septum is frequently not detected until late in childhood or in adolescence and is rarely diagnosed prior to 6 months of age. It is frequently encountered as an associated malformation in children with ventricular septal defect, pulmonic stenosis, tetralogy of Fallot, and many complex abnormalities. It permits a left-to-right shunt, which increases the flow through the right ventricle and pulmonary arteries. Occasionally, one or more of the pulmonary veins drain anomalously into the right atrium or superior vena cava.[18]

Signs and Symptoms The distinctive physical findings in children and young adults are an active right ventricular heave, a widely split and fixed second heart sound, and a systolic ejection murmur at the upper left sternal border, which often radiates widely and is a result of the increased flow through the normal right ventricular outflow tract and pulmonary arteries. A diastolic tricuspid flow rumble and third heart sound can be heard at the lower right sternal border. In infants and young children, the examination may be atypical, with wide but variable splitting of the second heart sound and limited radiation of the murmur. Mitral valve prolapse is sometimes present, especially in older patients, and results in a mid- or late systolic click and murmur. Congestive heart failure is rare in children, although it has been observed occasionally, even in infancy.

The electrocardiogram shows right axis deviation and right ventricular hypertrophy, frequently with an rsR′ pattern in V_1. There is cardiomegaly, a prominent pulmonary artery segment, and increased pulmonary vascularity on the chest film. The two-dimensional echocardiogram usually visualizes the atrial defect in the midportion of the septum and documents a dilated right ventricle (Figure 10-3). Failure to do so raises the possible diagnosis of partial anomalous pulmonary venous return with an intact atrial septum.

Management Elective surgical repair is usually done prior to school age or at the time of diagnosis. The unusual child with symptoms of congestive heart failure can undergo correction at any time. Because of the extremely low incidence of endocarditis, antibiotic prophylaxis is not recommended, even prior to corrective surgery. The prognosis after surgery in childhood is excellent, with a low incidence of dysrhythmias and mitral valve abnormalities.[19]

Endocardial Cushion Defects

Endocardial cushion defects represent a spectrum of lesions ranging from a complete AV canal to an ostium primum atrial septal defect.[20] They most commonly occur in association with Down's syndrome.[21]

Complete Atrioventricular Canal A complete atrioventricular canal is a large defect that includes the inferior portion of the atrial septum (ostium primum) and the superior, posterior aspect of the ventricular septum. The tricuspid and mitral valves share common leaflets that straddle the defect. An ostium primum atrial septal defect involves the atrial septum and often the anterior mitral leaflet.

Signs and Symptoms Congestive heart failure and pulmonary artery hypertension are almost uniformly present in the child with a complete AV canal defect, and thus the physical exam is similar to that of a large ventricular septal defect. Occasionally, mitral regurgitation is present as a result of the mitral valve abnormality.

The electrocardiogram for a complete AV canal shows left axis deviation and right and left ventricular hypertrophy. The left axis deviation is present at birth, and since it is virtually never a normal finding in infancy, it is an excellent clue to the presence of congenital heart disease. The chest film demonstrates cardiomegaly and increased pulmonary vascularity. The two-dimensional echocardiogram documents the posterior ventricular septal defect and the common AV valve.

Management Children with complete AV canal often fail to thrive despite maximal medical and nutritional therapy. Total correction in the first year, with closure of the septal defects and reconstruction of the valves, is almost always the only satisfactory treatment and must be performed to prevent the Eisenmenger syndrome. Mild mitral regurgitation is common following repair.[22]

Ostium Primum Atrial Septal Defect The physical findings of an ostium primum atrial septal defect are similar to those of a secundum atrial septal defect. The electrocardiogram, however, shows *left* axis deviation and *right* ventricular hypertrophy. The echocardiogram documents right ventricular dilatation and the atrial defect in the inferior portion of the septum adjacent to the AV valves. Elective surgical repair of these defects is usually undertaken by 5 years of age.

Aortic Valve Stenosis

Valvular aortic stenosis is a common disorder and represents a spectrum of disease, ranging from a bicuspid aortic valve with little or no obstruction to critical obstruction resulting from a severely deformed valve in a neonate.[23] Coarctation of the aorta is found as an associated lesion in 25% of children with aortic stenosis. The severity of the obstruction often increases with age. Aortic stenosis results in elevation of the left ventricular pressure, which in turn leads to left ventricular and left atrial hypertrophy. The degree of hypertrophy is usually proportional to the left ventricular pressure and thus to the severity of the obstruction. Cardiac output, especially at rest, is normal except in the most severe cases.

Signs and Symptoms The neonate with critical obstruction has congestive heart failure with pulmonary edema. Older children may complain of chest pain or experience syncopal attacks if the obstruction is severe. These are often precipitated by exercise and are a result of the inability to increase cardiac output or coronary blood flow to meet the demands of exercise. More commonly, an older child is entirely asymptomatic, and the diagnosis is established after the detection of a murmur.

The diagnosis of aortic stenosis and an assessment of severity can be made from the physical examination. The apical impulse is more forceful and sustained than normal. The first heart sound is normal and is followed by an ejection click. The second heart sound can be normal or narrowly split because of the delay in the aortic component. The murmur is typically a harsh systolic ejection murmur best heard at the upper right sternal border and radiating to the neck. As the stenosis becomes more severe, the murmur is louder and its intensity peaks later in systole. The peripheral pulses are normal in a child with mild obstruction; however, they are damped with a delayed upstroke in a child with severe obstruction. Rales resulting from pulmonary edema are unusual but can be found with severe obstruction.

The left ventricular hypertrophy on the electrocardiogram usually parallels the degree of obstruction in an unoperated patient, but it can be misleading in the child who has had previous surgery. The left ventricular hypertrophy in children with more severe obstruction is reflected by deep S waves in V_1 and V_2 or tall R waves in V_6. Severe obstruction is usually indicated by the additional finding of inverted T waves in V_6.

The echocardiogram shows the aortic valve thickening and anatomy and the degree of left ventricular hypertrophy. Peak aortic flow velocity by Doppler echocardiography correlates well with the pressure gradient across the obstruction measured by cardiac catheterization, providing another noninvasive means of assessing severity. The chest film is inferior to the electrocardiogram and echocardiogram in the assessment of ventricular size and hypertropy, although it can confirm the clinical findings of pulmonary edema.

Management Digoxin and furosemide may relieve the symptoms of the infant in congestive heart failure resulting from critical aortic stenosis. Surgical valvulotomy is effective in most infants and is indicated on an urgent basis in an infant with critical obstruction. Moderate stenosis, a 30 to 50 mmHg systolic pressure gradient, is usually an indication for elective valvulotomy in an older child. Aortic regurgitation is common following aortic valvulotomy for congenital aortic stenosis and can progress with time. Restenosis or an inability to relieve the stenosis are less common outcomes. Severe aortic regurgitation or persistent stenosis is an indication for aortic valve replacement.

Restrictions, with the exception of organized competitive school sports and especially contact sports for these children on anticoagulants, are not usually necessary in children after successful surgery or in those with mild gradients. Chest pain or dizziness during exercise usually indicates inadequate cardiac output or coronary blood flow and suggests reevaluation of a child previously thought to have mild obstruction. Since valvular aortic stenosis, even when initially mild, does progress with age, long-term follow-up is important. Bacterial endocarditis is relatively more common in children with aortic stenosis compared to other congenital heart defects, and the importance of antibiotic prophylaxis should be stressed.

Coarctation of the Aorta

Coarctation of the aorta is a common isolated lesion but is also frequently found in association with other defects including aortic stenosis, ventricular septal defect, and transposition of the great arteries.[24] There is typically a discrete, severe narrowing of the aorta distal to the left subclavian artery in the area of the ductus arteriosus. The proximity of the coarctation to the ductus arteriosus is of hemodynamic significance in that prior to ductal closure the obstruction may be partially relieved by the extra area of blood flow provided by the aortic end of the ductus. Following ductal closure this is lost and the obstruction becomes more severe, leading to the development of a pressure gradient, with hypertension in the vessels proximal to the obstruction (innominate, left carotid, and left subclavian) and hypotension with a dampened pressure wave distal to the coarctation. This leads to the development of large collateral vessels, including the internal mammary and long thoracic arteries, between the proximal and distal aorta.

Signs and Symptoms Infants with severe coarctation often have symptoms of congestive heart failure in the first months of life. Children who remain asymptomatic are usually diagnosed at routine physical examinations by the finding of absent femoral pulses or upper extremity hypertension. The hallmark of the physical examination in any child with coarctation is absence of or diminished and delayed lower extremity pulses. This can be confirmed by measuring upper and lower extremity blood pressures and calculating a pressure gradient. Some children have a systolic ejection murmur, which is best heard between the scapulae and represents the turbulent flow at the coarctation. Older children with well-developed collateral circulation have continuous murmurs heard bilaterally. The physical examination is otherwise modified by the presence of associated heart defects.

The electrocardiogram in the newborn with coarctation shows the normal finding of right ventricular hypertrophy. Some degree of left ventricular hypertrophy is usually found in older children. The coarctation and any associated abnormalities may be imaged by two-dimensional echocardiography. The chest film may be abnormal in the older child and show rib-notching from hypertrophied intercostal arteries and a "3 sign" at the aortic knob from the coarctation. Cardiac catheterization and aortography confirm the diagnosis and demonstrate the extent of the collateral circulation.

Management Medical management of the newborn with coarctation who is in congestive heart failure must be directed at improving the circulatory congestion with digoxin and furosemide and reducing the obstruction by dilatation of the ductus arteriosus with prostaglandin E_1.[9] These measures often lessen the associated metabolic acidosis and renal dysfunction and permit urgent surgical repair with the child in a more stable condition. Older children who are not hypertensive can be corrected electively at about 4 years of age or at the time of diagnosis. Children with hypertension proximal to the coarctation may respond to diuretics and propranolol, although surgery is the preferred treatment.

Late restenosis after surgical correction occurs in 20% to 30% of patients. Persistent hypertension has been found in a similar proportion of patients without evidence of restenosis.[25] Long-term complications of an untreated coarctation are well documented. Death prior to 50 years of age from atherosclerosis, rupture of cerebral aneurysms or the ascending aorta, and bacterial endocarditis occurs in 80% of such patients.

Idiopathic Hypertrophic Subaortic Stenosis

Idiopathic hypertrophic subaortic stenosis or asymmetric septal hypertrophy is a form of left ventricular outflow tract obstruction that can be inherited in an autosomal dominant fashion and tends to be progressive. The interventricular septum becomes thickened out of proportion to the left ventricular posterior wall. This results in narrowing of the area between the anterior leaflet of the mitral valve and the septum during systole. Changes that tend to decrease ventricular volume (standing position, Valsalva maneuver) or increase contractility (inotropic agents, tachycardia) intensify the obstruction. Conversely, increasing venous return or decreasing contractility diminishes the obstruction.

Signs and Symptoms This lesion can be distinguished from the other types of aortic obstruction by the changes in murmur intensity that occur with the maneuvers altering the volume or contractile state of the left ventricle. In addition, because the obstruction becomes more severe in late systole, the pulse contour is normal with mild obstruction and is double-peaked (bisferious) in the presence of severe obstruction.

The two-dimensional echocardiogram shows a thickened interventricular septum as compared to the posterior wall, a characteristic of idiopathic hypertrophic subaortic stenosis. The electrocardiogram indicates left ventricular hypertrophy.

Management Surgical therapy, including myectomy or myotomy of the interventricular septum, may fail to relieve the obstruction, resulting in conduction disorders. Propranolol has been useful in some patients to decrease myocardial contractility and thus the obstruction. The long-term prognosis is poor due to persistent severe obstruction, ventricular dysrhythmias, and sudden death.

Hypoplastic Left Heart Syndrome

The hypoplastic left heart syndrome is a frequent cause of profound congestive heart failure and shock in the first week of life. There is atresia or hypoplasia of the mitral valve, left ventricle, aortic valve, and the ascending aorta. In the days following birth, the ductus arteriosus usually closes, resulting in profound shock leading to metabolic acidosis and death.

Signs and Symptoms A physical examination done in the first 24 hours of life, while the ductus arteriosus remains patent, may be deceptively normal. As the ductus closes, poor feeding or tachypnea become evident. Examination at that time reveals a child with poor perfusion and pulses, hepatomegaly, single second heart sound, and a gallop rhythm. A murmur need not be present. The electrocardiogram shows the normal right axis deviation and right ventricular hypertrophy, but the chest film is often remarkable for cardiomegaly and evidence of pulmonary edema. The two-dimensional echocardiogram is diagnostic and reveals restricted or absent mitral valve motion, a small left ventricle, and a markedly hypoplastic ascending aorta. Cardiac catheterization is usually not necessary to confirm the diagnosis.

Management The prognosis for this defect is very poor, and death usually occurs by 2 weeks of age. Survival to 1 year of age has been reported but is extremely rare.

Pulmonic Valve Stenosis

The most common cause of right ventricular outflow tract obstruction is valvular pulmonic stenosis. The stenosis is usually due to thickening and fusion of the valve leaflets. The valve domes during systole, and the resulting jet of blood through the valve contributes to the development of poststenotic dilatation of the pulmonary artery. Some children have marked thickening and nodularity of the valve, with poor motion and underdevelopment of the pulmonary annulus, and are separately classified as having dysplastic pulmonary valves. These children conspicuously lack poststenotic dilatation and may have associated discrete coarctations of the branch pulmonary arteries (peripheral pulmonary arterial stenosis). An atrial septal defect is the most frequent associated lesion.

The stenosis results in increased right ventricular pressure and hypertrophy in proportion to the severity of the obstruction. In all but the most severe instances, the right ventricle is able to compensate for this load and the child is asymptomatic. In the presence of critical pulmonary stenosis, especially in the newborn, right ventricular failure may be present with right ventricular dilatation, tricuspid regurgitation, and cyanosis due to right-to-left atrial level shunting.

Signs and Symptoms The abnormalities on physical examination are related to the severity of the obstruction. A right ventricular heave is present in children with moderate obstruction and becomes more forceful as the severity of the stenosis increases. The first heart sound is normal and is followed by an ejection click; the absence of a click suggests a dysplastic pulmonary valve. The interval between the first heart sound and the click increases with severity. There is a harsh systolic ejection murmur that is best heard at the upper left sternal border. In a child with mild stenosis, the peak of the murmur is in midsystole. As the severity of the obstruction increases, the murmur becomes more intense and it peaks later in systole. The pulmonic component of the second heart sound is delayed and diminished in intensity, usually in direct relation to the severity of obstruction. In the absence of right ventricular failure, the liver size and pulses are normal.

The electrocardiogram may be normal in the child with mild stenosis; however, it shows right axis deviation and right ventricular hypertrophy in the child with moderate or severe stenosis. Usually this is manifested as an increase in the anterior forces, with a tall R wave in lead V_1. This varies from the electrocardiogram of a child with an atrial septal defect, which often shows an rsR′ pattern in lead V_1.

The two-dimensional echocardiogram shows the thickened pulmonic valve and poststenotic dilatation of the pulmonary artery. Doppler echocardiography identifies the turbulent and high-velocity main pulmonary artery blood flow and can be used to estimate the severity of obstruction. Cardiac catheterization demonstrates the pulmonary valve and arterial anatomy and documents the severity by directly measuring the pressure gradient across the pulmonary valve.

Management The medical and surgical treatment is dictated by the severity of the obstruction.[26] Most children with moderate or severe obstruction are now offered balloon dilatation of the pulmonary valve at the time of diagnostic catheterization. Preliminary data suggest that this results in long-term and nearly complete relief of the obstruction. Children in whom balloon valvuloplasty is ineffective require surgical valvotomy. After surgery the prognosis is usually excellent, the stenosis does not recur, and pulmonary regurgitation, if present, is well tolerated. Since mild pulmonic valve stenosis neither progresses nor causes symptoms in adulthood, treatment is unnecessary, and such patients should be encouraged to lead normal lives without restriction. There is a mildly increased risk of bacterial endocarditis, even after treatment, and thus prophylaxis is recommended.

Mitral Valve Prolapse

Mitral valve prolapse or Barlow syndrome may be detected incidentally on a routine physical examination or be diagnosed in a child with chest pain or supraventricular tachycardia.[27] It can be sporadic or inherited in an autosomal dominant fashion. Severe mitral valve prolapse is also frequently associated with Marfan's syndrome.

Signs and Symptoms The mitral valve is redundant and during ventricular systole it prolapses posteriorly, resulting in a click. Typically the click is at the apex and occurs in mid- to late systole. Mitral regurgitation may be present and have a honking quality. Positional changes such as sitting or standing, which tend to decrease left ventricular systolic volume, make the prolapse more prominent, causing the click to come earlier in systole or producing mitral regurgitation. The supine or squatting position has the opposite effect and can eliminate the prolapse.

The electrocardiogram is usually normal, although it may show T-wave inversion in leads I, II, aV_F, and V_6. The echocardiogram usually demonstrates the posterior prolapse of the mitral leaflets during systole.

Management Most children are asymptomatic and need not be restricted. Bacterial endocarditis prophylaxis is often prescribed; however, in the absence of mitral regurgitation, there is controversy as to its need. Some children complain of chest pain, which is usually not related to exercise. Although propranolol has been recommended in this situation, there is little evidence to support its efficacy. Supraventricular dysrhythmias are also more common in children with mitral valve prolapse and usually are treated with propranolol.

Essential Hypertension

Essential hypertension affects 2% to 9% of the pediatric population, and there is a growing literature suggesting that adult hypertension has its beginnings in adolescence and childhood.[28] Regular office screening has detected a group of asymptomatic children with consistent blood pressures above the 95th percentile for age and sex (Figure 10-4). An organized approach to the evaluation of these children clarifies the diagnosis and indicates management. The differential diagnosis of the child with hypertension is extensive (Exhibit 10-3) and includes renal, endocrine, and cardiovascular, as well as essential, hypertension. The risk factors for essential hypertension include a positive family history, obesity, high salt intake, a stressful life-style, and smoking.

Signs and Symptoms

Blood pressure should be measured on several occasions during multiple visits, with the patient in sitting position. Careful attention must be paid to technique, including appropriate cuff size, correct rate of inflation and deflation, and an accurate manometer. In addition to determining the blood pres-

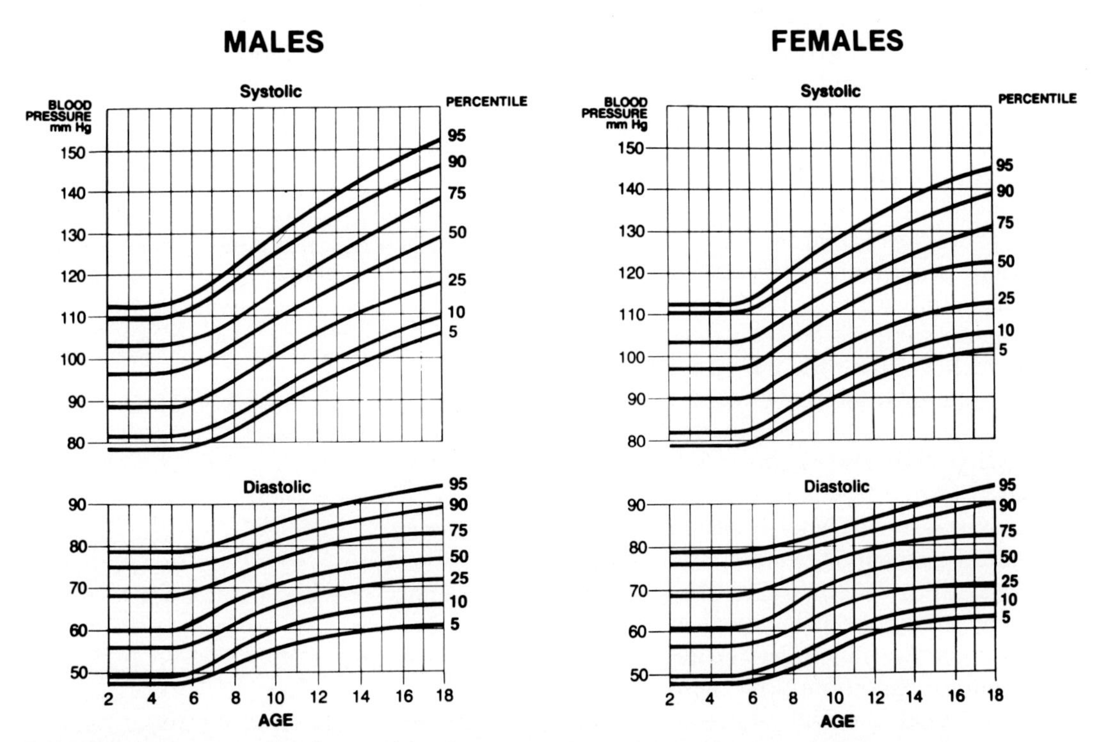

FIGURE 10-4 Normal values of blood pressure for males and females from age 2 to 18 years. Reprinted with permission from Report of NHLBI Task Force on Blood Pressure in Children. *Pediatrics* 59(Suppl.):803, 1977.

Exhibit 10-3 Differential Diagnosis of Hypertension in Childhood and Adolescence

Cardiovascular Causes
- Aortic regurgitation (systolic only)
- Coarctation of the aorta (proximal only)
- Essential hypertension

Renal Causes
- Glomerulonephritis
  - Hemolytic uremic syndrome
  - Lupus erythematosus
  - Periarteritis nodosa
  - Poststreptococcal
- Structural and vascular defects
  - Hydronephrosis
  - Polycystic disease
  - Pyelonephritis
  - Renal arterial stenosis
  - Renal vein stenosis
  - Trauma
  - Tumors

Endocrine Causes
- Congenital adrenal hyperplasia
- Exogenous corticosteroids or adrenocorticotropin
- Hyperthyroidism
- Pheochromocytoma
- Primary hyperaldosteronism

Central Nervous System Causes
- Encephalitis
- Intracranial pressure

sure in each extremity, the physical examination should seek evidence of end-organ involvement, including abnormal fundi oculi and a fourth heart sound. Further evaluation is indicated if the blood pressure on follow-up remains elevated above the 95th percentile for age and sex. Close follow-up is recommended for those children in the 90th to 95th percentiles.

Analysis of serum electrolytes, blood urea nitrogen, creatinine, and urine provides a rapid screen for renal dysfunction. A deep S wave in lead V_1 or V_2 on the electrocardiogram suggests left ventricular hypertrophy. On the echocardiogram, increased posterior wall thickness or an increase in the ratio of the left ventricular diastolic radius to the posterior wall thickness (greater than 3.0) also suggests left ventricular hypertrophy.[29] An intravenous pyelogram or renal scan further assesses renal function and structure. This limited work-up is usually adequate for the adolescent with hypertension. For the younger child a more complete search for renal or endocrine etiologies is warranted, including urine collections for catecholamine excretion, renal vein renin determinations, and renal arteriography.

Management

The therapy of essential hypertension begins with the elimination or amelioration, where possible, of risk factors. Alteration of diet and life-style and elimination of obesity require a major commitment from the patients, parents, and physicians. Pharmacologic treatment can be offered to those children with consistent blood pressure measurements above the 95th percentile, especially if left ventricular hypertrophy is present. A thiazide diuretic is commonly the first drug prescribed, with a β-blocker, usually propranolol or atenolol, added later if adequate lowering of the blood pressure is not achieved with a diuretic alone. A vasodilator such as hydralazine can then be tried in place of or in addition to the propranolol. These and some less frequently used drugs, with their dosages and side effects, are summarized in Table 10-7.

TABLE 10-7 Antihypertensive Agents

Drug	Dosage	Side Effects
Diuretics		
Chlorthiazide	10–20 mg/kg/d PO bid, maximum is 2 g/d	Hypokalemia, alkalosis, hyperglycemia
Hydrochlorthiazide	1–2 mg/kg/d PO bid, maximum is 200 mg/d	Hypokalemia, alkalosis, hyperglycemia
Spironolactone	1–3 mg/kg/d PO q6–8h	Hyperkalemia (contraindicated in renal failure)
Furosemide	3–6 mg/kg/d PO q8–12h or 1–2 mg/kg/dose IV	Hypokalemia, alkalosis, hypocalcemia, deafness
Adrenergic Blockers		
Propranolol	0.5–2.0 mg/kg/d PO q6h or 0.01–0.15 mg/kg/dose IV	Hypoglycemia, asthma, fatigue, congestive heart failure
Methyldopa	1.0 mg/kg/d PO q8–12h	False positive in Coombs' test, fever, leukopenia
Guanethidine	0.2 mg/kg/d PO	Postural hypotension, diarrhea, fluid retention
Vasodilators		
Hydralazine	0.75 mg/kg/d PO q4–6h	Nausea, diarrhea, lupus-like syndrome
Minoxidil	0.1–0.5 mg/kg/d PO bid	Fluid retention, tachycardia, hypertrichosis
Diazoxide	5 mg/kg IV	Hyperglycemia, hypertension
Nitroprusside	0.5–4.0 μg/kg/min IV	Hypotension, metabolic acidosis

Hypertensive crises are unusual in children with essential hypertension; they are more commonly a problem in hypertension due to renal disease. Administration of diazoxide usually produces a dramatic lowering of the blood pressure. Alternatively, sodium nitroprusside can be given as a continuous intravenous infusion, the dose titrated to the blood pressure.

Inflammatory Disease

Acute Rheumatic Fever

The incidence of acute rheumatic fever in the United States has fallen over the past century, in part because of the introduction of penicillin, but probably also as a result of the improvement in medical care and socioeconomic conditions. The cause, pathogenesis, and diagnostic criteria, including polyarthritis, chorea, erythema marginatum, subcutaneous nodules, fever, and evidence of a preceding streptococcal infection, are thoroughly discussed in many reviews.[30]

Signs and Symptoms The carditis associated with acute rheumatic fever results in mitral regurgitation and occasionally aortic regurgitation. Mitral regurgitation is recognized by a blowing holosystolic murmur that is best heard at the apex. In moderate-to-severe mitral regurgitation, the left ventricular impulse is increased and a third heart sound is present. The electrocardiogram may show PR-interval prolongation secondary to the rheumatic carditis or, if the regurgitation has been long-standing, left atrial and ventricular hypertrophy. The echocardiogram demonstrates left atrial and ventricular dilatation, which is usually proportional to the severity of the regurgitation.

Aortic regurgitation is characterized by a blowing decrescendo early diastolic murmur that is best heard at the left sternal border. The pulses are bounding if the regurgitation is hemodynamically significant, and the diastolic blood pressure is lowered. The echocardiogram shows left ventricular dilatation and mitral valve flutter. The electrocardiogram usually shows left ventricular hypertrophy.

Management Treatment of children with active carditis includes bed rest, aspirin (50 to 100 mg/kg/d) and, in severe cases, corticosteroids (prednisone, 1 mg/kg/d). The aspirin is continued for 6 weeks and the prednisone is tapered after 3 weeks. Patients should be placed on penicillin prophylaxis: either benzathine penicillin G, 1.2 million U/mo IM, or potassium penicillin G, 400,000 U/kg/d orally twice a day. Prophylaxis against subacute bacterial endocarditis should be added for those children with residual valvular regurgitation.

Children with chronic severe aortic or mitral regurgitation despite adequate anti-inflammatory treatment may be considered for valve replacement. Mitral or aortic stenosis can occur in the child who has had recurrent attacks, but otherwise the long-term prognosis is good in children with no residual murmurs.

Myocardiopathies

Myocardial inflammation or dysfunction is most frequently associated with systemic viral infections, usually from coxsackievirus A and B or echovirus. It also can be detected in children with severe systemic bacterial or fungal infections.[31] Endocardial fibroelastosis, a cause of congenital myocardial dysfunction, may be the end result of an intrauterine viral infection. Rare inborn metabolic errors, specifically carnitine deficiency and Pompe's disease, are associated with severe myocardial dysfunction. Drug-induced cardiomyopathies, usually from cyclophosphamide and doxorubicin hydrochloride, may be seen in children during cancer chemotherapy. Finally, myocardial ischemia and dysfunction may be signs of coronary artery anomalies, such as origin of the left coronary artery from the pulmonary artery.

Signs and Symptoms The diagnosis of viral myocarditis should be suspected in children with clinical evidence of left ventricular dysfunction, including dyspnea, tachycardia, tachypnea, and rales. A new finding of ectopic atrial or ventricular beats also can suggest subclinical myocarditis. The electrocardiogram is usually nonspecific, with PR-interval prolongation and ST segment T changes. In more severely affected cases, the echocardiogram shows a decreased ejection fraction and left ventricular dilatation.[11] Viral titers can indicate the infective organism. Myocardial dysfunction of nonviral etiology usually can be differentiated by the clinical setting or noninvasive studies.

Management Therapy of viral myocarditis is supportive and includes digoxin, diuretics, and afterload reduction when clinically indicated. Treatment of dysrhythmias, especially supraventricular and ventricular tachycardias, is important to decrease myocardial workload.

Mucocutaneous Lymph Node Syndrome

Originally described in Japan, mucocutaneous lymph node syndrome or Kawasaki syndrome is a systemic illness characterized by prolonged fever, conjunctival congestion, erythema of the oral cavity, a polymorphous exanthem of the trunk leading to desquamation, and nonpurulent cervical lymphadenopathy.[32]

Cardiac involvement has been reported to a varying degree in 20% of cases.[32] In the initial phase of the disease (0 to 9 days), acute pericarditis and myocarditis have been reported. Over the next 2 weeks, a panvasculitis can develop and result in the formation of coronary artery aneurysms or stenosis. In the ensuing weeks thrombosis and myocardial infarction can result, or involution of the aneurysms without infarction may occur. The cause is unknown.

Signs and Symptoms Diagnosis of the syndrome rests on the clinical features. Laboratory findings are usually nonspecific, although leukocytosis, thrombocytosis, and an elevated sedimentation rate are frequently seen.

Electrocardiographic abnormalities, including changes in PR and QTc prolongation and ST-T segment, are common but do not necessarily indicate coronary involvement. Two-dimensional echocardiography may demonstrate aneurysms of the proximal coronary arteries or any pericardial effusion. Coronary arteriography clearly identifies aneurysms and may be indicated in the child with evidence of ischemia.

Management Aspirin, 30 to 100 mg/kg/d, is the most frequent treatment. During the acute phase following resolution of fever, the dosage should be lowered to 5 to 10 mg/kg/d. This should be maintained until the sedimentation rate has returned to normal and the coronary arteries have been documented to be normal. Steroids may favor development of coronary artery aneurysms and should be avoided. Surgical treatment, including coronary artery bypass, is controversial and rarely performed.

Pericardial Diseases

Pericarditis and pericardial effusion are infrequent in childhood; they can occur as primary processes, usually infectious, or secondary to an underlying systemic illness.[33] Chest pain or fever can be the principal symptom of infectious pericarditis. The chest pain is often sharp, radiating to the neck, back, shoulders, and epigastrium, and is relieved by leaning forward. A friction rub is audible in some children and tends to be most prominent in children with small effusions. Large effusions impair cardiac function and result in venous distension and pulsus paradoxus. The typical electrocardiographic findings include ST-segment elevation without T-wave or QRS-complex abnormalities. Echocardiography delineates pericardial effusion if it is present.

Infectious pericarditis has viral, bacterial, and, rarely, tuberculous or fungal causes. Viral pericarditis is usually diagnosed in a child with a rub or effusion, fever, lymphocytosis, and no other source of infection. Pericardiocentesis can be useful to exclude other causes. Treatment is supportive. Aspirin may relieve the pain and reduce the inflammation; corticosteroids are rarely required.

Recurrent infectious pericarditis occurs in a minority of children. Staphylcoccal, streptococcal, pneumococcal, meningococcal, gonococcal, and *Haemophilus influenzae* pericarditis occur as primary infections or secondary to systemic infections. The diagnosis is made by pericardiocentesis, and surgical drainage is frequently necessary in addition to antibiotic therapy.

Noninfectious causes of pericarditis include systemic lupus erythematosus, rheumatoid arthritis, renal failure, metastatic tumors, and radiation therapy.

The postpericardiotomy syndrome is pericarditis or pericardial effusion following cardiac surgical procedures that require entering the pericardium. It is manifested usually by fever in the first postoperative week and may be diagnosed by the additional finding of a rub or pericardial effusion on echocardiogram. It occurs in one third of children over 2 years of age but is rare in infancy. Antiheart and antiviral antibody titers provide evidence of a dual viral and immunologic cause for this syndrome. It is usually self-limited. Treatment is supportive and includes aspirin.

Chest Pain

The differential diagnosis of chest pain includes disorders of the heart and blood vessels, chest wall, lungs, and gastrointestinal tract (Exhibit 10-4).

Myocardial ischemia in an otherwise normal heart is distinctly uncommon in children, in contrast to the adult population. Premature atherosclerosis as a complication of homozygous, type IIa familial hypercholesterolemia usually does not produce angina until the third decade. Subcutaneous xanthomas and a positive family history of myocardial infarction in early adulthood suggest this diagnosis. Structural defects producing myocardial ischemia include severe aortic stenosis and origin of the left coronary artery from the pulmonary artery. The former is readily diagnosed by physical examination; the latter is an unusual defect often manifest in infancy by severe myocardial failure.

As discussed previously, mitral valve prolapse

Exhibit 10-4 Differential Diagnosis of Chest Pain

- Cardiovascular
  - Mitral valve prolapse
  - Pericarditis
  - Premature ventricular contractions
  - Marfan's syndrome: aortic aneurysm
  - Pulmonary embolism
  - Premature atherosclerosis
    - Type IIa familial hypercholesterolemia
    - Progeria
  - Anomalous origin of left coronary artery from the pulmonary artery
  - Severe aortic stenosis
- Pulmonary
  - Pneumothorax
  - Pneumomediastinum
  - Pneumonia
  - Pleuritis
  - Mediastinal mass
  - Bronchial foreign body
- Chest Wall
  - Costochondritis
  - Trauma: rib fracture
  - Herpes zoster
- Gastrointestinal
  - Esophagitis
  - Diaphragmatic hernia

and pericarditis can be diagnosed on clinical and noninvasive grounds. Children with the Marfan syndrome have a distinctive body habitus. Echocardiography is useful in the Marfan syndrome as it frequently demonstrates a massively dilated aortic root and initial valve prolapse. Pulmonary embolism is extremely uncommon in childhood and could be recognized by sudden onset of severe chest pain, dyspnea, and right-sided heart failure. Lung scans and pulmonary angiography may confirm the diagnosis.

Pulmonary causes of chest pain are usually evident on the chest film. Local tenderness of the chest wall aids in the diagnosis of costochondritis or rib abnormalities. Gastrointestinal causes are suggested by pain relief after eating or aggravation in the supine position.

Syncope

The differential diagnosis of a child having a syncopal attack must include both cardiac and noncardiac causes. Cardiac conditions resulting in syncope include structural defects, usually left ventricular outflow tract obstruction; brady- and tachydysrhythmias; vasovagal attacks; and postural hypotension. Noncardiac causes include hypoglycemia, adrenocortical dysfunction, seizure disorders, and hyperventilation.

Signs and Symptoms

Syncope due to aortic valve stenosis, idiopathic hypertrophic subaortic stenosis, or discrete subaortic stenosis usually occurs in children with severe obstruction and is precipitated by exercise. In this setting the cardiac output cannot increase to meet the additional demand. Tachycardias, particularly ventricular tachycardia, can result in a rapid decrease in blood pressure, leading to dizziness or loss of consciousness. Children with chronic bradycardia as a result of congenital or postoperative complete heart block may remain asymptomatic because of a compensatory increase in the stroke volume, thus maintaining normal cardiac output. However, syncopal attacks can occur in such children, especially with exertion. Sick sinus syndrome is a dysfunction of the sinus node resulting in sinus or junctional bradycardia. The response of the heart rate to exercise may be normal; however, in the postexercise period the rate can drop below the resting rate as a result of further suppression of the sinus node and syncope can occur.

Vasovagal attacks are a frequent cause of syncope in an otherwise healthy child. Sharply increased vagal tone results in bradycardia, peripheral vasodilation, and syncope. Postural hypotension can be a side effect of antihypertensive medications or a manifestation of a variety of neurologic problems including familial dysautonomia and Guillain-Barré syndrome.

Supine and standing blood pressure measurements should be included in the physical examination of a child who has had a syncopal attack. Left ventricular hypertrophy or a dysrhythmia may be evident on the electrocardiogram. Frequently, 24-hour Holter monitoring is necessary to document brady- or tachydysrhythmias. An exercise test is particularly valuable for the child with sick sinus syndrome or exercise-induced syncope.

Management

Treatment is directed at the particular cause of the syncope. Children with left ventricular outflow tract obstruction should have it relieved if possible. Tachyrhythmias frequently can be managed medically with appropriate drugs. Bradyrhythmias may require implantation of a long-term artificial pacemaker.

Disorders of Conduction and Rhythm

First-Degree Heart Block

First-degree heart block is an electrocardiographic diagnosis and is defined as a PR interval greater than normal for age or heart rate. It can be found in otherwise normal children and be related to increased vagal tone. More commonly, it is associated with congenital heart defects, myocarditis, rheumatic fever, hyperthyroidism, hyperkalemia, and digoxin administration. There is no hemodynamic effect, and specific therapy beyond treatment of any underlying conditions is not indicated.

Second-Degree Heart Block: Wenckebach (Mobitz Type I)

In Wenckebach second-degree AV block, there is periodic failure of conduction from the atrium to the ventricle. The electrocardiogram shows progressive lengthening of the PR interval until the atrium fails to capture the ventricle, and the P wave is not followed by a QRS complex.

This condition is uncommon in normal children but can exist in children with congenital heart disease, especially after surgery. Children with Wenckebach periodicity are asymptomatic and no treatment is necessary. It can be an intermittent finding and is not prognostic of more severe conduction abnormalities.

Second-Degree Heart Block: Mobitz Type II

Mobitz type II second-degree AV block is never a normal finding and is seen principally in children after surgery or with electrolyte or central nervous system abnormalities. There is an abrupt failure of conduction from the atrium to the ventricle without any preceding prolongation of the PR interval. If every other P wave is blocked, it is a 2 : 1 AV block; blockage of every third P wave is a 3 : 2 AV block. If only one P wave of three is conducted, then a 3 : 1 AV block exists.

Children with higher grades of block (2 : 1, 3 : 1) may be symptomatic, and if the underlying cause cannot be corrected, therapy with atropine, isoproterenol, or pacing should be initiated. The administration of atropine alone carries some risk of increasing the sinus node rate, precipitating a higher degree of AV block. The net result is a lower ventricular rate. The addition of isoproterenol is useful in this circumstance to improve AV-node conduction.

Complete Heart Block

Complete heart block is the failure of conduction of the atrial depolarization into the ventricle, with a slower, unrelated junctional or ventricular rhythm (Figure 10-5). It can be a congenital abnormality, found particularly in children of mothers with collagen vascular disease. It also occurs as a transient or permanent problem after open heart surgery.

Children with complete congenital heart block without structural heart disease usually are initially asymptomatic. They generally have a relatively rapid (50 to 60 beats per minute) junctional pacemaker. However, with increasing age this junctional pacemaker gradually slows. At this time exercise intolerance, dizziness, or syncope may be evident. Children with associated congenital heart disease are more frequently symptomatic and may require treatment for both the anatomic and rhythm problems at an early age. Postoperative complete heart block, especially if not resolved in the first several weeks following operation, is often associated with a slower ventricular rather than junctional pacemaker. These children are thus more likely to be symptomatic if untreated.

A permanent ventricular pacemaker is the only reliable form of treatment for complete heart block. It is urgently indicated in any child who is symptomatic with dizziness or syncope. Documentation of slow ventricular rates (less than 40 beats per minute) on Holter monitoring, especially in younger children, also suggests the need for a pacemaker.

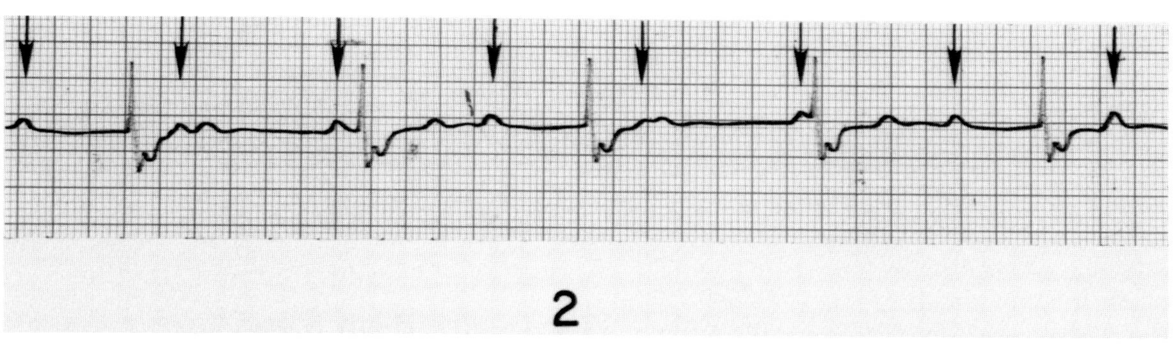

FIGURE 10-5 Electrocardiogram of a child with postoperative complete heart block showing an atrial rate of 68 beats per minute and a ventricular rate of 45 beats per minute.

Temporary pacing wires placed at surgery or transvenously are useful in the postoperative child while the need for permanent pacing is assessed. Permanent pacing with a demand pacemaker and epicardial leads placed by a limited thoracotomy is the preferred method in most children. Long-term follow-up for signs of battery or lead failure is essential.

Right Bundle-Branch Block

Right bundle-branch block is common in children after open heart surgery. The electrocardiogram shows prolongation (greater than 0.12 second) of the QRS duration and prominence of the right ventricular forces as a result of the muscle-to-muscle conduction to the right ventricle. There is an rsR′ pattern in V_1 and a deep, broad S wave in V_6 (Figure 10-6). Right bundle-branch block causes no symptoms and no treatment is indicated.

Left Bundle-Branch Block

Left bundle-branch block is very uncommon in children but occasionally is seen in children with cardiomyopathy or hemachromatosis. The pattern of left bundle-branch block—prolonged QRS duration with a wide, notched R wave in leads I and V_6, and a deep S wave in V_1—may be difficult to distinguish from severe left ventricular hypertrophy (Figure 10-7). No specific treatment is necessary.

Left Anterior Hemiblock

Left anterior hemiblock can occur after open heart surgery. The diagnosis is made by the new finding of left axis deviation on the electrocardiogram. Children with this condition are to be differentiated from those with congenital heart defects associated with left axis deviation; the latter are probably more accurately described as having an abnormal superior vector rather than true left anterior hemiblock. In the postoperative child left anterior hemiblock is often associated with right bundle-branch block. The QRS duration is normal in the absence of associated right bundle-branch block. The prognosis of isolated left anterior hemiblock is usually excellent, although some reports suggest an increased incidence of complete heart block or sudden death in children with postoperative right bundle-branch block and left anterior hemiblock.

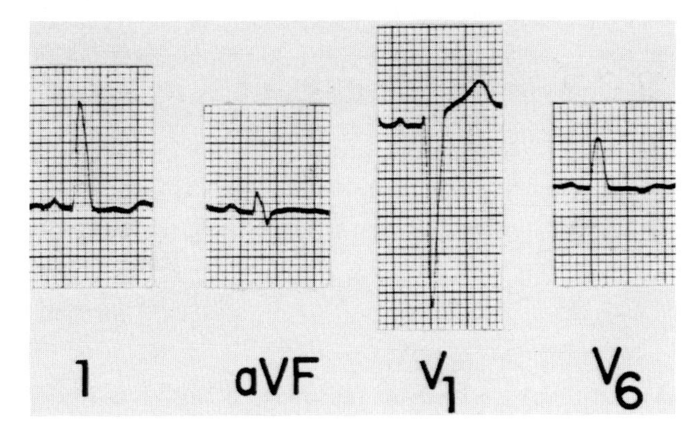

FIGURE 10-7 Left bundle-branch block with a QRS duration of 0.12 second and a broad R wave in V_6 and S wave in V_1.

Wolff-Parkinson-White Syndrome

Wolff-Parkinson-White syndrome is a preexcitation syndrome in which there is an accessory pathway bypassing the AV node. This results in a short PR interval, due to absence of the PR segment, and slurring of the upstroke and widening of the QRS complex on the electrocardiogram (Figure 10-8). The abnormal conduction does not alter the normal hemodynamics of the heart and the child is asymptomatic. There are two major types of Wolff-Parkinson-White syndrome: if the bypass tract is located posteriorly, then the QRS complex in lead V_1 is positive; conversely, if the bypass tract is anterior, the QRS complex in lead V_1 is predominantly negative.

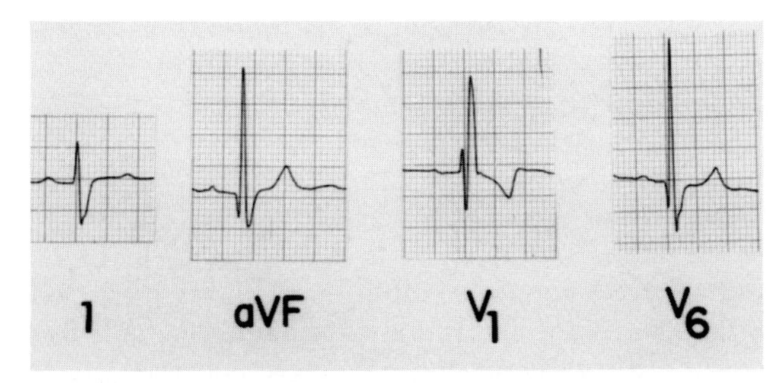

FIGURE 10-6 Broad S wave in leads V and V_6 with broad R′ in V_1 is characteristic of right bundle-branch block.

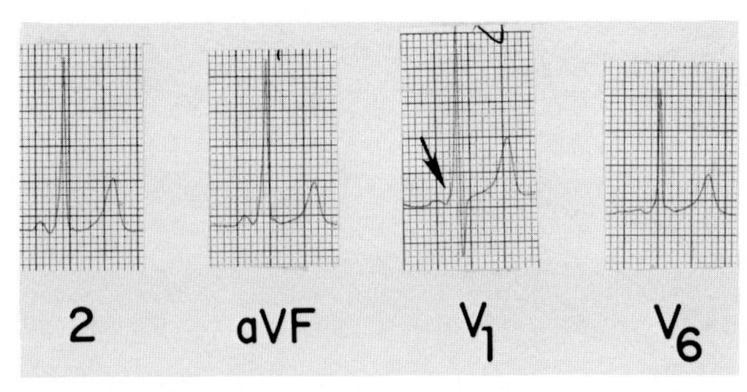

FIGURE 10-8 The delta wave (*arrow*) in this child with Wolff-Parkinson-White syndrome is best seen in lead V_1.

One third of the children with Wolff-Parkinson-White syndrome have congenital heart disease including ventricular septal defect, corrected transposition of the great arteries, and Ebstein's anomaly. Children with Wolff-Parkinson-White syndrome frequently, but not uniformly, develop episodes of supraventricular tachycardia resulting from reentry of the ventricular impulse into the ventricle via the accessary pathway.

Artificial Pacemaker

An artificial pacemaker results in a high-frequency electrical spike followed by a QRS complex on the electrocardiogram. Epicardial pacemakers placed on the left ventricle usually produce QRS complexes with a right bundle-branch block pattern (Figure 10-9). Endocardial, transvenous right ventricular pacemakers give rise to a QRS complex with a left bundle-branch block pattern. The RR interval is constant and fixed by the pacemaker's set rate. Failure of capture or suppression indicates pacemaker malfunction.

Sinus Rhythm

Sinus rhythm is the electrocardiogram diagnosis when the RR interval varies by less than 0.08 second and the P-wave axis is 0° to 90° (upright in leads I and aV_F)

Sinus Arrhythmia

Sinus arrhythmia is the normal increase of the heart rate with inspiration present in many children and adolescents. The diagnosis is made on the electrocardiogram when the RR interval varies without significant change in the P-wave configuration or PR interval. It results from changes in vagal tone and no treatment is indicated.

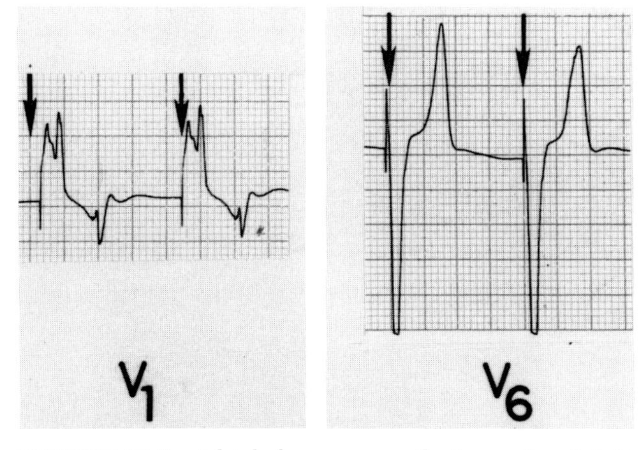

FIGURE 10-9 A high-frequency spike (*arrow*) and right bundle-branch pattern are found in children with left epicardial artificial pacemakers.

Sinus Bradycardia

Sinus bradycardia is a sustained slowing of the rate below the normal limits for age with a normal P-wave axis and PR interval. It can be found in normal, physically trained adolescents, usually long-distance runners, and is associated with a large stroke volume and mild cardiomegaly. In other children it indicates sinus node dysfunction. Twenty-four-hour ambulatory monitoring, exercise testing, and an electrocardiogram after atropine administration are useful in assessing the degree of sinus node impairment. Resumption of sinus rhythm after atropine suggests normal sinus node function with increased vagal tone. If the bradycardia is severe or symptoms of poor cardiac output are present, an artificial pacemaker is usually indicated.

Ectopic Atrial Rhythm

If the P-wave axis is consistently in a different quadrant than 0° to 90°, then the child is in an ectopic atrial rhythm. A P-wave axis of 90° to 180° (negative I, positive aV_F) suggests a high left atrial origin; 180° to 270° (negative I, negative aV_F) indicates a low left atrial focus; and 270° to 0° (positive I, negative aV_F) occurs with a low right atrial pacemaker. Although this may be a normal finding, an ectopic atrial rhythm can be the pacemaker in a child with the diagnosis of a sick sinus syndrome with abnormal slowing of the sinus node. Alternatively, abnormal automaticity of an ectopic atrial focus can produce an ectopic atrial tachycardia.

Wandering Atrial Pacemaker

Variation in vagal tone is also often responsible for a wandering atrial pacemaker. When sinus node slowing occurs, a second atrial focus, as indicated by a different P-wave axis, assumes the pacemaker role. The QRS morphology is unchanged. A wandering atrial pacemaker is differentiated from a premature atrial contraction by the increased RR interval of the former, in contrast to the RR interval of the latter, which is shorter than the underlying sinus rate. Usually this rhythm is found in asymptomatic normal children, although it can be seen in children with hyperkalemia or digitalis intoxication, or after cardiac surgery.

Premature Atrial Contraction

A premature atrial contraction is diagnosed when a normal QRS complex comes early and is preceded by a P wave with a different configuration and after shorter PR interval than the normal sinus beats (Figure 10-10). Similarly, a junctional premature beat occurs when a P wave cannot be identified or when it follows the premature beat. If the ectopic P

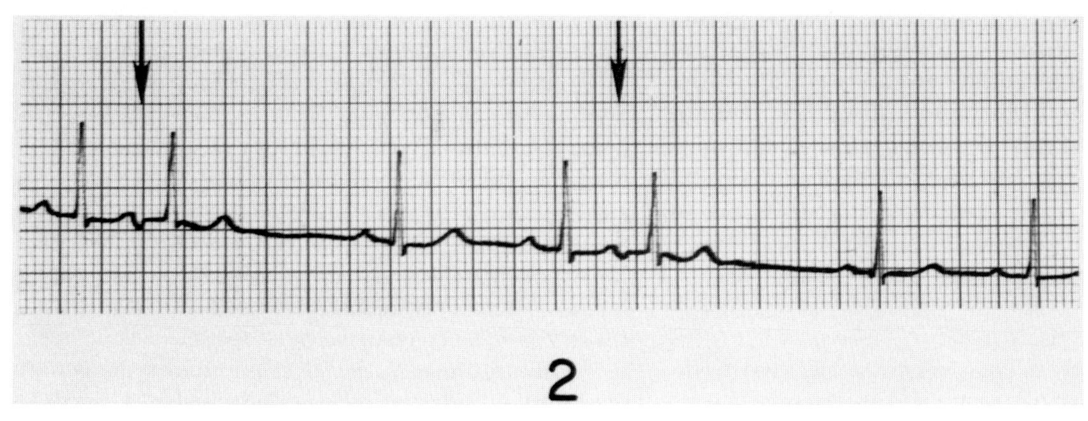

FIGURE 10-10 Short RR interval, biphasic P wave (*arrows*) and normal QRS morphology attributable to premature atrial contractions.

wave is very premature, it may find the ventricle refractory and a blocked premature atrial contraction results. The RR interval following the premature beat may be only slightly prolonged, and the interval between the preceding and following normal beats is less than twice the normal RR interval. Premature atrial contractions are found in normal children, including newborns, and in children with mitral valve prolapse, digitalis intoxication, or excessive sympathomimetic stimulation. The last can occur with asthma, cold medications, or caffeine-containing beverages. In general, with the exception of digitalis intoxication, isolated premature atrial contractions are benign and require no therapy. In the newborn they usually resolve spontaneously during the first few weeks of life.

Premature Atrial Contraction with Aberrancy

If an atrial or junctional focus depolarizes prematurely and the ventricles have not fully repolarized from the previous beat, the impulse may be conducted through the ventricles aberrantly. This results in a wide QRS complex, usually but not always with a right bundle-branch block pattern (Figure 10-11). On the surface electrocardiogram these

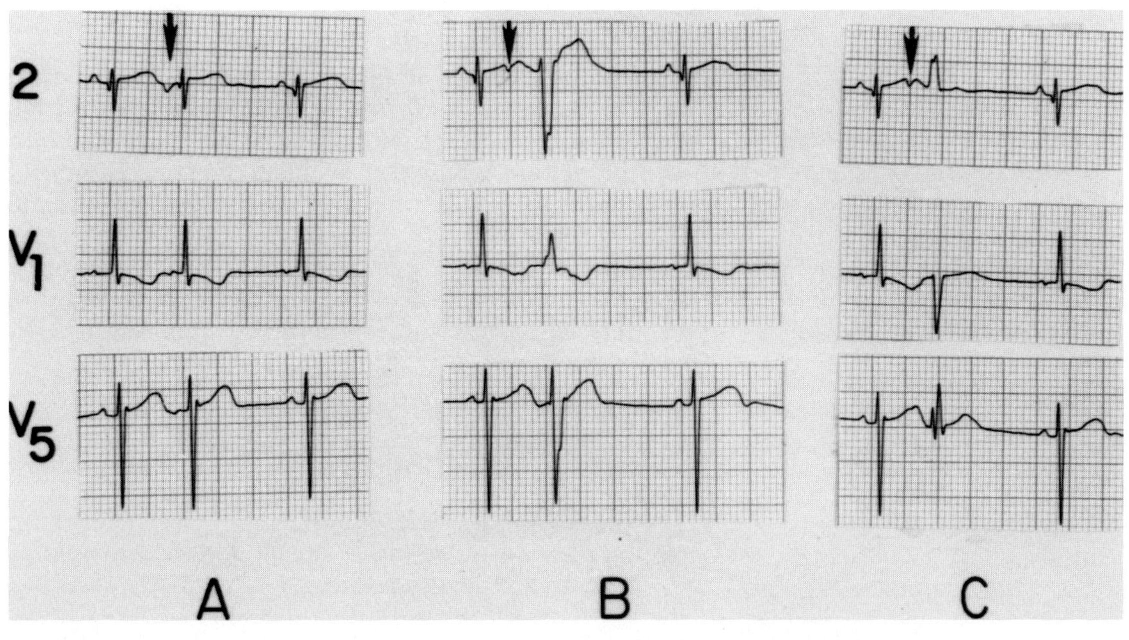

FIGURE 10-11 A, Premature contraction. B, Premature atrial contraction with right bundle-branch block aberrancy. C, Premature atrial contraction with left bundle-branch block aberrancy. P waves are best seen in lead II (*arrows*). Right ventricular hypertrophy is normal in this newborn.

beats can be difficult to differentiate from premature ventricular contractions. Premature P waves preceding the wide QRS complex suggest a supraventricular origin. Normally conducted premature atrial contractions on the same tracing also make premature atrial contractions with aberrancy a more likely diagnosis. The cause and management are similar to those of premature atrial contractions with normal conduction.

Junctional Rhythm

Junctional rhythm occurs when a site distal to the atria serves as the pacemaker. A normal QRS complex without identifiable P waves is found on the electrocardiogram. It may be seen for brief periods in normal children. An accelerated junctional rhythm occurs in some children after heart surgery. A slow junctional rhythm can suggest a sick sinus syndrome or increased vagal tone. In the latter case atropine (0.01 mg/kg IV or SC) or exercise returns the child to sinus rhythm, and either is a useful diagnostic test.

Atrioventricular Dissociation

AV dissociation is a form of junctional rhythm in which P waves are independent of the QRS complex (Figure 10-12). The junctional rate is slightly faster than the atrial rate, and the junctional impulse is not conducted retrograde into the atria. This is commonly seen in the postoperative child and is associated with an accelerated junctional pacemaker. Treatment is not necessary in the asymptomatic child.

Supraventricular Tachycardia

A sustained, rapid (up to 300 beats per minute) heart rate with normal QRS morphology, with or without identifiable P waves, is called supraventricular tachycardia (Figure 10-13). The RR interval is usually uniform. It should be differentiated from a sinus tachycardia resulting from fever or agitation, in which the heart rate is only mildly elevated, normal P waves are present, and some variability of the rate is documented.

Supraventricular tachycardia may be well tolerated for 12 to 24 hours by a child with a normal heart. In the child with structural heart disease or in the immediate postoperative period, it can result in signs and symptoms of poor cardiac output. Children at increased risk of developing supraventricular tachycardia include those with mitral valve prolapse, Wolff-Parkinson-White syndrome, and a history of extensive atrial surgery.

If the child is not critically ill, nonpharmacologic treatment is initially indicated. Some older children in supraventricular tachycardia respond to maneuvers that increase vagal tone, such as vagal stimulation, gagging, or the Valsalva maneuver. Infants frequently convert to sinus rhythm after facial stimulation with a cold, wet compress.

Digoxin is often an effective treatment within several hours for the asymptomatic child. For those children who are hemodynamically compromised, verapamil, 0.1 to 0.5 mg/kg by slow IV injection, is an effective short-term treatment for supraventricular tachycardia. It can produce severe hypotension and must be used with caution, especially in children under 1 year of age. Concern has been raised regarding the use of digoxin and verapamil in patients with Wolff-Parkinson-White syndrome since these drugs may enhance rapid ventricular conduction during atrial fibrillation or flutter. This, however, is rarely encountered in the pediatric patient. Alternative short-term treatments include propranolol, 0.05 to 0.1 mg/kg IV; phenylephrine, 0.01 to 0.1 mg/kg IV; or edrophonium, 0.2 mg/kg IV. Cardioversion with 0.25 to 1.0 W · s/kg or overdrive pacing should be utilized for critically ill children or when other modalities have failed.

Long-term therapy should be instituted if the episodes of tachycardia are frequent or disabling. Frequently children and their parents can be reassured that the episodes in the otherwise healthy child are not dangerous and are frequently self-limited. Di-

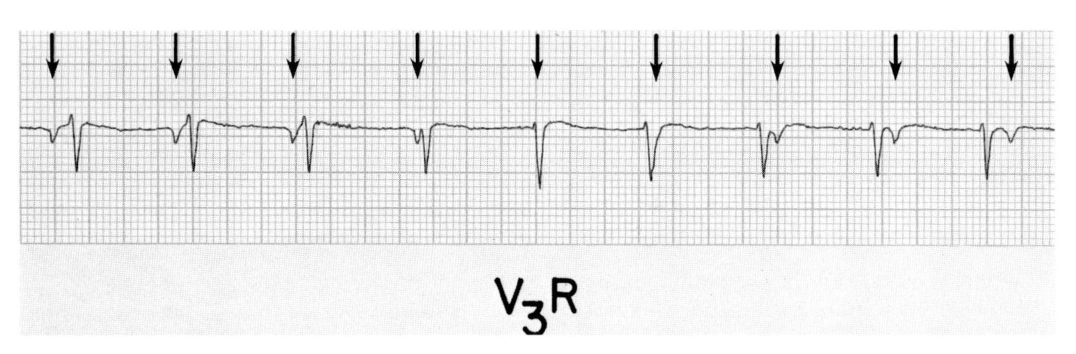

FIGURE 10-12 AV dissociation in a postoperative child.

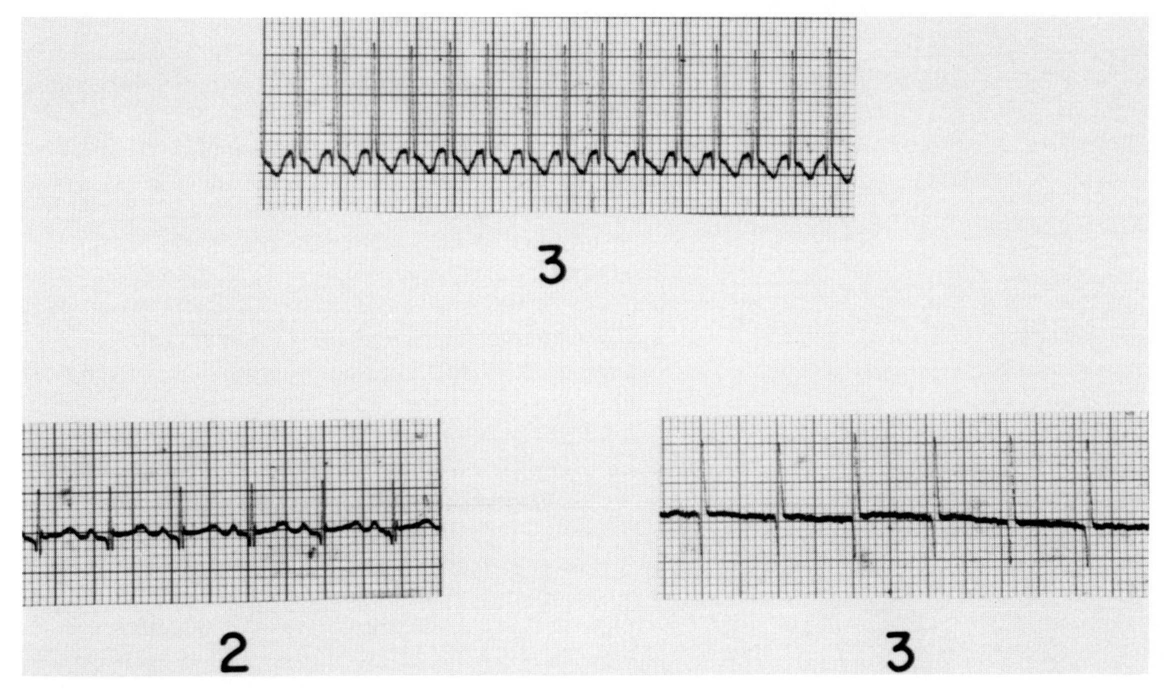

FIGURE 10-13 *Top,* Supraventricular tachycardia in a newborn with a rate of 300 beats per minute. *Bottom,* Following conversion, P waves are visible in lead II at a rate of 150 beats per minute.

goxin, 10 to 15 μg/kg/d orally, remains the drug of choice for supraventricular tachycardia in the first year of life. Frequently if the child remains tachycardia free at 1 year of age, the drug can be discontinued without recurrence of symptoms. Older children or those with resistant tachycardia can be started on propranolol, 0.5 to 1.5 mg/kg orally every 6 hours, or quinidine sulfate, 7.5 to 20 mg/kg orally every 6 hours. In selected cases verapamil, 1 to 5 mg/kg orally per dose every 8 hours, can also be effective. Serum drug levels, when available, and Holter monitoring should guide therapy. Ventricular function should be followed with echocardiography for those children with refractory tachycardia. Surgical ablation of accessory pathways can be offered to children with Wolff-Parkinson-White syndrome and refractory tachycardia.

Atrial Flutter

Rapid, regular atrial depolarization at a rate greater than 300 beats per minute is usually due to atrial flutter. It can follow atrial surgery, such as the Mustard operation for transposition of the great arteries, or can be seen less frequently in the first few months of life in an otherwise healthy child. Although each atrial impulse may be conducted and depolarize the ventricles, frequently 2 : 1 or 3 : 1 second-degree heart block occurs, resulting in a ventricular rate that is a fraction of the atrial rate. The diagnosis of atrial flutter with 2 : 1 block can be suspected on the physical examination in a child with a sustained tachycardia that does not vary with activity.

The "saw-toothed" baseline or flutter waves on the electrocardiogram of a child in atrial flutter are best recognized in leads II, III, aV_F, and V_1 (Figure 10-14). The RR interval depends on the degree of AV block and is a multiple of flutter wave interval.

Pharmacologic management of atrial flutter with digoxin and quinidine is frequently successful. The digoxin must be administered prior to the quinidine to increase the refractory period of the AV node. This prevents the 1 : 1 conduction that can result from the quinidine-induced decrease in the flutter rate and AV-node refractory period. If atrial flutter persists despite adequate blood levels of quinidine and digoxin, or if the child has signs of poor cardiac output, then DC cardioversion nearly always results in sinus rhythm. Long-term control is possible in some children with digoxin alone. If atrial flutter recurs on digoxin, then quinidine or propranolol can be added.

Atrial Fibrillation

Atrial fibrillation is an unusual rhythm in children. The atrial depolarization is extremely active and ir-

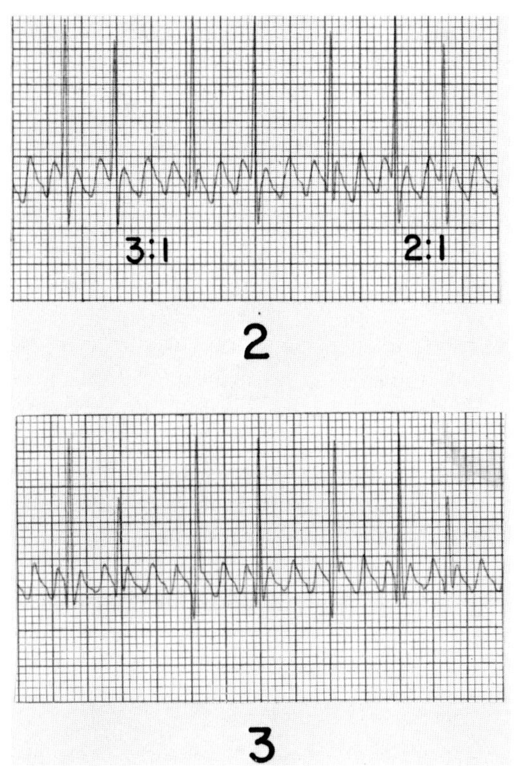

FIGURE 10-14 Atrial flutter with an atrial rate of 500 beats per minute and variable second-degree heart block.

regular. P waves cannot be identified on the electrocardiogram and the baseline is erratic. The ventricular response is variable and the RR interval is irregular.

Digoxin often shows the ventricular rate but does not usually result in sinus rhythm. Cardioversion can be effective in children without long-standing atrial fibrillation. Overdrive suppression is not successful.

Premature Ventricular Contraction

Premature ventricular contractions are common in children with structurally normal hearts as well as in children with congenital heart disease. They can be precipitated by medications such as aminophylline or epinephrine or by excessive consumption of caffeine-containing beverages.

The electrocardiographic features of a premature ventricular contraction are an early, wide QRS complex without preceding P wave; an abnormal T-wave axis; and a different direction of initial activation (Figure 10-15). If the ventricular depolarization is not conducted retrograde into the atria, then the interval between the previous and following complex is twice the normal RR interval (fully compensatory pause).

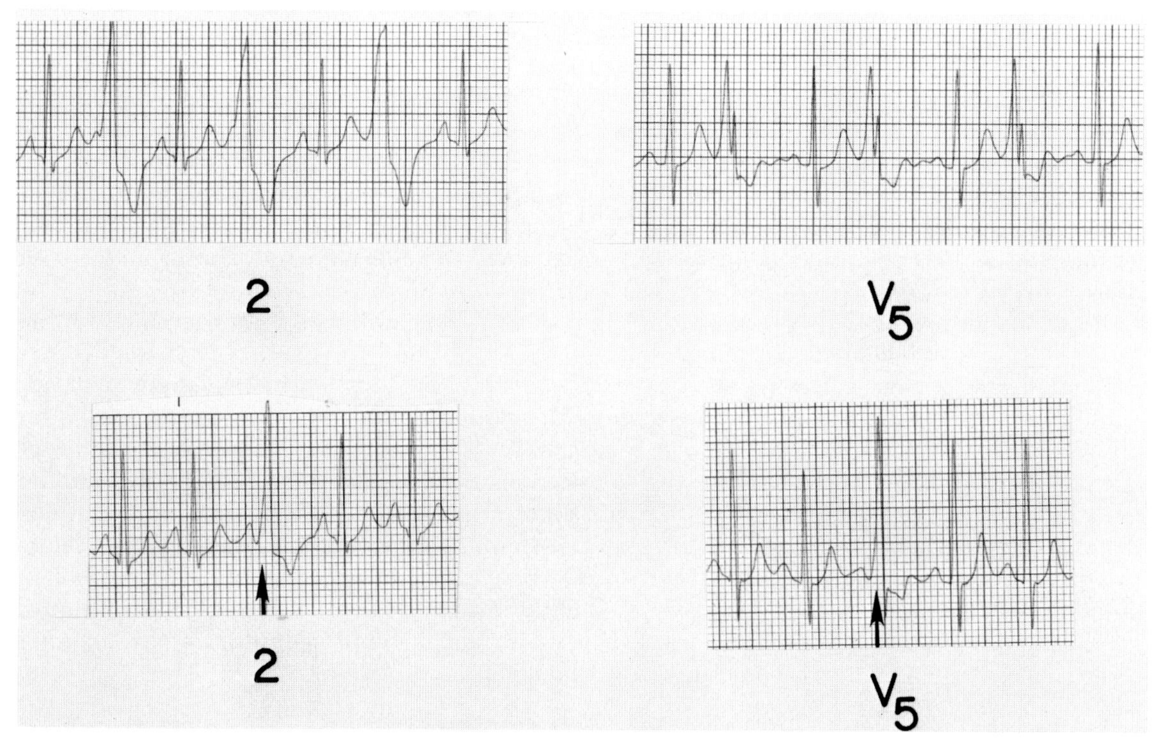

FIGURE 10-15 *Top,* Ventricular bigeminy with alternating sinus beats and premature ventricular contractions. *Bottom,* sinus rhythm with a fusion beat (*arrow*).

Most isolated premature ventricular contractions in children are benign and not associated with more serious ventricular dysrhythmias. Benign premature ventricular contractions are usually unifocal and decrease in frequency with exercise. The coupling interval between the previous normal heart beat and the premature ventricular contraction is fixed and longer than the QT interval. In contrast, premature ventricular contractions that can precipitate ventricular tachycardia or fibrillation are multifocal, variably coupled, and increased by exercise. Premature ventricular contractions after open-heart surgery, especially total correction of tetralogy of Fallot when there is persistent right ventricular hypertension, have been associated with sudden death and should be carefully evaluated.

Twenty-four-hour ambulatory monitoring provides an estimate of the frequency of premature ventricular contractions and identifies periods of ventricular tachycardia. Echocardiography can be useful as part of the assessment for children with structural heart disease, mitral valve prolapse, or cardiomyopathies.

The child with benign premature ventricular contractions should be reassured and permitted normal activity. Even frequent premature ventricular contractions including bigeminy, in the absence of myocardial ischemia, may be well tolerated and not require therapy. If further evaluation indicates a more serious dysrhythmia such as ventricular tachycardia, then specific therapy should be directed toward that dysrhythmia.

Ventricular Tachycardia

Ventricular tachycardia is a serious, and if sustained, life-threatening dysrhythmia. It is a result of rapid (120 to 200 beats per minute), regular depolarization of the ventricles. This is usually associated with a decreased stroke volume and thus a fall in cardiac output and blood pressure. It can occur in children with electrolyte imbalances such as hypokalemia, hyperkalemia, hypoglycemia, hypoxia, or acidosis, especially after cardiac surgery or during an episode of myocarditis. Drugs including isoproterenol, dopamine, and dobutamine can precipitate ventricular tachycardia, as well as toxic levels of digoxin or quinidine.

The electrocardiogram shows three or more wide (greater than 0.09 seconds) QRS complexes, usually with inverted T waves (Figure 10-16). The morphology of the complexes is most frequently a left bundle-branch block pattern, although right bundle-branch block may be seen. Although unusual in children, supraventricular tachycardia with aberrancy must be differentiated from ventricular tachycardia. Ventricular tachycardia is diagnosed by the presence of fusion beats (Figure 10-15) or AV dissociation. Documentation of premature atrial contractions with normal conduction in a child with wide QRS-complex tachycardia suggests a supraventricular origin. Similarly, isolated premature ventricular contractions support the diagnosis of ventricular tachycardia.

Acute ventricular tachycardia with hemodynamic instability should be treated with synchronized DC cardioversion, 1 to 2 W · s/kg, and correction, if possible, of any underlying cause. Alternatively, if the child's hemodynamic condition permits, lidocaine, 1 mg/kg by IV push followed by an IV infusion at 20 to 50 μg/kg/min, may terminate the tachycardia or prevent its recurrence after cardioversion. If these measures fail, brief ventricular pacing at a rate slightly higher than the tachycardia can be useful.

Chronic ventricular tachycardia can be an extremely difficult management problem requiring multiple drug therapies, including phenytoin, quinidine, and propranolol. The initial choice of drug can be guided by its effect during an invasive electrophysiologic study. Serial 24-hour Holter monitoring and measurement of serum blood levels

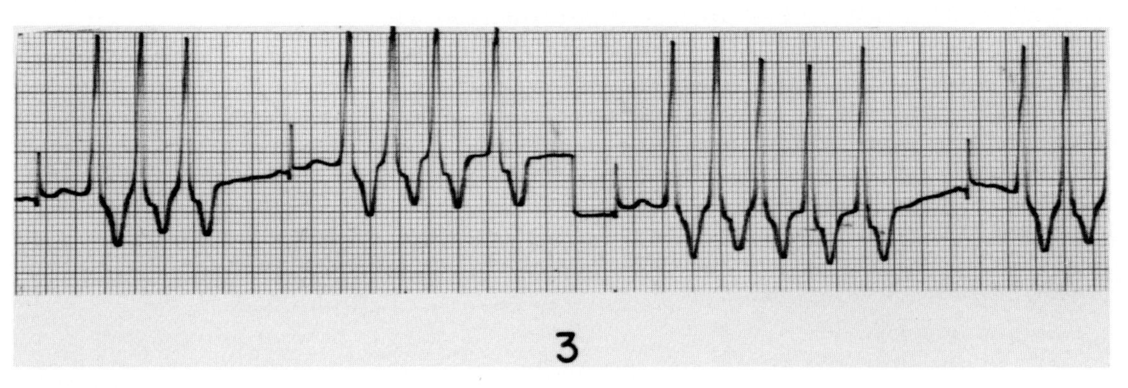

FIGURE 10-16 Repeated short bursts of ventricular tachycardia in an asymptomatic 4-year-old child.

are essential to assess the status of pharmacologic therapy.

MEDICAL MANAGEMENT OF HEART DISEASE AND ITS COMPLICATIONS

Cardiac Failure

Exhibit 10-2 summarizes the differential diagnosis of a child who has the signs or symptoms of congestive heart failure.

Digoxin

Digoxin traditionally has been administered to children with symptoms of congestive heart failure, either as a result of myocardial dysfunction or excessive pulmonary blood flow, although the latter indication is the source of recent debate. It is also the drug of choice in infants for the treatment of supraventricular tachycardia.

The loading dose of 40 μg/kg IV for IM (maximum, 1000 μg) is divided into an initial dose of 20 μg/kg and followed by 10 μg/kg every 8 hours for two doses. Maintenance therapy usually begins at 10 μg/kg IV or IM divided twice a day and can be increased to 15 μg/kg. Oral doses are approximately 20% greater than intravenous doses.

Side effects of digoxin include bradycardia, heart block, premature atrial and ventricular contractions, and vomiting; PR-interval prolongation or ST-segment changes are indications of digoxin effect, not toxicity. Toxicity can be precipitated by the simultaneous administration of quinidine. Digoxin levels are useful in the diagnosis of intoxication, although children with high levels (2.0 to 4.0 ng/mL) are frequently asymptomatic.

Digoxin intoxication should be treated by stopping the drug and correcting hypokalemia, if present. Phenytoin is administered for AV block or premature ventricular contractions. Bradycardia is treated with atropine or pacing.

Diuretics

Diuretics are useful in the management of fluid retention, especially in the lungs, as a result of left-to-right shunts or left ventricular failure. Furosemide, either orally or parentally, is most frequently used, beginning with 1 mg/kg as required and increasing as needed to 3 mg/kg every 6 to 8 hours. Electrolyte abnormalities, including hypokalemic hypochloremic alkalosis, must be carefully monitored and treated by dietary management or supplemental potassium chloride (1 to 3 mEq/kg/d). Alternatively, spironolactone is added to help limit furosemide-induced potassium loss. Other side effects of furosemide include ototoxicity, hyperuricemia, and nausea.

Inotropic Agents

Drugs to improve myocardial contractility and increase blood pressure or cardiac output are most frequently required in the postoperative period, although they can benefit children with left ventricular dysfunction at any time during the course of their disease.

Isoproterenol is a strong β-agonist, having both inotropic and chronotropic effects on the heart and stimulating peripheral vasodilatation. The usual net effect is an increase in heart rate and cardiac output and no change in blood pressure. It is administered by continuous IV infusion, beginning at 0.1 μg/kg/min. Tachycardia often limits the increase in the dose. Another important side effect is ventricular premature contractions, which resolve when the dose is lowered.

Dopamine is another endogenous catecholamine that in low doses (less than 5 μg/kg/min) increases renal blood flow by stimulating the dopaminergic receptors and improves urine output. At higher doses (5 to 10 μg/kg/min), it improves cardiac contractility and increases arterial pressure. Above 20 μg/kg/min, there is increased α-adrenergic receptor stimulation leading to vasoconstriction. This vasoconstriction includes the renal bed, and urine output may decrease. Tachycardia is usually less marked than that associated with isoproterenol.

Dobutamine is a synthetic catecholamine whose inotropic effects are similar to but whose chronotropic effects are less than dopamine and isoproterenol. It has a moderate peripheral effect resulting in vasodilatation. It is administered by continuous IV infusion at 2 to 10 μg/kg/min.

Vasodilators

Afterload reduction can benefit those children with congestive heart failure attributable to poor left ventricular function or mitral regurgitation. Sodium nitroprusside can be used intravenously for an acute problem, and hydralazine can be utilized for long-term management. Fluid retention often occurs and a diuretic also should be administered. Hypotension can limit the dosage of these drugs, especially in the case of nitroprusside.

The typical starting dose of nitroprusside is 1.0 μg/kg/min, which then can be adjusted according to the clinical status of the child. Oral hydralazine can be started at 0.75 mg/kg/d divided every 6 hours and increased slowly to 0.75 to 3.0 mg/kg/d as needed.

Prostaglandin E_1

Prostaglandin E_1 is an effective, palliative therapy in neonates with "ductus-dependent" defects—e.g., severe tetralogy of Fallot, tricuspid atresia, pulmonary atresia, and coarctation of the aorta arch interruption—who are symptomatic as a result of spontaneous ductal closure.[9] Administration of prostaglandin E_1, 0.1 μg/kg/min IV, results in rapid dilatation of the ductus arteriosus in almost all newborns less than 4 days old and occasionally in infants up to 2 weeks old. In infants with decreased pulmonary blood flow, ductal dilatation restores the pulmonary blood flow to a level that usually results in an increase of the Pa_{O_2} to 40 mmHg. This is often adequate to reverse the metabolic abnormalities resulting from hypoxia. Infants with coarctation of the aorta respond to prostaglandin E_1 administration and ductal dilatation by improvement of the blood flow distal to the coarctation, thus reversing the metabolic acidosis resulting from poor perfusion. Another group of newborns that can benefit from ductal dilatation are those with transposition of the great arteries. In these children, creating a shunt from the aorta to pulmonary artery increases the left-to-right atrial shunt after balloon septostomy. This is usually only necessary if the P_{O_2} falls below 25 mmHg.

The short-term side effects of prostaglandin E_1 include apnea, seizures, tremors, and fever. Bradycardia and hypotension are possible, especially after intra-aortic injection. Since prostaglandin E_1 inhibits platelet aggregation, bleeding complications are possible but rare.[34] These side effects may abate at a lower edge.

Administration of prostaglandin E_1 should be viewed as a short-term lifesaving therapy. Transport of the infant to a center equipped for neonatal cardiac catheterization and cardiovascular surgery should be arranged as promptly as possible.

Diet

A diet with an adequate caloric supply for growth and an appropriate balance of protein, carbohydrate, and fat is particularly important for children with congenital heart disease and symptoms of congestive heart failure. Congestive heart failure increases the caloric needs of the infant and at the same time tachypnea interferes with the infant's ability to consume even a normal volume of formula. Formulas with a high caloric density, up to 1 calorie/mL, must be used to provide these extra calories without an excessive fluid load. Actual fluid and salt restriction in the infant is usually not necessary, especially when diuretics are part of the medical management.

In the older child a no-added-salt diet without a fluid limit is usually well tolerated. Supplementing the normal diet with milkshakes can help maintain an adequate caloric intake.

Iron deficiency can occur, particularly in the child with cyanotic heart disease. In the absence of blood loss, anemia is unusual; however, iron deficiency diagnosed on the basis of microcytosis should be treated by iron supplementation.

Exhibit 10-5 Recommendations for and against Endocarditis Prophylaxis

High Risk Conditions: Endocarditis Prophylaxis Recommended
- Prosthetic cardiac valves including biosynthetic valves
- Most congenital heart defects
- Surgically constructed systemic-pulmonary shunts
- Rheumatic and other acquired valvular dysfunction
- Idiopathic hypertrophic subaortic stenosis
- Previous history of bacterial endocarditis
- Mitral valve prolapse with insufficiency

Low-Risk Conditions: Endocarditis Prophylaxis Not Recommended
- Isolated secundum atrial septal defect
- Isolated secundum atrial septal defect repaired without a patch at least 6 months earlier
- Patent ductus arteriosus ligated and divided at least 6 months earlier

Procedures for Which Endocarditis Prophylaxis Is Indicated
- All dental procedures likely to induce gingival bleeding (not simple adjustment of orthodontic appliances or shedding of deciduous teeth)
- Tonsillectomy and/or adenoidectomy
- Surgical procedures or biopsy involving the respiratory mucosa
- Bronchoscopy, especially with a rigid bronchoscope
- Incision and drainage of infected tissue
- Genitourinary/gastrointestinal (GI) procedures: cystoscopy, urethral catheterization (especially in the presence of infection), urinary tract surgery, colonic surgery, esophageal dilatation, colonoscopy, upper GI endoscopy with biopsy or protosigmoidoscopy with biopsy

Procedures for Which Endocarditis Prophylaxis Is Not Recommended, Especially for Low-Risk Patients
- Percutaneous liver biopsy
- Barium enema
- Uncomplicated vaginal delivery
- Brief bladder catheterization with sterile urine
- Uterine dilation and curettage*
- Cesarean section*
- Therapeutic abortion*
- Sterilization or insertion or removal of intrauterine devices*

* If infection is not suspected.

Complications

Cyanotic Spells

Cyanotic spells should be treated promptly by placing the child in the knee-chest position and administering morphine, 0.1 mg/kg SC or IV. If the spell continues, propranolol at a dose of 0.15 mg/kg IV, or phenylephrine at a dose of 0.1 mg/kg SC or IM or 0.01 μg/kg/dose IV can be given. Surgical palliation or correction should be undertaken at the earliest opportunity to prevent further spells. If this is not possible and the spells recur, then propranolol at 1 to 2 mg/kg orally every 6 hours may prevent further episodes.

Bacterial Endocarditis

All children with congenital heart disease, with the exception of an uncomplicated secundum atrial septal defect, are at increased risk of subacute bacterial endocarditis and should receive appropriate antibiotic prophylaxis at the time of dental, upper respiratory, gastrointestinal, and genitourinary procedures (Exhibit 10-5 and Table 10-8). This does not include the natural shedding of deciduous teeth, but care should be taken by the child and parents not to prematurely pull the tooth out and cause excessive bleeding.

The diagnosis of bacterial endocarditis is best made on the basis of fever; hepatosplenomegaly; evidence of vegetations, emboli, or immunologic reaction; and positive blood cultures. A change in the murmur is a late sign of endocarditis. Positive blood cultures without systemic signs do not necessarily make the diagnosis since a bacteremia can be associated with pneumonia or other localized infections. Echocardiography is useful to help localize vegetations, although in some lesions such as coarctation, ventricular septal defect, and many of the cyanotic defects with shunts, vegetations are not found on the valves.

TABLE 10-8 Prophylaxis against Bacterial Endocarditis

	Older Children and Adolescents	Children Less Than 60 lb (27 kg) (total dose not to exceed adult dose)
Dental and upper respiratory tract procedures		
Standard regimen	Penicillin V, 2.0 g orally 1 h before; then 1.0 g 6 h later For patients unable to take oral medications, 2 million U of aqueous penicillin G IV or IM 30–60 min before procedure; then 1 million U 6 h later	Penicillin V, 1.0 g orally 1 h before; then 0.5 g 6 h later For patients unable to take oral medications, aqueous penicillin G, 50,000 U/kg IV or IM 30–60 min before procedure; then 25,000 U/kg 6 h later
Special, regimens		
Parenteral regimen for use when maximal protection is needed, e.g., for patients with artificial valves or shunts	Ampicillin, 1.0–2.0 g IM or IV, plus gentamicin, 1.5 mg/kg IM or IV, 30 min before procedure; then 1.0 g oral penicillin V 6 h later. Alternatively, parenteral regimen can be repeated once 8 h later	Ampicillin, 50 mg/kg IM or IV, plus gentamicin, 2.0 mg/kg IM or IV 30 min before procedure; then 0.5 g oral penicillin V 6 h later. Alternatively, parenteral regimen can be repeated once 8 h later
Oral regimen for penicillin-allergic patients	Erythromycin, 1.0 g orally 1 h before; then 500 mg 6 h later	Erythromycin, 20 mg/kg orally 1 h before; then 10 mg/kg 6 h later
Parenteral regimen for penicillin-allergic patients	Vancomycin, 1.0 g IV slowly over 1 h, starting 1 h before. No repeat dose is necessary	Vancomycin, 20 mg/kg IV slowly over 1 h, starting 1 h before. No repeat dose is necessary
Gastrointestinal and genitourinary procedures		
Standard regimen	Ampicillin, 2.0 g IM or IV, plus gentamicin, 1.5 mg/kg IM or IV, 30–60 min before procedure. One follow-up dose can be given 8 h later	Ampicillin, 50 mg/kg IM or IV, plus gentamicin, 2.0 mg/kg IM or IV 30–60 min before procedure. One follow-up dose can be given 8 h later
Special regimens		
Oral regimen for minor or repetitive procedures in low-risk patients	Amoxicillin, 3.0 g orally 1 h before procedure; then 1.5 g 6 h later	Amoxicillin, 50 mg/kg orally 1 h before procedure; then 25 mg/kg 6 h later
Penicillin-allergic patients	Vancomycin, 1.0 g IV slowly over 1 h, plus gentamicin, 1.5 mg/kg IM or IV given 1 h before procedure. Can be repeated 8–12 h later	Vancomycin, 20 mg/kg IV slowly over 1 h, plus gentamicin, 2.0 mg/kg IM or IV given 1 h before procedure. Can be repeated 8–12 h later

Antibiotic therapy should be tailored to achieve bactericidal levels of an antibiotic directed at the documented or suspected pathogen for 4 to 6 weeks.

Central Nervous System Complications

Children with polycythemia, especially those with hematocrits greater than 65%, are at risk for strokes. Dehydration should be particularly avoided since it results in further hemoconcentration, and thus it should be treated promptly with fluid administration. Particular care must be taken to keep intravenous lines free of air because in children with right-to-left shunts, these air emboli can move from the systemic venous circulation into the cerebral arterial circulation.

A partial exchange transfusion with fresh frozen plasma can benefit children after a stroke or those who are suffering headache, chest pain, or dyspnea from polycythemia.

Brain abscess is another complication to which children with right-to-left shunts are prone. The diagnosis should be suspected in any child with fever and neurologic symptoms or signs. It can be confirmed by computed axial tomography. Treatment is by surgical drainage and appropriate antibiotic therapy.

Hemoptysis

Hemoptysis is a problem in adolescents and adults with pulmonary hypertension and cyanosis (Eisenmenger's complex). The bleeding can be brisk and is a recognized cause of death in some patients. Treatment is largely supportive. If bleeding continues and the site can be localized by pulmonary arteriography, then embolization of the vessel may be possible.

References

1. Nora JJ, Nora AH: The evolution of specific genetic and environmental counseling in congenital heart diseases. *Circulation* 1978;57:205–213.
2. Noonan JA: Syndromes associated with cardiac defects. *Cardiovasc Clin* 1980;11:97–116.
3. Lees MH: Cyanosis of the newborn infant: Recognition and clinical evaluation. *J Pediatr* 1970;77:484–498.
4. Keith JD, Rowe RD, Vlad P (eds): *Heart Disease in Infancy and Childhood*, ed 3. New York, Macmillan Publishing Co Inc, 1978.
5. Lange LW, Sahn DJ, Allen HD, et al: Subxiphoid cross-sectional echocardiography in infants and children with congenital heart disease. *Circulation* 1979;59:513–524.
6. Sahn DJ, Allen HD, Goldberg SJ, et al: Pediatric echocardiography: A review of its clinical utility. *J Pediatr* 1975;87:335–352.
7. Fyler DC (co-director): Report of the New England regional infant cardiac program. *Pediatrics* 1980;65(suppl):377–461.
8. Morgan BC, Guntheroth WG, Bloom RS, et al: A clinical profile of paroxysmal hyperpnea in cyanotic congenital heart disease. *Circulation* 1965;31:66–69.
9. Freed MD, Heymann MA, Lewis AB, et al: Prostaglandin E_1 in infants with ductus arteriosus-dependent congenital heart disease. *Circulation* 1981;64:899–905.
10. Liebman J, Cullum L, Belloc NB: Natural history of transposition of the great arteries: Anatomy and birth and death characteristics. *Circulation* 1969;40:237–262.
11. Bierman FZ, Williams RG: Prospective diagnosis of d-transposition of the great arteries in neonates by subxiphoid, two-dimensional echocardiography. *Circulation* 1979;60:1496, 1502.
12. Rashkind WJ: Balloon atrioseptostomy: A palliative measure for transposition of the great arteries and certain other critical congenital cardiac defects. *Adv Cardiol* 1974;11:2–10.
13. Delisle G, Ando M, Calder AL, et al: Total anomalous pulmonary venous connection: Report of 93 autopsied cases with emphasis on diagnostic and surgical considerations. *Am Heart J* 1976;91:99–122.
14. Calder L, Van Praagh R, Van Praagh S, et al: Truncus arteriosus communis: Clinical, angiocardiographic, and pathologic findings in 100 patients. *Am Heart J* 1976;92:23–38.
15. Alpert BS, Cook DH, Varghese PJ, et al: Spontaneous closure of small ventricular septal defects: Ten-year follow up. *Pediatrics* 1979;63:204–206.
16. Weidman WH, Blount SG Jr, DuShane JW, et al: Clinical course in ventricular septal defect. *Circulation* 1977;56(suppl 1):I-56–I-69.
17. Coggin CJ, Parker KR, Keith JD: Natural history of isolated patent ductus arteriosus and the effect of surgical correction: Twenty years' experience at The Hospital for Sick Children, Toronto. *Can Med Assoc J* 1970;102:718–720.
18. Bedford DE, Sellors TH, Somerville W, et al: Atrial septal defect and its surgical treatment. *Lancet* 1957;272:1255–1261.
19. Esscher E, Michaelsson M: Long-term results following closure of isolated ostium secundum atrial septal defect in children and adults. *Eur J Cardiol* 1977;6:109–116.
20. Bharati S, Lev M: The spectrum of common atrioventricular orifice (canal). *Am Heart J* 1973;86:553–561.
21. Park SC, Mathews RA, Zuberbuhler JR, et al: Down syndrome with congenital heart malformation. *Am J Dis Child* 1977;131:29–33.
22. Berger TJ, Kirklin JW, Blackstone EH, et al: Primary repair of complete atrioventricular canal in patients less than 2 years old. *Am J Cardiol* 1978;41:906–913.
23. Friedman WF: Congenital aortic valve disease: Natu-

ral history, indications, and results of surgery, in Morse DP, Goldberg H (eds): *Important Topics in Congenital, Valvular and Coronary Artery Disease.* New York, Futura Publishing Co Inc, 1975, pp 43–56.
24. Pennington DG, Liberthson RR, Jacobs M, et al: Critical review of experience with surgical repair of coarctation of the aorta. *J Thorac Cardiovasc Surg* 1979;77:217–229.
25. Nanton MA, Olley PM: Residual hypertension after coarctotomy in children. *Am J Cardiol* 1976;37:769–772.
26. Danilowicz D, Hoffman JIE, Rudolph AM: Serial studies of pulmonary stenosis in infancy and childhood. *Br Heart J* 1975;37:808–818.
27. Bisset GS III, Schwartz DC, Meyer RA, et al: Clinical spectrum and long-term follow-up of isolated mitral valve prolapse in 119 children. *Circulation* 1980;62:423–429.
28. Klein AA, McCrory WW, Engle MA: Hypertension in children. *Cardiovasc Clin* 1981;11:11–33.
29. Zahka KG, Neill CA, Kidd L, et al: Cardiac involvement in adolescent hypertension: Echocardiographic determination of myocardial hypertrophy. *Hypertension* 1981;3:664–668.
30. DiSciascio G, Taranta A: Rheumatic fever in children. *Am Heart J* 1980;99:635–658.
31. Wegner NK: Infectious myocarditis. *Cardiovasc Clin* 1972;4:168–185.
32. Yanagihara R, Todd JK: Acute febrile mucocutaneous lymph node syndrome. *Am J Dis Child* 1980;134:603–614.
33. Roberts WC, Spray TL: Pericardial heart disease. *Curr Probl Cardiol,* June 1977, vol 2, pp 1–71.
34. Lewis AB, Freed MD, Heymann MA, et al: Side effects of therapy with prostaglandin E_1 in infants with critical congenital heart disease. *Circulation* 1981;64:893–898.

Part IV

Disorders of the Central Nervous System

Raymond S. Kandt
Bernard J. D'Souza
Richard A. Kaplan
Howard E. Gendelman
Jerry S. Wolinsky
William C. Mobley

11 Disorders of the Central Nervous System

The signs and symptoms of neurologic disorders can result from a primary disease of the nervous system or occur secondary to other diseases. This chapter deals with acute disorders involving the central nervous system (CNS), emphasizing their presentation, diagnosis, and management.

COMA

Clinical Characteristics

Coma can be defined as an unarousable state of unconsciousness. It may or may not be accompanied by focal neurologic signs. Lesser degrees of altered consciousness should be described, e.g., "child opens eyes and moans in response to pain," rather than given labels such as stupor, obtundation, and the like. Descriptions of the state of consciousness enable subsequent examiners to accurately assess improvement or worsening.

Differential Diagnosis

Acute or subacute neurologic dysfunction is usually caused by drugs or poisons, trauma, infections, metabolic disorders, circulatory disturbances, or epilepsy. Many of these are treatable (Exhibit 11-1).

A clinical classification divides coma into three groups based on neurologic examination and characteristics of the cerebrospinal fluid (CSF):

1. *nonfocal coma with normal CSF:* toxic and metabolic comas
2. *nonfocal coma with abnormal CSF:* subarachnoid hemorrhage (see "Cerebrovascular Disease") and diffuse infections
3. *focal neurologic deficits with or without abnormal CSF:* localized infections, trauma, and most types of cerebrovascular disease

There may be some crossover among these groups, e.g., hypoglycemia can occasionally cause focal deficits.

Pathophysiology

The comatose state requires depression of the upper brainstem ascending reticular activating system or major dysfunction or destruction of both cerebral hemispheres.[1] Brainstem depression may be due to metabolic factors, intrinsic brainstem disease, or brainstem compression by local processess, supratentorial herniation, or pressure from cerebellar diseases.

Evaluation

Physical Examination

Blood pressure and vital signs are checked and stabilized. The patient is examined for evidence of illicit drug use (needle tracks), poisoning (cherry-red skin with carbon monoxide poisoning), trauma (including child abuse), systemic infections, and meningeal infections (nuchal rigidity). Further examination of the comatose patient includes a complete neurologic examination emphasizing

1. pattern and depth of respirations
2. mental status
3. funduscopic appearance, pupillary responses, and extraocular movements
4. asymmetry of muscle tone, movements, or reflexes

If the child does not respond to sound (call the child's name) with either speech, eye opening, or movement, then light touch, pressure, and painful stimuli should be applied sequentially to determine the level of responsiveness. Movements of the child that are intended to ward off obnoxious stimuli are a relatively favorable sign whereas flaccid unrespon-

Exhibit 11-1 Treatable Causes of Coma

- Drugs
  - Alcohol
  - Barbiturates
  - Opiates
  - Phenothiazines
  - Aspirin
- Poisons
  - Lead
  - Carbon monoxide
- Trauma
  - Subdural and epidural hematomas
  - Accessible parenchymal hematomas
- Infections
  - Meningitis (bacterial, tuberculous, fungal)
  - Subdural empyema
  - Brain abscess
  - Herpes simplex encephalitis
  - Severe systemic infections
- Metabolic disorders
  - Hypoglycemia
  - Diabetic acidosis
  - Hyperosmolar state
  - Uremia
  - Addisonian crisis
- Circulatory disturbances
  - Shock
  - Hypertensive encephalopathy
- Epilepsy
  - Major status epilepticus
  - Postconvulsive coma
  - Minor motor status epilepticus (spike-wave stupor)
- Immune-mediated (often parainfectious or postvaccinal)
  - Acute disseminated encephalomyelitis
  - Acute hemorrhagic leukoencephalitis

siveness to pain is an unfavorable sign.[2] Decorticate posturing (arms flexed) implies hemispheral dysfunction whereas decerebrate posturing (arms and legs extended) is a sign of deep hemispheral or upper brainstem dysfunction.

The constellation of a chaotic breathing pattern, increasing impairment of consciousness, and, especially, unilateral pupillary dilation is indicative of impending herniation of the temporal lobe (usually on the same side as the pupillary dilation). Deep coma with preserved pupillary responsiveness suggests a toxic or metabolic etiology for the coma. Spontaneous roving eye movements in the comatose patient testify to intact brainstem pathways extending from the nucleus of cranial nerve III in the midbrain down to the nucleus of cranial nerve VI in the pons. The doll's eyes maneuver can be performed if the cervical spine is intact. If the eye movements are full when the head is passively turned from side to side (intact doll's eyes or oculocephalic reflex), brainstem pathways are intact from the nucleus of cranial nerve III to the nucleus of cranial nerve VIII in the lower pons. If eye movements cannot be elicited with the doll's eyes maneuver, 30 to 90 mL of ice-cold water should be instilled separately into each external ear canal (after checking for intact tympanic membranes) with the head elevated 30° from the horizontal. A normal response in a comatose patient is tonic eye deviation to the side of the ice water.

Corneal reflexes are checked. Facial symmetry can be assessed if a facial grimace can be provoked by putting a cotton-tipped swab in the nostril. If the patient is intubated, the gag reflex can be checked by moving the endotracheal tube. If there is no response, one should press upon the larynx in the suprasternal notch. This will provoke a cough in all but the most severely compromised patients.

Diagnostic Tests

Blood is obtained immediately for determination of blood glucose. Tests are done to determine arterial blood gas measurements, blood chemistries (electrolytes, glucose, calcium, blood urea nitrogen), blood ammonia level, liver function (transaminases, bilirubin, albumin, prothrombin time), lead level and free erythrocyte protoporphyrin, and hematologic parameters. Urinalysis is performed to detect glucose and acetone. Blood, urine, and gastric aspirate are obtained for toxicologic analysis. A urine ferric chloride test can be performed in the emergency department to check for evidence of aspirin, phenothiazine, and other drug ingestions. The urine ferric chloride test can serve as a check on toxicologic studies which are sometimes inaccurate, in some cases due to logistical problems. If there is any question, repeat samples should be sent for analysis. An electrocardiogram and chest x-ray films are obtained.

A cranial computed tomography (CT) scan is the most useful way to detect a structural lesion. If a CT scanner is not available, radionuclide brain scanning to detect a brain abscess and cerebral arteriography to exclude a subdural, epidural, or intraparenchymal hemorrhage or mass should be performed.

Indications for lumbar puncture (LP) include suspicion of a CNS infection or any uncertainty about the cause of the coma. Relative contraindications to an LP include evidence of an intracranial mass or typical Reye's syndrome (see "Reye's Syndrome"). An electroencephalogram (EEG) may provide supplementary localizing information, demonstrate the triphasic waves of a metabolic encephalopathy (especially hepatic), or suggest subclinical status epilepticus. If herpes simplex encephalitis is suspected (see "Acute Viral Encephalitis"), a radionuclide brain scan and EEG should be performed quickly because they indicate the herpetic lesion earlier and with more specificity than CT scanning. Although controversial, decompressive craniotomy and cerebral biopsy of the clinically localized area of possible herpetic infection would be recommended by many for histologic and immunofluorescent studies and viral isolation.

Treatment

In the emergency department it is impossible to determine a child's ultimate prognosis. Therefore, full resuscitative measures should always be initiated. Treatment and evaluation are performed simultaneously. Breathing and circulation are stabilized, with endotracheal intubation, if necessary. After an intravenous line is established, blood is obtained for laboratory studies, and 25% dextrose is administered at a dosage of 2 mL/kg. If there is suspicion of opiate overdose (pupillary constriction, needle tracks, prior history, and so forth), naloxone (0.4 mg/mL) is given IV at a dosage of 0.01 mg/kg every 2 to 3 minutes for three doses. For example, the dose required by a 10 kg child is 0.1 mg (i.e., 10 kg × 0.01 mg/kg = 0.1 mg), which is equal to 0.25 mL. An individual weighing more than 40 kg should receive 0.4 mg per dose. Hypoxia and hypercapnia must be prevented since both cause dilation of intracranial vessels and increased intracranial pressure. Unilateral pupillary dilation indicates increased intracranial pressure, requiring urgent treatment by intubation, hyperventilation, and mannitol (see "Reye's Syndrome," Exhibit 11-11). Treatment for the specific disorders listed in Exhibit 11-1 is discussed in the corresponding sections of this chapter. Acute disseminated encephalomyelitis can improve with oral or IV dexamethasone or oral prednisone.

Long-term care is concerned with prevention of aspiration pneumonia, urinary tract infections, decubitus ulcers (turn the patient every 1 to 2 hours and pad bony prominences), fecal impaction (perform rectal examinations frequently), and corneal injury (treat with artificial tears or lubricating ointment). It also involves maintenance of fluid and electrolyte balance as well as good nutrition.

Neurologic Criteria for Death

A "Uniform Determination of Death Act" has been proposed by the American Bar Association, the American Medical Association, and other organizations and has been endorsed by the American Academy of Neurology. It reads: "An individual who has sustained either (1) irreversible cessation of circulatory and respiratory functions, or (2) irreversible cessation of all functions of the entire brain, including the brainstem, is dead. A determination of death must be made in accordance with accepted medical standards."[3]

The brains of infants and young children are more resistant to damage than those of adults. Therefore, the clinician must be extremely cautious in applying neurologic criteria for death to children younger than 5 years of age. Children who are comatose are cared for in intensive care units where a sense of urgency often prevails. This rapid-fire philosophy must never enter into the consideration of whether or not irreversible cessation of brain function exists.[4] Hypothermia or intoxication can temporarily abolish all evidence of brain function both clinically and by EEG. Shock also makes clinical tests unreliable. For the diagnosis of death, there must be, at the least, unreceptive and unresponsive coma, complete apnea, dilated and unreactive pupils, absence of all other brainstem reflexes, and a "flat" EEG (electrocerebral silence), all persisting for *at least* 6 hours without alterations. Even if these features are present, *death should not be declared* if (1) the cause of the coma is unknown; (2) hypothermia, intoxication, or shock is present; or (3) decerebrate or decorticate posturing or seizures are present. Neurologic consultation should be obtained.

Absence of blood flow to the brain, as determined by conventional arteriography or the radionuclide bolus technique, can complement the clinical diagnosis of irreversible cessation of brain function.

CEREBROVASCULAR DISEASE (STROKE)

Clinical Characteristics

Acute hemiparesis is the most frequent manifestation of a childhood stroke[5,6,7] and can be due to cerebral emboli, arterial or venous thrombosis, or hemorrhage. In contrast to adults, children rarely suffer from atherosclerosis. Abrupt coma can be caused by intracerebral hemorrhage, subarachnoid hemorrhage, or venous thrombosis. Other signs of possible cerebrovascular disease include hemianopsia, hemisensory deficit, and cranial nerve or cognitive dysfunction. These can occur alone or in association with hemiparesis or coma.

Acute infantile hemiplegia is the term used to designate the clinical picture of idiopathic, abrupt hemiplegia usually associated with fever, unilateral or generalized convulsions, and coma. The child is usually under the age of 2 years. Cerebral angiography may show occlusion of the supraclinoid portion of one or both internal carotid arteries or some other vascular abnormality. When supraclinoid occlusion is accompanied by telangiectasia of the basal ganglia, it is termed the moyamoya pattern. The moyamoya pattern is often idiopathic, but it has been associated with such diverse conditions as sickle cell anemia, neurofibromatosis, leptospirosis, bacterial and tuberculous meningitis, and following cranial radiation therapy. If a cause is found for the hemiplegia or vascular occlusion, the disorder is removed from the category of "acute infantile hemiplegia."

The key feature of cerebrovascular disease is the *abrupt* nature of the neurologic deficit. Absence of cognitive dysfunction or absence of a cranial nerve deficit (e.g., hemianopsia or facial weakness) does not exclude the diagnosis of stroke but leads one to consider alternative diagnoses such as spinal cord disease. CT scan or angiographic evidence for intracranial infarction, hemorrhage, or vascular occlusion should be obtained.

Differential Diagnosis

Childhood strokes can be divided into two general categories: (1) those associated with an underlying systemic disorder and (2) those without any underlying disorder (Exhibit 11-2). Further characterization should be made as to whether the cerebrovascular disease causes (1) a focal, neurologic deficit without alteration of consciousness; (2) coma associated with a focal neurologic deficit; or (3) a nonfocal, comatose state (see also "Coma"). This approach allows one to determine the nature and cause of a stroke and to exclude the disorders that mimic cerebrovascular disease (e.g., toxic, metabolic, infectious, and traumatic conditions). In general, an isolated arterial occlusion (usually thrombotic or embolic) causes focal neurologic signs, commonly hemiplegia, without alteration of consciousness. Intracerebral hemorrhage can cause abrupt alteration of consciousness with focal deficits. Extension of hemorrhage into the subarachnoid space or ventricles is likely to cause diffuse, nonfocal deficits, nuchal rigidity, and lethargy or

Exhibit 11-2 Causes of Childhood Strokes

- Strokes Associated with Underlying Systemic Disease
  - Cardiac disorders
    - Cyanotic congenital heart disease (often complicated by polycythemia and iron deficiency with microcytic, hypochromic red cell indices)
    - Bacterial endocarditis
    - Rheumatic heart disease
    - Atrial myxoma
    - Postsurgical or catheterization emboli
    - Coarctation of the aorta (associated with intracranial aneurysms)
    - Other valvular disease (e.g., mitral valve prolapse)
  - Purulent infections
    - Meningitis
    - Otitis media, mastoiditis, sinusitis
    - Scalp and face infections
    - Retropharyngeal abscess
    - Lung abscess or septic pneumonia
  - Other infections
    - Meningovascular syphilis
    - Tuberculosis
    - Some viral infections
  - Neck or intraoral trauma
  - Hematologic disorders
    - Sickle cell anemia
    - Thrombocytopenia (thrombotic thrombocytopenic purpura, leukemia, hemolytic-uremic syndrome, aplastic anemia, drugs)
    - Polycythemia
    - Hemophilia
    - Thrombocytosis
    - Vitamin K deficiency (hemorrhagic disease of the newborn)
    - Disseminated intravascular coagulation
    - Maternal anticonvulsant therapy in the neonate
    - Liver disease
    - Hypercoagulopathy
  - Homocystinuria
  - Connective tissue disorders
    - Systemic lupus erythematosus
    - Polyarteritis nodosa
    - Wegener's granulomatosis
  - Drugs
    - Birth control pills
    - Illicit intravenous drugs
    - Anticoagulants
  - Hypertension
  - Miscellaneous
    - Conditions associated with aneurysms (Marfan's syndrome, Ehlers-Danos syndrome, polycystic kidneys)
    - Fat emboli from long bone fractures
    - Lead encephalopathy
    - Severe dehydration
    - Hypercholesterolemia
    - Progeria
    - Hypoglycemia
    - Nonketotic hyperosmolarity
    - Recurrent complicated migraine
  - Prematurity (intraventricular hemorrhage)
- Strokes Not Associated with Underlying Systemic Disease
  - Acute infantile hemiplegia
  - Recurrent or alternating hemiplegias associated with the moyamoya vascular pattern (sometimes associated with underlying systemic disease)
  - Rupture of intracranial arteriovenous malformations or aneurysms

coma. Venous thrombosis or thrombophlebitis is often accompanied by fever, focal or generalized convulsions, increased intracranial pressure, nuchal rigidity, and coma, with or without focal neurologic deficits. This picture can be mimicked by bacterial meningitis, parainfectious encephalomyelitis (acute disseminated encephalomyelitis, acute hemorrhagic leukoencephalitis), or some viral encephalitides such as herpes simplex encephalitis. Cerebral angiography, demonstrating venous occlusions, is the only way of proving the diagnosis of venous thrombosis.

Pathophysiology

Vascular occlusion (venous or arterial) caused by emboli, thrombosis, vasospasm, or the compressive effects of hemorrhage or cerebral edema results in neuronal dysfunction because of the lack of metabolic substrates (especially glucose and oxygen). Vasospasm can occur in association with a vasculitis or several days after a subarachnoid hemorrhage. Cyanotic congenital heart disease, perioral infections, and severe dehydration are more likely to be associated with venous than arterial thrombosis.

Evaluation

To prevent progression of the stroke, the top priority is stabilization and support of cardiorespiratory function, followed by detection and treatment of any underlying systemic disorders. The most common disorders of childhood predisposing to stroke are (1) congenital heart disease; (2) infections of the scalp, face, oral cavity, sinuses, mastoids, and ears; (3) sickle cell anemia; and (4) neck or intraoral trauma. Bacterial meningitis must always be considered. Less common disorders that must be rapidly detected are other hematologic conditions predisposing to hemorrhage or thrombosis, cardiac disorders, and severe dehydration.

History and Physical Examination

With these considerations in mind, one must inquire about

- recent infections and medical conditions
- trauma
- symptoms of a bleeding diathesis
- chronic headaches or other neurologic deficits suggestive of a mass lesion
- an abrupt and severe headache followed by obtundation due to a ruptured arteriovenous malformation (AVM)[8] or aneurysm

A history of recurrent pulsatile or unilateral headaches associated with vomiting and relieved by sleep suggests the possibility that the hemiplegia is secondary to migraine. This is strengthened by a family history of hemiplegic migraine. Convulsive seizures may be followed by paralysis (postictal or Todd's paralysis) that resolves within 24 to 48 hours. Recent hematuria suggests the possibility of acute glomerulonephritis complicated by hypertensive encephalopathy or hemorrhage. In a child less than 2 years of age with cyanotic congenital heart disease, a focal neurologic deficit is commonly due to venous or arterial occlusion; in a child over 2 years of age, a brain abscess is a more likely cause. In the adolescent especially, drug use can predispose to a stroke, e.g., thrombosis related to birth control pills, embolization related to the endocarditis associated with illicit intravenous drugs, or cerebral vasculitis from the use of amphetamines and other drugs. A history of recurrent hemiplegias (unilateral or alternating) raises the possibilities of the moyamoya vascular pattern, hemiplegic migraine, multifocal seizures, a connective tissue disorder, homocystinuria, sickle cell disease, or a cardiac embolic disorder or arrhythmia.

Features to be noted on general physical examination include

- blood pressure
- evidence for intraoral, head, or neck trauma
- nuchal rigidity
- infections of the head or neck
- carotid or asymmetrical cranial bruits
- petechiae
- multiple café au lait spots
- cyanosis
- heart murmurs or clicks
- cardiac arrhythmias

Neurological examination should assess mental status and cranial nerve, motor, and sensory function. Special attention should be given to funduscopic evidence of papilledema or retinal hemorrhages. Blotlike preretinal hemorrhages are especially suggestive of subarachnoid hemorrhages. One should search for asymmetrical cranial nerve, motor, or sensory signs. Hemianopsia, aphasia, or a cortical sensory deficit suggests a cortical process whereas a crossed hemiplegia (e.g., ipsilateral facial weakness and contralateral arm and leg weakness) localizes the lesion to the brainstem. Hemiplegia and a dermatomal level below which sensation is altered in association with preserved cortical and brainstem functions typify a spinal cord lesion.

Exhibit 11-3 Laboratory Evaluation of Stroke

Blood studies
- Complete blood count (including platelets and coagulation profile)
- Hemoglobin electrophoresis
- Serologic test for syphilis
- Antinuclear antibody test
- Erythrocyte sedimentation rate
- Glucose, blood urea nitrogen, cholesterol and triglycerides
- Lipoprotein electrophoresis
- Blood cultures
- Liver function tests

Urine cyanide nitroprusside test for homocystinuria
Chest x-ray film
Electrocardiogram and echocardiogram
EEG
Cranial CT scan
LP
Cerebral arteriography

Diagnostic Tests

Laboratory tests should be chosen to detect an underlying illness (Exhibit 11-3) and define the disease process.

A cranial CT scan should be performed. Presence of subarachnoid blood on CT scan makes an LP superfluous. If subarachnoid blood or a mass (e.g., hematoma, tumor, brain abscess, local edema) is not visualized on CT scan, then an LP is performed to exclude meningeal infection or subarachnoid hemorrhage.

Cerebral arteriography should be performed if further definition of vascular anatomy will modify the treatment of the underlying disease. Additional strong indications for cerebral arteriography include a single, idiopathic stroke or a pattern of recurrent or alternating hemipareses. An AVM or aneurysm causing a subarachnoid hemorrhage may be detectable only by arteriography. Positron emission tomography (PET) is not used in the routine evaluation of a stroke but is likely to become very important in the future. Intravenous digital subtraction angiography is a noninvasive technique providing good visualization of a carotid artery in the neck but poor visualization of intracranial vessels. It is also able to detect large intracranial aneurysms. Technological advances are likely to improve this technique. Because cerebrovascular occlusive disease in children is more likely to be intracranial than cervical, conventional cerebral arteriography remains the procedure of choice at this time. Magnetic resonance imaging is difficult to use in emergency situations, and is not appropriate in the acute management of stroke.

Treatment

Cardiorespiratory support takes precedence. Treatment of an underlying process, seizures, and increased intracranial pressure are discussed elsewhere in this book. Cerebral fat embolism from fractures of the long bones should be treated with dexamethasone, 0.15 mg/kg IV every 4 hours, and cardiorespiratory support. Surgical thromboembolectomy should be considered as an emergency treatment for the child with traumatic carotid occlusion in the neck. With the possible exception of the rare adolescent with carotid atherosclerotic disease and transient ischemic attacks, surgical thrombectomy and anticoagulation for carotid or venous occlusion are not indicated. Anticoagulation with heparin is considered when an embolic source is present. Internal carotid to external carotid artery bypass grafts have been used in the treatment of supraclinoid carotid artery obstruction, but the natural history of the obstruction is variable enough that further evaluation of this treatment is needed. If surgically accessible, AVMs or aneurysms can be excised or ligated.

Treatment of neonatal intraventricular hemorrhages follows the same principles but also includes LP for immediate lowering of increased intracranial pressure.

Prevention of childhood strokes includes

- avoidance of hyperventilation during EEGs in children with sickle cell disease
- prohibition of the habit of walking around with a sharp object (lollipop) in the mouth
- treatment of severe dehydration or purulent infections of the head and neck
- treatment of polycythemia and hypochromic, microcytic anemia in children with cyanotic congenital heart disease
- correction of hematologic disorders

Posthemorrhagic hydrocephalus can complicate neonatal or childhood intracranial hemorrhages. In the neonate initial treatment includes serial LPs and administration of drugs that decrease CSF production (acetazolamide, furosemide). Ventriculoperitoneal (VP) shunting is performed in older children or in neonates who have failed medical therapy.

ACUTE ATAXIA

Coordination is a complex function requiring (1) sensory input from muscles and joints via the posterior columns and (2) intact motor output from the cortex and basal ganglia to the anterior horn cell, with the cerebellum exerting a modulating influence. "Ataxia" literally means lack of order, and refers most commonly to the pattern of incoordination associated with diseases at different levels of the nervous system. Clinically, it is manifested by a broad-based or unsteady gait, nystagmus, intention tremor, and impaired ability to perform rapid alternating movements. Thus ataxia can result from cerebellar dysfunction (cerebellar ataxia), sensory loss due to neuropathies or posterior column disease (sensory ataxia), weakness due to disease of the motor system, or vestibular dysfunction.

Cerebellar Ataxia

Ataxia can be acute, intermittent, or chronic; in the last instance, it can be progressive or static. Acute ataxia is a symptom of various disorders. In the majority of cases, prime consideration should be given to toxic and infectious causes.[9] Tumors in the posterior fossa may cause ataxia; however, it is rarely acute and usually progressive. In addition, patients with tumors frequently experience headache, vomiting, and signs of increased intracranial pressure; some have changes in personality, papilledema, and cranial nerve VI palsies. Children with brainstem tumors have multiple cranial nerve deficits in addition to ataxia without papilledema. In cases in which a diagnosis of a space-occupying lesion or increased intracranial pressure is suspected, an LP should be deferred and a CT scan should be obtained.

Intoxications

The most common toxic substances known to produce ataxia include anticonvulsant drugs, antihistamines, sedatives, tranquilizers, alcohol, and lead. These may be ingested by accident, as a result of error in dose administration, or in suicide attempts. Even without such a history, it is strongly recommended that a urine and serum drug screen be done. The signs and symptoms vary with the drug, quantity, and time elapsed since ingestion. Supportive care includes careful attention to the maintenance of adequate respiration and blood pressure and observation for changes in level of consciousness. Other measures include prevention of further absorption, use of appropriate antidotes, and methods to enhance elimination. The management of poisonings is discussed elsewhere (see Chapter 18).

Infections

"Acute cerebellar ataxia of childhood" is a syndrome seen in association with a wide range of viral infections, notably those caused by varicella-zoster, Epstein-Barr virus (EBV), and mumps virus. It can occur at any age but is seen most frequently between 1 and 4 years of age.[9,10]

Characteristically, there is the dramatic onset of incoordination, headaches, nausea, and vomiting. Less frequently, patients have nystagmus or cranial nerve deficits. CSF is usually normal but may reveal a mild lymphocytic pleocytosis in 25% of cases. The clinical course is self-limited, and complete recovery usually occurs within 1 to 2 weeks, although one third of patients may show residual deficits, including speech impairment, behavior and learning disabilities, and mild ataxia.[10] No specific therapy is available.

A more severe form of cerebellar ataxia of unknown etiology has been termed Kinsbourne's myoclonic encephalopathy or the "dancing eyes, dancing feet syndrome." The striking clinical features include chaotic, jerky eye movements (opsoclonus) and myoclonic jerks of the extremities. Intention tremor and truncal instability are also present. In severely affected individuals, improvement occurs with the use of adrenocorticotropin, and in many patients symptoms may recur with lowering the dosage or discontinuation of therapy.

Neuroblastoma

A nonresolving cerebellar ataxia with or without accompanying opsoclonus has been seen in association with neuroblastoma.[11] Since the neurologic symptomatology can precede the detection of this tumor, diagnostic studies should be done, including a urine screen for elevation of vanillylmandelic acid, serum enolase, and a CT scan extending from the neck to the pelvis. If the initial investigation is negative and symptoms persist, periodic studies at 6-month intervals for 18 months to 2 years are recommended. With the removal of the tumor or after antitumor therapy, the disorder may improve or resolve. If not, a trial of adrencorticotropin should be instituted at a dosage of 40 U/d IM for 1 to 2 weeks and then tapered over weeks to months, depending on clinical response. Despite resolution of the ataxia and abnormal movements, a significant number of patients are left with behavioral and intellectual deficits.

Familial Ataxia

Acute intermittent familial cerebellar ataxia is characterized by sudden onset of gait ataxia, dysarthria, and intention tremor. Some familial cases respond to acetazolamide, 10–20 mg/kg/d.

Sensory Ataxia

Dysfunction of the posterior columns, dorsal roots, or peripheral nerves also can produce ataxia. This disruption of sensory input results in difficulty in appreciating the position of the limbs, and movements are better performed with visual input. Consequently, the gait is characterized by lifting the feet high and stamping down vigorously with each step. Other accompanying signs include a positive Romberg sign, loss of position and vibration sense, and decreased deep tendon reflexes. The causes of posterior column dysfunction and neuropathy in children are usually hereditary, toxic, or rarely nutritional. Treatment is specific to the cause.

Motor Weakness

Myopathies, whether congenital or acquired, can be associated with ataxia. The proximal muscle groups usually are more involved, resulting in a waddling gait with lordotic posturing. Patients with spasticity secondary to cerebral or spinal cord lesions also may experience gait difficulties.

Metabolic Disorders

Acute intermittent ataxia can occur in Hartnup disease, the intermittent form of maple syrup urine disease, urea cycle defects, Leigh's encephalomyelopathy, and hyperalaninemia. Between attacks, the movements are relatively normal; however, the other signs and features associated with these disorders persist. Ataxia can last for days to weeks and frequently is precipitated by intercurrent infections. Patients repeatedly exposed to toxins can also exhibit acute intermittent ataxia. Metabolic disorders causing ataxia, depending on the specific defect, are variously treated with vitamin supplements such as nicotinamide or thiamine or with dietary restrictions.

Benign Paroxysmal Vertigo

This condition is characterized by recurrent attacks of vertigo associated with ataxia, vomiting, pallor, and nystagmus; the child may fall during an attack. Episodes usually last a few minutes and recur for weeks with decreasing severity. Consciousness is preserved, and with demonstrable abnormalities in labyrinthine function, it can be distinguished from temporal lobe seizures. Acute labyrinthitis also can create a similar symptomatology. Partly due to the brevity of attacks, treatment with antivertiginous agents such as meclizine or dramamine is rarely helpful for benign paroxysmal vertigo.

CEREBROSPINAL FLUID SHUNT MALFUNCTION

The standard treatment for hydrocephalus is shunting of the ventricular system, usually a lateral ventricle, with tubing extending from the ventricle to the peritoneum or, less commonly, the right atrium, via a right parietooccipital burr hole and then a subcutaneous tract down the right side of the neck and chest and thence into the peritoneum. Once inserted, at no point is any of the shunt apparatus exposed to external contamination. VP shunts are more commonly used in children because extra tubing can be coiled in the intestine to allow for growth in the height of the child. Most shunts now are installed with a flushing valve and reservoir (shunt bulb, pumping device) at the point where the tubing exits from the burr hole. In other cases, a one-way valve is incorporated into the tubing itself. Shunts have low-, medium-, or high-pressure valves, referring to the intracranial pressure required before CSF begins to exit via the shunt. Various permutations of shunt valves, tubing, and reservoirs are available for specialized purposes.

Clinical Characteristics

Malfunction is signaled by signs and symptoms of acute or chronic increased intracranial pressure or infection[12,13] that are usually associated with CSF abnormalities, elevated CSF pressure upon tapping of the shunt bulb, or increased ventricular size as indicated by cranial CT scan. In some individuals the ventricular walls have decreased compliance (i.e., they are stiffer), and rapid rises of intracranial pressure can occur *without* ventricular dilation.[14] Because the CT scan may appear unchanged or "normal" in this situation, clinical signs are of paramount importance, and if they are dismissed, the child may die.

Differential Diagnosis

The major alternative diagnostic consideration in a shunted child with fever, vomiting, and irritability is a benign viral infection. The coexistence of diarrhea is much more suggestive of a viral gastroenteritis than a shunt infection. A urinary tract infection in a child may have the same nonspecific features as a shunt infection, but it should be given special consideration in the shunted child with spina bifida, i.e., frequent urinary tract infections in these patients can mislead the clinician. When there are specific features of increased intracranial pressure or ventricular dilatation (e.g., papilledema, spastic legs with extensor plantar responses, palsy of cranial nerve VI), shunt malfunction should be given first consideration; however, recurrence of a possible primary tumor (e.g., medulloblastoma) that was treated at the time of shunt placement, subdural hematoma, pseudotumor cerebri, and brain abscess also should be considered. Minor head trauma with mild cerebral edema in a child with a marginally functional shunt can cause abrupt decompensation. An epidural, subdural, or intracerebral hematoma should be excluded in such an instance.

Pathophysiology

Shunt obstruction can be partial, complete, or intermittent. At the proximal (ventricular) end, the tip of the catheter can be occluded by pieces of the choroid plexus, brain parenchyma, blood clots, fibrin, or, uncommonly, the ventricular wall after excessive reduction to slitlike proportions. The atrial end of a ventriculoatrial (VA) shunt may be obstructed by a thrombus, and the peritoneal end of a VP shunt may be obstructed by omentum or coiled loops of bowel. Uncommonly, tubing becomes disconnected or the shunt tip is inserted or migrates into an area where drainage is blocked (e.g., the external abdominal wall muscles).

After shunt obstruction the ventricles typically dilate and intracranial pressure rises. In extreme cases pressure is transmitted to the medullary cardiorespiratory centers, with resultant bradypnea, bradycardia, increased pulse pressure, and, ultimately, cardiorespiratory arrest. Paralysis of upgaze is ascribed to dilation of the third ventricle and transmission of pressure to the vertical gaze centers in the rostral diencephalon. Stretching of the corticospinal fibers to the legs causes spasticity of the legs.

In children with "shunt dependency" due to decreased ventricular wall compliance or complete aqueductal stenosis, an excessively rapid rise of intracranial pressure can lead to rapid deterioration.

Evaluation

The most common causes of shunt malfunction are infection and blockage,[13] usually at the ventricular or peritoneal ends. Both causes may be present. Shunt infections occur in 6% to 25% of hydrocephalic patients with shunts. Most infections occur within the first week after shunting (often manifest as persistent fever), and 88% to 98% occur within 6 months.

In the immediate postoperative period, leakage of CSF from incisions or subcutaneous collections of CSF along the shunt pathway may signal shunt failure. Acute shunt malfunction should be suspected with any of the following symptoms (usually in combination but sometimes singly): fever, headache, vomiting, irritability, somnolence or other depression of consciousness, gait disturbance, and diplopia. On examination papilledema may be noted several hours after the increase of intracranial pressure but will be absent if optic atrophy exists or the sutures are open; palsy of cranial nerve VI can occur as a nonlocalizing sign. Paralysis of upgaze, spasticity of the legs, bulging of the anterior fontanel, and congestion of the scalp veins also may be noted. In children Cushing's triad of bradypnea, bradycardia, and increased pulse pressure can occur as intracranial pressure rises rapidly.

The reservoir can be tapped to measure the pressure and decrease it by removing CSF, which should be analyzed for cell count, glucose, and protein; cultured; and examined with Gram's stain. In the event of ventricular obstruction, the CSF pressure at the reservoir is usually normal or reduced whereas it is increased when the peritoneal end is blocked. If signs and symptoms are consistent with shunt obstruction, it is immaterial whether or not the reservoir pumps and refills well. Children without clinical or laboratory evidence of shunt obstruction may have abnormal pumping or refilling. Hence, a *change* in pumping or refilling in the context of a *change* in clinical condition has much more importance than isolated changes in the flushing valve.

When chronic partial shunt obstruction exists, the only signs may be a head circumference that is gradually enlarging to cross percentiles on a growth chart, gradual intellectual or scholastic deterioration, mild ataxia, spasticity of the legs, or chronic headache. This is often a difficult diagnosis to make with confidence. Serial psychometric testing and a CT scan of the head may help.

Secondary Shunt Complications

Numerous conditions, mostly abdominal, have been attributed to shunts:

- abdominal distention
- inguinal hernia
- inflammatory mesenteric pseudotumor
- peritonitis
- perforation of various organs or tissues: bladder, gall bladder, intestine, vagina, umbilicus
- intra-abdominal and omental cysts
- scrotal extrusion
- shunt migration through surgical incisions
- loss of peritoneal absorptive capacity and ascites
- intractable hiccups[15]

Too rapid decompression of chronic hydrocephalus can result in subdural hematomas. Shunt nephritis of immune-complex type and pulmonary embolization may complicate the use of a VA shunt.

Diagnostic Tests

An increased CSF cell count may be obtained from noninfected shunts.[12] Approximately 50% of patients with a CSF white blood cell count of less than 20/mm^3 have infected shunts, whereas approximately 90% of those with a CSF white blood cell count greater than 100/mm^3 are infected.[12] The CSF glucose level is often normal with shunt infections, in contrast to bacterial meningitis, in which it is commonly less than 50% of the blood glucose level. Organisms responsible for shunt infections are introduced at the time of surgical implantation of the shunt or during shunt taps. Therefore, as expected, *Staphylococcus* is the major infecting agent, with 50% of shunt infections attributable to *Staphylococcus epidermidis (albus)* and 25% to *Staphylococcus aureus*, and 25% to various other pathogens, including enteric organisms. When shunt CSF grows multiple enteric organisms, perforation of an abdominal viscus by the shunt tip should be suspected. Blood cultures are usually positive with VA shunt infections and uniformly negative with primary VP shunt infections. Positive blood cultures can arise from a primary infection when the VP shunt infection is secondary (e.g., *Haemophilus influenzae* meningitis). Only one third of patients with infected shunts have peripheral white blood cell counts greater than 20,000 mm^3.

A noncontrast CT scan of the head demonstrates enlarged ventricles in most cases of shunt obstruction. A baseline scan (performed several weeks after initial shunt placement) is necessary for comparison purposes. In patients with an open fontanel, ultrasound is useful in following infants with hydrocephalus. The ultrasonography is advantageous because it allows for rapid bedside examination without sedation, is less expensive than CT, creates no radiation exposure, and accurately assesses ventricular size.[16]

When a shunt is tapped, a pressure greater than 220 mm CSF is always abnormal, even in the presence of a high-pressure valve. A pressure greater than 140 to 150 mm CSF is abnormally high in the presence of most medium-pressure valves (the most commonly used pressure). If the obstruction is at the ventricular end of the catheter or at the valve inlet, the pressure is likely to be abnormally low, and often no additional CSF other than the few drops in the reservoir can be removed.

A more sophisticated analysis of shunt function involves the simultaneous assessment of shunt pressure with radionuclide clearance.[17] This type of study can be valuable in instances in which the CT scan does not show ventricular enlargement and isolated shunt taps show normal pressure, but the patient is clinically suspected of having intermittent or partial shunt obstruction.

Treatment

If rapid deterioration occurs, a long spinal needle should be inserted through the burr hole, bypassing the shunt apparatus, into the lateral ventricle by aiming toward the opposite inner canthus of the eye. Preferably this is done by a neurosurgeon, but in an extreme situation, it can be performed by the physician at hand. In most cases, however, a 25-gauge needle is aseptically introduced by the neurosurgeon into the shunt bulb, and CSF pressure is measured and removed to alleviate increased pressure. This should be performed before the CT scan if the patient's condition is serious.

An obstructed, noninfected shunt should be replaced. In the interim before surgery, critical observations include vital signs and state of alertness. Retapping of the shunt and medical therapy with acetazolamide (60 to 100 mg/kg/d orally or IV divided into three doses), furosemide (1 mg/kg/d orally or IV), or isosorbide dinitrate (1.5 mg/kg to 2.0 mg/kg every 6 hours orally) may be used as temporizing measures until surgery. When acetazolamide is used, the serum bicarbonate level should be monitored and kept above 18 mEq/L by utilizing Polycitra, Bicitra, or sodium bicarbonate (starting at 3 to 5 mEq orally or IV/kg daily and titrating upwards as needed).

When infection is suspected, 2 to 3 weeks of intravenous treatment with vancomycin, 40 mg/kg/d given every 6 h for children older than 1 month, or with meningitic doses of a penicillinase-resistant penicillin (e.g., nafcillin, 200 mg/kg/d) is instituted, usually together with chloramphenicol (100 mg/kg/d), pending culture results. In most centers the entire infected shunt is removed as soon as the infection is recognized; others wait 2 to 3 days, remove the entire shunt, and insert a new one in a different site. Combining systemic antibiotics with complete shunt removal can result in a 100% cure rate for shunt infections. Some authorities also institute several days of extraventricular CSF drainage before placing a new shunt and may also use intraventricular, as well as systemic, antibiotics. A controversial and currently less satisfactory method of treatment is the use of systemic and/or intraventricular antibiotics without removing the infected shunt. If intraventricular gentamicin is used for chloramphenicol-resistant coliforms, only the preservative-free, nonintravenous preparation should be administered.

FEBRILE SEIZURES

Febrile seizures occur in children between 3 months and 5 years of age in association with a fever but not because of infections of the CNS. Those with an underlying history of nonfebrile seizures are not included in this category. The majority of seizures are usually generalized, tonic-clonic, less than 15 minutes in duration, and not accompanied by a prolonged postictal state. However, complex seizures having one or more of the following characteristics occasionally occur: focal features, greater than 15 minutes' duration, and more than one seizure in a 24-hour period.[18,19]

In 60% to 70% of cases, the cause of the fever is related to a viral infection of the respiratory tract. Approximately 10% are related to gastrointestinal infections, and 5% are related to exanthems. There is frequently a strong family history of febrile seizures in parents and siblings of the patient.

Management

If the child is having a seizure, proper attention should be paid to maintaining an adequate airway and perfusion. As most seizures are brief, no anticonvulsant therapy is usually necessary. However, if a seizure is prolonged, diazepam in a dose of 0.3 to 0.5 mg/kg IV, not to exceed 10 mg, may be given and repeated after 5 minutes if needed (see "Status Epilepticus").

Otherwise, attempts should be made to reduce the temperature by tepid sponging and antipyretics. The work-up should include a detailed history, including characteristics of the illness, description of seizure, and degree of temperature elevation. A family and developmental history should also be obtained. Not infrequently, by the time the patient is seen, the temperature has diminished and is lower than the history indicates it was.

The physical and neurologic examination should include a careful search for the source of the fever. In children below 2 years of age, a stiff neck can be absent in the presence of a meningeal infection. Because of this possibility, an LP is indicated if a CNS infection is suspected.

Routinely obtaining other studies—a complete blood count, electrolytes, glucose, calcium, skull x-ray films, and CT scan—has limited value. Such studies should be ordered on an individualized basis according to the clinical picture. An EEG is optional; the presence of an abnormal study does not reliably predict the risk for epilepsy.

Hospitalization is rarely indicated. Parental anxiety about seizures rather than the associated illness is a frequent reason for hospitalization.

Anticonvulsant prophylaxis should be considered if there are two or more of the three major underlying risk factors for future epilepsy:[19]

1. the presence of abnormal neurologic or developmental history prior to the seizure
2. a prolonged or focal seizure
3. a positive family history of epilepsy

Seizures occurring in children less than 1 year of age or repeated seizures during the same illness are regarded as minor risk factors for recurrence.

Daily anticonvulsant therapy has been shown to reduce recurrence of febrile seizures, but there is no documented evidence that it prevents epilepsy. For effective prophylaxis drugs must be given daily and levels should be maintained in the therapeutic range. The drugs of choice are phenobarbital or sodium valproate. Phenobarbital is given orally at 4 to 6 mg/kg/d, half of the total dose every 12 hours. Sodium valproate therapy is begun at 10 to 15 mg/kg/d orally, half of the daily dose every 12 hours. The total daily dose is then increased if necessary for seizure control, in increments of 5 to 10 mg/kg/d at weekly intervals to a maximum of 60 to 100 mg/kg/d.

For the majority of children, febrile seizures represent a benign disorder. Sixty percent of children experience only a single seizure whereas 10% have more than three seizures. In 90% of the cases with recurrent seizures, they appear within 2 years of the first seizure and the patients are primarily in the high-risk group. More importantly, families should be educated about the benign nature of the problem, efforts used to control fever, and measures taken should seizure occur.[18]

ACUTE POLYNEURITIS

Clinical Characteristics

Guillain-Barré syndrome is the classic example of an acute inflammatory polyneuropathy characterized by progressive flaccid weakness of varying degree.[20] The early symptoms are often aching muscles and distal paresthesias; however, objective sensory findings are minimal. The motor weakness is often symmetrical and ascending. Facial, bulbar, and extraocular muscles can be involved. Progression of symptoms occurs over several days to weeks, reaching its peak within 2 weeks in 50% of cases and within 4 weeks in 90%. Usually sphincter function is not affected, but transient bladder paralysis can occur.

Other diagnostic features include an afebrile course and the characteristic CSF findings of protein elevation and a normal cell count. Nerve conduction studies can be normal, but approximately 80% of patients have evidence of slowing sometime during the course of the illness.[20] Distal latencies and F-wave responses also can be abnormal. The degree of abnormality may not correspond with the severity of weakness.

The Miller-Fisher syndrome is considered to be an atypical form of postinfectious polyneuritis in which, in addition to ataxia and areflexia, ophthalmoplegia is a prominent feature. The clinical course is usually benign.

Differential Diagnosis

Conditions that may share some of the features of the Guillain-Barré syndrome include

- exposure to paint vapors, glue (by sniffing), lead, organophosphates, nitrofurantoin, dapsone
- porphyria
- diphtheria, poliomyelitis, botulism
- tick paralysis

Pathophysiology

The existent hypothesis is that Guillain-Barré syndrome is an immune response, but its precise cause is not known. The majority of patients have a history of a preceding viral illness or immunization. It has been reported in association with bacterial infections, trauma, or surgery. The absence of preceding events does not rule out the diagnosis.

Treatment

The mainstay of treatment is maintenance of ventilatory and cardiovascular function.

Respiratory Support

Impaired respiratory function can result from involvement of the intercostal muscles and the diaphragm. In addition, the patient may have depressed swallowing, with pooling of secretions and the potential for aspiration. Postural drainage and mechanical suction should be used as needed. Sweating, persistent tachycardia, and restlessness are early warnings of hypoxia. It is essential to carefully monitor vital capacity, blood gases, respiratory rate, depth of respiration, and strength of voice during the acute phase.

If there are signs of deteriorating respiratory function, early institution of ventilatory support via endotracheal intubation and artificial ventilation is indicated. A tracheostomy should be performed if an endotracheal tube must be left in place for more than 3 or 4 weeks.

Chest physiotherapy is very important to avoid retention of secretions and segmental airspace collapse. Appropriate antibiotic therapy should be instituted if pneumonia develops.

Support of Cardiovascular-Autonomic Function

Acute pulmonary edema and arrhythmias can occur as a consequence of myocarditis, hypoxia, or fluid and electrolyte imbalance. Cardiac monitoring and frequent observation of vital signs are advised for all patients. In addition, there may be inappropriate secretion of antidiuretic hormone. Daily input and output should be recorded, as well as periodic serum electrolyte levels and urine specific gravity.

Despite the improvements in respiratory care, a few patients with Guillain-Barré syndrome die during the acute phase of the disease. It is now apparent that autonomic dysfunction can be life threatening. Hypertension, orthostatic hypotension, cardiac arrhythmias, ileus, and urinary retention are all manifestations of autonomic dysfunction.

Blood pressure measurements can fluctuate widely. It is advisable to treat hypertension with short-acting preparations. Postural hypotension can be corrected with intravenous fluids, vasopressors, leg stockings, and avoidance of rapid changes in posture. Bowel and bladder dysfunction can occur as a result of involvement of either the abdominal musculature or the autonomic nervous system. The Credé maneuver is helpful in emptying the bladder, and catheterization is rarely necessary.

Fever is not usually part of the syndrome and indicates infection, dehydration, or a disturbance in temperature regulation. In patients with prolonged disease, a nasogastric tube or feeding gastrostomy may be necessary to maintain adequate nutrition. Close attention must be paid to serum osmolality, volume of intake, and possible aspiration.

Acute glomerulonephritis has been reported in association with this syndrome. The clinical signs of nephritis may go undetected; therefore, serial chemical and microscopic urine examinations are advisable.

Skin care and frequent changes in position are needed to avoid decubitus ulcers. Psychologic support is also necessary, as patients often demonstrate changes in mood and behavior. Fatigue and irritability can persist after recovery of motor function. Diazepam (Valium) can be used cautiously to treat the anxiety. During convalescence (that is, when the neurologic status is stable), a graduated physical therapy program, including active and passive exercises, should be instituted to prevent contractures.

There is no convincing evidence that any specific drug therapy, including corticosteroids, alters the course of Guillain-Barré syndrome. Plasmapheresis is effective in improving patients with progressively worsening, severe Guillain-Barré syndrome, but is probably not useful for mild cases or for those that have either improved or failed to worsen for a week or more.[21]

BREATH-HOLDING SPELLS

Clinical Characteristics

The majority of breath-holding spells are of the cyanotic type (62%), followed by the pallid type (19%), and finally a combination of features from both types (19%). Eighty-four percent have their onset prior to 1½ years of age, with 8% starting in the neonatal period.[22]

Mental retardation and epilepsy are not sequelae, and the spells are felt to be benign. However, behavior problems occur more frequently in these children. In most cases (90%) the spells have ceased by the age of 6 years, although typical syncope may occur later (17% of cases). Children with breath-holding spells have a higher prevalence of anemia.[23]

Both types occur only while the patient is awake, usually in an erect posture, and do not create postictal confusion (but fatigue is common). Ocular compression (just below the supraorbital ridges) results in asystole lasting longer than 2 seconds in 61% to 78% of the pallid group (longer than 4 seconds in 55%), in 6% to 25% of the cyanotic group, and in 7% of controls (none longer than 4 seconds).[24]

In the cyanotic type, the child is angry or frustrated and, after a short period of crying, holds his breath in expiration, becomes cyanotic and limp, and occasionally has a few clonic jerks; after several seconds to a minute or so, the child recovers completely. The period of crying is precipitated by anger or frustration and followed by cyanosis and then unconsciousness, always occurring in that order.

The pallid type is provoked by fever (14% of cases) or a physical or emotional insult (the element of surprise has been stressed), and the child abruptly stops breathing, with accompanying bradycardia or asystole, and usually appears pale. This is followed by a deathlike limpness that may or may not be followed by generalized stiffening (the stiffening is an anoxic seizure and is dependent upon the duration of asystole). The child awakens after several seconds with an apparently clear sensorium (parents may feel that the child recognized them) and then seems tired and falls asleep. Spells can occur as often as one or more times per day (30% of cases) but usually occur at intervals of a week or longer.[25]

Differential Diagnosis

Seizures differ from breath-holding spells in that the tonic phase precedes the limpness, and there often is postictal confusion. Near-miss sudden infant death syndrome is characterized by apnea that usually occurs in a sleeping child under the age of 6 months and can be associated with nasopharyngitis. Such children may have a history of perinatal difficulties; however, this catastrophic illness still remains unexplained.

Pathophysiology

Cyanotic Type

The cerebral vasoconstriction secondary to the hyperventilation of a crying child combines with the decreased cardiac output secondary to the cessation of breathing in expiration to cause cerebral hypoxemia. The ventilatory response to hypoxia and hypercapnia in older children and adults who have a history of cyanotic breath-holding spells is normal.[26]

Pallid Type

Vagally mediated cardioinhibition causes bradycardia or asystole leading to cerebral hypoxemia.

Evaluation

A thorough history and normal physical exam are generally all that is needed to rule out other processes. In difficult cases ocular compression, with resuscitation equipment available, may show the asystole of breath-holding spells, or an EEG may show the definite spikes or spike waves of epilepsy. Exclusion of anemia is indicated.

Treatment

Immediate treatment is not needed, but a careful explanation of the episodes must be given to the parents. Although not thought to be causative, psychologic factors may exacerbate the problem, particularly with cyanotic spells; therefore, parental overindulgence and inconsistency should be avoided. For very frequent spells of the pallid type, atropine can be considered. However, long-term treatment with an anticholinergic drug has been questioned because of its possible deleterious effect on developing neurotransmitter systems. Anecdotally, spells have been halted by throwing cold water on the child or placing a cold compress on the child's forehead.

HEADACHES

Headache is a frequent symptom in children. The majority are infrequent and of little consequence. However, some are a manifestation of a systemic disorder or a result of a disturbance within the nervous system and associated head and neck structures. Chronic headaches constitute a challenge in diagnosis and management. A careful history and physical examination coupled with select laboratory tests aid in arriving at a proper diagnosis and treatment.[27]

The brain parenchyma, most of the dura and meningeal surfaces, and the ependymal lining of the ventricles are insensitive to pain. The intracranial pain-sensitive structures include the proximal portion of the large arteries, large venous sinuses, dural arteries, the part of the dura at the base of the skull, and certain structures innervated by cranial nerves V, IX, and X. Mechanisms that cause headaches include vasodilatation, inflammation, and traction and direct pressure on the intracranial structures. In addition, the scalp and neck muscles, sinuses, teeth, and orbits are pain-sensitive extracranial structures that can cause headache. Since the nerves innervating these structures are the same as those innervating the cerebral vessels and meninges, pain from extracranial structures can be perceived as a headache or as referred pain (Exhibit 11-4).

Exhibit 11-4 Classification of Headache

- Vascular Headaches of the Migraine Type
  - Classic migraine
  - Common migraine
  - Complicated migraine
    - Hemiplegic
    - Ophthalmoplegic
    - Basilar artery migraine
    - Acute confusional state
    - Alice-in-Wonderland syndrome
  - Migraine variants
    - Cyclic vomiting
  - Cluster headache
- Nonmigrainous Vascular Headaches
  - Systemic infection with fever
  - Convulsive states
  - Hypertension
  - Hypoxia
  - Miscellaneous
- Muscular Contraction Headaches
- Psychogenic Headaches
  - Depression
  - Conversion reaction or delusional state
  - Hypochondriacal state
- Traction Headaches
  - Tumor
  - Hematoma
  - Abscess
  - Post-LP
  - Pseudotumor cerebri
- Headaches with Cranial Inflammation
- Headaches Due to Diseases of Other Head or Neck Structures

Source: Adapted with permission from Dalessio DJ: *Wolff's Headache and Other Head Pain*. New York, Oxford University Press Inc, 1972.

Classification of Headaches

Migraine

Migraine is a vascular disorder affecting all age groups. There is a positive family history in 70% to 90% of cases. Vahlquist proposed criteria[28] that include paroxysmal headache separated by pain-free intervals and at least two of the following: unilateral pain, nausea, aura, and positive family history. Migraine occurs at any time of the day, lasts from 30 minutes to 2 or 3 days, and is often relieved by vomiting or sleep. Precipitating factors include stress, fatigue, exertion, head trauma, illness, or diet. Migraine can vary in intensity, frequency, and duration and is manifested in a variety of ways.

Muscle Contraction Headache

Muscle contraction headaches result from sustained contraction of the muscles of the neck and scalp. It is a most common form of headache in adolescents and adults. The pathophysiology is poorly understood. The patient describes a sensation of tightness or pressure in a bandlike distribution. Physical exam may reveal tenderness or tightness of the muscles in the occipital scalp or posterior cervical region. These headaches often last for weeks with varying degrees of intensity and do not interrupt regular daily activities.

Psychogenic Headache

A serious and overlooked cause of chronic headache in children is depression. Depression manifested as a headache is much less common in children than in adults but does occur. The child usually complains of a dull, constant headache that is generalized or localized to the occipital region. Other symptoms of childhood depression can often be elicited, including

- significant mood changes
- social withdrawal
- increasingly poor scholastic performance
- behavior problems at school
- sleep disturbances
- aggressive behavior
- persecution beliefs

- lack of energy
- weight loss and anorexia
- somatic complaints other than headache

Appropriate treatment depends on recognition of the underlying depression and can include environmental change, psychiatric intervention, antidepressant medications, or a combination of these. Good results have been obtained with antidepressants.

Traction Headache

As the name implies, a traction headache is caused by traction on the intracranial pain-sensitive structures. The traction may be exerted by a mass lesion such as a brain tumor, abscess, or subdural hematoma; by the weight of the brain after removal of CSF by LP; or by distortion of intracranial structures secondary to increased intracranial pressure as in hydrocephalus or pseudotumor cerebri. Although a relatively uncommon form of headache, it is often associated with serious intracranial pathology and hence warrants a careful evaluation.

Tumor Headache

Too often children with headaches are thought to have a brain tumor. Headache is often the first symptom of a brain tumor, but brain tumors are an uncommon cause of headache in childhood. Several characteristics help distinguish brain tumor headaches from other more benign varieties.[29] Headaches associated with brain tumors are usually traction headaches and are chronic and progressive in nature. Classically, the headaches are present in the morning on first arising and can be exacerbated by changes in position, coughing, or a Valsalva maneuver. The child is often not his usual self, even between attacks. Localization of the headache has only limited value since a mass lesion can distort a distant pain-sensitive structure. The patient's response to analgesics is also not a reliable clue. Brain tumor should be suspected when there is no previous history of headache or when there has been a recent change in the pattern of headache, particularly in the younger patient. It is important to note that headaches are rarely the only symptom of a progressing brain tumor. Associated symptoms such as vomiting, diplopia, weakness, ataxia, and personality changes are normally present. Physical exam often reveals papilledema, nuchal rigidity, irritability, focal neurologic deficits such as a visual field cut or hemiparesis, and signs of systemic disease. By the time medical attention is sought for these headaches, the child almost invariably has other signs that point to the presence of serious intracranial pathology.

Headache Associated with Other Head or Neck Structures

Refractive errors and eye muscle imbalance are common in children but only rarely do they cause headache. They can cause dull pain that is localized to the periorbital or frontal area and is clearly related to prolonged eye strain. Correction of the deficit leads to prompt resolution of the headache. Headache secondary to aural pathology is normally related to acute otitis externa, acute otitis media, or serous otitis media. The associated ear pain and the physical exam should make the diagnosis clear. Dental disease also can cause headache in association with severe local pain. Headache secondary to sinus disease is rare in young children because the sinuses are rather poorly developed.

Evaluation

History

The history is of paramount importance in establishing a correct diagnosis. Questions should be directed at both the patient and parents. Information should be sought regarding the character of the headache, its frequency and severity, the type of pain and its location, time of day during which attacks occur, and associated symptoms. A change in any of these parameters over time requires reevaluation. The location of a headache is often of little value in the pediatric age group. The severity of pain is not a reflection of the gravity of the underlying process and is best assessed by the degree of interference it causes in the activity level of the child.

Of particular importance is a detailed investigation of the triggering events and the events surrounding the first attack. This can provide a clue not only to the diagnosis but to the therapy. The history of a trauma and the nature of the insult, including the immediate consequences, should be part of the data base. The duration and frequency of the headache can indicate whether it requires urgent attention or simply an outpatient evaluation. A daily constant headache is most likely psychogenic in origin as opposed to recurrent morning headaches with vomiting. The presence of an aura can point to the diagnosis of migraine or temporal lobe seizures. Associated symptoms such as weakness, ataxia, personality change, and visual disturbances should make one suspect a mass lesion. The child's behavior between attacks is also important. A child who is well between attacks is much less likely to have organic disease than one with weight loss, fatigue, and irritability. These symptoms can also be found in childhood depression.

A family history of tension headache, migraine, seizures, and brain tumors should be elicited. Migraine in particular is a familial disorder, with a positive family history obtainable from 70% to 90% of patients. A family history of personality disorders, chronic abdominal pain, renal disease, collagen vascular disease, and hypertension also can be significant.

The type and number of medications used in the past is an indication of the perceived magnitude of the problem and can alert the physician to the potential for drug dependence or abuse. Sometimes a therapeutic response to a previously used agent is of diagnostic significance. Valuable insight into the family dynamics that often play an important role in childhood headache can also be gained by carefully observing the child's behavior and the parent-child interactions during the interview. At the end of the interview, the physician should have a good idea as to the type of headache present.

Physical Examination

Although findings are often normal in children and adults with headache, a complete general and neurologic examination is essential to rule out organic disease. In the general exam a blood pressure reading should be obtained. Disturbances in growth parameters, including head circumference, height, and weight, can indicate hydrocephalus, chronic disease, or the presence of a pituitary tumor. Particular attention should be given to the structure of the head and neck. One should palpate for scalp defects and for tenderness over the posterior cervical and occipital scalp area, percuss the sinuses, and auscultate for cranial bruits. Nuchal rigidity always should be excluded. Skin inspection can reveal evidence of a neurocutaneous disorder, such as café au lait spots or ash leaf lesions, or evidence of a metabolic disorder, such as Cushing's striae. The presence of muscle atrophy or wasting indicates chronic illness.

The neurologic exam should include a detailed evaluation of the visuomotor system, including a thorough funduscopic exam, testing of visual acuity and fields, and assessment of extraocular movements. Cranial nerve abnormalities and cerebellar findings can indicate a posterior fossa mass. Alterations of consciousness and personality change can be found in infectious and toxic encephalopathies. Gait disturbances and asymmetric motor findings point to possible structural abnormalities. When a properly done general and neurologic exam fails to reveal any significant abnormalities and the history is not atypical, one can usually rule out serious organic pathology without need for further work-up.

Diagnostic Studies

Illingworth[30] reports that of all children referred to a hospital for the evaluation of headache, an organic cause is found in only 5% or less. In these 5% the underlying abnormality can usually be suggested by a careful history and physical exam. Very rarely do laboratory tests reveal significant organic disease in the presence of a normal history and examination. Thus, in the majority of children with chronic headache, no laboratory studies are needed. When indicated, blood counts, sedimentation rate, urinalysis, blood lead level measurement, and sinus films may be of value. In select cases in which intracranial pathology is suspected, a variety of noninvasive and invasive neurodiagnostic procedures are available.

Skull X-Ray Films A skull film can be abnormal in a wide variety of conditions. In the evaluation of chronic headaches, it has been replaced by the CT scan.

Electroencephalography The EEG is minimally useful in the work-up of headaches. Even if the EEG is abnormal, one should always treat the patient and not the EEG.

Computed Tomography Scan CT is overutilized in patients with headache and is not indicated in the child with no other evidence of intracranial pathology. The CT scan does offer a safe, noninvasive, and sensitive means of detecting a variety of CNS structural lesions including brain tumor, hematoma, hydrocephalus, and hemorrhage. In the select group of children suspected of having a mass lesion or in the child with persistent neurologic deficit, a CT scan is mandatory.

Arteriography This procedure is rarely indicated in the diagnostic work-up of a child with headaches. Arteriography is indicated in the patient suspected of having an AVM or other vascular pathology.

Lumbar Puncture LP is seldom indicated in the work-up of chronic headache. However, it remains an invaluable tool in diagnosing the child with headache, nuchal rigidity, and signs or history suggesting CNS infection or bleeding. If papilledema is present or a mass lesion is suspected, the procedure should be done with caution.

Treatment

The treatment of childhood headaches should emphasize reassurance, removal of precipitating factors, and simple analgesics. Aggressive pharmacologic therapy should be avoided as much as possible. The parents and child are often more concerned about the possibility of a serious systemic illness or intracranial pathology than about the headache itself. Understanding that the pain is due to migraine or tension headaches and that these disorders are benign and have a good prognosis will relieve much of the anxiety. Nevertheless, a small number of children with chronic headache will require pharmacologic therapy.

Nonpharmacologic Therapy

A large number of external and constitutional factors play a role in triggering and exacerbating headaches in children. This is true of both migraine and tension headaches. Although these factors cannot be completely eliminated, their successful reduction significantly reduces the frequency and severity of symptoms. Foremost among these are the emotional stress of school, peer relations, and family tension. In adolescents the stresses of maturation, puberty, and the struggle to become independent are additional factors. For each child there is usually a particularly prominent area of tension that can be addressed. In selected cases family counseling or even psychotherapy may be indicated.

A change in living habits also can have a beneficial effect on the incidence of headaches. The irregular life-style of many adolescents contributes to their headaches, particularly in those with migraine. Fasting or missing meals, sleeping late or lack of sleep, and alcoholic consumption all have been implicated in triggering headache attacks. Other triggering factors include bright and flashing lights and heavy exertion. Dietary factors have not been conclusively implicated in migraine. However, in some patients there seems to be a correlation between ingestion of certain foods and headache, and in these patients dietary manipulation may be beneficial. In adolescent girls both migraine and tension headaches are often associated with menstrual periods. In addition, use of oral contraceptives can exacerbate headaches in many women.

Biofeedback and relaxation techniques are relatively new nonpharmacologic tools that have an increasingly important role in the management of chronic headaches, particularly in muscle contraction headaches and migraine. The safety of these techniques and the avoidance of drug dependency and the potential for abuse make it very attractive for use in adolescents with chronic headaches from all causes.

Short-Term Pharmacologic Treatment

For a large number of children with chronic headaches, both migrainous and tension related, therapy with a mild analgesic such as aspirin combined with rest in a quiet room offers adequate relief. For others a combination of aspirin and a mild sedative may be of help. Migraine attacks in children are generally of short duration, and reassurance and sedation, especially in the younger child, are often enough to get the child through the attack. With frequent migraine headache, prophylaxis may be necessary (Table 11-1).

Summary

Recurrent headaches are relatively common in children and adolescents. The majority of these are benign and do not reflect organic pathology. Diagnosis can usually be made by careful history and physical examination, and extensive laboratory investigations are rarely required. Most children can be managed with reassurance, simple analgesics, and mild sedation. For more severe cases, particularly of migraine, effective pharmacologic agents are available. The prognosis is favorable.

STATUS EPILEPTICUS

Although no universally accepted definition exists, status epilepticus can be defined as a state of recurring seizure activity lasting longer than 30 minutes, or recurrent convulsions without recovery of consciousness between episodes. Generalized (tonic-clonic) status epilepticus is a life-threatening condition, with a mortality rate as high as 20%, and requires prompt medical attention. Petit mal, complex partial, and focal motor status epilepticus is less life threatening.

Generalized status epilepticus produces systemic abnormalities including hypoxia, hypotension, acidosis, hyperthermia, and hypoglycemia. These factors in themselves contribute significantly to neuronal damage.

With this realization the rational approach in management should focus on (1) reversal of and prevention of systemic abnormalities, (2) cessation of seizures, and (3) determining the cause and prevention of further seizures[31,32,33] (Exhibit 11-5).

Immediate Therapy

The physician should promptly institute measures to stabilize the patient's vital functions, paying particular attention to an adequate airway and blood

TABLE 11-1 Drugs in Migraine Prophylaxis

Drug	Dosage: 6–12 yr	Dosage: Adolescents	Side Effects	Contraindications	Comments
Propranolol	5–10 mg tid; max, 20 mg qid	10–20 mg tid; max, 40 mg qid	Nausea, fatigue, bradycardia, hypotension, hypoglycemia	Congestive heart failure, insulin-dependent diabetes mellitus, asthma; use with caution in presence of family history of asthma	Very effective in all age groups and all forms of migraine
Phenobarbital	5 mg/kg/d; adjust to maintain serum levels 15–30 mg/L	3 mg/kg/d; adjust to maintain serum levels 15–30 mg/L	Drowsiness, impaired learning, idiosyncratic hyperactive response	Use with caution in hyperactive children	Probably more effective in younger age group
Phenytoin	5 mg/kg/d; adjust to maintain serum levels 10–20 mg/L	3–5 mg/kg/d; adjust to maintain serum levels 10–20 mg/L	Gingival hyperplasia, hirsutism, ataxia	Known allergy	Probably more effective in younger age group
Amitriptyline	Not approved	25–50 mg qhs; increase every 1–2 weeks to max 200–250 mg/d	Dry mouth, dizziness, fatigue, abdominal pain, mydriasis, urinary retention, constipation, weight gain	Known allergy	Especially useful in adolescents with combination of migraine and muscle contraction headache
Cyproheptadine	0.2–0.4 mg/kg/d in 2–3 divided doses	4–12 mg/d	Drowsiness, impaired learning, increased appetite, weight gain	Known allergy	Of limited use, primarily in younger children
Clonidine	0.01–0.02 mg/kg/d	Same	Nausea, fatigue, disturbed sleep patterns	Known allergy	Effective in adults; in controlled trial in children was not superior to placebo

Source: Reprinted with permission from Shinnar S, D'Souza BJ: Migraine in children and adolescents. *Pediatrics in Review* 1982;3:257–262.

pressure. The child is placed in the decubitus position, and pharyngeal secretions, if present, are suctioned and airway patency is reassessed. If ventilation remains inadequate, respiratory assistance with bag-and-mask or endotracheal intubation is instituted. Once the presence of adequate ventilation is established, oxygen is administered as needed. Gastric contents are aspirated through a nasogastric tube, and vital signs (pulse, blood pressure, and temperature) are monitored frequently. Measures are taken to protect the patient from injury during convulsive activity. An indwelling intravenous catheter is established and blood is drawn for determination of serum electrolytes, glucose, calcium, and blood urea nitrogen. It is also advisable to save blood for a toxicology screen. Anticonvulsant levels are determined if the patient was previously on such medication. A Dextrostix determination can be invaluable in ruling out hypoglycemia.

While these preliminary steps are being undertaken, the patient requires the prompt administration of *intravenous* anticonvulsants to arrest seizure activity[31,32,33] (see Exhibit 11-5 and Table 11-2). Cessation of such activity is frequently associated with return of airway patency and adequate spontaneous respiration. Failure to respond to anticonvulsants most often results from inadequate dosage or administration of drug intramuscularly, orally, or rectally. Another reason is failure to correct the underlying cause, be it metabolic-toxic or infectious.

Exhibit 11-5 Guidelines for Management of Status Epilepticus

I. Stabilization 0–10 min	Establish airway, blood pressure, nasal O_2; intubate if necessary. Collect blood for CBC,* electrolytes, BUN, drug levels, calcium, magnesium, toxic screen, glucose, and Dextrostix. Start IV with D5NS (if indicated, D25, push 1 mL/kg). Measure blood gas for O_2 + pH; if pH below 7.1, give bicarbonate. Monitor respirations, blood pressure, and electrocardiogram.
II. Control of Seizures 10–25 min	*Diazepam:* Give 0.3–0.5 mg/kg IV (10-mg maximum in one dose, to be given no faster than 2 mg/min). May repeat q10min for maximum of 3 doses. *Be prepared to intubate patient.* *Phenytoin:* Start after first dose of diazepam; give 18–20 mg/kg no faster than 50 mg/min. If bradycardia or hypotension occurs, slow infusion rate.
25–40 min	If seizures persist, intubate and then continue phenytoin infusion until seizures stop or to a maximum dose of 25 mg/kg.
40–60 min	If seizures continue, start infusion of *phenobarbital:* a loading dose of 15–25 mg/kg, no faster than 30 mg/min. Monitor respirations and blood pressure.
60–90 min	If seizures continue, start infusion of 4%–10% solution *Paraldehyde* diluted in normal saline (do not store in plastic bags). Administer at a rate fast enough to control seizures. A reasonable starting rate is 60–125 mL/h.
>90 min	If paraldehyde has not terminated seizures within 20 min from start of infusion, institute general anesthesia and EEG monitoring. Keep EEG near flat for at least 2 h, then begin slow withdrawal of anesthesia.
III. Diagnostic Evaluation	This should coincide with the control of seizures. It includes detailed history, physical examination, and consideration of further diagnostic work-up with special consideration for treatable diseases (e.g., meningitis, encephalitis, toxic-metabolic disorders, and mass lesions).

Source: Adapted with permission from Delgado-Escueta AV, Wasterlain C, Treiman DM, et al: Management of status epilepticus. *N Engl J Med* 1982;306:1337–1340; and from Barbosa E, Freeman JM: Status epilepticus. *Pediatrics in Review* 1982;4:185–189.

* Abbreviations: CBC, complete blood count; BUN, blood urea nitrogen; D5NS, 5% dextrose in normal saline; D25, 25% dextrose.

TABLE 11-2 Drugs in Status Epilepticus

Drugs	Intravenous Dosage	Side Effects	Comments
Diazepam (Valium)	0.3–0.5 mg/kg; maximum three doses	Respiratory depression, hypotension, thrombophlebitis	Insoluble in IV solution
Phenytoin (Dilantin)	18–25 mg/kg at a maximum rate of 50 mg/min	Bradycardia, hypotension, cardiac arrhythmias	Extreme caution with cardiac patients, toxicity secondary to rapid infusion rates
Phenobarbital	15–25 mg/kg at a maximum rate of 30 mg/min	Respiratory depression, hypotension	
Paraldehyde	4%–10% solution as rapidly as required to control seizures	Pulmonary hemorrhage, pulmonary edema, metabolic acidosis	Caution in patients with liver damage

Source: Reprinted with permission from Barbosa E, Freeman JM: Status epilepticus. *Pediatrics in Review* 1982;4:185–189.

Maintenance Therapy

Once the seizures are controlled, maintenance therapy (Table 11-3) is instituted to prevent recurrence. Serum drug levels are assayed to assure adequate therapeutic levels (Table 11-4).

The next step is determination of the cause. A variety of disorders can be incriminated as the precipitating cause of status epilepticus. Examination focuses on ruling out increased intracranial pressure, intracranial hemorrhage, and infection. Evidence of trauma or needle marks should be sought (diabetics, drug addicts). The most common causes (Exhibit 11-6) are identified through routine history and physical assessment in conjunction with appropriate laboratory studies.

Status epilepticus represents a true medical emergency. Management includes stabilizing the vital signs and the proper use of anticonvulsants. The assessment should detect the cause and thus determine appropriate treatment.

TABLE 11-3 Drugs Used in the Control of Seizure Disorders

	Generalized Tonic–Clonic (Major Motor)	Absence (Petit Mal)	Complex Partial	Simple Partial Seizures	Minor Motor
Phenobarbital	✓		✓	✓	
Phenytoin (Dilantin)	✓		✓	✓	
Primidone (Mysoline)	✓		✓	✓	
Carbamazepine (Tegretol)	✓		✓	✓	
Ethosuximide (Zarontin)		✓			
Clonazepam (Clonopin)		✓			✓
Valproic Acid (Depakene)	✓	✓			✓
Acetazolamide (Diamox)					✓
Adrenocorticotropin and corticosteroids					✓
Ketogenic diet					✓

TABLE 11-4 Therapeutic Antiepileptic Drug Regimens for Pediatric Patients

Drugs	Total Dose (mg/kg/d)	Form	Therapeutic Range	Half-Life (h)
Phenobarbital	4–8	Liquid: 20 mg/5 mL Tabs: 15, 30, 60, 100 mg	15–40 μg/mL	96
Phenytoin	4–10	Liquid (not recommended by authors) Tabs: 50 mg Caps: 30, 100 mg	10–20 μg/mL	24
Primidone	12–25	Tabs: 50, 250 mg Suspension: 250 mg/5 mL	6–12 μg/mL	12
Carbamazepine	20–30	Tabs: 100, 200 mg	5–12 μg/mL	12
Ethosuximide	20–40	Caps: 250 mg Liquid: 250 mg/5 mL	40–100 μg/mL	30
Clonazepam	0.03–0.2	Tabs: 0.5, 1, 2 mg	5–50 ng/mL (not reliable)	52
Valproic Acid	15–100	Caps: 250 mg Liquid: 250 mg/5 mL	>50 μg/mL	6–8
Acetazolamide	10–30	Tabs: 250 mg Syrup: 250 mg/5 mL	10–14 μg/mL (usually not available)	10–15

Exhibit 11-6 Common Causes of Status Epilepticus Excluding Antiepileptic Medication Withdrawal

- Infection (12%)
  - Meningitis
  - Encephalitis
  - Aseptic meningitis
- Trauma (1%)
- Toxic-Metabolic (11%)
  - Hypoxia
  - Dehydration
  - Electrolyte imbalances
  - Hypoglycemia
  - Uremia
  - Toxic ingestion
- Miscellaneous (77%)
  - Chronic encephalopathy (17%)
  - Idiopathic (25%)
  - CNS degenerative disease (4%)
  - Febrile seizures (28%)
  - Congenital abnormalities (3%)

Source: Adapted with permission from Barbosa E, Freeman JM: Status epilepticus. *Pediatrics in Review* 1982;4:185–189, and from Rawal K, D'Souza BJ: Status epilepticus. *Critical Care Clin* 1985;1:339–353.

REYE'S SYNDROME

Reye's syndrome, first described in 1963, is an acute, life-threatening, noninflammatory encephalopathy occurring most commonly after a viral illness and accompanied by fatty degeneration of the viscera.[34] Approximately 60% to 70% of cases of Reye's syndrome have been associated with respiratory illnesses, especially influenza B; 20% to 30% with varicella; and 5% to 15% with gastrointestinal illnesses, primarily diarrhea. Exhibit 11-7 lists the viruses associated with Reye's syndrome. Although infants and children of all ages are affected, the peak incidence occurs between 5 and 15 years; there is no clear sex predilection. Regional differences have been observed, with the highest incidence in Michigan, Ohio, Georgia, and a group of central and mountain states (Iowa, South Dakota, Nebraska, Colorado, Utah).[35] Because of the suspected link between aspirin and Reye's syndrome, the Committee on Infectious Diseases recommends that "aspirin not be prescribed under usual circumstances for children with varicella or those suspected of having influenza on the basis of clinical or epidemiologic evidence."[36] The association of Reye's syndrome and prior salicylate ingestion was confirmed in a Public Health Service pilot study published in 1985.[37]

Exhibit 11-7 Viruses Associated with Reye's Syndrome

- Influenza, types A and B
- Varicella
- Coxsackievirus
- EBV
- Echovirus
- Herpes simplex
- Parainfluenza
- Poliomyelitis
- Reovirus
- Rubella
- Rubeola
- Live virus vaccines

Pathophysiology

Pathologic changes of Reye's syndrome involve multiple organs. The liver is grossly enlarged and often yellow, reddish yellow, or white in appearance because of the 20% to 30% triglyceride content. Microscopically, the most important finding is diffuse microvesicular accumulation of lipid within the liver cell cytoplasm. No hepatic cellular necrosis or inflammatory infiltrates are seen. The ultrastructural changes are most prominent in the mitochondria, which are swollen and exhibit an outer membrane deformed by cytoplasmic invaginations. In addition, the mitochondrial matrix density is reduced.

The brain is edematous, with flattening of the gyri and increased weight. Microscopic changes consistent with hypoxia can be seen, specifically focal neuronal loss, eosinophilic changes in the neurons, and glial proliferation. The ultrastructural abnormalities include astrocytic swelling and other alterations that may be characteristic of Reye's syndrome, specifically swelling in the myelin sheaths (myelin bleb formation) and neuronal mitochondrial changes. The mitochondrial abnormalities are similar to those found in hepatocytes. Although the mitochondrial injury is reversible, the bleb formation results in permanent loss of myelinated fibers.

Fat droplets also have been found in the kidney tubule cells, skeletal muscle, and myocardium. Mitochondrial changes have been noted in myocardium and skeletal muscle.

The biochemistry and pathogenesis of Reye's syndrome is still incompletely understood. It appears that the multiple metabolic abnormalities arise from two processes: (1) a catabolic state caused by the viral illness, anorexia, and vomiting, and (2) mitochondrial dysfunction of unknown etiology. The catabolic process increases the mobilization of fat from adipose tissue, amino acids from muscle, and glycogen from liver and muscle. The metabolism of these substances by extrahepatic tissues is impaired by the mitochondrial injury, leading to an increase in substrate delivered to the liver. However, the liver cell mitochondria are similarly impaired, reducing the liver's ability to efficiently handle these substances. The increase in substrate mobilization combined with a decrease in hepatic clearance results in the marked elevation of a number of substances, in particular, blood ammonia, pyruvate, lactate, alanine, and free fatty acids.

Presently, there is active debate concerning the pathogenesis of the encephalopathy.[38] A combination of primary mitochondrial dysfunction in brain tissue along with the generalized metabolic derangement is likely responsible. The similar ultrastructural changes found in liver and brain mitochondria support the speculation that the mitochondrial injury is primary to both tissues. Different metabolites, especially ammonia and free fatty acids, have been implicated in the pathogenesis of the encephalopathy. The strongest evidence, however, appears to implicate ammonia. In patients with Reye's syndrome, both the blood level and the total duration of hyperammonemia correlate with the severity of the encephalopathy and mortality, whereas substantial elevations in free fatty acids can be seen in patients with inherited metabolic disorders without producing significant changes in mentation and awareness. Free fatty acids along with other substances may, however, act synergistically with ammonia to produce the encephalopathy.

Clinical Characteristics

The clinical features of Reye's syndrome in infants under 1 year of age differ from those in older children.[39] In infants, as in older children, the encephalopathy is almost always preceded by a prodromal viral illness. In infants, however, the prodrome is more commonly accompanied by diarrhea. This is followed by vomiting, which is usually mild; lethargy, marked respiratory abnormalities, especially hyperventilation; apneic episodes; and finally coma. Seizures frequently occur in the early stages of the disease in infants and can be grand mal, multifocal, or myoclonic. Hepatomegaly as well as hypoglycemia is found more frequently in infants than in older children.

In older children the prodromal illness is usually mild and lasts 5 to 7 days before the onset of the encephalitic phase, which begins with irritability, lethargy, and vomiting. Vomiting is a cardinal feature of the disease, occurring in greater than 90% of the cases, and the diagnosis should be questioned when it is absent. Low-grade fever may be present but is not a significant part of the illness initially. As noted recently, some if not most of the cases do not progress beyond this stage.[40] Other patients progress over hours to days (usually 24 to 48 hours) to stupor, coma, and death. More commonly, patients enter a hyperexcitable state characterized by

- restlessness
- inappropriate language and hallucinations
- disorientation
- combativeness
- slurred speech
- visual unresponsiveness
- sympathetic hyperactivity: fever, sweating, tachycardia, tachypnea, and sluggishly reactive and dilated pupils

The child may begin to recover or continue to deteriorate, with the CNS dysfunction following a rostral-to-caudal progression. Obtundation progresses to stupor and then coma. Normal posture is replaced by decorticate, then decerebrate, posturing and finally a flaccid areflexic state. The pupils that initially were large and sluggishly reactive become fixed and dilated. Apnea and circulatory collapse are the terminal events. Seizures are unusual in the early course of the disease but can occur later on. Papilledema is uncommon, although engorgement of retinal veins and loss of venous pulsations are frequently noted.

Studies indicate that the most important prognostic factor in outcome has been the stage of encephalopathy on admission. One of the more commonly used systems was suggested by Lovejoy et al. (Exhibit 11-8).[41] Recently, the National Institutes of Health (NIH) Consensus Conference proposed a system that it hopes will replace older rating systems (Table 11-5).[42]

Exhibit 11-8 Staging of Reye's Syndrome: Lovejoy Classification

I. Vomiting, lethargy, sleepiness, and laboratory evidence of liver dysfunction
II. Disorientation, delirium and combativeness, hyperventilation, hyperactive reflexes, appropriate response to noxious stimuli, and laboratory evidence of liver dysfunction
III. Obtundation, coma, hyperventilation, decorticate rigidity, preservation of pupillary light reaction and oculovestibular reflexes, and laboratory evidence of liver dysfunction
IV. Deepening coma, decerebrate rigidity, loss of oculocephalic reflexes (often asymmetric), large fixed pupils, dysconjugate eye movements in response to caloric stimulation of oculovestibular reflex, and minimal liver dysfunction
V. Absent deep tendon reflexes, seizures, respiratory arrest, flaccidity, and often normal hepatic function

Source: Reprinted with permission from Lovejoy FH, Smith AL, et al: Clinical staging in Reye syndrome. *Am J Dis Child* 128:36–41, 1974. Copyright © 1974, American Medical Association.

TABLE 11-5 Staging of Reye's Syndrome: NIH Classification

	I	II	III	IV	V
Level of consciousness	Lethargic, follows verbal commands	Combative, stupor, verbalizes inappropriately	Coma	Coma	Coma
Posture	Normal	Normal	Decorticate	Decerebrate	Flaccid
Response to pain	Purposeful	Purposeful, nonpurposeful	Decorticate	Decerebrate	None
Pupillary reaction	Brisk	Sluggish	Sluggish	Sluggish	None

Source: Reprinted from NIH Consensus Conference: Diagnosis and Treatment of Reye's Syndrome. *JAMA* 1981;246:2441–2444.

Diagnostic Tests

There are multiple laboratory abnormalities found in Reye's syndrome (Exhibit 11-9). Hyperammonemia is present in virtually all patients early in the course of the disease, and blood ammonia levels usually return to normal within 24 to 48 hours, regardless of treatment. Peak blood levels appear to be related to prognosis: peak ammonia levels greater than 300 μg/dL or five to six times the upper limit of normal are associated with increased mortality.

The prothrombin time is prolonged in 90% or more of the patients. Vitamin K administered to patients with Reye's syndrome usually is ineffective in correcting the coagulation abnormalities. The platelet count is usually normal and fibrin split products are usually absent. Patients under 4 years of age, especially infants, or those with an antecedent varicella or gastrointestinal illness have low blood sugar levels more commonly than older children or those with a prodromal respiratory illness.

Although there potentially is a small risk of provoking intracranial herniation, an LP should be performed when there is any uncertainty in the diagnosis.

Although most patients can be diagnosed without liver biopsy, in certain specific situations it may be helpful. Indications include

1. age under 1 year
2. recurrent episodes
3. family history
4. nonepidemic case without infection or vomiting, or when other illnesses with similar symptoms cannot be excluded
5. plans for a new and potentially dangerous therapeutic regimen

A CT scan is not necessary unless there is a clinical suspicion of some other disease process, for example intracranial hemorrhage, brain abscess, or infarction. Early in the illness the CT scan can be normal or show evidence of diffuse brain edema without evidence of shift or focal enhancement.

Exhibit 11-9 Laboratory Features of Reye's Syndrome

1. Serum transaminase levels at least three times the upper limit of normal
2. Elevated blood ammonia
3. Prolonged prothrombin time
4. Normal to slightly elevated bilirubin
5. Glucose low in infants but normal in older children.
6. CSF usually contains fewer than 8 cells/mm³ and normal protein and glucose except when there is hypoglycemia. The opening pressure can be normal or elevated.
7. Other laboratory abnormalities: mixed acid-base disturbance; leukocytosis; elevations in CPK,* uric acid, amylase, lactate, pyruvate, and BUN; hypophosphatemia; and elevations in serum amino acids and fatty acids
8. Liver biopsy shows diffuse microvesicular accumulation of lipid within cytoplasm of hepatocytes.
9. Appropriate tests show no evidence of toxin exposure or drug ingestion that could produce similar clinical findings.

* Abbreviations: CPK, creatine phosphokinase; BUN, blood urea nitrogen.

Differential Diagnosis

Exhibit 11-10 lists disorders that can mimic Reye's syndrome.

Treatment

Treatment depends on the stage of illness at the time the patient is admitted to the emergency department (Exhibit 11-11).

Prognosis

The mortality in 1963 was 80%.[34] More recently, the fatality rate has declined from approximately 41% in 1974 to 21% in 1980 and is probably approaching 10% in most university hospitals. The actual rate may even be substantially lower if, as recently reported,[40] the disease is more common than previously thought. The most likely explanation for the drop in mortality is greater awareness of the disease and thus earlier diagnosis coupled with improved intensive supportive therapy. The admission to the

Exhibit 11-10 Differential Diagnosis for Reye's Syndrome

Infections
- Viral or bacterial meningitis
- Viral encephalitis

Fulminant Hepatic Failure Secondary to Infection or Hepatotoxins

Toxins
- Salicylates
- Acetaminophen
- Valproic acid
- Methyl bromide
- Hypoglycin (Jamaican vomiting sickness)
- Aflatoxin (Udorn encephalopathy)
- Folk remedies: margosa oil
- Isopropyl alcohol
- Lead
- Trematol

Anoxic or Ischemic Encephalopathy

Inborn Errors of Metabolism
- Systemic carnitine deficiency
- Glutamic acidemia
- Ornithine transcarbamoylase deficiency
- Hereditary fructose intolerance
- Ketotic hyperglycinemia syndrome
- Medium chain acyl dehydrogenase deficiency

hospital of patients at earlier stages of Reye's syndrome and the decreasing death rates within each stage support this explanation.

Complete recovery can be expected in many, if not most, of the patients who survive the acute illness. However, between 30% and 60% may suffer either neurologic or psychologic sequelae including developmental delay, motor impairment, mental retardation, attentional and learning disorders, and anxiety and apprehension.[44] Younger children and those with the more severe encephalopathy are likely to have the more severe deficits.

CENTRAL NERVOUS SYSTEM INFECTIONS*

CNS infections constitute some of the most important disorders affecting man. In many instances emergency evaluation and care are indicated. This section provides guidelines for the approach to patients with CNS infections.[45,46,47] Symptom complexes are discussed, diagnostic work-up is outlined, and recommendations are made regarding

* Note: The authors wish to acknowledge very helpful suggestions regarding this section from Drs. Jay Tureen and E. Richard Moxon and the secretarial assistance of Elaine Langlois.

Exhibit 11-11 Therapy for Reye's Syndrome

1. Early diagnosis and referral to a center that has experience in managing patients with Reye's syndrome

2. Stage I or II
   a. Frequent monitoring of blood pressure, heart rate, respiratory rate, temperature, and neurological signs
   b. Administration of 5%–10% dextrose solution by intravenous infusion
   c. Correction of electrolyte abnormalities

3. Stage III or greater
   a. Monitoring: frequent arterial blood gases, continuous blood pressure, central venous or pulmonary artery/wedge pressure, cardiac output in critically ill children, accurate fluid balance, intracranial pressure, and temperature
   b. Intubation: pancuronium bromide, 0.1–0.2 mg/kg/dose, to control ventilation and intracranial pressure, if necessary
   c. Correction of metabolic abnormalities
      (1) Correction of electrolyte imbalances
      (2) Fluid administration adjusted to maintain adequate blood pressure and cardiac output without adversely affecting intracranial pressure
      *(3) Hypertonic glucose (10%–20% solution). Insulin can be administered at a dose of 1 U/5–10 glucose, by bolus or continuous infusion. Serum glucose should be maintained between 125 mg/dL and 175 mg/dL. Frequent monitoring of serum glucose and serum osmolality is mandatory.
      *(4) Lowering ammonia level
         (a) Neomycin by nasogastric tube at a dose of 100 mg/kg/d and/or lactulose, 1–2 g/kg/d, *OR*
         (b) Sodium benzoate or phenylacetate at a loading dose of 250 mg/kg, followed by 500 mg/kg/d, *OR*
         (c) Consider more invasive techniques—e.g., dialysis, exchange transfusion—for ammonia levels greater than 300 mg/dL or greater than 5–6 times upper limit of normal. Must weigh risk of procedure against unproven benefit.
   d. Reducing intracranial pressure
      (1) Muscle paralysis
      (2) Hyperventilation: maintain carbon dioxide pressure between 25 and 30 mmHg
      (3) Mannitol 0.25 g/kg/dose, if intracranial pressure rises above 20 mmHg. Serum osmolality should be monitored frequently and kept below 320 mosm/L. Watch for renal failure and hypotension.
      *(4) Barbiturate coma if above methods fail. Pentobarbital at a loading dose of 3–4 mg/kg, followed by 100–200 mg/h until a blood level of 3–4 mg/dL is obtained. Maintain burst-suppression EEG. Once coma is induced, clinical assessment is impossible. Complications include hypoxia, hypotension, and decreased cardiac output.[43]
      *(5) Decompressive craniotomy and hypothermia
   e. If significant bleeding occurs, or prior to invasive procedures, correct clotting abnormalities with fresh frozen plasma. Vitamin K is accepted therapy but usually does not work.

* Improved survival rates have not yet been demonstrated.

management. The focus is on those disorders most likely to be encountered in the emergency care setting.

CNS infection may create signs and symptoms that suggest primary meningeal involvement or meningitis. Headache, stiff neck, and Kernig's, and Brudzinski's signs are encountered. However, in children less than 2 years of age, signs of meningeal inflammation and fever can be absent; common findings include irritability, lethargy, seizures, vomiting, and poor feeding. Signs of CNS parenchymal involvement are due to tissue inflammation and necrosis or mass effect: headache, altered mental status or personality, convulsions, focal neurologic abnormalities, and signs of increased intracranial pressure. Encephalitis denotes inflammation of the brain parenchyma; myelitis, the spinal cord. In many patients the symptoms and signs of infection suggest involvement of both the meninges and the parenchyma. Nevertheless, it often proves useful during the initial evaluation of patients with CNS infections to attempt to characterize the process as primarily involving one or the other.

Examination of CSF can be especially important in guiding early management. Table 11-6 lists the findings generally encountered.

Initial Evaluation

The first minutes spent with a patient with a CNS infection can be the most informative and therapeutically important. First, the cardiorespiratory status is assessed, and, if necessary, appropriate support is arranged. The presence of coma or convulsions necessitates appropriate management (discussed earlier in this chapter). An intravenous line is inserted and laboratory studies are dispatched as indicated by the clinical context. Studies usually indicated in patients with suspected bacterial meningitis are given in Exhibit 11-12.

The nature and tempo of all neurologic symptoms must be detailed to establish the course as acute, subacute, or chronic. An evaluation of recent systemic infections and a search for those conditions predisposing to bacterial meningitis are included in the history. A history of fever, rash, cough, upper respiratory tract infection, recent gastrointestinal symptoms, and recent behavioral change should be noted. Paracranial infection may be indicated by symptoms related to otitis media, sinusitis, mastoiditis, osteomyelitis, or orbital cellulitis. Patients with dural defects (e.g., occipital or lumbar dermal sinus, basilar skull fracture, recent cranial trauma or craniotomy, CSF removal) or with intracranial appliances (e.g., VP shunt for hydrocephalus) are at increased risk for meningitis.

A number of preexisting conditions predispose to infection:

- congenital heart disease
- sickle cell anemia
- asplenia (or after splenectomy)
- hepatic cirrhosis
- hypogammaglobulinemia
- myeloproliferative disorders
- treatment with immunosuppressive agents
- collagen diseases

A recent travel history and unusual environmental and food exposures should be noted.

TABLE 11-6 CSF Patterns in CNS Infection and in Normal Patients*

	Pressure (mmH_2O)	Appearance	Protein (mg/dL)	Glucose (% of BS)†	Cells	PMN (%)
CNS infection						
Purulent	Usually ↑	Opalescent, turbid, or cloudy	Usually ↑	↓	>1000	>80
Granulomatous	N or ↑	Clear to opalescent	Usually ↑	Usually ↓	10–1000	<50
Lymphocytic (aseptic)	N or ↑	Usually clear	↑ or N	N	10–1000	<50
Normal values						
Preterm newborn infant		Clear to xanthochromic	60–200	70–80	0–15 (mean, 7)	60
Term newborn infant	90–110	Clear to xanthochromic	60–150	70–80	0–32 (mean, 8)	60
Child > 6 mo and adult	80–180 mm	Clear	≤45	50–60	≤5	0

* The values given should be used as guidelines for the evaluation of CSF samples. The final decision regarding the significance of CSF findings in the individual patient depends heavily on the clinical context.
† Abbreviations and symbols: BS, blood sugar; PMN, polymorphonuclear leukocytes; N, normal; ↑, increased, ↓, decreased.

Exhibit 11-12 Studies in Patients with Suspected Bacterial Meningitis

Usual Studies
- Complete blood count with differential and platelet count
- Urinalysis and urine culture (For children less than 1 year old, urine can be obtained by suprapubic aspiration.)
- Blood culture
- Prothrombin time
- Serum electrolytes, creatinine, blood urea nitrogen, and glucose
- Chest x-ray film
- Electrocardiogram
- LP and CSF examination. This includes recording of opening pressure, CSF appearance, complete cell count and differential, Gram stain for bacteria, acid-fast bacillus smear, and India ink preparation (all of these can be performed by the house officer). CSF should be sent to the laboratory for protein and glucose determinations, countercurrentimmunoelectrophoresis, latex agglutination test, and culture for bacteria (aerobes and anaerobes), fungi, and mycobacteria. A blood glucose reading should be obtained immediately prior to LP.
- Tuberculin skin test

Studies That May Be Indicated, Depending on Clinical Context
- Skull films
- Sinus and mastoid x-ray films
- Transillumination of the skull (infant)
- Cranial CT or magnetic resonance (MRI) scan
- Radionuclide brain scan
- EEG
- Toxicology screen
- Salicylate level
- Serum ammonia
- Liver function tests
- Partial thromboplastin time, serum fibrinogen, and factors V and VIII
- Blood and urine osmolarities
- Serum immunoglobulins
- Serum and CSF VDRL
- Specimens for viral isolation (e.g., stool, CSF, oropharyngeal secretions)
- Heterophile agglutinins
- Acute and convalescent phase sera to test for appropriate infectious agents

Source: Bell WE and McCormick WF: *Neurologic Infections in Children.* Philadelphia, WB Saunders, 1981.

A general physical examination helps to elucidate the nature and extent of coincident systemic illness. Cutaneous lesions are noted. Meningeal signs are sought, and the level of consciousness is assessed. Funduscopic examination is performed in all patients, including infants. The pattern of respirations is observed. Focal deficits are sought on cranial nerve, cerebellar, motor, sensory, and deep tendon reflex examinations; gait is tested, if possible. Signs of raised intracranial pressure include altered consciousness, papilledema, palsy(ies) of cranial nerve VI, tense anterior fontanel, altered pupillary light reflex, setting-sun sign or difficulty with upgaze, and ataxia. The characteristics of any attendant seizures are carefully noted. By this point in the evaluation of most patients, the physician can specify disease tempo and is usually prepared to classify the presentation as primarily meningeal or parenchymal in its manifestations. In the following sections CNS infections are discussed in the context of their usual clinical presentation.

Acute Bacterial Meningitis

Pathogenesis

Bacterial meningitis consists of an infection of the pia and arachnoid and of the fluid space they enclose, the subarachnoid space (SAS). Bacteria reach this location by hematogenous spread or by direct extension from a parameningeal focus. The SAS is continuous around the brain, optic nerves, and spinal cord. Once bacteria gain access to the SAS, they can enter the entire cerebrospinal space. The ventricles are reached either by direct spread or by reflux through the foramina of Luschka and Magendie. Once in the SAS, bacteria incite an inflammatory reaction in the pia, arachnoid, CSF, and ventricles. For the first few days, polymorphonuclear leukocytes (PMNs) are the principal inflammatory cell type migrating into the SAS. Mononuclear cells then increase in number. Foci of inflammation are present in the subarachnoid arteries and veins and may be associated with focal necrosis. These vascular changes and associated thrombosis, especially that occurring in veins, may explain some of the focal cerebral abnormalities encountered. Inflammation or vascular involvement of cranial nerve roots passing through the SAS may explain findings related to these structures (e.g., ocular palsies, facial weakness). Toxic by-products of bacterial infection may contribute to cerebral dysfunction and edema. As the infection is arrested, resolution ensues and inflammatory cells disappear in the same order as they arrived. The degree of resolution depends on the stage at which the infection is arrested.

Almost any bacterial agent can produce meningitis. However, in most cases the age of the patient dictates the organisms most frequently encountered (Table 11-7).

Neonatal Meningitis

Meningitis during the first month of life can be subtle and deceptive. Prematurity, maternal bacteremia, prolonged rupture of membranes, prolonged or traumatic labor, chorioamnionitis, and infection of the skin or the umbilical stump can all predispose to meningitis. Initial clinical findings may include irri-

TABLE 11-7 Most Common Causes of Bacterial Meningitis

Age Group	Organism
Birth to 4 wk	Group B streptococcus *Escherichia coli* *Listeria monocytogenes*
4–12 wk	Group B streptococcus *Streptococcus pneumoniae* *Salmonella* *Listeria monocytogenes* *Haemophilus influenzae*
3 mo to 10 yr*	*H. influenzae* *S. pneumoniae* *Neisseria meningitidis*
Over 10 yr	*S. pneumoniae* *N. meningitidis*

* Outside the US *Mycobacterium tuberculosis* is an important cause in this age group.

Source: Bell WE and McCormick WF: *Neurologic Infections in Children.* Philadelphia, WB Saunders, 1981.

tability, lethargy, poor feeding, vomiting, abdominal distention, respiratory distress, apnea, or unexplained jaundice. Fever may not be present, and in premature infants hypothermia can occur. The presence of even one of these findings is sufficient to suspect sepsis and meningitis. Seizures can occur and point to CNS involvement. Meningeal signs and symptoms are frequently absent. The bacteria most likely responsible for neonatal meningitis are group B streptococcus and *Escherichia coli.*

Group B streptococcus infections in the infant take two different forms: early onset and late onset. With early onset, clinical signs are present in the first hours to days after birth and reflect fulminating sepsis and pneumonia. Apneic spells, respiratory distress, shock, and coma can occur; meningitis is present in about 30% of such patients. The mortality rate among these infants is greater than 50%. Late onset infection begins between 10 days and 3 months of age and is frequently accompanied by meningitis. The clinical manifestations are those expected for meningitis in this age group, as discussed earlier. Mortality with this type is approximately 20%.

Less frequent causes of neonatal meningitis are other Gram-negative rods (family Enterobacteriaceae), *Pseudomonas, Streptococcus pneumoniae,* and *Listeria monocytogenes.* Rare causes are *Campylobacter fetus, H. influenzae,* and *Flavobacterium meningosepticum.* In infants 1 to 3 months old, group B streptococcus and *Streptococcus pneumoniae* are most often responsible for meningitis. *Salmonella* meningitis can occur in the infant, as well as during the first months of life. It is often associated with diarrhea, may be epidemic, and is rapidly progressive. Staphylococcal infection is an important cause of meningitis in infants shunted for hydrocephalus and in those with skin and umbilical stump infections. Congenital syphilis may be associated with acute or subacute meningitis.

The work-up of meningitis in infants consists of most of the usual studies (Exhibit 11-12), and any others that may reveal a source of systemic sepsis. In the case of neonates, the mother should be examined for signs of infection (amnionitis, endometritis, urinary tract infection, and sepsis). Diagnosis depends on the suspicion of meningitis and performance of an LP. The CSF abnormalities include PMN pleocytosis, reduced glucose, and elevated protein. Organisms are usually present on Gram stain and culture. As many as 50% to 75% of patients with neonatal meningitis die, and many of the survivors suffer sequelae including hydrocephalus, seizures, mental retardation, hyperactive behavior, and cranial nerve and long tract deficits.

Bacterial Meningitis in Older Infants, Children, and Adolescents

Between 3 months of age and adolescence, *Haemophilus influenzae,* type b, *Streptococcus pneumoniae,* and *Neisseria meningitidis* account for most cases of meningitis. *Haemophilus influenzae* meningitis occurs, chiefly, in patients under 5 years, but is also responsible for cases occurring in older children and adults.

***H. influenzae* Meningitis** *H. influenzae* meningitis usually results from infection with type b organisms. It is often preceded by an upper respiratory tract infection or otitis media.

The mortality rate in *H. influenzae* meningitis is 5% to 10%. Sequelae occur in approximately one third of survivors, with hearing loss being the most common deficit. Upon diagnosis of *H. influenzae* meningitis, rifampin prophylaxis should be provided to household members, including adults, in those households with at least one child less than 4 years old. The immunization (Haemophilus b vaccine) status of the latter may modify this recommendation (see reference 48). Prophylaxis is appropriate for nonresidents of the household who have been in repeated contact with the patient in the several days prior to illness.[48] Prophylaxis may also be appropriate for day-care and nursery school contacts.[48] The index case should also receive prophylaxis which should be given just prior to discharge. For prophylaxis, rifampin is given orally once a day for 4 days at 20 mg/kg/d (maximum dose, 600 mg/d). Prophylaxis is not recommended for pregnant women.

Subdural effusions occur in approximately 40% of cases of purulent meningitis due to *H. influenzae* and may complicate meningitis with other organisms. They often resolve without any intervention. Infrequently, they cause symptoms and require specific therapy. Suspicion of a potentially harmful subdural collection should be increased when (1) after 2 to 3 days of adequate therapy, recurrent fever, a tense anterior fontanel, seizures (particularly if focal), hemiparesis, or change in mental status develops; (2) there is an abnormal pattern of transillumination of the head; or (3) progressive suture spread is demonstrated. Subdural empyema occurs in about 2% of cases. CT scan confirms the diagnosis of a subdural fluid collection. An initial subdural tap can exclude subdural empyema. Otherwise, repeated tapping of the subdural space through the anterior fontanel, or through a burr hole if the fontanel is closed, is performed to relieve symptoms noted above. The fluid is allowed to drip freely, and the volume removed from both sides should not exceed 50 to 60 mL. Most spaces become dry after a few taps. Tapping should be discontinued when less than 5 mL is obtained. Persistent subdural effusions that increase in size when tapping is stopped or cause signs of increased intracranial pressure may require shunting. An infected subdural effusion requires surgical evacuation and drainage.

Pneumococcal Meningitis Almost half of all cases of pneumococcal meningitis occur in children between 1 month and 4 years of age. The onset is usually abrupt, with rapid progression of symptoms and signs. Although there may be cases without an obvious source of infection, in many patients a suppurative focus (e.g., pneumonia, otitis, sinusitis) is found. In some an underlying systemic defect (e.g., endocarditis, splenectomy, sickle cell anemia) may exist. Structural defects or basilar skull fractures that allow communication with the subarachnoid space also predispose to pneumococcal meningitis and to recurrent bouts of the disorder. Pneumococcal meningitis is associated with a disturbingly high mortality rate despite potentially curative antimicrobial therapy. The recent emergence of strains resistant to penicillin necessitates careful sensitivity studies of pneumococcal isolates.

Meningococcal Meningitis *Neisseria meningitidis* infection can occur in any age group. The clinical presentation of meningococcal disease can include septicemia with endotoxemia, as well as manifestations of hematogenous spread of the organism to various organs. A rash accompanies approximately half the cases of meningitis with this organism, and it varies from an erythematous maculopapular eruption to the more characteristic petechial or hemorrhagic lesions. Gram stain of skin lesions may reveal the organism. Similar lesions can occur in cases of sepsis or meningitis caused by *Neisseria gonorrhoeae*, *H. influenzae*, and staphylococci, as well as with Rocky Mountain spotted fever and echovirus and adenovirus infections. The onset of meningococcal meningitis can be quite abrupt, and the course fulminant. Death in fulminating cases can result from endotoxic shock or disseminated intravascular coagulation. Cases attended by adrenal hemorrhage (Waterhouse-Friderichsen syndrome) are clinically indistinguishable from those without hemorrhage. The mortality rate for all cases of meningococcal meningitis is 5% to 10% but may well be higher in infants and in those with signs of endotoxemia prior to receiving therapy. Household, nursery school, and day-care center contacts of patients with meningococcal disease should receive oral rifampin prophylaxis. The dosage for adults is 600 mg every 12 hours for four doses; for children ages 1 month through 12 years, 10 mg/kg (maximum dose, 600 mg) every 12 hours for 4 doses; and for children under 1 month, 5 mg/kg every 12 hours for 4 doses. Anyone directly exposed to the oral secretions of the patient should also receive prophylaxis. Rifampin prophylaxis would appear to be inappropriate for pregnant women.

Organisms Associated with Conditions Predisposing to Meningitis

Staphylococcal species are frequently responsible for meningitis in patients with ventricular shunts; Gram-negative organisms or staphylococcus may be found in cases of meningitis following penetrating head trauma or neurosurgery. *S. pneumoniae* often causes meningitis following closed head trauma; other organisms to be considered in this context and when paracranial infection is present are *S. aureus*, other streptococcal species, *H. influenzae* (especially in young children), *Bacteroides*, and other anaerobes. These same organisms, as well as Gram-negative organisms, may cause meningitis in immunocompromised patients. Anatomic (dural) defects predispose to meningitis with staphylococci, streptococci, and Gram-negative bacteria. Patients with sickle cell anemia, splenectomy, hepatic cirrhosis, and hypogammaglobulinemia are predisposed to *S. pneumoniae* meningitis.

Diagnosis and Treatment

Initial laboratory studies are suggested (see Exhibit 11-12). Acute meningitis is a bona fide medical emergency and demands immediate evaluation and initiation of therapy. Delay can result in significant sequelae or death. CSF should be obtained as soon as possible. Thus, with rare exception, LP must be expeditiously performed in all patients in whom meningitis is suspected. Indications for LP in a febrile patient are

1. headache and vomiting or severe headache alone
2. changes in mental status, including confusion and lethargy
3. signs of meningeal inflammation
4. signs of diffuse parenchymal involvement
5. cutaneous lesions suggesting meningococcemia (petechiae and purpura are classic, but other skin lesions are occasionally noted)
6. an acute "toxic" illness without apparent cause
7. new fever in a patient predisposed to CNS infection, as elucidated earlier
8. in the infant, any suggestion of sepsis

The only *absolute* contraindication to LP is evidence of brain herniation. In temporal lobe-tentorial herniation, there may be unilateral dilated unreactive pupil, hemiplegia ipsilateral to the herniating temporal lobe, or the triad of bradycardia, bradypnea, and increased arterial pulse pressure in the setting of altered consciousness. In cerebellar-foramen magnum herniation, there may be head tilt, arching or stiffness of the neck, extensor spasms, and alteration of consciousness with irregular respirations. For such patients LP is deferred and antibiotics are chosen empirically (Table 11-8). CT scan is indicated when the clinical course allows. Measures to monitor and treat raised intracranial pressure should be instituted. LP should be reconsidered after 8 to 24 hours of therapy, or earlier when the clinical context indicates that it can be safely performed.

There are several *relative* contraindications to LP. The first is evidence of an acute or progressive focal neurologic abnormality. This may suggest processes combining meningeal inflammation and focal abnormalities, such as

- brain abscess, subdural empyema, or epidural abscess
- herpes simplex encephalitis
- intracranial thrombophlebitis
- mycotic aneurysm with leakage
- intracranial hemorrhage
- CNS neoplasm
- acute hemorrhagic leukoencephalitis
- posterior fossa dermoid with congenital dermal sinus and associated meningitis

Because mass lesions substantially increase the likelihood of temporal lobe or cerebellar herniation following lumbar puncture, the patient with an acute or progressive focal neurologic deficit should have an emergent CT scan before the physician rules on the need for and advisability of LP. However, there should be no delay in initiating antibiotic therapy. Therefore, in some instances, it will be necessary to begin empiric therapy prior to LP.

The second relative contraindication is the *sudden* onset of severe headache or altered mental status; in such cases intracranial hemorrhage should be suspected. Emergent CT scan should precede a decision regarding LP. Again, there should be no delay in initiating therapy for suspected meningitis.

The third relative contraindication is evidence of increased intracranial pressure without focal findings. Diagnostic LP can precipitate temporal lobe or cerebellar herniation in some such patients. However, it is not possible at this time to predict which infants and children will herniate. A decision regarding LP and emergent CT scanning must be made within the clinical context. Generally, in the absence of focal signs and those suggestive of herniation, an LP should be performed as soon as possible. A small needle should be inserted with the bevel directed upward and a minimal volume of CSF removed. The physician must be aware of the possibility of herniation and be prepared to treat it. The neurosurgical consult should be aware of the patient's status. For selected patients, high-risk LPs may be preceded or accompanied by infusion of a hyperosmolar agent.

Other relative contraindications to LP are a coagulopathy and an infection of the overlying skin. CSF can be obtained by cisternal puncture in cases in which the lumbar region is seriously contaminated. The risk of hemorrhage due to coagulopathy may be obviated by administration of parenteral vitamin K and fresh frozen plasma.

TABLE 11-8 Initial Antimicrobial Therapy for Acute Bacterial Meningitis*

Age Group	Antibiotic
Infants > 2 mo	Ampicillin and aminoglycoside or ampicillin and cefotaxime
2 mo to 10 yr	Ampicillin and chloramphenicol, or cefuroxime or cefotaxime
10 yr and older	Penicillin G

* Systemic or structural factors that may require modification of these recommendations are discussed in the text.

The CSF pattern is purulent (Table 11-6) in the vast majority of patients with acute bacterial meningitis. Special circumstances in which the CSF formula may be modified include: (1) soon after the organisms enter the CSF or early in the course of an overwhelming infection, in which a poor PMN response and a normal CSF glucose may be seen; (2) in patients with leukopenia or who are immunosuppressed and cannot mount a brisk cellular response; and (3) in cases of partially treated meningitis. CSF Gram stain and culture may still be positive in these instances. Countercurrent-immunoelectrophoresis (CIE) of the CSF sample may identify antigens specific to one of the more common organisms. Its efficacy is increased by including samples of blood and urine. Other methods which may help to indicate a bacterial process within the CSF include latex particle agglutination, C-reactive protein determination in blood and CSF, limulus lysate test, and measurement of CSF lactic acid.

Treatment of bacterial meningitis includes prompt institution of *intravenous* antimicrobial therapy.[49,50] The goal of therapy is to achieve antibiotic concentrations in the CSF which are 10-fold the minimal bacterial concentration (MBC) for the organism responsible. The initial choice of antibiotics can be made on the basis of CSF examination and the patient's age. Table 11-8 gives recommendations for initial therapy. Coverage for other infectious agents may be indicated by CSF findings inconsistent with initial expectations or by the presence of structural or systemic factors predisposing to meningitis, as discussed earlier. Once culture results have identified the responsible organism and its sensitivities, antibiotic choices can be modified. The duration of antibiotic treatment varies from organism to organism but in general should be approximately 14 days. Longer courses may be indicated in certain contexts and for resistant organisms. For neonates the length of therapy is determined in part by the clinical and CSF response. Treatment should continue for 3 weeks, or for 2 weeks after bacteriologic cure, whichever is longer. Repeat LP after 24 to 48 hours to assess the result of therapy is particularly important in the neonate because few other parameters exist for assessing improvement. LP should be performed in neonates at intervals thereafter, at any time when the clinical course is unsatisfactory, and at the conclusion of therapy. Repeat LP is also recommended for any patient with meningitis due to Gram-negative enteric organisms. In older children and adults, prompt clinical improvement in an otherwise uncomplicated meningitis may obviate repeat LP.

Accepted antibiotic doses for different age groups are given in Table 11-9. They may need to be altered on the basis of the patient's ability to metabolize or excrete the drug, e.g., in those patients with hepatic or renal dysfunction. For such patients, as well as for infants, the serum concentration of the aminoglycosides and of chloramphenicol should be monitored and the dose adjusted accordingly. Routine monitoring of aminoglycoside levels is appropriate in all patients.

Gram-negative bacillary meningitis presents special therapeutic problems. Such organisms can be relatively insensitive to drugs that reach the CSF, while quite low CSF levels are achieved for aminoglycosides to which they are sensitive. Gram-negative bacillary meningitis is commonly encountered in neonates and may be found in the immunocompromised or neurosurgical patients. Recent reports indicate that third-generation cephalosporins are effective in the treatment of Gram-negative enteric bacillary meningitis in infants and children. These agents are making a significant contribution to the treatment of Gram-negative meningitis. Cefotaxime effectively penetrates inflamed meninges, and the combination of cefotaxime and ampicillin is an effective alternative for the treatment of neonatal meningitis. Cefotaxime or cefuroxime is also an alternative to ampicillin and chloramphenicol for treatment of bacterial meningitis in children[51] from the ages of two months to ten years.

Though uncommon, *Pseudomonas meningitis* is particularly difficult to treat effectively. Standard therapy in the past has included both intravenous and intrathecal antibiotics. Currently, combination systemic therapy with ceftazidime and an aminoglycoside may obviate the need for intrathecal antibiotic administration.

Though the new cephalosporins may obviate the need for intraventricular installation of aminoglycoside in many cases of Gram-negative meningitis, in some instances beyond the neonatal period this may still be necessary. Consultation with experts in treating infectious disease should be sought in all cases of bacillary meningitis which are suspected or proven to be due to Gram-negative bacillary organisms.

For all cases of meningitis vital signs must be carefully monitored, and adequacy of cardiorespiratory function must be assured. Other supportive measures include treatment of septic shock, disseminated intravascular coagulation, and inappropriate antidiuretic hormone secretion. Frequent reexamination of the patient aids in anticipating significant changes in the clinical course. Anticonvulsants are

TABLE 11-9 Antibiotic Dosages for Bacterial Meningitis*, †, ‡‡

Part A: Birth to 2 Mo.

Drug	Body Weight <2000 Gm		Body Weight >2000 Gm	
	Age 0–7 Days	**>7 Days**	**Age 0–7 Days**	**>7 Days**
Ampicillin	100 mg/kg/d (q12h)	150 mg/kg/d (q8h)	150 mg/kg/d (q8h)	200 mg/kg/d (q6h)
Penicillin G¶	100,000 U/kg/d (q12h)	150,000 U/kg/d (q8h)	150,000 U/kg/d (q8h)	200,000 U/kg/d (q6h)
Methicillin	100 mg/kg/d (q12h)	150 mg/kg/d (q8h)	150 mg/kg/d (q8h)	200 mg/kg/d (q6h)
Nafcillin	50 mg/kg/d (q12h)	75 mg/kg/d (q8h)	50 mg/kg/d (q8h)	75 mg/kg/d (q6h)
Carbenicillin	100 mg/kg/d (q12h)	100 mg/kg/d (q8h)	100 mg/kg/d (q8h)	100 mg/kg/d (q6h)
Ticarcillin	150 mg/kg/d (q12h)	225 mg/kg/d (q8h)	225 mg/kg/d (q8h)	300 mg/kg/d (q6h)
Mezlocillin	150 mg/kg/d (q12h)	225 mg/kg/d (q8h)	150 mg/kg/d (q12h)	225 mg/kg/d (q8h)
Kanamycin**	15 mg/kg/d (q12h)	22.5 mg/kg/d (q8h)	20 mg/kg/d (q12h)	30 mg/kg/d (q8h)
Gentamicin**	5 mg/kg/d (q12h)	7.5 mg/kg/d (q8h)	5 mg/kg/d (q12h)	7.5 mg/kg/d (q8h)
Tobramycin**	4 mg/kg/d (q12h)	6 mg/kg/d (q8h)	4 mg/kg/d (q12h)	6 mg/kg/d (q8h)
Amikacin**	15 mg/kg/d (q12h)	22.5 mg/kg/d (q8h)	20 mg/kg/d (q12h)	30 mg/kg/d (q8h)
Chloramphenicol	25 mg/kg/d (once daily)	25 mg/kg/d (once daily)	25 mg/kg/d (once daily)	50 mg/kg/d (q12h)
Cefotaxime	100 mg/kg/d (q12h)	150 mg/kg/d (q8h)	100 mg/kg/d (q12h)	150 mg/kg/d (q8h)
Ceftazidine	30 mg/kg/d (q12h)	30 mg/kg/d (q8h)	30 mg/kg/d (q12h)	30 mg/kg/d (q8h)
Vancomycin***	30 mg/kg/d (q12h)	45 mg/kg/d (q8h)	30 mg/kg/d (q12h)	45 mg/kg/d (q8h)

Part B: Children over 2 mo.‡

Drug		Maximum (adult) Dose§
Ampicillin	200–400 mg/kg/d (q6h)	6–12 gm/d
Penicillin G¶	250,000 U/kg/d (q4h)	10–20 million U/d
Methicillin	150–200 mg/kg/d (q4h)	4–12 Gm/d
Nafcilline	150–200 mg/kg/d (q4h)	4–12 Gm/d
Carbenicillin	400–600 mg/kg/d (q4h)	20–40 Gm/d
Ticarcillin	200–300 mg/kg/d (q4h)	12–24 Gm/d
Mezlocillin	200–300 mg/kg/d (q4h)	12–18 Gm/d
Kanamycin**	15–30 mg/kg/d (q8h)	1.5 Gm/d
Gentamicin**	††	300–400 mg/d
Tobramycin**	††	300–400 mg/d
Amikacin**	15–30 mg/kg/d (q8h)	15 mg/kg/d to a maximum of 1.5 Gm/d
Chloramphenicol	500–100 mg/kg/d (q6h)	4.0 Gm/d
Cefotaxime	200 mg/kg/d (q6h)	10.0 Gm/d
Ceftazidime	150 mg/kg/d (q8h)	6 Gm/d
Cefuroxime	240 mg/kg/d (q6h)	6 Gm/d
Vancomycin***	60 mg/kg/d (q6h)	4 Gm/d

* All antibiotics listed are given intravenously. Several, including kanamycin, gentamicin, and amikacin, may be given intramuscularly. The daily dose should be divided appropriate to the dosage interval listed within the parentheses.

† Doses may need to be modified in renal or hepatic failure. Chloramphenicol levels should be monitored in patients with hepatic insufficiency and in all infants. Aminoglycoside levels should be monitored in all patients (see below). Monitoring the levels of other agents may help to guide therapy, especially in infants.

‡ Antibiotics are prescribed on a mg/kg basis until children reach adult weight ranges, after which the adult maximum applies.

§ Adult doses are divided in the same fashion as for children over 2 months.

¶ For Group B streptococcus infections use: penicillin G 300,000–400,000 *units*/kg/d IV. Administer in divided doses (as indicated above) given over 20–30 minutes.

** Note that except for the newborn period, systemic aminoglycoside therapy is probably not effective in treating Gram-negative meningitis. See text. Note that the values given for the aminoglycosides may be considered as acceptable doses for initiating therapy; however, optimal treatment can only be achieved by adjusting the dose to reach acceptable peak levels. In all age groups, the dose should be adjusted to achieve these levels. Thus, it is possible that for some adults the levels may dictate that the suggested maximum be exceeded.

†† The doses for either gentamicin or tobramycin for children are: age 2 months to 5 years—7.5 mg/kg/d (q8h); age 5 to 10 years—6 mg/kg/d (q8h); and 4.5 mg/kg/d (q8h) for all patients older than 10 years. See maximum dose.

‡‡ See references 48, 49, 50, and 56 for any questions regarding dose.

*** Vancomycin dose should be given over 60 minute interval.

employed if seizures occur. In general, nondehydrated patients in the initial stages of therapy should have fluids restricted to two thirds of normal maintenance. In patients with severe brain swelling, and especially in those with evidence of herniation, the increased intracranial pressure should be treated aggressively (see Exhibit 11-11). Other treatment considerations include management of factors predisposing to meningitis, e.g., parameningeal infection. In patients with systemic foci of infection (e.g., bacterial endocarditis, osteomyelitis), the antimicrobial course must be prolonged. Infected intracranial shunts may need to be removed for the infection to be cured (see section on shunt malfunction).

Recurrence or persistence of fever is an indication for repeat LP. Causes for fever other than inadequate treatment of meningitis include phlebitis, a second source of bacterial infection (e.g., pneumonitis, otitis, sinusitis, subdural empyema), viral infection, or drug fever.

Partially Treated Meningitis Patients with meningitis frequently receive antibiotics before the diagnosis is suspected. In most instances of partial treatment, the CSF changes produced are not sufficient to alter confirmation of the diagnosis, but in a small number of patients this may be the case. In such situations CSF pleocytosis may be mainly lymphocytic; the glucose, normal; and the Gram stain, negative. The diagnosis of bacterial meningitis is thus obscured, suggesting instead a viral aseptic meningitis. The identification of the organism via culture also can be more difficult. Countercurrent immunoelectrophoresis, lactic acid measurement, latex particle agglutination, and limulus lysate tests on CSF, as well as serum or CSF C-reactive protein determination,[52] help to differentiate viral from bacterial meningitis. For these patients it is advisable to provide adequate therapy for the likely bacterial agents, according to age and to any conditions predisposing to meningitis.

Viral Meningitis

Many viruses can produce an aseptic meningitis.[53] The clinical picture is acute and includes fever, headache, photophobia, vomiting, neck stiffness, and other signs of meningeal irritation. Irritability may be found, as may mild lethargy or drowsiness. Seizures and focal neurologic deficits suggest an encephalitic component. The viruses most often associated are the mumps virus and the enteroviruses, especially the coxsackieviruses and the echoviruses. Enteroviruses cause sporadic and epidemic disease, with most cases occurring in the summer and early fall. Other viral causes include lymphocytic choriomeningitis (LCM) virus, herpes simplex type 2, arboviruses and EBV.

The disease course is typically benign. Symptoms last for a few days to two weeks. Sequelae are rare. The etiology may be suggested by history of prior infections, vaccinations, concurrent viral disease in family members or other contacts, and by the characteristics of systemic symptoms (e.g., parotitis with mumps or occasionally with coxsackie virus). Laboratory evaluation should include most of the studies usually obtained for cases of suspected bacterial meningitis (Exhibit 11-12). In addition to bacterial cultures, viral isolation may be attempted from the nasopharynx, stool, blood, and CSF. Acute and convalescent sera should be obtained. Other tests (e.g., serology for EBV) will be indicated by the clinical context.

Diagnosis requires that the CSF be proved aseptic. The CSF pattern is usually lymphocytic (Table 11-6). CSF protein may be elevated and glucose is normal. In mumps and LCM the glucose may be mildly decreased. Except early in the course, mononuclear cells usually predominate. In those instances in which PMNs are more numerous, the distinction between viral and bacterial meningitis may be blurred. The clinical context can help resolve treatment issues in such cases. In many instances the physician elects to treat such patients with antibiotics, pending culture results. In others, antimicrobial therapy is delayed pending a repeat LP 8 to 12 hours after the first. A worsening clinical course should prompt earlier repeat LP.

Of utmost importance in the context of aseptic meningitis is the exclusion of bacterial, mycobacterial, fungal, or parasitic agents. The differential diagnosis includes parameningeal foci of suppuration, partially treated bacterial meningitis, *Mycobacterium tuberculosis*, cryptococcosis, syphilis, and Rocky Mountain spotted fever. Special vigilance must be exercised with immunocompromised patients.

In addition to the disorders discussed above, a number of other infectious agents and conditions can suggest acute meningitis. These are given in Exhibit 11-13.

Subacute and Chronic Meningitis and Meningoencephalitis

Meningitis of more than 2 weeks' duration is considered subacute or chronic. A variety of signs and symptoms are associated with these disorders, but in most cases signs of meningeal inflammation and change in mentation and behavior are present. Cranial nerve and other focal neurologic deficits are frequent, resulting in the clinical picture referred to as meningoencephalitis. Hydrocephalus frequently complicates the course. The history and physical examination to be obtained are usually the same as for acute meningitis. Close attention should be paid to the nature and tempo of neurologic findings, and lingering systemic symptoms should be sought.

Diagnostic evaluation of such patients should proceed expeditiously (Exhibit 11-12). Contraindications to LP are the same as those cited under "Acute Bacterial Meningitis." The CSF pattern in chronic meningitis is usually of the granulomatous or lymphocytic type (Table 11-6). Cultures include

Exhibit 11-13 Disorders Suggesting Acute Meningitis

- Infectious Disorders
  - Bacterial
    - Partially treated meningitis
    - Parameningeal suppuration (e.g., brain abscess, subdural empyema, cortical vein thrombophlebitis)
    - Bacterial endocarditis
    - *Brucella* infections
    - Infections with anaerobes
    - Tuberculosis
    - Syphilis
    - Leptospirosis
    - *Borrelia* infections
    - Lyme disease
  - Rickettsial
    - Rocky Mountain spotted fever
    - Q fever
  - Fungal
    - *Candida* infections
    - Histoplasmosis
    - Blastomycosis
  - Helminthic
    - Toxocariasis
    - Trichinosis
  - Others
    - *Naegleria fowleri* infections
    - Trypanosomiasis
    - *Mycoplasma pneumoniae* infections
- Noninfectious Disorders
  - Subarachnoid hemorrhage
  - Acute hemorrhagic leukoencephalitis
  - Systemic lupus erythematosus
  - Mucocutaneous lymph node disease
  - Chemical meningitis
    - Pantopaque
    - Detergents
    - Chemotherapeutic agents
    - Leaking epidermoid dermoid, or craniopharyngioma cyst
  - CNS neoplasia
    - Leukemic and lymphomatous meningitis
    - Carcinomatous and gliomatous meningitis
  - Behçet's syndrome
  - Mollaret meningitis
  - Vogt-Koyanagi-Harada syndrome

those for aerobic and anaerobic bacteria, *Mycobacterium tuberculosis*, and fungus. CSF sediment is examined by Gram stain, acid-fast bacillus stain, wet mount, and India ink. A sample should be sent for cytological examination. Cryptococcal antigen can be sought in CSF as well as in blood and urine. CSF and serum should be examined for precipitin and complement-fixing antibody for *Coccidioides* and *Histoplasma*. CSF is also sent for VDRL testing and dark-field examination. A careful search should be made for extraneural evidence of tuberculosis and fungal infection. Cases are frequently encountered in which the clinical picture and CSF examination suggest chronic meningitis but for which a complete initial work-up is unproductive.

Tuberculous Meningitis

Meningitis caused by *M. tuberculosis* represents a complication of previous infection elsewhere in the body. The lung is the original focus in most cases. Meningeal tuberculosis occurs in all ages but is uncommon in children under 3 months of age. It usually occurs in association with miliary tuberculosis, but evidence of disease outside the CNS may be lacking. The onset of symptoms can be acute but in most cases is more gradual than for other forms of bacterial meningitis. Symptoms include fever, listlessness, irritability, headache, vomiting, and meningeal signs. Seizures can occur. Papilledema may be observed relatively early. Cranial nerve involvement (ocular palsies, facial paresis, and deafness) and altered mental status develop during the second week. Choroidal tubercules may be evident on funduscopic examination. Some patients exhibit hemiparesis or other major focal deficits. Without treatment the course relentlessly progresses to death within 3 to 5 weeks.

CSF findings are of a granulomatous nature (Table 11-6), though early in the course there may be more PMNs than mononuclear cells and the glucose may be normal. Smears of CSF sediment may reveal acid-fast bacilli, as may smears of the pellicle that forms after the fluid stands for a time. The diagnosis can be confirmed by culture.

Treatment begins immediately after a presumptive diagnosis is made and prior to the results of culture. One suggested treatment regimen includes:

1. isoniazid (INH): 10 to 20 mg/kg/d (up to 300 mg/d) orally
2. rifampin: 10 to 20 mg/kg/d (up to 600 mg/d) orally
3. pyrazinamide: 20 mg/kg/d (up to 2 G/d) orally.

A current recommendation is that INH and rifampin be given for 18 months and that pyrazinamide be given for the initial 2 months of treatment.[48] Pyridoxine prophylaxis for neurologic side-effects of INH has been recommended for children on meat- and milk-deficient diets[48] and should be given to all patients over age 12.

Corticosteroid treatment with dexamethasone is not routine and should be used only in conjunction with specific antituberculous therapy. Dexamethasone can be used for brief periods to treat the cerebral swelling that complicates cases of acute onset.

Mortality in tuberculous meningitis is 10% to 20%. Hydrocephalus can complicate the course. Sequelae occur in approximately one fourth of affected children and include intellectual, psychiatric, motor, and visual deficits.

Fungal Meningoencephalitis

Manifestations of fungal infections of the CNS include meningitis (acute, subacute, chronic), meningoencephalitis, abscess (solitary, multiple, microabscesses), granuloma (solitary, multiple, microgranulomas), and arterial thrombosis. Subacute or chronic meningitis and meningoencephalitis are common expressions of fungal neurologic infections. The immunocompromised patient is at special risk for fungal infections. The symptoms and signs of fungal meningoencephalitis and the CSF findings are often similar to those of tuberculous meningitis. Diagnosis is by examination of CSF sediment and by culture. Specific antigen and serologic studies are performed as well. The organisms most commonly infecting the CNS include *Cryptococcus, Candida, Coccidioides, Histoplasma, Aspergillus, Phycomycetes,* and *Blastomyces.* Primary antifungal therapy usually includes amphotericin-B, and in some cases 5-fluorocytosine is added.[53,55] Although *Nocardia* and *Actinomyces* are not true fungi, their clinical manifestations are similar. They are treated with antibacterial agents, sulfonamides for the former and penicillin for the latter. Other conditions that are suggested by the clinical pattern of subacute meningitis or meningoencephalitis are listed in Exhibit 11-14.

Exhibit 11-14 Disorders Suggesting Subacute or Chronic Meningitis or Meningoencephalitis

- Infections
  - Bacterial
    - Parameningeal suppuration
    - Partially treated bacterial meningitis
    - *Brucella* infections
    - Syphilis
    - Whipple's disease
  - Parasitic
    - Cysticercosis
    - Paragonimiasis
    - Trypanosomiasis
    - Toxoplasmosis
- Noninfectious Disorders
  - Neoplasia
    - Carcinomatous and gliomatous meningitis
    - Fourth ventricular tumor in children (medulloblastoma or ependymoma)
  - Other
    - Sarcoidosis
    - Granulomatous angiitis
    - Systemic lupus erythematosus
    - Vogt-Koyanagi-Harada syndrome

Disorders with Parenchymal Involvement

Acute Viral Encephalitis

The chief clinical features characterizing acute encephalitis are fever, headache, altered mental status (delirium, confusion, stupor, coma), convulsions, and symptoms and signs of diffuse or focal neurologic deficits.[52] Focal neurologic deficits include partial seizures, aphasia, hemiparesis, involuntary movements, ataxia, myoclonic jerks, nystagmus, ocular palsies, and facial weakness. Meningeal signs are frequently present (meningoencephalitis). The feature discriminating acute encephalitis from meningitis is the greater degree of parenchymal involvement, which is apparent by history and clinical examination. Numerous disorders can resemble acute viral encephalitis (Exhibit 11-15) and must be differentiated.

A large number of viruses can produce acute encephalitis. However, relatively few cause disease often enough to deserve routine diagnostic consideration. Mumps and LCM viruses, herpes simplex types 1 and 2, and the arboviruses are most frequently responsible. Epidemiologic considerations are pertinent to the last. Less frequent causes are enteroviruses, EBV, measles virus, and adenoviruses; rabies virus also causes encephalitis. It is especially important to arrive at a specific diagnosis because of the therapy currently available for herpesvirus encephalitis.

CSF examination in most cases of acute encephalitis demonstrates a predominantly mononuclear pleocytosis and a normal CSF-to-serum glucose ratio (>0.5). CSF glucose may be lowered to 20 to 40 mg/100 mL in some cases of mumps encephalitis and may be slightly reduced in encephalitis with herpes simplex and LCM. The CSF protein level is normal or elevated. On rare occasions CSF pleocytosis is low grade or lacking. The work-up is essentially the same as for bacterial meningitis (Exhibit 11-12). In addition, sera from acute and convalescent stages of illness are tested for appropriate agents and for heterophile agglutinins or other antibodies to EBV. Isolation of the virus should be attempted with samples from the CSF, nasopharynx, stool, and blood. Treatment for all viral agents includes excellent supportive care.

Herpes Simplex Encephalitis

Herpes simplex type 1 causes sporadic, year-round cases of an acute encephalitis in all age groups. The symptoms are those described above and evolve over several days. A predisposition for involvement of the orbital frontal and inferomedial temporal lobes is manifested in some patients by temporal lobe seizures, olfactory or gustatory hallucinations, bizarre or psychotic behavior, hemiparesis, or aphasia. Thus cerebral involvement can be focal and asymmetrical. Localized neurologic deficits, especially those pointing to temporal lobe involvement, should significantly increase suspicion of herpes simplex in cases of acute encephalitis. Herpes en-

Exhibit 11-15 Disorders Suggesting Acute Viral Encephalitis*

- Infectious or Parainfectious Disorders
  - Bacterial
    - Meningitis
    - Partially treated meningitis
    - Brain abscess
    - Endocarditis with multiple cerebral emboli
    - Tuberculous meningitis
    - Syphilis
    - Leptospirosis
    - Lyme disease
    - Legionnaire's disease
  - Fungal
    - *Candida* infections
    - Cryptococcosis
    - Histoplasmosis
    - *Mucor* infections
    - Nocardiosis
  - Rickettsial
    - Rocky Mountain spotted fever
    - Typhus
  - Helminthic
    - Toxocariasis
    - Trichinosis
    - Schistosomiasis
    - Paragonimiasis
  - Other
    - *M. pneumoniae* infections
    - Toxoplasmosis
    - Malaria
    - Trypanosomiasis
    - *N. fowleri* infections
    - Postinfectious and postvaccinal encephalomyelitis
    - Typhoid fever
- Noninfectious Disorders
  - Initial generalized convulsion
  - Acute encephalopathy accompanying certain systemic infections
  - Reye's syndrome
  - Drug overdose
  - Salicylate intoxication
  - Lead encephalopathy
  - Arsenic intoxication
  - Endocrine disturbances
    - Hypoglycemia
    - Adrenal insufficiency
    - Hyponatremia
  - Spontaneous intracranial hemorrhage
  - Systemic lupus erythematosus
  - CNS neoplasia

* AIDS Retrovirus infection is associated with a progressive encephalopathy which can demonstrate periods of marked deterioration over rather brief intervals (weeks).

cephalitis is a necrotizing hemorrhagic process, and CSF examination may reflect this via the presence of red blood cells and xanthochromia. Associated swelling of the brain can result in herniation of the temporal lobe, with coma, respiratory arrest, and death.

In patients suspected of having herpes simplex encephalitis, the physician must promptly attempt to obtain evidence for a focal component to the disease. The EEG, radionuclide brain scan, MRI scan and a CT scan performed with and without the administration of contrast material are useful in this regard. If a focus is apparent, then a decision must be made about the need for biopsy of the lesion to establish the diagnosis.

The issue of whether or not to biopsy such patients is controversial. Those in favor of biopsy point to the possibility of finding treatable processes which may masquerade as herpes encephalitis (e.g., brain abscess, tuberculosis, fungal infection, and Toxoplasmosis). Some physicians are opposed to biopsy of patients in whom clinical and laboratory evidence strongly support a diagnosis of herpes encephalitis, especially in view of the better outcome which is associated with early treatment. In general, it seems advisable to recommend biopsy early in the course and as soon as clinical and laboratory evidence indicate that herpes encephalitis is a significant possibility. Biopsy tissue must be sent for cultures (viral, bacterial, fungal, and tuberculosis), histology, electron microscopy, and immunofluorescence. It is often justifiable to begin early treatment with an antiviral agent such as acyclovir or vidarabine (Ara-A), even before a diagnosis is firmly established.

Herpes simplex type 2 infections in the neonate are usually acquired from an infected birth canal, either shortly before delivery or during passage. The mother is frequently asymptomatic. Dissemination of virus from the skin or eyes to multiple organs, including the brain, is frequent; cerebral involvement produces encephalitis. Unlike the herpes simplex type 1 encephalitis of older patients, there is less selectivity for the orbital frontal and temporal lobes. Onset of symptoms in affected infants is within 12 days after birth. The earliest clues to diagnosis are skin or ocular lesions. Early encephalitic manifestations can include lethargy and vomiting. Disease progression results in convulsions, tense fontanel, nystagmus, and rigidity or flaccidity. Coma may ensue. The CSF often contains red blood cells and shows a mild-to-moderate lymphocytic pleocytosis. Glucose is normal or low whereas protein is elevated. Brain biopsy is indicated when the diagnosis is not firmly established by the clinical context. The presence of a maternal genital herpetic infection lends support. The virus may be isolated from vesicular skin lesions, the conjunctivae, urine, stool, nasopharynx, blood, and possibly CSF. Electron microscopic examination of exfoliated cells in vesicular fluid may identify herpetic virions. External lesions provide material for other morphologic observations including

Tzanck smear and immunofluorescence. Disseminated herpes virus infection in the newborn is a life-threatening illness, and cerebral sequelae can be severe.

Outside of the neonatal period, acyclovir is the treatment of choice for herpes simplex encephalitis at a dose of 30 mg/kg/d IV for 10 days.[55] The daily dose is divided into equal q8h doses which are each administered over 1 hour. For neonates, acyclovir and Ara-A may be equivalent in efficacy.[55] Treatment of neonates with Ara-A is with 15 to 30 mg/kg/d administered IV by slow infusion over 12 hours. The agent is given in standard IV solutions at a concentration not exceeding 0.7 mg/mL. The dose of acyclovir for neonates is the same as listed above. If cultures are positive for herpes or no reasonable alternative diagnosis is provided, acyclovir or Ara-A is continued for 14 to 21 days. Other aspects of care include careful attention to fluid and electrolyte management to avoid fluid overload. Intracranial pressure monitoring may be needed, as may anti-edema agents including dexamethasone.

The prognosis of untreated herpes simplex encephalitis is dismal; the mortality rate is 70% and significant sequelae are found in most survivors. Mortality is reduced to 28% by treatment with acyclovir, and 54% with Ara-A.[54] Prognosis is significantly improved in patients who are treated before marked compromise of mental status, but sequelae are frequent.

Neonatal Viral Encephalitis

The fetal brain can be invaded by rubella and cytomegalovirus. Congenital rubella has a variety of manifestations, some systemic (growth retardation, thrombocytopenia, cardiac malformations, ocular defects, hepatosplenomegaly, jaundice) and others involving the CNS, including mental retardation, deafness, and chronic meningoencephalitis. Infants infected with cytomegalovirus in utero may have encephalitis. Though the CNS is usually only one of many organ systems affected, in some cases it is selectively involved. Echovirus or group B coxsackievirus infections in the neonate may produce the picture of acute encephalitis. Associated clinical findings in neonatal enterovirus encephalitis are those expected for sepsis in this age group. In addition to encephalitis, group B coxsackievirus often causes prominent myocardial dysfunction (encephalomyocarditis).

Acute Viral Myelitis

Poliovirus causes destruction of the anterior horn cells of the spinal cord, with resulting paralytic disease. Poliovirus myelitis is now an infrequent occurrence. Coxsackieviruses and echoviruses can produce a very similar but usually less severe clinical picture. Typically, pain in the neck, back, and legs is associated with meningeal signs and an aseptic meningitis. Muscle weakness may develop rapidly. Findings are frequently asymmetric and vary in severity from case to case. Bulbar and respiratory involvement may occur. Significant recovery of function occurs in many cases.

To be distinguished from the above are cases of acute transverse myelitis in which there is involvement of the whole thickness of the spinal cord. An autoimmune pathogenesis may be responsible for the acute transverse myelitis which has been described in association with a number of viral infections (usually exanthematous) or with vaccination for rabies and smallpox. Weakness and numbness of the feet and legs (and less often the upper extremities), and difficulty voiding develop over a few days. There may be a sensory level established. Patients may complain of leg or back pain and there may be headache and meningeal signs. CSF may show a mild lymphocytic pleocytosis. Isolation of virus should be attempted but is frequently unsuccessful. Recovery occurs but significant residua are not uncommon.

It is important to note that other infectious and noninfectious causes may also produce the picture of acute transverse myelitis. In suspected cases of transverse myelopathy, it is essential to rule out a space occupying lesion which may require neurosurgical intervention. Acute spinal epidural abscess must be considered in a child with this clinical picture. Myelography or other radiographic studies are essential for diagnosis (see below). Myelitis may also develop as a result of bacterial (including syphilis and tuberculosis), fungal, parasitic, and *Mycoplasma pneumoniae* infections of the meninges and spinal cord. Appropriate laboratory studies must be performed. Noninfectious causes include: (1) ischemic myelopathy, possibly in association with vasculitis; (2) ischemia or hemorrhage associated with a spinal vascular malformation; (3) spinal or epidural hemorrhage complicating a bleeding diathesis; and (4) demyelinating disease.

Focal Suppuration

Suppurative foci produce primarily parenchymal symptoms. These result from either mass effect or tissue inflammation and necrosis.

Brain Abscess

The clinical presentation of brain abscess can vary greatly. In some patients the course is marked by swiftly emerging manifestations while in others it is subacute or even indolent. Abscesses can be solitary or multiple and are less common in infants than in older children. In infants they can become quite large before becoming clinically apparent via vomiting, excessive head growth, and seizures. In older patients, the clinical presentation usually includes headache, drowsiness, confusion, and evidence of increased intracranial pressure and focal neurologic dysfunction. Seizures may occur. Fever may or may not be present. Signs of increased intracranial pressure may be prominent with cerebellar abscess and ataxia may be present. Sudden deterioration of the clinical status of a patient with an abscess suggests herniation of the brain, rupture of the abscess into the ventricular system, or hemorrhage into the abscess.

Brain abscess is frequently associated with an extracranial suppurative focus; important sites include the paranasal sinuses, middle ear, and mastoid cells. Other sources include the heart (bacterial endocarditis), pulmonary infections, suppurative skin lesions, and abscessed teeth. Associated conditions include congenital heart disease, especially of the cyanotic type in children over 2 years of age; pulmonary arteriovenous fistula; and immune-deficient states.

The location of the abscess can reflect the suppurative focus. Otitis and mastoiditis spread to the cerebellum and temporal lobe. Cerebellar abscess may follow infection of a dermoid cyst at the end of a posterior fossa dermal sinus. Frontal and temporal lobe abscesses are associated with sinusitis. In congenital heart disease abscesses are usually solitary and located in frontal, temporal, or parietal lobes. Abscesses that occur in the setting of acute bacterial endocarditis are frequently multiple.

The organisms most often isolated from brain abscesses are *Streptococcus* species (many of which are anaerobic or microaerophilic), anaerobic bacteria, *Staphylococcus* species, and Gram-negative rods. Gram-negative bacilli are especially frequent in neonates. Mixed infections are encountered in some abscesses. *Nocardia* and *Actinomyces* may cause cerebral abscesses. In addition to bacterial pathogens, cerebral abscess may be found in infections with *M. tuberculosis*, fungus (e.g., *Candida*, *Aspergillus*), and parasites.

The initial stage of abscess formation consists of a focus of septic cerebritis. Subsequent necrosis centrally results in production of an abscess cavity encapsulated by fibroblastic and gliotic activity. Edema is found in cerebral tissues next to the encapsulated mass.

LP in patients with cerebral abscesses is hazardous and can predispose to herniation. Emergency CT scan should precede a decision regarding the need for and advisability of LP in patients suspected of having a brain abscess (see earlier discussion regarding contraindications to LP). CSF findings can be normal but usually include increased pressure, mild pleocytosis, elevated protein and normal glucose levels. The work-up of patients suspected of harboring a cerebral abscess includes those studies listed in the top part of Exhibit 11-12 (excluding LP). In addition, a paracranial or systemic focus of suppuration should be sought. The CT scan pattern for an encapsulated abscess is a region of hypodensity that is central to an enhancing ring after injection of contrast material. On occasion, cystic tumors or infarcts with neovascularized rims give the same appearance. EEG may reveal a focus of high-voltage slow activity. When clinical and laboratory findings do not rule out other lesions (e.g., primary or metastatic tumor, herpes simplex encephalitis, intracranial thrombophlebitis with infarction), the diagnosis of brain abscess can be made only by biopsy.

Treatment of brain abscess includes surgical drainage or extirpation of the abscess and antibiotic therapy. Recent data suggest that surgery may be avoided for selected patients. In awake patients who are judged not to be suffering from increased intracranial pressure or mass effect and who are neurologically stable, it may be possible to initiate treatment with antibiotics alone. Nonsurgical treatment is especially attractive when stable patients have multiple abscesses, have an abscess in a deep or critical brain area, or are poor surgical candidates. Repeated CT scans should be performed to document the response of the abscess to therapy. Surgery is indicated for neurological deterioration or if the abscess and surrounding edema do not respond to 2 to 3 weeks of antibiotic therapy. CT scan surveillance is continued for all patients until the abscess resolves and, at intervals, through 1 year to rule out recurrence.

The appropriate initial choice of antibiotics for most cases of cerebritis and brain abscess includes intravenous penicillin and chloramphenicol in the doses suggested for meningitis (Table 11-9). When *S. aureus* is a possible organism, and this is frequently the case, nafcillin must be added to the regimen. When the abscess is a complication of trauma or neurosurgery, coverage must be broad. Nafcillin and gentamicin are appropriate in this context. *Pseudomonas* infection of the ear or lung indicates that ticarcillin (ormezlocillin) and gentamicin (or tobramycin) should be used. Metronidazole may provide an alternative to chloramphenicol for treatment of anaerobic bacteria. For infants and for other patients predisposed to Gram-negative bacillary infection, initial empiric therapy should include coverage for these organisms. Third generation cephalosporins may be shown to play a role in the treatment of brain abscess. The duration of antibiotic therapy will be determined by details of the individual case. In surgically treated patients, the antibiotics course averages 4 weeks. Nonsurgical approaches have included antibiotic courses of 6 to 8 weeks.

Careful fluid management must be practiced for patients with cerebritis and abscess. Antiedema therapy with dexamethasone and mannitol may be required; the dose for the latter is given in the section on Reye's syndrome (Exhibit 11-11). Dexamethasone is given as a loading dose of 1.0 mg/kg IV followed by a maintenance dose of 0.25 mg/kg/d divided q6h IV for 5 days. The dose is tapered if clinical and CT signs of intracranial pressure are resolving.

Mortality with brain abscess is significantly lessened by antimicrobial therapy and surgery. Residua of brain abscess include intellectual and focal neurologic deficits, including focal epilepsy.

Subdural Empyema

This intracranial suppurative process is localized to the space between the dura and arachnoid and is usually present on one side only. A very serious infection, it is characterized by an acute-to-subacute clinical course with fever, malaise and signs of increased intracranial pressure, meningeal irritation, and focal cortical dysfunction. The infectious source is usually a frontal or ethmoid sinusitis and, less often, otitis or mastoiditis. Intracranial spread follows thrombophlebitis of perforating cerebral veins and the venous sinuses. Subdural empyema can also follow from direct spread of infection from the suppurative focus through bone and then dura, from penetrating head injury, from orbital cellulitis or, rarely, from spread of organisms from lungs or blood. On occasion, subdural empyema will be due to spread from a brain abscess. The most common predisposition to subdural empyema in patients less than 1 year old is meningitis.

When subdural empyema results from sinus or mastoid disease, as is the usual case in patients beyond infancy, the organisms encountered are streptococci (aerobic or anaerobic), *Bacteroides*, staphylococci, *E. coli*, *Proteus*, and *Pseudomonas*. In infants in whom subdural empyema complicates meningitis, the most frequent bacterial agents are *H. influenzae*, *Streptococcus pneumoniae*, and Gram-negative bacilli.

Clinical signs are produced by the pressure of the mass lesion and by the effects on underlying brain of thrombophlebitis, arteritis, and cortical venous thrombosis with resulting hemorrhagic infarction and edema. Meningeal signs are produced by the irritative effect of the lesion. The onset of symptoms can be associated with complaints related to a preexisting suppurative focus (i.e., sinusitis, otitis, mastoiditis). New onset of malaise, fever, vomiting, and headache can indicate intracranial spread. These symptoms are joined in one to several days by meningeal signs, drowsiness, increasing stupor, and focal neurologic deficits. The latter include hemiplegia, unilateral seizures, cortical sensory deficits, and aphasia. Intracranial hypertension may be present. Unidentified and untreated, subdural empyema is usually rapidly fatal.

LP should be avoided when subdural empyema is a diagnostic consideration since it can predispose to herniation. Emergency CT scan should be performed to attempt to demonstrate the lesion. Otherwise, work-up of these patients includes the studies shown in Exhibit 11-12. Skull films may demonstrate a paracranial focus

Treatment includes immediate surgical drainage coupled with antimicrobial therapy. The antibiotics are chosen in the same manner as suggested for brain abscess and should be initiated prior to surgery. Initial therapy in infants less than 2 months old should include ampicillin and gentamicin or, possibly, ampicillin and a third generation cephalosporin. Subsequent decisions regarding therapy will be guided by bacteriologic findings. The course of antimicrobial therapy should be at least 3 weeks, longer if an associated osteomyelitis is discovered. Antiedema measures may be indicated. Recovery in promptly treated patients can be quite good.

Intracranial Epidural Abscess

This lesion is usually associated with a source of infection in the ear or paranasal sinuses but can follow neurosurgical procedures. Rarely, an extracranial septic focus or spread from a dural sinus thrombophlebitis is involved. The clinical course is usually not as aggressive as that of subdural involvement. Typically, signs of local inflammation in the ear or sinuses are associated with fever. Increased intracranial pressure can produce headache and vomiting. Localizing signs are usually absent. The diagnosis is made by CT scan; LP can be hazardous. Treatment consists of prompt antimicrobial therapy and surgical drainage. Initial antibiotic treatment is chosen in the same manner as specified for brain abscess and should include coverage for S.

aureus. The treatment course should be at least 3 weeks, longer when osteomyelitis is associated.

Spinal Epidural Abscess

Acute spinal epidural abscess represents an extremely important neurologic infection which demands immediate attention to appropriate diagnostic studies and therapy. Spinal epidural abscess results from hematogenous spread from furuncles or direct spread from vertebral osteomyelitis. It is most often located at the midthoracic and lower lumbar levels. The most frequent agents are *S. aureus*, streptococci, Gram-negative bacilli, and anaerobes. Initial clinical symptoms are fever and back pain, followed in one to several days by radicular pain, headache, and neck stiffness. Several days later a rapidly progressive paraparesis ensues, together with sensory loss in the lower body and urinary and fecal retention resulting from sphincter paralysis. Examination reveals tenderness at the site of infection and evidence of cord and/or root dysfunction. Spinal films may reveal osteomyelitis.

When spinal epidural abscess is suspected, a neurosurgeon should be called in and neurologic studies initiated to define the abscess. These may include an MRI scan, CT scan after introduction of a contrast agent intrathecally, or myelography. It is desirable that CSF be sampled in order to identify an associated meningitis, but care must be taken to avoid introducing organisms in the abscess into the SAS. The CSF usually has fewer than 100 cells per cubic millimeter, CSF protein is elevated, and glucose is normal. CSF should be cultured and stained for anaerobic and aerobic bacteria, *M. tuberculosis*, and fungus.

Acute spinal epidural abscess is a neurosurgical emergency and requires laminectomy and drainage as soon as possible. Abscess material should be sent for appropriate cultures and stains. Empiric antibiotic therapy should be given preoperatively. Coverage for *S. aureus* must be included. One regimen would be nafcillin, ampicillin, and gentamicin. Antimicrobial therapy should be guided by culture results and should continue for 3 to 4 weeks; longer in the case of vertebral osteomyelitis.

Disorders with manifestations similar to those of spinal epidural abscess are acute disc space infection and acute transverse myelitis. Plain films, CSF examination, and neuroradiographic studies will differentiate these disorders.

Sinus Thrombophlebitis

The dural sinuses usually involved by infection are the lateral, cavernous, and longitudinal (sagittal). Infection of these structures usually extends from an infection in the facial skin, ear, mastoid, or paranasal sinuses. Occasionally they are infected by direct trauma. Intracranial thrombophlebitis can result in large areas of hemorrhagic infarction and constitutes a potentially life-threatening illness. The organisms most frequently encountered are streptococci and staphylococci. Thrombophlebitis is frequently associated with other intracranial suppurative processes including meningitis, subdural empyema, epidural abscess, and brain abscess. Clinical signs include fever, headache, signs of increased intracranial pressure, and focal neurologic deficits.

Lateral sinus thrombosis often follows chronic otitis and mastoiditis. Symptoms expected of these conditions precede, by days to weeks, onset of fever, headache, signs of toxemia, and papilledema. Spread of the clot to the jugular foramen can produce dysfunction of cranial nerves IX, X, and XI. Involvement of the superior longitudinal (sagittal) sinus causes seizures and focal cerebral signs.

Cavernous sinus thrombosis results from infections of the face, paranasal sinuses, and orbit. Headache, fever, and toxemia are complemented by local effects. Ophthalmic vein obstruction causes chemosis, proptosis, and facial edema. Retinal vein engorgement may be followed by retinal hemorrhage and papilledema. Ptosis, ocular palsies, and pain and sensory loss around the eye and forehead are due to involvement of cranial nerves III, IV, ophthalmic division of V, and VI. Bilateral symptoms indicate spread to the opposite side. A similar clinical picture can be produced by mucormycosis and *Aspergillus* infections and by carcinomatous or sarcomatous invasion of sphenoid bone or by sphenoid wing meningioma.

Superior longitudinal sinus thrombosis is associated with headache, increased intracranial pressure, and papilledema. Signs include unilateral hemiplegia and seizures, first on one side and then on the other. Bilateral leg weakness and sensory loss can occur, as well as other neurologic deficits.

Diagnosis of intracranial thrombophlebitis can often be made on clinical grounds and may be confirmed by MRI scan or CT scan with and without contrast. LP may be hazardous with focally increased intracranial pressure. When LP must be performed to rule out bacterial meningitis, CT scan should be obtained on an emergent basis. The results of the scan will help to determine whether an LP may be safely performed. A CT scan is otherwise indicated in all cases of intracranial thrombophlebitis to investigate other foci of intracranial suppuration. Extracranial suppurative foci must also be documented. Treatment includes prompt initiation of high dose antibiotics. The regimen for brain abscess is appropriate for initial treatment; coverage for *S. aureus* should be included. Other treatment choices may follow from consideration of organisms identified in a presumed focus.

Antiedema therapy may be indicated for cerebral edema. Surgical decompression should be considered in cases in which a severe increase in intraorbital pressure threatens retinal or optic nerve function. Pituitary insufficiency may follow cavernous sinus thrombosis in children and should be assessed during convalescence.

References

1. Plum F, Posner, JB: *The Diagnosis of Stupor and Coma,* ed 3. Philadelphia, FA Davis Co, 1980.
2. Margolis LH, Shaywitz BA: The outcome of prolonged coma in childhood. *Pediatrics* 1980;65:477–483.
3. Report of the medical consultants on the diagnosis of death to the President's Commission for the Study of Ethical Problems in Medicine and Biomedical and Behavioral Research: Guidelines for the determination of death. *Neurology* 1982;32:395–399.
4. Freeman JM, Rogers MC: On death, dying, and decisions. *Pediatrics* 1980;66:637–638.
5. Gold A: Stroke in children, in Rowland LP (ed): *Merritt's Textbook of Neurology,* ed 7. Philadelphia, Lea & Febiger, 1984, pp 172–177.
6. Mueller SM, Golden GS, Swaiman KF, et al: Vascular diseases of the brain and spinal cord, in Swaiman KF, Wright FF (eds): *The Practice of Pediatric Neurology,* edition 2. St. Louis, CV Mosby Co, 1982, pp 765–793.
7. Solomon GE: Strokes in children. *Pediatr Ann* 1978;7:32–53.
8. Kelly JJ, Mellinger JF, Sundt TM: Intracranial arterial venous malformations in childhood. *Ann Neurol* 1978;3:338–343.
9. Cottom DG: Acute cerebellar ataxia. *Arch Dis Child* 1957;32:181–188.
10. Weiss S, Carter S: Course and prognosis of acute cerebellar ataxia in children. *Neurology (NY)* 9:711–721, 1959.
11. Solomon GE, Chutorian AM: Opsoclonus and occult neuroblastoma. *N Engl J Med* 1968;279:475–477.
12. Schoenbaum SC, Gardner P, Shillito J: Infections of cerebrospinal fluid shunts: Epidemiology, clinical manifestations, and therapy. *J Infect Dis* 1975;131:543–552.
13. Yogev R, Davis TA: Neurosurgical shunt infections. A review. *Child's Brain* 1980;6:74–81.
14. Freeman JM, D'Souza BJ: Pediatrics editorial: Obstruction of CSF shunts. *Pediatrics* 1979;64:111–112.
15. Karian JM, Buchheit WA: Intractable hiccup as a complication of ventriculoperitoneal shunt: Case report. *Neurosurgery* 1980;7:283–284.
16. Skolnick ML, Rosenbaum AE, Matzuk T, et al: Detection of dilated cerebral ultrasound and computed tomography. *Radiology* 1979;131:447.
17. Hayden PW, Rudd TG, Shurtleff DB: Combined pressure-radionuclide evaluation of suspected cerebrospinal fluid shunt malfunction: A seven-year clinical experience. *Pediatrics* 1980;66:679–684.
18. Freeman JM: Febrile seizures: A consensus of their significance, evaluation and treatment. *Pediatrics* 1980;66:1009.
19. National Institutes of Health Consensus Report: Febrile seizures: Long-term management of children with fever-associated seizures. *Pediatrics* 1980;66:1009–1012.
20. Asbury AK: Diagnostic considerations in Guillain-Barré syndrome. *Ann Neurol* 1981;9(suppl):1–5.
21. McKhann GM: The Guillain-Barré syndrome study group: Plasmapheresis and acute Guillain-Barré syndrome. *Neurology* 1985;35:1096–1104.
22. Lombroso CT, Lerman P: Breathholding spells (cyanotic and pallid infantile syncope). *Pediatrics* 1967;39:563–581.
23. Holowach J, Thurston DL: Breath-holding spells and anemia. *N Eng J Med* 1963;268:21–23.
24. Stephenson JBP: Reflex anoxic seizures ('white breath-holding'): Nonepileptic vagal attacks. *Arch Dis Child* 1978;53:193–200.
25. Livingstone S: Breath-holding spells in children. *JAMA* 1970;212:2231–2235.
26. Anas NG, McBride JT, Boettrich C, et al: Ventilatory chemosensitivity in subjects with a history of childhood cyanotic breath-holding spells. *Pediatrics* 1985;75:76–79.
27. Shinnar S, D'Souza BJ: The diagnosis and management of headaches in childhood. *Pediatr Clin North Am* 1982;29:79–94.
28. Vahlquist B: Migraine in children. *Int Arch Allergy* 1955;7:348–355.
29. Honig PJ, Charney EB: Children with brain tumor headaches. *Am J Dis Child* 1982;136:121–124.
30. Illingworth RS: *Common Symptoms of Disease in Children,* ed 5. Oxford, Blackwell Scientific Publications, 1975, p 98.
31. Barbosa E, Freeman JM: Status epilepticus. *Pediatrics in Review* 1982;4:185–189.
32. Delgado-Escueta AV, Wasterlain C, Treiman DM, et al: Current Concepts in neurology: Management of status epilepticus. *N Engl J Med* 1982;306:1337–1340.
33. Rawal K, D'Souza BJ: Status epilepticus. *Crit Care Clin* 1985;1:339–353.
34. Trauner DA: Reye's syndrome. *Curr Probl Pediatr* 1982;12:1–31.
35. Hurwitz ES, Nelson B, Davis C, et al: National Surveillance for Reye Syndrome: A five-year review. *Pediatrics* 1982;70:895–900.
36. Committee on Infectious Diseases: Aspirin and Reye syndrome. *Pediatrics* 1982;69:810–812.
37. Hurwitz ES, Barrett MJ, Bregman D, et al: Public Health Service study on Reye's syndrome and medications. Report of the pilot phase. *N Engl J Med* 1985;313:849–857.
38. DeLong GR, Glick TH: Encephalopathy of Reye's syndrome: A review of pathogenic hypotheses. *Pediatrics* 1982;69:53–63.
39. Huttenlocher PR, Trauner DA: Reye's syndrome in infancy. *Pediatrics* 1978;62:84–90.
40. Heubi JE, Daugherty CC, Partin JS, et al: Grade I Reye's syndrome—outcome and predictors of progression to deeper coma grades. *N Engl J Med* 1984;311:1539–1542.
41. Lovejoy FH, Smith AL, et al: Clinical Staging in Reye syndrome. *Am J Dis Child* 1974;128:36–41.
42. NIH Consensus Conference Statement: The diagnosis and treatment of Reye's syndrome, March 2–4, 1981. *Oklahoma State Med J* 1982;75:118–123.
43. Marshall LF, Shapiro HM, et al: Pentobarbital therapy for intracranial hypertension in metabolic coma: Reye's syndrome. *Crit Care Med* 1978;6:1–5.
44. Shaywitz SE, Cohen PM, et al: Long-term consequences of Reye syndrome. *J Pediatr* 1982;100:41–46.
45. Bell WE, McCormick WF: *Neurologic Infections in Children.* Philadelphia, WB Saunders Co, 1981.
46. Murphy FK, Mackowiak P, Luby J: Management of infections affecting the nervous system, in Rosenberg RN (ed): *The Treatment of Neurological Diseases.* New York, SP Medical and Scientific Books, 1979, pp 249–376.
47. Sagar SM: Infectious disease, in Samuels MA (ed): *Manual of Neurologic Therapeutics.* Boston, Little Brown & Co, 1982, pp 137–198.
48. *Report of the Committee on Infectious Diseases,* ed. 20. EIK Grove Village, IL, American Academy of Pediatrics, 1986.
49. Rhodes KH, Johnson CM: Antibiotic therapy for severe infections in infants and children. *Mayo Clin Proc* 1983;58:158–164.
50. Bell WE: Treatment of bacterial infections of the central nervous system. *Ann Neurol* 1981;9:313–327.
51. Jacobs RF, Wells TG, Steele RW, et al: A prospective randomized comparison of cefotaxime vs ampicillin and chloramphenicol for bacterial meningitis in children. *J Pediatr* 1985;107:129–133.
52. Peltola H, Valmari P: Serum C-reactive protein as detector of pretreated childhood bacterial meningitis. *Neurology* 1985;35:251–253.
53. Johnson RT: *Viral Infections of the Nervous System.* New York, Raven Press, 1982.
54. Bell WE: Treatment of fungal infections of the central nervous system. *Ann Neurol* 1981;9:417–422.
55. Whitley RT, Alford CA, Hirsch MS, et al: Vidarabine versus acyclovir therapy in herpes simplex encephalitis. *N Engl J Med* 1986;314:144–149.
56. Nelson J: 1985 *Pocketbook of Antimicrobial Therapy.* Baltimore, Williams & Wilkins, 1985.

John D. Ward

12 Central Nervous System Injuries

Head injury is an affliction of the younger patient; in fact, a good portion of these patients are below the age of 15 years.[1] Therefore, those involved in the emergency care of patients need to be skilled in the evaluation and care of the child with a CNS injury. To accomplish this goal, it is necessary to understand the types of injuries sustained, the nervous system's response to this injury, and its reaction to various types of therapeutic measures upon which treatment is based.

The first part of the chapter concentrates primarily on the general approach to the child with a head injury rather than on specific types of injury. The later section briefly discusses specific types of head injury and concludes with a discussion of spinal cord injuries.

PATHOPHYSIOLOGY

At the moment of impact, the brain sustains a number of injuries in a variety of locations. These include contusions, lacerations, shearing injuries,[2] and, in the more severe cases, brain stem injury.[3] There is little one can do about these primary injuries once they have occurred. However, it is felt that further damage to injured neural tissue does occur in the form of secondary insults from hypoxia, ischemia, and other metabolic derangements. It is in preventing these secondary insults that those caring for children with CNS trauma have a role.

There is little doubt that secondary insults occur. In one study hypoxia was present in about a third of patients arriving at the emergency department while hypotension was present in about 15%.[4] In addition to ischemia from hypotension, the brain can become ischemic if the intracranial pressure (ICP) is allowed to rise to unacceptable levels. This is based on the fact that the cerebral perfusion pressure (CPP) is dependent on the mean arterial blood pressure (MAP) as well as the ICP (CPP = MAP − ICP).[5] Therefore it is important to prevent elevations in ICP. This is accomplished by the prompt diagnosis of mass lesions and the aggressive treatment of intracranial hypertension.

Thus it is the job of the person caring for the head-injured child to (1) prevent hypoxia, (2) preserve cerebral perfusion by the prevention of hypotension, and (3) control intracranial hypertension by the rapid diagnosis of mass lesions.

RESUSCITATION

Figure 12-1 outlines the overall approach to a patient with a head injury. The treatment of a child with a head injury properly begins at the scene of the accident. This is done with the establishment of

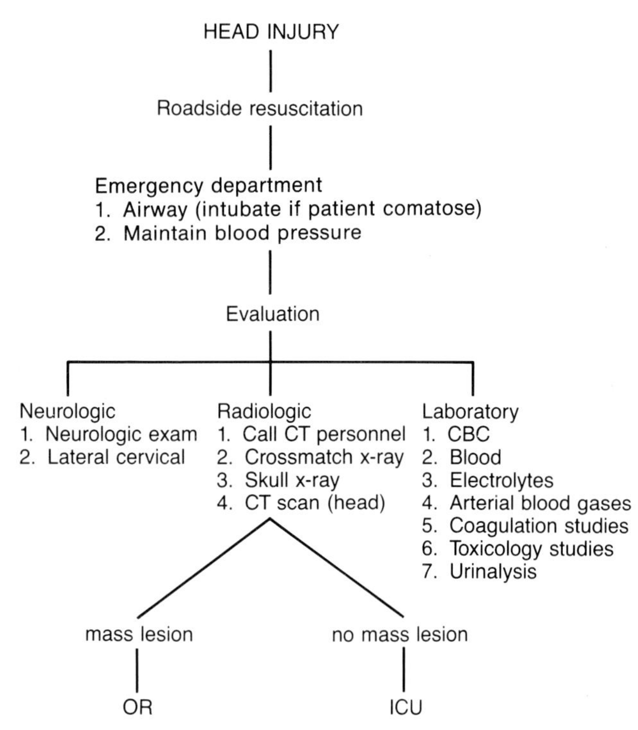

FIGURE 12-1 Care of acute head injuries.

an adequate airway and the administration of oxygen. When the patient arrives at the emergency department, resuscitation is carried out in the same fashion as for any multiply injured patient.[6] An unconscious child should be intubated to prevent hypoxia, which can occur even if the child appears to be adequately ventilating.[4]

Intubation should be performed by someone skilled in handling children. It must be done with a minimum of trauma and coughing. If necessary, to accomplish this end, the child is paralyzed with pancuronium bromide (0.1 mg/kg). Obviously, this is done only after a quick but adequate neurologic assessment and only when qualified personnel with appropriate equipment are present to handle the required intubation.

After intubation the child is then hyperventilated to maintain an arterial carbon dioxide pressure in the range of 25–30 mmHg. This causes cerebral vasoconstriction of sufficient magnitude to compensate temporarily for elevated intracranial pressure but not enough to compromise cerebral blood flow.

After the airway is secured, at least two intravenous lines are inserted. Sufficient crystalloid, colloid, or blood is given to maintain a normal circulating blood volume and pressure for age. Adequate cerebral perfusion pressures depend on an adequate blood pressure. It is therefore important to maintain volume expansion. There is no place for initial fluid restriction in the patient with a head injury. However, the use of hypotonic fluids is to be avoided as this may result in a shift of free water into the brain tissue.

When the vascular lines are inserted, blood samples are sent for: complete blood count, typing, and cross-matching, determination of electrolyte and arterial blood gas levels, toxicological screening, and coagulation studies. A Foley catheter is inserted to evaluate urine output and to collect samples to test for the presence of blood.

EVALUATION

The neurologic evaluation tries to answer three questions: (1) What is the extent of neurologic damage? (2) Is there a mass lesion present? (3) What is the patient's course, i.e., is the patient getting better, worse, or staying the same since the accident?

To answer these questions it is not necessary, nor is it practical to perform a full detailed neurologic examination. The pertinent points of the examination consist of the mental status evaluation, assessment of pupils and brainstem function, motor examination, as well as an overall examination of the soft tissues of the head and neck.

Examination of mental status is patterned after the Glasgow Coma Scale.[7] This is an assessment of eye opening, verbalization, and response to stimulation. If the patient is unable to respond to verbal stimulation, then sufficient painful stimulation should be applied to provide an adequate estimation of the patient's response to noxious stimuli.

It is important to look for any asymmetry of movement since this can indicate the presence of a mass lesion. Pupils are then assessed with light of sufficient intensity to produce an adequate stimulation. A unilaterally dilated pupil can indicate either ipsilateral uncal herniation from a mass lesion or direct injury to cranial nerve III. Both eyes should be stimulated to examine the direct and consensual light responses.

Oculocephalic or doll's eyes response is then evaluated by turning the head. This is performed only after the possibility of a spine or spinal cord injury has been excluded by appropriate x-ray studies. If the neck cannot be manipulated or oculocephalic responses are absent, then caloric responses are checked by injecting ice water into each ear. Prior to this the eardrum has to be evaluated; if there is a perforation, then this test is not performed.

The limbs are then checked for the presence and symmetry of movement. If there is hemiparesis, then the possibility of a mass lesion should be considered. If monoparesis is present, then a plexus injury is more likely. If there is little or no movement bilaterally, then a possible spinal cord injury should be considered. It is uncommon for a patient with a head injury to be flaccid unless drugs, alcohol, barbiturates, or paralyzing agents are present; the patient is neurologically dead; or there is a spinal cord injury.

Once resuscitation, intravenous line insertion, blood sampling, and neurologic and systemic examinations have all been accomplished, then x-ray films are obtained. There has been much controversy about what x-ray studies are appropriate in a patient with a head injury. In the patient who is unconscious with a severe head injury, the procedure of choice is a CT scan.[8] The capacity to perform this test should exist in any major center that deals with head injuries.

Once the patient has been quickly evaluated, appropriate radiology personnel should be notified so that they are standing by when the patient is stabilized and ready for transfer to the CT suite. The scan is especially helpful in depicting mass lesions, estimating the amount of shift, and evaluating intracerebral contusions, cerebral swelling, and the degree of penetration of any depressed fractures that may be present.

There is more controversy about the need for obtaining plain skull films. Exhibit 12-1 lists indications for obtaining skull films. The general principle is not to delay the CT scan in an unconscious child in order to get plain films of the skull. The CT scan helps in evaluating whether or not there are any significant depressed fractures or other intracranial abnormalities. If, however, there is time to obtain plain skull films in a child with severe head injury, they occasionally are of benefit in detecting fractures and the distribution of bone fragments.

Before obtaining x-ray films of the skull and the rest of the body, we immediately get a cross-table lateral cervical spine film on any child that comes in with a severe head injury. This is done promptly while the child is being resuscitated so that subsequent maneuvers can be performed safely without aggravating a preexisting spine injury. If the cross-table lateral cervical spine x-ray film is normal, then we proceed with the chest film, abdominal films, and extremity films, as indicated.

If the CT scan is not available and if the child is comatose, angiography or ventriculography can be useful in establishing the presence or absence of the mass lesion.

Exhibit 12-1 Indications for Skull Film in Head Trauma

1. Obvious defect in skull
2. Possibility of intracranial foreign body
3. Significant soft tissue injury
4. Significant history of severe trauma
5. Sign of basilar skull fracture
6. Presence of CSF leak

MULTIPLE INJURIES

Although multiple injuries have been discussed elsewhere, a word is in order about priorities in evaluating and treating a child with multiple injuries. The general principle is that stabilization of the vital signs, i.e., of the airway and vascular integrity, should take priority over management of all other injuries. Once this has been accomplished, then diagnosis and evaluation of the head injury should be the next priority.

If major systemic injuries such as uncontrolled intra-abdominal bleeding, lung injuries, and soft tissue injuries are of such a magnitude that they prevent the child's vital signs from being stabilized, then these must be addressed promptly, even if they require sending the child to surgery without a CT scan. If this occurs, the people who are evaluating the head injury should follow the child to surgery and perform an appropriate evaluation while the child is being stabilized. Although ventriculography is awkward in the presence of other ongoing procedures, it can be done and provides an indication of the child's ICP as well as the presence or absence of a mass lesion.

The main thing to remember in the child with multiple injuries is that the need for cooperation is paramount. The child should be resuscitated in the normal way, in an orderly, systemic fashion so that problems are dealt with in order of importance.

CONTROL OF ELEVATED INTRACRANIAL PRESSURE

Elevated ICP occurs in almost all patients with significant mass lesions, which can occur from 10% (9) up to 23% which we observed in our patients. In addition, a certain number of patients with diffuse injury also have elevated ICP.[9] When intracranial hypertension is suspected, it should be treated promptly.

With the airway under control, the first step is to hyperventilate patients to an arterial carbon dioxide pressure of 20 to 50 mmHg. In addition, mannitol is delivered in doses between 0.5 to 2.0 g/kg. The rationale behind this is to use hyperventilation and osmotic diuretics to protect the brain while further evaluation and, if necessary, surgery is performed.

MEDICATIONS

Several medications are routinely used in the treatment of head injury. The most common of these are the corticosteroids. The exact role that steroids play in the treatment of head injury is unclear. Some literature indicates that corticosteroids are of great benefit;[10] other research indicates that the benefits have not been proven.[11] Despite this lack of agreement, their use is widespread. The usual dose given is equivalent to 10 mg of dexamethasone by IV bolus and then 4 mg IV every 6 hours. Obviously, this has to be adjusted in the very young children.

In addition to the use of mannitol, which has already been discussed, furosemide has also been advocated in doses of 0.5 to 1.0 mg/kg.[12]

The use of anticonvulsants as prophylaxis also is somewhat controversial. Generally, our policy is to give prophylactic anticonvulsants to those patients who demonstrate focal neurologic deficits or evidence of structural damage on their CT scans. Older children receive phenytoin in a loading dose of 15 to 25 mg/kg; younger children are given phenobarbital in a loading dose of 15 to 25 mg/kg. The child that arrives while having seizures receives short-term treatment with diazepam (0.3 mg/kg) and then is given phenytoin or phenobarbital, depending on age.

Antibiotics are indicated only for an associated systemic injury or a compound skull fracture. If there is concern about intracranial contamination, treatment with chloramphenicol and penicillin is initiated. These two antibiotics enter the CNS and provide coverage for the most common infecting organisms.

SPECIFIC INTRACRANIAL PROBLEMS

Mild Head Injuries

Probably the most common head injury in a child is a mild head injury. The typical story is that of a child who has fallen or been hit over the head and has a brief episode of unconsciousness, followed by wakening and perhaps vomiting. Being lethargic, the child is then brought to the emergency department. On arrival the child may be either neurologically normal or slightly lethargic.

The two decisions to be made at this point are (1) how far to evaluate the child and (2) whether or not to admit the child. It is important to adequately evaluate these children. A detailed history of the injury is obtained. The neurologic examination includes an assessment of mental status, cranial nerves, reflexes, motor and sensory function, and gait and balance. If there is any indication that the child has received any significant trauma or if any other indications are present, skull films are obtained (Exhibit 12-1).

If the child is awake and neurologically intact, then performance of a CT scan is deferred. Exhibit 12-2 lists the criteria for hospital admission of patients with head injuries. If the child has any neurologic deficit or if there is significant alteration of consciousness, a CT scan is obtained. The child should be watched closely for 24 to 48 hours and be allowed to go home when neurologically normal and without symptoms of significant headache or dizziness.

Skull Fractures

Skull fractures can be divided into (1) linear versus depressed and (2) open versus closed. The presence of a linear skull fracture merely indicates that the child has had sufficient trauma to cause fracture of the skull and is therefore a candidate for admission. The parents generally are told that a skull fracture exists, indicating a severe blow to the head, and that the fracture itself has caused little damage.

On the other hand, depressed fractures present interesting problems. If the fracture is closed, then the diagnosis can be made because of either the presence of an actual indentation or, if there has been subgaleal or subperiosteal hemorrhage, the presence of significant swelling. The diagnosis is generally made with skull films.

Surgery is indicated if the bone fragment is depressed below the inner table to a depth greater

Exhibit 12-2 Criteria for Admission Following Head Injury

Loss of significant alteration of consciousness
Memory deficit
Focal neurologic signs
Post-traumatic seizures
Persistent vomiting
Fever
Severe headache
Skull fracture
Circumstances of head injury cannot be obtained

than the thickness of the skull. CT scans of the head are obtained on all patients with skull fractures severe enough to require surgical intervention. Patients with depressed fractures that have a laceration over them (i.e., open depressed fractures) receive antibiotics and undergo surgical repair.

Hospitalization is mandatory for all children who have signs and symptoms of a basilar skull fracture. These include bruising behind the ear (Battle's sign), CSF otorrhea or rhinorrhea, periorbital ecchymoses, or air on the plain skull films. Antibiotics are not started unless there is a CSF leak. Although the use of antibiotics in basilar-skull fractures is controversial,[13] in the presence of an active leak, we generally institute penicillin treatment for at least 48 to 72 hours. Patients are kept in a head-up position and watched closely for the signs and symptoms of meningitis.

Mass Lesions

Mass lesions in head injury can be divided into epidural, subdural, and intracerebral hematomas; cerebral contusions; or a combination of any of these. The diagnosis is generally based on the neurologic examination and a CT scan. Treatment is usually surgical decompression.

Intracerebral hematomas and contusions are operated upon if they are causing (1) significant neurologic deficit or (2) elevation of ICP.

As is mentioned earlier, patients with these lesions must be evaluated carefully and quickly. The diagnosis of these mass lesions should be made promptly, and surgery, if indicated, should be performed before further neurologic deterioration.

SPINAL CORD INJURIES

Fortunately, spine and spinal cord injuries are not as common in children as in adults. Automobile accidents appear to be the most common cause, followed by falls and other injuries.[14] It should be remembered that there is approximately a 10% incidence of significant neck injuries with head injuries. As with the head injuries, spinal cord injuries should be handled in an orderly and appropriate sequence.

Resuscitation

In patients with known spinal cord injuries, establishment of an airway is a more difficult problem. If the injuries are in the cervical spine, the patient may have only diaphragmatic breathing, or if they are above C5, the patient may have little respiratory action. In addition, when a cervical spine injury is present, the neck should be manipulated as little as possible. Therefore, the care and time taken to secure an airway depends on the clinical situation. If the patient is apneic or very hypoxic, intubation needs to be done with minimal manipulation but also as rapidly as possible so that the patient has an adequate airway. If intubation is required, the head should be moved as little as possible and have traction applied in the longitudinal plane. It does little good to avoid manipulation of the neck if the patient ends up with hypoxic brain injury.

However, if ventilation and oxygenation are adequate, the patient can be monitored by measuring arterial blood gases and tidal volume. If these parameters deteriorate, then elective intubation can be performed carefully while the patient is in traction and preferably nasally over a fiberoptic scope.

While an adequate airway and oxygenation are being established and appropriate intravenous lines are being inserted, it is imperative to stabilize the neck until adequate x-ray films are obtained. This is usually accomplished by placing sandbags on either side of the neck and then securing the chest and the head so that the patient is unable to flex or extend the neck. If only the head is immobilized, then the patient may attempt to sit up or move causing further neurologic damage. Therefore, one must not only secure the head but also the chest. An alternative is to fit the patient with a firm collar, with appropriate measures to prevent the patient from moving.

In moving a child with a spinal cord injury, it is important that a sufficient number of people be used so that the entire body and head can be raised as a unit while someone is applying general traction on the head in a longitudinal direction. At no time should the child be allowed to flex or extend the neck.

Evaluation

Neurologic evaluation of a child with a spinal cord injury consists of an assessment of mental status, pupillary response, reflexes, and sensory and motor function. Oculocephalic testing is deferred.

As mentioned earlier, lack of movement below the neck is a clear clinical clue that a spinal cord injury may be present. In evaluating the patient or getting the patient to move, it should be mentioned that shrugging of the shoulders is mediated by the spinal accessory nerve and not the cervical roots from the cervical spinal cord.

Motor evaluation of the patient is done in sequential fashion, starting at the high cervical roots and then going through each muscle group in a descending fashion until the level of the lesion has been adequately demonstrated. Sensory function is determined by starting in an area of anesthesia and proceeding upward slowly until areas of sensation are encountered. Reflexes are checked in both arms and legs, and there should be assessment of rectal tone as well as of the presence or absence of a bulbocavernosus reflex.

This evaluation can be complicated by the presence of spinal shock, a complete flaccid paralysis with loss of tone and reflexes below the level of the lesion. The duration of this condition varies from a few hours to several days. Incomplete lesions can create a confusing picture, with partial sensory and motor loss. In evaluating a patient neurologically, it is of the utmost importance to get a very good and complete assessment of the patient's motor and sensory function so that subsequent improvement or deterioration can be documented adequately.

In the patient who has no neurologic deficit, a spine injury may still be present. One of the clues for this clinical situation is the presence of pain, either expressed by the patient or elicited on examination of the neck. It is extremely uncommon for a patient to have a significant spine injury with no neck pain. The obvious corollary to this is that any patient complaining of neck pain should be presumed to have a spine injury until proven otherwise.

As mentioned earlier, the radiologic evaluation of the patient with a spinal cord injury consists first of obtaining a cross-table lateral cervical spine film. All seven cervical vertebrae should be demonstrated; it may be necessary to pull down on the arms or get a swimmer's view to accomplish this goal. If the film is completely normal and the patient has no neurologic deficits or pain, then it is reasonably safe to proceed with other views of the spine. However, if there is any abnormality at all on the cervical spine film or if the patient complains of any significant neck pain or if there is any neurologic deficit associated with a spinal cord injury, the patient's neck is immobilized and further radiologic evaluation is deferred until appropriate tomography can be obtained.

Lower spine injuries can be more difficult to assess. If the patients are stable, they need to be transported to the x-ray department to obtain better films of the lumbar and thoracic spine. As in the patient with a neck injury, care should be taken in moving these patients to avoid further damage.

It has been demonstrated that the child's spine is much more mobile than the adult's spine. Therefore, care must be taken to avoid overinterpreting the pediatric spine film.[15] If there is any question at all during any phase of evaluation, the patient is presumed to have a spine injury and is treated as such until further, more sophisticated radiologic assessment is undertaken.

Once a spine injury is diagnosed, the next step is to immobilize the spine so that further injury cannot occur. In the older child and adolescent, Gardner-Wells tongs are used for skeletal traction. In the infant with a very thin skull, this may be more difficult initially and some type of collar arrangement or traction through more elective surgical procedures[16] may have to be provided.

Patients who have spinal cord damage require urinary catheterization because of bladder dysfunction. A nasogastric tube is also necessary since the incidence of ileus is quite high in these patients.

Complications

Several complications can occur in the patient with a spinal cord injury. Hypotension resulting from decreased vascular tone and pooling can be a real problem. Sufficient fluids should be given to maintain good intravascular volume. Bradycardia is another problem that can occur from lack of sympathetic input in the presence of the complete cervical spine injury. It is not usually necessary to treat bradycardia unless the blood pressure is affected. If this happens, periodic doses of atropine will maintain the heart rate adequately enough to sustain a normal blood pressure.

SUMMARY

Emergency care of the child with CNS trauma demands adherence to the principles basic to the care of any patient with multiple trauma. Vital signs are stabilized, neurologic dysfunction is rapidly but adequately assessed, and steps to remedy any treatable cause of neurologic damage are immediately instituted. Children have a remarkable recuperative power; however, if they are allowed to harbor damaging neurologic injuries without appropriate evaluation and treatment, the results can and will be discouraging. It is only with proper understanding of the pathophysiology of CNS trauma and appropriate, aggressive evaluation and treatment that the best possible results can be obtained in the child with a CNS injury.

References

1. Kalsbeek WD, McLaurin RL, Harris BSH, et al: The national head and spinal cord injury survey: Major findings. *J Neurosurg* 1980:53(suppl):S19–S31.
2. Graham DI, Adams H: The pathology of blunt head injuries, in Critchley M, O'Leary JL, Jennett B (eds): *Scientific Foundations of Neurology.* London, William Heinemann Medical Books Ltd, 1972, pp 478–491.
3. Rosenblum WI, Greenberg RP, Seelig JM, et al: Midbrain lesions: Frequent and significant prognostic feature in closed head injury. *Neurosurgery* 1981;9:613–620.
4. Miller JD, Sweet R, Narayan R, et al: Early insults to the injured brain. *JAMA* 1978;240(5):439–447.
5. Miller JD, Stanek A, Langfitt TW: Concepts of cerebral perfusion pressure and vascular compression during intracranial hypertension, in Meyer JS, Schadé JP (eds): *Progress in Brain Research.* Amsterdam, Elsevier Publishing Co, 1972, vol 35: *Cerebral Blood Flow,* pp 411–432.
6. Ward JD: Emergency treatment of major head trauma. *Hosp Med* 1980;16:55–65.
7. Teasdale G, Jennett B: Assessment of coma and impaired consciousness. *Lancet* 1974;2:81–84.
8. French BN, Dublin AB: The value of computerized tomography in the management of 1,000 consecutive head injuries. *Surg Neurol* 1977;7:171–183.
9. Bruce D, Raphaely RC, Goldberg AJ, et al: Pathophysiology, treatment and outcome following severe head injury in children. *Childs Brain* 1979;5:174–191.
10. Faupel G, Reulen HJ, Muller D, et al: Double-blind study on the effects of steroids on severe closed head injury, in Pappius HM, Feindel W (eds): *Dynamics of Brain Edema.* Berlin, Springer-Verlag, 1976, pp 337–343.
11. Cooper R, Moody S, Clark WK, et al: Dexamethasone and severe head injury: A prospective double-blind study. *J Neurosurg* 1979;51:307–316.
12. Cottrell JE, Robustelli A, Post K, et al: Furosemide and mannitol induced changes in intracranial pressure and serum osmolality and electrolytes. *Anesthesiology* 1977;47:28–30.
13. Haines SJ: Systemic antibiotic prophylaxis in neurological surgery. *Neurosurgery* 1980;6:355–361.
14. Anderson MJ, Schutt AH: Spinal injuries in children: A review of 156 cases seen from 1950 through 1978. *Mayo Clin Proc* 1980;55:499–504.
15. Fielding JW: The cervical spine in the child, in O'Brien MS (ed): *Pediatric Neurological Surgery.* New York, Raven Press, 1975, pp 147–171.
16. Gaufin LM, Goodman SJ: Cervical spine injuries in infants: Problems in management. *J Neurosurg* 1975;42:179–184.

Perry W. Stafford
Thomas V. Whalen
J. J. Tepas III

13 Craniofacial Injuries

Traumatic injury to the head and neck exacts a harsh toll on children and their families. Studies have estimated that one child in ten will suffer head trauma severe enough to cause loss of consciousness and that one in two will require medical attention for facial injury during the preteen years. Because these injuries rarely cause the death of a child prior to arrival at the emergency department, they are commonly considered to be minor trauma. When they appear as part of a complex of more severe, life-threatening injuries, proper care is appropriately delayed until resuscitative measures have stabilized the patient. Unfortunately, the pressing concern for these more immediately life-threatening injuries can overshadow these seemingly more minor problems, causing them to remain unnoticed or inadequately treated until irreversible damage has occurred. The ability of these seemingly minor facial injuries to maim or disfigure a child can never be underestimated. Indeed, no discussion of trauma to a child's face and major sensory organs—the eyes, ears, nose, and mouth—would be complete without stressing their importance in the youngster's subsequent physical and psychologic development. A disfiguring injury—or one merely perceived as disfiguring by the child, peers, or family—will have a devastating effect on the psychosocial emergence of the child as a well-adjusted and fully functional adult.

Against this background, this chapter discusses cervicofacial injury to children with particular emphasis on initial evaluation of facial trauma, including maxillofacial skeletal injury, and an anatomic approach to soft tissue injury to specific organs of the face and neck. The chapter specifically excludes consideration of injury to the neurocranium and the cervical spine, topics covered more completely and appropriately in Chapter 12. It must be stressed at the outset and remembered throughout this discussion that any trauma severe enough to cause significant cervicofacial injury must be assumed to have injured underlying CNS structures. These injuries must be specifically excluded prior to further evaluation.

INITIAL EVALUATION

The initial evaluation of a child with cervicofacial injury is best carried out in a well-staffed emergency department and in conjunction with appropriate specialists. Obviously, life-threatening injuries must be diagnosed and treated prior to further evaluation of specific injuries to the face or neck. Adherence to the well-proved sequence of emergency care with initial establishment of an adequate airway is of paramount importance. The child's smaller upper airway must be quickly cleansed of blood, mucus, saliva, teeth, and all foreign material. If the child is unconscious or if an airway cannot be maintained with an oropharyngeal or nasopharyngeal airway, endotracheal intubation must be considered. Rarely will emergency tracheostomy be required in childhood trauma.

Exsanguinating hemorrhage is unusual in uncomplicated cervicofacial trauma, and the presence of shock should alert the examiner to search elsewhere for hidden sources of bleeding. In most instances hemorrhage from the face can be controlled with direct pressure, elevation of the head, or packing with sterile gauze. An exception to this rule would be hemorrhage from scalp lacerations in infants, which can cause severe systemic hypotension. A rapid general physical examination should disclose significant chest, abdominal, pelvic, or extremity injury. The possibility of craniocerebral and cervical spine injury should be investigated in *all* patients with major facial injury, and the neck should be protected until adequate radiologic evaluation can be obtained. Exhibit 13-1 summarizes the initial management of cervicofacial trauma.

The importance of obtaining a good past medical history and the exact circumstances of the injury cannot be overemphasized and is particularly important in childhood trauma. A child may be unable or reluctant to volunteer information to a stranger, and therefore all sources of information—parents, paramedical personnel, and any available witnesses—must be questioned prior to their leaving the emergency room. The child's pediatrician can be an invaluable source for both medical history and background information on the child and family and should be informed of the child's status as soon as possible.

Exhibit 13-1 Initial Management of Pediatric Craniofacial Trauma

Airway
- Stabilize the neck—assume instability.
- Cleanse the mouth of blood, clots, teeth, and foreign material.
- Establish nasotracheal-orotracheal airway and mask ventilation with oxygen; use an endotracheal tube or cricothyroidotomy if needed. Tracheostomy is rarely required except in laryngotracheal injury.
- Evaluate the larynx carefully.

Hemorrhage
- Control with digital pressure.

Shock (unlikely in pure cervicotracheal injury)
- Suspect other injury—abdomen.

Soft Tissue
- Replace displaced flaps.
- Protect with moist saline dressing.

Transportation
- Have the patient accompanied by experienced medical personnel.
- Keep the patient prone.
- Watch tongue-mandible position.

Tetanus Prophylaxis and Antibiotics

INJURY TO THE FACIAL SKELETON

Most injuries to the soft tissues and the facial skeleton of children can be treated in the same manner as those of the adult. Special consideration, however, must be given to the effect of these injuries on the proportional transformation of the developing juvenile facial skeleton. Although the facial skeleton grows during the entire period of childhood, the period of maximal enlargement of the midface occurs during the sixth and seventh years. The size of the facial skeleton increases during childhood more than three times that of the neurocranium, major development of which is finished by three years. The facial proportions are themselves mainly influenced by the development of the midface and eruption of the teeth; once permanent dentition has erupted, the definitive skeletal development of the face is complete. Thus evaluation and treatment of facial skeletal injury after adolescence differs little from that of the adult. However, treatment of the preadolescent must reflect the stage of facial development as well as the long-term effects that may occur with later disturbed growth.

Any combination of signs and symptoms is possible in a patient with multiple facial injuries, and only by methodically evaluating each bony complex can an accurate diagnosis be made. The majority of adult facial fractures are compound and most are impacted; the child's more pliable facial bones, however, are subject to incomplete "greenstick" fractures, and definitive radiologic evaluation may be impossible. In general, loss of facial landmarks and facial deformity not due to edema indicate displacement of fracture fragments, which when unilateral produce loss of facial symmetry. The evaluation of facial skeletal trauma in children is thus difficult both clinically and radiologically, but the potential sequelae of the injuries are so disfiguring and functionally debilitating that prompt assessment and expeditious referral to specialists are necessary.

The facial skeleton is anatomically and physiologically designed to withstand considerable trauma while protecting the delicate neurocranium. It is not designed, however, to withstand nonphysiologic force. Yarington[1] has developed a classification of maxillofacial injury based on the mechanism of trauma, which delineates the most likely source of bone injury and provides purposeful direction for further evaluation.

Frontonasal Injuries

In frontonasal injuries (class 1), the head is minimally extended at the neck, and the velocity of impact is minimal. The primary site of injury/impact is the area of the frontal bone to the columella, including both lateral aspects of the nose. The primary bony structures to be investigated include the nasal bones, the frontal sinus, and the nasal processes of the maxilla. Suggested x-ray films include a Waters' view, a dental occlusion view, and an evaluation of the lateral nasal bones. Physical examination and diagnosis in children is difficult, and adequate examination frequently requires vasoconstrictors and anesthesia. One must examine the nasal septum with particular care to rule out septal displacement or septal seroma or hematoma formation prior to cartilaginous resorption. It is extremely important to diagnose and refer these children promptly since childhood healing occurs so quickly.

Zygomatico-Orbital Injuries

In zygomatico-orbital injuries (class 2), the head is slightly turned to one side, and the impact area involves the orbit, lateral orbital wall, malar prominence, or superior aspect of the maxilla. The sites of suspected fracture include the orbital margin, malar complex, zygomatic arch, or orbital floor. X-ray films should include orbital views: laminograms (if necessary), "bucket-handle" views, and/or a submental view. Although these fractures occur far less frequently in children than adults, the potential for long-term deformity is high, and immediate referral to a specialist for restoration of normal skeletal anatomy and evaluation of ocular function is vitally important.

Maxillo-Occlusal Injuries

In maxillo-occlusal injuries (class 3), the head is moderately extended by inertia of the nuchal extensors and the force of impact is significantly increased. The scope of injury includes the area of class 1 injuries as well as the entire anterior aspect of the upper alveolar ridge, the anterior maxilla, and the mandible. The expected injuries include isolated fractures of the maxilla and mandible and the variations of the LeFort fractures. The mechanism of injury, occlusive problems, and mobility of the midface should alert the examiner to search for these fractures. The most common isolated mandibular fracture in children is the subcondylar fracture, either unilateral or bilateral, and close attention must be directed to the radiologic examination of this area. Confirmatory x-ray films must be taken early, before edema and opacification of the paranasal sinuses preclude accurate diagnosis; initial x-ray films should include a complete set of sinus films and either a mandibular series or a panoramic view. Findings from the ocular exam—specifically regarding the integrity of the globe, visual function, and extraocular movements—must be accurately assessed and recorded. In this instance nasal packing to treat epistaxis should be avoided. Obviously, immediate referral to a specialist is required.

Other Injuries

Larygotracheal injuries (class 4) are discussed later in this chapter, and cerebrospinal injuries (class 5) are discussed fully in Chapter 12. However, two additional fracture groups need to be briefly discussed: frontobasilar and temporal bone fractures. In younger children the only pneumatized paranasal sinus is the ethmoid. In injuries to the skull or upper facial skeleton (class 1), the examiner should be especially alert for pneumocranium or CSF rhinorrhea, both signs of an open fracture between the neurocranium and upper airways. Untreated, this fracture can lead to recurrent meningitis and severe neurologic damage. Similarly, trauma to the occipital or occipitomastoid region can fracture the temporal bone either transversely or longitudinally, more often the latter. These patients may have bleeding from the external auditory canal, hemotympanum, facial nerve paralysis, collections of blood in the mastoid area (Battle's sign), or CSF otorrhea.

INJURIES TO FACIAL SOFT TISSUES

Repair of soft tissue injuries should be addressed only after appropriate disposition of facial fractures. The soft tissue defects often allow visualization of the underlying fracture fragments and allow direct surgical access for reduction and fixation. Even if surgery must be delayed, the "bone first, soft tissue second" sequence should be followed. Thus when facial soft tissue injury is complicated by fracture, the emergency department physician should not embark on lengthy plastic closure of wounds and should concentrate instead on compulsive wound cleaning while awaiting consultant evaluation.

Simple soft tissue injuries, not associated with fractures, can be appropriately handled if they are not extensive, contaminated, or more than 24 hours old. Cardinal surgical principles must always be observed, and the same care must be expended in the emergency department as would be expected in the operating room. Appropriate equipment should be available in a clean, well-lighted area where wound preparation and unhurried closure can be accomplished; if these conditions cannot be met, the wound should be cleaned, tetanus immunization given if indicated by the child's history, and the child referred promptly for surgical treatment.

Closure of simple facial lacerations is not difficult. Meticulous concern for preservation of viable tissue is absolutely paramount. Gentle initial handling and judicious debridement can determine whether the child undergoes a simple, expeditious repair or a multistaged, prolonged reconstruction.

Local anesthesia is used to provide analgesia and hemostasis; lidocaine (0.5% or 1.0%) with epinephrine (1:200,000), supplemented with appropriate sedatives, is the usual choice. The maximum pediatric dose of lidocaine is 7 mg/kg (3.2 mg/lb) when used with epinephrine and 4.5 mg/kg (2.0 mg/lb) without epinephrine. Regional blocks require less anesthetic agent and do not distort the anatomy, but they provide no hemostasis. General anesthesia is preferred for patients with extensive facial wounds or fractures and those who are unwilling or unable to cooperate. Children frequently fall into this category and should be quickly referred if any question arises concerning the advisability of either examination or repair under local anesthesia. There are several useful regional blocks in the head and neck that are described in the appropriate subsection later in this chapter.

After satisfactory anesthesia all wounds should be cleansed thoroughly with a dilute saline solution of mild antiseptic soap (PhisoHex, povidone-iodine), including scrubbing with a surgical brush or sterile toothbrush, and irrigated copiously with warm, sterile saline until all foreign material is washed away. Oil or tar can be removed with small amounts of ether or acetone, being careful to avoid inadvertent injury to the eyes. Shaving scalp hair may be necessary to provide adequate exposure, but the eyebrows should never be shaved. In addition to providing an accurate line of approximation, they occasionally do not regrow after being shaved.

Facial wounds should be debrided conservatively, with judicious trimming limited to obviously necrotic skin edges, and undermined carefully to decrease tension during closure. In general the amount of undermining should equal or double the width of the gap at its widest point. The amount of undermining necessary is determined to some extent by the orientation of the laceration to relaxed skin tension lines; when the laceration is perpendicular to the tension lines, undermining must be more vigorous than when the laceration lies more parallel. Undermining should be limited to the subcutaneous layer, using either the belly of a number 15 Bard-Parker blade, multiple connecting stab incisions with a number 11 Bard-Parker blade, or appropriate scissors.

Although suturing techniques are discussed in Chapter 30, a few points unique to facial trauma are worth reiterating. On first appearance a fresh facial wound may seem formidable because of the apparent complexity of the structures involved and the natural tendency of the skin to contract, expanding the surgical defect. Identification of known landmarks and approximation of known fixed points are the first steps; this may restore order to the entire operative field. The most effective landmarks include the nasolabial fold, the eyebrow, wrinkles (particularly on the forehead), and the white line immediately outside the vermilion border of the lips. The physician must take time to make careful stitches, using fine sutures and delicate instruments, such as small skin hooks and tissue forceps (Castroviego or Adson) to hold the tissue gently and needle holders designed for fine needles (Webster or Gillies). Skin edges on the face should be approximated with 6-0 or 7-0 nonabsorbable suture material (nylon, polypropylene, or Dacron). Subcutaneous or dermal sutures are usually 4-0 or 5-0 catgut, chromic, Dexon, or Vicryl. The oral mucosa is best sutured with 3-0 or 4-0 chromic on a cutting needle. All facial lacerations should be closed in layers, placing sutures in each anatomic plane that has been incised. In layers below the skin, all knots should be inverted so that they are buried in the depths of the wound. Subcutaneous sutures should be carefully placed equally on both sides of the wound and spaced approximately every 5 mm. They hold the wound surfaces together so that the skin sutures merely coapt the epithelial edges. The skin is usually closed with a simple, running suture, with stitches placed approximately every 2 mm, not tied too tightly, and everting the skin edges. Obviously, repair of a child's facial laceration is time-consuming and tedious; approximately three quarters of an hour per inch is required to close severe facial lacerations.[2] If this time is not available in the emergency department, the child should be referred rather than undergoing a compromised repair.

SCALP TRAUMA

As has been discussed, the vast majority of pediatric head trauma involves only the extracranial soft tissue and not the neurocranium proper; however, it cannot be overemphasized that CNS injury must be suspected and specifically excluded in each case, particularly in children with posterior head injuries. The management of a simple scalp laceration is not difficult, but several principles must be recognized. First, scalp lacerations in infants can result in profound hypotension, and control of bleeding should be promptly attained at the accident site, if possible. This usually only requires digital pressure along the laceration margin. Bulky loose dressings that simply absorb and hide the source of bleeding must be avoided. Second, scalp lacerations need digital or instrumental exploration prior to closure; oftentimes small fractures or debris are otherwise overlooked. Finally, even a small scalp laceration if improperly managed can be a portal that leads to major intercranial infection with obvious mortality and morbidity.

The scalp has five layers:

1. the thick and highly vascular skin
2. the dense and tough subcutaneous tissue containing the major arteries
3. the strong galea aponeurotica running between the bellies of the occipitalis and frontalis muscles
4. the subgaleal connective tissue space, the emissary veins of which provide the potential pathway for extension of infection into intracranial sites
5. the periosteum or pericranium that is adherent to the skull and has little clinical importance

To obtain adequate levels of local anesthesia, the anesthetic agent should be deposited above the galea in the subcutaneous tissues where the majority of the nerves and blood vessels are located (Figure 13-1); lidocaine 0.5% with epinephrine 1 : 200,000 is the usual choice. Obviously, if the subgaleal area alone is infiltrated, neither effective anesthesia nor hemostasis will be obtained. A field block of the anterior two thirds of the scalp can be obtained by blocking the supraorbital and supratrochlear nerves bilaterally. These nerves are both branches of the frontal nerve and exit along the upper border of the orbit. They are easily and satisfactorily blocked by raising a weal on the forehead over the root of the nose and advancing a long, fine needle under the skin immediately above and along the entire eyebrow while injecting 3 to 6 mL of lidocaine 1% with epinephrine. Anesthesia of the other side can be produced similarly from the same skin weal (Figure 13-2).

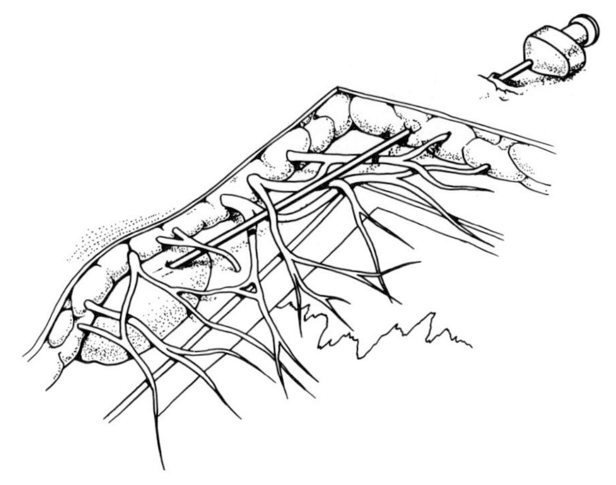

FIGURE 13-1 Technique for infiltration of local anesthetic. In anesthetizing an open wound, infiltration through the wound is often less painful for the child.

Only obviously devitalized tissue should be debrided; many scalp lacerations are burst injuries that split along tension lines and spare the hair follicles, leaving a linear bald spot that parallels the wound (Figure 13-3). Hair may be shaved if it interferes with the closure, but a few strands of cleansed

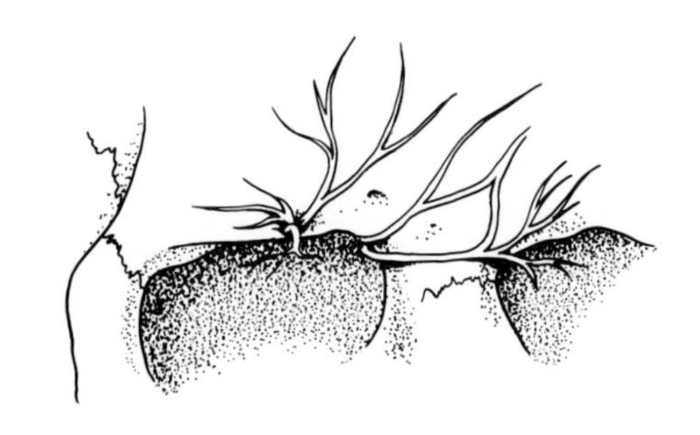

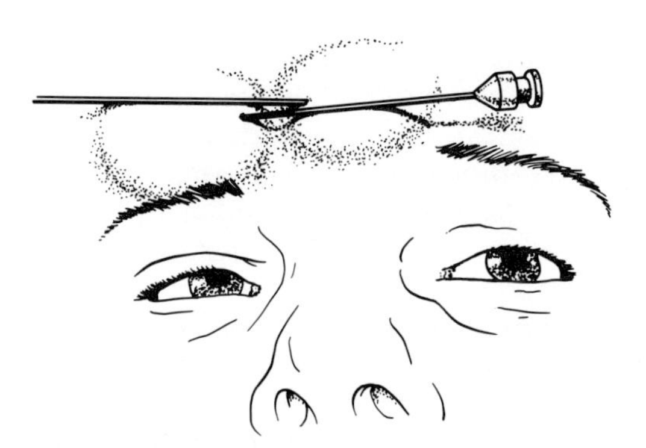

FIGURE 13-2 Infiltration technique for forehead block.

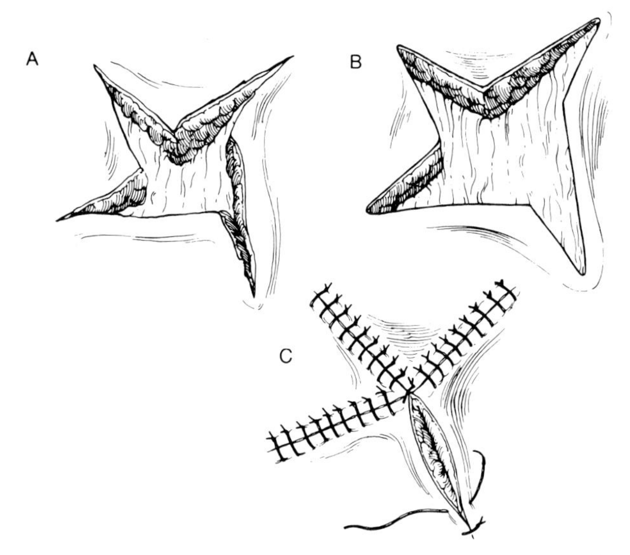

FIGURE 13-3 Operative strategy for closing stellate scalp lacerations. (Courtesy of Drs. T. R. Weber, D. W. Vane, and J. L. Grosfeld)

hair sutured along the wound margin do not significantly impair wound healing. Most scalp lacerations will require a layered closure if the galea has been opened. The galea is customarily closed with a 3-0 or 4-0 suture that is either nonabsorbable or very slowly reabsorbed. The skin and subcutaneous tissue layers are closed together with a suture technique that provides hemostasis as well as skin closure; interrupted mattress or figure-of-eight stitches or a running, locked stitch using 4-0 or 5-0 nylon serve quite well. If a single-layer closure including the galea is employed, the sutures should be removed later than the customary 7 to 10 days for layered scalp repairs.

EYE TRAUMA

Initial management begins with a careful history specifically detailing the mechanism of injury, the injuring agent, and any visual disturbance noted immediately after the accident. Unfortunately, the possibility of child abuse needs to be considered.[3] A rapid and reproducible check of visual acuity is absolutely essential at this point. Most emergency departments have pediatric Snellen charts available, but a pocket chart, a newspaper, counting fingers, or recognizing a favorite toy can be used to assess both acuity and extent of visual fields. The child's parents and pediatrician can be sources to document any preexisting acuity problems. A child with an injured eye is usually crying and frightened, and an organized, precise ophthalmologic examination is frequently impossible. If CNS involvement has been excluded and cooperation is unattainable, sedation with diazepam, 0.05 mg/kg IV or IM, is usually sufficient to allow an adequate assessment.[4]

Exhibit 13-2 is a checklist that should be completed for every eye injury. The external ocular examination is not detailed but is extremely important. The eyelids must be carefully examined for lacerations, disruption of lid margins, and paralysis. The size, shape, and reactivity of the pupils must be determined. Extraocular motion is checked in all directions to specifically look for paralysis or entrapment. Finally, the integrity of the globe itself must be assessed. The presence of blood within or under the conjunctiva, the condition of the sclera, and the suggestion of a penetrating injury with extrusion of the intraocular contents must all be investigated.[5]

Initial ophthalmoscopic examination in a child may be limited to a brief glimpse of the fundi, determination of lens position and integrity, and search for possible hyphema. A large hyphema will produce the classic "eight ball" sign created by blood in the anterior chamber, whereas a more limited collection of blood, although no less devastating, may require careful ophthalomoscopic examination

Exhibit 13-2 Checklist for Assessment of Ocular Injury

- History
  - Mechanism of injury
  - Injuring agent
  - Previous visual problems
- Physical Examination
  - Gross visual acuity check
  - Orbital examination
    - Fractures (step off), entrapment motion
    - Edema
  - Eyelid
    - Lash, margin intact
    - Ptosis, function
  - Extraocular motion
    - Full range of motion
- Globe
    - Intact
    - Consistency
    - Hyphema (eight ball sign)
  - Pupils
    - Round
    - Equal
    - Reactive
- Funduscopic Examination
    - Hyphema
    - Lens clear
    - Fundi normal
  - Cornea
    - Slitlamp, ultraviolet light

for diagnosis. Any time corneal trauma is suspected, the eyes should be examined under an ultraviolet light after fluorescein staining.

Bony injuries of the orbit can often be palpated before the onset of soft tissue edema, and if they are suspected, radiologic examination should include a Waters' view to assess the orbital floor. The frequency of ocular injury associated with a blow-out fracture can be as high as 40%.[6] There is also an especially high incidence of retinal tears associated with both orbital blow-out fractures and malar complex fractures with orbital extension.[7] This problem is particularly acute in myopic children, who are more prone to retinal damage.[8] The diagnosis of orbital blow-out fracture is made by noting that the child has double vision and restricted eye movement in one or more directions. Exophthalmos is also usually present. These injuries should be promptly referred.

Penetrating Ocular Injuries

Sedation is usually required for the initial evaluation and care of a child suspected of having a penetrating or disrupting eye injury. A hysterical, agitated child can easily raise central venous and intraocular pressure enough to extrude the intraocular contents from the injured globe. Excessive extraocular motion stimulated by the movement of the uninjured eye can increase the severity of the initial injury. Once a penetrating injury is identified, both eyes are patched, and intravenous broad-spectrum antibiotics are immediately started; no drops or ointment is placed in the eye. The patient should remain lightly sedated in a quiet, dark room, with the parents present for security and immediate ophthalmologic referral obtained. If pain is severe, analgesia should be given systemically rather than locally.

Chemical Ocular Injury

The most important initial therapy for any chemical eye injury is copious irrigation. Mild irritation, as may arise from excess chlorine in swimming pool water, can be treated with a prophylactic antibacterial agent such as 10% sulfacetamide sodium solution or ointment. More serious chemical injury, however, requires copious saline irrigation for several minutes. Once this therapy has begun, the remainder of the eye examination can be performed while the irrigant washes through the conjunctival sac. This may require both restraint and sedation so that a thorough lavage can be accomplished. Accurate assessment of visual acuity remains paramount and should be performed as soon as possible. Regardless of whether the injuring agent is an acid (capable of causing coagulation necrosis) or an alkali (capable of causing liquefaction necrosis), the possibility of corneal damage and resultant scarring must be considered. At the completion of lavage, evaluation of conjunctival fluid with litmus paper will confirm the nature of the injuring agent as well as provide an estimate of the effectiveness of initial therapy. Immediate ophthalmologic consultation must be obtained, especially in cases of alkaline burns, which commonly cause devastating tissue injury.

Foreign Bodies

Foreign bodies within the conjunctival sac produce severe pain and reflex tearing. In an upset child adequate control to expose and attempt to dislodge the material often requires 0.5% tetracaine drops and mild sedation. Both lids must be everted to search for residual foreign matter. Copious lavage is often effective in dislodging the foreign body. Manual extraction, using a cotton swab, forceps, or needle tip, can only be attempted in a completely cooperative child. Corneal examination using fluorescein staining and ultraviolet light is then performed to assess the status of the corneal epithelium. Since the sensation of a foreign body can persist after removal, patching of the involved eye after instillation of a polymyxin B-bacitracin ointment (Polysporin) and two drops of 5% homatropine may be necessary to provide temporary symptomatic relief. If symptoms persist unabated after 24 hours, a careful reevaluation, including fluorescein staining and slitlamp examination should be performed.

A child with a corneal abrasion will complain of a painful, red, tearing eye. Ptosis is often present and is usually unilateral. Instant and dramatic relief from this severe pain can be obtained by placing several drops of 0.5% tetracaine or proparacaine solution on the involved cornea. The eye should be quickly checked to record visual acuity and then examined with an ophthalmoscope or preferably a biomicroscope (slitlamp) to remove any residual foreign body. This should be followed by fluoroscein staining and ultraviolet light examination. Exhibit 13-3 details the treatment of a corneal abrasion.

Lid Lacerations

Although they are the frequent site of minor lacerations that seemingly require minimal surgical expertise to close, the eyelids must always be viewed

Exhibit 13-3 Treatment of Corneal Abrasion

1. Dilate the pupil and relax the ciliary muscles.
   a. Instill mydriatic and cycloplegic drops:
      (1) Cyclopentolate hydrochloride (Cyclogyl) 1%—cycloplegia
      (2) Phenylephrine (Neo-Synephrine) hydrochloride 10%—fast, short-acting mydriasis
      (3) Homatropine 5%—slower, longer-acting (up to 48 h) mydriasis
   b. Avoid atropine drops. Both mydriasis and cycloplegia may last for 2 weeks.
2. Apply topical antibiotics.
   a. Instill several drops of sulfacetamide sodium 10%.
   b. If the patient is allergic to sulfa, use polymyxin B-bacitracin-neomycin (Neosporin) or chloramphenicol (Chloromycetin).
3. Patch the eye. Close the lid and apply a secure, tight patch over the eye so that the eyelid remains closed.
4. Give systemic analgesics. Choose the analgesic according to the patient's need; range can be from aspirin to codeine drops.
5. Never prescribe topical anesthetics for home use.

as the complicated protective organs that they are. The action of the orbicularis oculi and levator palpebrae muscles on the fragile framework of the tarsal plates produces a shutter mechanism with the primary function of enclosing and protecting the eye. Any laceration or skin avulsion that affects this system should be assessed and treated in light of restoring the accurate function of these components. Even the smallest of lacerations must be adequately examined to assess depth and involvement.[9] Skin and subcutaneous injuries that do not involve tissue loss can be closed primarily if they are clean and uncontaminated. However, any injury that disrupts the lid margin or traverses the tarsal plate requires precise closure in proper anatomic layers to minimize any residual lid dysfunction.[10] In children this is usually best accomplished in the quiet control of the operating room. Accordingly, any laceration to the lids or orbital contents that appears to involve extensive tissue loss or damage to components other than skin or subcutaneous tissue should be covered with sterile saline-moistened gauze and referred for more definitive surgical repair.

Triage

Figure 13-4 is a triage protocol applicable to most eye injuries. Those that produce disruption of the globe, hyphema, lid laceration superiorly through the tarsal plate or medially through the lacrimal drainage system, or direct trauma to the cornea should be initially managed by coverage with a sterile dressing, sedation, tetanus booster injection if

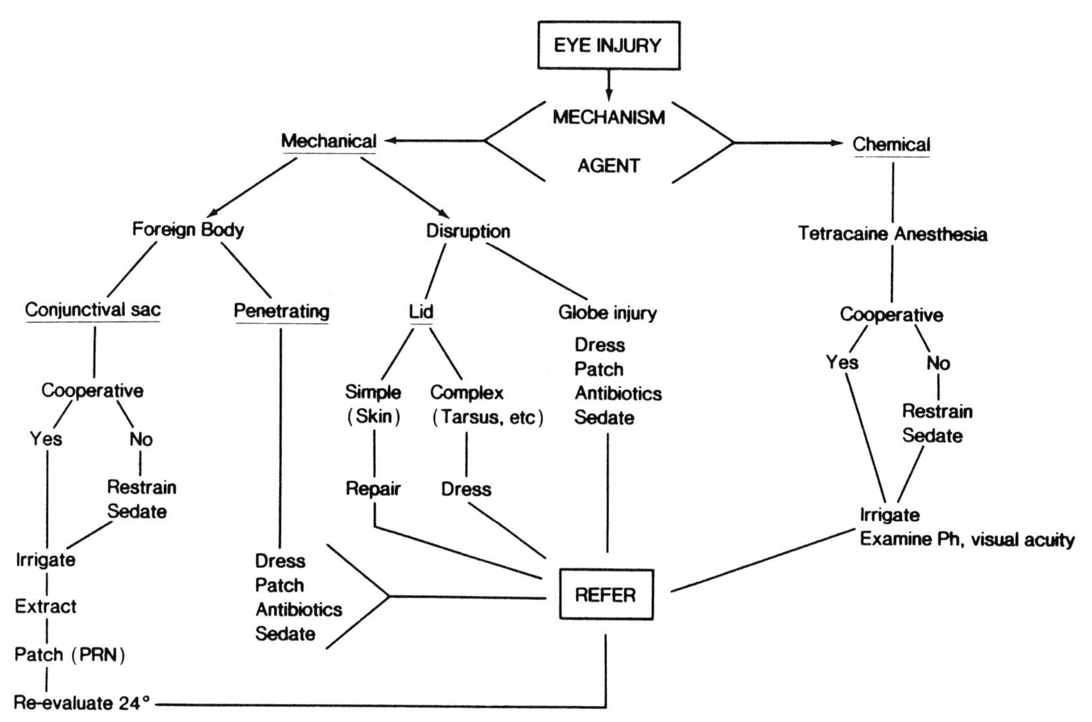

FIGURE 13-4 Triage and treatment of pediatric eye injuries. (Reprinted with permission from Stafford PN, Tepas JJ: Triage and treatment of injuries of the eyes, ears, nose and mouth in children. *Top Emerg Med* 1982;4:19–26.)

necessary, systemic antibiotics, and immediate referral to an ophthalmologist.[11] Eye injuries that require more definitive initial management in the emergency department include chemical burns, foreign bodies, and minor periorbital lacerations. Regardless of the nature of the injury, no child should be released from an emergency department with topical anesthetic and no patient should be treated with topical corticosteroids until appropriate ophthalmologic consultation has been obtained. Ideally, every eye injury should be referred, some for definitive therapy and all for ultimate follow-up.

EAR TRAUMA

Examination of a child with an injured ear includes assessment of the external elements and suspicion of injury to the more important internal elements. A gross hearing check can be conducted using a watch, tuning fork, or the snap of a breaking applicator stick. In situations in which a closed head injury is suspected, evaluation should include a careful search for retroauricular ecchymosis (Battle's sign), hemotympanum, radiologic evidence of a basilar fracture, and lateralized hearing loss. Eighty percent of temporal bone fractures are longitudinal to the axis of the petrous pyramid and cross the middle ear, with possible disruption of the tympanic membrane.[12] Otorrhea should always alert the examiner to a possible disruption of the bony architecture of the inner ear, with resultant leak of CSF.

Common soft tissue injuries to a child's pinna can usually be handled conservatively. The pinna normally achieves near-adult size by 5 years of age; so any injury that involves major tissue loss must be assessed in light of this subsequent limited regenerative potential. Direct trauma can produce a shearing effect, causing hemorrhage and hematoma between the cartilage and perichondrium. If extensive enough, this produces an avascular necrosis of the cartilaginous skeleton of the pinna, resulting in a "cauliflower ear" deformity.[13] Whenever a hematoma is large enough to involve the entire pinna, sterile surgical drainage should be considered and appropriate consultation should be obtained.

Ear Lacerations

Trivial injuries to the external auditory meatus commonly follow the use of a sharp instrument to remove wax or soothe an itch. Apart from some minimal pain and perhaps bleeding, these injuries are of little significance.

Lacerations of the pinna are potentially more dangerous and require treatment with the goal of avoiding septic complications involving the delicate elastic cartilage skeleton. Closure of skin defects must be meticulously performed, both to ensure a good cosmetic result and to prevent breakdown of the skin covering the auricle and exposure of the cartilage, with resultant perichondritis and chrondritis. The excellent blood supply of the auricle allows both primary closure of the wound up to 24 hours after injury and surgical reattachment of avulsed portions of the ear connected by a narrow pedicle. As elsewhere, good surgical principles apply to auricular repair: minimal debridement and copious irrigation followed by sterile draping and meticulous surgical repair.

Good anesthesia can be obtained with infiltration or field block. With a sedated or cooperative child, an easy and effective ear block can be obtained by blocking the posterior auricular nerve and the auriculotemporal branch of the mandibular nerve. The posterior auricular nerve is blocked by injecting 1 to 2 mL of 0.5% to 1.0% lidocaine with epinephrine at several sites posterior to the pinna over the mastoid process; the auriculotemporal nerve is blocked anteriorly with infiltration of skin and periosteum around the incisura terminalis over the auditory canal in front of the ear.

After adequate levels of anesthesia are obtained and the laceration has been thoroughly irrigated, repair of the laceration should begin with placement of initial key sutures at well-defined anatomic points. In older children the cartilage is repaired with a few anchoring sutures through the cartilage and more frequent perichondrial sutures; in younger children the cartilage is so delicate that the perichondrial sutures alone are sufficient. Most references suggest the use of plain 4-0 catgut for this repair. The skin is then closed with closely spaced 6-0 synthetic nylon sutures that are removed on the fourth or fifth day (Figure 13-5). Lacerations in the region of the external auditory meatus require gentle packing of the canal after suture repair. Iodoform gauze that has been impregnated with antibiotic ointment is useful in this regard; it should be left in the canal for 2 weeks to prevent canal or meatal stenosis. The repaired pinna should be splinted with a benzoin cotton mold, and systemic antibiotics effective against staphylococci should be given for at least 10 days.

Tympanic Membrane Injuries

Traumatic perforations tend to occur in healthy children; generally the prognosis is excellent, and

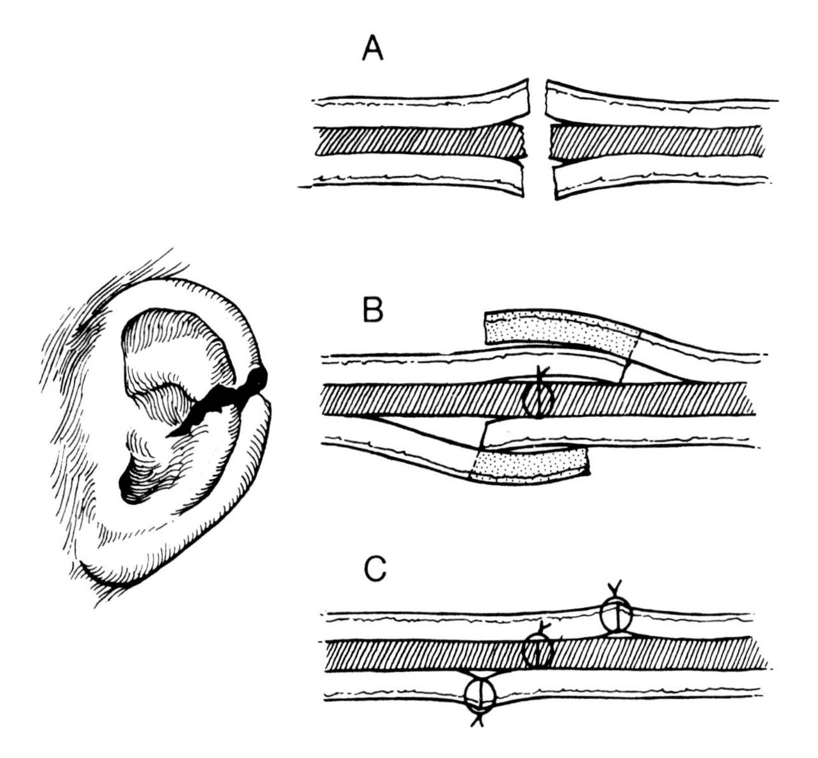

FIGURE 13-5 Technical aspects of closure of ear lacerations. Note proper approximation of anatomic layers with overlap of soft tissue. (Courtesy of Drs. T. R. Weber, D. W. Vane, and J. L. Grosfeld)

disruption of the tympanic membrane from either mechanical or acoustic trauma almost always heals spontaneously within 6 weeks. Prophylactic therapy is therefore the most effective management. Initial evaluation must consider the possibility of a disrupted ossicular chain or residual foreign material in the ear, especially in the pediatric population. After initial evaluation sterile cotton should be loosely packed in the outer canal, and the child should be referred to an otolaryngologist for follow-up.

NASAL TRAUMA

Fractures

Because of the relatively smaller size relationship of midface to cranium, a child's nose does not become as vulnerable a leading part of the face until the end of the first decade of life. Nevertheless, almost half of all nasal fractures occur in children and adolescents.[14] A direct blow severe enough to disrupt the mucous membrane and produce bleeding must always be suspected of having fractured part of the nasal skeleton. Unfortunately, even nasal x-ray films of the highest caliber are sometimes inadequate in documenting a fracture. As a rule, radiolucent lines that run parallel to the nasal bones are nutrient vessels, whereas those that are perpendicular or oblique are fractures.[15] As with adult fractures, if treatment is sought before development of edema and ecchymosis, most fractures can be reduced and splinted. If such is not the case, most children will require reduction under general anesthesia after the edema has subsided.[16]

Epistaxis

Epistaxis in children is commonly the result of incidental trauma to nasal mucous membrane and should be approached conservatively.[17] Allergies, overdry air, or septal deviation can predispose the child to this problem. Since 95% of bleeding originates from the anterior inferior aspect of the septum, control can usually be achieved by 5 minutes of pressure applied by compressing the anterior aspect of the nose between the examiner's thumb and forefinger. Application of a topical vasoconstrictor followed by cauterization with silver nitrate usually controls any bleeding that does not respond to direct pressure.

Whether the epistaxis is primary or traumatic, once the bleeding has been controlled, the nasal septum must be carefully examined from both nares. A bilateral septal hematoma must be surgically drained before packing so that avascular necrosis of the septal cartilage does not occur. Failure to consider and treat this problem can cause complete destruction of the cartilage, resulting in a "saddle nose" deformity in later childhood or adolescence.[18]

Epistaxis in a child that does not respond to these modalities can be the harbinger of a congenital or neoplastic disorder within the nose and should be referred to an otolaryngologist for further evaluation and treatment.

Lacerations

Immediate application of ice to a soft tissue injury of the nose may delay swelling so that definitive repair can be accomplished without delay. If the injury is limited to an abrasion or a simple laceration without cartilaginous involvement, closure in the emergency department is appropriate after thorough irrigation and minimal debridement. Tissue preservation is again the paramount consideration, and aggressive lavage with normal saline and scrubbing with a mild aseptic solution should remove all foreign material from the wound. Abrasions, even those that appear minor, must always be considered a source of tattooing. If adequate cooperation cannot be obtained in the emergency department, more aggressive debridement under general anesthesia should be considered. Material that is not removed from a fresh wound will be incorporated into the resultant scar and may disfigure the child for life.

Lacerations of the nose frequently expose cartilage that may be lacerated or anatomically displaced. These injuries should be addressed prior to wound closure; therefore, the wound should be covered with moist, sterile gauze and referred immediately. Similarly, any laceration along the lateral nasal border that suggests involvement of the lacrimal apparatus must be immediately referred. Simple lacerations can be closed with an excellent cosmetic result using 5-0 or 6-0 nonabsorbable suture; subcutaneous sutures are rarely needed. Sutures should be removed in 5 to 7 days. Avulsion injuries to a child's nose can be approached in a similar fashion: all avulsed tissue and the wound should be cleansed carefully, and the tissue should be replaced primarily. If the tissue loss is extensive, the child should be referred. As with any nasal injury in a child, septal hematoma must be ruled out.

ORAL TRAUMA

Intraoral Lacerations

The inclination of young children to chew on almost anything they can fit into their mouths predisposes them to intraoral trauma. Should a child be hit or fall with a foreign body within the mouth, lacerations of the palate, gingiva, or tongue are likely to occur. Profuse bleeding, more a threat to parental equanimity than to the child's life, is commonly the presenting complaint. On initial examination, calm reassurance and an ice-water mouth rinse are the most effective therapeutic tools. Having the child sit up while rinsing with the ice water usually slows the bleeding enough to allow an adequate oral examination. It is important that the child be encouraged to expectorate the rinse rather than swallow it so that the stomach will remain empty should general anesthesia be required for repair. Specific attention should then be paid to the palate and tongue. The possibility of aspiration or ingestion of the foreign body also must be considered and excluded.

Most small lacerations spontaneously cease bleeding and require no further treatment. A large flap or avulsion injury may require accurate reapproximation under anesthetic control and should be referred to a specialist for evaluation. Deep lacerations of the tongue usually stop bleeding because of muscular contraction. Occasionally a child requires sedation and closure, using absorbable 4-0 under local anesthesia with a 1% lidocaine solution.

Lip Lacerations

Lacerations of the lips and perioral area are a common sequelae of childhood accidents because of their location and the underlying teeth that frequently cause through-and-through lacerations. Because of the circumferential and radial nature of the perioral musculature, these injuries often gape and appear to involve tissue loss. Adequate anesthesia usually can be obtained with local infiltration although mental nerve blocks work well for chin and lower lip injuries. The mental nerve arises in the mandibular canal as a branch of the inferior alveolar nerve and exits from the mental foramen on a level with the second premolar. The mental foramen can be palpated intra- or extraorally, and the nerve is blocked by injecting 1 to 2 mL of 2% lidocaine with epinephrine at a point just posterior to the first premolar, in close proximity to the neurovascular bundle that usually can be felt quite easily. The wound then must be explored for tooth fragments and other foreign debris and be thoroughly irrigated.

The mucosal surface need not be sutured unless the wound is extensive or irregular because the mucosal laceration allows good drainage and will heal nicely without sutures. The two most important facets of the cutaneous repair are absolutely precise apposition of the cut edges of the vermilion border and repair of the orbicularis oris muscle (Figure 13-6). Marking the appropriate spots along the vermil-

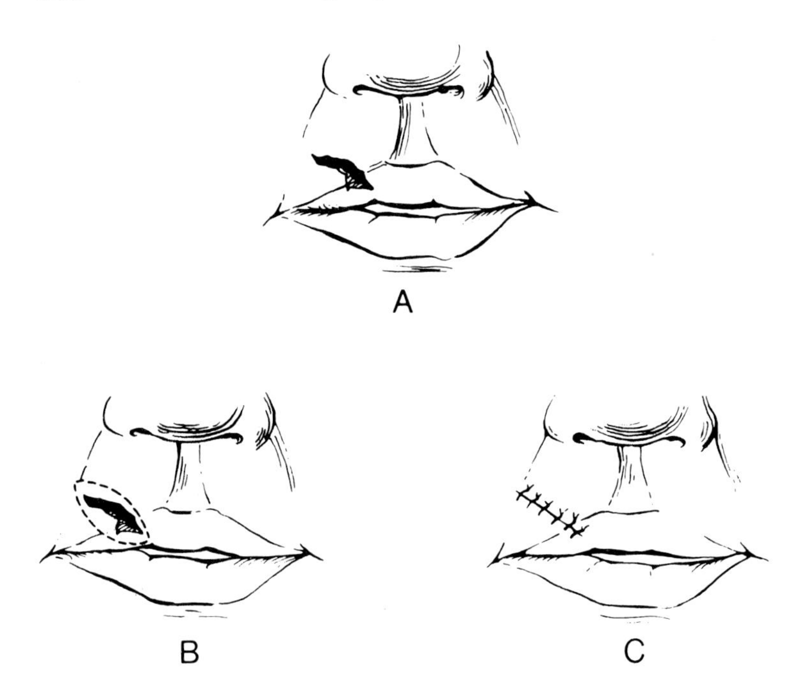

FIGURE 13-6 Technique for closure of lip laceration. Accurate approximation of vermilion border is absolutely necessary. (Courtesy of Drs. T. R. Weber, D. W. Vane, and J. L. Grosfeld)

ion border with methylene blue before anesthetic infiltration distorts the anatomy ensures an accurate closure. If the vermilion border appears indistinct, moistening the area may highlight the mucocutaneous margin and facilitate the repair. The muscle fibers and mucosa should be approximated with 4-0 absorbable sutures while the lip and cutaneous repair should be accomplished with 6-0 synthetic or silk suture. The skin sutures should be removed in 3 or 4 days. Dressings are generally not used since they become wet and mascerate the area, increasing the incidence of wound infection. Avulsed portions of the lip are placed back into normal position, even if the blood supply appears deficient; their ample vascularity allows an amazing survival capacity. If possible, the patient should be kept in a semisitting position until perioral edema has subsided. Ice compresses may aid in decreasing edema. Because of the bacterial flora of the human mouth, any patient with lacerations involving the oral cavity should be treated with penicillin or an appropriate substitute until healing is complete.

Electrical Burns

Another injury common to the pediatric population occurs when a child bites an electrical cord, causing a burn that usually involves the corners of the mouth and exhibits an eschar at the point of electrical contact. The coagulation necrosis that occurs is frequently much more extensive than it initially appears, and when slough occurs 72 hours later, profuse bleeding from the labial artery can result. Before the patient is released from the emergency department, parents must be made aware of this possibility and instructed that simple compression of the artery usually controls the bleeding. Fortunately, despite the extensive initial appearance of the injury, complete healing with a good cosmetic and functional result usually occurs. Nevertheless, appropriate surgical follow-up is required so that any additional necessary treatment can be provided.

TRAUMA TO THE MALAR OR PREAURICULAR AREA

Injuries to these areas present a different and challenging problem. Although these injuries do not require restoration of mobile or functional projecting structures, both the parotid gland and facial nerve can be injured, either in the accident or during the repair. Likewise, injuries in this area are frequently caused by animal bites, usually dog bites, and may require adjunctive antibiotic coverage. Both cat and dog bites often require penicillin V potassium for protection against *Pasteurella multocida.* These wounds should be thoroughly irrigated and closed primarily. Parents must be cautioned that these wounds have a high incidence of infection that may require the child's early return to the emergency department for suture removal and wound drainage.

Injuries that are suspected to involve either the facial nerve or parotid gland require referral. Preexisting facial nerve injury must be determined before anesthesizing and cleansing the wound. Although present microsurgical techniques allow primary repair and interposition grafting of the facial nerve, repair statistics are directly related to the promptness of referral. Traumatic injuries of the parotid gland are often complicated by wound infection, sialadenitis, salivary fistulas, and sialocele formation. These problems can only be avoided if they are considered during the initial evaluation.

TRAUMATIC INJURIES TO THE UPPER RESPIRATORY TRACT

Laryngeal trauma is usually seen in a patient with severe multisystem injuries. Any sharp compression of the larynx, hyoid bone, and upper trachea between two immobile structures, most commonly the dashboard anteriorly and the cervical spine posteriorly, can result in significant injury. The larynx and trachea are protected from minor trauma by the elasticity of the fibrous connective tissue, by the strength of the supporting intracartilaginous tracheal ligaments, and by the mandible. The cervical spine limits the posterior mobility of the larynx and the trachea. In major anterior cervical trauma, the neck is extended, elevating the mandible, and the larynx and trachea are crushed between the cervical vertebrae and the impacted object. The most common injury is a vertical fracture of the thyroid cartilage, with or without accompanying cricoid cartilage fracture. The tetrad of symptoms and signs of laryngotracheal fracture comprise dysphonia or aphonia, hemoptysis, persistent pain, and stridor with subcutaneous emphysema. The finding of a flattened thyroid cartilage with loss of the thyroid notch confirms the diagnosis (Exhibit 13-4). Other important symptoms include pain on swallowing or protrusion of the tongue, wheezing, inspirating retractions, and cervical swelling.[8]

The immediate management of laryngotracheal injury is based on (1) recognition and (2) establishment of a safe airway. This is perhaps the only time in pediatric head and neck trauma when tracheotomy is preferable to endotracheal intubation and also one of the few times that treatment must precede cervical spine evaluation and x-ray films, despite the high incidence of injuries to this area. If the airway is inadequate, the head is maintained in a neutral position and the tracheostomy is performed without delay. The most consistent sign of laryngeal fracture is a complete loss of palpable landmarks.[19] If the cervical area is completely flat and the thyroid cartilage appears to float or "crunch" on palpation, airway protection while awaiting consultant evaluation is absolutely essential.

Exhibit 13-4 Diagnosis of Laryngeal Fracture

Problem
Recognition
Tetrad
Dysphonia or aphonia
Hemoptysis
Pain
Stridor or subcutaneous emphysema
Most Consistent Sign
Complete loss of palpable and visible landmarks

CONCLUSION

The lesions discussed occur commonly as the result of everyday accidents in a child's life. Most are not immediately life threatening, although they can be perceived as such by distraught parents. A calm hand and a cool head on the part of the examining physician will go a long way in reassuring patient and parent alike. Most importantly, proper initial evaluation and treatment, based on a thorough knowledge of the characteristics of these injuries, will provide the child with the best possible care, shortest recovery, and least damage from an unfortunate mishap.

References

1. Yarington CT Jr: The initial evaluation in maxillofacial trauma. *Otolaryngol Clin North Am* 1979;12:293–301.
2. Cairus AB: Soft tissue injuries of the face. *Otolaryngol Clin North Am* 1969;2:251–263.
3. Harley RD: Ocular manifestations of child abuse. *J Pediatr Ophthalmol Strabismus* 1980;17:5–13.
4. Biller JA, Yeager AM (eds): *The Harriet Lane Handbook,* ed 9. Chicago, Year Book Medical Publishers Inc, 1981.
5. Freeman HF, McDonald PR, Scheie H: Examination of the traumatized eye and adnexa, in Freeman HD (ed): *Ocular Trauma.* New York, Appleton-Century-Crofts, 1979, pp 1–15.
6. Evans JGN, Fenton PJ: Blow-out fractures of the orbit. *J Laryngol Otol* 1971;83:1127-1145.
7. Fradkin AH: Orbital floor fractures and ocular complications. *Am J Ophthalmol* 1971;72:699–700.
8. McGuirt WF (ed): *Pediatric Otolaryngology Case Studies.* New Hyde Park, NY, Medical Examination Publishing Co Inc, 1980, pp 397–422.
9. Ballin PH: Trauma of the eyelids, orbit, and adnexa, in Gomkos GH (ed): *Handbook of Ophthalmologic*

Emergencies. New Hyde Park, NY, Medical Examination Publishing Co Inc, 1973, pp 153–173.

10. Paton D, Goldberg MF: *Management of Ocular Injuries.* Philadelphia, WB Saunders, 1976, pp 163–172.
11. Fox SA: Trauma, in Leibman S, Gellis S (eds): *The Pediatrician's Ophthalmology.* St Louis, The CV Mosby Co, 1966, pp 264–273.
12. Snow JB: Surgical disorders of the ears, nose, paranasal sinus, pharynx, and larynx, in Sabiston (ed): *Textbook of Surgery,* ed 10. Philadelphia, WB Saunders Co, 1972, pp 1207–1208.
13. Tanzer RC, Bellucci RJ, Converse JM, et al: Deformities of the auricle, in Converse JM, McCarthy JG, Littler JW (eds): *Reconstructive Plastic Surgery. Principles and Procedures in Correction, Reconstruction and Transplantation,* ed 2. Philadelphia, WB Saunders Co, 1977, vol 3, p 1732.
14. Goode RL, Spooner TR: Management of nasal fractures in children. *Clin Pediatr* 1972;11:526–529.
15. Moran WB: Nasal trauma in children. *Otolaryngol Clin North Am* 1977;10:95–101.
16. Bailey BJ: Management of soft tissue trauma of the head and neck in children. *Otolaryngol Clin North Am* 1977;10:193–204.
17. Barelli PA: The management of epistaxis in children. *Otolaryngol Clin North Am* 1977;10:91–93.
18. Strumpler W: Traumatology of the face in children, in Jazbi B (ed): *Pediatric Otorhinolaryngology: A Review of Ear, Nose, and Throat Problems in Children.* New York, Appleton-Century-Crofts, 1980, pp 253–263.
19. Shumrick DA: Traumatic injuries of the upper respiratory tract. *Otolaryngol Clin North Am* 1969;2:403–410.

Part V

Gastroenterologic Disorders

Michael B. Andorsky

14 Gastroenterologic Disorders

CLINICAL MANIFESTATIONS OF GASTROINTESTINAL DISEASE

Gastrointestinal (GI) symptoms frequently accompany acute illness in infants and children. The first part of this chapter is devoted to a discussion of these signs and symptoms and of the diseases they may reflect; the latter part considers specific GI disorders, with emphasis on diseases of a nonsurgical nature.

Failure to Thrive

For the purposes of this chapter, failure to thrive means failure to gain weight as well as expected. Linear growth and ultimately brain growth may be eventually but not primarily affected. Inadequate weight gain occurs secondary to inadequate caloric intake, increased caloric loss from vomiting or malabsorption, or increased caloric needs.

History

Inadequate Caloric Intake For growth in the first 4 months of life, a baby requires at least 115 kcal/kg/24 h and a protein intake of approximately 2.2 g/kg/24 h.[1,2] For bottle-fed babies determine the calories per ounce of formula and the ounces of formula consumed versus ounces offered. Find out who feeds the baby most of the time and if the baby is held or bottle "propped" during feedings. Severely malnourished breast-fed babies are being reported with increasing frequency. Paradoxically, the baby sucks well, appears content between feedings, and the mother usually says her "milk is in"; however, the baby is often constipated (fewer than two stools daily) and urinates infrequently (fewer than six times daily). Weighing the baby before and after feeding reveals inadequate intake. For older infants and children, the prolonged use of elimination diets or of vegetarian diets that exclude milk and eggs may reduce caloric intake.

Feeding time should be about 30 minutes. Suspect a problem if the mother reports that it takes her over 45 minutes to feed the baby. Sucking and swallowing difficulties can reflect neuromuscular disease, esophageal anomalies, and malformations of the oropharynx. Inadequate intake because of fatigue is associated with pulmonary and cardiovascular disease. Lethargy and irritability are associated with metabolic problems such as hypothyroidism and urea cycle defects. Anorexia can reflect occult infections, malignancies, or chronic pain.

Increased Caloric Loss Regurgitation, even after every feeding, usually does not cause weight loss. Projectile vomiting suggests upper intestinal obstruction, metabolic derangements with acidosis, increased intracranial pressure, or milk protein intolerance. Various malabsorption syndromes are usually accompanied by diarrhea. Carbohydrate malabsorption usually is manifested as dehydration, not failure to thrive. Fat malabsorption accounts for most GI causes of failure to thrive and can occur without diarrhea. In fact, even constipated children may malabsorb fat.

The following diseases should be considered as causes of increased caloric loss:

- cystic fibrosis
- celiac disease
- giardiasis
- immunodeficiency states
- inflammatory bowel disease
- milk protein intolerance
- dissacharidase deficiencies

Signs and symptoms associated with these entities may include chronic cough, irritability, diarrhea, foul-smelling stools, unusual infections, and blood passed via the rectum. Inquire about introduction of wheat and rye cereals, addition of fruits and juices, use of cow's milk formula, and a family history of milk intolerance.

TABLE 14-1 Outpatient Approach to Failure to Thrive

Signs and Symptoms	Studies
Vomiting	Upper GI series with small-bowel follow-through
No vomiting or vomiting with normal upper GI series	Blood tests CBC,* ESR, Na, Cl, K, HCO_3, Ca, serum protein and albumin, blood glucose, SGPT, BUN, creatinine, IgM, IgA, IgG, carotene
	Urine tests Urinalysis, ferric chloride, reducing substances, urine culture
	Stool tests Occult blood; Gram's stain for PMNLs, ova and parasites (for *Giardia*); culture for enteric pathogens
	Others Sweat chloride, 72-h fecal fat (normal value may reflect decreased fat intake)

* Abbreviations: CBC, complete blood count; ESR, erythrocyte sedimentation rate; SGPT, serum glutamic-pyruvic transaminase; BUN, blood urea nitrogen; IgM, immunoglobulin M; PMNLs, polymorphonuclear leukocytes.

Increased Caloric Needs Properly digested and absorbed sources of calories may not be utilized at the cellular level, as is the case in diabetes mellitus, glycogen storage diseases, galactosemia, fructose intolerance, and phenylketonuria. Hypermetabolic states consume energy without allowing growth, as in hyperthyroidism, diencephalic syndrome, malignancies, anemias, chronic renal disease, and occult infections.

Physical Examination

Signs of malnutrition include a protuberant abdomen, hepatomegaly, and scant fat in buttocks and thighs. Patients may be irritable or lethargic. Older children may have delayed dentition or horizontal white lines on fingernails (Murphy's lines), which reflect episodes of growth arrest. Observe both the mother and baby during a feeding for the following:

- appropriate feeding techniques
- appropriate mothering
- uncoordinated or poor sucking
- visible peristalsis over the baby's abdomen
- a palpable "olive" just to the right of the midline above the umbilicus
- vomiting during or after feeding
- increased and high-pitched bowel sounds

When the diagnosis is not apparent after a careful history and physical examination, begin the outpatient work-up outlined in Table 14-1. If these screening tests do not suggest a cause, hospitalize the patient for further studies.

Dysphagia

Difficulty in swallowing is described as "something sticking in the throat" or "heartburn" in older children. Newborns and infants exhibit weak or uncoordinated sucking, choking on fluids, slow feeding, or vomiting. Congenital malformations of the oral cavity, esophageal obstruction, disordered peristalsis, inflammation of the oropharynx or esophagus, and psychogenic factors all produce dysphagia.

History

Dysphagia always occurs during swallowing. Associated findings in the history help narrow the diagnostic possibilities. Recurrent wheeze or pneumonia can indicate a tracheoesophageal fistula or partial obstruction associated with mediastinal masses. Neck posturing while swallowing may be a maneuver to empty a Zenker's diverticulum or to propel the food bolus across an area of disturbed peristalsis: posturing may also suggest gastroesophageal reflux (Sandifer's syndrome). Gradual and progressive dysphagia occurs secondary to the abnormal peristalsis of neuromuscular disease (e.g., Werdnig-Hoffmann disease, scleroderma). Midline chest pain or hematemesis indicates esophagitis, distal esophageal stricture, and other causes of distal obstruction. Pain in the oropharynx occurs with ingestion of corrosives and infectious pharyngitis. Fear of swallowing in an adolescent girl suggests anorexia nervosa.

Physical Examination

Feed the patient to confirm the presence of dysphagia. Observe the general state of nutrition. Inspect the oropharynx for cleft palate, inflammation, and signs of trauma. Palpate the neck for diverticula as the patient first swallows fluids and then solids. Observe respiration and listen for wheezing and rales. Test the patient for cranial nerve deficits, and elicit gag and deep tendon reflexes.

Ancillary Data

A chest film and barium swallow remain the most useful initial studies in determining the cause. Look for pneumonia, chronic lung disease, a right-sided or double aortic arch, tracheoesophageal fistulas, and hiatal and paraesophageal hernias. Observe the peristalsis; foreign bodies, webs, extrinsic masses pressing on the esophagus, and distal strictures are usually obvious. Always obtain a hemoglobin and examine several stools for occult blood. Screen the patient for connective tissue disorders by determining the erythrocyte sedimentation rate (ESR) and assaying for antinuclear antibodies. In selected cases cinefluoroscopy, manometric studies, and esophagoscopy with biopsy may provide a diagnosis.

Vomiting

Vomiting is the forceful ejection of stomach contents by mouth. Acute infectious diseases, increased intracranial pressure, toxic ingestions, food intolerances, mechanical obstruction of the GI tract, metabolic diseases of infancy, and functional disorders are all causes of vomiting.

History

Focus on three questions: Is the child in fact vomiting? What is the cause? Is the child dehydrated? Difficulty swallowing solids but not liquids, choking, cyanosis, posttussive emesis, and emesis at the onset of feeding and swallowing all suggest dysphagia. "Gushing" or projectile emesis indicates vomiting. "Spitting up" and "dribbling," however, indicate regurgitation (i.e., nonforceful emesis), which frequently occurs in healthy young infants. Note the age of the child, duration of the problem, and frequency. A school-age child who has vomited twice every Monday morning for the past 3 months is unlikely to have organic disease. However, the school-age child who has chronic, random bouts of vomiting may have malrotation with intermittent volvulus or mesenteric artery syndrome. In an infant this history suggests recurrent intussusception.

Vomiting can cause profound dehydration within 24 hours, especially when associated with diarrhea. Note the frequency of urination. A 2-year-old fills the bladder about every 2 hours. No urination within 12 hours in patients of any age suggests dehydration. Conversely, increased frequency of urination with vomiting and dehydration may indicate diabetic ketoacidosis or diabetes insipidus, and, in the neonate, the adrenogenital syndrome.

Inquire about the color and consistency of the vomitus. Children under 2 years of age often vomit yellow bile, but yellow, bilious vomiting beyond this age or green, bilious vomiting at any age signals bowel obstruction distal to the second portion of the duodenum. Curdled stomach contents, mucus, or fatty foods (e.g., milk, cheese, eggs) ingested up to 8 hours previously usually reflect an atonic stomach, not anatomic obstruction. The greener the bile, the more distal the obstruction.

Hematemesis often arises from inconsequential esophageal tears produced by forceful emesis, but it also can result from esophagitis, gastritis, peptic ulcer disease, heavy metal poisoning, and ingestion of red foods (e.g., gelatin desserts, beets). If vomiting is related to ingestion of foods or medicine, consider contaminated food (e.g., staphylococcal food poisoning, salmonellosis), specific food intolerances (e.g., cow's milk, soy, gluten-induced enteropathy), and such known offenders as erythromycin, theophylline, and codeine.

Associated signs and symptoms help pinpoint the diagnosis. Fever suggests infection; diarrhea, gastroenteritis or food intolerance; constipation, an anatomic obstruction. Localized abdominal pain often occurs with appendicitis, hepatitis, cholecystitis, pancreatitis, peptic ulcer disease, inflammatory bowel disease, or urinary tract infection. Generalized abdominal discomfort is less helpful because vomiting itself produces muscle soreness. An associated change in the level of consciousness suggests central nervous system and metabolic causes. Head trauma can cause postconcussive vomiting lasting up to 8 hours. Vomiting from subdural bleeds may not occur until months after the initial injury. Intracranial tumors, Reye's syndrome, aminoacidopathies, and urea cycle disorders cause vomiting and lethargy or irritability.

Physical Examination

Evaluate the patient for signs of dehydration. Observe for irritability, waxing and waning of consciousness, or marked lethargy. Inspect the skull for trauma, the eyes for anisocoria or third nerve palsy, and the tympanic membranes for hemotympanum. Note any localized infection as a possible extragastrointestinal cause for vomiting. Examine the abdomen for signs and symptoms of an acute abdomen: guarding, tenderness, absent bowel sounds, and obturator and psoas signs. Palpate to detect hepatosplenomegaly, hydrops of the gall bladder, a pyloric "olive," and other abdominal masses. Also inspect the perianal area for a rash produced by diarrhea, and perform a digital rectal examination to rule out abdominal, rectal, and pelvic masses, as well as tenderness referred to the abdomen.

Ancillary Data

Vomiting in children usually reflects a brief, mild, self-limiting disease that responds to symptomatic therapy. Further investigation is indicated under the following conditions: dehydration, progressively severe vomiting, persistent vomiting of all fluids for more than 24 hours despite symptomatic management, and whenever the history and physical examination suggest a specific diagnosis. A useful screen consists of the following: complete blood count (CBC); ESR; serum electrolytes, alanine aminotransferase/aspartate aminotransferase (ALT/AST); urinalysis; and a flat plate film of the abdomen. This suggested screen can be abridged or expanded depending on information available from the history and physical examination.

Symptomatic Outpatient Therapy for Vomiting

Offer small amounts of sugared, clear fluids. Sugar causes sodium and potassium absorption, and oxidation of sugar reverses the ketosis that predisposes to vomiting. Sucrose, glucose, and fructose are all adequate. Avoid fat-containing foods, such as milk, because these remain in the stomach longest. Instruct the parents in home care, as indicated in Exhibit 14-1.

Hospitalize the child whenever significant dehydration occurs or whenever the outpatient work-up suggests life-threatening disease (e.g., Reye's syndrome, appendicitis).

Exhibit 14-1 Outpatient Management of Vomiting

1. Give cola syrup on cracked ice, 1 tablespoon every 5 min for 5 doses; then,
2. Give any sugared, clear fluid (e.g., soda pop, weak tea with sugar, apple juice), 1 tablespoon every 5 min for 5 doses; then,
3. Give sugared, clear fluids in amount and frequency as determined by child's thirst.
4. If steps 1 and 2 are not tolerated, offer wet lollipops (from bowl of water) to be sucked and frequently exchanged for another wet lollipop.
5. For children on solid foods: after 12 h without vomiting, add gelatin dessert, popsicles, bread, crackers, dry cereals.
6. Gradually introduce regular diet as the acute illness resolves.

Diarrhea

Diarrhea is the passage of stools that are too loose and too frequent. Derangements of intraluminal digestion, mucosal absorption, and peristalsis prevent water resorption and stimulate water secretion.

History

Establish the presence of diarrhea and determine its pattern: acute, recurrent, or chronic. Up to ten bowel movements daily within the first 3 months of life, six daily through 18 months of age, and three or fewer daily after toilet training can be normal. Normal stools are mustardlike for newborns, variably progressing to oatmeal-like by the age of 6 months and formed by the age of 2 years. Explosive, watery bowel movements are always abnormal. Parents often mistake green feces, movements with food particles, and foul-smelling morning diapers for diarrhea. Green bile reflects a decreased transit time. Food particles and odor change more often relate to diet changes (e.g., vegetables, meats). Mucus has no significance unless copious. Bloody, unformed stools and tenesmus indicate a colitis. Recent exposure to others with flulike or diarrheal illness suggests infection or food poisoning. Ask about ingestion of heavy metals (e.g., lead), recent antibiotics, vomiting, and fever. A history of eczema, colic, and early feeding problems suggests cow's milk protein intolerance. Diarrhea can be related to recent introduction of cow's milk, fruits, or wheat. Chronic constipation can precede diarrhea in Hirschsprung's enterocolitis and irritable bowel syndrome; functional constipation can result in overflow diarrhea.

Physical Examination

Estimate the water, electrolyte, and nutrient depletion. Chronically malnourished children may have potbellies and wasted extremities and buttocks. Look for extragastrointestinal signs of infection. Examine extremities for joint swelling (e.g., inflammatory bowel disease) and edema (e.g., lymphangectasia). On abdominal and rectal examination, rule out an "acute abdomen." Listen for bowel sounds.

Ancillary Data

For acute diarrhea, stain a stool specimen with methylene blue and look for polymorphonuclear leukocytes. Also examine the specimen for occult blood. Neither appears with acute viral diarrhea. Both can be present in bacterial gastroenteritis and inflammatory bowel disease. Copious mucous secretions suggest a colitis. When fever (body temperature > 38.8° C) or signs of colitis are present, obtain a stool specimen for enteric pathogens (*Salmonella, Shigella, Yersinia enterocolytica, Campylobacter*), ova, and parasites (*Giardia, Ascaris, Amoebas*); a CBS; and an ESR. If clinical dehydration has occurred, obtain blood urea nitrogen (BUN) and serum electrolyte measurements. Collect a urine specimen for protein, specific gravity, and for culture.

For chronic or recurrent diarrhea associated with poor weight gain or constitutional symptoms, evaluate bowel absorption as well. The serum D-xylose concentration 1 hour after 5 g are ingested measures jejunal absorption; a level exceeding 20 mg/dL is a normal response. Assess fat absorption with serum carotene and 72-hour fecal fat collection.

In children with chronic diarrhea, serial stool specimens for ova and parasites may reveal *Giardia*; however, absence of *Giardia* in the stool does not rule out this infestation. A stool pH below 6 and the presence of reducing substances reflect sugar malabsorption. A low serum albumin level screens for protein-losing enteropathies, and the ESR is elevated in 85% of children who have Crohn's disease or ulcerative colitis.[3]

Dietary Treatment

Dietary treatment of acute diarrhea has a sound physiologic basis and is approached in stepwise fashion, as outlined in Exhibit 14-2. Failure to respond to this regimen may necessitate hospitalization.

Exhibit 14-2 Outpatient Management of Acute Diarrhea

Objective: Stop the diarrhea by limiting diet and decreasing the bowel's work of absorption.

Day	Diet
1*	Give clear fluids only (commercial 2% glucose-electrolyte solutions, weak tea with sugar, diluted apple juice [1:1], flat soda pop).
2	Add carbohydrate solids (bread, toast, crackers, jelly, gelatin dessert, rice cereal, bananas, applesauce).
3	Add milk products (cottage cheese, processed cheese) and egg whites.
4**	Add lactose-free formula (Prosobee, Isomil) or half-strength cow's milk formula or half-strength cow's milk.
5	Return to full-strength formula or cow's milk.
6	Return to full diet for age.

* Breast-fed babies may continue breast-feeding.
** As the physician directs.

Constipation

Constipation is the infrequent passage of hard, pellet-like, or very viscous stool. Infrequent means fewer than two bowel movements daily in infants and missed days in children over 2 years of age.

History

Constipation is usually functional. Inquire about the frequency, consistency, shape of the bowel movement, age of onset, and the parents' definition of constipation. Is there abdominal pain, encopresis, or episodic diarrhea? Also ask about the child's bowel habits within the first 48 hours of life, family history of functional GI disease, and intake of constipating foods or medicines.

Physical Examination

Record the child's weight and height, listen for bowel sounds, and palpate the abdomen for organomegaly, masses, and guarding. Inspect the anus for fissure. Elicit a "perianal wink" (constriction of the anus) by stroking the perianal skin to confirm an intact sacral innervation. By digital rectal examination ascertain sphincter tone, size of the ampulla, and presence or absence of stool, and note whether or not removal of the finger from a full rectum stimulates a bowel movement.

Treatment

Unless the history and physical examination suggest a specific cause, treat mild constipation with a bulk cathartic and stool softener. Chronic constipation without vomiting in an apparently well and growing child may be treated as functional for 1 to 2 weeks before contemplating any diagnostic tests. Consider anatomic obstruction or Hirschsprung's disease in the child who appears chronically ill on initial examination, vomits, or does not respond to a vigorous anticonstipation regimen (Exhibit 14-3).[4]

Abdominal Pain

Abdominal pain in children is usually self-limited and often functional. However, serious organic disease of the abdominal viscera, genitourinary tract, lungs, or pharynx also causes abdominal pain.

History

Determine whether or not the child has an acute abdomen. In the acute abdomen, distension of the involved organ followed by parietal peritoneal inflammation adjacent to that organ causes two kinds of pain. The initial stretching produces a deep, dull, and sometimes crampy discomfort referred to the midline. Where in the midline depends on the organ involved. For supraumbilical pain, consider the liver, biliary tree, pancreas, stomach, and proximal small bowel. For periumbilical pain, suspect the distal small bowel, cecum, appendix, and ascending colon. For suprapubic pain, consider the descending and sigmoid colon, rectum, urinary tract, and pelvic organs. When the inflammation progresses to the peritoneum, sharp, well-localized pain over the involved organ occurs. A child with an acute abdomen usually feels generally unwell, has progressively more intense pain, and develops an ileus with nausea, vomiting, and constipation.

Physical Examination

The child often walks hunched forward and will not hop when asked. Fever is variably present. Palpate the abdomen for guarding and rebound tenderness. Psoas and obturator signs are elicited by pressing the inflamed peritoneum between viscera and muscle. Examine the abdomen for distension, loss of bowel sounds, and masses. Rectal examination may produce pain referred to the area of involved viscera or reveal a mass or blood. Examine the ovaries and cervix by bimanual palpation.

In the nonacute abdomen, pain may be marked, but peritoneal signs are never present. Gastroenteritis is the most commonly identified cause. However, consider early appendicitis whenever the patient has nausea or vomiting without passage of a bowel movement or has diarrhea with localized abdominal pain.

Ancillary Data

When an acute abdomen is suspected clinically, obtain a CBC, urinalysis, and abdominal flat plate film. Look for polymorphonuclear leukocytes in the blood, protein and white blood cells in the urine, and air-fluid levels, absence of air in the distal bowel, and appendiceal fecaliths on the roentgenogram.

Chronic, Recurrent Abdominal Pain

Chronic, recurrent abdominal pain occurs in about 10% of school-age children[5] and is usually functional. Try to separate the functional from the organic etiologies by a careful history and physical examination, with a minimum of laboratory work-up.

Obtain a complete description of the pain including its *location* and *character*. Is the pain epigastric, periumbilical, suprapubic, or lateralized? Specific disorders sometimes have particular qualities: *gnawing* peptic ulcer, *burning* esophagitis, *cramping* colonic disease. Consider an acute surgical problem when the pain is sharp and lateralized.

Exhibit 14-3 Vigorous Management of Chronic Constipation

Do the following after dinner every evening:

1. Have the child sit on toilet for 15 min.
2. For each of the first 7 days administer a mineral oil enema, 4 oz (adult size).
3. Beginning in second week administer a phosphate enema, 4 oz (adult size) whenever child fails to defecate on toilet for 2 days.

Medicines

1. Senna (e.g., Senekot granules): 1 teaspoon before breakfast; 1 teaspoon before dinner.
2. Docusate sodium (Colace): 1 teaspoon or 1 capsule with each dose of Senekot.
3. Give only half dose of Senekot if this medicine causes abdominal discomfort. Double dose if enemas are still required by the end of week 3 of treatment.

Diet

1. Encourage raw vegetables; raw fruits, especially prunes, figs, dates, apricots; raw bran, bran muffins, bran cereals.
2. Discourage milk—no more than 16 oz daily; cheese, yogurt, and ice cream—no more than 1 serving of 1 of these daily; pears and rice—avoid.

Determine the *frequency* and *timing* of the pain. Constant pain or pain that disturbs sleep is more likely to be organic than functional. Infrequent but severe pain is usually functional but sometimes indicates intermittent obstruction. Important dietary factors which may cause pain include lactose, fatty foods, and medicines such as theophylline and erythromycin. *Alleviation* of pain by eating indicates peptic disease. Pain relieved by passage of bowel movement suggests constipation, and relief of pain by flexing the hips indicates peritoneal inflammation.

Assess *growth* and *constitutional symptoms*. Weight loss, failure to thrive, delayed appearance of secondary sexual characteristics, malaise, anorexia, disturbed sleep, or recurrent fever requires further evaluation for organic disease. Review of systems should include questions referable to the genitourinary tract, the major extra-intestinal source of abdominal pain. [See Exhibit 14-4 for a partial differential diagnosis.]

Children with functional abdominal pain are usually of school age, good students, and emotionally intense. Their pains are intermittent, periumbilical, and may be severe. Repeated physical examinations are unrevealing, sleep is never disturbed, growth is uniformly excellent, and constitutional symptoms are never present.

Hematemesis

Bleeding from the mouth or rectum in infants or children is often benign but always alarming.

Exhibit 14-4 Causes of Chronic, Recurrent Abdominal Pain

Most Common

- Functional abdominal pain
- Constipation
- Urinary tract infection

GI

- Intussusception
- Volvulus
- Polyp
- Superior mesenteric artery syndrome

- Crohn's disease
- *Yersinia* enterocolitis

- Meckel's diverticulum
- Peptic ulcer disease

- Milk protein intolerance
- Lactose intolerance

- Cholecystitis
- Chronic pancreatitis
- Pancreatic pseudocyst
- Ruptured viscus

Gynecologic

- Premenstrual cramps
- Mittelschmerz
- Pelvic inflammatory disease

History

Verify that hematemesis has occurred. Vomitus containing beets, artifically flavored cereals, red beverages, or crayons can easily be mistaken for blood. Breast-fed babies may suck, then vomit significant quantities of maternal blood from cracked nipples. Consider factitious hematemesis in a disturbed adolescent. Attempt to estimate the volume of bleeding, and try to determine the source of blood. Hematemesis always indicates a lesion proximal to the ligament of Treitz. If there is pain, determine the location and character. Table 14-2 lists the types of pain classically associated with various causes of upper GI bleeding. Nosebleeds remain the most common cause of hematemesis in childhood.

TABLE 14-2 Pain Associated with Hematemesis

Cause	Location	Character
Esophagitis	Substernal	Burning
Gastritis	Epigastric	Gnawing
Gastric ulcer	Epigastric	Gnawing
Duodenal ulcer	Periumbilical	Gnawing
Pancreatitis	Shoulder, back	Gnawing

Physical Examination

Signs of significant, acute blood loss include tachycardia, postural hypotension, pallor, and lethargy. Examine the nasopharynx and gingiva for bleeding sources and the teeth for remnants of foreign red materials (e.g., crayons). Abdominal examination is often benign, even in the presence of gastritis or peptic ulcer disease. Look for signs of mechanical obstruction and ileus, as well as for evidence of chronic liver disease (e.g., hepatomegaly, splenomegaly, caput medusae). On rectal examination check for referred pain and blood. Although melena is the rule with upper GI tract lesions, bright red blood may be passed via the rectum when there is brisk bleeding from as high as the esophagus. Examine the skin: petechiae extending below the nipple line or purpura suggest generalized bleeding disorders.

Ancillary Data

The hematocrit is usually normal at onset of bleeding but falls within 6 hours as hemodilution occurs. The initial work-up is shown in Table 14-3.

TABLE 14-3 Initial Work-up for Hematemesis

Condition	Laboratory Tests
Hematemesis present?	Guaiac test of emesis
	Wright's stain
	Apt test
	Blood type (emesis or venous blood)
Minor bleeding	Hematocrit
Severe bleeding	CBC, estimate of platelets
	ESR
	BUN
	Electrolytes
	ALT,* AST
	PT, PTT

* Abbreviations: ALT, alanine aminotransferase; AST, aspartate aminotransferase; PT, prothrombin time; PTT, partial thromboplastin time.

Hematochezia, Melena, and Occult Blood

Rectal bleeding can originate from lesions anywhere in the GI tract. The gross appearance of the blood helps to localize the source. Bright red blood (hematochezia) on the stool, not mixed in, indicates a bleeding source in the bowel distal to stool formation (i.e., between rectum and perianal skin). Differential diagnosis includes anal or rectal fissures, polyps, and proctitis; hemorrhoids are rare in children without portal hypertension. Bright red blood from urine or the vagina sometimes mimics rectal bleeding. Bright red blood mixed into stool usually originates in the descending colon and suggests colitis or polyps. Occasionally, it may come from as high as the duodenum during a massive hemorrhage. In general, the higher the lesion, the darker the blood; suspect colonic or ileal sources or Meckel's diverticulum. Melena, the tarry, foul-smelling, digested products of hemoglobin, usually indicates gastric and duodenal bleeding. Since at least 50 mL of digested blood is needed to detect melena,[6] its appearance always indicates a major hemorrhage with volume depletion. Conversely, occult blood, as determined by a guaiac slide test (e.g., Hemoccult), can represent a loss of as little as 2 mL of blood from anywhere in the GI tract.[7]

History

Get a description of the blood. Inquire about constipation, diarrhea, rectal pain, recent oral antibiotics, and constitutional symptoms. Suspect intussusception in an infant with recurrent irritability but no fever, and suspect infection in any child with fever. If black stools are reported, ask about bismuth-containing medications, iron, raisins, and beets. All can produce black stools and a false-positive guaiac slide test.

Physical Examination

Estimate blood loss as for upper GI bleeding. Direct special attention to the abdominal and rectal examinations; look for hard stool, anal fissures, and perianal rashes.

Ancillary Data

Obtain a CBC with a platelet count, ESR, BUN, serial hematocrits, and a stool specimen for enteric pathogens, ova and parasites. Selected cases of nonemergent bleeding require sigmoidoscopy, double-contrast barium enema, and small-bowel series with follow-through, in that order.

SPECIFIC DIAGNOSES

Achalasia

Achalasia is the inability of the morphologically normal gastroesophageal sphincter to relax. This rare disorder causes chronic, often intermittent, dysphagia and vomiting. It is rarely seen in children under 5 years of age. Barium swallow reveals a dilated esophagus that narrows distally. Lower esophageal sphincter pressure, as determined by esophageal manometrics, is at least twice the normal value and remains elevated when the patient swallows.[8] Cinefluoroscopy after the administration[9] of metacholine (2.5 mg sc) reveals disorganized esophageal motility. Esophagoscopy rules out esophagitis, distal stricture, and Zenker's diverticulum. At present, pneumatic dilatation is the treatment of choice.

Gastroesophageal Reflux

Reflux of stomach contents into the esophagus is usually secondary to a functionally incompetent lower esophageal sphincter. Infants vomit, regurgitate feedings, and may experience apneic episodes. The history and physical examination may reveal failure to thrive, persistent cough, wheezing, or dysphagia. A diagnostic work-up is indicated to demonstrate reflux and its severity, and to rule out hiatal hernia, esophagitis, and other causes of vomiting. Work-up includes a CBC, stool guaiac test, chest film, barium swallow and upper GI series, and an esophageal pH probe. If esophagitis or stricture is suspected, even with a normal barium swallow, do an esophagoscopy with biopsy.

Management of thriving "spitters" under the age of 9 months consists of giving them thickened feedings and maintaining them in a 30° elevated prone position for a full hour after feeding.[10] Vigorous medical management of the ill infant also includes treatment with anticholinergic drugs and administration of antacids after feedings for 6 weeks. Those patients who show no clinical improvement after 1 month are candidates for a surgical cure with a Nissen fundoplication.

Hiatal Hernia

Protrusion of part of the stomach into the thoracic cavity creates a hiatal hernia. Most are *sliding hiatal hernias* in which the gastroesophageal junction and a portion of the stomach intermittently rise above the diaphragm and into the thorax. This contributes to gastroesophageal reflux, as discussed earlier.

A *paraesophageal hernia* is the protrusion of a knuckle of stomach into the thoracic cavity; the gastroesophageal junction is normally positioned. This unusual hernia causes acute esophageal blockage by incarceration. The clinical manifestations are severe chest pain and dysphagia, rather than recurrent vomiting. It is diagnosed with a barium swallow and requires surgical correction.

Peptic Ulcer Disease

Peptic ulcer disease remains the most common cause of upper GI blood loss in children. Hydrochloric acid and pepsin secretion cause edema, mucosal erosion, and, finally, bleeding. In gastric ulcers the primary problem appears to be a patch of mucosa unable to protect itself from physiologic levels of gastric secretions. Conversely, duodenal ulcers are caused by abnormally increased acid and pepsin secretions. In general, peptic ulcer disease causes solitary lesions. Although peptic ulcers occur in all age groups, be especially suspicious of the school-age child with GI bleeding, recurrent abdominal pain, recurrent vomiting, or unexplained melena.

Younger children have acute hematemesis and vague abdominal pain. In children older than 9 years of age, recurrent, gnawing epigastric pain relieved by eating often precedes hematemesis by many months. Swallowed blood or pyloric stenosis can cause nausea and vomiting. Gastric ulcers, more frequently found in preschoolers, are usually secondary to infections and other causes of organic stress. They do not recur following treatment. However, duodenal ulcers, usually noted in school-age children, are primary and often recur.

On physical examination look for signs of anemia and volume loss. Abdominal examination generally remains benign, despite complaints of pain. The two exceptions are duodenal perforation (acute abdomen) and pyloric stenosis associated with antral or pyloric ulcers (ileus, distension). Rectal examination may reveal blood.

Ancillary data should include a hematocrit and guaiac slide test. An upper GI series may provide the definitive diagnosis. Always request a "small-bowel follow-through" to avoid missing Crohn's disease. Arrange an upper endoscopic examination, when available, for acute, ongoing upper GI bleeding. Endoscopy is also in order when roentgenography fails to reveal a strongly suspected lesion. This procedure remains more sensitive than roentgenography, not only for peptic ulcer disease but also for esophageal varices, esophagitis, and gastritis.

Initial therapy for massive bleeding includes gastric suction and lavage with iced normal saline through a nasogastric tube until acute bleeding ceases, maintenance of vital signs with intravenous fluids, and fresh whole blood transfusions. In selected patients who continue to bleed briskly, infuse vasopressin (Pitressin) into the mesenteric artery.

Treatment of choice for peptic ulcer disease without active bleeding is frequent antacids and a histamine Hz receptor antagonist. A magnesium-aluminum hydroxide suspension (e.g., Maalox liquid), given after meals and at bedtime, effectively neutralizes hydrochloric acid. Cimetidine or ranitidine prevents acid secretion. Restrict caffeine-containing foods (e.g., soda pop, coffee, tea) to prevent stimulation of acid secretions, but encourage a full diet otherwise. Propantheline or hyoscyamine preparations help alleviate pain. After 6 weeks of treatment, repeat the upper GI series. If the x-ray film reveals healing and if the patient is asymptomatic, discontinue treatment. Follow children with apparently healed peptic ulcers with serial stool guaiac tests for 6 months.

Lactose Intolerance

Lactose, or milk sugar, cannot be absorbed by the human GI tract. However, lactase, a brush border enzyme found throughout the small bowel, with greatest concentration in the jejunum, catalyzes the splitting of this disaccharide into two readily absorbed monosaccharides, glucose and galactose.

Failure to digest lactose causes an osmotic diarrhea with bloating, flatus, and abdominal cramps. Lactase deficiency is classified as congenital, secondary, or acquired. Congenital lactase deficiency, an inherited and persistent lack of enzyme from the time of birth, probably does not exist. However, preterm infants commonly have a transient, physiologic lactase deficiency. Secondary lactase deficiency refers to the temporary loss of enzyme because of an insult involving the brush border of the small-bowel mucosa. Acute infectious diarrhea is the most common cause of secondary lactase deficiency in the pediatric age group, and postinfectious lactase intolerance can last for 4 months.[11] Other causes of secondary lactase intolerance include oral broad-spectrum antibiotics, celiac disease, and cystic fibrosis.

Acquired lactase deficiency is the loss of enzyme activity that occurs with increasing age. The prevalence of clinical lactose intolerance is highest among Blacks, Jews, and Asians (70%) and lowest among those of Northern European heritage (10%). Although lactase activity drops off sharply in all populations by 1 year of age, clinical symptoms of acquired lactose intolerance never occur before the age of 5 years and usually not before adolescence.

Resolution of symptoms on a 1-week lactose-free diet and recrudescence upon reintroducing milk and milk products provide a presumptive diagnosis. A stool pH of less than 6 and reducing substances in the stool are also suggestive. In questionable cases obtain a standard lactose tolerance test or a breath hydrogen assay. Both tests measure absorption of a 5-g bolus of lactose. To make the diagnosis, both studies must correlate with clinical signs of osmotic diarrhea. Delayed gastric emptying yields false-negative results in up to 25% of cases.[12] Measurement of the lactase concentration in a jejunal biopsy is not helpful since criteria for normal levels have not been determined.

Treat the patient by limiting that amount of dietary lactose which produces symptoms. Most patients tolerate a lactose-free soy formula and acidophilus milk. Also, suggest the consumption of processed cheese, cheddar, cottage cheese, and yogurt—all of which have less lactose than other milk products.

Milk Protein Intolerance

Various GI, respiratory, and allergic symptoms have been associated with ingestion of specific cow's milk proteins. Clinical features vary. Life-threatening nonspecific colitis or chronic, intractable diarrhea can occur during the first 6 months of life. Vomiting or regurgitation, mild diarrhea, and colicky abdominal pain are considered the three most common GI manifestations. Wheezing, rhinorrhea, and rashes have also been attributed to cow's milk ingestion. Mean age at onset is 3 months, and spontaneous resolution usually occurs between the ages of 12 to 15 months. A family history for atopic eczema makes milk protein intolerance more likely. All clinical features are thought to represent an immunologic response to foreign protein.[13]

The clinical diagnosis is made if symptoms subside after withdrawal of cow's milk protein from the diet and then recur within 48 hours of a challenge on three separate occasions.[14] Most practitioners appropriately settle for a presumptive diagnosis based upon one challenge.

Treat the patient by substituting soy formula for cow's milk formula during the first year of life. A greater than expected frequency of children with "cow's milk allergy" are also intolerant of soy[15] and require one of the more expensive hydrolyzed (e.g., Nutramigen, Progestimil) or meat-based formulas. The most common reason for a poor response to multiple formula changes remains an incorrect initial diagnosis.

Celiac Disease

The gluten-induced enteropathy known as celiac disease ranks second only to cystic fibrosis as a GI cause of failure to thrive in the United States. The world-wide incidence ranges from 1 in 6500 live births in Sweden[16] to 1 in 300 in western Ireland.[17] When gluten, a protein found in wheat, barley, and rye, is ingested by susceptible individuals, the gliadin fraction of gluten causes a toxic, presumably allergic reaction within the small bowel. This leads to villous atrophy, fat malabsorption, and malnutrition.

Failure to thrive and foul-smelling stools in an anorexic, irritable 18-month-old child with a protuberant abdomen and wasted buttocks strongly suggests the diagnosis. The older the child, the less pronounced is the clinical presentation. Failure to thrive occurs secondary to decreased caloric intake and malabsorption. Chronic diarrhea appears more frequently in younger infants, and up to 10% of patients are constipated.[18] Steatorrhea, usually related to the length of bowel involved, is absent in 25% of children with celiac disease.[19] Abdominal pain or vomiting occur occasionally. Signs and symptoms resolve within days after gluten has been eliminated from the diet, but bowel morphology requires months to return to normal. Celiac crisis, a rare manifestation of the disease, is characterized by intractable diarrhea, vomiting, and dehydration.

Definitive diagnosis requires jejunal biopsy, which should reveal complete villous atrophy. Gluten-free diets should not be started before the initial biopsy, since partial resolution of villous atrophy masks the definitive tissue diagnosis. For those patients initially seen on a gluten-free diet, reintroduce gluten and arrange a biopsy 6 months later or whenever symptoms recur, whichever comes first.

Dietary treatment consists of a lactose-free diet until the brush border has returned (about 8 weeks) and a gluten-free diet for life. Treat the celiac crisis with intravenous hydrocortisone as well.

Never reintroduce gluten once the diagnosis has been established. After the linear growth spurt of adolescence, patients with celiac disease often fail to develop frank malnutrition on a gluten-containing diet; however, villous atrophy, mineral malabsorption, and anemia do recur.[20] The most compelling reason for remaining on a gluten-free diet for life is the increased frequency of GI cancers among adults with poorly controlled celiac disease.[21]

Ulcerative Colitis

Ulcerative colitis refers to an idiopathic, recurrent colitis. Onset is before the age of 16 years in 15% of cases. The peak incidence in childhood occurs between the ages of 10 to 19 years,[22] although this illness can attack preschool children. Classic signs include bloody diarrhea, mucoid stools, tenesmus, crampy abdominal pain, and low-grade fever. However, the disease often begins insidiously. Suspect ulcerative colitis in the child who fails to "get over" the viral gastroenteritis that the rest of the child's family had. Malaise and anorexia often go unrecognized by the patient because the symptoms have been present for so long. Arthralgias occur in up to 25% of cases. Weight loss, almost always present, may be ascribed incorrectly to restricted diets used to curb the diarrhea.

Examine the patient for fever, weight loss, poor height growth velocity, and delay of secondary sexual characteristics. Check for pallor and signs of dehydration. Bowel sounds may be increased, and the abdomen may be slightly tender without guarding. The perianal region remains free from disease. Sigmoidoscopy reveals frank bleeding, friability, and granularity of mucosa. Disease extends proximally and without interruption for a variable distance.

Laboratory studies usually reveal a microcytic, hypochromic anemia; polymorphonuclear leukocytes; an elevated ESR; and a depressed serum albumin. Examine a methylene blue stain of stool for leukocytes and red blood cells. Ova, parasites, and enteric pathogens are absent. Obtain a barium enema to determine the length of colon involved and an upper GI series with follow-through to rule out small-bowel disease. Fine spicules or a blurred column of barium reflect mucosal disease of the colon. A "backwash ileitis" often appears when the entire length of colon is involved. During sigmoidoscopy obtain a biopsy specimen of an involved area of the colon. In ulcerative colitis the inflammatory process is confined to the mucosa. Crypt abscesses are pathognomonic when present.

Patients with ulcerative colitis have recurrent episodes of clinical illness. Remissions may last from months to years and appear to be independent of the initial clinical manifestation or age of onset. Cancer of the colon eventually occurs if the colon is not surgically removed, or if the colonic mucosa is not stripped by a Souve procedure. The incidence of carcinoma, 3% in the first decade after onset, rises to 20% per decade thereafter. Early onset and more extensive disease are correlated with earlier onset of cancer.[23]

Sulfasalazine (60 mg/kg/d up to 4 g qd as 3 divided doses) is the drug of choice. Prednisone (2 mg/kg/d up to 60 mg qd) should be added for severe cases. Prednisone should be gradually tapered and discontinued within 6 weeks.

Crohn's Disease

Crohn's disease is an idiopathic, full-thickness, chronic inflammation of segments of bowel, small and/or large. Fever, abdominal pain, and failure to grow are the principal manifestations in children. Diarrhea is uncommon, although involvement of the colon produces a colitis often indistinguishable from ulcerative colitis. In recent years Crohn's disease appears to occur more frequently than ulcerative colitis in childhood and has an insidious onset.[22] Physical examination may reveal a pale, undergrown child, with abdominal tenderness and delayed secondary sexual development. More often, the physical examination is unremarkable. Isolated perianal disease may appear months before detectable GI tract inflammation. Sigmoidoscopy often reveals patchy involvement, with bleeding, friability, and aphthous ulcers. The biopsy specimen always shows full-thickness involvement. Granulomata, when present, are pathognomonic. Barium enema and upper GI series with follow-through usually reveal terminal ileal involvement. Look for small-bowel fistulas, linear ulcerations, and edematous small-bowel segments.

Crohn's disease in children tends to be chronic and continuous, not intermittent as is ulcerative colitis. Patients are initially managed with a tapering dose of prednisone, but almost all will eventually require year-round steroids. Sulfasalazine helps when symptoms of Crohn's colitis flare but neither provides prophylaxis nor gives dramatic relief as it does in ulcerative colitis. The incidence of GI carcinoma with long-standing disease is only fourfold greater than that for the general population.[24] Prophylactic colectomy is contraindicated since surgical intervention often stimulates new disease. Thus surgery is avoided except for draining fistulas, obstruction, or perforation with abscess formation which fail to respond to medical and nutritional management.

Gastroenteritis

Several bacteria and viruses cause acute infectious diarrheas through the release of enterotoxins or by invasion of bowel mucosa. (For a summary of appropriate antibiotic therapy, see Table 14-4.)

Viral Agents

Rotovirus Rotovirus is a double-stranded RNA virus that accounts for more than 50% of acute viral gastroenteritis in infancy.[25] The virus invades duodenal and jejunal mucosa. Villi are flattened and absorption fails. Villi remain abnormal for up to 1 month after the clinical illness has ceased, and intestinal disaccharidases may be reduced. Most commonly seen in winter months, the disease begins with an abrupt onset of vomiting, followed by watery diarrhea, crampy abdominal pain, and fever, all after a 48-hour incubation period. Pharyngeal ery-

TABLE 14-4 Antibiotic Treatment for Bacterial GI Infections

Infection	Antibiotic	Dosage
Campylobacter infections*	Erythromycin	50 mg/kg/d po in 3 divided doses for 5 d
Cholera	Tetracycline or trimethoprim-sulfamethoxazole or chloramphenicol	50 mg/kg/d po in 4 divided doses for 3 d
Enteropathogenic *Escherichia coli* infections*	Neomycin or ampicillin	100 mg/kg/d po in 3 divided doses for 10 d 100 mg/kg/d IV in 4 divided doses for 10 d
Salmonellosis*	Ampicillin	50 mg/kg/d po or IV in 4 divided doses for 7 d
Enteric fever	Ampicillin or chloramphenicol	200 mg/kg/d IV in 4 divided doses for 14 d 50 mg/kg/d IV in 4 divided doses for 14 d
Shigellosis	Trimethoprim-sulfamethoxazole	10–50 mg/kg/d po in 2 divided doses for 5 d
Staphylococcal enterocolitis	Vancomycin	40 mg/kg/d IV in 4 divided doses for 5 d
Yersina enterocolitica infections*	Trimethoprim-sulfamethoxazole	10–50 mg/kg/d po in 2 divided doses for 5 d

* Treat selected cases only (see text).

thema and rhinitis may be seen. Vomiting stops before diarrhea begins; the latter lasts 7 days. Stool and vomitus remain contagious as long as clinical illness persists. Infants become more ill than toddlers. There is no carrier state, and exposure confers long-lasting immunity. A complement-fixation test or enzyme-linked immunosorbent assay (ELISA) confirms the diagnosis; however, with a clinical diagnosis, symptomatic treatment should be started for the vomiting or diarrhea (Exhibits 14-1 and 14-2).

Norwalk Agent The infection caused by the Norwalk agent appears as an epidemic of vomiting and diarrhea in school-age children. The chief clinical differences between the illnesses caused by the Norwalk agent and rotovirus are the older age group affected and the shorter duration of illness with the Norwalk agent. Routine laboratory confirmation is not available.

Adenoviruses These viruses primarily affect children under 2 years of age. Symptoms consist of self-limited fever, vomiting, and diarrhea. Stools do not contain blood or mucus. There also may be respiratory tract involvement. Diagnosis by ELISA is available.

Bacterial Agents

Campylobacter fetus The most common cause of bacterial diarrhea in childhood may be *C. fetus*.[26] Peak incidence is between the ages of 1 and 5 years. Infection is contracted from poultry, dogs, and contaminated water. *Campylobacter* invades small-bowel mucosa, but the pathophysiology of the diarrhea remains unclear. After a 2- to 11-day incubation period, the disease causes high fever, chills, malaise, headache, and periumbilical pain followed by mild, watery, blood-streaked diarrhea. Pain sometimes returns after the stools become firm, and fewer than a third of affected children vomit. Recovery is complete within 2 weeks. A mild polymorphonuclear leukocytosis supports a definitive diagnosis made by blood and stool cultures. Although erythromycin effectively eradicates *Campylobacter*, the need for an antibiotic in this mild, self-limited gastroenteritis has not been established.

Yersinia enterocolitica This Gram-negative rod causes diarrhea in infants and toddlers, and severe right lower quadrant abdominal pain without diarrhea in older children. Although most frequently confined to the mucosa of the ileocolic region, this organism can invade the bowel from stomach to rectum and cause transmural necrosis. When the colon is the chief area affected, the disease may cause a florid colitis with bloody diarrhea and high fever. In most cases, however, watery stools containing occult blood last less than 2 weeks. Occasionally, the disease causes chronic, recurrent diarrhea or a polyarthritis. The diagnosis is made by stool culture. Therapy for this self-limited disease is usually symptomatic, although trimethoprim-sulfamethoxazole or tetracycline should be considered for severe or prolonged cases.[27]

***Shigella* Species** *Shigella*, a genus of Gram-negative bacilli, causes colitis by invasion of large-bowel mucosa and intramucosal release of enterotoxin. After a 1- to 3-day incubation period, high fever, crampy abdominal pain, and headache begin. Tenesmus and bloody suppurative diarrhea follow 1 day later. Symptoms resolve within 10 days from onset, and the stool is usually clear of *Shigella* within 2 weeks. In infants, prostration, seizures, and meningism without diarrhea may delay diagnosis.

Within the pediatric population, shigellosis most frequently occurs in toddlers and preschool children in summertime. Transmission occurs through contact with contaminated stool and can be water- and foodborne.

Diagnosis requires (1) methylene blue stain of the stool for polymorphonuclear leukocytes and (2) stool culture. Blood cultures are rarely positive. Leukopenia occurs in fewer than 20% of patients. Treatment includes hydration and trimethoprim-sulfamethoxazole or ampicillin for 5 days.[28]

Vibrio cholerae *V. cholerae,* a Gram-negative curved rod, releases enterotoxin into the small-bowel lumen, inducing a marked secretory diarrhea. After an incubation period of less than 1 week, profuse watery diarrhea without tenesmus begins. Vomiting, periumbilical pain, and fever are mild. However, dehydration and metabolic acidosis occur rapidly because of the voluminous fluid and electrolyte loss. Diarrhea lasts 7 days even when oral feedings are withheld, then ceases abruptly. There is no carrier state in children. The chief modes of transmission are water and shellfish contaminated by adult carriers or by stool of people with mild illness. In the United States cholera has occurred in epidemics with no special prevalence in the young.

Diagnosis is suggested by the clinical feature of profuse "rice-water" stools without tenesmus or high fever. Methylene blue stains reveals few, if any, polymorphonuclear leukocytes or erythrocytes. Stool culture makes the definitive diagnosis. Treatment consists of isotonic rehydration and antibiotics. Tetracycline is the treatment of choice for children aged 8 years or older (50 mg/kg/d orally in four divided doses for 3 days). Also effective are furazolidone, trimethoprim-sulfamethoxazole, and chloramphenicol.[29]

***Salmonella* Species** *Salmonella,* a genus of Gram-negative rods, causes several diseases, two of which involve the GI tract: (1) acute gastroenteritis, which is limited to the bowel; and (2) enteric fever, which reflects *Salmonella* sepsis. Each has its own pathophysiology.

Acute Gastroenteritis In acute gastroenteritis, various *Salmonella* species produce endotoxins that also invade small-bowel mucosa. Onset of symptoms varies between a few hours to 3 days after ingestion of contaminated food and drink. Common sources are poultry, eggnog, beef, pork, and foods with mayonnaise. Domestic animals, such as Easter chicks, pet turtles, cats, and dogs also transmit disease by contaminated feces. Even cockroaches are suspected vectors.

Nausea, vomiting, and severe abdominal cramps precede fever and mucoid, foul-smelling, diarrhea. Bloody diarrhea is uncharacteristic but occurs with colonic involvement. The clinical illness resolves within 3 to 10 days, but salmonellae continue to be shed for 2 weeks to 3 months. A chronic carrier state sometimes occurs in adolescents and adults.

A history of recent exposure and a methylene blue stain of stool demonstrating polymorphonuclear leukocytes suggest the diagnosis. The white blood count may be normal or low. Stool culture provides a definitive diagnosis.

In general, only treat symptoms and correct dehydration when present. Reserve ampicillin (50 mg/kg/d in four divided doses for 7 days, IV or orally) for clinically ill infants below the age of 3 months and for patients with bacteremia. Ampicillin does not shorten the duration of illness in older infants and children and may predispose to a carrier state in adolescents.

Enteric Fever Enteric fever, caused by *S. typhosa* (typhoid fever) and several other species of *Salmonella* (paratyphoid fever) occurs after organisms invade the small bowel, enter the blood stream, and multiply in spleen, liver, and lymph nodes. These organisms then reseed the blood stream, causing sepsis and infecting other organs, including the gall bladder. The cycle is completed when *Salmonella* organisms return to the small bowel in increased numbers via the gall bladder and cause gastroenteritis. In older children enteric fever secondary to *S. typhosa* has a 10- to 40-day incubation period, followed by the insidious onset of frontal headache, cough, myalgias, and fever. The fever peaks and body temperatures remain above 40° C during the second week. By this time abdominal pain, vomiting, and diarrhea are present. Diarrhea, however, is not a sine qua non for enteric fever.

Physical examination at the height of illness reveals a tender, distended abdomen, large spleen, and sometimes "rose spots," a maculopapular, erythematous eruption. Active disease resolves within 1 month, but, typically, a second month is needed to convalesce.

The CBC reveals a normal to low white blood count and normochromic, normocytic anemia. Blood cultures are positive during the first week of clinical illness, and febrile agglutinins become elevated during the second and third weeks. Stool culture remains negative until the third week.

In children under the age of 2 years, typhoid fever occurs variably as a mild gastroenteritis that persists for 2 weeks, sepsis without prodrome, or fever of unknown origin. The white blood count may be normal or elevated. The disease is usually suspected because of exposure to an adult with classic typhoid fever.

Chloramphenicol (50 to 100 mg/kg/d in four divided doses for 14 days) is the treatment of choice for enteric fever. Ampicillin (200 mg/kg/d in four divided doses for 14 days) can be used instead.[27] Administer the antibiotic intravenously until the patient has improved clinically (usually 3 to 6 days), then switch to the oral route for the duration of the 14-day course.

Escherichia coli Epidemiologic and laboratory studies demonstrate that some strains of *E. coli* can sometimes cause gastroenteritis.[30] However, appropriate diagnostic tools remain unavailable to the practitioner. Three disease patterns have been described.

Enteropathogenic *E. coli* Enteropathogenic strains are noninvasive and cause watery diarrhea and sometimes vomiting with low-grade fever lasting for 5 to 8 days. Serotyping reveals the organism. Since these organisms also can be found in the formed stools of well children, the relationship between serotype and cause of sporadic diarrhea remains unclear. A presumptive diagnosis of enteropathogenic *E. coli* (EPEC) in an infant under the age of 18 months with diarrhea requires a history of acute onset, positive EPEC serotype, and isolation of a pure, single strain of EPEC from stool culture. The treatment of choice includes fluids and neomycin (100 mg/kg/d in three divided doses for 5 days). Infants under 3 months of age with systemic signs of infection require ampicillin (100 to 200 mg/kg/d IV in four divided doses).

Enterotoxigenic *E. coli* Following 1 to 2 days' incubation, enterotoxigenic *E. coli* (ETEC) strains release an enterotoxin that adheres to mucosal cells of the upper jejunum. This causes a secretory diarrhea similar to but much less severe than that associated with cholera. Watery diarrhea lasts 3 to 4 days and is not usually accompanied by fever. ETEC is thought to be the chief cause of "turista," traveler's diarrhea. Diagnosis is usually presumptive and based on a history of recent travel. Treatment of choice is bismuth subsalicylate (Pepto-Bismol), which in large doses selectively inhibits the activity of ETEC enterotoxin (1 oz every ½ h × 8). Trimethoprim sulfasoxazole may be used if diarrhea persists.

Enteroinvasive *E. coli* Certain strains of *E. coli* invade the mucosa of the colon to cause a *Shigella*-like dysentery; fortunately, this disease appears to be rare in the United States and has never been documented in infants. High fever, tenesmus, headaches, and purulent, bloody diarrhea occur after a 1-day incubation. Since no commercial diagnostic tests are available, rule out other causes of colitis to make this diagnosis. The treatment of choice is fluids and intravenous ampicillin.

Staphylococcus Species Staphylococcal enterocolitis is a rare, fulminant disease, found in some patients who have had recent abdominal surgery or have been exposed to massive doses of broad-spectrum antibiotics. The microbe replaces normal bowel flora and invades mucosa. The criteria for diagnosis are demonstration of a florid, acute colitis and a pure growth of *Staphylococcus*, phage type 3, from the stool. Treatment of choice is oral vancomycin.[30]

Food Poisoning

Various species of *Clostridium* and of *Staphylococcus* cause food poisoning and enterocolitis.

Clostridium perfringens Type A

C. perfringens type A elaborates a toxin in unrefrigerated meat and poultry. Within 24 hours of ingestion of contaminated food, this toxin induces a violent secretory diarrhea. Tissue invasion by clostridia plays a secondary role. Patients experience sudden onset of diarrhea and abdominal cramps in the absence of fever or vomiting. Recovery is complete within 2 days. Make the diagnosis by isolating the microbe or its toxin from stool, serum, or the contaminated food. Only symptomatic treatment is indicated.

Clostridium botulinum

C. botulinum, which grows in improperly canned foods, excretes a powerful curare-like neurotoxin. Within 12 hours after consumption of contaminated food, the patient develops nausea and vomiting, a distended abdomen, diminished bowel sounds, and either diarrhea or constipation. Progressive paresis of cranial nerves and respiratory muscles make the diagnosis obvious.

Once the diagnosis is suspected, treat the child promptly. All patients suspected of botulism require hospitalization. Support respirations and blood pressure. Induce vomiting if a gag reflex is present. Remove the remaining neurotoxin by gastric lavage and by purging with charcoal and magnesium sulfate administered via a nasogastric tube. Also administer two phosphate enemas. Administer penicillin G (50,000 U/kg/d orally in six divided doses for 7 to 10 days) to prevent further proliferation of clostridia. Administer polyvalent antitoxin, which is available from the Center for Disease Control pending identification of the botulinum toxin.[27]

Staphylococcus Species

Coagulase-positive staphylococci are commonly responsible for food poisoning but rarely for enterocolitis. Several species produce an enterotoxin that causes secretory diarrhea. The organism proliferates and produces toxin in mayonnaise- and custard-containing foods at or above room temperature. Between 3 and 6 hours after ingestion of contaminated food, violent vomiting, watery diarrhea, and abdominal cramping begin. The patient is left prostrate but recovers within 24 hours. Diagnosis, usually suspected because of exposure and illness in contacts, can be confirmed by culturing the suspected food source. Treat the patient symptomatically.

Irritable Bowel Syndrome

Chronic, nonspecific diarrhea in a thriving child between the ages of 6 months and 3 years is common and has characteristic clinical features. Episodes of watery diarrhea, four to six times daily, begin between 6 to 20 months of age. The foul-smelling stools contain particles of mucus, which adhere to the buttocks. All the day's stools are often passed within a few hours. Stool consistency varies from day to day, and the patient may occasionally be constipated. Often associated with minor physical stresses, these episodes are neither prevented nor effectively treated by restrictive diets. In fact, a full diet containing fat (at least 4 g/kg/d) can contribute toward fewer and firmer stools.[31] Despite diarrhea the child continues to thrive and appears happy. By the age of 3 years, the recurrent diarrhea resolves. Past medical history often reveals constipation or colic during the neonatal period. Also, one of the parents usually has or perceives himself to have a functional bowel disorder.

Treatment consists of reassuring the parents and offering the child an unrestricted diet. Parents accept their toddler's diarrhea more easily after they realize that growth is normal, nutrients are not being evacuated, dehydration will not occur, no underlying disease exists, and the problem is common, self-limited, unrelated to specific foods, and more inconvenient to the parents than to the child.

Aganglionic Megacolon

Aganglionic megacolon, also known as Hirschsprung's disease, is a congenital disorder of large-bowel peristalsis. Lack of ganglion cells within a segment of colon interrupts the peristaltic movement of feces and results in obstruction. Aganglionosis begins in the distal rectum and does not extend above the sigmoid colon in 75% of cases.[32] Total colonic involvement occurs rarely. The lesion is always continuous, never multifocal. The patient's neonatal history provides a useful diagnostic clue. Ninety-five percent of infants later shown to have Hirschsprung's disease do not pass meconium by 24 hours of age, whereas 94% of healthy term infants do.[32] This disease, which occurs in 1 of 5000 births in the general population, is 50 times more frequent among the relatives of an identified case.[33] Infants have marked constipation, abdominal bloating, vomiting, and poor feeding. Spontaneous bowel movements almost never occur. Older children usually have intractable constipation without encopresis. Enterocolitis, a life-threatening complication of undiagnosed Hirschsprung's disease in infancy, develops secondary to partial obstruction. This is manifested as a watery diarrhea at about 6 weeks of age and is rapidly followed by fever, abdominal distension, and bloody diarrhea. Mortality approaches 50%.[33]

In Hirschsprung's disease, rectal examination reveals an empty anal ampulla of normal or small caliber. If the examining finger crosses the aganglionic segment, diarrheal stool and flatus spurt out as the finger is withdrawn. In long segment disease rectal stimulation does not stimulate a bowel movement.

Diagnosis is made by biopsy, barium enema, or rectal manometry. A rectal suction biopsy specimen reveals the absence of ganglion cells. This painless outpatient procedure is accurate in over 95% of cases[34] and is usually the only study needed to confirm the disease. Alternatively, a barium enema can show "the transition zone," a sharp line of demarcation separating the distally narrowed aganglionic bowel from the proximally dilated normal colon. Also, persistence of barium on a 48-hour postevacuation film strongly suggests Hirschsprung's disease. Always obtain this late film since the transition zone often fails to appear before the age of 2 months and never develops with aganglionosis of the entire colon. Rectal manometry reveals failure of the internal anal sphincter relaxation and rectal distension. Obtain an intravenous pyelogram in all cases of documented Hirschsprung's disease to rule out an associated megaloureter.

Management aims to relieve obstruction and restore normal peristalsis to the GI tract. Infants require a transverse colostomy or, for total colonic aganglionosis, an ileostomy. After the child reaches 1 year of age, the bowel is reanastomosed, and one of several rectal pull-through operations is performed.

Polyps

Juvenile polyps, benign retention cysts, usually present as bright red blood on formed stools in a well-appearing 4- or 5-year-old child. Onset rarely occurs before 1 year of age. The intermittent, painless bleeding spontaneously resolves within 6 months as the polyp's stalk separates from the bowel wall. Polyps, usually solitary, occur more frequently in the colon than in the small bowel. Seventy-five percent are found within the rectosigmoid area.[35]

Polyps must be distinguished from other causes of rectal bleeding including Meckel's diverticulum, colitis, and anal fissure. Make the diagnosis by rectal examination, sigmoidoscopy with biopsy or removal of the polyp, and by double-contrast barium enema in selected cases. Obtain a hematocrit to rule out an associated anemia.

Treatment consists of reassuring the parents and child that the polyp is benign and will pass spontaneously within 6 months. Indications for removal of a juvenile polyp are iron deficiency anemia in a child receiving adequate dietary iron, intussusception or rectal prolapse with the polyp as the lead point, significant colicky abdominal pain, or rectal bleeding lasting for more than 6 months.

Four rare syndromes of multiple polyps, inherited through autosomal dominant transmission, classically result in thousands of small polyps. Multiple juvenile polyposis classically is confined to the colon but sometimes extends into small bowel. Chronic blood loss, recurrent intussusception, and protein-losing enteropathy present major problems. Peutz-Jeghers syndrome is characterized by increased perioral pigmentation and hamartomatous polyps throughout the bowel. Ovarian and colon cancers occur slightly more frequently among these patients during adulthood. Familial adenomatous polyposis coli presents during adolescence, and colectomy is usually done before 20 years of age. Without prophylactic colectomy the risk of carcinoma of the colon developing before the age of 40 years is 50%.[36] Gardner's syndrome consists of adenomatous polyps of the colon with benign soft tissue and bone tumors. Soft tissue tumors first appear during adolescence. Since the risk for carcinoma of the colon is the same as for familial adenomatous polyposis coli, a prophylactic colectomy is indicated.

Bleeding Meckel's Diverticulum

Meckel's diverticulum is a fingerlike outpouching of the ileum that is often lined with gastric mucosa. Ulceration leads to bleeding. Suspect this diagnosis in a child under 2 years of age who has an episode of painless but massive hemorrhage. Intractable episodes of vomiting secondary to intussusception or volvulus occur less commonly. Also, suspect Meckel's diverticulum in a child of any age who has hematochezia with iron deficiency anemia and a past medical history suggestive of bleeding via the rectum. Rule out other sources of bleeding (e.g., peptic ulcer, polyp, inflammatory bowel disease), then attempt to make a definitive diagnosis by roentgenographic imaging. A technetium scan sometimes demonstrates the ectopic gastric mucosa; computed tomography scans and mesenteric angiography have also been used. These procedures often fail to reveal the diagnosis, however, and laparotomy usually is required.

Lymphoid Hyperplasia

Lymphoid hyperplasia occurs when lymphoid follicles rapidly multiply into a blanket of tiny submucosal nodules. Usually found in the rectum, these nodules sometimes involve the entire colon and uncommonly are found in the small bowel as well. Lymphoid hyperplasia probably reflects the bowel's response to infection, allergens, and nonspecific irritation. The typical manifestation is hematochezia in a child between the ages of 1 and 3 years. Uncomplicated lymphoid hyperplasia lasts up to 3 months, resolves spontaneously, and is not associated with anemia or constitutional symptoms.

Make the diagnosis by double-contrast barium enema. If lymphoid hyperplasia is confirmed, do an upper GI series with small-bowel follow-through. If the small bowel is involved also, rule out an associated hypogammaglobulinemia or giardiasis.

Anal Fissures

Anal fissures are the most common cause of bright red rectal bleeding in infancy. Pain with defecation is typical. Diarrhea, hard stools, and water used for cleansing the diaper area can all produce a painful longitudinal slit in the anal mucosa. Pain is usually out of proportion to the mild pathology found. Bleeding, which may appear profuse, is always bright red and is on, rather than mixed into, the bowel movement. If not the primary cause of the fissure, constipation occurs secondary to pain associated with passage of bowel movements across a fissure. Diagnosis is made by inspecting the anus while the infant's buttocks are spread apart.

Treatment includes correction of constipation with hexylresorcinol-hydrocortisone (e.g., Anusol-HC) suppositories twice daily for 1 week and careful diaper care. Wipe perianal area clean with lanolin-containing wipes (e.g., Tuck's), not water. Dry with powder and apply a thin layer of petroleum jelly.

Cystic Fibrosis

Cystic fibrosis[37] is the most common GI cause for failure to thrive in infants and children. The disease occurs in approximately 1 of 2000 white live births; the incidence is appreciably lower in blacks. Inherited as an autosomal recessive disease, cystic fibrosis has a dismal prognosis, with 25% of clinically affected youths dying before the age of 18 years; 50% before the age of 25 years. Cystic fibrosis is primarily a disease of the exocrine glands. Abnormally viscous secretions block the ductules and prevent normal function. This causes chronic pulmonary disease, pancreatic insufficiency, and increased sodium chloride in sweat. Neonates have meconium ileus. More than 80% of older infants and children have complete achylia with fat malabsorption. Other GI complications include rectal prolapse in 20% of infants and large-bowel obstruction secondary to inspissated feces (i.e., meconium ileus equivalent), intussusception, and cirrhosis in less than 5% of patients. Edema and hypoalbuminemia associated with malabsorption of soy formula can occur in infants.

To make the diagnosis, demonstrate elevated sweat chloride by pilocarpine iontophoresis. Fat malabsorption can be demonstrated by a 72-hour fat balance test; chronic lung changes, by roentgenography.

Dietary therapy consists of dessicated pancreatic extract, a high-calorie diet rich in fat and protein, fat-soluble vitamins, and medium-chain triglyceride supplements. Pulmonary therapy attempts to loosen secretions with acetylcysteine and postural drainage and to control infection with antibiotics.

Pancreatitis

Inflammation of the exocrine pancreas, an unusual cause of abdominal pain in children, appears as either an acute or a chronic, relapsing disease. Acute pancreatitis, usually idiopathic, may also be associated with mumps, rubeola, hepatitis B, gallstones obstructing the sphincter of Oddi, a pseudocyst following blunt abdominal trauma, and chronic steroid use. Chronic, relapsing pancreatitis sometimes occurs with Schwachman syndrome and may herald cystic fibrosis. Also consider hyperparathyroidism, hyperlipoproteinemia (types I and V) in adolescents, and hereditary pancreatitis, an autosomal dominant disease.

The corrosive action of pancreatic digestive enzymes upon the pancreas and adjacent structures accounts for the dramatic symptomatology. Older children with acute pancreatitis complain of midepigastric, boring pain with radiation to the back; younger children just appear irritable. The disease progresses to signs of an acute abdomen with fever, vomiting, and dehydration. Pleural effusion may be seen. Severe intractable ascites can occur with a leaking pseudocyst. Dehydration is out of proportion to the vomiting because of third-space losses and enzymatically induced peripheral vasodilation. Chronic, relapsing pancreatitis is manifested as episodes of acute pancreatitis or as failure to thrive with steatorrhea.

Laboratory evaluation helps monitor the course of the illness and determine its cause. Serum amylase rises within 2 to 12 hours after onset of symptoms, returns to normal within 4 days, and is the best marker of active disease. Urine amylase from a 24-hour urine collection remains elevated for 2 weeks; serum lipase also is elevated. The CBC reveals a marked polymorphonuclear leukocytosis with a shift to the left. A serum calcium level below 7 mg/dL, depressed because of calcium soap formation by the enzymatically active extravasated fluid, indicates severe peritoneal involvement. Also, obtain blood glucose, SGPT, serum electrolytes, BUN, and bilirubin. To determine etiology, obtain the following: hepatitis B surface antigen (HB_sAg), mumps and rubella titers; serum triglycerides, cholesterol, and lipoprotein electrophoresis; sweat chloride. On chest films look for effusions, a raised hemidiaphragm on the left, chronic lung disease, a mediastinal pseudocyst, and pneumonia. On an abdominal flat plate film, look for ileus and pancreatic calcifications. Obtain an ultrasonogram to rule out a pseudocyst.

Control the pain with analgesics, support hydration with intravenous fluids, and decrease the activity of the pancreas with intermittent gastric suction and anticholinergic drugs. The patient usually recovers within 1 week. If fever is greater than 39° C or persists for more than 5 days, suspect an abscess.

When a pseudocyst is present, medical management followed by surgical correction 4 to 6 weeks later is advised.

Acute Viral Hepatitis

Although several viruses cause acute inflammation of the liver, acute viral hepatitis refers to hepatitis A, hepatitis B, and non-A, non-B hepatitis. Hepatitis in childhood most frequently is caused by hepatitis A virus (HAV). In all these illnesses swelling and necrosis of hepatocytes interferes with their metabolic functions, disturbs the normal liver architecture, and promotes cholestasis. All cause a similar clinical illness. The prodrome lasts between 1 and 3 weeks and is characterized by low-grade fever, headache, malaise, anorexia, nausea, vomiting, and mild abdominal pain. A cholestatic phase follows, lasting from days to weeks, and is characterized by hepatomegaly, dark urine, acholic stools, and right upper quadrant tenderness. An erythematous, macular rash; arthralgias; and lymphadenopathy sometimes occur. Although affected adolescents always become jaundiced, over half of the affected preschool children fail to develop icterus. Paradoxically, patients feel better as they become more jaundiced. Complete convalescence may require months, with malaise persisting after the other clinical signs and laboratory evidence of disease have resolved. In general, the younger the child, the shorter and less severe the illness.

Hepatitis A

Hepatitis A, caused by a single-stranded RNA virus, has a short incubation period of 15 to 50 days. Saliva and stool are infectious from 2 to 3 weeks prior to the onset of symptoms to 1 week after the onset of jaundice. Hepatitis A is abrupt in onset, and SGPT usually exceeds 1000 U within 4 days. Full recovery occurs within 2 to 3 weeks, and no carrier state exists. Fulminant hepatic failure, aplastic anemia, and myocarditis are unusual but life-threatening sequelae.

Hepatitis B

Hepatitis B is caused by a double-stranded DNA virus (HBV). The incubation period lasts between 45 to 160 days. With hepatitis B, unlike hepatitis A, patients remain contagious for as long as they are viremic. Contamination of mucous membranes or the broken skin barrier of contacts with infected blood accounts for most secondary cases. Fecal transmission does occur but requires a much larger inoculum than does hepatitis A. Onset of clinical illness is insidious, liver enzymes commonly remain elevated for up to 2 months after onset, and convalescence takes months. Complications include arthritis, glomerulonephritis, chronic persistent hepatitis, chronic active hepatitis, and a chronic carrier state.

Non-A, Non-B Hepatitis

Non-A, non-B hepatitis is a diagnosis of exclusion. HAV, HBV, cytomegalovirus, Epstein-Barr virus infections must be ruled out. The responsible agent remains to be identified. At present, this illness accounts for 90% of cases of postransfusion hepatitis. Jaundice and hepatomegaly appear after a 6- to 10-week incubation period. The chronologic course appears to be intermediate between those of hepatitis A and hepatitis B.

Laboratory Evaluation

Initial laboratory evaluation for all patients suspected of having acute viral hepatitis includes

- measurements of fractionated bilirubin, serum glutamic-oxaloacetic transaminase, SGPT, prothrombin time, partial thromboplastin time, and serum protein and albumin
- complete blood, reticulocyte, and platelet counts
- assays for HB_sAg and anti-HAV-immunoglobulin
- Infectious mononucleosis spot test

Several serologic markers for acute viral hepatitis A and B have been isolated. These markers are the antigenically active parts of the virus or the antibodies formed in response to these various antigens. Hepatitis B has three antigens: the lipoprotein envelope or surface antigen (HB_sAg), the electron-dense core (HB_cAg), and a third antigen, the "e" antigen (HB_eAg), manufactured by the virus. Hepatitis A acts as a single antigen. These four antigens stimulate four specific antibody responses. Commercial tests now detect anti-HAV, all the HBV antibodies, and the HBV antigens except HB_cAg, which does not exist in serum without its coat, HB_sAg. These various antigens and antibodies, appearing at various times during the course of HBV infection, have improved accuracy of diagnosis and prediction of outcome. Nomenclature and interpretation of tests are summarized in Table 14-5.

TABLE 14-5 Significance of Serologic Tests for Hepatitis B

Test	Description	Significance
HB_sAg	Hepatitis B surface antigen	Active infection Carrier state Chronic active hepatitis
anti-HB_s	Antibody to hepatitis B surface antigen	Convalescence Persistent infection Past infection
anti-HB_cAG	Antibody to hepatitis B core antigen	Present infection Past infection
HB_eAg	Hepatitis B "e" antigen	Highly infectious Increased risk for congenital adrenal hyperplasia Fetus and newborn at risk
anti-HB_e	Antibody to hepatitis B "e" antigen	Noninfectious Fetus and newborn not at risk

Prophylaxis against Viral Hepatitis

For sexual or household exposure to HAV, prophylaxis with standard immune serum globulin is indicated.[38] For reliable prophylaxis, administer immune serum globulin, 0.02 mg/kg IM (up to 2 mL) within 7 days of exposure.[38]

Postexposure prophylaxis with hepatitis B immune globulin is indicated after exposure via needle stick or direct mucous membrane contact with HBV-infected blood and for the newborn of an HB_sAg-positive mother.[38] Do not immunize patients who already have titers of anti-HBV since this may produce an iatrogenic disease secondary to immune complexes.

α-1-Antitrypsin Deficiency Disease

Deficiency of α-1-antitrypsin is the most commonly identified cause of chronic liver disease in infants. α-1-Antitrypsin is a glycoprotein usually found in the α-2-globulin peak on serum protein electrophoresis and is so named because it inhibits the action of trypsin and certain other serum enzymes. Absence of an α-1-globulin peak reflects deficiency of the most common of many forms of α-1-antitrypsin. These several forms are identified by characteristic migration patterns on electrophoresis.

In one large study 10% of infants with this deficiency had obstructive jaundice.[39] Although clinical remission within 2 months usually occurred, 2% progressed to cirrhosis. The eventual prognosis is unknown but guarded, since half of the children still have abnormal liver function tests by the age of 4 years[40] and 10% of adults developed hepatic carcinoma.[41]

Suspect α-1-antitrypsin deficiency disease in any infant or child with unexplained cholestasis or hepatomegaly, abnormal liver function tests, and no α-2-globulin peak or on serum protein electrophoresis. Order an α-1-antitrypsin assay to make a definitive diagnosis. Treatment is expectant. Phenobarbital and cholestyramine help relieve cholestasis; corticosteroids are of no value.

References

1. Food and Nutrition Board: *Recommended Dietary Allowances.* Washington, DC, National Academy of Sciences–National Research Council, 1980.
2. Vaughan VC III, McKay RJ: *Nelson Textbook of Pediatrics,* ed 10. Philadelphia, WB Saunders Co, 1975, p 254.
3. Ehrenpreis T, Gierup J, Lagercrantz R: Chronic regional enterocolitis in children and adolescents. *Acta Paediatr Scand* 1971;60:209–215.
4. Illingworth RS: *The Normal Child: Some Problems of the Early Years and Their Treatment,* ed 8. Edinburgh, Churchill Livingstone, 1983, pp 256–270.
5. Apley J: *The Child with Abdominal Pains,* ed 2. Oxford, Blackwell Scientific Publications, 1975.
6. Glober GA, Peskoe SM: Outpatient screening for gastrointestinal lesions using guaiac-impregnated slides. *Am J Dig Dis* 1974;19:399–403.
7. Sleisenger MH, Fordtran JS: *Gastrointestinal Disease: Pathophysiology, Diagnosis, Management.* Philadelphia, WB Saunders Co, 1973.
8. Azizkhan RG, Tapper D, Eraklis A: Achalasia in childhood: A 20-year experience. *J Pediatr Surg* 1980;15:452–456.
9. Lawson EE, Grand RJ, Neff RK, et al: Clinical estimation of liver span in infants and children. *Am J Dis Child* 1978;132:474–476.
10. Orenstein SR, Whitington PF: Positioning for prevention of infant gastroesophageal reflux. *J Pediatr* 1983;103:534–537.
11. Lifshitz F, Coello-Ramirez P, Guitierrez-Topete G, et al: Carbohydrate intolerance in infants with diarrhea. *J Pediatr* 1971;79:760–767.
12. Newcomer AD, McGill DB: Lactose tolerance tests in adults with normal lactase activity. *Gastroenterology* 1966;50:340–346.
13. Lebenthal E: Cow's milk protein allergy. *Pediatr Clin North Am* 1975;22:827–833.
14. Goldman AS, Anderson DW Jr, Sellers WA, et al: Milk allergy: I. Oral challenge with milk and isolated milk proteins in allergic children. *Pediatrics* 1963;32:425–443.
15. Whitington PF, Gibson R: Soy protein intolerance: Four patients with concomitant cow's milk intolerance. *Pediatrics* 1977;59:730–732.
16. Borgfars I, Selander P: The incidence of coelic disease in Sweden. *Acta Paediatr Scand* 1968;57:260.
17. Mylotte M, Eagen-Mitchell B, McCarthy CF, et al: Incidence of coeliac disease in the West of Ireland. *Br Med J* 1973;1:703–705.
18. Eagan-Mitchell B, McNicholl B: Constipation in childhood coeliac disease. *Arch Dis Child* 1972;47:238–240.
19. Lebenthal E, Branski D: Childhood celiac disease—a reappraisal. *J Pediatr* 1981;98:681–690.
20. Young WF, Pringle EM: 110 children with coeliac disease, 1950–1969. *Arch Dis Child* 1971;46:421–436.
21. Selby WS, Gallagher ND: Malignancy in a 19-year experience of adult celiac disease. *Dig Dis Sci* 1979;24:684–688.
22. Grand RJ, Homer DR: Approaches to inflammatory bowel disease in childhood and adolescence. *Pediatr Clin North Am* 1975;22:835–850.
23. Devroede GJ, Taylor WF, Sauer WG, et al: Cancer risk and life expectancy of children with ulcerative colitis. *N Engl J Med* 1971;285:17–21.
24. Weedon DP, Shorter RG, Ilstrup DM, et al: Crohn's disease and cancer. *N Engl J Med* 1973;289:1099–1103.
25. Bishop RF, Davidson GP, Holmes IH, et al: Detection of a new virus by electron microscopy of faecal

extracts from children with acute gastroenteritis. *Lancet* 1974;1:149–151.
26. Rettig PJ: *Campylobacter* infections in human beings. *J Pediatr* 1979;94:855–864.
27. Gellis SS, Kagan BM (eds): *Current Pediatric Therapy,* ed 10. Philadelphia, WB Saunders Co, 1982, p 545.
28. Chang MJ, Dunkle LM, Van Reken D, et al: Trimethoprim-sulfamethoxazole compared to ampicillin in the treatment of shigellosis. *Pediatrics* 1977; 59:726–729.
29. Hirschhorn N, McCarthy BJ, Ranney B, et al: Ad libitum oral glucose-electrolyte therapy for acute diarrhea in Apache children. *J Pediatr* 1973;83:562–571.
30. Silverman A, Roy CC (eds): *Pediatric Clinical Gastroenterology,* ed 3. St. Louis, The CV Mosby Co, 1983, pp 204, 342.
31. Cohen S, Mathis R, Walker WA: Chronic non-specific diarrhea: Role of dietary management in control, abstract no. 412. *Pediatr Res* 1978;12:432.
32. Swenson O, Sherman JO, Fisher JH: Diagnosis of congenital megacolon: An analysis of 501 patients. *J Pediatr Surg* 1973;8:587–594.
33. Ehrenpreis T: Hirschsprung's disease. *Am J Dig Dis* 1971;16:1032–1052.
34. Campbell PE, Noblett HR: Experience with rectal suction biopsy in the diagnosis of Hirschsprung's disease. *J Pediatr Surg* 1969;4:410–415.
35. Silverberg S: "Juvenile" retention polyps of the colon and rectum. *Am J Dig Dis* 1970;15:617–625.
36. Bussey H Jr: Gastrointestinal polyposis. *Gut* 1970;11:970–978.
37. Wood RE, Boat TF, Doershuk CF: Cystic fibrosis. *Am Rev Respir Dis* 1976;113:833–878.
38. Recommendation of the Immunization Practices Advisory Committee: Immune globulins for protection against viral hepatitis. *MMWR* 1981;30:423–435.
39. Sveger T: Liver disease in alpha-1-antitrypsin deficiency detected by screening of 200,000 infants. *N Engl J Med* 1976;294:1316–1321.
40. Sveger T, Thelin T: Four-year-old children with alpha-one-antitrypsin deficiency: Clinical follow-up and parental attitudes towards neonatal screening. *Acta Paediatr Scand* 1981;70:171–177.
41. Eriksson S, Hagerstrand I: Cirrhosis and malignant hepatoma in alpha-one-antitrypsin deficiency. *Acta Med Scand* 1974;195:451–458.

Bibliography

Andorsky M, Finley A, Davidson M: Pediatric gastroenterology 1/1/69–12/31/75: A review: I. Hollow viscera and the pancreas. *Am J Dig Dis* 1977;22:56–68.

Andorsky M, Finley A, Davidson M: Pediatric gastroenterology 1/1/69–12/31/75: A review: II. The liver and biliary tract. *Am J Dig Dis* 1977;22:155–167.

Davidson M, Wasserman R: The irritable colon of childhood (chronic nonspecific diarrhea syndrome). *J Pediatr* 1966;69:1027–1038.

Friedland GW, Sunshine P, Zboralske FF: Hiatal hernia in infants and young children: A 2- to 3-year follow-up study. *J Pediatr* 1975;87:71–74.

Grady GF, Keusch GT: Pathogenesis of bacterial diarrheas, Parts 1 and 2. *N Engl J Med* 1971;285:831–841, 891–900.

Grand RJ, Watkins JB (eds): Symposium on gastrointestinal and liver disease. *Pediatr Clin North Am* 1975;22:1–1009.

Walker-Smith J: Cow's milk protein intolerance: Transient food intolerance of infancy. *Arch Dig Dis Child* 1975;50:347–350.

Stephen A. Wolf
Dennis W. Shermeta

15 Abdominal Pain

One of the most important and perplexing problems facing the emergency physician is the accurate assessment of the child with abdominal pain. Because so many diseases of childhood can produce symptoms of abdominal pain, it is absolutely essential that the individual initially evaluating these children be aware of many of the potential causes of abdominal pain that would require emergency surgical intervention, inpatient hospitalization, or judicious outpatient care.[1–3] This chapter is intended to provide a means of assessing the child with abdominal pain so that the intensity of the child's disease process and the appropriate initial therapy can be determined. Rather than being a compendium of all the different disease entities that can produce abdominal pain in childhood, this chapter intends to provide a rational approach, allowing insights into some of the pathophysiologic processes that are at work in this clinical situation.

SIGNS AND SYMPTOMS

A history of pain, anorexia, nausea and vomiting, and changes in bowel habits indicates potential intra-abdominal disease. Pain may be most helpful in characterizing and localizing the problem. Important findings upon physical examination include tenderness to palpation, involuntary guarding, and an abdominal mass. Distension and changes in bowel sounds are more difficult to interpret because of extra-abdominal influences.

Pain

Abdominal pain results from two sources of stimuli: visceral and somatic. Stretching of nerve endings in the wall of a hollow viscus or capsule of a solid organ, as may be seen in bowel obstruction, early appendicitis, or acute hepatomegaly, is frequently the earliest stimulus. Such pain is mediated by parasympathetic pathways and is perceived as deep and poorly localized. It may be projected to the surface in the cutaneous distribution of the spinal segment where the fibers integrate into the central nervous system. The sympathetic fibers accompanying the vascular tree mediate visceral ischemic pain, most commonly occurring with inflammation and somewhat better localized.

Somatic pain originates in the abdominal wall, particularly in the peritoneum, the diaphragm, and the root of the mesentery. It is well localized. Stretching, ischemia, and inflammation are the most common stimuli. Somatic pain is generally of later onset than visceral pain.

In the nonverbal child, abdominl pain is manifested by crying and drawing the legs up onto the abdomen. These observations are of greater significance than the subjective complaint "my tummy hurts."

Anorexia, Nausea, and Vomiting

Anorexia, nausea, and vomiting are nonspecific responses occurring in many pathophysiologic states, including metabolic and central nervous system disorders. When originating within the abdomen, they are usually associated with distension of a hollow viscus or mesenteric stretching and are a secondary response to low-level painful stimuli mediated by the parasympathetic system. Poor feeding is the equivalent of anorexia or nausea in the nonverbal infant. Vomiting occurs in response to the same painful stimuli. Vomiting associated with poor or refused feedings is also a manifestation of ileus resulting from neurogenic or ischemic stimuli and occurs in the young infant with generalized sepsis or the child with localized intra-abdominal sepsis. It is very important to differentiate the lack of interest in feeding from vomiting of feedings with eager acceptance of the next feeding. The latter is characteristic of gastric outlet obstruction as occurs in hypertrophic pyloric stenosis and may not be the result of any painful stimuli within the abdomen.

Changes in Bowel Habits

Bowel evacuation is usually coordinated with feeding, particularly in younger children. Changes in the pattern frequently accompany intra-abdominal or systemic disease. Neurogenic stimuli resulting in ileus, as seen in sepsis, usually curtail lower bowel activity. Conversely, increased defecation results from an irritative process within the lumen of the GI tract. Mucosal inflammation from viral or bacterial infection increases mucous secretion and net transfer of water into the bowel lumen, producing diarrhea. Blood in the intestinal tract stimulates peristalsis. The mixture of blood and increased mucous secretion is an important sign of intestinal ischemia and can be seen in ileocolic intussusception.

Tenderness

The abdominal examination represents a systemic manipulation of the abdomen to ascertain the voluntary and involuntary responses of the patient and to determine what elicits tenderness (increased pain).

Guarding

Another important "peritoneal" sign is involuntary guarding. If one envisions the abdomen as having two halves separated by the linea alba, the patient's response to light pressure on one side and then the other often supplies useful objective information. In the relaxed or distracted child, asymmetry in the muscular behavior between the sides of the abdominal wall is caused by involuntary guarding and must be interpreted as an objective sign of localized intra-abdominal pathology. Generalized peritonitis produces generalized involuntary guarding and eventually a rigid abdomen. Differentiation from voluntary guarding can be difficult but is greatly aided by distracting the patient.

Presence of a Mass

Recognition of an abdominal mass is facilitated by minimal pressure on the relaxed abdominal wall. Once stimulated painfully, the child voluntarily contracts the entire abdominal wall, making it difficult to define an abnormal mass. If the mass is not associated with tenderness, it is important to determine its characteristics, including location, size, shape, and mobility. A large bolus of stool can be expected to move with the bowel that contains it in a horizontal or vertical plane. Similarly, an ileocolic intussusception with the lead point within the transverse colon is felt as a very superficial mass in the upper abdomen and has vertical mobility. A large ovarian cyst or teratoma may be movable in a transverse plane within the hypogastrium or upper pelvis. The need for abdominal relaxation in palpation of a mass is best illustrated by comparing the apparent size of an appendiceal abscess determined in the emergency department with its size under general anesthesia. Complete muscular relaxation usually can greatly magnify the size of the mass or even reveal a mass that had not been appreciated previously.

Distention

Abdominal distension must be viewed in relation to overall appearance and judged within the context of normal variations. Children from 2 to 6 years of age usually have a protuberant abdomen and when lying supine may have a greatly exaggerated lumbar lordosis. The muscular tone of the anterior abdominal wall must be considered as well. The child who has little muscular resistance to moderate pressure but demonstrates a tight abdomen has significant abdominal distension. Such distension reflects gas or liquid within the intestinal tract or free within the peritoneal cavity. It is important to remember that accumulation of intraluminal air and fluid can occur with ileus from any cause. There are also many causes for ascites. Conversely, free intraperitoneal air always requires immediate surgical consultation.

Bowel Sounds

Changes in bowel sounds are of relative value because of the many generalized factors that influence abdominal autonomic tone. Auscultation is best employed to differentiate mechanical obstruction and intraluminal irritation, which tend to increase peristaltic activity and bowel sounds, from diseases that result in an adynamic ileus and "quiet abdomen."

EVALUATION

Evaluation of the child with abdominal pain must start with a careful history. The onset of pain and its relation to anorexia, nausea and vomiting, and trauma are important differentiating factors. The nature, quality, duration, severity, and location of pain must be determined, as well as factors that increase or decrease it. A history of similar symptoms in other family members or friends should be sought. One may then proceed to examine the entire child. However, discussion of only abdominal examination follows.

Abdominal examination is an organized process to determine both the response of the patient to stimulation of the abdomen and the presence of structural abnormalities. It begins with inspection for symmetry, distension, cutaneous lesions, and, in particular, evidence of inguinal or umbilical hernia. Auscultation is performed next. Only then can palpation begin. It is important to avoid the initial voluntary muscular response by starting with a slight stimulus. Gentle stroking of the skin over the anterior abdominal wall should be the first step in determining whether there is abdominal tenderness. Light pressure can then be applied in all four quadrants, gradually progressing to deeper palpation. It is wise to avoid areas of obvious tenderness until the end to minimize the child's voluntary anticipatory contraction of the entire abdominal wall. This provides more objective information about the degree and localization of abdominal tenderness. Palpation also allows identification of organomegaly and masses and aids in assessing the degree of distension. A greatly distended stomach or urinary bladder should be emptied before proceeding with the examination; percussion may be helpful in recognizing this. It is essential to palpate for inguinal and umbilical hernias and to inspect the external genitalia.

Rectal examination should be considered part of the evaluation. This is best accomplished with the child supine rather than in a decubitus or prone position. Cooperation can usually be obtained by gently displacing the perineum posteriorly and pausing until the child relaxes. Palpation is then performed for stool, masses, tenderness, and, in the female, the internal genitalia. The stool also must be evaluated.

Interpretation of persistent abdominal tenderness or distension after completing the physical examination usually is assisted by obtaining supine and decubitus abdominal roentgenograms. Decubitus films of the abdomen differentiate intraluminal from extraluminal distension and usually also demonstrate free air or fluid. Abnormal calcification or evidence of peritoneal inflammation may also be seen (Figure 15-1).

Initial laboratory evaluation of the child with abdominal pain should be minimal and directed by history and physical findings. Complete blood count and urinalysis, including microscopic examination, are generally sufficient. Determination of

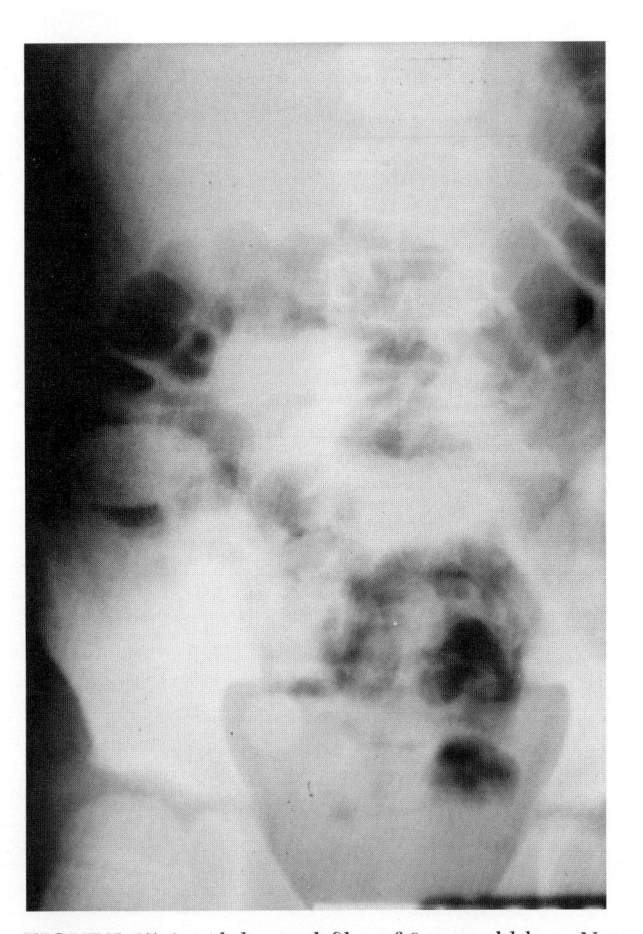

FIGURE 15-1 Abdominal film of 9-year-old boy. Note appendicolith in the right lower quadrant.

serum electrolyte levels is appropriate in the dehydrated child. Tests of hepatic, pancreatic, or renal function should be obtained only upon strong clinical indications.

DISEASES THAT DO NOT REQUIRE SURGERY

When evaluating children with abdominal pain, the emergency physician must recognize complaints and findings that indicate further surgical consultation. The physician is frequently confronted with conditions that mimic the clinical appearance of those requiring surgical intervention. It is therefore pertinent to briefly discuss the most important of these.

Enteric Infections

The most frequent abdominal complaint seen in the emergency department is a viral enteritis syndrome. These children may be febrile, complain of abdominal pain, and have a distended abdomen. Although most patients eventually have vomiting or diarrhea, both signs may be absent initially. Abdominal palpation usually reveals a soft, distended abdomen. If present, tenderness tends to be generalized rather than localized and is nonspecific. Involuntary guarding is absent. The severe crampy episodes of abdominal pain seen prior to the onset of diarrhea may be identical to those seen with intussusception. In some cases differentiation of a viral syndrome from an "acute abdomen" is difficult and may require surgical consultation.

Nonviral enteric infections also can produce a picture mimicking an acute abdomen. Gastroenteritis caused by staphylococci, salmonellae, and shigellae produces distension with abdominal pain. Bowel sounds are hyperactive, and the child usually has diarrhea, often bloody. Leukopenia with a relative lymphocytosis if often found. Occasionally, differentiation from intussusception is difficult and requires barium enema examination, but surgical consultation should precede this.

Sepsis

Generalized sepsis often produces signs and symptoms compatible with a primary intra-abdominal disorder, particularly in the neonate or young infant. These patients are distended and may have bilious vomiting. Other signs of sepsis such as hypotension, tachycardia, and tachypnea may be present. In septic patients abdominal distension is secondary to reflex ileus and is unassociated with abdominal tenderness or involuntary guarding. Bowel sounds are decreased or absent. The differential diagnosis of sepsis in the young child must consider sources in the central nervous system and the urinary tract, as well as sepsis originating within the abdomen.

Hematologic Disorders

Many hematologic disorders, including sickle cell disease, hemophilia, and neoplasm, can be complicated by episodes of acute abdominal pain. Most important is sickle cell disease, which affects 1 of every 500 blacks. Abdominal complications include pain crisis, ileus secondary to remote osteomyelitis, cholelithiasis, and congestive hepatomegaly. Abdominal crisis often is characterized by acute colicky pain, distension, and, possibly, nausea and vomiting. Distension and ileus can be secondary to vertebral body infarction or sepsis arising at a remote site. Physical examination reveals a soft abdomen with voluntary guarding that can be overcome. A history of sickle cell disease is essential for accurate diagnosis. Abdominal pain in the right upper quadrant may accompany passive distension of Glisson's capsule of the liver in patients with cardiomyopathy and congestive heart failure. This must be differentiated from abdominal pain accompanying complications of cholelithiasis, such as cholecystitis, choledocholithiasis, or pancreatitis.

Children with hemophilia or other bleeding disorders also may have abdominal distension and pain. Most often these are due to a retroperitoneal hematoma with secondary ileus and require only symptomatic treatment and specific attention to the underlying disorder. Children with neoplastic diseases can undergo rapid splenic or hepatic enlargement that produces upper abdominal discomfort. This is analogous to passive hepatomegaly in congestive heart failure and requires symptomatic measures only.

Metabolic-Collagen Disorders

A variety of metabolic, collagen, and vascular diseases can produce significant abdominal discomfort. In the adult, diabetic neuropathy is included in the differential diagnosis of the acute abdomen, but this is unusual in children. Other metabolic abnormalities such as porphyria are seen only rarely. Serositis associated with collagen disorders can result in alarming abdominal findings. Past history helps clarify the diagnosis.

Conditions of Uncertain Etiology

Henoch-Schönlein purpura and hemolytic-uremic syndrome represent two complex problems frequently confused with acute diseases that require surgical intervention. Many of these patients undergo exploratory laparotomy. Patients with these syndromes may have crampy abdominal pain, distension, and tenderness. Henoch-Schönlein purpura can follow a chronic course over a number of weeks. Colicky abdominal pain may precede development of the characteristic rash on the lower extremities and buttocks, making diagnosis difficult. Diffuse rectal bleeding can occur. Similarly, hemolytic-uremic syndrome often causes acute abdominal pain and rectal bleeding initially. Development of the characteristic hematologic abnormalities and evidence of renal failure usually occur later. Both conditions can produce alarming abdominal symptomatology, partially confirmed by physical examination. Differential diagnosis must include intussusception, and an emergency barium enema may be required for resolution; surgical consultation should be obtained during continued observation.

Trauma

Blunt abdominal and thoracic trauma must be included in the differential diagnosis of the acute abdomen. A history may be completely lacking. Evidence of trauma, including signs of child abuse, should be sought. A small amount of intraperitoneal bleeding can produce ileus, abdominal discomfort, tachycardia, and fever. Traumatic pancreatitis and pseudocyst also can occur.

DISEASES THAT REQUIRE SURGERY

In the sections that follow, the most important diseases that require surgery are ordered according to the common age of presentation, from infancy to adolescence. It is important to remember that some can be seen at any age.

Inguinal Hernia

Inguinal hernia is one of the most common congenital anomalies seen by pediatric surgeons. The hernia is frequently recognized during the early weeks or months of life, and the child often is brought to the emergency department because of a swollen inguinal area. The risk of incarceration is greater for younger children, 65% of incarceration cases occur during the first year of life. The child is often irritable and the inguinal bulge is easily diagnosed. If incarceration is of sufficient duration, abdominal distension and vomiting may be noted. Plain roentgenograms may have the appearance of a small-bowel obstruction. Air is occasionally seen in the scrotum. An incarcerated hernia can progress to ischemic compromise of the hernial contents, usually small bowel and a tender, erythematous scrotum. Immediate surgical exploration is indicated for this complication. More frequently, the hernial contents are not compromised and can be reduced. After successful reduction the child should be hospitalized for semielective repair within the next 48 to 72 hours. Even in the absence of strangulation, immediate surgical exploration is required if the hernia cannot be reduced.

Midgut Volvulus

Anomalous rotation of the small bowel with subsequent midgut volvulus is the most devastating surgical catastrophe occurring in children. The majority of patients become symptomatic during the first month of life, although midgut volvulus can occur at any age, including adulthood. A previously well child has the onset of abdominal distension, colicky pain, and bilious vomiting. Mesenteric vascular compromise rapidly leads to intestinal ischemia and can progress to loss of the entire intestinal tract unless prompt surgical intervention is undertaken. Similar episodes with spontaneous resolution may be reported by older patients. Immediate surgical consultation must be sought before any additional evaluation is performed.

Hirschsprung's Enterocolitis

Hirschsprung's enterocolitis is a potentially fatal complication of Hirschsprung's disease (aganglionic megacolon). Ten percent of newborns with unrecognized Hirschsprung's disease develop this complication during the first month of life; the incidence increases to 30% during the second month and an additional 30% during the third month. Children have abdominal distension and often vomiting. Obstipation or passage of liquid stools can occur. When seen in the emergency department, these patients have severe intravascular dehydration and hypovolemic shock. Differentiation from septic shock is difficult. In the latter a quiet abdomen is found rather than the hyperactive obstructive bowel sounds found with enterocolitis. A history of poor bowel evacuation since birth is helpful in the diagnosis. Radiologic evaluation suggests small-bowel obstruction with multiple airfluid levels. Enterocolitis produces rapid sequestration of fluid in the lumen and wall of the functionally obstructed "normal" bowel. Immediate supportive measures include large volumes of intravenous fluids and nasogastric and rectal intubations. Neonatal diagnosis and appropriate diversion of the intestinal tract prevent enterocolitis until definitive reconstructive surgery can be performed.

Intussusception

Intussusception is the most important acute surgical problem in older infants and preschool-age children. Classically, these children are between 6 and 24 months of age and are robust and healthy. Boys are affected more commonly than girls. There is sudden onset of crampy abdominal pain characterized by drawing of the legs up onto the abdomen. The pain spontaneously disappears only to occur again in a short while. Vomiting may be associated. The classic "currant jelly" stools formed by mucus mixed with blood do not appear until significant intestinal ischemia has occurred. Except during episodes of pain, abdominal examination can be misleading. The child is quiet and relaxed, the abdomen soft and nontender. The classic midepigastric sausage-shaped mass may be palpated. However, while the leading edge of the intussusception is posterior to the edge of the liver, it will not be palpable. Plain films of the abdomen may reveal absence of gas in the right lower quadrant of the intussusception itself. Barium enema reduction is curative in the majority of cases but should never be attempted without prior surgical consultation. Intussusception in a very young child is generally not associated with a demonstrable lead point. Intussusception occurring later, beyond 6 years of age, is likely to have a pathologic lead point. Intussusception is also commonly seen in children with cystic fibrosis, secondary to thickened intestinal secretions causing "meconium ileus equivalent."

Appendicitis

In school-age children acute appendicitis begins to play the prominent role it will continue to display throughout the remainder of the first and second decades of life. The classic symptoms begin with anorexia, followed by nonspecific midabdominal discomfort and pain. Vomiting frequently occurs but is not a continuous symptom in most cases. The initial pain is visceral in origin in response to distension of the obstructed appendix. Because of its visceral nature, it is poorly localized and is perceived as generalized and midabdominal. Once localized inflammation of the peritoneum and mesentery develop, the pain shifts toward the right lower quadrant as somatic stimuli become more dominant. At this time cutaneous hypesthesia and localized tenderness in the right lower quadrant develop.

Laboratory findings in a child with acute appendicitis include a mild leukocytosis with a shift toward immature forms. Determination of serum electrolyte levels is rarely indicated unless prolonged vomiting or diarrhea have been part of the clinical features. Radiologic evaluation is often nonspecific, perhaps showing signs of peritoneal inflammation with loss of the right fat stripe or scoliosis of the lumbar spine. A fecalith may be present. Prior to taking a child to the operating room, it is important to eliminate the possibility that pneumonia in the right lower lobe is producing abdominal symptoms.

The classic history and physical findings of acute appendicitis are not frequently seen in the emergency department. Children with an unusually placed appendix, particularly a rectocecal appendix, have an atypical history with a long delay in localization of somatic pain. Rectal examination is frequently essential to help differentiate between acute appendicitis and the many causes of abdominal pain that are treated medically. If any doubt exists concerning the diagnosis, surgical consultation is mandatory. It is quite appropriate to admit these children for observation rather than discharge them for observation at home by the family.

Biliary Tract Disorders

Cholelithiasis begins to play a more prominent role in adolescents. Gallstones occur in teenagers without other illnesses but are most common in children with hematologic disorders, particularly sickle cell disease. Complications of cholelithiasis include acute cholecystitis, choledocholithiasis, and pancreatitis. Pain in the right upper quadrant, frequently making the patient extremely restless, is characteristic. Serum bilirubin levels are elevated, even above the common mild elevation of patients with chronic hemolysis. Obstructive patterns of hepatic enzyme elevation are often seen, as well as leukocytosis. Surgical complications of cholelithiasis should be handled according to the guidelines appropriate for older patients with gallstones.

Gynecologic Disorders

Torsion of an ovarian cyst, particularly on the right side, may be indistinguishable from acute appendicitis. Surgical consultation and possibly ultrasonography may be necessary to establish the diagnosis. Acute pelvic inflammatory disease is seen with increasing frequency in pediatric emergency departments. A history of sexual activity may not always be obtained. Examination in these patients should include cervical culture, and treatment should follow guidelines for older patients with pelvic inflammatory disease. Dysmenorrhea and mittelschmertz also first appear in the adolescent girl. Finally, some young girls are seen with monthly abdominal pains of recent onset but no history of menarche. Examination may reveal a suprapubic mass confirmed on rectal palpation. An imperforate hymen with hematocolpos must be considered.

Peptic Ulcer Disease

Peptic ulcer disease occurs in the teenage population and can lead to perforation without an antecedent history. These patients have a rigid, boardlike abdomen that eventually demonstrates free intraperitoneal air. Surgical intervention is essential. Less dramatic complications of peptic ulcer disease also occur in younger children, including penetrating ulcer and bleeding. Emergency surgical intervention is infrequently indicated but appropriate consultation should be obtained.

Trauma

Abdominal trauma must be considered as a cause for surgical intervention in a child of any age. Penetrating trauma always requires surgical consultation and frequently abdominal exploration. Blunt abdominal trauma is more difficult to manage but requires surgical intervention less frequently, although conservative nonsurgical management must be carried out by the surgical service.

CONCLUSION

The emergency physician must frequently evaluate children who have acute abdominal pain. The majority of these patients have diseases that do not require surgery, and many can be managed on an outpatient basis. The role of the emergency physician is to recognize those children with more serious medical and surgical problems requiring admission and specialized consultation.

Many pathophysiologic states can produce abdominal distension, ileus, and pain. In the young infant these are frequently infectious in origin, and early recognition can prevent overwhelming, catastrophic complications. Recognition of emergencies that require surgery can be facilitated by familiarity with historical and clinical patterns. The most important step in diagnosis is abdominal examination. Involuntary guarding, peritoneal irritability, and an abdominal mass are all strong indications for surgical consultation. The surgeons should make the final differentiation between illnesses requiring emergent surgical intervention and those in which either medical or surgical observation is appropriate.

References

1. Valman HB: ABC of 1 to 7: Acute abdominal pain. *Br Med J* 1981;282:1858.
2. Knight J, Vassy E: Specific diseases mimicking appendicitis in childhood. *Arch Surg* 1981;116:74.
3. Cope Z: *The acute abdomen in rhyme*, ed 5. London, HK Lewis & Co Ltd, 1972.

Richard J. Andrassy

16 Gastrointestinal Bleeding

The physician confronted by a child with GI bleeding and anxious parents frequently encounters a diagnostic and management dilemma. Despite the availability of many sophisticated diagnostic techniques, these are not generally of much value in early diagnosis and management. The exact cause of the bleeding may often go undetermined, but fortunately, repeat bleeding in these patients is rare. In truth, other than the small size of the patient, the frequently poor history, and the overestimation of blood loss by the parents, the approach to diagnosis is quite clear. It is based on a firm understanding of the few truly surgical emergencies, thus leading to early diagnosis and to medical management or operative intervention, whichever is appropriate.

INITIAL MANAGEMENT

Children have the ability to maintain their blood pressure despite significant blood loss because of their ability to vasoconstrict. Correction of moderate hypovolemia based on urine output and monitoring of vital signs is perhaps the most accurate and simplest means of early management. Severe hypovolemia may require central venous pressure monitoring in selected cases. Urine output should be maintained at approximately 1 to 2 mL/kg/h in the small child and 1 mL/kg/h in the older child. Initial bolus replacement with lactated Ringer's solution at 20 mL/kg, followed by blood replacement with packed red cells at 5 mL/kg or whole blood at 10 mL/kg, is appropriate when significant bleeding and hypovolemia are present. A nasogastric tube is placed temporarily to help determine the level of bleeding. The aspiration of gross blood or "coffee-ground" material immediately localizes the bleeding point to the esophagus, stomach, or duodenum. If the nasogastric tube should drain clear or bile-stained material, the source of hemorrhage is distal to the ligament of Treitz. Physical examination may reveal some clues related to rare causes of bleeding, such as hemangiomas or melanin spots on the skin. Bruises and petechiae on the skin or nasal bleeding can indicate some systemic bleeding disorders. Examination for evidence of an enlarged spleen, abdominal masses, or anal fissures can also aid in limiting the differential diagnosis. By following an organized rational approach and utilizing diagnostic procedures as needed, physicians can undoubtedly decrease the number of "undetermined" causes of GI bleeding in children.

UPPER GASTROINTESTINAL BLEEDING

A general approach to the initial evaluation of the infant or the child with upper GI bleeding is shown in Exhibit 16-1.

Exhibit 16-1 Evaluation of Upper GI Bleeding

1. History for bleeding disorders, skin lesions, and aspirin or steroid ingestion
2. Physical examination for presence of enlarged liver, spleen, masses, ascites, or evidence of trauma or portal hypertension
3. Bleeding studies
4. Treat; if no response—endoscopy
5. Contrast studies if bleeding stops
6. Persistent bleeding or recurrence—endoscopy

Neonates

Upper GI bleeding in the neonate is a relatively common occurrence, but fortunately it is generally limited in nature, and only rarely does massive bleeding occur. The majority of babies with either hematemesis or blood-tinged nasogastric aspirate can be treated by simple medical therapy without extensive evaluation or surgical intervention. It is important to obtain an adequate history regarding the volume of blood passed as well as the length of time the baby has been bleeding. Bleeding during the first 24 hours of life is most often due to ingested maternal blood. This is easily confirmed by the Apt test, which measures reduced fetal hemoglobin (Figure 16-1).[1] Hemorrhagic disease of the newborn is relatively rare since most newborns are given vitamin K in the delivery room. Its presence may be suggested by ecchymoses or petechiae or a history of maternal medication shortly before delivery. Blood studies, including complete blood count, prothrombin time, partial thromboplastin time, and platelet count, can be obtained or the baby can be empirically treated with vitamin K. A baby under 1 week of age should be admitted for evaluation, while babies over 1 week of age who have minor bleeding can be observed closely as outpatients. If a normal prothrombin time has ruled out hemorrhagic disease of the newborn and a negative Apt test eliminates swallowed maternal blood as a cause, the baby most frequently has stress gastritis or ulcers as a cause of bleeding and should be initially treated without further diagnostic intervention. A flow diagram for the evaluation of upper GI bleeding in neonatal patients is shown in Figure 16-2.

In a review of 94 neonates with GI bleeding, Sherman and Clatworthy[2] reported that 50% had hematemesis, 33% had bright red rectal bleeding, and 17% had melena. In this study no babies had a lesion requiring urgent surgical intervention, and 49 patients had "unexplained" bleeding. However, patients with obstruction, peritonitis, sepsis, or other disease states were not included in their review. In the children for whom a diagnosis was made, most upper GI bleeding was due to swallowed blood or hemorrhagic disease of the newborn, and most lower GI bleeding was due to anorectal trauma (fissures). There were no deaths in patients with unexplained bleeding. All patients were admitted to the hospital; therefore, this study does not include patients treated as outpatients. Serious massive hemorrhage requiring surgical consultation may be seen infrequently and should be considered in any neonate with persistent or recurrent bouts of bleeding. Bleeding duodenal ulcer or stress gastritis has been seen and can lead to rapid exsanguination if not rapidly treated.[3]

Mix 1 part stool or vomitus with 5 parts H_2O
Centrifuge the mixture and remove 5 mL (pink)

Add
1 mL 1% NaOH
Wait 2 minutes

Remains pink
(Fetal blood)

Turns brown-yellow
(Maternal blood)

FIGURE 16-1 Apt-Downey test used to distinguish maternal from fetal hemoglobin. (Reprinted with permission from Apt L, Downey WS Jr: "Melena" neonatorum: The swallowed blood syndrome. A simple test for the differentiation of adult and fetal hemoglobin in bloody stools. *J Pediatr* 1955;47:6.)

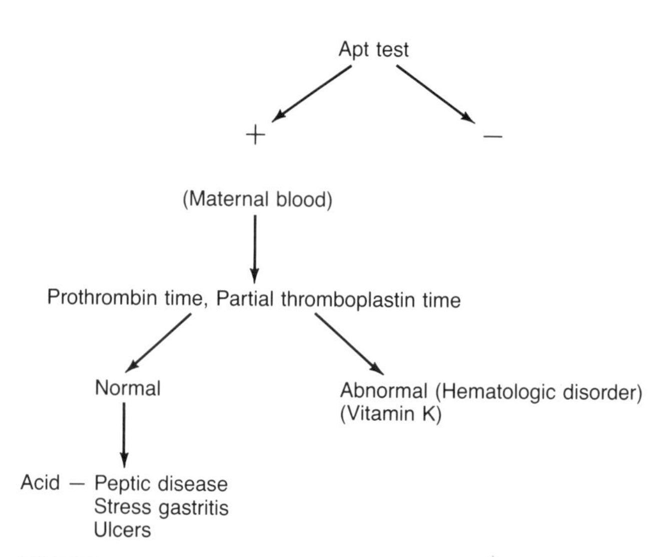

FIGURE 16-2 Evaluation of upper GI bleeding in the neonate.

Children under 1 Year of Age

The causes of GI hemorrhage in children under 1 year of age are shown in Table 16-1. Upper GI bleeding was seen in only 18 of 158 patients in this group. This study was done prior to the advent of endoscopy, and since superficial ulcerations and erosions are not visualized by conventional radiologic studies, many lesions may have been missed. Today, with experience, endoscopy can be performed in small infants and children. With more frequent use of endoscopy, esophagitis secondary to reflux (Figure 16-3) and leading to anemia has been recognized more frequently, although complications of esophagitis are more often seen in the somewhat older patient. Variceal bleeding does not generally occur until the child is approximately 2 to 3 years of age or older. Children less than 1 year of age who have hematemesis can generally be suspected of having ulcer disease and are managed very similarly to the adult patient. Prevention of stress ulceration by using antacids, defined formula diets, and perhaps cimetidine is warranted for the seriously ill child at risk for stress gastritis or ulceration.[4]

Children over 1 Year of Age

The most common causes of GI hemorrhage in children over 1 year of age are shown in Table 16-2.[3] Esophageal variceal bleeding secondary to portal hypertension is the most common cause of serious upper GI bleeding in this age group, followed by peptic ulcer disease. Variceal bleeding most frequently occurs unexpectedly and massively in patients who have been previously in apparent good health. Frequent occurrences during a several year period are not uncommon. This diagnosis should be considered when rapid bleeding occurs and a large

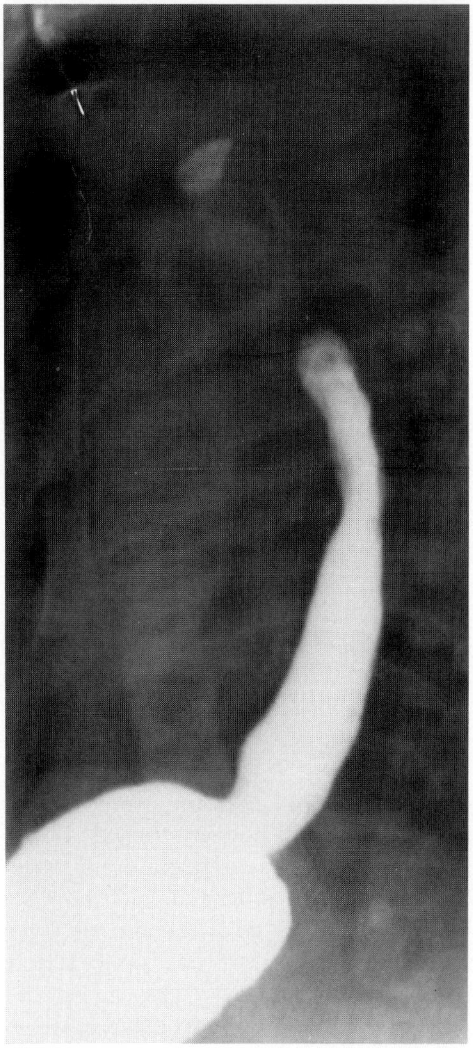

FIGURE 16-3 Gastroesophageal reflux in a 6-month-old child with failure to thrive and anemia secondary to esophagitis.

TABLE 16-1 Causes of GI Hemorrhage in 158 Patients under 1 Year of Age

Disorder	No. of patients
Anal fissure	68
Intussusception	50
Gangrenous bowel	14
Duodenal ulcers	10
Gastric ulcers	8
Meckel's diverticulum	6
Ileal hematoma	1
Duplication—colon	1
Colonic polyps	0
Esophageal varices	0

Source: Adapted with permission from Spencer R: Gastrointestinal hemorrhage in infancy and childhood: 476 cases. *Surgery* 1964;55:719.

TABLE 16-2 Causes of GI Hemorrhage in 119 Patients over 1 Year of Age

Disorder	No. of patients
Colonic polyps	59
Anal fissure	15
Intussusception	11
Esophageal varices	11
Gastric ulcers	9
Duodenal ulcers	7
Ulcerative colitis	3
Meckel's diverticulum	2
Regional enteritis	1
Hemorrhoid	1

Source: Adapted with permission from Spencer R: Gastrointestinal hemorrhage in infancy and childhood: 476 cases. *Surgery* 1964;55:719.

spleen is palpated on physical examination. The liver function tests are generally normal since the block is prehepatic in the portal vein. A barium esophagram to demonstrate portal varices may be helpful. Splenoportography to demonstrate the anatomy can be done after hospitalization and stabilization.[5] The enlarged spleen and thrombocytopenia have led many an unwary physician to consider splenectomy. This is definitely not to be done as a means of treatment for portal hypertension. The acute bleeding is usually tolerated and stops with conservative management.[6] This includes admission to the intensive care unit, correction of hypovolemia, and establishment of a good urine output. Mild sedation is generally helpful, and, on occasion, a pediatric Sengstaken-Blakemore tube can be used to tamponade the bleeding. The frequency and occurrence of bleeding are generally unpredictable but usually decrease with age and the development of natural collateral decompressing vessels. Occasionally, portal decompression by a variety of shunt techniques or injection of the varices with sclerosing agents is necessary. Most children, however, can be managed conservatively in the short-term situation.

Another cause of esophageal bleeding that is more frequently recognized now by the use of endoscopy is the Mallory-Weiss syndrome. This lesion has been reported in a 15-year-old patient.[7] Mallory-Weiss syndrome can go unrecognized if not suspected and if the patient is not subjected to esophagoscopy for diagnosis.

Anemia or stricture secondary to esophagitis is seen most commonly in the patient over 3 years of age. Although reflux is more common in the younger patient, the complications of reflux related to the esophagus are seen in the somewhat older patient. An outline of the most common causes of upper GI bleeding in children is shown in Exhibit 16-2.

Exhibit 16-2 "Common" Causes of Upper GI Bleeding in Children over 1 Year of Age

- Esophagus
  - Varices
  - Esophagitis
  - Mallory-Weiss syndrome
  - Duplication cyst
- Stomach
  - Gastric erosions
  - Ulcer
  - Duplications
  - Tumor
  - Hematoma
  - Pyloric stenosis
- Duodenum
  - Duodenitis
  - Duodenal erosions
  - Ulcer
  - Hemobilia
  - Hematoma
- Nonspecific
  - Swallowed maternal blood
  - Hemorrhagic disease
  - Nosebleed

Source: Adapted with permission from Gryboski J, Walker WA: *Gastrointestinal Problems in the Infant,* ed 2. Philadelphia, WB Saunders Co, 1983, p 86.

RECTAL BLEEDING

Neonates

A flow diagram for the initial evaluation of rectal bleeding in the neonate is shown in Figure 16-4. The three most common causes of lower GI bleeding in the neonate include fissures, necrotizing enterocolitis, and malrotation with volvulus. Fissures are seen by gently spreading the buttocks and are treated symptomatically with stool softeners and sitz baths. Necrotizing enterocolitis is diagnosed by abdominal films and physical examination and is initially treated medically. Obvious signs of obstruction or bilious vomiting in conjunction with rectal bleeding should suggest the possibility of malrotation, volvulus, and early mucosal ischemia. This is truly an urgent condition requiring immediate intervention. Eight of 74 babies with malrotation at the Children's Hospital at Los Angeles had bloody stools, while only 1 had frankly necrotic bowel at celiotomy.[8] This condition generally involves vomiting as well as rectal bleeding and should lead to an early diagnosis, which is generally made by barium enema and/or upper GI barium studies. Duplications of the intestine may be associated with massive rectal bleeding, either from mucosal ulceration or intussusception with ischemia. This is a rather rare occurrence. Bleeding from Meckel's diverticulum is more frequently seen in babies over 1 month of age, although it too has been reported in the neonate. Other causes of rectal bleeding in the neonate are shown in Exhibit 16-3.

Children under 1 Year of Age

The major causes of GI hemorrhage in 158 patients from one reported study are shown in Table 16-1.[3] A complete list of the causes of rectal bleeding, in

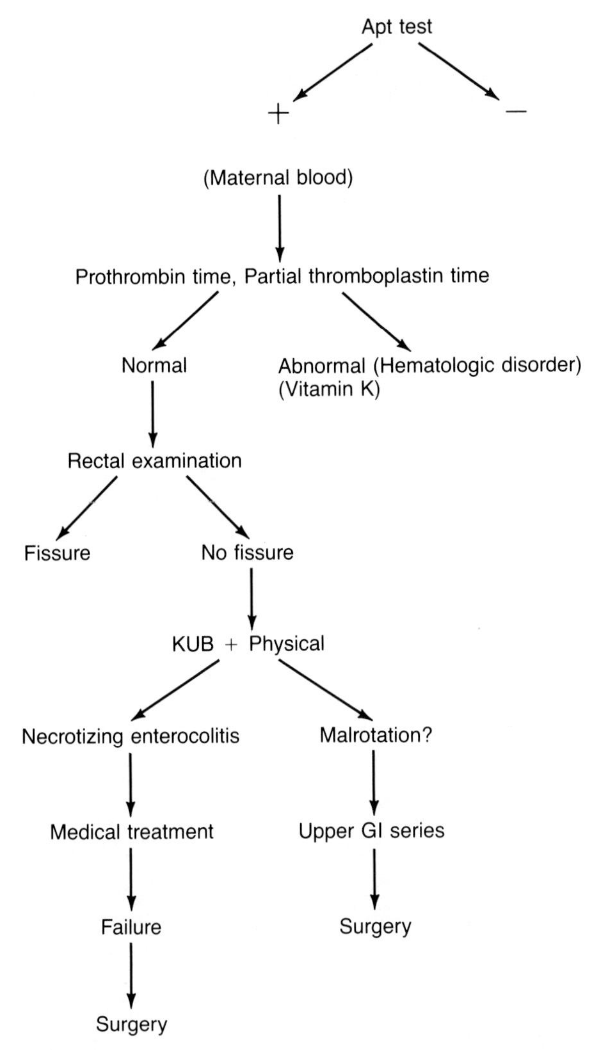

FIGURE 16-4 Evaluation of rectal bleeding in the neonate.

Exhibit 16-3 Causes of Rectal Bleeding in the Neonate

Swallowed maternal blood
Anal fissure
Gangrenous bowel
Infection
Milk allergy
Antibiotics
Peptic ulcer
Meckel's diverticulum
Duplication cyst
Intussusception
Arteriovenous malformation
Colitis of immune deficiency
Tumor
Entercolitis of Hirschsprung's disease

Source: Adapted with permission from Gryboski J, Walker WA: *Gastrointestinal Problems in the Infant,* ed 2. Philadelphia, WB Saunders Co, 1983, p 89.

order of frequency in children under 1 year of age, is shown in Exhibit 16-4. During the first year of life, the major causes of rectal bleeding leading to surgical consultation include anal fissure, intussusception, and gangrenous bowel. Volvulus may be seen in this group but is much less common than in the neonate. Meckel's diverticulum is occasionally observed in the 6- to 12-month age group but most commonly is seen in the child 1 to 2 years of age. As in the neonate, anal fissures are treated symptomatically with stool softeners and warm sitz baths. Chronic fissures can be treated with dilatation or lateral sphincterotomy.

Intussusception is a relatively common cause of lower GI bleeding in the child under 1 year of age. The greatest incidence occurs in infants 4 to 10 months of age. The majority of these infants are well-nourished, healthy boys. Many such children have a recent history of upper respiratory tract infection, otitis media, or gastroenteritis. Intermittent attacks of severe crying, stiffening, vomiting, and straining may be reported. The baby typically has normal resting periods between bouts of pain. As the course progresses, the stools may be tinged with blood, or bloody mucoid clots—"currant jelly" stools—are passed. On physical examination there may be a sausage-shaped mass present within the abdomen and signs of partial bowel obstruction. On rare occasions the intussusception appears as a prolapse of the bowel through the anal opening. This should not be mistaken for simple rectal prolapse and reduced. A lubricated tongue blade or cotton-tipped applicator should be passed along the side of

Exhibit 16-4 Causes of Rectal Bleeding in the Child under 1 Year of Age

Anal fissure
Infection
Milk or soy allergy
Antibiotics
Intussusception
Lymphoid hyperplasia—colon
Gangrenous bowel
Meckel's diverticulum
Polyp
Hematoma
Duplication cyst
Arteriovenous malformation
Peptic ulcer
Foreign body
Tumor
Gastric heterotopia in ileum

Source: Adapted with permission from Gryboski J, Walker WA: *Gastrointestinal Problems in the Infant,* ed 2. Philadelphia, WB Saunders Co, 1983, p 89.

the protruding mass before reduction is attempted. If the applicator can be inserted more than a centimeter or two into the anal ring, the diagnosis of intussusception should be considered. While routine laboratory studies are obtained, the surgeon and radiologist should be notified. An early attempt at barium reduction under fluoroscopy, with the surgeon in attendance, is warranted. If the patient is acutely ill or has signs of peritonitis, this can be forgone and early surgical intervention employed. Otherwise the patient can have a barium enema for diagnosis; as many as 50% to 80% of patients may have the intussusception reduced by barium pressure. The barium must reflux into the terminal ileum to be sure that the reduction is complete. This study can be repeated if recurrent intussusception occurs. Approximately 5% to 10% of patients, particularly in the older age group, have a lead point, whereas most children less than 1 year of age have no definite lead point. If hydrostatic reduction is unsuccessful, the patient should be started on antibiotics, provided adequate hydration, and taken immediately to the operating room for manual reduction.[9,10]

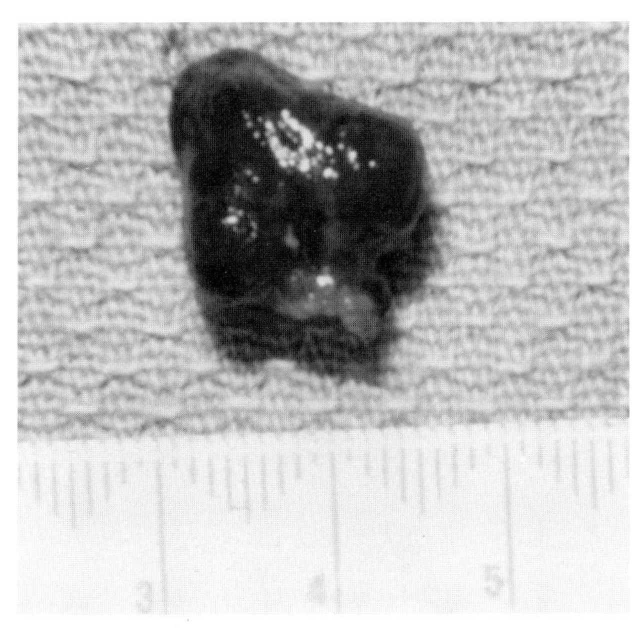

FIGURE 16-5 Juvenile polyp resected with the colonoscope.

Children over 1 Year of Age

In the child over 1 year of age, the most common cause of rectal bleeding, as reported by Spencer,[3] is juvenile polyps (Table 16-2). This type of polyp accounts for about 80% of childhood polyps, whereas lymphoid polyps rank a distant second. True adenomatous polyps are very rare and occur in less than 3% of children with polyps. Another rare polyp in childhood is the hamartomatous polyp associated with the Peutz-Jeghers syndrome. The most common age for children who have bleeding rectal "juvenile" polyps is 3 to 10 years, with a peak at approximately 5 to 6 years of age.[11] Occasionally, the polyp prolapses out of the anus or can be palpated simply by rectal examination. Others are seen with the proctoscope or on colonoscopy. The majority of patients undergo colonoscopy to rule our other polyps and to endoscopically remove these lesions (Figure 16-5).[12] Barium enemas given at 6-month intervals are used to follow unresected polyps (Figure 16-6). Juvenile polyps generally cause intermittent, recurrent, bright to dark red bleeding with stools, but it is rare to see massive rectal bleeding. Occasionally, these polyps outgrow their blood supply and pass spontaneously.

Anal fissure remains a common cause of rectal bleeding in the child over 1 year of age but is less common beyond 2 to 3 years of age. Massive bleed-

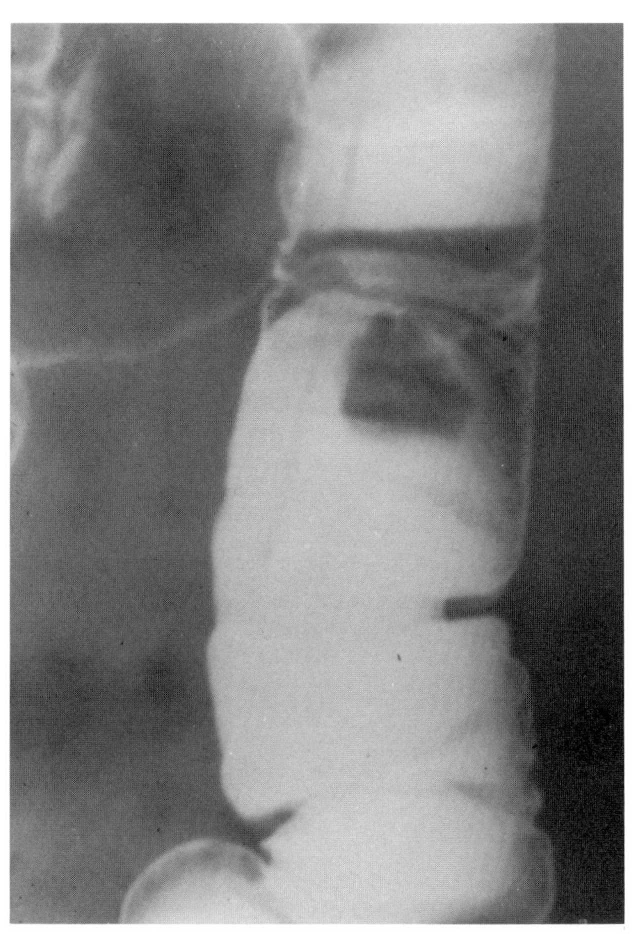

FIGURE 16-6 Barium enema showing a polyp in a 6-year-old child with rectal bleeding.

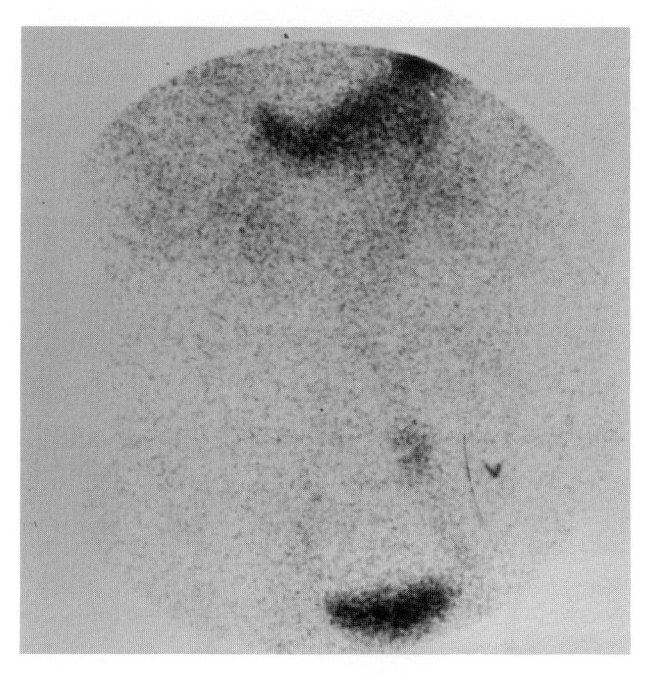

FIGURE 16-7 Scan with technetium-99m pertechnetate showing presence of Meckel's diverticulum with gastric mucosa.

ing via the rectum is most frequently associated with Meckel's diverticulum.[13,14] The majority of patients that are symptomatic from Meckel's diverticulum are seen in early childhood as a result of hemorrhage, obstruction, or diverticulitis. Bleeding is usually painless but on occasion is associated with crampy, midabdominal pain. The diverticulum can be demonstrated by technetium-99m pertechnetate injection and imaging (Figure 16-7).[15] If results are positive, this technique is very helpful, but there is a high incidence of false-negative. Barium contrast studies are completely unreliable. Persistent bleeding in the absence of positive diagnostic studies warrants surgical exploration. Other causes of rectal bleeding in the child over 1 year of age are shown in Exhibit 16-5.

Exhibit 16-5 Causes of Rectal Bleeding in the Child over 1 Year of Age

Anal fissure
Infection
Intussusception
Polyp
Lymphoid hyperplasia—colon
Meckel's diverticulum
Milk allergy
Antibiotics
Hematoma
Arteriovenous malformation
Colitis
Tumor
Gastric heterotopia in ileum

Source: Adapted with permission from Gryboski J, Walker WA: *Gastrointestinal Problems in the Infant,* ed 2. Philadelphia, WB Saunders Co, 1983, p 89.

CONCLUSION

A careful, orderly approach to resuscitation and diagnosis usually eliminates life-threatening causes of GI bleeding. Early consultation and a cooperative approach with the pediatric surgeon can lead to rapid evaluation and treatment. Fortunately, most pediatric patients with bleeding can be managed medically, but early surgical consultation can prevent delays in operative intervention if rapid bleeding persists.

References

1. Apt L, Downey WS Jr: "Melena" neonatorum: The swallowed blood syndrome. A simple test for the differentiation of adult and fetal hemoglobin in bloody stools. *J Pediatr* 1955;47:6–12.
2. Sherman NJ, Clatworthy HW Jr: Gastrointestinal bleeding in neonates: A study of 94 cases. *Surgery* 1967;62:614–620.
3. Spencer R: Gastrointestinal hemorrhage in infancy and childhood: 467 cases. *Surgery* 1964;55:718–734.
4. Cox K, Ament ME: Upper gastrointestinal bleeding in children and adolescents. *Pediatrics* 1979;63:408–413.
5. Weitzman JJ, Stanley P: Splenoportography in the pediatric age group. *J Pediatr Surg* 1978;13:707–712.
6. Fonkalsrud EW, Myers NA, Robinson MJ: Management of extrahepatic portal hypertension in children. *Ann Surg* 1974;180:487–491.
7. Countryman D, Norwood S, Andrassy RJ: Mallory-Weiss syndrome in children. *South Med J* 1982;75:1426–1427.
8. Andrassy RJ, Mahour GH: Malrotation of the midgut in infants and children. *Arch Surg* 1981;116:158–161.
9. Ein SH, Stephens CA: Intussusception: 354 cases in 10 years. *J Pediatr Surg* 1971;6:16–27.
10. Rosenkrantz JG, Cox JA, Silverman FN, et al: Intussusception in the 1970s: Indications for operation. *J Pediatr Surg* 1977;12:367–373.
11. Louw JH: Polypoid lesions of the large bowel in children with particular reference to benign lymphoid polyposis. *J Pediatr Surg* 1968;3:195–209.
12. Gleason WA Jr, Goldstein PD, Shatz BA, et al: Co-

lonoscopic removal of juvenile colonic polyps. *J Pediatr Surg* 1975;10:519–521.
13. Rutherford RB, Akers DR: Meckel's diverticulum: A review of 148 pediatric patients, with special reference to the pattern of bleeding and to mesodiverticular vascular bands. *Surgery* 1966;59:618–626.
14. Mequid M, Canty T, Eraklis AJ: Complications of Meckel's diverticulum in infants. *Surg Gynecol Obstet* 1974;139:541–544.
15. Jewett TC, Duszynski DO, Allen JE: The visualization of Meckel's diverticulum with 99m Tc-pertechnetate. *Surgery* 1970;68:567–570.

J. J. Tepas III

17 Abdominal Trauma

The two most common causes of traumatic death in childhood are neurologic, from closed head injuries, and hemorrhagic, from thoracoabdominal injuries.[1] Significant abdominal injuries are characteristically present with some degree of hypovolemia, and, unless expeditiously identified and treated, may rapidly progress to death. An organized, logical approach to the evaluation of the child with abdominal trauma is an absolute necessity if any improvement in the survival rate for these injuries is to be expected.

CHARACTERISTICS OF THE CHILD AS A TRAUMA VICTIM

Before childhood injuries can be intelligently assessed, consideration must be given to some of the unique anatomic characteristics of the child. Of major significance is the increased size ratio of the head and trunk to the extremities. This ratio is at its greatest in early childhood and progressively decreases to adult proportions as the child reaches adolescence. As a result there is an accumulation of vital organs close to the ground, where bumpers and fenders can exert maximum force on impact. Likewise, the small size of the child's abdomen places many vital organs in close proximity, through which impacting forces must dissipate. This increases the incidence of multiple-organ injury, which is of paramount importance in the evaluation of the injured child.

The relative size of a child's abdominal organs is somewhat different than the adult's and changes more significantly with growth and minor disease processes. The liver is larger in relation to the rest of the abdominal cavity, contains less fibrous stroma, and is therefore more vulnerable to applied force. In addition, the rib cage, which in the adult provides rigid protection, is less calcified and more horizontally flared. This provides a more resilient, less encompassing cover that is capable of transmitting more force to underlying organs.

Children generally have less body fat than adults, are less well insulated, and usually have a greater degree of mobility in supportive ligaments and connective tissue. All of these characteristics produce a "target" in which more energy will be efficiently transmitted to more tissues than a similar injury in an adult.

CLINICAL FEATURES

By definition abdominal injuries involve damage or disruption of solid or hollow viscera. The effect of peritoneal contamination by spilled contents of hollow viscera, while potentially life-threatening, is usually not manifest immediately after injury. Peritonitis and sepsis that proceed from rupture of the

GI tract evolve over a matter of hours and demand careful evaluation and reevaluation for timely diagnosis. By far the most important, immediate threat to the life of a child with an abdominal injury is hemorrhage.[1,2] Triage and treatment must therefore proceed in a rapid and orderly manner as soon as these patients arrive in the emergency department.

IMMEDIATE ASSESSMENT

The cool, pale patient in obvious shock with hypotension, tachycardia, and absent capillary refill is rarely missed. Immediate management goes without saying and should be automatic for the emergency physician.

Of a more insidious nature, however, is "evolving shock." This occurs in the child whose injury produces a rate of hemorrhage that can be temporarily negated by the normal reflex vasoconstriction that occurs in response to hemorrhage. These children initially may have a slight tachycardia as the only sign of their progressing hypovolemia. Erroneously reassured by these otherwise "stable" vital signs, the unwary physician may initially underestimate the child's condition. As the amount of blood loss begins to exceed the ability to maintain mean arterial pressure, the child rapidly plunges into profound shock from which resuscitation may be impossible. Tragically, this can occur when the patient is awaiting some minor diagnostic test at a location remote from the primary treatment area. It is absolutely essential, therefore, that the pediatric trauma patient be placed in an environment where adequate observation and close monitoring of time are provided by personnel experienced in the resuscitation of children.[2] No child's vital signs should be considered stable until multiple evaluations have established a reliable pattern.

Large-volume hemorrhage is the prime concern in children with abdominal injuries.[2,3] Lesions resulting in this degree of blood loss commonly produce signs of an enlarging accumulation of blood within the abdomen. Distension, then, is one of the first signs of major abdominal injury. Since the presence of even small amounts of blood within the peritoneum can produce irritation, tenderness is another commonly associated feature of these injuries. Finally, any superficial injury to the trunk, such as abrasions or ecchymoses, can indicate a significant injury within. Here again, the initial assessment of the child's abdomen should be viewed as only the first point on a curve. Repeat physical examinations, preferably by the same examiner, remain the most reliable means of identifying increasing abdominal tenderness and distension.

INITIAL MANAGEMENT

The same priorities of management that apply to any life-threatening emergency apply to the child with severe abdominal injury. An adequate airway with appropriate ventilation and oxygenation must be confirmed or established. What little circulating volume may be present on admission is of no value if adequate oxygenation is not possible.

Intravenous Access

The major priority in treatment of severe abdominal trauma is adequate treatment of hemorrhagic shock. At least two large-bore intravenous lines must be established immediately. While this one thing is frequently considered the most difficult aspect of the immediate care of the severely injured child, it need not be so if a few basic principles are remembered. Since the abdominal cavity is most commonly the site of severe, exsanguinating injury, the first and most important principle to be considered is the possibility that intravenous fluid given below the diaphragm may not reach the right atrium. The vessels in the neck or upper extremities are therefore the most efficacious means of immediate venous access. Most children of the age group likely to sustain severe trauma have well delineated antecubital veins, which can be easily cannulated by even the most inexperienced house officer. If, after placing the patient in Trendelenburg position, these are inaccessible, transcutaneous insertion of either an internal or external jugular catheter is indicated. Subclavian catheterization, so easy and popular in the adult, is frequently an invitation to disaster in the uncooperative, frightened child. Because of the small size of the child's neck and the height of the apices of both lungs, a misguided attempt at subclavian catheterization is more likely to produce harm than good.

Children in frank shock rarely have enough of a circulating volume to distend the peripheral veins, even with the help of the Trendelenburg position.[2,4] The application of military antishock trousers (MAST trousers), if they have not been previously used, may help in this situation. Because of the anatomy of the vein wall, an empty vessel collapses to a ribbon-shaped structure with an elliptical cross section. Even if successfully impaled by an intravenous needle, the vein is more likely to allow the

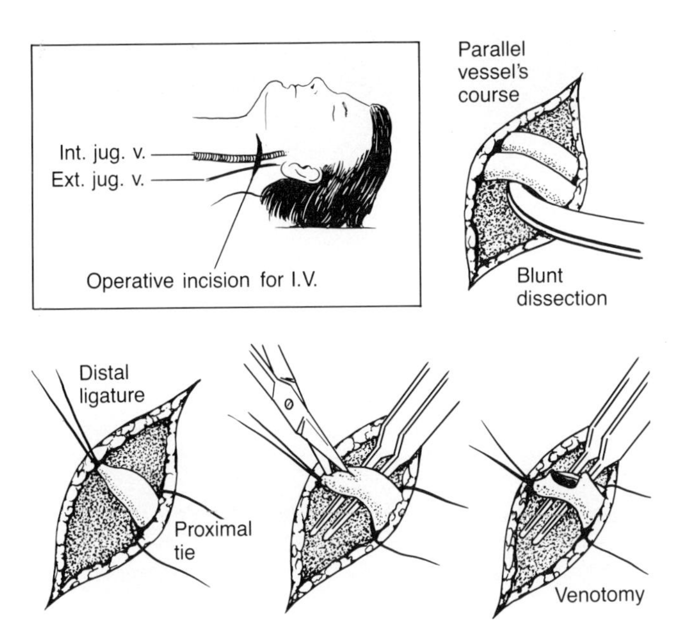

FIGURE 17-1 Technique for venous cutdown.

needle to pass straight through rather than accept a cannula within the lumen. For this reason any child in severe shock in whom venous cannulation cannot be readily accomplished percutaneously should be immediately prepared for a surgical cutdown to provide good, reliable venous access.[2,4] Figure 17-1 illustrates a commonly accepted technique for venous cutdown.

Fluid Replacement

Once adequate venous access has been established, a bolus of lactated Ringer's solution (40 mL/kg) should be given. The timing and appropriateness of using glucose-containing solutions in pediatric resuscitation remains somewhat controversial.[4] On the one hand, it must be remembered that the child's glycogen stores are nowhere near those of the adult. Rapid depletion as a result of the stress response can render the very small child hypoglycemic in a relatively short period of time. On the other hand, the detrimental effect of high-glucose loads resulting from high-volume infusion of glucose-containing solutions must be constantly considered. The provision of adequate glucose stores always must be weighed against the potential electrolyte imbalance and an "artificial" diuresis induced by glycosuria. In cases of severe, ongoing bleeding, type-specific blood must be given as soon as possible.

Ancillary Measures

The final aspect of immediate care of the child with a severe abdominal injury involves placement of other devices required to assess specific organ systems and the patient's response to therapy.[5] A nasogastric tube is placed to assess the stomach contents and to provide adequate decompression. Once a rectal examination has confirmed normal prostatic position, a urinary catheter is inserted to measure urine output and to decompress the bladder. Blood samples for a complete battery of laboratory tests, including typing and cross-matching, hemogram, coagulogram, and arterial blood gas measurement, are dispatched as soon as possible.

SECONDARY ASSESSMENT

Secondary assessment begins as soon as all aspects of primary treatment are completed. The first goal is to determine the effect of any initial resuscitative effort. In the absence of a thoracic or major extremity injury, a lack of response to resuscitation efforts indicates a major abdominal injury and demands immediate surgical intervention. Unlike the patient with an exsanguinating chest wound, in whom an urgent thoracotomy performed in the emergency department may be lifesaving, rarely are patients with these types of abdominal injuries helped by injudicious exploration in areas away from a well-equipped operating room. Adequate lighting, good suction, and proper instrumentation are all essential to the proper care of the major abdominal injury. Despite even a meager response to resuscitation, some tamponade effect is usually being exerted by the abdominal contents and is best maintained until the patient can be delivered into the appropriate setting for exploration. Inflation of both leg and abdominal portions of MAST trousers may help stabilize the patient until appropriate surgical intervention is possible. Emergency department thoracotomy for aortic cross-clamping, although conceptually appealing, has not been effective in management of the child with blunt trauma.[6,7]

A complete physical examination should be performed, identifying and cataloging even the most minor of injuries. Regarding the abdomen, the examination should determine the presence and quality of bowel sounds. Their absence may mean nothing since aerophagia, crying, pain, and fright can all produce an adynamic state. Their presence, on the other hand, can frequently be construed as an indication that the intestinal tract has no major injury.

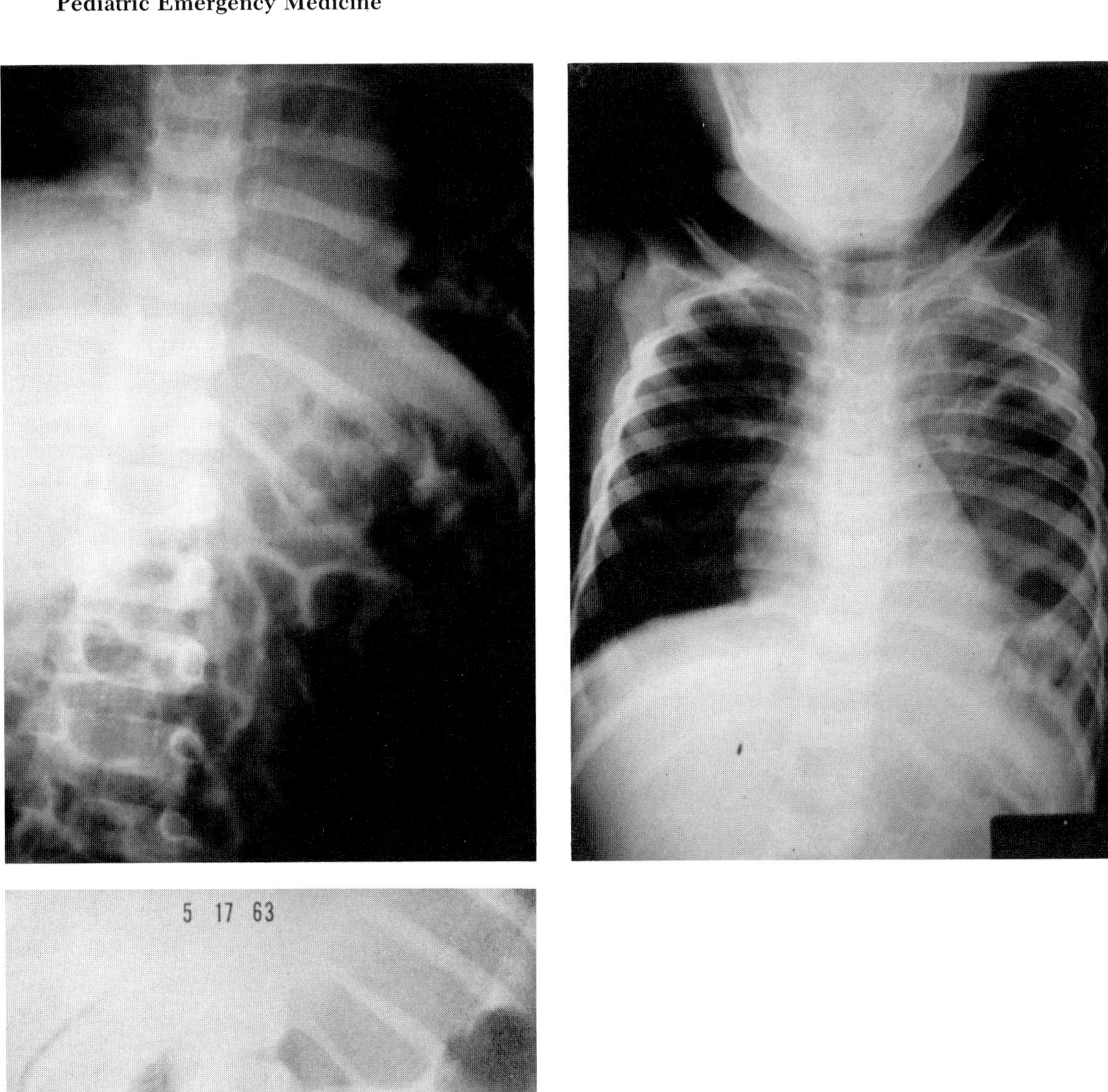

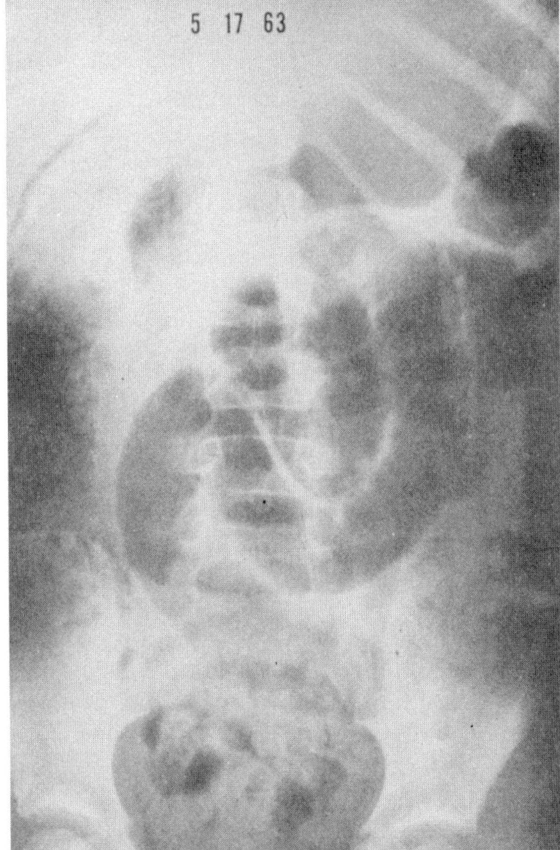

FIGURE 17-2 A and B (top right and left): X-ray films of a diaphragmatic hernia sustained from blunt abdominal trauma. C (bottom): X-ray film of a duodenal perforation with air outlining the right kidney.

Careful palpation of the abdomen can elicit areas of tenderness, muscular spasm, and any masses that may be present. A thorough rectal examination is essential to rule out the presence of blood within the rectum, to assess the sphincter tone, and to ensure that there has been no disruption of the lower urinary tract.

In the child whose injury has not produced profound shock or who has responded to resuscitation and is stable, the findings of the first complete abdominal examination will be the most important data produced during the patient's emergency department care.

Assuming the patient has not demonstrated the need for immediate surgical intervention, it is at this point that the first set of x-ray films should be requested. Cervical spine films can exclude the possibility of neck injury. A chest film helps rule out the existence of a major thoracic injury and provides information concerning the diaphragm and upper abdominal contents. Anteroposterior and cross-table lateral views assess the distribution of gas, the presence of free air, and possibly the existence of increased amounts of fluid or blood within the peritoneal cavity.[3,5] Figure 17-2 illustrates some typical radiologic findings that can result from abdominal trauma.

FURTHER ASSESSMENT

The presence of blood within a child's peritoneal cavity is no longer an automatic indication for surgical exploration. Consequently, peritoneal lavage is frequently superfluous and, by producing an area of tenderness and pain on the child's abdomen, may actually be counterproductive to an accurate assessment. In the patient whose findings do not warrant immediate exploration, frequent physical examinations by personnel familiar with previous findings are the most reliable way to assess the status and progress of the injured child. Peritoneal lavage should be reserved for those children whose neurologic status renders a reliable examination impossible. Children with associated injuries requiring a general anesthetic also may be considered acceptable candidates, although many surgeons prefer the security of knowledge gained through a minilaparotomy over the somewhat sketchy data gained from a simple lavage.

Other ancillary studies that can be helpful at this time are the intravenous pyelogram, liver-spleen scan, and abdominal computed tomography (CT) scan.[8,9] In patients with major abdominal trauma, especially those in whom the exact mechanism of injury is unknown, confirmation of the integrity and function of both renal units must be obtained as soon as possible. Any lesion that disrupts renal blood flow should be repaired within hours of occurrence if there is to be any hope of success. After a test dose of contrast medium, a dose of 1 to 3 mL/kg (maximum, 40 mL) is rapidly infused. The function of both units as well as the anatomy of the lower collecting systems provides important information not only about the urinary tract but also about the retroperitoneum and the pelvis.

Radionuclide scans are rapidly becoming available in emergency departments as a result of the development of portable γ-ray cameras. These provide exceptionally high quality imaging of hepatic and splenic injuries and enable early and accurate diagnosis of these lesions. CT scanning is becoming a major tool in the evaluation of abdominal injuries. The imaging is usually precise enough not only to delineate the presence of blood within the abdomen but also to identify the exact characteristics of the injuries to various organs.[8,9] Figure 17-3 illustrates the effectiveness of CT scan and scintiscan in assessing the nature of a splenic injury and documenting gradual resolution over subsequent months.

DIAGNOSIS OF SPECIFIC ORGAN INJURIES

The preceding principles of management are intended to identify the severely injured child and to delineate the abdomen as the site of this potentially or immediately life-threatening injury. Once initial assessment and treatment have stabilized the patient, information about the state of specific organs must be evaluated.

Hepatic Injuries

As it is the largest organ in the child's abdomen, the liver is frequently the site of major, exsanguinating injury.[1,3,5,10] The diagnosis of the more severe variety is usually evident on presentation and constitutes a management problem for the surgeon, who must deal with it expeditiously in the operating room. As has been discussed, the emergency physician's primary responsibility is initiation of proper resuscitation. The less severe lesions that cause mild or minimal hemorrhage may not pose an immediate threat to life and must be identified as soon as possible so that proper disposition can be made. Other than some distension and tenderness in the right upper quadrant, physical examination of these children is nonspecific. There is no reliable pattern

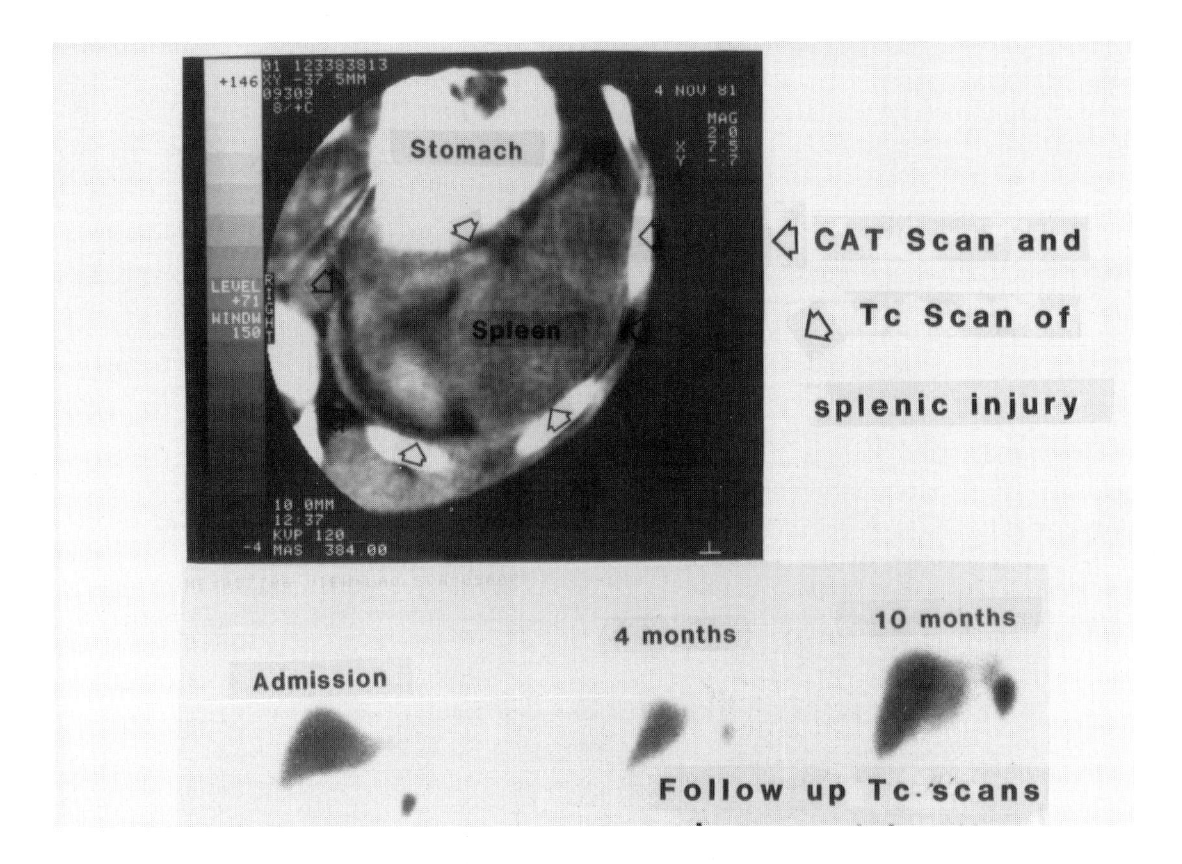

FIGURE 17-3 Combined CT scan and liver-spleen scintiscan evaluation of splenic injury. Arrows indicate borders of splenic hematoma. The lower portion shows healing over the subsequent 8 months.

to bowel sounds, and a mass effect is usually not appreciable.

Biochemical analysis of liver function may show abnormal values. Against a background of potential multiple-organ injury, however, these tests may not be specific enough for adequate assessment. Abdominal films can show the ground-glass appearance of blood or fluid in the peritoneal cavity; otherwise they are nonrevealing. By far the best means of evaluating the liver in acute injury is by radionuclide scintiscan. This not only demonstrates disruption of hepatic parenchyma but also shows intraparenchymal lesions that can produce hemobilia or abscess later on. The CT scan may likewise provide this information, although it is usually more expensive and more complicated than the liver-spleen scan.[5]

Once a liver injury of any sort has been identified, proper management dictates admission to a facility where careful ongoing observation and care can be provided. The absence of severe hemorrhage requiring immediate exploration does not guarantee that surgical intervention will not be required within the next few hours or days. Frequent examination and reevaluation is consistently the best means of determining this and requires the patient's admission to an appropriate care area.

Splenic Injuries

No organ has generated more debate over the last decade than the spleen. This organ was long thought to be physiologically expendable; thus the traditional surgical therapy for an injured spleen was removal. The report of King and Schumacher[11] in 1952 on the association of splenectomy with overwhelming sepsis in infants focused attention on the possible role of the spleen in maintaining immunologic integrity. Subsequent reports have sufficiently confirmed this association so that most pediatric surgeons now advocate splenectomy only when no other alternatives exist.[12] In addition to the many techniques for splenic repair that have been recently described, there have been an increasing number of reports of successful nonsurgical management of these injuries.[13]

Accurate physical examination remains one of the most reliable means of diagnosing splenic injury. The patient's abdomen may be distended, and there is usually tenderness in the left upper quadrant. Palpation of this area may produce pain in the left shoulder (Kehr's sign). A plain film of the abdomen sometimes demonstrates extrinsic compression of the stomach from the expanded mass of injured spleen and hematoma in the left upper quadrant.

An excellent way of confirming a suspected splenic injury is by radionuclide scan. A liver-spleen scan not only provides accurate information about the nature of the splenic injury but also serves as a baseline against which subsequent studies can determine healing. A CT scan frequently is as helpful in this regard, and the combination of both studies can usually provide exact data about the nature of the injury, the distribution of the hematoma, and the viability of the injured segments. Again it must be emphasized that these tests are appropriate only in a stable patient accompanied by an adequately trained attendant.

Retroperitoneal Injuries

Injuries of retroperitoneal organs are the only other lesions in which hemorrhage is likely to be the initial clinical feature. Genitourinary injuries are well described in Chapter 22. Vascular and pelvic injuries, however, do merit some discussion as their occurrence in children is not infrequent.

Because of its resiliency and usual lack of atherosclerotic changes, the aorta of a child is rarely disrupted as a result of blunt trauma. When these injuries do occur, they are usually thoracic and frequently result in rapid death. Aortic injuries stable enough to allow transport to the emergency department usually have been controlled by spontaneous tamponade. Hypovolemia or shock is a common feature. Physical examination may demonstrate discoloration of the flank or a palpable mass. Lateral x-ray films frequently show anterior displacement of bowel loops. Whenever these lesions are suspected, ultrasound examination of the abdomen can provide rapid, noninvasive confirmation.[5] If the patient is stable enough, definitive information can then be sought by arteriogram.

Caval injuries can likewise lead to exsanguinating hemorrhage[3,5] and are usually associated with hepatic injuries. The most common site of injury is at the insertion of the hepatic veins into the inferior vena cava just below the diaphragm. This is almost always associated with a major hepatic parenchymal injury. The large volume of bleeding from the confluence of the systemic and splanchnic venous return in an area of limited access produces a lesion that is commonly fatal. Because of this these children usually are in profound shock and require immediate resuscitation and intervention.

Pelvic fractures are a frequent occurrence in children and can produce extensive blood loss into the retroperitoneum. They are frequently identifiable by palpable instability of the pelvis on physical examination. Abdominal x-ray films can confirm the existence and location of the fracture and may indicate the need for further studies to evaluate the urinary or GI tracts. Although these injuries do not usually require urgent surgical intervention, they can cause extensive bleeding and must be referred to an appropriate care unit as soon as possible.

Pancreatic Injuries

Blunt abdominal injuries in children frequently involve direct trauma to the epigastrium.[3,5,14] Falls onto bicycle handlebars, sports injuries, and many recreational activities can produce a direct blow to the abdomen in which the pancreas may be suddenly compressed against the vertebral column. The resultant injury may involve complete disruption of the pancreas or produce a localized area of parenchymal damage. Release of activated pancreatic enzymes produces an inflammatory response characterized by signs and symptoms of severe peritonitis. Occasionally, a pseudocyst develops and is manifested as a tender mass in the epigastrium. Unlike the immediate effects of hemorrhage, this process usually evolves over the first 12 hours after injury and this possibility mandates that any child with severe blunt abdominal trauma be observed for at least 24 hours. The definition of "severe" requires the consideration of a careful history, a thorough physical examination, assessment of parental reliability, and common sense. Any child hurt badly enough to warrant a visit to the emergency department must be assumed to have sustained a degree of injury somewhat beyond usual child's play.

The most important laboratory test for the diagnosis of pancreatic injuries is the assay for serum amylase. Serial assays should be obtained at 12-hour increments, since the first samples frequently reflect normal preinjury values. Ultrasound and CT scans can also be of help in evaluating the extent and degree of injury.

Gastrointestinal Injuries

Injuries of the GI tract can occur either as an avulsion of the gut from its mesentery or as a disruption of its integrity. In the former case, bleeding into the peritoneum is frequently the first finding. If the avulsion is extensive enough to devitalize a segment of bowel, the child may have severe tenderness and guarding.

Perforation of the GI tract results in peritoneal contamination and evolves into a picture of severe peritonitis and sepsis within a few hours of injury. The primary characteristic of the physical examination in these injuries is the overwhelmingly tender, often rigid, abdomen. Abdominal x-ray films usually show a collection of free air under the diaphragm and should be the only confirmatory examination needed to indicate immediate surgical exploration.

Because of their retroperitoneal location, injuries to the duodenum present unique diagnostic problems.[3,5] Hemorrhage within the duodenal wall can produce a hematoma large enough to obstruct its lumen. Children with duodenal hematoma usually have a history of injury and signs of upper GI obstruction. The diagnosis is frequently missed in the acute phase and can be made only if it is considered and the child is observed.

Duodenal perforation may initially be very subtle. There is little or no free air on x-ray films. Pain is nonspecific and diffuse. Careful evaluation of a cross-table lateral film may show a rim or some bubbles of air within the area of the second or third portion of the duodenum. Usually, however, a contrast study with a water-soluble agent is required to confirm the diagnosis.

Anorectal Injuries

Trauma to the anus and rectum in children is frequently the result of sexual abuse. When a child comes to the emergency department with a history of multiple trauma, the initial evaluation should include careful assessment of the status of the anorectum. In addition to careful inspection of the external anus, examination should include palpation for sphincter tone and a search for the presence of foreign material or blood within the rectal vault. The most important factor for appropriate triage at this point is the determination as to whether or not the integrity of the bowel has been violated. Penetration or perforation of the wall of the colon or rectum usually produces signs of evolving peritonitis within hours of occurrence. Flat plate and upright x-ray films of the abdomen should be obtained to rule out the possibility of free air or radiopaque foreign material. In the absence of overt signs of peritonitis where there is a high index of suspicion of significant rectal trauma, careful proctoscopy can be performed in the emergency department or, if the child is uncooperative, under general anesthesia in the operating room.

When evaluating a child with any type of anorectal injury, either in association with other injuries or as an isolated complaint, it is most prudent to consider admission to the hospital for observation for at least 24 hours. This permits a more careful and thorough assessment of the status of the anorectum and, most importantly, allows for early recognition of signs and symptoms of penetration of the bowel wall.

SUMMARY OF THE SYSTEMATIZED APPROACH

The approach to a child with abdominal trauma can only be effective if it is based on a rational, logical disposition of prioritized problems. Figure 17-4 illustrates a logical sequence of decision making oriented to initial evaluation and care of these problems.

First and foremost is the initial resuscitation of the patient. This proceeds along established guidelines, which are well discussed in preceding chapters, and should be a reflex for any emergency physician. Part of this phase is the identification of the abdomen as a site of injury and the assessment of hemorrhage, the most serious immediate result of abdominal injuries.

Once resuscitation has begun, attention can be focused on the abdomen. If resuscitative efforts are unsuccessful or only marginally successful, preparations for immediate surgical intervention must begin. If the child responds to resuscitation, then more data as to the nature and location of the injury can be gathered. The nature of material returned from the nasogastric tube, the digital rectal examination, and the urinary catheter all help evaluate the status of abdominal organs. A thorough physical examination specifically looking for distension, tenderness, rigidity, or guarding can further elucidate the situation. Laboratory tests done at this point establish a cross-match for transfusion, determine any coagulation abnormalities, evaluate oxygenation, and provide a baseline for later comparison.

If the patient is stable enough, a basic set of x-ray films of the neck, chest, and abdomen can be obtained. If the situation so warrants, a quick-infusion intravenous pyelogram can likewise be performed at this time. With this much data specific organ injuries can be identified, and decisions about further tests or disposition can be made. Proper consultative assistance can be requested, and appropriate preparations for safe conduct of any further evaluation can be made.

The emergency physician who understands these principles and the unique characteristics of

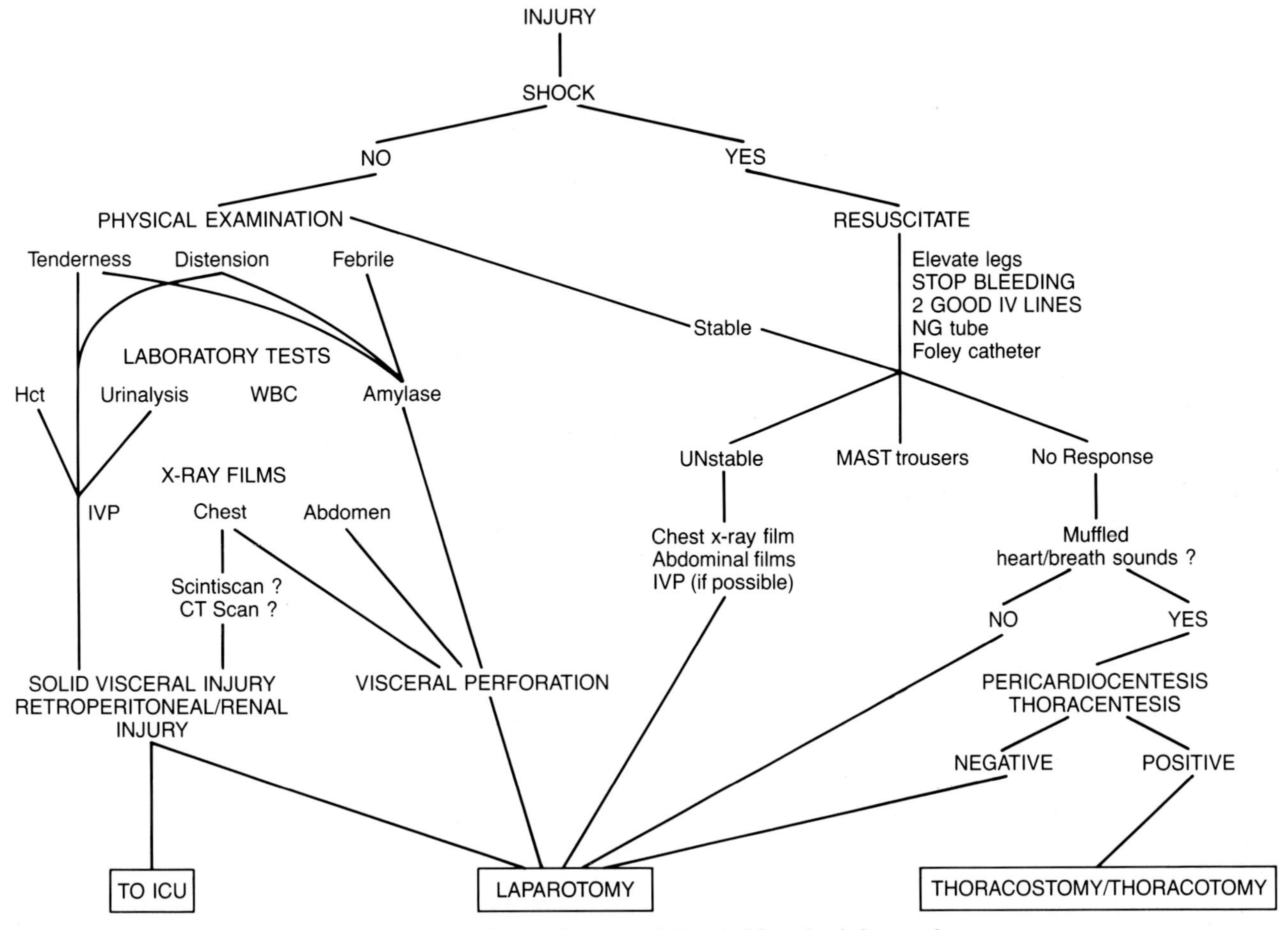

FIGURE 17-4 Decision-making protocol for evaluation of the child with abdominal trauma, Hct, Hematocrit; IVP, intravenous pyelogram; NG, nasogastric; WBC, white blood cell count.

the injured child is by far the best hope for improved care of what is frequently a preventable tragedy.

References

1. Eichelberger MR, Randolph JG: Pediatric trauma: An algorithm for diagnosis and therapy. *J Trauma* 1983;23:2, 91–97.
2. Welch KJ: Abdominal injuries, in Randolph JG, et al (ed): *The Injured Child.* Chicago, Yearbook Medical Publishers, 1979, pp 155–205.
3. Shandling B: Hemorrhage and Shock, in Toronto Hospital for Sick Children: *Care for the Injured Child.* Baltimore, Williams & Wilkins, 1975, pp 10–14.
4. American College of Surgeons Committee on Trauma: Shock, in Advanced Trauma Life Support Syllabus. Chicago, American College of Surgeons, 1984, pp 179–204.
5. Tepas JJ: Pediatric trauma. *Audio-Digest Emergency Medicine* 1985;2:6.
6. Dupak V, Simoni E, Smith R, et al: Resuscitative thoracotomy for patients with traumatic injury. *Surgery* 1983;94:4, 554–561.
7. Bodai BS: Emergency thoracotomy: Who should perform it, and where? *Hosp Phys* February, 1985;9–10.
8. Federle M: Radiologic evaluation of blunt abdominal trauma. *Trauma Quart* May, 1985;59–68.
9. Jones TK, Walsh JW, Maull KI: Diagnostic imaging in blunt trauma of the abdomen. *SG&O* 1983;157:389–397.
10. Giacomautonio M, Filler R, Rich H: Blunt hepatic trauma in children: Experience with operative and nonoperative management. *J Pediatr Surg* 1984; 19:5, 519–522.
11. King H, Shumaker HB: Susceptibility to infections after splenectomy performed in infants. *Ann Surg* 1952;136(2):239–242.
12. Llende M, Santiago-Delpin EA, Lavergne J: Immunobiological consequences of splenectomy: A review. *J Surg Res* 1986;40:1, 85–92.
13. Wesson DE, Filler RM, Ein SH, et al: Ruptured spleen—When to operate? *J Pediatr Surg* 1981; 16:324–326.
14. Weber TR, Grosfeld JL: Abdominal injuries in children. *Top Emerg Med* 1982;4:3, 41–55.

Francis T. Ferry
Andrew M. Yeager

18

Poisonings and Ingestions

Poisoning is the most common medical emergency in children. Over two million poisoning events are reported each year, with 80% to 90% involving preschool children. In fact, 6% to 12% of all children less than 5 years of age will ingest a poison at some time.

Traditionally, childhood poisoning has been classified as a subgroup of "accidents," although its occurrence is often related to potentially controllable developmental and circumstantial factors. A less common though disturbingly increasing phenomenon is the incidence of self-poisoning among older children and adolescents. All poisonings in adolescents and in children over the age of 6 years should be considered potential suicides. These patients require immediate psychiatric intervention, with many requiring hospitalization.

Poisons can be ingested, inhaled, injected, or absorbed through the skin. Oral ingestion is the most common route, with drugs causing 44% of all poisonings. Household products rank second.

Many ingested substances are potentially quite toxic, and their aggressive management is discussed in detail; others are usually nontoxic and do not require aggressive therapy. This distinction is important since inappropriately aggressive management of poisoning can lead to iatrogenic morbidity and even death. To qualify as nontoxic, an ingestion must meet the criteria shown in Exhibit 18-1.

ASSESSMENT AND DIAGNOSIS OF ACUTE POISONINGS

The assessment of a patient with acute poisoning must be rapid and thorough, and give the physician substantial information about the substance ingested and the patient's clinical status. Ingestions by children usually involve substances found within the home, and the ingested agent is generally known. Evidence of the poison is often brought in with the patient, e.g., empty containers or tablets found near the victim. Identification of the poison may be obscure in the older patient, and a multiple-drug overdose must be considered. The emergency management of the patient must take precedence over the identification of the poison.

The initial questions must include the following:

- type of exposure (e.g., ingestion, inhalation, transcutaneous absorption)
- identity of the agent (if known)
- time of ingestion of the agent
- amount of the agent ingested

Whenever possible, the remainder of the suspected poison and the container from which it came should be obtained; however, this can be misleading, since the contents may not be in their original container. If the patient vomited before arriving at the hospital, the vomitus should be placed in a clean con-

Exhibit 18-1 Criteria for Nontoxic Ingestions

Absolute identification of the product
Assurance that only a single product was ingested
Absence of a signal word (danger, poison, warning, caution) on the container
A good approximation of the amount ingested
Absence of symptoms
Ability to call back and check on the victim's status
Victim under 5 years of age

Source: Adapted with permission from Mofenson HC, Greensher J: Controversies in the prevention and treatment of poisonings. *Pediatr Ann* 1977;6:725.

TABLE 18-1 Glasgow Coma Scale*

Category	Response	Score
Eyes	Open spontaneously	4
	Open to verbal command	3
	Open to pain	2
	No response	1
Motor response	Obeys verbal command	6
	Responds to painful stimulus:†	
	Localizes pain	5
	Flexion—withdrawal	4
	Flexion—abnormal (decorticate rigidity)	3
	Extension (decerebrate rigidity)	2
	No response	1
Verbal response‡		
Older children	Oriented, converses	5
	Disoriented, converses	4
	Inappropriate words	3
	Incomprehensible sounds	2
	No response	1
Infants and young children without language skills	Recognizable words	5
	Cry or moan	2
	No response	1

* Lowest total score = 3; highest score = 15.
† Apply knuckles to sternum and observe arms.
‡ Arouse patient with painful stimulus, if necessary.
Source: Adapted with permission from Jennett B, Teasdale G: Aspects of coma after severe head injury. *Lancet* 1977;1:878.

tainer for toxicologic analysis. By examination of the container from which a known agent was taken, the physician may be able to make immediate identification of the poison and to estimate the amount taken (e.g., a prescription bottle with name of drug and number of tablets included). In the case of household or industrial products, the ingredients may be obtained from the label, or a manufacturer's product information telephone number may be found. Tablets and capsules can be identified with product identification charts in the *Physicians' Desk Reference* or other similar publications.

The largest possible amount should be estimated when assessing the amount of poison ingested. In the situation in which two or more children are involved in the ingestion of a toxic agent, it must be assumed that *each* child took the maximum (total) amount of substance available, and all of the children should be managed according to this estimate.

The poison information center is an invaluable aid. Its telephone number should be readily available.

Signs and Symptoms

A rapid but meticulous physical examination is the basis for initial supportive management of the poisoning victim and provides a baseline against which to compare the subsequent clinical course. Attention to vital signs and mental status is critical. The degree of obtundation is best assessed with the Glasgow coma scale (Table 18-1), which can be used for the serial evaluation of mental status as the clinical course unfolds and as treatment is administered.

Other aspects of the physical examination include pupillary reflexes, condition of the skin and mucous membranes, status of the nervous system, breath odor, and the color and odor of body fluids (blood, urine, vomitus). A listing of the symptoms and signs associated with specific poisonings is presented in Table 18-2.

Laboratory Tests

The definitive analysis of a poison is usually made by its isolation from blood, urine, or vomitus, and samples of these fluids should be sent to the laboratory for emergency toxicologic analysis as soon as possible after the patient is stabilized. However, these tests often require several hours to perform, and the physician must rely heavily on clinical judgment for the initiation of therapy.

Samples should be sent to the laboratory for the following tests:

1. complete blood count: look for neutropenia, leukopenia, anemia, and/or thrombocytopenia. Note that the color of whole blood may indicate the toxin (cherry red in carbon monoxide or cyanide poisoning, chocolate brown in methemoglobinemia).
2. serum electrolytes and serum urea nitrogen.
3. blood glucose: may be decreased in salicylate poisoning and plumbism. A rapid estimate can be made at the bedside with Dextrostix reagent strips.
4. qualitative and quantitative toxicologic analysis.
5. routine and microscopic urinalysis.

A few basic tests can be done by the physician in the emergency department. For the *urine ferric*

TABLE 18-2 Signs and Symptoms of Poisonings

Sign or Symptom	Poison
Eyes	
Pupillary dilatation	Belladonna alkaloids, atropine, meperidine, sympathomimetics, parasympatholytics, antihistamines, cocaine, camphor, benzene, botulinus toxin, cyanide, carbon monoxide, LSD,* mescaline, thallium
Pupillary constriction	Opiates, sympatholytics, parasympathomimetics, barbiturates, cholinesterase inhibitors, chloral hydrate, phenothiazines, ethanol, organophosphate insecticides, phencyclidine
Nystagmus	Phenytoin, propoxyphene
Ptosis	Botulinus toxin, phenytoin, propoxyphene
Strabismus	Botulinus toxin, thallium
Face and Scalp	
Alopecia	Arsenic, radioactive agents, cancer chemotherapeutic agents, vitamin A, lead, boric acid, thallium
Skin and Mucous Membranes	
Sweating	Cholinergics, arsenic, mercury, bismuth, organophosphate insecticides, fluoride, nicotine
Hot, dry skin	Atropine, belladonna alkaloids, botulinus toxin
Flushing	Sympathomimetics, anticholinergics, boric acid, carbon monoxide, alcohol, snake bites, atropine, antihistamines, phenothiazines
Salivation	Caustics, arsenic, mercury, bismuth, cholinergics, organophosphate insecticides, muscarine-containing mushrooms, salicylates, nicotine, fluoride
Dry mouth	Atropine, belladonna alkaloids, botulinus toxin, antihistamines, sympathomimetics, narcotics, anticholinergics
Burns	Corrosives, thallium, boric acid
Stomatitis	Cancer chemotherapeutic agents
Discoloration	Lead, mercury, thallium, bismuth, arsenic
Gray color	Lead, phenacetin
Cyanosis	Carbon monoxide, barbiturates, opiates, aniline dyes, nitrates, nitrites, methylene blue
Pink color	Cyanide
Jaundice	Arsenic, acetaminophen, mushroom toxins, naphthalene and other potentially hemolytic agents, carbon tetrachloride, phosphorus
Nervous System	
Ataxia	Lead, organophosphate insecticides, antihistamines, thallium, alcohol, phenytoin, propoxyphene, dextromethorphan
Obtundation and coma	Narcotics, barbiturates, phenothiazines, benzodiazepines, chloral hydrate, bromides, alcohols, lead, cyanide, carbon monoxide, nicotine, benzene, atropine, belladonna alkaloids, organophosphate insecticides, insulin, aniline dyes, mushrooms, salicylates, hydrocarbons, mercury, boric acid, antihistamines, arsenic, iron, digitalis, theophylline, phenytoin
Delirium	Atropine, belladonna alkaloids, cocaine, alcohol, lead, marijuana, arsenic, amphetamines, antihistamines, camphor, LSD, PCP, benzene, barbiturates, DDT, aniline dyes, theophylline, digitalis
Convulsions	Strychnine, camphor, cocaine, atropine, belladonna alkaloids, organophosphate insecticides, amphetamines, nicotine, lead, mushrooms, caffeine, theophylline, cyanide, tricyclic antidepressants, salicylates, narcotics, barbiturates (withdrawal), boric acid, mercury, phenothiazines, antihistamines, arsenic, DDT, hydrocarbons, fluoride, digitalis, thallium, alcohols, PCP, propoxyphene, phenytoin
Headache	Atropine, organophosphate insecticides, carbon monoxide, benzene, anilines, lead, indomethacin
Muscle spasms	Atropine, strychnine, lead, spider and scorpion bites, phenothiazines, camphor, fluorides
Paresthesias, weakness, paralysis	Carbon monoxide, botulinus toxin, alcohols, curare, DDT, nicotine, cyanide, mercury, lead, arsenic, thallium, organophosphates, fluorides
GI Tract	
Nausea, vomiting, diarrhea, abdominal pain	Arsenic, iron, corrosives, lead, spider bites, boric acid, organophosphates, phosphorus, nicotine, fluorides, thallium, methanol, mushrooms, digitalis, opiates, DDT, botulinus toxin, cocaine, salicylates, theophylline, snake bites, food poisoning, mercury, naphthalene
Dysphagia	Caustics, botulinus toxin, camphor, iodine, arsenic
Hematemesis	Caustics, fluoride, iron, arsenic, salicylates, theophylline, warfarin, phosphorus
Ear	
Tinnitus	Salicylates, quinine, quinidine, aminoglycosides, camphor, nicotine, methanol
Urinary Tract	
Proteinuria	Arsenic, mercury, phosphorus
Hematuria and/or hemoglobinuria	Arsenic, mercury, naphthalene and other potentially hemolytic oxidizers
Blood	
Anemia	Lead, naphthalene and other potentially hemolytic agents, snake venom
Hemorrhage	Warfarin, thallium
Methemoglobinemia	Nitrates, nitrites, aniline dyes, methylene blue

TABLE 18-2 *(continued)*

Sign or Symptom	Poison
Respiratory System	
Respiratory depression and failure	Opiates, fluorides, cyanide, barbiturates, alcohols, snake venom, carbon monoxide, benzodiazepines, phenothiazines, organophosphates
Tachypnea and hyperpnea	Atropine, belladonna alkaloids, cocaine, amphetamines, strychnine, salicylates, camphor, hydrocarbons, snake venoms, cyanide, carbon monoxide, talc, caustics
Cardiovascular System	
Bradycardia	Digitalis, mushrooms, quinine, quinidine, lead, barbiturates, opiates, organophosphates
Tachycardia	Amphetamines, atropine, cocaine, sympathomimetics, caffeine, aminophylline
Hypertension	Amphetamines, sympathomimetics, lead, nicotine, mercury
Hypotension	Chloral hydrate, phenothiazines, iron
Cardiovascular collapse (shock)	Arsenic, boric acid, iron, phosphorus, food poisoning, lead, caustics
Arrhythmias	Digitalis, tricyclic antidepressants, theophylline, narcotics, amphetamines, phenothiazines, solvents
Breath Odor	
Alcoholic	Phenols, chloral hydrate, alcohol
Sweet	Chloroform, acetone, ether
Bitter almond	Cyanides
Pears	Chloral hydrate
Garlic	Phosphorus, arsenic, organophosphate insecticides
Wintergreen	Methyl salicylate
Violets	Turpentine
Pine	Pine oil
General	
Agitation	Caffeine, theophylline
Fever	Atropine, salicylates, food poisoning, antihistamines, phenothiazines, camphor, alcohols, theophylline, quinine, belladonna alkaloids

* Abbreviations: LSD, lysergic acid diethylamine; PCP, phencyclidine; DDT, dichlorodiphenyltrichloroethane.
Source: Adapted with permission from Arena JM: *Poisoning: Toxicology, Symptoms, Treatments,* ed 4. Springfield, IL, Charles C Thomas Publisher, 1979, pp 6–9. Copyright © 1979 Charles C Thomas Publisher.

chloride test, two drops of 10% ferric chloride are added to 1.0 mL of fresh urine, and the color is observed immediately and again after a few minutes. With the exception of salicylate, high concentrations of the reacting metabolite are required. Thus, a negative ferric chloride test *does not* exclude the ingestion of an agent known to cause a positive reaction (Table 18-3). To test for suspected salicylate poisoning (Table 18-4), a drop of serum from the patient is placed on a Phenistix reagent strip (Ames Company).

Radiologic Studies

Radiopaque particles in the GI tract can be seen on a plain film of the abdomen and suggest the inges-

TABLE 18-3 Clinical Conditions Associated with a Positive Ferric Chloride Test in the Urine

Clinical Condition	Reacting Compound	Color Produced
Normal urine	Phosphates	Brownish, whitish, or yellowish
Salicylate ingestion	Salicylates	Deep purple, stable
p-Aminosalicylic acid ingestion	*p*-Aminosalicylic acid	Red-brown
Antipyrine and acetophenetidin ingestion	Antipyrine and acetophenetidin derivatives	Cherry red
L-Dopa ingestion	L-Dopa metabolites, dopylacetic acid	Green (vanishes then reappears) or stable emerald green
Isoniazid ingestion	Isoniazid	Yellowish green to gray
Phenothiazine ingestion	Phenothiazine derivatives	Blue-purple
Ketosis	Acetoacetic acid	Purple to red, fades in minutes
Hyperbilirubinemia (direct)	Conjugated bilirubin	Green, stable
Hepatic failure	*p*-Hydroxyphenylactic and *p*-hydroxyphenylpyruvic acids	Transient blue-green

Source: Adapted with permission from Taylor GA: Metabolic tests, in Biller JA, Yeager AM (eds): *The Harriet Lane Handbook: A Manual for Pediatric House Officers,* ed 9. Chicago, Year Book Medical Publishers Inc, 1981, pp 45–47. Copyright © 1981 Year Book Medical Publishers.

TABLE 18-4 Test for Salicylate Poisoning

Phenistix Color	Salicylate Level (mg/dL)
Tan	<40
Brown	40–90
Purple	>90

Source: Adapted with permission from Ferry FT: Poisonings, in Biller JA, Yeager AM (eds): *The Harriet Lane Handbook: A Manual for Pediatric House Officers*, ed 9. Chicago, Year Book Medical Publishers Inc, 1981, p 215. Copyright © 1981 Year Book Medical Publishers.

tion of metallic compounds such as lead, iron, bismuth, thallium, or arsenic. The presence of radiodense lines in the proximal fibula and the distal radius and ulna is consistent with chronic poisoning from either lead or fluoride.

Diagnostic Therapeutic Procedures

The empiric administration of selected toxin antagonists can be of diagnostic importance as well as therapeutic benefit. However, these drugs are given only in situations in which the clinical suspicion is high for poisoning with a particular agent. Examples of diagnostic therapeutic agents include atropine for cholinergic overdosage, deferoxamine for iron poisoning, naloxone for narcotic overdosages, and physostigmine for anticholinergic poisoning.

GENERAL MANAGEMENT

Initial Management

Stabilization of the patient must take precedence over identification of the poison. Maintenance of airway patency, adequate ventilation (with endotracheal intubation and assisted ventilation, if necessary), replacement of volume losses, administration of pressors, correction of hyperpyrexia or hypothermia (best accomplished with a temperature-controlled blanket), and control of seizures may be necessary. The insertion of a large-bore intravenous catheter is an essential early step in the management of the poisoned patient. Blood samples for diagnostic tests should be obtained before any intravenous fluids or medications are administered. When available, devices to monitor cardiac and respiratory function should be employed. Patients in whom hemodynamic impairment exists may benefit from monitoring of central venous pressure via a central intravenous catheter and from placement of a radial arterial line for effective ongoing measurement of blood pressure and arterial blood gases.

Prevention of Systemic Absorption

The removal of ingested poisons from the GI tract and the inhibition of further absorption of these agents from the gut are of paramount importance in most poisonings. These procedures should be instituted as soon as possible after the ingestion has occurred, since many drugs are absorbed from the GI tract within 2 to 4 hours after the ingestion, by which time peak blood levels may be attained. However, some agents such as enteric-coated tablets are absorbed more slowly, and delayed GI absorption can occur if GI motility is inhibited (e.g., by anticholinergics, opiates, or coma). Therefore, one should generally take measures to prevent systemic absorption of the poison, even though several hours may have elapsed from the time of the ingestion. These measures include emesis, gastric lavage, administration of activated charcoal, and cathartics.

Emesis

For most ingestions the induction of emesis with syrup of ipecac is a safe and effective procedure. Contraindications to ipecac-induced emesis include stupor or coma, hematemesis, caustic ingestions, and diminished or absent gag reflex. A controversial area is the advisability of ipecac administration in hydrocarbon ingestions (see "Hydrocarbons" in this chapter).

Ipecac is available without a prescription, and parents should be advised to keep it available for emergency use at home. Its long shelf life makes this economically feasible. The following doses of ipecac syrup are appropriate:

- 9 to 12 months of age: 10 mL
- 1 to 12 years of age: 15 mL
- over 12 years of age: 30 mL

The dose of ipecac is followed by 100 to 500 mL of clear fluids, according to the age of the child. If emesis does not take place within 20 minutes after administration of ipecac, the dose is repeated and more fluids are administered. If the patient fails to vomit after the second dose of ipecac, another dose *should not* be given; instead, gastric lavage is performed. The reason for this is not the toxicity of syrup of ipecac, which is negligible, but rather the need to remove the toxin for which the ipecac was given.

Gastric Lavage

Gastric lavage is indicated in infants under the age of 9 months (in whom ipecac-induced emesis is contraindicated), in patients who have not responded to ipecac, and in stuporous or comatose patients. Gastric lavage is contraindicated in caustic ingestions and in most hydrocarbon ingestions (see the section on hydrocarbons for guidelines on treatment of hydrocarbon ingestions). In patients with altered mental status or a depressed gag reflex, the insertion and inflation of a cuffed endotracheal tube prior to performing gastric lavage decreases the risk of aspiration pneumonitis as a complication of the lavage procedure.

The technique of gastric lavage is as follows:

1. The patient is positioned on the left side with the head slightly lower than the body.
2. A large-bore nasogastric tube is inserted into older children and adults (at least a no. 24 French), an orogastric tube in infants and young children (at least a no. 12 French).
3. Lavage is performed with normal saline (0.9% NaCl), 20 to 50 mL per pass, depending on the size of the patient, until the gastric contents are clear. This may require several liters of lavage fluid in the larger patients. The initial "pass" is saved for toxicologic analysis.
4. Before the gastric tube is removed, activated charcoal and, if indicated, a cathartic are instilled.

Activated Charcoal

Activated charcoal is a nontoxic, nonabsorbable black powder that adsorbs a wide variety of poisons and other toxins by virtue of its extremely small particle size and resultant voluminous surface area.[1] Thus, administration of activated charcoal prevents systemic absorption of poisons from the GI tract, inhibits the effects of drugs that exhibit enterohepatic or enterogastric circulation, and allows excretion of the poison as a stable charcoal complex in the stool. Other forms of carbon, e.g., barbecue charcoal or burned toast (the latter a component of the worthless "universal antidote"), lack the fine particle size and should never be substituted for activated charcoal.

Activated charcoal is not useful in poisonings with acetaminophen, alcohols, boric acid, caustics, cyanide, hydrocarbons, and iron. However, the lack of toxicity and the potential benefit from activated charcoal warrant its administration after emesis or lavage in all ingestions except the aforementioned. A slurry of 30 mL of activated charcoal in 240 mL of clear fluid is prepared; cola or fruit punch is useful in disguising the color and in making the slurry more palatable. The slurry is administered in a dose of 5 mL/kg by mouth or by gastric tube. Activated charcoal should *never* be given before or immediately after administration of ipecac, since the charcoal adsorbs ipecac and prevents its emetic effect. Appearance of charcoal in the stool is an indicator of GI motility and of elimination of ingested poison from the body.

Cathartics

Specific ingestions may cause decreased GI motility, e.g., anticholinergic overdoses and narcotic poisonings, and therefore predispose the patient to absorption of the drug over a prolonged period of time. In these situations administration of cathartics can enhance the elimination of the poison or toxin from the GI tract. After the administration of activated charcoal, sodium sulfate or magnesium sulfate is given at a dose of 250 mg/kg, either orally or by gastric tube. The dose is repeated every 3 hours until stool is produced. Sodium or magnesium sulfate should not be administered to patients with renal insufficiency. Irritant cathartics such as aloe or cascara should never be used in the poisoned patient.

Other Techniques

Drugs excreted by renal mechanisms can be eliminated more rapidly with forced diuresis. Ion trapping (urinary acidification or alkalinization) may be employed to increase the amount of ionized drug in the urine and thus enhance excretion and inhibit renal reabsorption.

Dialysis may be required in severe poisonings for which rapid removal of the agent is essential. Hemodialysis, peritoneal dialysis, hemoperfusion over charcoal or resin columns, and exchange transfusions have all been used for a variety of poisonings. However, the only poisonings for which dialysis is *absolutely* indicated are methanol and ethylene glycol ingestions. Dialysis can be considered in patients with renal, hepatic, and/or cardiac failure; in the face of significant underlying illnesses; or in severe and overwhelming poisonings.

ACETAMINOPHEN

Acetaminophen is widely used as an aspirin-free analgesic and antipyretic. There is scant evidence of fatal acetaminophen poisoning in infants and young children. Conversely, fatalities in young adults from acetaminophen overdosage are well recognized, in the form of delayed fulminant hepatic failure.

Pathophysiology

Acetaminophen is converted by hepatic enzyme systems to two major metabolites: the sulfate and glucuronide conjugates.[2-4] Neither acetaminophen nor either of these conjugates is directly toxic to the liver, suggesting that minor metabolites of acetaminophen are responsible for the hepatotoxicity seen in overdosage of the drug. It is likely that these minor metabolites, formed by the mixed-function (cytochrome P-450) oxidase system, are the hepatotoxic agents that cause damage to the liver through utilization and depletion of hepatic stores of glutathione. The hepatic damage, which pathologically is a centrilobular necrosis, may not be clinically apparent until several days after the ingestion; however, it is a type of fulminant hepatic failure with a 5% to 10% case-fatality rate.

The dearth of fatal acetaminophen poisonings in childhood suggests that pediatric patients may exhibit alterations in the production of minor metabolites of acetaminophen or may have relatively greater heptic glutathione stores, thus enjoying an innate protection against the hepatotoxicity of acetaminophen metabolites.[5] However, the precise metabolic pathways of acetaminophen are not well delineated in children, and it is not clear at what age children begin to manifest evidence of the hepatic toxicity of overdosage with acetaminophen. Therefore, the physician must pursue the specific therapy of acetaminophen poisoning, regardless of the age of the patient.

Clinical Features

The toxic dose of acetaminophen in adolescents and adults is greater than or equal to 140 mg/kg.[1,3] Within hours after ingestion of a toxic quantity of acetaminophen, the patient may experience nausea and vomiting. Diaphoresis and malaise are usually present. However, there are no specific early clinical indicators of acetaminophen toxicity. After an apparent improvement in symptoms over the next 48 to 72 hours, hepatic dysfunction is evidenced (tender hepatomegaly, icterus, and elevation of transaminases), with a wide variation in severity. Excitation, delirium, and then stupor and coma portend a particularly grave outcome. Hypothermia, hypoglycemia, and metabolic acidosis reflect hepatic dysfunction and metabolic derangements. Dyspnea, tachycardia, and arrhythmias may also occur.

Diagnostic Tests

The plasma level of acetaminophen should be determined as soon as possible, since the drug is rapidly absorbed from the GI tract. Peak levels occur at 30 minutes after ingestion of acetaminophen elixir and at 60 minutes with tablets. Plasma levels of acetaminophen that exceed 300 μg/mL at 2 hours after ingestion are frequently associated with hepatotoxicity; plasma acetaminophen levels can be correlated with the likelihood of hepatic toxicity by using the nomogram devised by Rumack (Figure 18-1).[3]

Hepatic enzymes (the serum transaminases) should be determined initially and should be followed as the clinical course unfolds. Generally, the transaminases are maximally elevated at 3 to 4 days after the ingestion. In cases of suspected hepatic coma, blood ammonia levels should be measured. If hepatic damage is significant, the patient's coagulation status should be monitored by measuring the fibrinogen level, prothrombin time, and partial thromboplastin time.

Therapy

Induction of emesis or, in the comatose patient, gastric lavage is indicated in all cases of acetaminophen overdose. In significant ingestions (i.e., total dose ≥140 mg/kg), activated charcoal *should not* be administered since it adsorbs acetylcysteine, which is useful in treatment of the poisoning.[6,7]

Acetylcysteine (Mucomyst) is a glutathione substitute that can ameliorate the hepatotoxicity in acetaminophen overdose, but it is only of value if given within 24 hours of the ingestion. A 20% solution of acetylcysteine is administered in four volumes of a carbonated beverage, as a loading dose of 140 mg/

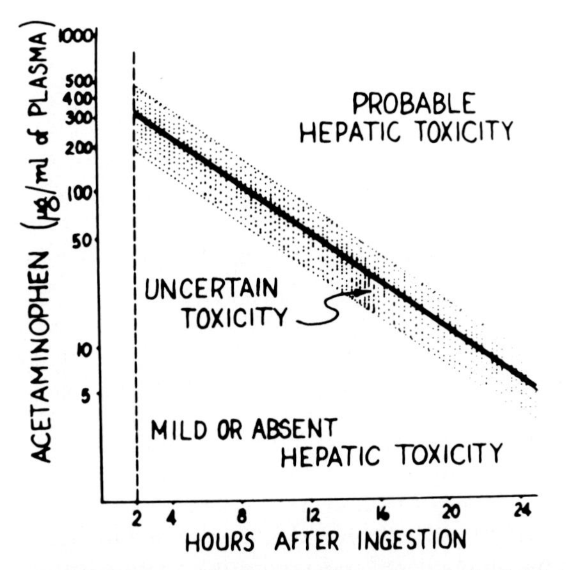

FIGURE 18-1 The "Rumack nomogram," which relates the plasma level of acetaminophen to the probability of hepatic toxicity. See text for explanation. (Reprinted with permission from Rumack BH, Matthew H: Acetaminophen poisoning and toxicity. *Pediatrics* 1975;55:873. Copyright American Academy of Pediatrics 1975.)

kg orally or by gastric tube. Therapy with acetylcysteine should be continued with a dose of 70 mg/kg orally every 4 hours, for a total of 18 doses. If vomiting makes oral therapy impossible, then intravenous protocols for acetylcysteine therapy are available from regional poison control centers or duodenal intubation may be considered.

During therapy for acetaminophen poisoning, the plasma acetaminophen levels should be monitored regularly. Hepatic enzymes, bilirubin, electrolytes, and prothrombin time also should be followed. In patients who exhibit signs of hepatic failure, the administration of oral neomycin and lactulose, imposition of protein restriction, provision of sufficient carbohydrates, and injection of supplemental vitamin K are indicated.

Follow-up

In cases of hepatic dysfunction with acetaminophen overdosage, the hepatic enzyme levels return to the normal range within 4 to 6 weeks after the ingestion. Chronic hepatitis and cirrhosis are extremely uncommon complications, usually limited to those with preexisting liver disease. Therefore, the prognosis for full recovery of hepatic function is excellent. Liver biopsy is seldom required in patients convalescing from acetaminophen-associated hepatic failure.

ALCOHOL AND GLYCOLS

Ethanol remains the major drug of abuse in this country and worldwide. The incidence of alcoholism among teenagers continues to increase, and the acute ingestion of a large quantity of ethanol can be potentially life-threatening. Numerous drugs and household products contain ethanol as the major solvent and thus pose a risk to younger children as well. Isopropyl alcohol, methanol, and ethylene glycol are related compounds commonly found in the home as solvents, cleaning fluids, rubbing alcohols, and antifreeze. These have toxic effects on the central nervous system (CNS) and respiratory system similar to the effects of ethanol, as well as severe metabolic, ocular, and renal toxic effects of their own.

Pathophysiology

Alcohol is readily absorbed from the stomach and intestinal tract. It has a direct irritant and toxic effect on the GI mucosa that can result in severe hemorrhagic gastritis. This effect is even more pronounced with isopropyl alcohol, methanol, and ethylene glycol. Acute pancreatitis is another common complication.[8,9]

Inhalation and skin absorption also occur. Poisoning from alcohol sponge bathing is well documented.[10]

After absorption, ethanol is oxidized by the hepatic enzyme alcohol dehydrogenase to acetaldehyde. Acetaldehyde, ethanol itself, and a few minor end products produce toxic effects. Further oxidation through acetyl coenzyme A leads to carbon dioxide and water.[8,9] Methanol and ethylene glycol are oxidized incompletely by alcohol dehydrogenase. Methanol metabolism leads to production of formaldehyde and formic acid, substances much more toxic than the methanol itself.[8,9] These products are responsible for the severe metabolic acidosis and ocular, hepatic, renal, and myocardial damage characterizing methanol ingestion. Glycolaldehyde, glycolic acid, glyoxylic acid, and oxalic acid are end products of ethylene glycol metabolism and are responsible for the acidosis and CNS impairment.[8,11] Renal failure can result from oxalate deposition in the kidneys. Isopropyl alcohol is a direct CNS toxin; it can also produce a necrotizing, hemorrhagic bronchopneumonia since it is excreted by the lungs to a greater extent than other alcohols. Its metabolism to acetone can provide a diagnostic clue to its ingestion.[8,9]

Initial euphoria and uninhibited behavior are due to effects on the reticular activating system. Further effects on the cortex and medullary centers result in deepening coma and eventual respiratory failure and autonomic instability, although direct myocardial toxicity and metabolic acidosis play a role.

Hypoglycemia is a common complication of alcohol ingestion, especially in young children. Its pathophysiology is obscure.

Clinical Features

Disorientation, ataxia, slurred speech, and alcoholic breath odor are early signs. Ethylene glycol is odorless; isopropanol can produce an acetone odor. Nausea, vomiting, and abdominal pain may be early indicators of gastritis or pancreatitis; hematemesis, melena, and hypovolemic shock may occur. Hypoglycemia and acidosis can lead to coma or convulsions. Direct neurotoxic effects are coma, respiratory arrest, and vasomotor collapse. Methanol produces a papillitis that can result in optic atrophy and blindness. Flank pain, hematuria, oliguria, and renal failure occur with ethylene glycol ingestions. Hemoptysis and pneumonitis are seen with ingestions of isopropyl alcohol, but aspiration pneumonitis can occur with all of these ingestions, in which vomiting, coma, and depressed gag reflex coexist.

Diagnostic Tests

Quantitative blood alcohol levels are useful for determining prognosis and in planning therapy. Blood ethanol levels above 300 mg/dL produce coma, and death is likely with levels greater than 400 mg/dL. Methanol ingestions are usually lethal when blood levels exceed 50 mg/dL. Isopropyl alcohol levels greater than 150 mg/dL produce deep coma.

Laboratory studies of use in guiding therapy measure serum electrolytes, glucose, blood urea nitrogen, creatinine, hepatic transaminases, and arterial blood gases. Oxalate crystals found in urine during microscopic examination are characteristic of ethylene glycol poisoning; their disappearance correlates with final clearance of toxic metabolites. Acetonuria without glycosuria is found in isopropanol poisoning.

Therapy

The level of coma determines the magnitude of cardiopulmonary support required. Use of endotracheal intubation, mechanical ventilation, invasive monitoring, and fluid and pressor therapy is guided by careful evaluation of clinical and laboratory parameters. Protection of the airway is essential, as vomiting and aspiration are constant dangers.

Attempts should be made to remove ingested poison and to limit its adsorption. Syrup of ipecac should be used in the alert patient, but early neurologic effects are the rule, and gastric lavage is often necessary. Airway protection with an inflated, cuffed endotracheal tube is essential. Activated charcoal and magnesium sulfate cathartics further inhibit absorption. Isopropyl alcohol is excreted in part by the salivary glands and gastric mucosa, and repeated use of lavage and/or activated charcoal can shorten the comatose period.

Erosive gastritis is best diagnosed by endoscopy and is treated with fluid and blood product support. The therapy of pancreatitis is likewise supportive. Hypoglycemia requires intravenous glucose-containing solutions, and metabolic acidosis is best handled by continuous infusion of sodium bicarbonate solutions. Careful monitoring of the patient's fluid status is imperative. Methanol and especially ethylene glycol are nephrotoxic, and renal failure may supervene.

Many of the ocular, renal, and other toxic effects of methanol and ethylene glycol poisoning are the result of toxic metabolites. Oxidation of these substances can be competitively inhibited by ethanol, allowing excretion of the unchanged and less toxic parent compounds.[11] Oral doses of 50% ethanol at 0.5 g/kg can be administered every 2 to 4 hours, or an IV infusion of 5% ethanol at 0.1 mL/kg/h can be initiated. Blood ethanol levels of 100 to 200 mg/dL must be maintained for 3 to 4 days to be effective. This therapy is not of value in isopropyl alcohol poisoning.

In addition to ethanol therapy, osmotic diuresis with intravenous fluids and mannitol may minimize oxalate nephropathy in ethylene glycol poisoning.[8] Urine output and overall fluid status must be carefully monitored if this modality is tried.

Alcohols and glycols are removed very effectively by hemodialysis. Peritoneal dialysis is also effective but slower. These therapies are indicated when potentially lethal blood levels are documented or when supportive measures fail to control the acidosis or cardiovascular instability.

Follow-up

Prognosis is good if prolonged hypotension or hypoxia have been avoided. Methanol poisoning often leaves permanent visual impairment. Most of the renal toxic effects of ethylene glycol poisoning are reversible. The prognosis in the management of chronic ethanol abuse is not so favorable.

ANTICHOLINERGICS

Several groups of agents produce signs and symptoms of anticholinergic poisoning: antihistamines, atropine, homatropine, scopolamine, propantheline, belladonna alkaloids, tricyclic antidepressant drugs (e.g., imipramine, nortriptyline, amitriptyline) and a variety of plants (jimson weed, nightshade).

Pathophysiology

Anticholinergic agents act at the neuromuscular junction to antagonize acetylcholine at the receptor level. As a result smooth muscle, exocrine glands, and myocardium are most significantly affected by these drugs. Therapeutic intervention in anticholinergic poisoning is directed at increasing the levels of acetylcholine at the neuromuscular junction or nerve synapse, thus overriding the blockade by the drug.[12]

Clinical Features

Patients with anticholinergic overdose are usually symptomatic within 3 hours after the ingestion, although the onset of symptoms may be delayed for 12 to 24 hours. Neurologic findings predominate, notably those referable to the autonomic nervous system. Agitation, irritability, disorientation, delirium, and hallucinations occur; stupor, coma, and seizures may be present in severe cases.[13] In very young children, especially after overdosage with antihistamines, an initial hyperexcitable state is observed, followed by CNS depression.[14] Tachycardia, vasodilatation, muscle twitching, tremors, mydriasis (with resultant blurring of vision), decreased GI motility, urinary retention, dry mouth, and hot, red, dry skin are all indicative of anticholinergic poisoning. In patients with tricyclic antidepressant poisoning, disorders of cardiac rhythm may be prominent; conduction defects and bigeminy can occur. Recurrences of cardiac findings during the first week of recovery from the ingestion have been described.

Diagnostic Tests

There are no rapid bedside screening tests to detect anticholinergic agents. Toxicologic analysis of blood and urine may identify the compound. Baseline measurements of serum electrolytes, urea nitrogen, and glucose; complete blood count; and urinalysis should be obtained. An electrocardiogram with a long rhythm strip may provide valuable information on cardiac rate and rhythm. Findings on the electrocardiogram that suggest anticholinergic poisoning include widening of the QRS complex, depression of the ST segment, and abnormal T waves.[12]

Therapy

Ipecac-induced emesis or gastric lavage, administration of activated charcoal, and a cathartic to prevent further systemic absorption of the anticholinergic agent and to hasten its removal are all indicated. Supportive care of the patient includes careful monitoring of cardiac and respiratory status, supplemental intravenous fluids with additional bicarbonate or acetate to correct acidosis, ventilatory assistance if required, and maintenance of normal core body temperature. If seizures are present, they may be controlled with intravenous diazepam and/or phenytoin. Intermittent or indwelling catheterization of the bladder may be required if acute urinary retention is present.[12]

Physostigmine salicylate, a tertiary amine, is an effective antidote that leads to increased levels of acetylcholine by inhibition of the enzyme acetylcholinesterase, thus preventing the breakdown of neural acetylcholine.[14,15] Results can be seen within minutes after its injection by the intravenous route. Physostigmine crosses the blood-brain barrier and thus is capable of reversing both the central and peripheral anticholinergic effects.[16] Neostigmine and pyridostigmine are analogous to physostigmine but do not enter the CNS and, therefore, cannot alter the central manifestations of anticholinergic poisoning.[14,15]

Symptomatic patients, especially those with serious signs or symptoms (e.g., coma or arrhythmias), can be given physostigmine empirically. Physostigmine is administered by slow intravenous injection. Children should receive 0.5 mg over 2 to 3 minutes, whereas adolescents and adults should receive 2.0 mg over 2 to 3 minutes. If no effect is observed, the dose can be repeated every 5 minutes until a cumulative dose of 2 mg in children or 4 to 6 mg in adolescents and adults has been reached. Once the desired effect is reached, the lowest effective dose can be repeated every 30 to 60 minutes, as anticholinergic signs or symptoms recur, since physostigmine has a half-life of approximately 2 hours.[14]

Physostigmine is toxic and must be infused slowly because seizures can occur following its rapid injection.[17] If the patient develops signs and symptoms of physostigmine poisoning (vomiting, salivation, miosis, urination, and diarrhea), the drug should be discontinued, and atropine, at a dose half that of physostigmine, should be administered to reverse the cholinergic symptoms.

Hemodialysis, peritoneal dialysis, and forced diuresis are ineffective in poisoning with anticholinergic agents.

Cardiac arrhythmias and conduction disorders are commonly seen in patients with tricyclic antidepressant poisoning and less commonly in other anticholinergic overdoses. These dysrhythmias are, in part, attributable to losses of intracellular potassium. Alkalinization of the blood (to pH 7.45 to 7.50) with intravenous sodium bicarbonate or by hyperventilation has been recommended in the past, but has not been considered effective by some experts. Supplemental intravenous potassium chloride (40 mEq/L of intravenous fluids), is indicated in the treatment of arrhythmias *after* the use of physostigmine has failed to abort cardiac dysfunction. Low doses of propranolol for severe ventricular tachydysrhythmias appear to be satisfactory. Lidocaine and phenytoin can also be used but only after satisfactory trials of physostigmine, and potassium chloride. Quinidine and procainamide are contraindicated in arrhythmias caused by the overdose of tricyclic antidepressants, since these agents have actions that are similar to the tricyclics and thus could further impede cardiac contractility and conduction.

Patients with anticholinergic poisoning are usually better within 24 to 48 hours but should be monitored for an additional 1 or 2 days after resolution of all symptoms and signs of the overdose.

Follow-up

Late arrhythmias and deaths, occurring 7 to 10 days after ingestion of an anticholinergic, have been described in patients who manifested early cardiotoxic effects. Therefore, patients who exhibit cardiac dysfunction after anticholinergic poisoning, despite apparent resolution of symptoms, should be observed for a prolonged period after ingestion.

BENZODIAZEPINES

Benzodiazepines include diazepam (Valium), chlordiazepoxide (Librium), flurazepam (Dalmane), oxazepam (Serax), and clorazepate (Tranxene).

Pathophysiology

The precise mechanism of action of the benzodiazepines is not well known. These agents apparently can inhibit arousal of the CNS upon stimulation of the reticular formation in the brain stem. Benzodiazepines also may exert their tranquilizing effect through action on the limbic system.

The benzodiazepine drugs potentiate the toxicities of alcohol, barbiturates, and narcotics. Concomitant abuse of two or more of these agents presents significant risks of morbidity and mortality.

Clinical Features

The major toxicity of the benzodiazepines is CNS depression. There are no primary autonomic or cardiovascular side effects. The most dangerous complications are respiratory depression and hypoxia.

Diagnostic Tests

Blood levels of the substance are of little value in management. However, identification of other toxins is important.

Therapy

Therapy largely involves support of respiration. Hypotension is unusual and easily treated with fluids. Dialysis is not indicated.[18]

Follow-up

Prognosis is determined more by the presence or absence of other poisons. Psychologic, but not physical, dependency can result.

CHOLINERGICS

Several classes of agents are toxic by virtue of their cholinergic properties, acting either as analogs of the neurotransmitter acetylcholine or as inhibitors of acetylcholinesterase, the enzyme that inactivates acetylcholine. Examples of the former include nicotine, pilocarpine, methacholine, and bethanechol. In the latter group are neostigmine, physostigmine, pyridostigmine and insecticides of both carbamate and organophosphate types, including such compounds as TEPP (tetraethylpyrophosphate), OMPA (octamethyl pyrophosphoramide), malathion, parathion, Di-Syston, Diazinon and Systox, Baygon, carbaryl (Sevin), aldicarb (Temik), and some plants and poisonous mushrooms. Since nicotine is poorly absorbed from ingested tobacco, most children who swallow cigarettes or other forms of tobacco do not develop significant nicotine poisoning.

Pathophysiology

Acetylcholine is the biochemical mediator of synaptic transmission at the endings of postganglionic parasympathetic nerves, the sympathetic and parasympathetic preganglionic nerve fibers, the neuromuscular junction of skeletal muscle, and also within areas of the CNS. Cholinergic overdosage leads to overstimulation of receptors at these sites by acetylcholine (in cases of anticholinesterase poisoning) or by its analogs (e.g., nicotine, muscarine). Symptoms of cholinergic poisoning are attributable to stimulation of "nicotinic" receptors in smooth muscle, heart, and exocrine glands, and of cholinergic pathways within the CNS.[19,20]

Both the organophosphate and carbamate insecticides are potent inhibitors of acetylcholinesterase. In particular, organophosphates cause phosphorylation and thus "irreversible" inhibition of acetylcholinesterase; with carbamate insecticides the inhibition of cholinesterases is fairly rapidly reversible. This peculiar pharmacology of the organophosphate insecticide group must be taken into account in the management of poisoning with those compounds, since the administration of pralidoxime chloride (2-PAM) is indicated (see "Therapy"), in addition to other measures.

Clinical Features

Patients with cholinergic overdose demonstrate symptoms referable to overstimulation of cholinergic receptors. The "muscarinic" effects include

- miosis
- bronchospasm (with wheezing and complaints of chest tightness)

- increased lacrimation, salivation, and bronchorrhea
- diaphoresis
- increased GI tone with nausea, vomiting, diarrhea, and abdominal cramps
- bradycardia
- urinary incontinence caused by detrusor contraction

"Nicotinic" effects are manifested by muscle weakness, easy fatigability, cramping, and fasciculations. Respiratory failure, with dyspnea and cyanosis, can result from both weakness of the respiratory muscles and bronchoconstriction. Other nicotinic effects may be seen at the level of the sympathetic ganglion and can override or mask some of the muscarinic effects described above. Thus tachycardia, hypertension, pallor, and hyperglycemia can occur.[19,20]

Accumulation of acetylcholine in the CNS is responsible for the symptoms of anxiety, nausea, insomnia, emotional lability, and confusion. Slurring of speech, ataxia, depression of CNS respiratory and circulatory centers, and coma may be seen as central effects of cholinergic overstimulation.

The most common symptoms are weakness, headache, abdominal pains, and dyspnea. Respiratory failure is the single most important cause of morbidity and death in cholinergic poisoning. Bronchoconstriction, increased tracheobronchial secretions, weakness of the muscles of respiration, and depression of the CNS respiratory center are additive factors in the development of hypoxia, hypercarbia, and respiratory arrest.

Diagnostic Tests

Since the history and physical examination often provide sufficient information to make a presumptive diagnosis of cholinergic poisoning, the physician should *not* wait for the results of laboratory studies before initiating therapy in most cases. However, selected routine laboratory tests (complete blood count; measurement of electrolytes, serum urea nitrogen, blood glucose, and arterial blood gases) should be obtained before instituting therapy. Blood samples for determination of plasma and erythrocyte cholinesterase levels should also be obtained before the administration of any antidotes; the erythrocyte acetylcholinesterase level appears to be identical to that found in neural tissue and is a sensitive test to assess the degree of cholinergic poisoning.[21] Normal levels of erythrocyte and plasma cholinesterase rule out significant poisoning with a cholinergic agent; however, the depression of erythrocyte cholinesterase to 30% to 40% of normal values and the total inhibition of plasma cholinesterase may be observed in the absence of clinical symptoms.

Routine urinalysis is indicated in all patients with cholinergic poisoning. Toxicologic analysis of the urine may identify some organophosphorus compounds or disclose the presence of urinary paranitrophenol, which is a product of the metabolism of organophosphate insecticide.

Therapy

Establishment of airway patency with endotracheal intubation, if necessary; suctioning of copious secretions; and assisted ventilation may all be required. Supplemental oxygen is indicated, especially if the patient appears cyanotic. In addition to general measures for the removal of the poison from the GI tract (emesis or lavage, activated charcoal, catharsis), particular attention should be paid to the skin, which can be a major route for absorption of some cholinergics (e.g., insecticides). Areas of contaminated skin should be cleansed with mild soap and water; the addition of baking soda to the water has been advocated as a method of hastening the hydrolysis of organophosphate esters. Cleansing of the eyes by irrigation may be required if absorption from the conjunctiva is suspected.

All significant poisonings with cholinergics can be managed initially with the intravenous administration of atropine.[19–22] Atropine blocks the action of acetylcholine or its analogs at the postsynaptic receptors, thereby blocking the effects of cholinergic overstimulation. Large doses of atropine are necessary to overcome cholinergic effects: in the infant and child, a dose of 0.05 mg/kg is appropriate, whereas a dose of 2 to 3 mg may be given to an adolescent or adult. These doses should be repeated every 5 to 10 minutes until the patient is fully "atropinized," i.e., when pupillary dilatation; increasing pulse rate; dry, flushed skin; dry mouth; and decreased bowel sounds are all present. Doses of atropine should then be repeated as necessary to maintain full atropinization.

In patients with poisoning due to organophosphate insecticides, atropine does not restore the levels of tissue cholinesterases, which have been "irreversibly" phosphorylated into an inactive state. In organophosphate poisoning *only*, the administration of 2-PAM (Protopam) reverses the organophosphate-induced inactivation of cholinesterases by accelerating the hydrolysis of the phosphorylated enzyme.[22] 2-PAM should be given only after the patient is fully atropinized. It is administered by slow push intravenously; a dose of 250 mg is recommended for infants and children, and 0.5 to 1 g may be given to adolescents and adults. These doses can be repeated in 1 hour if needed and again in 8 to 12 hours. 2-PAM is of value only within the first 24 hours after exposure to organophosphates, and it is of no value in the management of poisonings due to carbamate insecticides or other cholinergic agents.

Certain drugs are contraindicated in patients with organophosphate insecticide poisoning: aminophylline, theophylline, succinylcholine, and morphine. Chlorpromazine and other tranquilizing drugs should be avoided. Occasionally, the patient with cholinergic poisoning may have seizures, in which case ventilatory support should be provided and intravenous diazepam or thiopental can be administered.

Since symptoms of cholinergic poisoning usually last from less than 24 to up to 48 hours, the therapy described above should continue for 24 hours, followed by observation for 48 to 72 hours, ideally in an intensive care setting. In those patients who demonstrate a recurrence of cholinergic symptoms and signs, immediate reinstitution of atropinization is indicated.[20]

Follow-up

Patients treated for cholinergic overdosage caused by pesticide poisoning should avoid reexposure to the offending agent for several weeks after the episode of poisoning, because of increased sensitivity to those agents during the recovery period.

HALLUCINOGENIC DRUGS

Drugs in this group include lysergic acid diethylamide (LSD), psilocybin, mescaline, marijuana, amphetamine, derivatives such as STP (dimethoxymethylamphetamine), phencyclidine (PCP), and cocaine.

Pathophysiology

Most of the initial clinical findings with these drugs are related to their sympathomimetic effects. However, the consciousness-altering manifestations often last from hours to days. Some data suggest that these latter changes are due to effects on brain serotonin levels. "Flashbacks," recurrences of the consciousness-altering effects, have not been explained. These phenomena do not occur with cocaine or PCP.

Clinical Features

Sympathomimetic effects include tachycardia, dry mouth, pupillary dilatation, hypertension, and hyperthermia.[23,24] With cocaine and PCP, hypertension may be so intense as to produce intracranial hemorrhage and stroke. The so-called "mind-altering" effects include visual illusions, feelings of euphoria and detachment, and altered sense of time and space.[23,24] These are generally the sought-after effects from use of the drug; however, in large doses and in certain susceptible individuals, these effects can lead to feelings of depersonalization, loss of control, fear of losing one's mind, and paranoid ideations. During these "panic attacks," the users can be dangerous to themselves and others.[25] PCP seems especially likely to produce an aggressive, combative, paranoid state.[23]

Diagnostic Tests

Emergency drug screens should be obtained, although many of these agents are difficult to detect or continue to produce derangements of consciousness even after clearance from the circulation. The common substitution of anticholinergics, amphetamines, and PCP for other hallucinogens sold "on the street" also makes this important.

Therapy

In most cases calm reassurance, a quiet environment, and help with reality testing is all that is required to "talk down" the panicking user.[24,26] Physical restraints are often counterproductive, but sedation with diazepam[27] or chlordiazepoxide is helpful and can often be given orally. Phenothiazines should be avoided since they can produce hypotension and paradoxical effects when used with STP or PCP. Forced emesis and gastric lavage are rarely useful and may reinforce the patient's feelings of paranoia. In PCP ingestions, however, this may be required, and continuous gastric suction may enhance elimination. Acid diuresis, as described for amphetamine intoxication (see "Sympathomimetics"), also hastens elimination of PCP.[23] Severe hypertension, if present, should be treated with phentolamine, propranolol, or other antihypertensive agents.

Follow-up

"Flashbacks," which are common in chronic users, can also occur with one-time use and can be managed as described previously. LSD can produce chromosomal aberrations. Chronic rhinitis and even nasal septal perforation are sequelae of chronic "snorting." An apathetic withdrawal from the world can occur in the chronic abuser.[24,26]

HYDROCARBONS

Hydrocarbons are second only to medications as a cause of poisoning. Ingestion is the most common route, but poisoning by inhalation also occurs because of the volatility of many of these compounds. Although sometimes accidental, this occurs more often as a sequela of deliberate inhalation, so-called "glue-sniffing."

Pathophysiology

Most of the morbidity and mortality of hydrocarbon poisoning is due to the resultant pulmonary changes. Experimental evidence suggests that hydrocarbon pneumonitis results from direct chemical injury to the alveolar lining and pulmonary capillaries. Even small amounts can produce marked damage. These substances may be aspirated during ingestion or with subsequent vomiting; many reach the pulmonary parenchyma by direct extension from the hypopharynx because of their viscosity, volatility, and surface tension characteristics. Surfactant is disrupted by the solvent action, and the resulting pathologic change is a fibrinous, hyaline-membrane exudate that fills the alveoli. Edema, inflammatory cell infiltration, and hemorrhage also can occur.

Toxic CNS effects often accompany pulmonary symptomatology. This may be due to hypoxic cerebral damage or to a direct effect from absorbed toxin. Much of this absorption may be across the alveolar-capillary membrane, since GI absorption is generally poor. The pulmonary and CNS complications caused by some common hydrocarbons are listed in Table 18-5.

Hepatic and renal necroses are uncommon but may accompany severe poisoning. Halogenated hydrocarbons, such as carbon tetrachloride and trichloroethane, can severely injure these organs. Mycardial depression and ventricular arrhythmias are other major complications. Intravascular hemolysis also has been described.

TABLE 18-5 CNS and Pulmonary Complications Caused by Poisoning with Common Hydrocarbons

Product	Synonym	Main Use	CNS Depression	Pulmonary Pathology
Benzene	Benzol	Paint thinner	4+	1+
Toluene		Paint remover	4+	1+
Xylene (aromatic hydrocarbons)		Solvent, plastic, rubber cement	4+	1+
Turpentine (volatile oil)	Oil of turpentine	Paint thinner, paint remover	3+	1+
Petroleum ether	Benzine (*not* benzene)	Rubber solvent	4+	0
Gasoline	Petroleum spirits	Fuel	3+	2+
Petroleum naphtha	Ligroin	Cigarette lighter fluid	3+	3+
VMP naphtha	Varnish naphtha, painter's naphtha	Paint or varnish thinner	3+	3+
Mineral spirit	Stoddard solvent, white spirits, varsol, mineral turpentine, petroleum spirits	Dry cleaner, paint thinner, solvent	3+	3+
Kerosene	Coal oil	Charcoal lighter fluid; solvent; fuel for stoves, lamps	1+	2+
Fuel oil	Home heating oil	Fuel	1+	1+
Diesel oil	Gas oil	Fuel	1+	1+
Mineral seal oil	Signal oil	Furniture polish	1+	4+
Mineral oil (nontoxic)	Liquid petrolatum	Laxative, suntan oil	0	1+
Lubricating oils (nontoxic)	Motor oil, household oil, cutting oil, transmission fluid	Lubricants	0	1+
Triorthocresyl phosphate	Machine oil	Machine oil	Paralysis	
Shellac (5% methanol, 1% gasoline in ethanol)	Solox		3+	0
Asphalt	Asphalt, tar		0	0

Source: Reprinted with permission from Done AK: The toxic emergency: The fuel shortage—a dangerous spinoff. *Emerg Med* 1974;6:291.

Clinical Features

Early symptoms include a burning sensation in the mouth and throat, choking and gagging spells, cough, nausea, and often vomiting. Hydrocarbon odor of the breath is always a diagnostic clue. Worsening pulmonary involvement may become evident within an hour of ingestion, with cyanosis, grunting, flaring, retracting, rales, and even hemoptysis. Fever is often present. CNS symptoms include weakness, dizziness, delirium, agitation, coma, and convulsions. A euphoric phase may precede these, especially with inhalation poisoning.

Diagnostic Tests

A chest x-ray film must be obtained on all patients with a possible history of hydrocarbon ingestion. A follow-up film at 24 hours after ingestion may also be indicated, especially if the initial film was taken less than 12 hours after the ingestion occurred. Up to 75% of the patients have radiologic abnormalities, although only 25% to 40% are symptomatic. These abnormalities consist of fine, mottled densities extending from the perihilar regions to the lung bases, often with peripheral hyperaeration. This may progress to areas to form consolidation or atelectasis with surrounding emphysema. Pleural effusions, pneumothorax, pneumomediastinum, and pneumatoceles are unusual but do occur. Resolution is variable, within days to several weeks.

Leukocytosis is often present. Some specific hydrocarbons and large ingestions may produce transaminase elevations, cholestasis, azotemia, renal tubular acidosis, albuminuria, and cylindruria. Careful attention to blood gas parameters is more important with pulmonary involvement.

Therapy

Symptomatic patients, patients with a history of symptoms, and patients with abnormal chest films should be hospitalized. Asymptomatic patients films can be discharged from the emergency department after 6 to 8 hours of observation.

The role of emesis and gastric lavage in the treatment of hydrocarbon ingestions remains controversial. In the asymptomatic patient who has ingested less than 1 mL of a hydrocarbon per kilogram of body weight, emesis and lavage are unnecessary and should be avoided. (This group, no doubt, represents the bulk of patients.) However, the hydrocarbon should be removed from the stomach if

1. The hydrocarbon has significant intrinsic CNS, hepatic, renal, or myocardial toxic effects (e.g., triorthocresyl phosphate, benzene, toluene, turpentine, pine oil).
2. The amount ingested (greater than 1 to 2 mL/kg) may produce such toxic effects.
3. An additive (e.g., camphor, naphthalene, heavy metals, nitrobenzene, pesticides, or trichloroethane) is toxic.

In the alert patient with an intact gag reflex, induction of emesis with syrup of ipecac seems at least as safe as gastric lavage if it is carried out under careful supervision and in an upright posture. In the patient with any significant symptoms, gastric lavage should be performed *after* a cuffed endotracheal tube has been inserted and inflated. Patients requiring endotracheal tubes too small to be cuffed can be managed with external cricoid pressure during the lavage procedure.

Gastric instillation of olive oil or mineral oil is of no benefit and may increase GI absorption of the hydrocarbon. Lipoid pneumonia is another potential complication of this outmoded therapy.

Careful attention to oxygenation and ventilation is the mainstay of therapy in this disorder. Positive-pressure assisted ventilation is used to normalize blood gas parameters.

Controlled studies show no benefit from the use of corticosteroids in hydrocarbon pneumonia. Likewise, prophylactic antibiotics do not reduce the incidence of secondary bacterial infections but can lead to the emergence of resistant strains. However, the usual signs of bacterial infection are mimicked by hydrocarbon pneumonitis and may justify the use of antibiotics.

Epinephrine and other adrenergic agents may provoke life-threatening arrhythmias in these patients and are contraindicated. Dopamine or dobutamine are the pressor agents of choice if required in this situation.

Follow-up

The long-term prognosis for patients who survive the acute pneumonitis appears good, provided significant hypoxic CNS damage has not been done. Most are asymptomatic, although some roentgenographic and pulmonary function abnormalities may persist. The long-term risk for the development of chronic obstructive pulmonary disease is unknown.

IRON

The accidental ingestion of medicinal iron is common in children, and the intentional overdosage of iron-containing compounds can be seen in young adults. The availability of iron tablets poses a significant threat to children, who may mistake the colored, enteric-coated tablets for candy. There are very few cases of serious poisonings caused by children's iron-supplemented multivitamins or iron drops. The amount of elemental iron varies with different preparations, and this factor must be taken into account when one estimates the total potential dose that the patient might have taken. For example, ferrous sulfate contains 20% elemental iron; ferrous fumarate, 33%; and ferrous gluconate, 11.5%. In addition, the awareness of the clinical stages in iron poisoning is important for the optimal assessment of the patient and the institution of specific therapy.

Pathophysiology

After its absorption from the GI tract, iron causes vasodilation and increased capillary permeability, which leads to hypotension, hypoperfusion, and acidosis.[28,29] When sufficient quantities of iron are absorbed, serum transferrin becomes saturated and free iron appears in the circulation. Free iron is taken up by the liver, where it induces mitochondrial dysfunction, perhaps by the peroxidation of lipids within the mitochondrial membranes. The electron transport system, which is essential for aerobic respiration, is impaired as a result of mitochondrial damage. The shunting of electrons to the accumulated iron, which acts as an "electron sink" within the mitochondria, further inhibits electron transport, uncouples oxidative phosphorylation, and leads to losses in production of adenosine triphosphate. The end result is hepatocellular dysfunction and necrosis. In the GI tract the contact of iron with the mucosa causes ulcerations and bleeding.

Clinical Features

The toxic dose of elemental iron is greater than or equal to 80 mg/kg; however, signs and symptoms of poisonings (e.g., nausea, vomiting, and hematemesis) can be seen with lower doses (50 mg/kg). One must assume that the *greatest potential amount* available to the patient was ingested and employ that amount to estimate the severity of the ingestion (on the basis of body weight). The exact identity of the compound is also important, since the amount of elemental iron varies with the type of ferrous salt in the preparation.

The patient with iron poisoning demonstrates four clinical stages.[28–30] The *first stage* occurs within the first 6 hours after ingestion and is manifested by direct GI toxic effects (nausea, vomiting, diarrhea, and abdominal pain). Hematemesis and, on rare occasions, melena are due to hemorrhagic gastroenteritis, which may lead to life-threatening blood loss in severe cases. Evidence of impaired perfusion includes hypotension, peripheral vasoconstriction, and mental status abnormalities (irritability, drowsiness, or coma).

The *second stage* of iron poisoning lasts from 24 to 48 hours after the ingestion and is characterized by an apparent improvement in the clinical status. It is crucial that the clinician should not enjoy a false sense of security at this time, during which free iron is present in the circulation and is beginning to exert toxic effects on the liver. Failure to recognize this "quiescent interlude" in the evolution of iron poisoning can result in inadequate therapy or inappropriate lack of monitoring of the patient.

The *third stage* represents the expression of the toxic effects of free iron in the circulation. Metabolic acidosis, hepatocellular damage, hyperpyrexia, shock, decreased perfusion, and hypoglycemia may be present. Pulmonary edema, cyanosis, and elevated total leukocyte count can also be seen at this stage. Even at this juncture, serum iron levels may be normal or only slightly elevated.

The *fourth stage* accounts for the late sequelae observed in survivors of acute iron poisoning. Weeks to months after the ingestion, hepatic necrosis or fibrosis, GI strictures or obstruction, and damage to the CNS may be observed.

Diagnostic Tests

Patients with a history of iron ingestion should have the following studies: determination of serum electrolytes and urea nitrogen, complete blood count, urinalysis, and guaiac tests on vomitus and stool. Serum iron and total iron-binding capacity (TIBC) should be determined initially and several hours later, since peak levels of iron are reached between 2 and 4 hours after the ingestion. Free iron is present when the serum iron concentration exceeds the TIBC. Patients in whom the TIBC is reduced (e.g., chronic disease states, hypoproteinemia) manifest toxic effects at lower iron levels because the TIBC is rapidly saturated and relatively more free iron is present.

Other diagnostic procedures may help in assessing the severity of the ingestion. Since iron-containing tablets are radiopaque, a plain x-ray film of the abdomen may demonstrate intact pills and pill fragments. This film is especially useful after induction of emesis, since it serves as an indicator of residual iron in the GI tract.

A valuable and important diagnostic and therapeutic test is the deferoxamine challenge test.[28] This procedure relies on the ability of deferoxamine

(Desferal) to chelate iron and on the excretion of this chelated iron, as ferrioxamine, in the urine. Since ferrioxamine is a colored compound, its appearance as a salmon pink or "*vin rosé*" color in the urine indicates a significant ingestion of iron. Two grams of deferoxamine is administered IM, and all subsequent urine output is observed for a change in color.

Therapy[31]

Emesis should be induced with ipecac if no contraindications to its administration exist. Activated charcoal does not adsorb iron and therefore should not be given. Following emesis, *all patients* should have gastric lavage performed with a solution containing 2 g deferoxamine in 1 L of water, to which is added sufficient sodium bicarbonate to raise the gastric pH above 5.0. After lavage the patient should receive via gastric tube 10 g deferoxamine in 50 mL of water that has been alkalinized with sodium bicarbonate to maintain a gastric pH above 5.0. An abdominal x-ray film should be obtained to detect intact pills and large pill fragments. Serum iron levels and TIBC should be determined. Intravenous fluids must be administered to ensure satisfactory urine output, and all urine should be observed for the characteristic *vin rosé* color of chelated iron.

The patient should be observed for at least 6 hours after ingestion. A patient who is completely asymptomatic at that time and has no evidence of residual pill fragments or of ferrioxamine excretion in the urine may be discharged with close follow-up. However, patients who, at any time during the period of observation, demonstrate signs or symptoms of acute iron poisoning, pass characteristic *vin rosé* urine, and/or have radiologic evidence of residual iron-containing pills in the GI tract should be treated with a continuous IV infusion of deferoxamine at a dose of 15 mg/kg/h. The deferoxamine can be added to normal saline or lactated Ringer's solution; administration rates should not exceed 15 mg/kg/h because hypotension can occur at higher doses. Continue the intravenous deferoxamine therapy until the urine color is normal and the patient is asymptomatic for at least 24 hours.

The comatose, hypotensive patient with anuria is rarely seen but this may be evidence of severe iron poisoning. In this situation hemodialysis along with concurrent intravenous administration of deferoxamine is warranted. Peritoneal dialysis is not effective in the hypotensive patient with poor perfusion.

Follow-up

The patient who has ingested a toxic amount of iron should be followed up within a few weeks of the poisoning.[30,31] The local effects of iron on the GI tract mucosa warrant follow-up contrast studies (barium enema, upper Gi series with small-bowel follow-through) since strictures and obstruction can develop, especially at antral and pyloric locations. The toxic effects of free iron on the liver may cause cirrhosis and hepatic fibrosis; therefore, serial measurement of liver size (span) by physical examination and tests to determine hepatic function should be done. Some patients who survive severe iron ingestions may require liver biopsy to ascertain the degree of resultant hepatic cirrhosis.

Finally, the chelation therapy utilized in iron poisoning, along with GI blood losses, can deplete normal iron stores, which may be marginal in the child. Therefore, measurements of the hemoglobin level and mean corpuscular hemoglobin concentration as well as a reticulocyte count are necessary in the follow-up of patients after treatment for iron ingestion. If evidence of iron deficiency is present on these tests, a therapeutic trial of iron is indicated.

LEAD

Symptomatic lead poisoning has become an unusual disorder. However, asymptomatic increased lead burden is a major public health problem. Increasing evidence suggests that "asymptomatic" lead poisoning plays a role in cognitive deficits and behavioral disorders in children.[32] The recognition and management of plumbism in its early stages are important to minimize sequelae.

Pathophysiology

Lead has no known biologic function in man. Environmental sources of lead contamination, such as house dust and automobile exhaust, have been linked to moderate blood levels detected in asymptomatic individuals. Pica for lead-based paint and plaster is no doubt the major source of lead in symptomatic cases. Uncommon environmental sources, such as lead smelting, burning of battery casings, ingestion of lead weights or shot, and contamination from leaded pipes, pottery, and canned goods should be ruled out. The removal of the patient from sources of environmental contamination is always the first step in management.

Deficient dietary intake of calcium, magnesium, zinc, and copper, as well as excessive dietary fat, increase the absorption, retention, and toxicity of lead. Iron deficiency usually accompanies lead poisoning.

The principal tissues affected by lead poisoning are the erythroid cells of the bone marrow, the central and peripheral nervous systems, and the kidney. Erythroid cells are most sensitive; lead interferes with the biosynthesis of heme at several steps. Alterations in levels of heme precursors and degradation products are important in the diagnosis of plumbism.[33,34]

Clinical Features

Signs and symptoms include

- pica
- anorexia
- abdominal pain
- vomiting
- irritability
- developmental delay or regression
- hyperactivity
- behavioral problems
- seizures
- ataxia

Asymptomatic individuals may demonstrate "lead lines" on x-ray films obtained for other reasons or may have a microcytic anemia. Peripheral neuropathy, gingival lead lines, and gouty manifestations are unusual in children.

Acute encephalopathy usually has a prodrome of several weeks' duration, consisting of insidious anorexia, apathy, irritability, incoordination, developmental regression, and vomiting. Gross ataxia, persistent and forceful vomiting, stupor, coma, and convulsions are manifestations of increased intracranial pressure and cerebral vasculitis.

Symptomatic cases are more common in the warmer months of the year, as blood lead levels tend to rise at this time. While increased exposure is postulated as one cause, no true explanation has been found.

Diagnostic Tests

Whole blood lead concentration is the most widely used index of current and recent lead absorption. Erythrocyte protoporphyrin (EP) levels, indicative of abnormalities in heme synthesis, are now widely used in screening for asymptomatic plumbism and can be determined from capillary blood samples. EP is also a rough measure of the chronicity of exposure. Table 18-6 lists the classes of plumbism, as defined by EP levels. Two tables are given as the classes vary depending upon the method used to measure EP. This classification merely suggests the relative risk and the priority for medical evaluation and environmental intervention. The tables should be used only as general guidelines. Children 12 to 36 months old should be given priority over older ones, and children whose EP and blood lead levels are in the upper range of a class should be given priority over those whose levels fall in the lower range. Children in Class IV—at urgent risk for lead toxicity—should be medically evaluated within 24 hours. Children in Class III are at high risk, Class II at moderate risk, and those in Class I at low risk. Children with symptoms should be referred for immediate evaluation, regardless of their risk classification, but if the blood lead concentration is less than 50 μg/dl, other diagnostic possibilities should be vigorously sought. EP levels fall slowly with termination of exposure. They may even rise transiently during treatment. EP is a rough measure of the chronicity of exposure. It is also elevated in iron deficiency, hemolytic anemias, and acute illnesses.

δ-Aminolevulinic acid determinations are rarely used clinically. The urine coproporphyrin test, although sensitive in symptomatic cases, is also little used today. The calcium disodium versenate ($CaNa_2$-EDTA) provocative test is useful in asymptomatic cases.[34A] $CaNa_2$-EDTA is administered at a dose of 500 mg/m^2 IV in 250 ml/m^2 of 5% dextrose, infused over 1 hour. (A painful but practical alternative is to administer the same dose IM mixed with

TABLE 18-6

Zinc Protoporphyrin (ZnPP) by Hematofluorometer
Risk Classification of Asymptomatic Children for Priority Medical Evaluation

	Erythrocyte Protoporphyrin (EP) #			
Blood Lead #	**<35**	**35–74**	**75–174**	**>175**
Not done	I	*	*	*
<24	I	Ia	Ia	EPP+
25–49	Ib	II	III	III
50–69	**	III	III	IV
>70	**	**	IV	IV

Erythrocyte Protoporphyrin (EP) by Extraction
Risk Classification of Asymptomatic Children for Priority Medical Evaluation

	Erythrocyte Protoporphyrin (EP) #			
Blood Lead #	**<35**	**35–109**	**110–249**	**>250**
Not done	I	*	*	*
<24	I	Ia	Ia	EPP+
25–49	Ib	II	III	III
50–69	***	III	III	IV
>70	***	***	IV	IV

= Units are in μg/dl of whole blood.
* = Blood lead test needed to estimate risk.
EPP+ = Erythropoietic protoporphyria. Iron deficiency may cause elevated EP levels up to 300 μg/dl, but this is rare.
** = In practice, this combination of results is not generally observed; if it is observed; immediately retest with whole blood.
*** = In practice, this combination of results is not generally observed; if it is observed, immediately retest with venous blood.
NOTE: Diagnostic evaluation is more urgent than the classification indicates for—
1. Children with any symptoms compatible with lead toxicity.
2. Children under 36 months of age.
3. Children whose blood lead and EP levels place them in the upper part of a particular class.
4. Children whose siblings are in a higher class.
These guidelines refer to the interpretation of screening results, but the final diagnosis and disposition rest on a more complete medical and laboratory examination of the child.

Source: Reprinted with permission from Centers for Disease Control: *Preventing lead poisoning in young children.* Atlanta: U.S. Department of Health and Human Services, 1985.

0.5% Procaine.) All urine must be collected with lead-free equipment over 8 hours. The total urinary excretion of lead in micrograms is dived by the amount of $CaNa_2$-EDTA given in milligrams to obtain the "lead excretion ratio." The $CaNa_2$-EDTA provocation test is considered positive if the lead excretion ratio exceeds 0.60. This test is contraindicated in symptomatic patients and in patients with blood lead levels greater than 55 μg/dl because it may unmask encephalopathy.

Basophilic stippling of bone marrow normoblasts is characteristic of plumbism; stippling of erythrocytes in the peripheral blood is less consistent. A hypochromic, microcytic smear mimics iron deficiency, although plumbism and iron deficiency often coexist. X-ray films of the abdomen may reveal radiopaque foreign matter. Metaphyseal lead lines in long bones are a function of the duration and degree of excessive lead absorption but are not related to the severity of symptoms. The levels of lead in hair or fingernails are not well correlated with blood lead levels; therefore, tests for these levels are not considered useful in diagnosis. Renal abnormalities in plumbism may include Fanconi's syndrome (hypophosphatemia with hyperphosphaturia, glycosuria, and generalized aminoaciduria), albuminuria, hematuria, and renal failure.

Lumbar puncture should be avoided in acutely symptomatic cases unless other causes of increased intracranial pressure must be excluded. In those situations the minimum amount of cerebrospinal fluid should be collected through the smallest needle possible. In acute lead encephalopathy the cerebrospinal fluid shows mild pleocytosis, a normal glucose level, and moderate elevation of protein.

Therapy[31]

The patient must be removed from the lead-contaminated environment immediately. Asymptomatic individuals should receive a low-fat, lead-free diet, with adequate calcium, magnesium, zinc, iron, and copper. After chelation therapy, iron deficiency should be treated. Exhibit 18-2 lists the chelation protocols.

All symptomatic patients should be treated as if they have impending encephalopathy. Symptomatic or frankly encephalopathic patients are treated as follows: Patients are given nothing orally and receive a 10% glucose solution, 10 to 20 mL/kg IV, to establish urine output. Mannitol, at a dose of 1 to 2 g/kg IV, may also be required. Fluids are then restricted to minimize increased intracranial pressure yet still maintain adequate urine output (0.5 to 1.0 ml/kg/h). Invasive intracranial pressure monitoring, controlled hyperventilation, hypothermia, and pentobarbital coma may be indicated. The role of corticosteroids is controversial. Seizures, if present, are best controlled with intravenous diazepam and paraldehyde; phenobarbital and phenytoin are less useful here but may be required later for long-term seizure control. Renal failure may require dialysis.

Chelation in the symptomatic patient involves two drugs: British anti-Lewisite (BAL) and $CaNa_2$-EDTA. The side-effects of BAL include vomiting, hypertension, and tachycardia. It is available only as an IM preparation. $CaNa_2$-EDTA is given by continuous IV drip in dextrose and water or 0.9% saline solution. The concentration of $CaNa_2$-EDTA should not exceed 0.5% in the parenteral fluid. In the treatment of acute encephalopathy, restriction of parenteral fluids takes precedence, so that $CaNa_2$-EDTA may have to be given intramuscularly with 0.5% Procaine if fluid overload is to be avoided. $CaNa_2$-EDTA is contraindicated in the anuric patient. If it is used alone in the symptomatic patient, $CaNa_2$-EDTA may exacerbate increased intracranial pressure. Combined BAL-$CaNa_2$-EDTA therapy is given for a total of 5 days. During treatment, renal and hepatic function and serum electrolyte levels should be monitored daily.

Asymptomatic children with increased body burden of lead may also require chelation therapy based on their blood lead concentration and/or $CaNa_2$-EDTA provocation test. If the blood lead level is greater than 69 μg/dl, BAL and $CaNa_2$-EDTA should be given in the same doses and with the same guidelines as for the treatment of symptomatic lead poisoning. At lower blood lead levels treatment should be limited to $CaNa_2$-EDTA alone. This is best given by continuous IV infusion, though divided IV doses are also effective. As a less preferred option, $CaNa_2$-EDTA may be administered IM with 0.5% procaine in a single daily dose. This is a practical but painful alternative. During treatment, blood lead, renal, and hepatic function, and serum electrolyte levels must be monitored.

D-Penicillamine is an experimental chelating agent for the treatment of lead poisoning. It is not licensed by the FDA for this indication.

Follow-up

Patients with acute encephalopathy often have residual neurologic deficits and seizure disorders. Neurologic abnormalities in less severely affected patients may be reversible. Renal lesion generally resolve, but chronic renal failure can result. Iron deficiency must be corrected. Most importantly, reexposure to lead must be eliminated or minimized.

Exhibit 18-2 Choice of Chelation Therapy Based on Symptoms and Blood Lead Concentration

Clinical presentation	Treatment		Comments
Symptomatic children			
Acute encephalopathy	BAL $CaNa_2$-EDTA	450 $mg/m^2/day$ 1500 $mg/m^2/day$	Start with BAL 75 mg/m^2 IM every 4 hours. After 4 hours start continuous infusion of $CaNa_2$-EDTA 1500 $mg/m^2/day$. Therapy with BAL and $CaNa_2$-EDTA should be continued for 5 days. Interrupt therapy for 2 days. Treat for 5 additional days, including BAL if blood Pb remains high. Other cycles may be needed depending on blood Pb rebound.
Other symptoms	BAL $CaNa_2$-EDTA	300 $mg/m^2/day$ 1000 $mg/m^2/day$	Start with BAL 50 mg/m^2 IM every 4 hours. After 4 hours start $CaNa_2$-EDTA 1000 $mg/m^2/day$, preferably by continuous infusion, or in divided doses IV (through a heparin lock). Therapy with $CaNa_2$-EDTA should be continued for 5 days. BAL may be discontinued after 3 days if blood Pb <50 μg/dl. Interrupt therapy for 2 days. Treat for 5 additional days, including BAL if blood Pb remains high. Other cycles may be needed depending on blood Pb rebound.
Asymptomatic children			
Before treatment, measure venous blood lead.			
Blood Pb >70 μg/dl	BAL $CaNa_2$-EDTA	300 $mg/m^2/day$ 1000 $mg/m^2/day$	Start with BAL 50 mg/m^2 IM every 4 hours. After 4 hours start $CaNa_2$-EDTA 1000 $mg/m^2/day$, preferably by continuous infusion, or in divided doses IV (through a heparin lock). Treatment with $CaNa_2$-EDTA should be continued for 5 days. BAL may be discontinued after 3 days if blood Pb <50 μg/dl. Other cycles may be needed depending on blood Pb rebound.
Blood Pb 56 to 69 μg/dl	$CaNa_2$-EDTA	1000 $mg/m^2/day$	$CaNa_2$-EDTA for 5 days, preferably by continuous infusion, or in divided doses (through a heparin lock). Alternatively, if lead exposure is controlled, $CaNa_2$-EDTA may be given as a single daily outpatient dose IM or IV. Other cycles may be needed depending on blood Pb rebound.
Blood Pb 25 to 55 μg/dl			
Perform $CaNa_2$-EDTA provocation test to assess lead excretion ratio (see text).			
If ratio >0.70	$CaNa_2$-EDTA	1000 $mg/m^2/day$	Treat for 5 days IV or IM, as above.
If ratio 0.60 to 0.69			
Age <3 years of age	$CaNa_2$-EDTA	1000 $mg/m^2/day$	Treat for 3 days IV or IM, as above.
Age >3 years of age	No treatment		Repeat blood Pb and $CaNa_2$-EDTA provocation test periodically.
If ratio <0.60	No treatment		Repeat blood Pb and $CaNa_2$-EDTA provocation test periodically.

Source: Reprinted with permission from Piomelli S, Rosen JF, Chisolm JJ Jr, Graef JW: Management of childhood lead poisoning. *J Pediatr* (1984;105:523–532), Copyright © 1984, CV Mosby Company.

MUSHROOM POISONING

Mushroom poisoning is an unusual but potentially lethal phenomenon. To all but the most expert, all wild mushrooms should be considered potential poisons. If ingestion occurs, exact identification by a competent mycologist is very useful.

Pathophysiology

Mushrooms may contain several different toxins. These include choline, muscarine, atropine and other alkaloids, hallucinogens such as psilocybin and psilocin, various GI toxins, and the very deadly complex polypeptides amanitin and phalloidin. Symptomatology depends upon the type and amount of toxin present.

Clinical Features

Immediate onset of signs and symptoms suggests that the poisoning is not likely to be serious. The early cholinergic symptoms of muscarine-like compounds include salivation, bradycardia, miosis, gastroenteritis, ataxia, and muscle twitching. Atropine-like symptoms may also occur. Delayed onset of symptoms, more than 6 hours after ingestion, is suggestive of potentially fatal poisoning with a phalloidin-type toxin. Signs and symptoms are those of gastroenteritis with nausea, vomiting, abdominal pain, and bloody diarrhea. Jaundice and hepatorenal failure develop 3 to 4 days after ingestion.

Therapy

Gastric evacuation should be performed. Activated charcoal and a cathartic can further limit absorption. The severity and preponderance of cholinergic or anticholinergic symptoms guide the use of physostigmine or atropine. In delayed-onset poisoning, hemodialysis or charcoal hemoperfusion is indicated. Antidotal therapy with thioctic acid, although still experimental, is available from the nearest poison control center.

Follow-up

Fatalities are common in delayed-type poisonings. Immediate-onset symptoms are usually amenable to supportive therapy.

OPIATES AND NARCOTICS

Narcotic overdose is usually the result of pediatric accidental ingestion, an overdose of street drug, or a medication error. Common narcotics are

- heroin
- morphine
- meperidine (Demerol)
- codeine
- diphenoxylate (with atropine; Lomotil)[35]
- propoxyphene (Darvon, Darvocet)[36]
- pentazocine (Talwin)
- loperamide (Imodium)
- butorphanol (Stadol)
- hydromorphone (Dilaudid)
- oxycodone (Percodan)
- methadone
- paregoric

Routes of exposure are ingestion, inhalation, or injection.

Pathophysiology

The GI absorption of narcotics is variable and depends on the preparation involved. Oral doses of heroin are poorly absorbed but it is the most potent addictive drug when used parenterally or by inhalation. Methadone is well adsorbed by the oral route and is increasingly a cause of childhood poisoning, being available in households through some drug treatment programs.

The apparently random phenomenon of sudden death immediately following intravenous injection of heroin is poorly understood but may be related to arrhythmias or an acute pulmonary hypersensitivity reaction. Acute pulmonary edema also can occur as a less sudden but life-threatening toxic effect.

Acute narcotic poisoning produces profound depression of the CNS. Sleep, analgesia, and respiratory depression are direct effects of its action on the cerebral cortex and medulla. Occasionally, stimulation of the medullary vomiting center causes severe nausea and vomiting. Hypotension, hypothermia, and cardiovascular collapse are secondary to severe hypoxia.

Clinical Features[8,24]

Stupor or coma has usually supervened by the time the physician first sees the patient with a narcotic overdose. Respirations are slow and shallow, and cyanosis is often evident. Blood pressure is at first maintained but then falls if hypoxia is not corrected. Pupils are usually pinpoint but may begin to dilate with profound coma or as a terminal event. Meperidine may produce pupillary dilation directly. Hypothermia is common, and the musculature is flaccid, often creating airway obstruction from local tissues. Codeine and heroin may initially produce excitement. Convulsions occur more commonly in children and with codeine or propoxyphene overdose. Itching and urticaria may be present because of histamine release. With Lomotil poisoning, symptoms of atropinization are often most prominent.[35]

Diagnostic Tests

Drug screens of the blood and urine should be carried out to identify the causative agent. Several drugs may be involved because of multiple-drug use or the presence of adulterants.

Therapy

Careful attention to airway patency and oxygenation is the critical first step. Cardiovascular instability often resolves with correction of hypoxia. If ingestion has been the mode of exposure, gastric lavage, activated charcoal, and cathartics are indicated, while protecting the airway at all times.[8]

A specific pharmacologic antagonist is available. Naloxone (Narcan), at a dose of 0.01 mg/kg IV, should be administered in all cases in which narcotic overdose might be involved.[24,37] Any improvement in mental status or pupillary findings confirms this. At least three doses given at 3-minute intervals should be tried before ruling out narcotic involvement. In severe intoxications doses up to 0.1 to 0.2 mg/kg have been required to produce a response.

Even at these doses naloxone has no known adverse side effects or contraindications.[37]

Any patient who demonstrates improvement with naloxone should continue to receive the drug as often and in as large a dose as required until mental status remains improved and respirations are normal and stable. This may require administration every 5 minutes, with continuation of the drug for up to several days. Naloxone has a very short half-life in comparison to most narcotics, and careful monitoring and maintenance of respiration and oxygenation must be continued until the depressant effect of the narcotic is clearly resolved.[24,37]

Follow-up

If respiratory support and naloxone administration have been optimal, recovery from the acute intoxication should be uneventful. Symptoms of withdrawal may supervene, however, and must be dealt with, although they are usually not life-threatening. Similarly, infants of addicted mothers may show early withdrawal symptoms if naloxone resuscitation was required.

PLANT POISONING

As reported to the National Clearinghouse for Poison Control Centers, plant poisoning is now the most frequent type of ingestion in children under 5 years of age. Plant poisonings are rarely fatal but are responsible for a great deal of morbidity.

Pathophysiology

Poisonous plants can be categorized according to their toxic constituents. These include alkaloids, glycosides, resins, phytotoxins, and oxalates.[38] Toxic plant products may be present in all of the plant or in only a portion.

Clinical Features

About 75% of plant poisonings involve toxic effects in the GI tract, with nausea, vomiting, and diarrhea. In addition, ingestion of toxic plants can produce a variety of other local and systemic reactions such as dermatitis, mucous membrane irritation, CNS symptoms, hepatic dysfunction, renal failure, and cardiac arrhythmias.[38,39]

Therapy

Treatment is largely symptomatic and supportive. Removal of the substance from the GI tract should be attempted by forced emesis with syrup of ipecac. Activated charcoal and cathartics are also useful. Symptoms and treatment for some of the more common plants are listed in Table 18-7.

Follow-up

Overall prognosis is generally good with supportive care because the magnitude of the ingestion is usually small.

SALICYLATES

Aspirin is one of the most common drugs accidentally ingested by children and accounts for the largest number of childhood deaths caused by poisoning. In addition to standard (325 mg) and "baby" (75 mg) aspirin tablets, acetylsalicyclic acid is a component of many prescription drugs and over-the-counter remedies. Methyl salicylate, more commonly known as oil of wintergreen, is found in many liniments and ointments. Because of its high concentration of salicylate, a small volume of oil of wintergreen can be highly toxic: 1 teaspoonful (5 mL) has been reported lethal in a 2-year-old child.

Pathophysiology

The toxic effects of salicylate are manifested at several levels.[40] Initially, stimulation of the respiratory center in the CNS leads to increased depth and rate of respirations; the attendant decrease in alveolar and arterial carbon dioxide pressure results in elevation of blood pH and respiratory alkalosis. However, increased renal excretion of bicarbonate, in response to the respiratory alkalosis, causes a decrease in total body buffering capacity and metabolic acidosis. Salicylates uncouple oxidative phosphorylation, leading to increased oxygen demand, decreased production of adenosine triphosphate, increased production of carbon dioxide, and increased total endogenous heat production. Tissue glycolysis and glucose utilization increase in salicylate poisoning and are especially significant in the CNS. Breakdown of glycogen, lipolysis, and inhibition of dehydrogenase enzymes in the Krebs cycle also occur. The formation of organic acids and ketone bodies as a result of these metabolic derangements causes metabolic acidosis, aciduria, and ketonuria. Glycosuria and ketonuria are accompanied by substantial fluid losses due to polyuria.

Clinical Features

The toxic single dose of salicylate is 150 mg/kg. If patients are evaluated soon after an ingestion, the serum levels of salicylate may not be elevated, and,

TABLE 18-7 Common Plant Poisonings

Plant	Toxic Part	Toxin	Symptoms	Treatment
Philodendron	All parts	Oxalates	Mouth and throat pain and swelling, with possible airway obstruction; abdominal pain; renal failure; hypocalcemia	Airway management, aluminum-magnesium hydroxide solutions, calcium supplements, adequate hydration
Yew	All parts	Taxine (alkaloid)	GI upset, mydriasis, weakness, bradycardia	Emesis, lavage, charcoal; cardiorespiratory support
Nightshade	Green fruit and spoiled sprouts	Solanine and atropine (alkaloids)	Gastroenteritis, hyperthermia, headache, CNS depression, delirium	Emesis, lavage, charcoal; supportive care; physostigmine
Holly	Berries	Ilicin, ilexanthin	Nausea, vomiting, diarrhea, stupor	Emesis, lavage, charcoal; supportive care
Poinsettia	White latex exuding from all parts of plant when broken	Not identified	Similar to oxalates	As for oxalates
Dieffenbachia	All parts	Oxalates	See philodendron	See philodendron
Black elder	All parts except berries	Cyanogenic glycoside sambunigrin	Dyspnea, excitation, ataxia, paralysis, seizures, coma, death	Lavage with sodium thiosulfate solution; amyl nitrite inhalation; IV sodium nitrite and sodium thiosulfate
Oleander	All parts	Cardiac glycosides nerioside and oleandroside	Mucous membrane irritation, gastroenteritis, arrhythmias	Emesis, lavage, charcoal; antiarrhythmic agents
Jerusalem cherry	Berries	Solanine (alkaloid)	See nightshade	See nightshade
Jimsonweed	Seeds	Atropine alkaloids	Pupillary dilatation, tachycardia, hyperthermia, delirium	Emesis, lavage, charcoal; physostigmine
Mistletoe	All parts, especially berries	Tyramine and β-phenylethylamine	Gastroenteritis bradyarrhythmias, hypertension	As for cardiac glycosides

Source: Adapted with permission from Burton D, Hanenson IB: Plant toxins, in Hanenson IB (ed): *Quick Reference to Clinical Toxicology.* Philadelphia, JB Lippincott Co, 1980, pp 243.

therefore, signs of poisoning may be minimal or absent. These patients merit a full evaluation, despite lack of symptomatology, to assess the potential severity of the ingestion and to institute therapeutic intervention (inhibition of further absorption of the ingested salicylate).[41,42]

Patients who exhibit toxic effects may have fever, tachypnea ("air hunger"), tachycardia, diaphoresis, and polyuria. Signs of dehydration may be present. Evidence of GI distress includes vomiting, diarrhea, and hematemesis. CNS manifestations include restlessness and irritability, and some patients may demonstrate delirium and hallucinations. Worrisome findings are those of seizures and coma.

The metabolic derangements referable to salicylate poisoning are more pronounced in younger children, i.e., under the age of 3 to 4 years.[41,43] In this group, metabolic acidosis is commonly encountered. Persistence of acidosis in these patients can enhance the uptake of salicylate into the CNS, leading to prolonged depressions of glucose in the CNS, despite normal or elevated blood glucose levels. It is felt that acidosis and low glucose concentrations within the CNS are factors in the clinical course, morbidity, and mortality of salicylism in young children.[40–42] In contrast, older children and adults with salicylate poisoning may manifest only a mild respiratory alkalosis and tend to have a smooth clinical course in the absence of underlying disease states. Hypoglycemia and hyperglycemia are also seen in patients with salicylate poisoning, although the former is more likely to occur in younger patients.

The loss of water and electrolytes, because of polyuria and excess sweating, leads to dehydration. Abnormalities in serum sodium potassium and bicarbonate are observed. Serum sodium levels tend to be elevated but may be normal or low. Although serum potassium levels may be in the normal range, total body potassium stores are usually depleted in severe salicylate poisoning. Depression of the serum bicarbonate concentration reflects the metabolic acidosis and the loss of total body buffering capacity.

Diagnostic Tests

Baseline studies in all patients with suspected salicylate ingestion should include measurement of serum electrolytes, blood glucose, serum urea nitrogen, and arterial blood gases; complete blood count; and urinalysis. Since salicylate can impair synthesis of prothrombin, inhibit platelet adhesiveness, and directly cause bleeding from mucosal surfaces, the evaluation of prothrombin time and guaiac tests for occult blood in the vomitus and stool are also indicated.

The quantitative determination of serum salicylate levels is imperative.[44] A semiquantitative rapid estimate of the serum salicylate level can be made with Phenistix reagent strips (Ames Company). Ferric chloride testing of urine yields positive results with very small concentrations of salicylate; thus, a positive urine ferric chloride test does not reflect the amount of salicylate ingested. Correlation of the severity of intoxication with the salicylate level can be made with the Done nomogram (Figure 18-2).[44] Note, however, that the nomogram starts at 6 hours after ingestion, to assure that peak levels have been obtained. The nomogram can be used earlier than 6 hours after an ingestion of salicylate, but *only* if other subsequent determinations are made to document declining levels of the substance.[44]

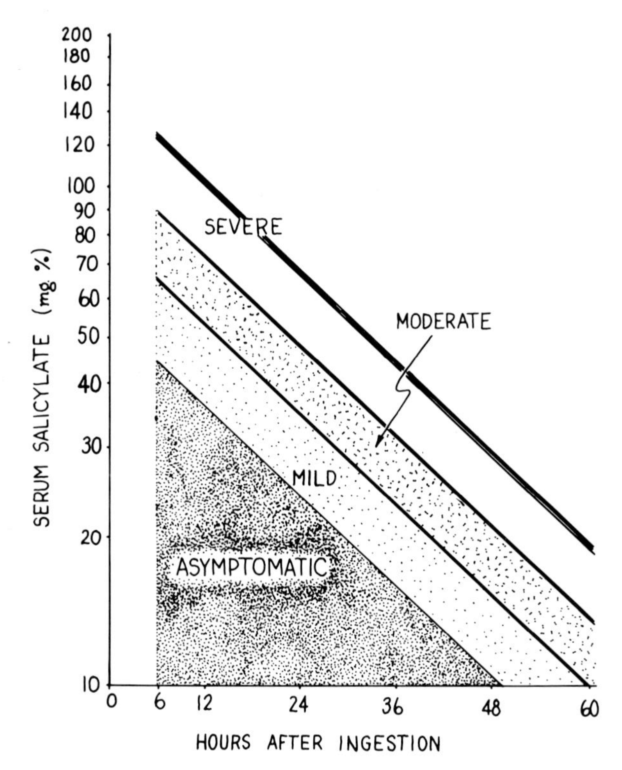

FIGURE 18-2 The "Done nomogram," which relates symptomatology to the serum salicylate level. See text for explanation. (Reprinted with permission from Done AK: Salicylate intoxication: Significance of salicylate levels in blood in cases of acute ingestion. *Pediatrics* 1960;26:805. Copyright American Academy of Pediatrics 1960.)

Therapy

Initial steps in the management of salicylate poisoning are those taken with most ingestions: rapid assessment of the type and amount of salicylate ingested, and measures to prevent further systemic absorption. The age of the patient must be taken into account, since younger children (under the ages of 3 to 4 years) are especially at risk for the significant metabolic complications of salicylate poisonings.

The induction of emesis with syrup of ipecac is indicated in all patients who have ingested salicylate, unless the patient is obtunded or comatose or unless hematemesis is present. Although most aspirin is well absorbed from the GI tract within 4 hours,[45] methyl salicylate (oil of wintergreen) may not be absorbed for 6 to 8 hours, and delayed absorption can also occur in other salicylate-containing products, such as enteric-coated aspirin. Thus evacuation of any residual salicylate in the stomach is warranted.

If the patient is obtunded, comatose, or having seizures, gastric lavage is performed with a solution of half-normal (75 mEq/L) sodium bicarbonate solution to dissolve the aspirin tablets and thus enhance their removal. After emesis or gastric lavage, a slurry of activated charcoal is instilled, and either sodium or magnesium sulfate is administered as a cathartic.

The patient with salicylism can demonstrate striking hyperpyrexia, and core temperatures can exceed 41.0°C. The judicious use of a cooling blanket is indicated in the management of hyperpyrexia resulting from salicylate poisoning.

Fluid status and fluid therapy demand close attention, since dehydration and acidosis aggravate the toxic effects of salicylate and also lead to disorders of body electrolyte composition. Insertion of a large-bore intravenous catheter is one of the single most important procedures in the management of these patients. In addition to monitoring blood pH and electrolytes and acquiring urine samples for urinalysis, strict and scrupulous measurement of intake and output is essential. The insertion of an indwelling (Foley) catheter into the bladder should be done for more exact measurements of urinary output. Furthermore, data about the clinical status (e.g., level of consciousness, vital signs) and from the laboratory results should be entered on a flow sheet along with notation of pertinent therapeutic maneuvers (e.g., content and rate of intravenous fluids administered). This flow sheet becomes a valuable adjunct to patient care, and it should be posted near the patient's bedside so that staff can keep track of the patient's progress "at a glance."

If the patient is hypotensive or appears to be in hypovolemic shock, a volume expander should be infused. Either 5% plasma protein fraction (Plasmanate, Albumisol), normal saline in 5% dextrose, or lactated Ringer's solution in 5% dextrose can be infused at 10 to 15 mL/kg/h over 1 hour. Infrequently, there is substantial blood loss because of hematemesis, in which case whole blood can be administered at 10 to 15 mL/kg over 1 hour.

The provision of sufficient volumes of parenteral fluids and adequate amounts of extracellular buffer is necessary to achieve satisfactory flow of alkaline urine, in which the salicylate ion is trapped and excreted.[40–42] Alkalinization of the urine can only occur after the replenishment of potassium deficits, which are commonplace in salicylism. Maintenance of alkalinity in the blood and urine also prevents entry of salicylate ion into the CNS. Fluid therapy in salicylate poisoning should begin with a solution that will initiate diuresis and alkalinization. For this purpose 5% dextrose, to which is added 50 mEq of sodium bicarbonate per liter, should be infused at 400 mL/m^2 for 1 hour, by which time urine output should be established (at least 2 mL/kg/h). If urine output is not established by the end of the first hour, the same solution is continued at 200 to 250 $mL/m^2/h$.

After sufficient urine output is achieved, potassium is added to the infusion: 5% dextrose with 50 mEq sodium bicarbonate and 40 mEq potassium chloride per liter. The solution is infused at a rate of 3 to 5 $L/m^2/d$ to maintain adequate urine output. Electrolytes, blood gases, and urine pH should be monitored, and the composition of the intravenous fluid should be modified according to the results of these tests. Avoidance of hypokalemia and maintenance of urine pH above 7.0 are the two most important aspects of fluid and electrolyte therapy in salicylate poisoning. The alkalinity of the urine, rather than its volume, is important for the excretion of salicylate ion. Fluid therapy should be continued until the patient has been asymptomatic for several hours. Serial determinations of serum salicylate levels should fall progressively as therapy continues.

In severe ingestions of salicylate, prothrombin synthesis may be impaired. The empiric administration of vitamin K by either the intramuscular or (with caution) the intravenous route is warranted in these severe cases.

Dialysis removes salicylate; however, it is indicated in only a limited number of situations. Convulsions (attributable to the salicylate poisoning and not to the complications of therapy), renal failure, and acidosis refractory to vigorous fluid and electrolyte therapy are all indications for institution of dialysis. Hemodialysis is generally employed in older children, whereas peritoneal dialysis is useful in younger children. In infants and very young children, exchange transfusion is the procedure of choice in severe salicylate poisoning.

Follow-up

The patient who has ingested a significant amount of salicylate should be elevated for neurologic status and renal dysfunction in the posttreatment period. Appropriate physical examination and laboratory tests should be performed to assess cardiorespiratory and electrolyte status. Attempts should be made to enforce and stress poison prevention at home.

SEDATIVES AND HYPNOTICS

Barbiturates are the most widely available drugs in this class. Numerous preparations are available, and their various durations of action have pathophysiologic importance. Most commonly abused are the short- to intermediate-acting drugs, especially secobarbital and amobarbital.

Common nonbarbiturate sedatives are chloral hydrate, glutethimide, meprobamate, methaqualone, methyprylon, and ethchlorvynol. While very similar in toxicity to the barbiturates, several of these have additional adverse effects and clinical findings. All of these drugs, as well as the barbiturates, can produce a severe, potentially life-threatening withdrawal syndrome.

Pathophysiology

The major life-threatening toxic effects of these drugs involve the CNS, the cardiovascular system, and the respiratory system. Temperature regulation, the GI tract, the renal system, and the skin are also affected.

CNS depression is the predominant feature of sedative and hypnotic poisonings, resulting in coma and, more importantly, central respiratory depression at the medullary centers.[24,46] The resulting hypoxia causes further, often irreversible, CNS deterioration and many of the cardiovascular and renal effects. In the absence of hypoxic or ischemic damage, the direct CNS effects, although profound, are usually reversible.

The cardiovascular system is affected directly, with myocardial depression, vasodilatation, and venous pooling. Pulmonary edema can occur. These events, plus the hypoxia, cause the blood pressure to fall. Renal function deteriorates because of poor perfusion and often also because of hypothermia secondary to exposure and peripheral vasodilation. However, hyperpyrexia also can occur, especially early in recovery. With more severe stages of coma, GI motility diminishes and then ceases, with resultant ileus. Barbiturates and some of the other sedatives have a toxic effect on the sweat glands, causing necrosis and formation of bullae. The drug can often be detected in fluid from these bullae.

Several of the nonbarbiturate drugs have other specific effects. Methaqualone can produce CNS hyperexcitability, hyperreflexia, and convulsions. Glutethimide has significant anticholinergic effects. Chloral hydrate causes myocardial irritability, with supraventricular and ventricular arrhythmias.

Clinical Features

Accurate clinical assessment of the level of coma is, in practice, the most useful means of assessing the severity of the poisoning itself. The system of Reed and coworkers[47] is commonly used. In this system the response to pain, presence or absence of deep tendon reflexes, and the integrity of vital signs allow grading from I through IV. Alternatively, the Glasgow scale (Table 18-1) can be used. The standard painful stimulus is rubbing of a clenched fist on the patient's sternum.

Coma may be longer lasting in poisonings caused by long-acting barbiturates, but the grade of coma most often remains stable. With short-acting drugs rapid progression to grade IV can supervene, and the most aggressive and vigilant management may be required.

Pupillary responses, considered by some to be a good index of poisoning severity, are in fact quite variable. Classically, barbiturate poisoning produces small, poorly reactive pupils; however, this is often not the case, especially with nonbarbiturate hypnotics. With deep coma the pupils may be quite dilated. With the anticholinergic effects of glutethimide, pupillary dilatation is more often the rule. Peripheral limb reflexes also can be very variable.

Other clinical features of sedative poisoning include

- cyanosis
- shallow or ineffective respirations
- hypotension
- poor peripheral perfusion
- weak pulses
- temperature instability
- diminished or absent bowel sounds
- absent or poor urine output

Additional neurologic findings may include absent corneal and gag reflexes. Corneal ulcerations can occur, and the potential for aspiration pneumonitis is real and life-threatening. Bullous lesions suggest severe intoxication, and pressure necrosis is also common.

The withdrawal syndrome occurs mainly in patients habituated to barbiturates but can occur with other sedatives as well, even when taken for a relatively short time.[24] Manifestations can occur as early as 8 to 12 hours after the last dose of drug, and anxiety, sleep disturbances, nausea, vomiting, and tremulousness are common. Deterioration into convulsions, hypotension, psychosis, hyperpyrexia, and death may occur. Treatment with a tapering schedule of phenobarbital is well described and can be used for nonbarbiturate sedatives as well.

Diagnostic Tests

Measurement of blood drug levels in barbiturate and sedative overdose is suggested but is of limited usefulness. Clinical assessment remains the major guide to therapy. However, levels of short-acting barbiturates greater than 35 μg/mL and levels of long-acting barbiturates greater than 100 μg/mL are correlated with severe and often fatal poisoning and may be indications for dialysis or other therapy beyond the usual supportive measures. Clinical severity out of proportion to blood levels should suggest the possibility of multiple-drug ingestion, and other toxins should be sought by a general drug screen. Importantly, alcohol can worsen the clinical severity of sedative ingestions, by its own toxicity and by enhancing absorption of other drugs, especially glutethimide.

Standard laboratory parameters of supportive care should be monitored, with special attention to arterial blood gas values. Surveillance for secondary respiratory and urinary tract infections is also important.

Therapy

The level of coma should dictate the course of therapy. Careful attention to the adequacy of oxygenation is essential. Airway patency must be ensured, and assisted ventilation should be utilized as required. In most cases hypotension can be managed with intravenous fluids alone, although dopamine and/or dobutamine may be necessary in the most severe cases. Effective cardiopulmonary management leads to a favorable outcome in the vast majority of cases.[24,46]

Removal of the drug from the GI tract or inhibition of its absorption should be attempted. Unfortunately, with the exception of glutethimide, these drugs are rapidly and well absorbed, although their own effect on gut motility may retard absorption for a time. In the alert patient with an intact gag reflex, forced emesis with syrup of ipecac is the preferred method. However, most patients with sedative overdose are stuporous or comatose and require gastric lavage. Ideally, this should be undertaken only after insertion and inflation of a cuffed endotracheal tube to prevent aspiration of gastric contents. The addition of sodium bicarbonate or activated charcoal to the lavage solution may increase recovery of the drug. After lavage, instillation of activated charcoal or castor oil absorbs the drug and further limits its GI absorption. This is especially important for drugs that undergo enterohepatic recirculation, such as glutethimide. Repeated doses of charcoal may be of further benefit since renewed absorption can occur in recovery as GI motility returns. This phenomenon may explain the waxing and waning course of many of these patients.

Phenobarbital, because of its lower pK, can be significantly mobilized by forced alkaline diuresis with intravenous fluids containing sufficient bicarbonate and potassium to maintain a urinary pH greater than 8.0.[46] However, some experts feel this therapy is not as effective as previously believed.

Hemodialysis and, to a lesser extent, peritoneal dialysis are useful and indicated in rare cases of sedative poisoning in which normal excretory mechanisms are impaired or cardiopulmonary parameters cannot be adequately maintained. Charcoal hemoperfusion, a recently developed technique, is more effective than the former two modalities but is rarely available as yet.

Stimulant medications are of no value in the therapy of sedative poisonings.

Follow-up

If cardiopulmonary management is effective, the prognosis for recovery from the acute event is good, with mortality less than 5%. Unfortunately, the incidence of subsequent suicide attempts, often with the same drug, is high. Psychiatric care should be initiated before hospital discharge and kept ongoing.

SYMPATHOMIMETICS

Sympathomimetics affect the CNS in addition to the autonomic nervous system; hence the term "stimulant drugs" is often applied to this group.

Poisoning with certain sympathomimetics may be iatrogenic, such as in the inadvertent overdosage of epinephrine in a hospital setting. Infants and young children may be encountered in the emergency department for accidental ingestion of nasal sprays (which can contain ephedrine, tetrahydrozoline, phenylephrine, or naphazoline) or amphetamines. The use of stimulant drugs (dextroamphetamine, methylphenidate, pemoline) in the treatment of attention-deficit disorders in children provides another source for accidental or intentional ingestions of these agents by young patients. Adolescents and young adults are most commonly seen for acute amphetamine poisoning as a result of substance abuse and experimentation with illicit drugs.[48] Both accidental and intentional ingestions of over-the-counter allergy and cold remedies, which may contain antihistamines as well as sympathomimetics, are encountered in all age groups.

Pathophysiology

Sympathomimetics stimulate the autonomic nervous system by direct action on adrenergic receptors (ephedrine, epinephrine, phenylephrine) or by stimulating the release of norepinephrine from nerve endings and inhibiting reuptake of norepinephrine from the synaptic cleft (e.g., amphetamines). Presumably, similar modes of action exist in the CNS to account for the central stimulatory effects observed after administration of these drugs.

The clinical effects of sympathomimetics are diverse and depend on the differential stimulation of α-adrenergic and β-adrenergic receptors by the particular drug. The α-adrenergic effects include mydriasis and vasoconstriction (in skin and viscera). The β-adrenergic effects are modulated at two separate receptor sites (β_1 and β_2) and include enhancement of myocardial contractility and rate (β_1), vasodilatation in muscles (β_2), relaxation of bronchial smooth muscle (β_2), glycogenolysis, and release of fatty acids in the blood. Both α-adrenergic and β-adrenergic effects inhibit GI motility.[49,50]

Clinical Features

Signs of sympathetic overstimulation are present: tachycardia, hypertension, perspiration, and peripheral vasoconstriction (with coolness and blanching of the skin). Occasionally, fever, chills, and palpitations are observed. Pupillary dilatation is usually significant and accounts for the symptom of blurry vision. Arrhythmias or chest pain also may be encountered.[8]

Effects on the CNS are especially common in poisonings with ephedrine, epinephrine, and the amphetamines. Irritability, insomnia, and anxiety are present. Tremors, tics, increased muscle tone, and hyperactive deep tendon reflexes are frequently observed. The patient is often hyperactive and talkative and may demonstrate repetitive, often purposeless, movements or rituals (automatisms). Dyskinesias, similar to those seen with phenothiazines, have been described in sympathomimetic poisoning.[48] Hostility and aggressive behavior may be encountered. Paranoid ideation, free association, and visual hallucinations are common. In particular, some amphetamines (dimethoxymethylamphetamine, trimethoxymethylamphetamine and their congeners) are especially hallucinogenic. In *chronic* amphetamine poisoning resulting from drug abuse and dependency, the patient may exhibit behavior consistent with paranoid schizophrenia. Bruxism, lip-smacking, and jerky choreiform movements are also observed in this situation, along with the alterations in mental status.[48,50]

Patients with severe sympathomimetic poisoning may develop delirium and convulsions. Pulmonary edema, myocardial failure, and circulatory collapse can supervene. In some cases these factors contribute to a fatal outcome.

Diagnostic Tests

There is no single, specific laboratory test for sympathomimetic poisoning. Toxicologic analysis of blood and urine may identify amphetamines and some other agents. Measurement of baseline electrolyte levels, complete blood count, urinalysis, and an electrocardiogram are indicated. Glycosuria is a common feature of ingestions of sympathomimetic agents.

Therapy

The remaining poison should be removed by ipecac-induced emesis or by lavage. Subsequently, activated charcoal and a cathartic should be administered. If the patient is agitated or psychotic, treatment in a quiet, "nonthreatening" environment may be calming. If seizures are present, intravenous diazepam or short-acting barbiturates can be given.

Renal excretion of some sympathomimetics, especially amphetamines, is a major pathway of elimination. Therefore, adequate hydration with intravenous fluids (2 to 4 $L/m^2/d$) is important in management. The excretion of amphetamines is facilitated in an acid urine, and the oral administration of sufficient ammonium chloride to maintain a urine pH below 5.5 has been advised in the past. However, some experts currently feel this therapy is ineffective. Patients with significant cardiovascular manifestations of sympathetic overstimulation (e.g., tachycardia, hypertension) may benefit from the judicious use of adrenergic blocking agents such as propranolol (β-antagonist) or phentolamine (α-antagonist). Alternatively, chlorpromazine (Thorazine), 1 to 2 mg/kg/d IM or slowly IV, has been widely used to control both CNS excitation and hypertension. Good results have been obtained with haloperidol (Haldol) or droperidol (Inapsine), although the experience with these agents has been limited.

Follow-up

Attention to psychopathology is important in the follow-up of the patient with sympathomimetic abuse. Patients with chronic amphetamine poisoning may require either chlorpromazine or haloperidol as an antipsychotic drug. Most important, enrollment of the patient in a detoxification and rehabilitation program is strongly advised following the initial therapy of chronic amphetamine ingestions.[48]

XANTHINES

Xanthines are the mainstay of oral therapy for bronchial asthma and also have been employed in chronic obstructive pulmonary disease in adults and in apnea of the premature infant. Occasionally, parental errors in administration of oral bronchodilators (incorrect amount, frequency, or route of administration) to children has led to significant toxic effects from aminophylline and theophylline preparations. Iatrogenic xanthine poisoning during the management of status asthmaticus and apnea of prematurity has been reported.[57] Poisoning from other xanthines, such as caffeine (No-Doz) and theobromine, is observed much less frequently and is usually associated with a milder clinical course.

Pathophysiology

The xanthines have effects on the CNS, myocardium, GI tract, smooth and skeletal muscles, and kidney. These diverse effects may be linked to the inhibitory action of xanthines on the enzyme phosphodiesterase, which catabolizes cyclic adenosine monophosphate (cAMP) to 5′-AMP; thus intracellular levels of cAMP are increased after pharmacologic doses of xanthines. Endogenous catecholamines (epinephrine, norepinephrine) also raise intracellular concentrations of cAMP by stimulation of the membrane-linked enzyme adenyl cycla-

The resultant increase in cellular cAMP that follows xanthine administration not only mimics but also potentiates the physiologic effects of the catecholamines.

In therapeutic doses xanthines act as a CNS stimulant. Caffeine has the most stimulatory effects on the cortex, while both caffeine and theophylline stimulate the cardiac, respiratory, and vasomotor centers in the medulla, as well as increase reflex excitability in the spinal cord. Xanthines increase myocardial contractility (inotropic effect) and at higher doses also increase the cardiac rate (chronotropic effect). These drugs cause smooth muscle relaxation, hence their therapeutic value in bronchospastic processes. Increased tone in skeletal muscle, probably independent of the CNS actions of the xanthines, also occurs. Xanthines increase gastric secretion of both hydrochloric acid and pepsin. Finally, the xanthines act as mild diuretics, apparently by action at the level of the renal tubular cells.

Clinical Features

Since there is substantial patient-to-patient variability in the pharmacokinetics of the xanthines, the toxic dose range for theophylline and its congeners is wide.[51–54] Fatalities due to aminophylline have been reported in children who have received as little as 100 mg IV, 25 to 100 mg/kg by rectal suppository, and 8.4 mg/kg orally. However, some of these fatalities may be attributable to hypersensitivity to the drug, with immediate (1 to 2 minutes after injection) hypotension and cardiac arrhythmias. In most cases of xanthine poisoning, symptomatology is well correlated with serum levels of the drug.[55,56]

Irritability, restlessness, tremors, headache, and, on occasion, a "maniacal" state are characteristic of the CNS manifestations of acute xanthine poisoning. Seizures (focal or generalized) and obtundation or coma may be observed, usually with higher drug levels, e.g., serum theophylline levels exceeding 50 μg/mL.[52,54]

The cardiac findings in xanthine poisoning include sinus tachycardia, hypotension or hypertension, and, in more severe cases, ventricular tachyarrhythmias and multiple premature ventricular contractions. Xanthines increase myocardial contractility and lower the fibrillation threshold. One of the earliest signs of xanthine poisoning is GI toxic effects, which are apparent when blood levels of theophylline exceed 20 μg/mL. Nausea and vomiting occur most commonly; hematemesis, because of a Mallory-Weiss syndrome (esophageal ulcerations and tears caused by persistent retching and vomiting) and possibly gastric acid secretion, may also be present. Dehydration may be observed as the result of vomiting and, to a lesser extent, of the diuretic effects of the drug; in young infants the urinary fluid losses can be especially significant.[54,57]

Diagnostic Tests

Serum levels of theophylline are important in assessing the severity of the poisoning. The therapeutic range is 10 to 20 μg/mL. GI manifestations are common above 20 μg/mL, and significant CNS findings (seizures, obtundation) usually occur when levels exceed 50 μg/mL.[55,56] Other initial routine laboratory studies may indicate hyperglycemia, glycosuria, ketonuria, slight proteinuria, metabolic acidosis, hypokalemia, and anemia.

Therapy

Induction of emesis with ipecac is contraindicated in patients with hematemesis and profound vomiting. In such situations gastric lavage should be performed. An activated charcoal slurry should be administered either by mouth or by gastric tube. Intravenous fluids should be given to correct any electrolyte imbalances or dehydration and to ensure adequate urine output. If seizures are present, intravenous phenobarbital or phenytoin (loading doses followed by maintenance) is indicated. Hematemesis is an indication for the oral administration of an antacid, e.g., aluminum hydroxide gel. Limited experience suggests that oral or parenteral cimetidine may be of value in the suppression of gastric acid secretion in patients with xanthine poisoning and hematemesis.

In severe cases of theophylline poisoning (theophylline levels exceeding 60 to 70 μg/mL), hemoperfusion over an activated charcoal column has been very effective. However, this technique must be limited to tertiary care centers that possess the equipment and expertise necessary to provide this modality.[58] Hemodialysis and peritoneal dialysis, two techniques that are generally more available, have also been used with success in severe xanthine poisoning.

Follow-up

Close attention should be paid to the neurologic, cardiac, and GI status of patients after xanthine poisoning. Patients who require xanthines for bronchodilator therapy must be warned about the potential for overdosage, the importance of appropriate administration of the xanthine preparation, and the need for poison prevention to reduce the likelihood of subsequent xanthine poisoning in the patient or inadvertently in other family members.

References

1. Levy G, Houston JB: Effect of activated charcoal on acetaminophen absorption. *Pediatrics* 1976;58:432–435.
2. Ameer B, Greenblatt DJ: Acetaminophen. *Ann Intern Med* 1977;87:202–209.
3. Koch-Weser J: Drug therapy: Acetaminophen. *N Engl J Med* 1976;295:1297–1300.
4. Rumack BH, Matthew H: Acetaminophen poisoning and toxicity. *Pediatrics* 1975;55:871–876.
5. Peterson RG, Rumack BH: Pharmacokinetics of acetaminophen in children. *Pediatrics* 1978;62(suppl):877–879.
6. Prescott LF, Park J, Sutherland GR, et al: Cysteamine, methionine, and penicillamine in the treatment of paracetamol poisoning. *Lancet* 1976;2:109–113.
7. Rumack BH, Peterson RG: Acetaminophen overdose: Incidence, diagnosis, and management in 416 patients. *Pediatrics* 1978;62(suppl):898–903.
8. Arena JM: *Poisoning: Toxicology, Symptoms, Treatments*, ed 4. Springfield, Il, Charles C Thomas Publisher, 1979.
9. Ritchie JM: The aliphatic alcohols, in Gilman AG, Goodman LS, Gilman A (eds): *Goodman and Gilman's The Pharmacologic Basis of Therapeutics*, ed 6. New York, Macmillan Publishing Co Inc, 1980, pp 376–390.
10. Senz EH, Goldfarb DL: Coma in a child following use of isopropyl alcohol in sponging. *J Pediatr* 1958;53:322–323.
11. Parry MF, Wallach R: Ethylene glycol poisoning. *Am J Med* 1974;57:143–150.
12. Callaham M: Tricyclic antidepressant overdose. *JACEP* 1979;8:413–425.
13. Petit JM, Biggs JT: Tricyclic antidepressant overdoses in adolescent patients. *Pediatrics* 1977;59:283–287.
14. Rumack BH: Anticholinergic poisoning: Treatment with physostigmine. *Pediatrics* 1973;52:449–451.
15. Wang SF, Marlowe CL: Treatment of phenothiazine overdosage with physostigmine. *Pediatrics* 1977;59:301–303.
16. Burks JS, Walker JE, Rumack BH, et al: Tricyclic antidepressant poisoning: Reversal of coma, choreoathetosis, and myoclonus by physostigmine. *JAMA* 1974;230:1405–1407.
17. Mofenson HC, Greensher J: Physostigmine as an antidote: Use with caution. *J Pediatr* 1975;87:1011–1012.
18. Greenblatt DJ, Allen MD, Noel BJ, et al: Acute overdosage with benzodiazepine derivatives. *Clin Pharmacol Ther* 1977;21:497–514.
19. Goldfrank L, Kirstein R: Toxicologic emergencies: SLUD. *Hosp Physician*, November 1976, pp 20–33.
20. Zavon MR: Poisoning from pesticides: Diagnosis and treatment. *Pediatrics* 1974;54:332–336.
21. Milby TH: Prevention and management of organophosphate poisoning. *JAMA* 1971;216:2131–2133.
22. Namba T, Nolte CT, Jackrel J, et al: Poisoning due to organophosphate insecticides: Acute and chronic manifestations. *Am J Med* 1971;50:475–492.
23. Aronow R, Done AK: Phencyclidine overdose: An emerging concept of management. *JACEP* 1978;7:56–59.
24. Bourne PG: *A Treatment Manual for Acute Drug Abuse Emergencies*. Washington, DC, US Government Printing Office, 1975.
25. Solursh LP, Clement WR: Hallucinogenic drug abuse: Manifestations and Management. *Can Med Assoc J* 1968;98:407–410.
26. Diagnosis and management of reactions of drug abuse. *Med Lett Drugs Ther* 1977;19:13–16.
27. Solursh LP, Clement WR: Use of diazepam in hallucinogenic drug crises. *JAMA* 1968;205:644–645.
28. Robotham JL, Lietman PS: Acute iron poisoning: A review. *Am J Dis Child* 1980;134:875–879.
29. Whitten CF, Brough AJ: The pathophysiology of acute iron poisoning. *Clin Toxicol* 1971;4:585–595.
30. Fischer DS, Parkman R, Finch SC: Acute iron poisoning in children: The problem of appropriate therapy. *JAMA* 1971;218:1179–1184.
31. Ferry FT: Poisoning, in Biller JA, Yeager AM (eds): *The Harriet Lane Handbook: A Manual for Pediatric House Officers*, ed 9. Chicago, Year Book Medical Publishers Inc, 1981, pp 219–220.
32. Needleman HL, Rabinowitz M, Leviton A, et al: Deficits in psychologic and classroom performance of children with elevated dentine lead levels. *N Engl J Med* 1979;300:689–95.
33. Chisolm JJ Jr, Barltrop D: Recognition and management of children with increased lead absorption. *Arch Dis Child* 1979;54:249–262.
34. Klein R: Lead poisoning. *Adv Pediatr* 1977;24:103–132.

34A. Markowitz ME, Rosen JF: Assessment of lead stores in children: Validation of an 8-hour $CaNa_2$-EDTA provocative test. *J Pediatr* 1984;104:337–341.

35. Rumack BH, Temple AR: Lomotil poisoning. *Pediatrics* 1974;53:495–500.
36. Sturner WQ, Garriott JC: Deaths involving propoxyphene. *JAMA* 1973;223:1125–1130.
37. Moore RA, Rumack BH, Conner CS, et al: Naloxone: Underdosage after narcotic poisoning. *Am J Dis Child* 1980;134:156–158.
38. Burton D, Hanenson IB: Plant toxins, in Hanenson IB (ed): *Quick Reference to Clinical Toxicology*. Philadelphia, JB Lippincott Co, 1980, pp 242–251.
39. Hardin JW, Arena JM: *Human Poisoning from Native and Cultivated Plants*, ed 2. Durham, NC, Duke University Press, 1974.
40. Temple AR: Pathophysiology of aspirin overdosage toxicity, with implications for management. *Pediatrics* 1978;62(suppl):873–876.
41. Done AK: Aspirin overdosage: Incidence, diagnosis, and management. *Pediatrics* 1978;62(suppl):890–897.
42. Pierce AW Jr: Salicylate poisoning. *Pediatrics* 1974;54:342–347.
43. Buchanan N, Rabinowitz L: Infantile salicylism—a reappraisal. *J Pediatr* 1974;84:391–395.
44. Done AK: Salicylate intoxication: Significance of measurements of salicylate in blood in cases of acute ingestion. *Pediatrics* 1960;26:800–807.
45. Levy G: Clinical pharmacokinetics of aspirin. *Pediatrics* 1978;62(suppl):867–872.
46. Matthew H: Barbiturates. *Clin Toxicol* 1975;8:495–513.
47. Reed CE, Driggs MF, Foote CC: Acute barbiturate intoxication: A study of 300 cases based on a physiologic system of classification of the severity of the intoxication. *Ann Intern Med* 1952;37:290–303.
48. Goldfrank L, Kirstein R: Toxicologic emergencies: Stop the noise! *Hosp Physician*, May 1976, pp 22–25.
49. Weiner N: Norepinephrine, epinephrine, and the sympathomimetic amines, in Gilman AG, Goodman LS, Gilman A (eds): *Goodman and Gilman's The Pharmacological Basis of Therapeutics*, ed 6. New York, Macmillan Publishing Co Inc, 1980, pp 138–175.
50. Rumack BH, Peterson RG: Clinical toxicology, in Doull J, Klaassen CD, Amdur MO (eds): *Doull's Toxicology: The Basic Science of Poisons*, ed 2. New York, Macmillan Publishing Co Inc, 1980, pp 677–698.
51. Hendeles L, Weinberger M: Poisoning patients with intravenous theophylline. *Am J Hosp Pharm* 1980;37:49–50.
52. McDonald JM, Ladenson JH, Turk J, et al: Theophylline toxicity. *Clin Chem* 1978;24:1603–1608.
53. Van Dellen RG: Theophylline: Practical application of new knowledge. *Mayo Clin Proc* 1979;54:733–745.
54. Vaucher Y, Lightner ES, Walson PD: Theophylline poisoning. *J Pediatr* 1977;90:827–830.
55. Jacobs MH, Senior RM, Kessler G: Clinical experience with theophylline: Relationships between dosage, serum concentration, and toxicity. *JAMA* 1976;235:1983–1986.
56. Zwillich CW, Sutton FD Jr, Neff TA, et al: Theophylline-induced seizures in adults: Correlation with serum concentrations. *Ann Intern Med* 1975;82:784–787.
57. White BH, Daeschner CW: Aminophylline (theophylline ethylenediamine) poisoning in children. *J Pediatr* 1956;49:262–271.
58. Russo ME: Management of theophylline intoxication with charcoal-column hemoperfusion. *N Engl J Med* 1979;300:24–26.

E. Stevers Golladay
J. J. Tepas III

19 Caustic Ingestion

Exploration by young boys and suicidal attempts by adolescent girls constitute the predominant source of the annual 5000 cases of corrosive ingestion by children in this country.[1] The problem will continue because legislative attempts to make packages with safety caps or warnings do not protect against an inquisitive toddler nor a determined adolescent. Parental disregard for maintenance of a proper container is highly contributory to toddler ingestions and requires enhanced efforts in public education. Strong alkalis packaged as oven cleaners or drain cleaners are most often responsible for the severe esophageal injury,[2] but ammonia, wax matrix potassium chloride, bleach, nonphosphate detergent, Clinitest® tablets, batteries, and sodium carbonate have also injured the esophagus. Acid products such as swimming pool cleaners, denture cleaners, and toilet bowl cleaners also cause damage.

PATHOPHYSIOLOGY

Proper care of these children requires a thorough understanding of the effects of these agents. Alkalis produce liquefactive necrosis and consequent transmural damage to the esophagus, but the neutralizing effect of the gastric acid and the protective effect of the mucous usually limits the effect of an alkali on the stomach.[3] Strong acids produce a coagulative necrosis that limits the depth of injury in the esophagus but can cause gastric injury from long exposure. The adage, "Acid licks the esophagus and bites the stomach while alkali bites the esophagus and licks the stomach" is helpful in remembering this important difference. Alkali ingestion may cause acute airway compromise through inflammation or direct aspiration. No less devastating are the long-term effects of dense scarring that occurs and can rapidly produce an intractable stricture. Because of the long-term effects of alkaline ingestion, every child must be thoroughly evaluated following a history of ingestion.[4]

EXAMINATION AND TREATMENT

An irrefutable history of ingestion is not necessary. Presumptive evidence supplied by an opened, spilled container should warrant full investigation. Drooling, dysphagia, refusal to eat or drink, and burns about the face, neck, chest, or hands are often found. The severity of the burn is dictated by the agent, its concentration, the volume, the duration of contact, and the postprandial state of the stomach; this information as well as any treatment or substernal, back, or abdominal pain indicating possible perforation and vomiting should be carefully sought in the history. The examiner must be alert for tenderness in the chest or abdomen, as well as for the hoarseness, stridor, or dyspnea indicative of laryngeal edema secondary to aspiration; if elicited, these findings are harbingers of a stormy course.[4] The presence of any of these signs or symptoms requires immediate referral.

A protocol for management of caustic ingestions is shown in Figure 19-1. Although transmural esophageal burns are necessary to produce stricture, there is no accurate means of determining the depth of injury. Every child must have an upright chest x-ray film with a lateral view to assess pneumonia, pneumomediastinum, or pneumoperitoneum. A contrast esophagram is not reliable in documenting esophageal burns. Accordingly, all children with suspected caustic ingestion should be admitted and undergo esophagoscopic evaluation within 24 hours.[3] The efficacy of corticosteroids in diminishing stricture formation remains unclear; however, most studies suggest that whatever benefits there are occur only when therapy is begun within hours of injury. Dexamethasone (0.25 mg/kg/d IV or IM) or prednisone (2 mg/kg/d) are appropriate medications and should be started in the emergency department. Antibiotic administration is essential to prevent infectious complications and should be concurrent with the corticosteroid therapy. Corticosteroids are tapered over a 3-week period and a repeat esophagram obtained. If a definite stricture is present, then corticosteroid therapy is stopped and retrograde dilatations via gastrostomy are performed.[3,4]

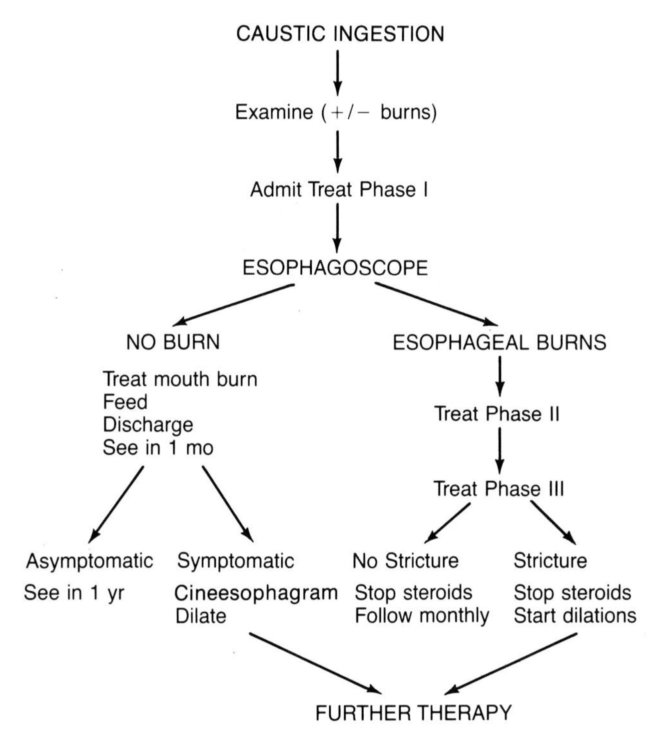

TREATMENT

Phase I
Admit — notify GPS, ENT
Nothing orally, IVs
Ampicillin, Prednisone
CBC, Chest x-ray film, UA
Permit for esophagoscopy
Esophagoscopy within 12 hr

Phase II
Continue antibiotics, steroids
IVs until patient can swallow
Advance diet as tolerated
Cinefluoroscopy at 3 wk

Phase III
Stop steroids
Esophagram:
Stricture — Begin dilation
No stricture — Follow for 1 mo

FIGURE 19-1 Treatment of caustic injuries of the esophagus. CBC, complete blood count; ENT, ear, nose, and throat department; GPS, pediatric surgical service; UA, urinalysis.

CONCLUSION

Accidental ingestion of caustics continues to be a major threat to the pediatric population. The injury can range from an immediate threat to life to inconsequential oral burns. Acute mediastinitis or airway obstruction requires aggressive management to save the patient's life. Prevention of a strictured, dysfunctional esophagus requires timely initiation of therapy and thus a high index of suspicion by the initial physicians.

References

1. Holinger PH: Management of esophageal lesions caused by chemical burns. *Ann Otol Rhinol Laryngol* 1968;77:819–829.
2. Borja AR, Ransdell HT Jr, Thomas TV, et al: Lye injuries of the esophagus. Analysis of 90 cases of lye ingestion. *J Thorac Cardiovasc Surg* 1969;57:533–538.
3. Haller JA Jr, Andrews HG, White JJ, et al: Pathophysiology and management of acute corrosive burns of the esophagus: Results of the treatment in 285 children. *J Pediatr Surg* 1971;6:578–584.
4. Haller JA Jr: Corrosive strictures of the esophagus, in Ravitch MM, Welch KJ, Benson CD, et al (eds): *Pediatric Surgery*, ed 3. Chicago, Year Book Medical Publishers Inc, 1979, vol 1, pp 472–475.

Randall W. Powell

20 Foreign Bodies in the Gastrointestinal Tract

Foreign bodies in the GI tract occur mainly in young children and are related to that exploratory phase of childhood when much of the exploring involves placing objects in the mouth. Significant morbidity or mortality from such foreign bodies is unusual. In his book *The Surgery of Infancy and Childhood* (1953), Robert Gross[1] describes a series of 766 swallowed foreign bodies with one death related to perforation of the esophagus by a pin, which resulted in bacterial pericarditis. Gans and Austin[2] report no deaths in a series of 106 patients. Benson and Lloyd[3] report that approximately 150 children per year are seen in their emergency department with ingestion of foreign bodies. Unlike respiratory tract foreign bodies, GI tract foreign bodies require hospitalization of only 25% to 30% of the children involved.

CLINICAL FEATURES

The child usually has a history of being observed swallowing the object or having confessed to the act, either from pride or fear. Occasionally, the child exhibits symptoms related to a complication of foreign body ingestion, e.g., esophageal or gastric outlet obstruction, and the object is later noted on radiographs. Many episodes of ingestion are heralded by gagging or choking. If the foreign body passes through the esophagus, symptoms usually cease. If the object impacts in the esophagus, symptoms such as cough, gagging, excessive salivation, inability to swallow, and pain will persist.[4] In unrecognized cases the child may exhibit mainly respiratory symptoms such as stridor, wheezing, or chronic pneumonia related to repeated bouts of aspiration.[5] One infant with failure to thrive was discovered to have a large bolt impacted in the hypopharynx, causing feeding difficulties and some respiratory distress.[6]

Another important aspect of the history concerns the known presence of congenital anomalies that can predispose the child to foreign body impaction. The classic example is the child who has undergone repair of an esophageal atresia. Many of these children have varying degrees of narrowing at the anastomosis and all have some degree of esophageal dysmotility,[4] both of which contribute to foreign body impaction. Often the offender is poorly chewed meat.[3]

Once in the stomach 90% to 95% of ingested foreign bodies pass through the GI tract without complications.[1,7] The usual complications include obstruction (of the pylorus, duodenum, ligament of Treitz, ileocecal valve, and rectosigmoid),[7] perforation with resulting peritonitis, and hemorrhage from trauma to the bowel wall. Perforations in the stomach and duodenum often produce symptoms similar to a perforated ulcer, whereas perforations in the ileocecal area often have symptomatology similar to that of acute appendicitis. Occasionally, objects perforate the GI tract and lodge in solid organs in the abdominal cavity (spleen, liver, kidney) where they may incite symptoms.[4] Other complications include intraperitoneal and retroperitoneal abscesses and intestinal fistulas.[2]

The peak age group for foreign body ingestion lies between 6 months and 4 years.[1,3] In the series reported by Gross,[1] 85 patients were less than 1 year of age; 131, age 1; 178, age 2; 124, age 3; 86, age 4; 56, age 5; 29, age 6; and 76 between 7 and 15 years of age.

The type of foreign bodies, like those discussed in aspiration (see Chapter 9), are limited only by the child's imagination and ability to reach the object. The most common objects include coins, open and closed safety pins, bobby pins, straight pins, marbles, toys or parts of toys, buttons, nails, tacks, and screws. Of 766 foreign bodies described by Gross,[1] the most common were pennies (154), open safety pins (88), nickels (61), closed safety pins (60), bobby pins (56), straight pins (33), quarters (23), tacks (21), and nails (20). Objects requiring special consideration include aluminum tabs from disposable cans, batteries, objects containing lead, and excessively long objects in relation to the child's size. Aluminum tabs have been implicated in several severe complications.[8] Burrington[8] described seven children with aluminum tab tops lodged in the esophagus. Two patients had abscesses following esophageal perforation, and one died as a result of exsanguination from a fistula from the aortic arch to the esophagus. Aluminum absorbs x-rays poorly and is difficult to visualize if overlying a vertebral body. The sharp edges of the tops contribute to the ease with which they seem to perforate the esophagus. Blunt objects left in the esophagus can also cause perforation by pressure necrosis and lead to mediastinal or cervical abscesses or tracheoesophageal fistulas.[9,10] A history or documentation of the ingestion of batteries or objects containing lead changes the management of these children. Because of their corrosive contents, batteries may require surgical or endoscopic removal if not promptly passed through the GI tract (within 48 to 72 hours).[2] Objects containing lead should not be left in the stomach beyond 6 to 7 days or in the small intestine more than 14 days.[3]

Diagnosis

Diagnosis depends on a good history, physical examination (invariably normal unless the foreign body lodges in the esophagus), and appropriate radiologic studies. Radiographs should include posteroanterior and lateral views of the neck and chest; a flat plate film of the abdomen should be acquired if the former are negative. Unlike airway foreign

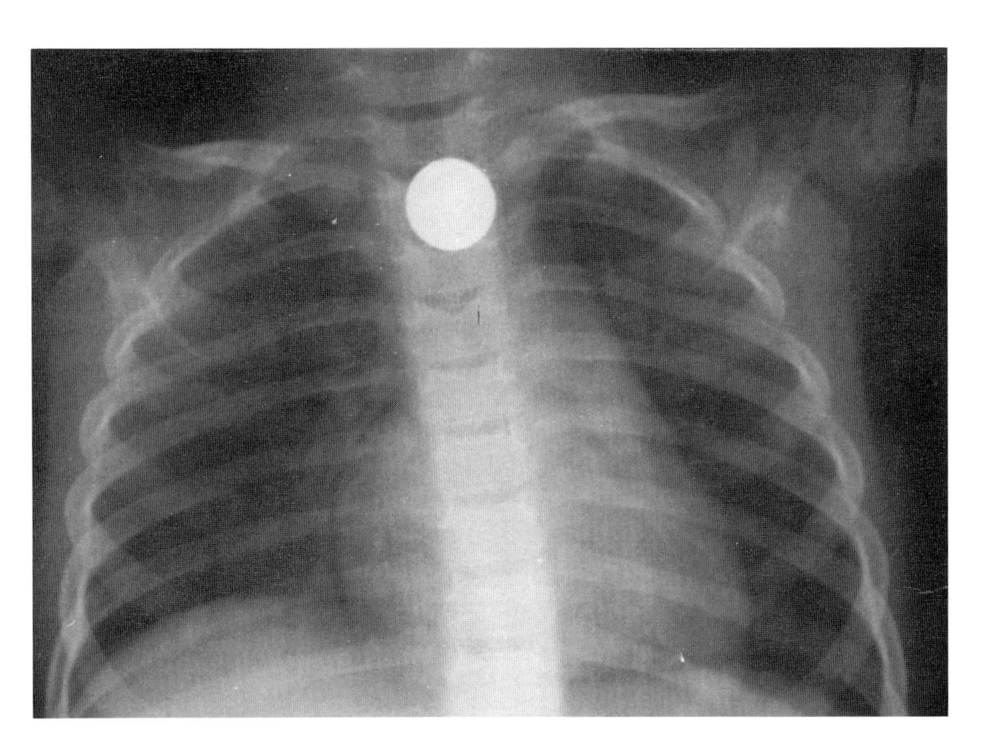

FIGURE 20-1 Swallowed coins often lodge in the upper esophagus near the aortic arch as shown.

bodies most GI tract foreign bodies are radiopaque. This facilitates diagnosis, localization, and follow-up of these children. If the object is radiolucent, a barium swallow examination of the esophagus can document foreign body impaction. Figures 20-1 and 20-2 illustrate typical GI tract foreign bodies.

Management

Management of children with ingested foreign bodies depends mainly on the site of lodgment, the type of foreign body, or complications induced by the foreign body. Objects lodging in the esophagus require removal because of the possibility of aspiration pneumonia and perforation. The preferred technique for removal is rigid tube esophagoscopy under general anesthesia.[1–4] Gross[1] removed 151 esophageal foreign bodies with one death, which was related to esophageal and pericardial perforation by the foreign body. Esophageal foreign bodies usually lodge at the level of the cricoid cartilage, aortic arch, or esophagogastric junction,[4] all sites of physiologic narrowing. All of these sites are easily accessible to the rigid esophagoscope, and the safety of this approach has been well documented.[1,11]

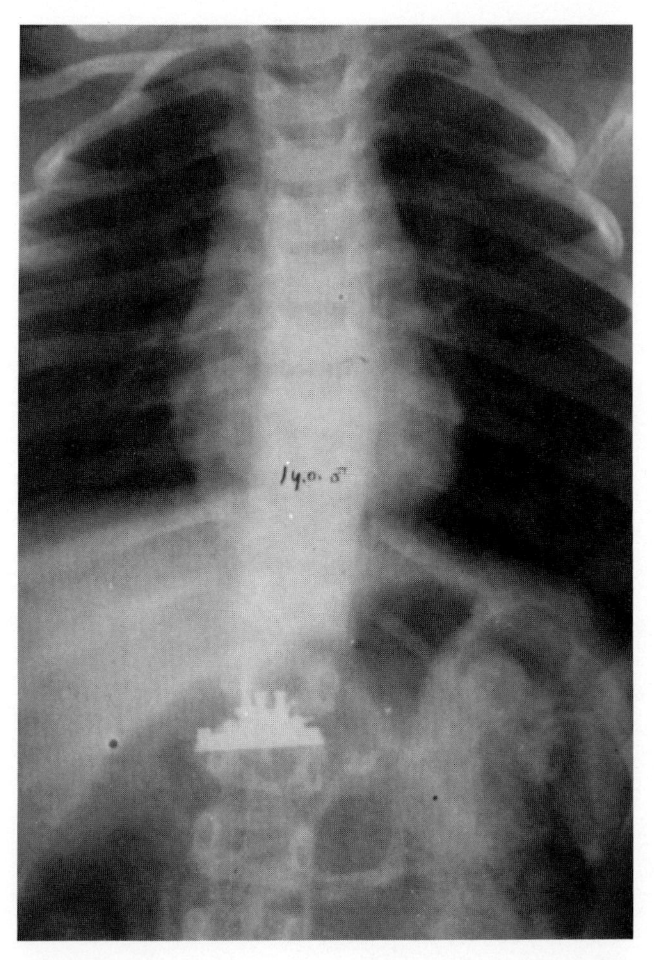

FIGURE 20-2 The toy ship sailing through this child's stomach safely transversed the GI tract without difficulty. Most objects reaching the stomach experience little problem navigating the remainder of the GI tract.

Alternative forms of management include Foley catheter extraction or extraction with the flexible endoscope. There are several reports of good results with the Foley catheter technique.[12–14] This technique involves the use of fluoroscopy and an appropriate size Foley catheter. The child is immobilized on the fluoroscopy table with the head down to prevent aspiration. (One physician utilizes the prone oblique position.[13]) The Foley catheter is passed beyond the foreign body, and the catheter balloon is filled with contrast material. The catheter is slowly withdrawn, bringing the foreign body with it. This technique has been utilized mainly with blunt radiopaque objects (mainly coins) and in the absence of esophageal disease. Nixon[14] has expanded the technique to include radiolucent objects and has performed this type of extraction in patients with esophageal anomalies. Although the technique has been described as an emergency department procedure,[15] this application is to be discouraged. Lodging the foreign body in the larynx is definitely a possible complication. Only persons experienced in the management of the obstructed pediatric airway should attempt Foley catheter extraction.

The flexible panendoscope offers another mode of removing esophageal foreign bodies, and good results have been reported.[7,16] General anesthesia appears necessary to control the airway and prevent aspiration from the obstructed esophagus. The flexible panendoscope offers no distinct advantages over the rigid esophagoscope for the removal of esophageal foreign bodies.

Most of the literature discourages the use of various enzyme preparations to digest food particles, especially a meat bolus, lodged in the esophagus in small children.[3] The risks of esophageal damage, aspiration into the lungs, and electrolyte abnormalities outweigh any possible benefits.[3]

Foreign bodies that successfully pass through the esophagus usually pass through the remainder of the GI tract without difficulty (90% to 95%). The management of these objects usually depends on their character. Blunt objects such as coins, marbles, and closed safety pins usually pass through, causing no problems. A child may be sent home after radiologic confirmation of the object's location is obtained. The child's diet should not be altered except for the possible addition of mineral oil and/or bran to increase stool bulk and decrease transit time. No cathartics should be utilized to speed elimination of the foreign body. Parents should check or strain the stools for the foreign body. If it is not passed in 4 to 5 days, a return visit for a radiograph of the abdomen is recommended. Most objects pass in 3 to 7 days, but some may require 3 to 4 weeks. With blunt, rounded objects the conservative approach invariably prevails. If the object remains in the stomach or causes a gastric outlet obstruction, removal with the panendoscope should be attempted before surgical exploration.

Sharp objects require more attention, and either daily outpatient follow-up or hospitalization is recommended until the object passes through the GI tract or is extracted.[2] Mineral oil and bran may be helpful in promoting passage. Cathartics are absolutely contraindicated. If a sharp object causes progression for a 3 to 5-day period, intervention is recommended.[2–4] Again, if the object is in the stomach, extraction with the panendoscope should be attempted prior to surgical removal.

When a child is being followed as an outpatient, the parents must be instructed to return to the hospital if the child experiences hematemesis, melena, hematochezia, persistent abdominal pain, vomiting (especially if bilious), or persistent fever. All of the above indicate a probable complication related to the foreign body that would require surgical intervention.

If the foreign body possesses a relatively long axis in relation to the size of the child, e.g., a 3- to 4-inch nail in a 2-year-old, the likelihood of the object passing through the GI tract decreases. The duodenal loop and ligament of Treitz offer a significant course to be traversed. If the child has such a foreign body still in the stomach or upper duodenum, extraction with a panendoscope would eliminate any possible need for operative intervention.

Trichobezoars represent a relatively frequent complication of foreign body ingestion in children.[1,3,4] The history of trichophagia (hair eating) and the common finding of patchy alopecia in the presence of a child with epigastric pain, vomiting, early satiety, and often an epigastric mass form the usual clinical picture. Plain radiographs usually confirm a mass in the area of the stomach, and the bezoars can be seen easily with barium studies. Surgical removal is recommended,[1,2,4] but the use of the panendoscope and papain irrigations may obviate surgery.

Rectal foreign bodies may occur in infants, small children, and adolescents. In small infants the usual object is a broken thermometer. Inspection of the anus is usually unrewarding; radiographs can confirm the presence of the broken thermometer. A suitable examination under general anesthesia is recommended to remove the foreign body, inspect the anal canal and lower rectum for injuries, and repair any damage. Rectal foreign bodies in young children may indicate child abuse, and appropriate work-up should be performed, i.e., radiographs to look for old fractures and a careful physical examination for other signs.

Removal of the foreign body in the operating room under general anesthesia allows for atraumatic extraction and permits adequate inspection to rule out rectal injuries. Rectal foreign bodies in adolescents, often secondary to sexual acts,[7] usually require general or spinal anesthesia for removal. Careful inspection for rectal injuries after removal is mandatory to prevent the serious complications that can occur when such injuries are missed.

References

1. Gross RE: *The Surgery of Infancy and Childhood: Its Principles and Techniques.* Philadelphia, WB Saunders Co, 1953, pp 246–252.
2. Gans SI, Austin E: Foreign bodies, in Holder TM, Ashcraft KW (eds): *Pediatric Surgery.* Philadelphia, WB Saunders Co, 1980, Chap 57.
3. Benson CD, Lloyd JR: Foreign bodies in the gastrointestinal tract, in Ravitch MM, Welch KJ, Benson CD, et al (eds): *Pediatric Surgery.* Chicago, Year Book Medical Publishers Inc, 1979, pp 897–902.
4. Raffensperger JG: Foreign bodies in the gastrointestinal tract, in Raffensperger JG (ed): *Swenson's Pediatric Surgery,* ed 4. New York, Appleton-Century-Crofts, 1980, Chap 23.
5. Newman DE: The radiolucent esophageal foreign body: An often forgotten cause of respiratory symptoms. *J Pediatr* 1978;92:60–63.
6. Buckler JMH, Stool SE: Failure to thrive: An exogenous cause. *Am J Dis Child* 1967;114:652–653.
7. Roseman DM: Foreign bodies in the gut and upper airway, in Sleisenger MH, Fordtran JS (eds): *Gastrointestinal Disease: Pathophysiology, Diagnosis, Management.* Philadelphia, WB Saunders Co, 1978, pp 605–611.
8. Burrington JD: Aluminum "pop tops": A hazard to child health. *JAMA* 1976;235:2614–2617.
9. McLaughlin RT, Morris JD, Haight C: The morbid nature of the migrating foreign body in the esophagus. *J Thorac Cardiovasc Surg* 1968;55:188–192.
10. Yee KF, Schild JA, Holinger PH: Extraluminal foreign bodies (coins) in the food and air passages. *Ann Otol Rhinol Laryngol* 1975;84:619–623.
11. Jackson C, Jackson CI: *Diseases of the Air and Food Passages of Foreign Body Origin.* Philadelphia, WB Saunders Co, 1936.
12. Shackelford GD, McAlister WH, Robertson CL: The use of a foley catheter for removal of blunt esophageal foreign bodies from children. *Radiology* 1972;105:455–456.

13. Campbell JB, Davis WS: Catheter technique for extraction of blunt esophageal foreign bodies. *Radiology* 1973;108:438–440.
14. Nixon GW: Foley catheter method of esophageal foreign body removal: Extension of applications. *AJR* 1979;132:441–442.
15. Dunlap LB: Removal of an esophageal foreign body using a foley catheter. *Ann Emerg Med* 1981;10:101–103.
16. Christie DI, Ament ME: Removal of foreign bodies from esophagus and stomach with flexible fiberoptic panendoscopes. *Pediatrics* 1976;57:931–934.

Part VI

Genitourinary Disorders

Fred J. Heldrich
Charles R. Medani

21 Genitourinary Disorders

Diseases of the genitourinary tract frequently come to the attention of the physician because of abnormal urinary findings noticed by the patient or discovered on routine urinalysis. This chapter begins with a discussion of such findings. Specific diseases that produce these symptoms or are commonly seen in a primary care setting at onset are then discussed individually.

LABORATORY EVALUATION OF RENAL FUNCTION

The outpatient laboratory evaluation of renal function begins with the examination of the urine. Much information can be gleaned from the macroscopic and microscopic examination, combined with urine culture and measurement of serum levels of urea and creatinine.

Urinalysis

Collection of Specimens

Collection of urine from older children usually presents no difficulty, as long as the assisting adult is instructed properly in the methods of obtaining a clean-caught midstream specimen. For younger children it is usually necessary to use a plastic bag applied to the perineum, with removal of the specimen as soon as it is obtained. This urine is also acceptable for a screening culture if done immediately.[1]

The first morning specimen is ideal since it is usually the most concentrated urine of the day. However, random urine specimens are usually acceptable for most screening purposes.

In cases in which it is important to accurately document infection or obtain urine as soon as possible, suprapubic puncture in infants and in very small children is the method of choice. Urethral catheterization is not indicated for routine urine examination or culture but is very helpful in obtaining a "clean" specimen in the case of equivocal culture results. Urine may be refrigerated up to 48 hours after collection and still be useful for culture, although cellular elements may begin dissolution soon after urine is obtained, despite refrigeration.[1]

Color and Specific Gravity

The appearance of normal urine is clear, pale yellow to deep amber, varying with the concentration and presence of certain foods and drugs, urobilinogen, bilirubin, and carotene. Turbid urine may indicate the precipitation of phosphates or urates, or the presence of particles such as cells or chyle.

The specific gravity of the urine reflects the combined weight of all particles in solution. It is a rough indicator of the concentration of the urine, which is more accurately indicated by urinary osmolarity; however, in most cases specific gravity can be used for determination of concentrating power. The specific gravity of normal urine ranges from 1.001 to 1.035 and depends upon the state of hydration, concentrating ability of the kidneys, presence of antidiuretic hormone or diuretics, renal maturity, and nutrition. In general, a specific gravity of at least 1.017 implies that the urinary concentrating mechanism is intact. However, dehydration without maximum concentration of urine requires further investigation.

Chemical Analysis

Proteinuria is an important indicator of renal disease, especially in childhood. The dipstick impregnated with tetrabromphenol blue is used to indicate the presence of albumin, down to approximately 5 mg/dL. Sulfosalicylic acid (SSA) is more sensitive and detects albumin and nonalbumin proteins, as may be present in renal parenchymal disease. It is important to remember that the level of proteinuria indicates the concentration of protein at one particular point in time. Although it can indicate abnormal amounts of protein, it may be elevated to "trace-1+" in concentrated urine without the existence of underlying pathology.

The dipstick measures the presence of hemoglobin or myoglobin with orthotolidine-impregnated squares, which turn blue in the presence of oxidizing agents. False-positive reactions may be due to microbial peroxidase, occasionally present with large numbers of certain types of bacteria. Other oxidizing agents may also cause a false-positive reaction. Myoglobinuria and hemoglobinuria can coexist.

The presence of glucose in the urine is measured with a glucose oxidase-impregnated square, which is glucose specific. With this method there is no measurable glucose in the normal urine. A positive reaction for glucose indicates abnormal levels, possibly secondary to diabetes mellitus or renal tubular defects.

Normal urinary pH ranges from 4.5 to 8, depending upon the systemic acid-base status, state of hydration, presence of urease-producing bacteria in the urine, electrolyte balance, and acidifying capacity of the urine. Accurate pH values can be obtained from fresh urine, before significant loss of CO_2 or significant production of bacterial urease has occurred.[1]

Microscopic Examination

Microscopic examination of the urine evaluates the presence of cells, casts, crystals, and other noncellular elements of the urine. Ten to fifteen milliliters of urine should be centrifuged for 5 to 10 minutes at 1500 to 2500 rpm. The supernatant fluid is then discarded, and the remaining pellet is resuspended, placed on a clear microscopic slide, and covered with a coverslip. The slide should be examined under low power, with the microscope condenser in the low position and the iris diaphragm partially closed. The examiner should look for casts, which tend to be found near the edges of the coverslip. Under high-dry power, cells, crystals, and the specific cast type can be identified.[1]

More than five leukocytes per high-power field in a centrifuged urine specimen may suggest (but *not* diagnose) a urinary tract infection. Leukocyturia also may be present as a result of viral cystitis, acute or chronic renal disease, urethritis, foreign body, urinary tract tuberculosis, local external irritation, or lower abdominal inflammatory disease.

The presence of renal casts (cylindruria) is an important finding in renal parenchymal disease. Casts are shaped by the tubular lumen of the nephron and reflect the form of the tubule. They can be physiologic or pathologic and are classified according to the material imbedded in their matrix (Figure 21-1). Their width and composition give clues to the disease process. They degenerate quickly in nonacidic or dilute urine. The basic matrix is Tamm-Horsfall mucoprotein.[2]

Hyaline and granular casts are generally considered nonpathologic. Factors favoring hyaline cast formation include decreased urine flow, low pH, and high protein or solute concentration. Granular casts are from plasma proteins and degenerating cells. There is a gelation of urinary protein and incorporation of particulate matter. They may increase in number after exercise. Granular casts imply some degree of stasis in the nephron, and large numbers may be associated with renal parenchymal disease. There is no advantage to differentiating coarse and finely granular casts. It is generally thought that fine granular casts are a result of further degeneration of coarse granular casts; this may imply prolonged intrarenal stasis.

The presence of renal tubular epithelial casts can indicate renal parenchymal disease and tubular damage.

White cell casts indicate an inflammatory reaction in the kidney that is generally tubulointerstitial in nature. White cells usually enter from the interstitium of the kidney, not from the glomerular capillary loops.

The presence of red cell casts indicates bleeding within the nephron and is generally diagnostic of glomerular disease. A blood cast is a degenerated red cell cast that appears granular because of cell breakdown products and hemoglobin. The red cell

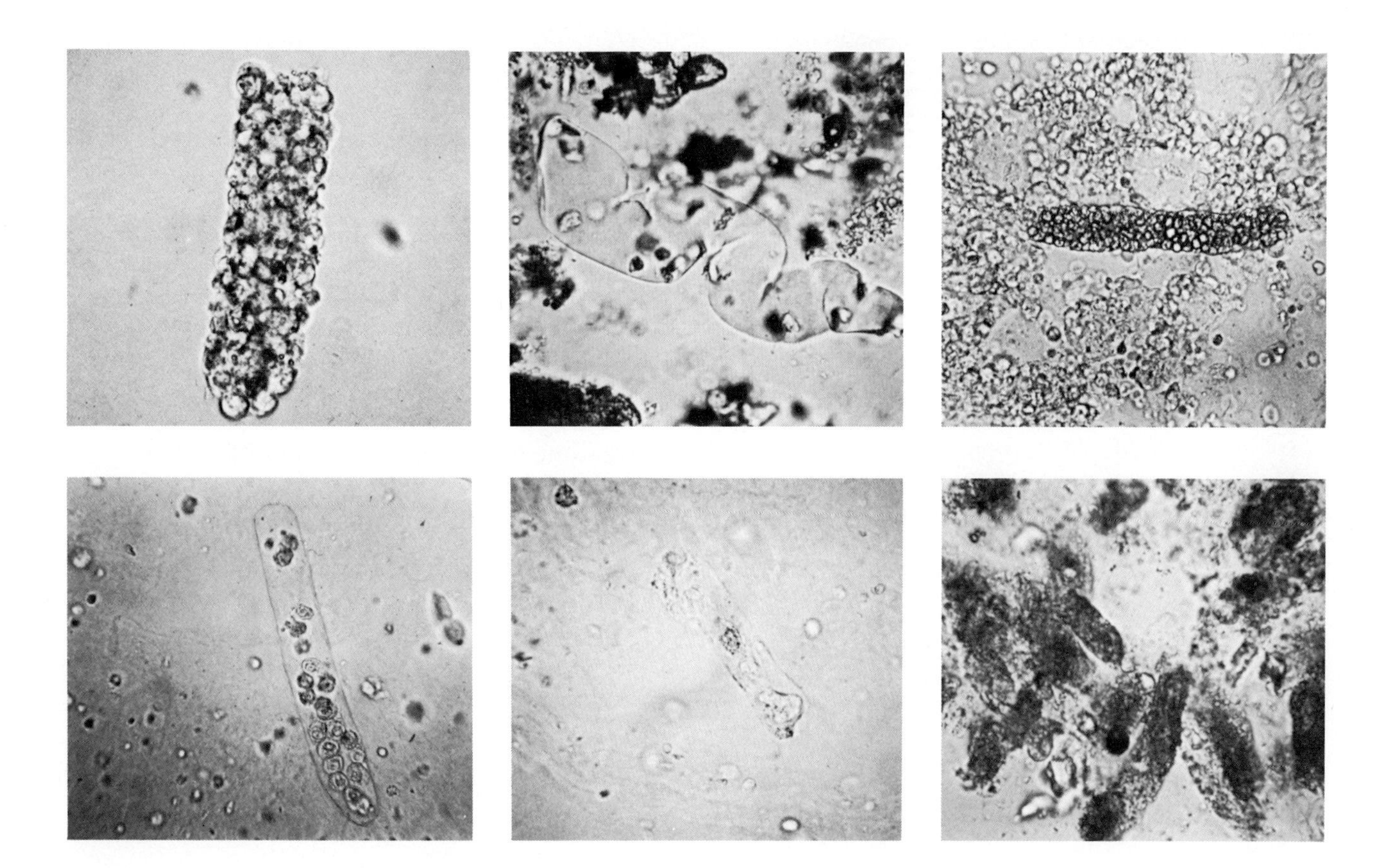

FIGURE 21-1 Renal casts. A, Hyaline cast with degenerating cellular inclusions. B, Coarsely granular casts. Sediment taken from a patient with acute tubular necrosis. C, Leukocyte cast. D, Erythrocyte cast. E, Epithelial cell cast. F, Waxy cast. (Reprinted with permission from Kassirer JP, Gennari FJ: Laboratory evaluation of renal function, in Early LE, Gottschalk CW (eds): *Strauss and Welt's Disease of the Kidney*, ed 3. Boston, Little Brown & Co, 1979, pp. 75–79. Copyright © 1979, Little Brown & Co.)

cast is generally rusty to reddish brown. Hemoglobin or myoglobin casts may have a similar appearance.

A waxy cast is the last stage in cellular degeneration and implies local nephron obstruction. Such casts are frequently associated with tubular inflammation and degeneration, and broad waxy casts are frequently indicative of chronic renal disease with tubular atrophy and dilatation.[2]

Blood Tests

When the question of possible renal disease arises, measurements of blood urea and creatinine are useful screening tests for evaluating a child's renal status. Blood urea nitrogen (BUN) is the major end product of protein-nitrogen metabolism. Normal values are less than 15 mg/dL but may be significantly lower in growing children. Many factors can influence the level of BUN, including the state of hydration, urine flow rate, renal function, dietary protein, liver function, and other causes of protein catabolism or anabolism. Although the BUN is commonly used as a parameter that varies directly with renal function, the many factors influencing its production and excretion must be considered when interpreting abnormal levels in the blood.

Serum creatinine is derived from the enzymatic degradation of creatinine in skeletal muscle. It is freely filtered by the glomerulus, and a small amount is secreted by the renal tubules. The production and release of creatinine is constant and is only minimally dependent upon physical activity, protein intake, and protein metabolism. Secretion varies little throughout the day. Normal serum values vary with age and sex (Table 21-1). Serial measurements are frequently more useful than absolute values, which may vary according to type and accuracy of analyzer. The urinary creatinine clearance is a rough measure of the renal filtration rate, and al-

TABLE 21-1 Serum Creatinine Concentrations for Boys and Girls 1 to 20 Years of Age

	Creatinine (mg/dL)	
Age (yr)	Girls	Boys
1	0.35	0.41
2	0.45	0.43
3	0.42	0.46
4	0.47	0.45
5	0.46	0.50
6	0.48	0.52
7	0.53	0.54
8	0.53	0.57
9	0.55	0.59
10	0.55	0.61
11	0.60	0.62
12	0.59	0.65
13	0.62	0.68
14	0.65	0.72
15	0.67	0.76
16	0.65	0.74
17	0.70	0.80
18–20	0.72	0.91

Source: Adapted with permission from Schwartz GJ, Haycock GB, Spitzer A: Plasma creatinine and urea concentration in children: Normal values for age and sex. *J Pediatr* 1976; 88:829.

though not as accurate as inulin clearance, it is frequently used because of its convenience. Normal values are greater than 100 mL/min/1.73 m^2 after the age of 1 year.[3]

The hematocrit, platelet count, and red cell morphology are also useful in distinguishing among diseases associated with hematuria (Table 21-2).[4]

HEMATURIA

In the differential diagnosis of red urine, the dipstick test detects red cells, hemoglobin, myoglobin, and other oxidizing substances that produce a positive reaction. The microscopic examination detects the presence of cells and casts (Table 21-3).

Hemoglobinuria can be the result of systemic hemolysis from any cause or of urinary hemolysis; the latter occurs in dilute, alkaline, or old urine. In hemoglobinuria the serum remains pink after centrifugation because of the presence of the hemoglobin-binding molecule, haptoglobin.

Myoglobinuria also results in a positive dipstick test and is frequently due to trauma, strenuous exercise, or other causes of muscle breakdown. In contrast to hemoglobinuria, the serum in myoglobinuria is clear after centrifugation. Myoglobinuria can be confirmed by laboratory analysis.[5,6]

Some other preliminary aids in localizing the site of bleeding are outlined in Table 21-4.

Etiology

Acute Renal Disease

Acute glomerulonephritis (AGN) is the most common cause of gross hematuria in childhood. Other syndromes that must be considered, however, include Henoch-Schönlein purpura, hemolytic-uremic syndrome (HUS), acute tubular necrosis, vascular thrombosis, subacute bacterial endocarditis, and other types of glomerulonephritis.[5]

Chronic Renal Disease

Chronic renal disease may cause microscopic or macroscopic hematuria. The diseases included in this category are all those chronic renal diseases with or without decreased function, such as

- membranoproliferative glomerulonephritis
- focal segmental glomerulosclerosis
- systemic lupus erythematosus
- renal dysplasias
- cysts
- malformations
- hereditary nephritis
- benign recurrent hematuria
- benign familial hematuria

TABLE 21-2 Complete Blood Count in the Differential Diagnosis of Several Types of Renal Disease

	Hematocrit	Red Blood Cell Morphology	Platelets
Acute glomerulonephritis	Normal to slightly decreased	Normal	Normal
Henoch-Schönlein purpura	Normal to slightly decreased	Normal	Normal
Hemolytic-uremic syndrome	Decreased	Fragments	Decreased
Chronic renal failure	Decreased	Normal	Normal to slightly decreased
Hemoglobinopathy	Decreased	Dependent upon type of hemoglobinopathy	Normal

TABLE 21-3 Use of Dipstick and Microscopic Examination in the Differential Diagnosis of Red Urine

	Dipstick	Microscopy
Erythrocytes	+	Erythrocytes
Hemoglobin	+	No erythrocytes
Myoglobin	+	No erythrocytes
Dyes	−	No erythrocytes
Bacterial peroxidase	+	No erythrocytes

TABLE 21-4 Preliminary Aids in Localizing the Source of Hematuria

	Extrarenal	Renal
Color	Frequently pink or red	Usually brown, "smoky," tea-colored, "Coke colored"
Variance in color of stream	Frequent	No variance
Casts	None	If seen, localizes site as renal

Infection of the Urinary Tract

Urinary tract infections from bacteria or viruses frequently cause hematuria. Hemorrhagic cystitis caused by adenovirus and other agents can produce gross hematuria; systemic viral or bacterial infections (including mumps, rubeola, varicella) may cause transient hematuria. Schistosomiasis and tuberculosis are other causes of hematuria in childhood, although they are uncommon in the United States.[7]

Urinary Tract Neoplasms

Urinary tract neoplasms, such as Wilm's tumor, may cause isolated hematuria, and any type of genitourinary tumor or polyp can produce microscopic or macroscopic hematuria. It is very uncommon to have hematuria as the presenting sign of neuroblastoma.

Trauma

Traumatic causes of hematuria include foreign bodies, manipulation or masturbation, and circumcision. In the presence of hydronephrosis or tumor, seemingly insignificant trauma can result in hematuria.

Hematologic Disorders

Hematologic disorders usually produce signs and symptoms other than those referable to the urinary tract. Leukemia, hemoglobinopathies, clotting factor deficiencies, and platelet deficiencies can cause hematuria, but this is associated with other symptoms and signs of the underlying disorder.

Miscellaneous Causes

Other causes of hematuria include

- drugs (especially methicillin and cyclophosphamide)
- strenuous exercise
- menstrual bleeding
- urinary tract stones (may be asymptomatic)
- scurvy
- malignant hypertension
- "pseudohematuria" because of iodine cleansing solution
- hypercalciuria.[5–7]

Differential Diagnosis

With the aforementioned categories in mind, one must approach the diagnosis of hematuria with a careful history, physical examination, and appropriate screening laboratory tests. The history is notable especially for trauma, drugs, antecedent illnesses, "lower tract symptoms," family history, previous episodes, and abdominal pain. The physical examination can also be revealing. Purpura can be seen in severe infection, Henoch-Schönlein purpura, HUS, and thrombocytopenic states. Growth failure can indicate chronic disease; fever and a murmur, endocarditis. The presence of an abdominal mass can suggest renal pathology such as hydronephrosis, polycystic kidneys, or tumor. Hypertension and edema accompanying hematuria may indicate acute or chronic glomerulonephritis or other renal disease.

Because the history and physical examination are frequently unrevealing, a few basic laboratory studies are usually necessary. The urinalysis can be very helpful. A high specific gravity indicates good tubular function and speaks against chronic renal disease. However, it is compatible with AGN, in which the glomeruli are relatively more affected than the tubules. Significant proteinuria points to renal parenchymal disease, as does the presence of red or white cell casts. An elevated pH can suggest infection with urease-splitting bacteria.

Blood tests also have a role in determining the cause of hematuria. Elevated levels of BUN and creatinine may be gross indicators of significant dehydration and acute or chronic renal disease. A complete blood count can help differentiate several types of acute or chronic pediatric diseases. In addition, blood from blacks, Puerto Ricans, and Mediterraneans should be tested for sickle cell anemia.

In all cases of suspected AGN, blood samples for antistreptococcal enzyme titers (antistreptolysin O [ASO]) should be sent to the laboratory. A useful confirmatory measure of AGN is the level of complement component C3, which may be decreased in AGN, systemic lupus erythematosus, membranoproliferative glomerulonephritis, serum sickness, and shunt or subacute bacterial endocarditis nephritis. It is most useful in identifying the first three of these disease entities.[5–7]

Management

A child with hematuria and an abdominal mass or with mild trauma requires an intravenous pyelogram (IVP). A child with hypertension, edema, azotemia, and red cell casts probably has acute or chronic nephritis and may require hospitalization, depending upon the severity of these findings. Red cell fragments, anemia, and thrombocytopenia should indicate immediate admission for presumed HUS. If there is a suspicion of coagulopathy, appropriate studies should be obtained and the child admitted to the hospital. Urine cultures should be done for all children with hematuria.[7]

If the urine culture is positive, the patient should be treated and then reevaluated in 1 to 2 weeks. If the culture is negative, the other studies are normal, and the hematuria persists more than 2 to 3 weeks, an IVP should be performed. If this radiologic study is normal and the urine clears of blood, it is advisable to follow the child closely with repeat urinalyses; however, if the IVP is normal and *gross* hematuria persists, without evidence of a renal origin, cystoscopy should be planned. If all the results of these studies are normal and the hematuria persists, a renal biopsy should be considered. However, it has been found that isolated hematuria, without significant proteinuria or the development of renal functional impairment, is usually benign and probably does not require aggressive diagnostic studies, only periodic monitoring of renal function, blood pressure, and growth.[5,6]

PROTEINURIA

Significant, persistent proteinuria is generally interpreted as a sensitive, yet nonspecific, indicator of renal disease. Although there is usually a small amount of protein in the urine, the upper limit of normal for children is approximately 100 $mg/m^2/24$ h. In normal proteinuria 60% of the protein originates from normal plasma and 40% from "tissue" proteins. Although the one-time detection of proteinuria by urine dipstick is a common occurrence in pediatric patients, the persistence of significant levels of proteinuria is uncommon. Protein can enter or exit the urinary fluid as a result of high serum protein levels (as seen in multiple myeloma), increased permeability of the glomerular capillary wall, or decreased absorption of normal amounts of filtered protein or protein from damaged tubular cells.

Measurement

The urinary dipstick indicator is tetrabromphenol, which is very sensitive to small amounts of protein, especially albumin. The SSA method is slightly more sensitive and particularly good for detecting nonalbumin proteinuria. Causes of false-positive reactions with the dipstick method include an elevated urinary pH. With the SSA method a false-positive reaction can occur in the presence of acetic acid, nitric acid, radiologic contrast material, penicillin, tolbutamide, and sulfisoxazole (Gantrisin). Elevated urinary pH causes a false-negative reaction with the SSA method.

Orthostatic proteinuria, the presence of abnormal amounts of protein in the urine during the active parts of the day, with very little proteinuria during the sleeping hours, is particularly common in adolescence. However, it is usually not greater than 1 g/24 h. On long-term (30 years) follow-up, it has not been shown to indicate the presence of renal disease.[8]

Diagnostic Approach

When one has determined that there is significant protein in the urine, it is important to document its persistence. This can be done over several weeks. Initially, the history and physical examination are directed at uncovering evidence of conditions associated with transient proteinuria, such as fever, vigorous exercise, epinephrine injections, and false-positive reactions, as noted previously. A urinalysis should be done. Elevated levels of BUN and creatinine indicate the need for further investigation.

When significant proteinuria is first discovered, a urine culture should be performed, despite the absence of lower urinary tract symptoms. Orthostatic proteinuria can be screened by having the child or the parents check for morning and evening proteinuria. If there is any question, a nighttime and a daytime collection should be tested for protein and creatinine, giving a measure of creatinine clearance and degrees of proteinuria in the resting and active states.

If the proteinuria persists throughout the day over a period of several weeks, and if the urine culture is negative, an IVP is indicated, as well as determination of the serum complement level. The IVP may show evidence of renal pathology, but it can also be normal despite the presence of chronic renal disease. The serum complement, if low, indicates the presence of unsuspected AGN, membranoproliferative glomerulonephritis, systemic lupus erythematosus, serum sickness, and other rather rare causes of decreased complement. Renal biopsy should be considered if the proteinuria is unexplained, persistent, and accompanied by abnormal test results. If the proteinuria persists but the IVP and complement level are normal, it is reasonable to wait several months before considering renal biopsy. If the IVP is abnormal, further management depends upon the type of renal pathology present.

In the presence of a normal 24-hour protein excretion, urinary tract infection, orthostatic proteinuria, or transient proteinuria, follow-up urinalyses are indicated to detect persistence or increases in the degree of proteinuria, or the development of other urinary abnormalities. In this event further diagnostic work-up is indicated.

If hematuria occurs with proteinuria, the chances of significant renal disease are greatly increased, and evaluation should not be delayed.[5,6]

Nephrotic Syndrome

The nephrotic syndrome or "nephrosis" is a clinical state characterized by the presence of proteinuria, hypoalbuminemia, edema, and hyperlipidemia. It is sometimes accompanied by hematuria, hypertension, or azotemia. It may be "primary" or "secondary." Primary nephrotic syndrome is associated with primary glomerular disease. Secondary nephrotic syndrome is associated with a recognized systemic disease or condition, frequently immunologic in nature, that results in glomerular damage.

Seventy to eighty percent of the cases of primary nephrotic syndrome are "minimal change" or "lipoid" nephrosis. Minimal change nephrosis is characterized histopathologically by the absence of major structural changes. The incidence varies from 1.5 to 2 cases per 100,000 children per year, with a prevalence of approximately 13 cases per 100,000 children. There is no geographic, ethnic, or socioeconomic predisposition. The incidence of minimal change nephrosis is highest in the first few years of life and declines thereafter.[9]

Etiology

The etiology of minimal change disease is unknown. Relapses occurring in a significant proportion of children have been associated with allergic rhinitis and immunizations, suggesting an immunologic mechanism. The success of immunosuppressive drugs in the treatment of the disease is also suggestive. Although immunologic mechanisms seem to be a prime suspect in a pathogenesis of minimal change disease, biopsy material is, by definition, negative for immune complex deposition, and the serum complement level is within normal limits.

The separate roles of genetics and environment have yet to be elucidated. It appears that there is a genetic component involved, with familial cases being greater than expected. The male-to-female ratio is 1.7 : 1, and there is a high degree of concordance, i.e., if one sibling has minimal change disease and another also develops a nephrotic syndrome, it will almost always be minimal change disease. It has been estimated that approximately 3.5% of minimal change nephrosis is familial.[8]

Pathophysiology

Proteinuria is generally accepted as the primary abnormality. Protein in the urine far exceeds the normal value of 100 mg/m^2/d. The major protein lost in most childhood nephrotic syndromes is albumin. The major defect in the primary glomerular nephrotic syndrome is an increased glomerular permeability to proteins.

Molecular size, shape, and electrical charge are major determinants of the passage of macromolecules across the capillary wall. One factor thought to be partly responsible for maintaining appropriate negative charge of the glomerular capillary wall is sialic acid, which is found on the basement membrane itself and on the cell membrane of the epithelial prodocytes. In those individuals with nephrotic syndrome, there is a decrease in the content of sialic acid, which may decrease electrostatic hindrance to the passage of albumin.[9]

Plasma protein abnormalities include marked hypoalbuminemia and decreases in α-globulins and fibrinogen. Massive urinary loss is the major cause but probably not the only reason for hypoalbuminemia. There are conflicting data regarding the rate of albumin metabolism at nonrenal sites; however, renal losses of protein probably are greater than nonrenal losses in the gastrointestinal tract.

Hyperlipidemia is a frequent accompaniment of the nephrotic syndrome, with increased low-density lipoproteins, very low density lipoproteins, and triglycerides. Two mechanisms have been suggested for this increase in serum lipids: (1) nonspecific liver activity in response to hypoalbuminemia, causing elevated serum lipids, lipoproteins, and triglycerides; and (2) decreased lipoprotein lipase activity in blood vessel walls.

The development and perpetuation of edema involves two factors: (1) a decrease in plasma oncotic pressure secondary to urinary losses of protein, and (2) excessive renal tubular reabsorption of sodium and water secondary to a decreased renal blood flow and other ill-defined factors. Intravascular volume depletion leads to increased aldosterone and antidiuretic hormone secretion, further promoting the reabsorption of sodium and water.[9,10]

Clinical Features

The primary clinical manifestations of the disease include edema, gastrointestinal disturbances, poor appetite, and, occasionally, respiratory distress. The edema is first noted around the eyes, where there is loose subcutaneous tissue. The parents usually note the edema before the physician can detect it. The edema may be persistent and progressive or may subside and reappear. The development of edema can be rapid or insidious and is frequently attributed to a "cold" or "allergies." Eventually, the child's shoes become tight, the waistline grows, and the child gains weight despite the poor appetite. Eventually, the parents seek the physician's help, frequently after it is noted that there is genital edema. When seen by the physician, the child may have a round face with eyelids that are so edematous they are closed, massive ascites, labial or scrotal edema, presacral and pretibial edema, an umbilical hernia, dilated abdominal wall veins, and even rectal prolapse. The children are most commonly anorectic and fatigued. The gastrointestinal disturbances, which are very common, are probably secondary to bowel wall edema. The anorexia, also presumably secondary to gastrointestinal edema, helps to perpetuate the edema through decreased protein intake combined with continued urinary losses. If the abdominal distension is marked, there may be respiratory distress secondary to ascites.

Diagnostic Studies

The history, physical examination, and laboratory studies are aimed at discovering evidence of associated disease states, such as Henoch-Schönlein purpura, systemic lupus erythematosus, AGN, renal vein thrombosis (RVT), sickle cell disease, and hepatitis, and the presence of nephrotoxins. The likelihood of minimal change disease decreases with evidence of systemic illness, which may be a causative factor in the development of nephrotic syndrome; persistent significant hypertension; or persistent hematuria.

Response to an initial intensive course of corticosteroids provides the single most useful noninvasive technique to discriminate among the primary glomerular diseases. More than 90% of children with minimal change nephrotic syndrome respond to corticosteroids within 8 weeks. Failure to respond forms the basis for recommending renal biopsy and can identify other histologic patterns of primary nephrosis, including focal segmental glomerulosclerosis, membranoproliferative glomerulonephritis, membranous glomerulopathy, mesangial proliferative glomerulonephritis, and focal proliferative glomerulonephritis. Each of these has a prognosis and management that may be quite different from that of minimal change disease. Therefore, unless minimal change nephrotic syndrome is strongly suspected, diagnostic renal biopsy should be considered.

In addition to the history and physical examination, the following laboratory studies should be done initially: urinalysis; complete blood count; measurement of serum levels of electrolytes, urea, nitrogen, creatinine, calcium, phosphorus, total protein, albumin, cholesterol, triglycerides, C3, and hepatitis B surface antigen; and screening for connective tissue disease. A 24-hour urine specimen should be obtained for determination of protein and creatinine levels, as well as another urine specimen to culture. An intradermal test with purified protein derivative (PPD) should be given.[9,10]

Treatment

Prednisone, at 60 mg/m^2/d (maximum dose, 60 mg/d), is administered for 4 weeks. This is followed by "intermittent" therapy: 40 mg/m^2/d on 3 consecutive days in a week for 4 weeks. Chlorambucil and cyclophosphamide should be reserved for children with severe corticosteroid-dependent or relapsing nephrotic syndrome with significant corticosteroid side effects, such as uncontrollable hypertension, cataracts, significant growth retardation, disabling emotional changes, bone disease, and diabetes.

Children with active nephrosis should have a low-salt diet with a high biologically available protein intake. It is important that these children have no fluid restriction, which would tend to augment their hypercoagulable state.

Activity for the nephrotic child should be as tolerated. Bed rest is not necessary for the management of acute nephrotic syndrome, although in some children with severe anasarca, bed rest may help to mobilize some of the edema fluid.

Mild diuretics, such as thiazides, can be used for gradual removal of excess fluid. The major function of diuretics is to remove excess salt, after which water will follow. Overly aggressive diuresis depletes plasma volume, which may lead to hypotension, shock, and vascular thrombosis.

Children who are initially hospitalized with severe nephrosis and are quite uncomfortable with the excess fluid accumulation can be treated with albumin and furosemide. An infusion of salt-poor albumin, 1 g/kg over 2 hours, followed by an intravenous injection of furosemide, 0.5 to 1.0 mg/kg 1 hour after the infusion is started and again at the completion of the infusion, will cause diuresis in most individuals with severe edema. However, one must take appropriate precautions with this regimen. Acute hypervolemia with pulmonary edema and/or hypertension may occur if albumin is infused too rapidly or in large amounts. Vigorous diuretic therapy can result in hypovolemia and electrolyte imbalance with their attendant risks.[9,10]

Complications

The major complications involved with the nephrotic syndrome include hypercoagulability, infection, and impaired physical and psychosocial growth.[8]

There may be excesses and deficits of most clotting factors. This is due to their loss in the urine, coupled with the aforementioned nonspecific synthetic activity of the liver. The sum of these abnormalities leads to a hypercoagulable state. In addition, this hypercoagulability may be augmented by intravascular hypovolemia, hemoconcentration, and possibly changes in vascular structure secondary to hyperlipidemia. This hypercoagulability has important implications for treatment, necessitating adequate intravascular hydration of all nephrotics. Therefore, water should not be restricted in a child with nephrotic syndrome.

Increased susceptibility to infection is common in those children undergoing relapse. Suggested mechanisms include a decreased resistance secondary to edema, low immunoglobulin levels, generalized protein deficiency, immunosuppressive therapy, and decreased phagocytosis and chemotaxis of leukocytes. Sepsis and peritonitis caused by Gram-positive and Gram-negative organisms are uncommon, but they still occur and must be treated vigorously to avoid preventable deaths. The usual signs and symptoms are fever with abdominal pain. Localizing signs of abdominal pathology are often lacking. It is recommended that prophylactic antibiotics not be used routinely, although aggressive broad-spectrum antibiotics are indicated for suspected infections. Pneumococcal vaccine has been recommended for nephrotics, but its efficacy in these children has yet to be confirmed.

With the advent of corticosteroids, impaired growth has become a major consideration in the therapy of the nephrotic syndrome. Growth diminishes markedly and may cease in patients with uncontrolled nephrotic syndrome or in those children who are on high-dose corticosteroids for a prolonged period of time. There may be decreased linear growth and delayed bone maturation, especially when the dose is greater than 5 $mg/m^2/d$.

The physical growth impairment and the physical changes frequently induced by long-term corticosteroid therapy add disturbances in psychosocial functioning to the other complications of the nephrotic syndrome. These psychosocial problems must be dealt with as aggressively as the other complications of nephrosis to avoid having a child in complete prolonged remission but with a decreased ability to function adequately in society.

Prognosis

The course and prognosis depend upon the type of underlying disease and are not directly related to the severity at onset. In fact, there may be an inverse relationship between the apparent severity of the disease and its ultimate prognosis. Minimal change disease tends to be more severe initially, with the more rapid development of edema, the more common occurrence of anasarca, a lower level of serum albumin, and a larger amount of urinary protein. This is in contrast to the other primary forms of nephrotic syndrome, in which the onset tends to be more insidious and less severe, but the ultimate outcome is frequently much worse than minimal change disease.

The good prognosis of minimal change nephrotic syndrome sets it apart from other glomerular diseases that may cause nephrosis. In the preantibiotic era, there was a 60% to 70% mortality from the nephrotic syndrome; with the advent of antibiotics, mortality declined to 30% to 40%. Currently, since the introduction of corticosteroid therapy, there is less than 1% mortality in minimal change disease. The duration of the active disease averages 2 to 3 years, although there is a wide range of variability. Minimal change nephrotics do not progress to renal failure; deaths are due mostly to infection and thrombosis.[8]

ACUTE GLOMERULONEPHRITIS

AGN is a renal disease characterized by cellular proliferation and inflammation in the glomerulus mediated by an immunologic mechanism. Varying degrees of hematuria, proteinuria, azotemia, and hypertension occur.

The true incidence of AGN is unknown, yet it is still considered to be the most common nonsuppurative renal disease of childhood. The peak incidence is in children 5 to 10 years of age; the disease is uncommon in children less than 3 years of age. The male-to-female ratio is 2:1. Family studies have indicated a high incidence of unrecognized disease.[10]

Etiology

The commonly recognized preceding infection associated with AGN is caused by group A β-hemolytic streptococci, but other infectious agents have been implicated: staphylococci, pneumococci, and viruses, including coxsackie, ECHO, influenza, and mumps. Nephritogenic strains of streptococci have been identified, especially types 12, 1, and 4 after nasopharyngeal disease and types 49, 2, 55, 57, and 60 after cutaneous infection. The occurrence of AGN after nasopharyngeal infection tends to be sporadic and clusters in the winter and spring months. Impetigo-related disease tends to be epidemic and clusters in the summer and fall months.

Pathophysiology

In AGN there is a decrease in the glomerular filtration rate and renal blood flow. Tubular function is not compromised as much as glomerular function, resulting in a relative glomerulotubular imbalance that leads to retention of sodium and water and expansion of the extracellular fluid volume. Sparing of tubular function results in a more concentrated urine and the kind of low urinary sodium level frequently seen in prerenal failure, despite the parenchymal nature of this disease.

Clinical Features

The "typical" case has a latency of 5 days to 3 weeks after apparent infection, with an average of 10 days. The most common sign is edema, frequently accompanied by hematuria. The edema is usually periorbital first, but it may progress to the extremities, genitals, and abdominal cavity and may even produce signs of extracellular fluid overload with congestive heart failure. The urine is frequently "tea-colored" because of hematuria, which usually decreases by 4 to 5 days, although it can last as long as 4 weeks after the initial episode. Hypertension may occur secondary to fluid retention and an abnormality of the renin-angiotensin system. Pallor is a manifestation of edema and mild anemia; the latter is partially dilutional and also due to decreased erythropoiesis. Urine output is diminished but rarely to the point of total anuria. Although proteinuria is usually present, it is generally not of the magnitude seen in the nephrotic syndrome. Patients may have seizures secondary to a hypertensive encephalopathy.

Diagnostic Studies

Serologic Tests

Extracellular antigens of the infecting agent stimulate an antibody response in the host. ASO titers rise approximately 10 to 14 days after infection, peak at 3 to 5 weeks, and decline slowly over the next several months. However, the ASO titer rises in only 70% to 80% of individuals after nasopharyngeal disease and less often after cutaneous infection. In addition, a rise in ASO titer is prevented by the early administration of penicillin. Anti-DNase B is probably the single most sensitive indicator of significant streptococcal infection. There is no direct correlation between the magnitude of serologic response and either severity or prognosis of the glomerulonephritis.

The major evidence for the role of immune complexes in poststreptococcal glomerulonephritis is the nodular deposition of immunoglobulin G (IgG) and C3 in the subepithelial areas of the glomeruli. Serum levels of C3 decrease in 80% to 90% of patients and return to normal levels within 8 weeks in 90% to 95%.[10]

Urinalysis

Urinalysis is a valuable adjunct to diagnosis of glomerulonephritis. Although urinalysis results are occasionally normal, there is usually microscopic or macroscopic hematuria, with the presence of red cells and red cell casts. Significant proteinuria is generally present, specific gravity is relatively high, and there is no glycosuria.

Other Diagnostic Aids

Other diagnostic aids include measurement of serum electrolytes, urea nitrogen, and creatinine; complete blood count; erythrocyte sedimentation rate; urine culture; and measurement of antistreptococcal antibodies. An abdominal film helps to determine kidney size, which is usually increased in states of acute inflammation.

Exacerbation of an underlying chronic glomerulonephritis, such as membranoproliferative glomerulonephritis (hypocomplementemic glomerulonephritis), Henoch-Schönlein purpura, systemic lupus erythematosus, familial nephritis, IgA nephropathy, and nephrosis, must be excluded.

Treatment

There is no specific treatment for acute postinfectious glomerulonephritis.[10] Children with AGN require hospitalization if there are signs of circulatory overload, hypertension, severe edema, severe oliguria, or encephalopathy, or if there is biochemical evidence of severe renal failure (azotemia, hyperkalemia, metabolic acidosis). Diuretics may improve edema and circulatory overload, but generally only moderate fluid restriction is necessary for the usual degrees of fluid retention. Hypertension usually responds well to diuresis but may occasionally require aggressive pharmacologic intervention. The specific drugs used depend upon the circulatory status of the child, the degree of hypertension, and the speed with which the blood pressure must be lowered (see "Hypertensive Emergencies"). In cases of moderate to severe renal failure, the characteristic fluid and electrolyte abnormalities should be treated appropriately. In the uncommon instance of severe renal failure, with marked circulatory overload unresponsive to diuretics, hypertension, severe azotemia, or acidosis, dialysis should be strongly considered.

Prognosis

The course and prognosis of children with poststreptococcal glomerulonephritis is excellent. Although there may be a persistent microscopic hematuria, with gross hematuria supervening during the periods of subsequent infection (such as with viral syndromes), the hematuria is not an indicator of recurrent or progressive disease. Proteinuria may persist for up to a year or more but generally fades quickly. Poststreptococcal glomerulonephritis rarely leads to chronic renal failure. Although most cases of postinfectious AGN have an uncomplicated course, certain atypical presentations may indicate the need for renal biopsy (Exhibit 21-1).[11]

Exhibit 21-1 Indications for Considering Renal Biopsy in AGN*

"Atypical" Presentation
- Etiology
  - Absence of infection prior to onset
  - Onset of renal symptoms coincident with infection
  - Absence of serologic evidence of streptococcal etiology (using appropriate tests)
  - Absence of depression of serum complement, or C3
- Early clinical course
  - Anuria
  - Presence of nephrotic syndrome
  - Azotemia out of proportion to other clinical findings
- Miscellaneous factors
  - Age less than 2 yr and over 12 yr
  - Prior history of renal disease
  - Abnormal growth data
  - Family history of nephritis
  - Significant systemic symptomatology

Delay in Rate of "Resolution"
- Early
  - Oliguria and/or azotemia persisting past 2 wk
  - Hypertension persisting past 3 wk
  - Gross hematuria persisting past 3 wk
  - C3 continues low beyond 6 wk
- Late
  - Persistent proteinuria and hematuria past 6 mo
  - Persistent proteinuria past 6 mo
  - Persistent hematuria past 12 mo

* One or more of these indications may cause the physician to *consider* whether biopsy is, or is not, indicated.
Source: Reproduced with permission from Travis LB: Acute postinfectious glomerulonephritis, in Edelmann CM Jr (ed): *Pediatric Kidney Disease.* Boston, Little Brown & Co, vol 2, p 623. Copyright © 1978 Little Brown & Co.

HEMOLYTIC-UREMIC SYNDROME

HUS is the association of acute renal failure, hemolytic anemia, and thrombocytopenia. It is seemingly provoked by a variety of presumed causes and pathogenic mechanisms. Geographic surveys have demonstrated epidemic and endemic areas, familial-genetic cases, seasonal trends, and recurrences. The recognition that HUS is not a result of a single clinicopathologic entity may explain conflicting results regarding that prognosis of the disease and the efficacy of different forms of therapy.[12]

Etiology

The clinical picture in many patients suggests that HUS (especially in childhood) is the consequence of an infectious process. There is a prodrome, which frequently is an upper respiratory tract infection or gastroenteritis with vomiting and diarrhea. This is often followed by a silent period of several days, and finally there is the appearance of the full-blown syndrome. Numerous viral and bacterial agents, as well as rickettsiae, have been associated with HUS. A few of the organisms associated are

- coxsackievirus
- influenza virus
- echovirus
- mumps virus
- myxovirus
- *Pseudomonas*
- *Escherichia coli*
- *Salmonella*
- *Shigella*
- *Bacteroides*
- *Rickettsia*
- *Streptococcus pneumoniae*
- group A β-hemolytic streptococci
- *Haemophilus influenzae*

Presumably, infectious agents account for the epidemics of HUS.

The pathogenesis of HUS remains speculative. A number of immunologic factors have been associated, including immunizations, transplant rejections, thymic dysplasia, and combined immunodeficiency, as well as the use of oral contraceptives, pregnancy, postpartum malignant hypertension, metastatic carcinoma, arsenic ingestion, and the onset of diabetes mellitus. In general, these associated conditions tend to be single case reports.

A number of studies have reported HUS in families, implicating both genetic and environmental factors. The natural history of HUS reported from different areas of the world suggests different causes manifested in a final common pathway of vascular injury.

Pathophysiology

Although the exact pathogenesis of HUS continues to be controversial, there seems to be an abnormality or injury to the endothelial cells of the glomerular capillary tuft. Many different initiating events can lead to this endothelial cell damage.

The frequent association of infection has led to the suggestion that there is some circulating substance, such as an endotoxin or vasoactive amine, that causes the syndrome. Based on the available evidence, disseminated intravascular coagulation is not the initiating event, although there is the possibility of local intravascular coagulation. IgM, C3, and IgG have occasionally been noted in early biopsies, and a transient decrease in complement has been reported, suggesting an immunologic mechanism. Soluble immune complexes can produce vascular lesions in which the endothelium is altered.[13]

Clinical Features

HUS occurs most frequently in children under 4 years of age. Boys and girls are affected equally. A prodromal illness, generally mild but sometimes severe, is manifested as nonspecific gastroenteritis or upper respiratory tract infection. Within several days to 2 weeks, there is the abrupt appearance of pallor, weakness, petechiae, purpura, bloody stools, icterus, and dark-colored urine. There may be colicky abdominal pain (usually periumbilical), vomiting, diarrhea, and hematemesis. Oliguria or anuria may lead to congestive heart failure with edema and hepatosplenomegaly. Hypertension is common and is related to volume overload and, in many cases, excess renin production. There may be neurologic manifestations, including seizures and coma.[14]

Abdominal symptoms may suggest intussusception, acute appendicitis, ulcerative colitis, or acute enterocolitis. Therefore, HUS may pose a therapeutic dilemma for the surgeon. Valid indications for surgical intervention exist, but failure to recognize the underlying problem of impending renal failure may result in inappropriate fluid and electrolyte management. Hazardous conditions for laparotomy include hypertension, anemia, and thrombocytopenia. If, after careful and repeated observations of the patient, surgery is deemed necessary, an awareness of the potential fluid and electrolyte imbalances will serve the child best. Laparotomy also makes subsequent peritoneal dialysis impossible.

The course of HUS is variable. The prognosis bears some relationship to initial severity in that prolonged oliguria or anuria for more than 3 weeks is associated with increased morbidity and mortality. Persistent hypertension also suggests a poor prognosis.[15]

It may take weeks to months to recover renal function, and in some patients, especially those with prolonged oliguria, varying degrees of renal failure persist. There may be recurrences, mild or severe, independent of the severity of the initial episode.

Fortunately, most children recover. They follow the typical pattern of acute renal failure, and within several weeks have recovered adequate glomerular and tubular function. With improved management, including earlier recognition and earlier dialysis to avoid the complications of hyperkalemia and fluid overload and to enable earlier nutrition, mortality in children has decreased to 5% to 10%.[12]

Diagnostic Studies

Abnormal laboratory results include a microangiopathic hemolytic anemia, a blood smear that contains red cell fragments (Burr or helmet cells), thrombocytopenia, reticulocytosis, and hyperbilirubinemia secondary to hemolysis. Urine, which may be scanty, contains blood, protein, and usually abnormal cellular casts. Electrolyte disorders characteristic of acute renal failure include hypernatremia or hyponatremia, hyperkalemia, hypocalcemia, hyperphosphatemia, metabolic acidosis, azotemia, and an elevated serum creatinine level. Some patients with HUS have evidence of hepatocellular injury, with abnormal transaminase levels and decreased serum albumin.

Abdominal x-ray films demonstrate ascites and bowel wall edema. Barium enemas reveal the "thumbprint sign" suggestive of bowel wall edema. Proctoscopy reveals a denuded, friable rectal mucosa with edema and possible loss of sphincter tone.

Treatment

It is of utmost importance to control the potentially lethal abnormalities as soon as possible. Severe hypertension, hyperkalemia, fluid overload, acidosis, azotemia, seizures, and anemia should be treated in standard fashion. Although the conservative management of acute renal failure may be adequate in any particular case, dialysis should be readily available. It should be used to prevent severe complications of acute renal failure and not as a method of last resort. The early use of dialysis has helped to reduce mortality to 5% to 10%.[12]

Various other forms of treatment have been proposed for the HUS, including corticosteroids, heparin, streptokinase, aspirin, dipyridamole, and plasma exchange. The role of these other therapies has not been well defined and must await more definitive studies.

RENAL VEIN THROMBOSIS

RVT is a vascular complication of the kidney leading to hemorrhagic infarction of renal tissue. It is seen most frequently in children during the first year of life, and especially within the neonatal period.[16]

Etiology

RVT should be suspected in any acutely ill baby whose condition is complicated by hyperosmolarity or dehydration, or who develops hematuria, an abdominal mass, thrombocytopenia, or a reduction in renal function. Predisposing conditions include

- maternal diabetes mellitus
- cyanotic heart disease
- exposure to radiologic contrast substances
- dehydration
- diarrhea
- hemoconcentration
- hypercoagulability
- disseminated intravascular coagulopathy
- a history of asphyxia

Presumably, the decreased renal blood flow seen in many of these conditions, with increased sludging in an intrinsically slow capillary system, predisposes the renal vein to thrombosis.

Pathophysiology

The common sites for initial thrombosis are the smaller renal vessels, including the interlobular and arcuate veins and the vasa recta. From here, thrombi may extend into larger or smaller vessels. Rarely, this thrombosis may progress to the renal vein and even to the inferior vena cava. The thrombosis may be unilateral or bilateral; if bilateral, it may be symmetrical or asymmetrical. Anatomic findings vary widely, depending upon the extent and duration of the thrombosis. Grossly, the kidney(s) may appear only minimally affected or markedly enlarged, or may be lobulated, scarred, and contracted with calcifications.

Clinical Features

The diagnosis of RVT must be suspected with the sudden onset of hematuria or appearance of a flank mass in an infant who is "sick" or dehydrated, whose serum is hyperosmolar, or whose history includes any of the aforementioned predisposing conditions. A high index of suspicion must be maintained since RVT may be relatively minor and cause only hematuria. A flank mass is palpable in approximately 66% of children with RVT; hematuria is seen in approximately 66%, and anemia, in approximately 33%. Other diagnostic indicators include thrombocytopenia, which is present in 90% of cases; severe proteinuria; disseminated intravascular coagulopathy; and a microangiopathic blood smear. Decreases in renal function—oliguria, anuria, and other fluid and electrolyte disorders characteristic of renal failure—support the diagnosis. Serial observations are important to confirm the diagnosis and evaluate the severity.[16]

Diagnostic Studies

The differential diagnosis includes hydronephrosis, multicystic kidneys, polycystic kidneys, renal or adrenal tumors, retroperitoneal hemorrhage, and other intra-abdominal catastrophes. Initial laboratory evaluation to make the diagnosis and evaluate the degree of renal failure should include the determination of serum electrolytes, urea nitrogen, glucose, creatinine, total protein and albumin, calcium, phosphorus, and uric acid; complete blood count with platelet count and blood smear; and a screen for disseminated intravascular coagulopathy.

There are other diagnostic tools that, if available, can be extremely useful. Renal ultrasonography, which is noninvasive, may detect hydronephrosis, cystic kidneys, intrarenal and pararenal masses, and the number and size of the kidneys and their location. A renal scan gives a measure of individual renal function and position. It also may indicate obstruction. An IVP should be avoided, if possible, because the contrast material increases hypertonicity, further damaging the kidneys or even inducing renal failure. It also causes an osmotic diuresis which leads to dehydration and further complicates evaluation of the infant's renal status. An inferior venacavagram is of little use and, like the IVP, is potentially very hazardous to the child with RVT.[16]

Treatment

The mainstay of therapy is adequate hydration, correction of electrolyte imbalances, and supportive treatment of underlying conditions such as shock and sepsis.[16] This supportive therapy also helps to decrease further thrombosis within the kidney. Conservative therapy for renal failure in cases of intractable fluid and electrolyte imbalances, congestive heart failure, severe azotemia, acidosis, and hypertension is also important to the successful resolution of RVT. Dialysis may be necessary.

Anticoagulant and fibrinolytic therapy has not been adequately evaluated and offers no significant advantage at this time. Complications of this type of therapy are significant, including induction of bleeding.

Surgical therapy for RVT is no longer utilized routinely. Thrombectomy is generally of no help since most thrombi begin in smaller vessels, beyond the access of the surgeon. Nephrectomy, which was used in the past, is no longer indicated unless the child clearly has an infected kidney refractory to treatment or intractable hypertension. Additionally, major surgery in a sick infant with fluid, electrolyte, and acid-base abnormalities, thrombocytopenia, and renal failure is especially hazardous.

Prognosis

The overall prognosis of RVT is improving with more rapid diagnostic and supportive treatment. The ultimate level of recovery is not predictable simply on the basis of initial results of laboratory studies. Thrombosed vessels frequently recanalize, and poorly functioning kidneys may recover almost completely. Careful support may be necessary for several weeks. Functionally adequate renal status usually returns, although hypertension and chronic renal failure may be the sequelae for survivors of RVT.

ACUTE RENAL FAILURE

Acute renal failure can be defined as an abrupt decline in renal function sufficient to result in retention of nitrogenous wastes and fluid and electrolyte derangement. The normal kidney has a variety of special functions, including excretion of wastes, controlling fluid and electrolyte balance, mediating blood pressure, and erythropoiesis; it also has a central role in vitamin D metabolism. Any or all of these functions can be deranged in acute renal failure. Acute renal failure should be considered when the BUN or serum creatinine level is elevated. From that point it is important to identify reversible causes of these abnormalities and provide appropriate, immediate treatment. A standard approach to the differential diagnosis of renal failure is to identify possible prerenal, renal parenchymal, and postrenal causes, directing the history, physical examination, and laboratory studies appropriately.[17]

Etiology

Prerenal azotemia occurs after inadequate perfusion of the kidneys or a metabolic event resulting in increased urea production. Prerenal azotemia may occur with any condition that decreases blood flow to the kidney, including severe or prolonged vomiting, diarrhea, inadequate fluid intake, blood loss, hypotension or shock, burns, surgery, or asphyxia. Prerenal azotemia also may be caused by protein loading, especially in small infants, and by states of increased catabolism, e.g., those induced by corticosteroid therapy.

Postrenal azotemia is obstructive and is uncommon in the pediatric age group after the newborn period. Posterior urethral valves, functional disorders such as neurogenic bladder or prune belly syndrome, or any extrinsic or intrinsic obstruction to urine flow can effectively produce elevation in creatinine and urea nitrogen. Many causes of prerenal azotemia and postrenal azotemia can lead to permanent renal parenchymal damage; therefore, little time should be lost before initiating appropriate corrective medical or surgical therapy.

The most common causes of parenchymal renal failure in pediatric patients are intrinsic diseases of the glomeruli, vessels, interstitium, or tubules, such as AGN, HUS, RVT, and "vasomotor nephropathy" (acute tubular necrosis).

Clinical Features

The diagnosis of acute renal failure requires appropriate consideration of the history, physical examination, and laboratory evaluation.[18] The history should be directed at finding evidence for volume loss or redistribution, heart failure, and symptoms of systemic disorders such as lupus erythematosus and Henoch-Schönlein purpura. A history of preexistent renal disease, hypertension, or growth failure may suggest the presence of a chronic underlying condition. Potentially nephrotoxic medications should be identified, and a history of streptococcal infections or bloody stools should be sought.

The physical examination is directed at defining the state of hydration and discovering reversible causes of inadequate renal perfusion, including dehydration, congestive heart failure, and shock. Evidence of postrenal obstruction (enlarged bladder) is also sought. During the physical examination, physical signs of chronic illness or systemic disease are also identified.

Diagnostic Studies

Urinalysis can be extremely helpful in deciding whether apparent renal failure is due to parenchymal or prerenal problems. A high specific gravity, a dipstick test that is negative for blood or trace to 1+ for albumin, and the absence of cellular casts suggest the presence of prerenal azotemia, although rarely, such a "negative" urine may be seen with AGN or acute obstruction. Conversely, a low specific gravity, significant proteinuria or hematuria, and the presence of cellular casts suggest renal parenchymal disease and/or chronic obstructive disease.

Urinary volume is unreliable as a diagnostic indicator of renal failure. Although in the past a decrease in urine volume was considered important for the diagnosis of acute renal failure, it has become increasingly clear that nonoliguric renal failure is not an uncommon entity and in some instances may be more prevalent than oliguric failure. Oliguria can be defined as less than 250 mL of urine per square meter in a child and less than 1 mL/kg/h in an infant weighing less than 10 kg. Oliguria is compatible with either prerenal, postrenal, or renal parenchymal disease. The quality, not the quantity, of the urine must be stressed. Anuria is very uncommon and may indicate a catastrophic renal disease such as renal cortical necrosis, RVT, or complete obstruction.

Tests of tubular function can be useful in the differential diagnosis of prerenal and parenchymal renal failure. Assuming that the tubules respond appropriately, the renal response to hypoperfusion is to avidly conserve sodium and water. This results in an elevated specific gravity and, frequently, an elevated urine-to-plasma ratio of osmolarity, urea nitrogen, and creatinine. One of the best measures of prerenal versus renal failure is the fractional excretion of sodium (see Table 21-5).

The normal level of BUN is less than 20 mg/dL; however, significant changes in the level of BUN can occur in small, normally anabolic children who may experience a doubling of the urea nitrogen without the absolute value appearing abnormal. Adults may increase their level of BUN from 15 to 30 mg/d, depending upon their metabolic and nutritional state. Infants may only increase their level of BUN from 5 to 10 mg/d after renal shutdown. Steroid therapy or protein loading also can effect a rise in BUN without a decrease in renal function.

Serum creatinine in children is normally less than 1.0 mg/dL and varies according to the size of the child. A significant, progressive rise in creatinine is much more accurate an indicator of decreased renal functional capacity than a single, questionably elevated level.

Other laboratory findings that may also suggest the diagnosis of decreased renal function include hypernatremia or hyponatremia, hypercalcemia, metabolic acidosis, hyperphosphatemia, and anemia (as seen in HUS).

A plain abdominal film may indicate the size of the kidneys and the presence of stones. Large kidneys can indicate glomerulonephritis; small kidneys, renal asymmetry, or staghorn calculi strongly suggest a chronic problem.

TABLE 21-5 Laboratory Aids in the Differential Diagnosis of Acute Renal Failure

	Prerenal Oliguria		Low-output Acute Tubular Necrosis	
	Adult	Infant	Adult	Infant
Urine Na (mEq/L)	<20	<10	>25	>40
FeNa (%)	<1	<1.8	>3	>10
U/P* osmolarity	>2	>2	<1.1	<1.1
U/P area (mg/dl)	>20	>5	<10	<5
U/P creatinine (mg/dl)	>40	>20	<10	<5
Urine sediment casts	Hyaline and granular		Cellular	

* Abbreviations: U, urine: P, plasma; FeNa, fractional sodium excretion.
Source: Reproduced with permission from Medani CR, Davitt MK, Huntington DF, et al: Acute renal failure in the newborn. *Contrib Nephrol* 1979:15;49.

An IVP attempted in a patient with renal failure frequently results in poor visualization and risks a contrast-induced nephropathy. On the other hand, renal ultrasonography is noninvasive and can identify obstruction or hydronephrosis and the size and internal morphology of the kidney, bladder, and ureters. If available, it is the procedure of choice in the differential diagnosis of acute renal failure.

Radionuclide studies are of particular importance in neonatal acute renal failure. They can determine the presence and location of functional renal tissue. These studies may also be useful in older patients with renal failure.

Arteriography and venography are generally not indicated for initial workup of the azotemic patient. The diagnosis of renal artery thrombosis and RVT is made on clinical grounds. Contrast-induced renal failure is a potential side effect of such studies, and venography is not accurate for the diagnosis of neonatal RVT.

Treatment

Once the diagnosis of renal failure is suspected, adequate hydration (20 mL/kg/h) and perfusion should be maintained if there is no cardiac compromise. This should lead to an increase in urine output in the patient with prerenal oliguria. Lower tract obstruction is bypassed, if possible, with a urinary catheter, and a spot sample of urine is obtained for further diagnostic studies, if necessary. If urine flow does not increase with these measures, a trial of furosemide, 1 to 2 mg/kg IV, is indicated. This occasionally has the effect of changing oliguric renal failure to a nonoliguric type, with subsequently easier management and less morbidity and mortality. Mannitol also has been used instead of furosemide but carries the potential for acute circulatory overload.

If these maneuvers are not successful in increasing urine flow in the oliguric patient, the diagnosis of renal failure must be strongly considered.

Although advances are being made in attempts to develop specific therapy for acute renal failure (e.g., infusion of adenine nucleotides and, in the case of potential toxin-induced failure, discontinuing the toxin and possibly inducing diuresis), the mainstay of therapy is to support the patient until the kidneys have recovered enough function to maintain life or until it is decided that chronic dialysis is indicated. A delay in appropriate management can result in clinically significant long-term renal functional impairment.

The following is a discussion of the main considerations in therapy.

Sodium and Water

The body weight, obtained at least daily, is the most important guide to adjusting fluid needs. The initial prescription for water should be equal to urinary output plus 30 to 35 mL/100 calories metabolized (insensible water loss minus water of oxidation minus preformed water). In the properly managed patient, there should be approximately 0.5% to 1% loss of body weight per day, reflecting loss of carbohydrate and fat. Maintenance of a stable weight reflects gradual overhydration of the patient. Sodium should be added for initial rehydration or ongoing losses. Hyponatremia and hypernatremia generally reflect water excess or water deficit, respectively, and should be treated as such.

Potassium

Serum potassium levels are of immediate importance. Since acute renal failure is a catabolic state, potassium is released from the breakdown of cells. In addition, dietary potassium and endogenous potassium from hemolysis or necrotic tissue may add to the potential problem. Oral potassium should be restricted unless there are excessive potassium losses, which may be seen with high-output renal failure, and the serum potassium level is less than 2.5 to 3 mEq/L. Significant potassium excess is reflected in the electrocardiogram by peaked T waves, widening of the QRS complex, decreasing amplitude of the P waves, and eventually a sine-wave pattern as the QRS complex merges with the T wave.

Depending on the severity, treatment of hyperkalemia (>5.0 mEq of potassium per liter) should include one or more of the following:

- exchange resin (Kayexalate), 1 g/kg orally or rectally
- sodium bicarbonate, 2 to 3 mg/kg IV
- glucose, 0.5 to 1.0 g/kg IV, with regular insulin added to the infusion at a dose of 1 U for every 3 to 4 g of glucose
- calcium gluconate, 0.5 mL/kg of 10% solution, given slowly IV
- dialysis

Acidosis

Acidosis can be controlled with dietary restriction of proteins and buffer correction (sodium bicarbonate, 1 mEq/kg, if allowed by the cardiovascular status). Excess sodium and fluids cause eventual fluid overload and congestive heart failure, especially in oliguric renal failure.

Nutrition

The main thrust of nutritional support for a child with acute renal failure is to decrease waste products and increase the caloric intake. This is accomplished by decreasing the protein intake to 0.5 g of protein with high biological availability per kilogram of body weight. The dietary prescription should also take into account sodium and potassium restrictions and provide for a very high nonprotein caloric intake to prevent as much endogenous protein catabolism as possible and to speed recovery from the catabolic state.

Hypertension

Hypertension is usually a result of fluid overload, although hyperreninemic states may contribute to hypertension in renal failure. If the elevation in blood pressure is severe, emergency treatment is indicated. Diazoxide, 3 to 5 mg/kg in a rapid IV push, is indicated for severe hypertension, followed by more standard drug therapy such as oral propranolol, 1 mg/kg/d divided into four doses, or parenteral hydralazine, 0.2 to 0.5 mg/kg/dose four times daily.

Congestive Heart Failure

Heart failure is generally the result of fluid overload and should be treated with fluid restriction or dialysis if the child is in a critical state. Digitalis is difficult to use in a uremic individual since it is excreted by glomerular filtration; in addition, the abnormal levels of calcium, potassium, and sodium may increase the likelihood of digitalis intoxication.

Azotemia

The rate of increase in urea nitrogen can be retarded by appropriate dietary restriction of proteins or by infusion of essential amino acids if the oral route is contraindicated. Dialysis should be strongly considered if the BUN is greater than 100 mg/dL or if the rise is extremely rapid.

Seizures

Seizures may be secondary to hyponatremia, hypernatremia, hypocalcemia, uremia, or water intoxication. These seizures can be treated immediately without regard to cause, which should be sought during subsequent therapy.

Hyperphosphatemia

Hyperphosphatemia occurs with acute renal failure when the kidney is unable to excrete large amounts of dietary phosphates that are normally ingested. This is generally treated with phosphate binders such as aluminum hydroxide, at a dose of 100 mg/kg/d in divided doses with meals.

Hypocalcemia

Hypocalcemia is secondary to hyperphosphatemia, and generally does not cause tetany since there is usually systemic metabolic acidosis. Calcium, either oral or parenteral, is not indicated in renal failure except in the rare instance of hypocalcemic tetany. Increasing calcium levels will increase the incidence of metastatic calcifications, especially renal.

Anemia

Anemia in acute renal failure is usually dilutional or secondary to blood loss. Although uremia may depress marrow erythropoiesis, this is generally not a clinically important problem in acute renal failure. Transfusions in renal failure can lead to the acute onset of congestive heart failure, hypertension, and pulmonary edema secondary to hypervolemia.

Dialysis

The liberal use of peritoneal dialysis or hemodialysis, depending upon availability, to *prevent* uremic symptomatology rather than to reverse it, has improved the survival rate in acute renal failure. Dialysis is indicated in the following instances:

- intractable electrolyte disorders
- severe hypertension
- congestive heart failure with pulmonary edema
- acidosis refractory to buffer correction
- azotemia of greater than 100 to 120 mg/dL
- hyperuricemia of greater than 15 mg/dL
- bleeding diathesis of uremia
- to provide a route of excretion for metabolic products of adequate nutritional support
- for the removal of nephrotoxic drugs or drugs with serum levels in the toxic range.

Course

In oliguric renal failure the duration of oliguria may last from a few days to several weeks. As renal function recovers, osmotic diuresis coupled with a tubular concentrating defect causes an increased urine flow, even to the point of causing dehydration or severe electrolyte imbalance. It is particularly important during this phase that fluids and electrolytes be carefully controlled to avoid a relapse of renal failure.

Infection is a major cause of death in individuals with renal failure. Avoidance of urethral catheters on a prolonged basis, careful monitoring of intravenous catheter sites, correction of pulmonary stasis, and prevention of malnutrition are critical to the rapid, uncomplicated recovery of the child. Fever is frequently absent, but hypotension, tachycardia, and evidence of continued hypercatabolism may be early signs of sepsis. Prophylactic antibiotics are to be avoided.

It is clear that the appropriate and adequate therapy of acute renal failure requires great care and effort from physicians, nurses, and other members of the health team in a setting that is designed for the care of children. Since most occurrences of acute renal failure in children are reversible, it is important to be meticulous in the daily management of this syndrome, which can cause complex systemic disorders.[17,18]

HYPERTENSIVE EMERGENCIES

Blood pressure determination in children is an integral part of the child's medical evaluation. Hypertensive children, once thought to be rare, are being identified more frequently as a result of routine measurement of blood pressure. The treatment of hypertension is rarely an emergency, and such children can usually be evaluated on an outpatient basis. However, markedly elevated blood pressure in a child is a medical emergency that, if untreated, may cause heart failure, cerebral dysfunction, renal failure, cerebrovascular accidents, coma, and even death.

Children's blood pressure levels are lower than adult standards, and the evaluation of blood pressure requires the use of standard nomograms (Figure 21-2). Markedly elevated blood pressure is a diastolic pressure greater than 110 mmHg in the older child and adolescent; in younger children a diastolic blood pressure of greater than 20 mmHg above the 95th percentile should be considered severe and treated accordingly.[19]

Etiology

The most common causes of severe hypertension in children are renal.[13] All of the following can result in hypertension:

- acute or chronic glomerulonephritis
- acute or chronic renal failure
- glomerular disease associated with systemic illnesses such as Henoch-Schönlein purpura or systemic lupus erythematosus
- renal artery thrombosis or embolus
- HUS
- chronic pyelonephritis, congenital hypoplasia, dysplasia
- cystic disease of the kidney.

Vascular causes of hypertension include coarctation of the aorta and renal artery stenosis. Metabolic disorders such as hypercalcemia and cystinosis, and adrenal disorders, such as pheochromocytoma and hyperadrenocorticism, may cause extreme elevations in blood pressure. Substances implicated include methamphetamines, phencyclidine, extreme amounts of licorice, corticosteroids, and many of the decongestant products used in children. Renin-secreting tumors have also been reported as a cause of severe hypertension (Exhibit 21-2).[20]

Pathophysiology

Fibrinoid necrosis develops in arteriolar walls of the brain, kidneys, and other organs. Either severe arteriolar spasm or the development of cerebral edema underlies the development of hypertensive encephalopathy.

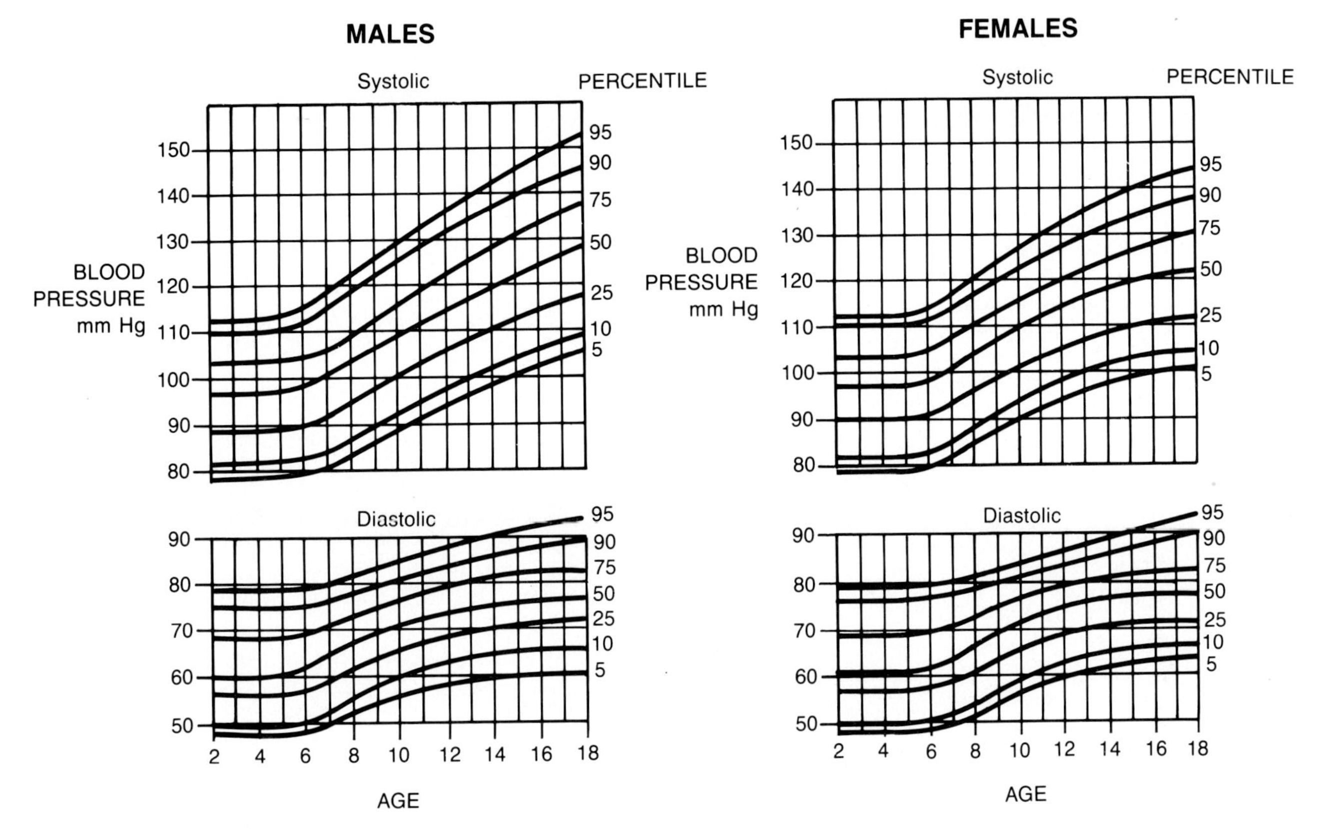

FIGURE 21-2 Percentiles of blood pressure measurement in boys and girls aged 2 to 18 years. (Adapted with permission from Blumenthal S, Epps RP, Heayenrich R, et al: Report of the task force on blood pressure control in children. *Pediatrics* 1977;59(Suppl):797. Copyright © American Academy of Pediatrics 1977.)

Clinical Features

The child with severe hypertension may or may not be symptomatic. Various nonspecific signs and symptoms may be present, including malaise, lethargy, vomiting, headache, visual disturbances, or central nervous system abnormalities. Epistaxis may be a presenting sign.

On physical examination the blood pressure should be measured with an appropriately sized cuff, covering at least half of the upper arm. The child should be in the seated position, calmed if necessary and if possible, and several measurements should be done over the period of the examination.[19]

Signs of congestive heart failure, abnormalities in the neurologic examination, or abnormal funduscopic findings may be present. Papilledema, retinal hemorrhage, and exudates (signs of "malignant" hypertension) are uncommon in children.

Diagnostic Studies

Initial laboratory evaluation of the child with severe hypertension should assess renal status via urinalysis and measurement of BUN, serum creatinine, and electrolyte levels (Exhibit 21-3). The urinalysis results may be abnormal, either from primary renal disease or as a result of the hypertension, and reveal hematuria, albuminuria, and cellular casts. The degree of elevation of BUN and serum creatinine indicates the severity of renal failure, as do abnormal serum electrolyte levels. Either an IVP or a renal ultrasonogram with an isotope scan can assess the urinary tract from both a structural and functional standpoint. Obstruction of urine flow, renal masses, and glomerular filtration can be evaluated by these studies. Arteriography may eventually be necessary to define the presence of renal artery stenosis. Cardiac status should be evaluated with a chest film, electrocardiogram, and possibly an echocardio-

Exhibit 21-2 Causes of Acute Hypertension in Childhood

- HUS
- Acute postinfectious glomerulonephritis
- Other nephritides:
  - Henoch-Schönlein purpura nephritis
  - Systemic lupus nephritis
  - Membranoproliferative nephritis
- Chronic pyelonephritis
- After genitourinary surgery
- Renovascular disease
  - Renal artery stenosis
  - Segmental hypoplasia
- End-stage renal disease—during dialysis
- Renal transplantation
- Elevated central nervous system pressure
  - Meningitis
  - Encephalitis
  - Trauma
  - Tumor
  - Hydrocephalus
  - Respiratory acidosis (CO_2 retention)
  - Familial dysautonomia
  - Quadriplegia (micturitional crises)
- Burns
- Drugs
  - Steroids
  - Phenylephrine
  - Drug-drug interaction
  - Clonidine rebound
  - Reserpine overdose
  - Amphetamines
  - Phencyclidine
- Quadriplegia
- Food ingestions—toxins
  - Licorice
  - Lead
- Tumors
  - Pheochromocytoma
  - Renin-secreting tumors
- Essential hypertension
- Thalassemia crisis
- Polycythemia vera

Source: Reproduced with permission from Ingelfinger JR: *Pediatric Hypertension.* Philadelphia, WB Saunders Co, 1982, p 219. Copyright © 1982 WB Saunders Co.

gram. Central nervous system dysfunction may suggest the need for a computed tomography scan of the brain.

Treatment

Eradication of the cause of the hypertension is the ultimate goal. A sustained diastolic blood pressure of greater than 110 mmHg or greater than 20 mmHg above the 95th percentile for age is an indication for immediate hospitalization and parenteral antihypertensive medications (Table 21-6), plus a comprehensive investigation for the underlying cause. A child who has sustained pressures exceeding the 95th percentile but less than 110 mmHg and who has symptoms of cerebral dysfunction (hypertensive encephalopathy) also needs immediate hospitalization and treatment. If the child has moderately severe hypertension but has diastolic pressures less than 110 mmHg and is asymptomatic, hospitalization may not be necessary, provided good follow-up is guaranteed. Treatment may begin with oral medication as the evaluation of the underlying mechanism is carried out.

It must be stressed that a sustained markedly elevated blood pressure, although occasionally asymptomatic, will lead to irreversible renal, central nervous system, cardiac, and ophthalmologic complications. The need to treat overrides the need for time-consuming diagnostic procedures in this potentially life-threatening circumstance. The blood pressure must be decreased within a few hours of the discovery, preferably in an intensive care environment.

Exhibit 21-3 Phased Approach to the Diagnosis of Hypertension

- Phase I: Broad Screening (may be outpatient)
  - Urinalysis: 24-h protein excretion
  - Urine culture
  - BUN
  - Creatine and creatinine clearance
  - Electrolytes and TCO_2
  - Electrocardiogram
  - Chest x-ray film
  - IVP
- Phase II: Specific Screening and Diagnoses—Noninvasive
  - Renal scan, adrenal scan
  - Ultrasonogram
  - Voiding cystogram
  - Plasma renin profiling
  - Plasma catecholamines
  - Plasma dopamine β-hydroxylase
  - 24-h urine samples for:
    - Vanillylmandelic acid (VMA) and catecholamines
    - 17-Keto- and 17-hydroxysteroids
    - Aldosterone excretion
- Phase III: Specific Diagnoses—Invasive
  - Arteriography
    - Renal
    - Adrenal
  - Venography
    - Renal vein renins
    - Caval catecholamines
  - Saralasin infusion*
- Phase IV
  - Renal biopsy
  - Split renal function studies

* Experimental in children

Source: Adapted with permission from Ingelfinger JR: *Pediatric Hypertension,* Philadelphia, WB Saunders Co, 1982, p 12. Copyright © 1982 WB Saunders Co.

TABLE 21-6 Agents Used in the Treatment of Severe Hypertension

Name	Mechanism	Dose	Onset	Advantages	Disadvantages	Comments
Diazoxide (Hyperstat)	Direct vasodilator	3–5 mg/kg rapid IV push over several seconds	Within seconds	Hypotension uncommon Tolerance does not develop Secondary increase in cardiac output	Reflex tachycardia Concomitant therapy with propranolol may block cardiac output Fluid retention Mild hyperglycemia, hyperuricemia	Agent of choice for most hypertensive emergencies Add diuretic
Nitroprusside (Nipride)	Direct vasodilator	0.5–10.0 μg/kg/min	Within seconds	Most potent drug available Increases cardiac output Decreases left ventricular filling pressure	Constant supervision required Continuous infusion necessary Nausea	Potential for thiocyanate toxicity, tinnitus, delirium, blurred vision Cautious use with increased intracranial pressure
Hydralazine (Apresoline)	Direct vasodilator	0.2–0.6 mg/kg/dose IV or IM; maximum, 20 mg	15 min	May be used parenterally	Reflex tachycardia Increased cardiac output, sodium, water retention blunts effectiveness Headache, flushing	Usually used with drug that limits cardiac output, and with diuretic
Methyldopa (Aldomet)	Central effect	20–40 mg/kg/d in 4 doses; maximum, 65 mg/kg/d or 3 g/d, whichever is less	2–3 h	May be used parenterally	Somnolence Delayed onset Highly variable response	CNS* side effects may mask pathologic changes in CNS status
Phentolamine (Regitine)	α-Adrenergic blockade	1–2 mg IV	1 min	See comments	Short half-life; dosing interval 5–10 minutes	Specifically for use with pheochromocytoma, other catecholamine-releasing states

* CNS, Central nervous system.

After the initial parenteral therapy with diagoxide or nitroprusside for severe hypertension, oral medication should be initiated, if possible. The use of standard therapy, with oral agents such as diuretics, vasodilators, and β-blockers (Table 21-7), is preferable to medications with a primarily central mechanism of action. The centrally acting drugs, which have the common side effects of lethargy, sleepiness, personality change, or other symptoms related to the central nervous system, may confuse the clinical picture of a child who has had hypertensive encephalopathy and the unsuspected compli-

TABLE 21-7 Drugs Frequently Used in Treating Hypertension

Diuretics	Vasodilators	Adrenergics
Thiazides	Reserpine	Captopril
Chlorthalidone	Minoxidil	Propranolol
Furosemide		Guanethidine
Spironolactone		Methyldopa
		Clonidine

cations of stroke or hemorrhage. These oral medications should be started as soon as the controlled blood pressure begins to rise from normal levels. If the blood pressure continues its upward course, augmentation with parenteral medications may be necessary.[21]

In the case of hypertensive encephalopathy, diagnostic studies must be delayed until the hypertension is brought under control. However, the studies previously outlined should be performed as soon as possible to identify correctable causes and complications of severe hypertension.

URINARY TRACT INFECTIONS

Infections of the genitourinary tract are a common problem in the pediatric age group, ranking second in frequency only to infections of the respiratory tract. While frequently seen on an outpatient basis, patients with urinary tract infections often are ill enough to require hospital admission; such patients account for 3% to 5% of admissions to pediatric hospital wards.[14,22]

Epidemiology

The incidence of urinary tract infection varies within different pediatric age groups and with the sex of the patient.[23–28] It is slightly higher for boys in the neonatal period, but at all other ages in childhood, it is higher for girls. In the neonatal period asymptomatic infections occur with similar frequency in both sexes, but symptomatic infections occur more often in males. Preterm infants have a threefold greater incidence of infection than term infants. In all other age groups (preschool, school-age, and adolescent), girls are affected more often than boys by approximately 10 to 1, whether symptomatic or asymptomatic. The overall prevalence of urinary tract infections in girls after the neonatal period is from 1% to 2%.

A longitudinal study has revealed that 5% of schoolgirls became bacteriuric during their elementary and high school years. For all schoolgirls with bacteriuria, the probability of recurrence is significantly increased when they become sexually active or pregnant.[19]

Pathophysiology

Urinary tract infections in the neonate are felt to be the result of hematogenous spread. The high incidence of positive blood cultures found in neonates with urinary tract infection supports this concept; however, recent evidence indicating non-circumcised male infants are at higher risk of acquiring a urinary tract infection may invalidate this theory. Beyond the newborn period, urinary tract infection, which occurs predominantly in females, usually begins with the ascent of bacteria up the urethra into the bladder. The orifice of the relatively short female urethra is easily contaminated with fecal bacteria, which may ascend into the urinary bladder; the organisms that are responsible for urinary tract infections are usually part of the rectal flora. Normal body defense mechanisms may clear these organisms, or, instead, bacteria may remain and multiply, producing a cystitis. Infected urine may then ascend to the pelvis of the kidney, facilitated by reflux caused by ureterovesicle valve incompetence. This incompetence is secondary to infection in the bladder involving the vesicoureteral valve orifice or is the result of an anatomic abnormality. Bacterial motility allows organisms to ascend, and endotoxins elaborated by the bacteria may assist the ascent by impairing ureteral peristalsis. The renal medulla, an area in which leukocyte function and complement activity are reduced because of hypertonicity and low pH, is the initial site of parenchymal invasion. Invasion of the renal cortex follows. Experimental data have shown that in the progression of untreated pyelonephritis, there is a phase of sequestration during which viable bacteria can be recovered from parenchymal tissue in the absence of bacteriuria.[29] Depending on the organism producing the pyelonephritis, this period can vary from 4 to 12 weeks before ultimate recovery, or, in some instances, the bacteria may remain viable for longer periods and progressively destroy tissue, with scarring and compromised renal function. Although renal scarring is not infrequent, renal failure secondary to infection in an otherwise normal urinary tract is quite rare in childhood.[23]

Other factors influence which individuals become infected; some are known, while others remain to be identified. Among those felt to influence susceptibility is the bacteria's ability to adhere to uroepithelial cells. Serotypes of *E. coli* with little ability to adhere have been identified with bacteriuria of minimal clinical severity. Adherence predisposes to more severe disease.[30] The defense mechanism of the bladder, mediated by secretory immunoglobulins, may be less efficient in some patients and allow bacteria to adhere and multiply. Retention of residual urine in the bladder creates a culture medium in which bacteria can multiply. Additional factors known to correlate with an increased incidence of urinary tract infection are sexual activity and pregnancy.[16] Still, our knowledge concerning why some patients develop urinary tract infections and others do not is far from complete.

Clinical Features

Urinary tract infections can be classified as symptomatic or asymptomatic. It should not be concluded, however, that children with asymptomatic urinary tract infections are always totally free of symptoms. Retrospective evaluation of patients so classified has indicated that symptoms were present in the majority of them but either had not been severe enough to prompt medical attention or had not been considered indicative of urinary tract infection.[31] Thus the majority of patients with urinary tract infections are symptomatic.

As originally defined by Kass,[32] "asymptomatic bacteriuria" is an operational definition to define a finding in patients who were not considered by the physicians who saw them to have sufficient evidence of urinary tract infection to warrant a diagnosis, a treatment, or a culture of the urine. If the physician has a high index of suspicion and realizes that symptoms are frequently nonspecific, the number of patients with "asymptomatic" infections should be very small. Furthermore, renal damage may occur in patients who have infections with either minimal or no symptoms. Symptoms vary depending on the age of the patient and are most apt to be nonspecific in the younger patients. They may be acute or chronic and insidious.

In the neonate the infection may be fulminant, with the infant appearing toxemic. Severe signs and symptoms are probably related to an endotoxin. Less severe and nonspecific symptoms include hyperthermia or hypothermia, poor feeding, lethargy, vomiting, diarrhea, irritability, jaundice, and abdominal distension. On palpation there may be abdominal tenderness, and in the presence of an obstructive uropathy, a mass may be palpable. Cultures of both blood and urine are usually positive.

During infancy, crying and irritability, a diaper that is constantly wet, diarrhea, constipation, fever, vomiting, and failure to thrive are signs and symptoms associated with urinary tract infection. A diaper rash with foul-smelling or even bloody urine may be noted. Seizures may result from the hyperpyrexia.

In children and adolescents the signs and symptoms classically associated with urinary tract pathology are observed: urinary urgency, frequency, dysuria, enuresis, and abdominal or flank pain. Fever with chills correlates reasonably—but not absolutely—with pyelonephritis. Enuresis after continence has been accomplished may be an early sign. At any age unexplained fever requires a careful search for urinary tract infection.

Diagnostic Studies

The clinical picture alone is not sufficient to confirm the diagnosis of urinary tract infection; this can only be made by urine culture. The method used to collect the urine sample establishes the criteria to be used in confirming the diagnosis. Acceptable methods of collection include a clean-caught midstream sample, a specimen obtained by catheterization, or one obtained by suprapubic aspiration. The number of organisms necessary to establish a diagnosis varies with the method of collection, as does the number of positive specimens required. The criteria are suggested in Table 21-8.

Obtaining a noncontaminated specimen is crucial and necessary to make an accurate diagnosis. Bag urines are more often confusing than helpful in establishing the diagnosis, but they are useful in following patients after diagnosis has been confirmed and therapy has been initiated. A negative culture is of greatest significance; positive cultures frequently contain multiple organisms because of contamination.

There are exceptions to these guidelines. For example, persistent recovery of a single organism at less than 100,000 colonies per milliliter is certainly compatible with infection. In other instances, such as the presence of an abnormal urinary tract, multiple organisms may be present. Thus decisions must be made on an individual basis. In cases in which

TABLE 21-8 Criteria for Diagnosis of Urinary Tract Infection

Method of Collection	No. of Colonies	No. of Specimens
Clean-caught midstream	>100,000/mL	2
Catheterization	>1,000/mL	1
Suprapubic aspiration	Any growth	1

immediate antibiotic therapy is warranted on clinical grounds, it is important that the specimen be obtained in the most precise manner, by either catheterization or suprapubic aspiration. When these are properly performed, there can be no confusion, and complications of these procedures are quite rare.

Care in obtaining the urine specimen is mandatory, regardless of the method used. In obtaining a clean-caught midstream specimen in girls, the genital area must be cleaned with sterile water, the labia minora must be separated, and a sample of urine must be caught after voiding has been initiated. In uncircumcised boys the foreskin should be retracted before the glans is cleansed. Catheterization, once popular and then abandoned because of the risk of introducing bacteria into the bladder, is being used more frequently and with apparent safety. Identification of the urethral orifice prior to attempting catheter insertion, cleansing the area carefully, and using sterile gloves when inserting the small, sterile polyvinyl catheter are all mandatory if contamination is to be avoided. When performing a suprapubic aspiration, the skin should be cleansed with alcohol and then an iodine solution should be used prior to aspiration. In all instances, since preparation of the skin prior to obtaining the specimen may provoke urination, obstructing urination by inserting a finger in the rectum and exerting upward pressure, pushing the urethra against the symphysis pubis, will allow recovery of urine before premature emptying of the bladder has occurred. In boys the same result can be obtained by exerting lateral pressure on the penile urethra.

Once the urine specimen is obtained, it should be cultured promptly, using a quantitative method. If the specimen cannot be cultured within 30 minutes, it should be stored at 4° C until inoculation on culture media can be performed; however, even this delay is undesirable because both false-negative and false-positive values have been reported following this procedure.[33]

Only the urine culture is diagnostic, but other laboratory findings may be useful in making the diagnosis. A Gram stain of a drop of fresh, uncentrifuged urine may reveal organisms and is very strong presumptive evidence of infection. Pyuria is so variable that it must be considered unreliable, although clumps of white blood cells or leukocyte casts are highly suggestive. Hematuria is a frequent finding in urinary tract infections but may be present for other reasons, as may proteinuria.

Localization of the infection in the upper urinary tract cannot be done with certainty unless a positive specimen of urine is obtained by ureteral catheterization, the bladder wash-out technique, or renal biopsy. None of these procedures is infallible, and none is usually performed in an outpatient setting or on hospital wards. Their use is reserved either for research studies or in a most unusual clinical setting. Attempts have been made to use other laboratory procedures, but all fail to absolutely differentiate patients with pyelonephritis from those with only lower urinary tract infection. These include determination of C-reactive protein levels, titration of serum antibodies, erythrocyte sedimentation rate, measurement of renal concentrating capacity, labeling with immunofluorescent antibodies, and tests for urinary lactic dehydrogenase.[34–35] Positive blood cultures plus positive urine cultures should be considered evidence of pyelonephritis. Clinical evaluation remains an important consideration.

Identification of the organism further refines the diagnosis and aids in selecting therapy. *E. coli* is the organism most commonly recovered from patients with urinary tract infections (Table 21-9).

All patients, both boys and girls, should have a radiologic evaluation of the genitourinary tract with the first infection. Severity of illness bears no relationship to the probability of abnormal radiologic findings. Abnormalities have been found in 30% to 50% of all patients studied. Radiologic studies provide a way to demonstrate renal damage, congenital abnormalities, stasis of urine, and vesicoureteral reflux. Results of these studies are used to determine the appropriate duration of treatment and the need for urologic consultation.

Both an IVP and a voiding cystourethrogram are indicated. Failure to do both studies will allow some pathology to be missed. The voiding cystourethrogram is extremely important if ureteral reflux is to be diagnosed. We perform the radiologic

TABLE 21-9 Bacteria Cultured from Urine Specimens*

Bacteria	No. of Patients
E. coli	199
Klebsiella	21
Staphylococcus	13
Proteus	7
Enterobacter	5
S. fecalis	3
Pseudomonas	3
Serratia	1
Salmonella	1
Total	253

* Specimens were obtained from patients during their first visit to the renal clinic.

studies as soon as the patient is asymptomatic and find that the incidence of abnormalities is no different from when studies are performed in patients after therapy has been completed. An additional advantage of early investigation is the prompt identification of those patients who require immediate urologic consultation.

Reflux in the youngest patients increases the risk of developing upper tract disease and renal damage. Stated another way, older patients with reflux are those most likely to exhibit renal scarring.[36] It is important to maintain a sterile urine as long as reflux persists for it is the reflux of infected urine that leads to damage of the renal parenchyma. Cystoscopy or urologic consultation is not often necessary but is indicated if an obstructive uropathy, ectopic ureter, or severe reflux is identified.

Baseline blood studies that should be performed to evaluate renal function include measurement of serum urea nitrogen, creatinine, and electrolyte levels, and a complete blood count. The blood pressure should always be determined.

TABLE 21-10 Drug Therapy for Urinary Tract Infections*

Drug	Dosage (mg/kg/24 h)	Maximum (mg/24 h)	Prophylaxis (mg/kg/single dose/24 h)
Ampicillin	100	4,000	—
Cephalexin	50	1,000	—
Gentamycin†	3–5		
Carbenicillin†	400		
Nitrofurantoin	5–7	400	1–2
Sulfisoxazole‡	150	4,000	—
TMX			
Trimethoprim	8–10	320	2
Sulfamethoxazole	40–50	1,600	10

* Give a bactericidal drug for 2 w, then follow with a bacteriostatic drug.
† Hospital drug.
‡ Not for patients less than 2 months of age, with glucose 6-phosphate dehydrogenase deficiency, or near term.

Treatment

Antimicrobial Therapy

Choice of an antibiotic, the dosage, and the duration of therapy are decisions to be made. The ultimate basis for choosing an antibiotic and continuing it is its ability to sterilize the urine. If symptoms are not too severe, treatment can be delayed until results of the urine culture are available, to allow selection of the most appropriate antibiotic. If therapy is started before the organism is identified, an antibiotic likely to be effective against *E. coli* should be chosen. Ampicillin or amoxicillin, both of which are bactericidal, is our preference, although one of several bacteriostatic antibiotics (sulfisoxazole or nitrofurantoin) can be chosen as the initial drug. A change to one of them is made 2 weeks after controlling the infection with the bactericidal drugs. Patients ill enough to be hospitalized are begun on intravenous ampicillin unless they are allergic to the drug. Those most severely ill may be presumed to have bacteremia, and an aminoglycoside should be added (Table 21-10).

Treatment of the acute infection requires full therapeutic doses. In long-term therapy a full therapeutic dose of antibiotic is given for 6 weeks, followed by one half to one quarter of the therapeutic dose of a bacteriostatic drug for suppression of infection during the remainder of the treatment period.

Duration of treatment remains controversial and, judged from the frequency of recurrent infections, not well established. The decision to determine duration is based on results of the radiologic study of the genitourinary tract and a history of presence or absence of previous infection. Either short-term or long-term therapy is chosen. Short term varies from 2 to 6 weeks; long term is for 6 months or more. Very short term therapy in children, 1 to 4 days, cannot be recommended on the basis of present data.[37]

Patients placed on short-term therapy are those with first or second infections plus a normal IVP and voiding cystourethrogram. Long-term therapy is prescribed for patients with more than two prior infections or a radiologically abnormal genitourinary tract, especially with evidence of urinary stasis or reflux.

Six months of treatment is considered long term, provided there is no evidence of urinary stasis or reflux after that period of time. Should these abnormalities persist, then therapy may be continued until the radiologic studies are normal. Nuclear screening with technetium can be used when performing subsequent voiding cystourethrograms and greatly reduces radiation exposure. While not providing the detail obtained with the conventional voiding cystourethrogram, it does provide an adequate measure of reflux and is very useful in follow-up studies. Five or more recurrences would be an indication for suppressive therapy for 2 years (Figure 21-3).

The choice of 6 weeks of treatment is based on the inability to localize the urinary tract infection with methods immediately available, and the realization that organisms in the renal parenchyma may persist for several weeks.[29,34,35]

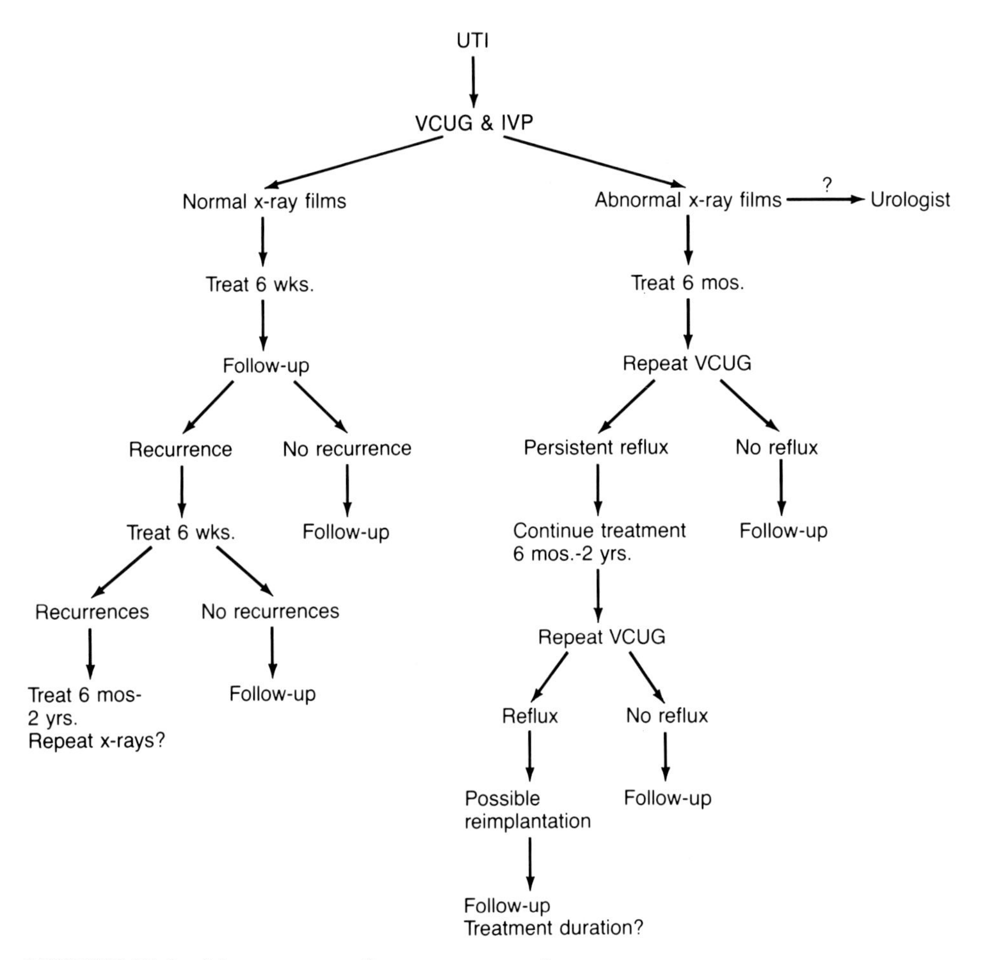

FIGURE 21-3 Management of urinary tract infection. UTI, Urinary tract infection; VCUG, voiding cystourethrogram.

Nonspecific Treatment

Nonspecific treatment includes those measures designed to alleviate conditions associated with, or suspected of being associated with, an increased likelihood of urinary tract infection.

Perineal Hygiene. Girls should be instructed in the proper use of toilet tissue to reduce the likelihood of contamination of the urethral orifice. Diaper rashes should be treated appropriately. Pinworm infestation can produce perianal and perineal irritation and requires specific medication. A vaginal discharge should be cultured and treated, and there should be an examination for foreign bodies.

Hydration. The liberal use of liquids is encouraged, especially while the patient is receiving medication.

Voiding. Patients should be encouraged to void as necessary. It may be necessary to intervene with school teachers on behalf of patients to ensure that they are excused as necessary.

Constipation. This should be corrected because fecal impaction may impede emptying of the bladder at micturition, resulting in residual urine.

Bathing. Shower baths, rather than tub baths, are advised. Bubble bath is to be avoided.

Follow-up

Although the appropriate duration of therapy remains uncertain, there is no disagreement on the importance of adequate follow-up. Regardless of the type of therapy, the rate of recurrent infection remains high, ranging from 25% in neonates to 75% in those who have experienced frequent infections in the past.[25] Reinfection is most apt to occur within the first year after therapy, and the risk decreases with each succeeding year that the patient is free of infection. After 3 years infection free, the risk of reinfection is approximately 5%. Periods of increased likelihood of reinfection include the onset of sexual activity and pregnancy.[38]

The sine qua non of adequate follow-up is urine culture. Rapid slide or dipstick cultures tests are available for ambulatory screening. A dipstick test based on the ability of Gram-negative bacilli to convert nitrate to nitrite may also be useful. None of these tests is as accurate as a quantitative urine culture, and this should be used if the screening tests are questionable or contrary to clinical impression. Because reinfections are apt to occur soon after treatment, follow-up visits should be scheduled monthly in the first year, every 3 months the second year, and every 6 months thereafter or at any time symptoms occur. All reinfections should be treated.

References

1. Goldsmith DI: Clinical and laboratory evaluation of renal function, in Edelmann CM Jr (ed): *Pediatric Kidney Disease*. Boston, Little Brown & Co, 1978, pp 213–224.
2. Schumann GB: *Urine Sediment Examination*. Baltimore, Williams & Wilkins, 1980.
3. Schwartz GJ, Haycock GB, Spitzer A: Plasma creatinine and urea concentration in children: Normal values for age and sex. *J Pediatr* 1976;88:828–830.
4. Kassirer JP, Gennari FJ: Laboratory evaluation of renal function, in Early LE, Gottschalk CW (eds): *Strauss and Welt's Disease of the Kidney*, ed 3. Boston, Little Brown & Co, 1979, pp 41–90.
5. West CD: Asymptomatic hematuria and proteinuria in children: Causes and appropriate diagnostic studies. *J Pediatr* 1976;89:173–182.
6. Dennis VW, Kreuger RP, Robinson RR: Hematuria, leukocyturia, and cylindruria, in Edelmann CM Jr (ed): *Pediatric Kidney Disease*. Boston, Little Brown & Co, 1978, pp 312–315.
7. James JJ: Proteinuria and hematuria in children: Diagnosis and assessment. *Pediatr Clin North Am* 1976;23:807–816.
8. Royer P, Habib R, Mathied H, Broyer M: Proteinuria, in Schaffer AJ (ed): *Major Problems in Clinical Pediatrics: Pediatric Nephrology*. Philadelphia, WB Saunders Co., 1974, Vol 11, pp 247–252.
9. Arant BS, Singer SA, Bernstein J: Steroid-dependent nephrotic syndrome. *J Pediatr* 1982;100:328–333.
10. The primary nephrotic syndrome in children. Identification of patients with minimal change nephrotic syndrome from initial response to prednisone. A Report of the International Study of Kidney Disease in Children. *J Pediatr* 1981;98:561–564.
11. Travis LB: Acute postinfectious glomerulonephritis, in Edelmann CM Jr (ed): *Pediatric Kidney Disease*. Boston, Little Brown & Co, 1978, Vol 2, 611–631.
12. Fong JSC, de Chadarevian JP, Kaplan BS: Hemolytic-uremic syndrome: current concepts and management. *Pediatr Clin North Am* 1982;29:835–856.
13. Koster F, Levin J, Walker L, et al: Hemolytic-uremic syndrome after shigellosis: Relation to endotoxemia and circulating immune complexes. *N Engl J Med* 1978;298:927–933.
14. VanWierengen PMV, Monnens LAH, Schretlen: Haemolytic-uremic syndrome. Epidemiological and clinical study. *Arch Dis Child* 1974;49:432–437.
15. Kaplan BS, Katz J, Lurie A, et al: An analysis of the results of therapy in 67 cases of the haemolytic-uremic syndrome. *S Pediatr* 1971;78:420–425.
16. Arneil GC: Renal venous obstruction, in Edelmann CM Jr (ed): *Pediatric Kidney Disease*. Boston, Little Brown & Co, 1978, pp 1098–1104.
17. Dobrum RS, Larsen CD, Holliday MA: Acute renal failure, in Smith CA (ed): *The Critically Ill Child*. Philadelphia, WB Saunders Co, 1972, pp 113–123.
18. Schrier RW: Acute renal failure: Pathogenesis, diagnosis, and management. *Hosp Prac* 1981;16:93–112.
19. Ingelfinger JR: *Pediatric Hypertension*. Philadelphia, WB Saunders Co, 1982.
20. Londe S: Causes of hypertension in the young. *Pediatr Clin North Am* 1978;25:55–65.
21. Goldring D, Robson AM, Saintiago J: Systemic hypertension, in Gellis K (ed). *Current Pediatric Therapy*. Philadelphia, WB Saunders Co, 1986, pp 150–157.
22. Michie AJ: Pediatric urology: Summary of a round table. *Pediatrics* 1959;24:1118–1122.
23. Heptinstall RH: *Pathology of the Kidney*, ed 2. Boston, Little Brown & Co, 1974, vol 2, pp 877–927.
24. Kunin CM: Epidemiology and natural history of urinary tract infection in school age children. *Pediatr Clin North Am* 1971;18:509–528.
25. Hellerstein S: Recurrent urinary tract infections in children. *Pediatr Infect Dis* 1982;1:271–281.
26. Riley HD Jr: Pyelonephritis. *Adv Pediatr* 1968; 15:191–269.
27. Gillenwater JY, Harrison RB, Kunin CM: Natural history of bacteriuria in schoolgirls: A long-term case-control study. *N Engl J Med* 1979;301:396–399.
28. Wiswell TE, Smith FR, Bass JW: Decreased incidence of urinary tract infections in circumcised male infants. *Pediatrics* 1985;75:901–903.
29. McCabe WR, Jackson GG: The natural course of retrograde infections of the urinary tract of rats with different serotypes of *Escherichia coli* or *Enterococcus*, in Quinn EL, and Kas EH (eds): *Biology of Pyelonephritis*. Boston, Little Brown & Co, 1960, pp 39–58.
30. Lomberg H, Hellström M, Nodal N, et al: Virulence associated traits in *Escherichia coli* causing first and recurrent episodes of urinary tract infection in children with or without vesicoureteral reflux. *N Inf Dis* 1984;150:561–569.
31. Savage DCL, Wilson MI, McHardy M, et al: Covert bacteriuria of childhood: A clinical and epidemiological study. *Arch Dis Child* 1973;48:8–20.
32. Kass EH: Asymptomatic infections of the urinary tract. *Trans Assoc Am Phys* 1956;69:56.

33. Scheinman JI, Hester DJ, Integlia SS, et al: Antibiotic treatment of asymptomatic bacteriuria. *Am J Dis Child* 1973;125:349–352.
34. Carvajal HF: Kidney and bladder infections. *Adv Pediatr* 1978;25:383–413.
35. Jodal U, Lindberg U, Lincoln J: Level diagnosis of symptomatic urinary tract infections in childhood. *Acta Paediatr Scand* 1975;64:201–208.
36. Kincaid-Smith P, Becker G: Reflux nephropathy and chronic atropic pyelonephritis: A review. *J Infect Dis* 1978;138:774–780.
37. Durbin WA Jr, Peter G: Management of urinary tract infections in infants and children. *Pediatr Infect Dis* 1984;3:564–574.
38. Naeye RL: Causes of the excessive rates of perinatal mortality and prematurity in pregnancies complicated by maternal urinary tract infections. *N Engl J Med* 1979;300:819–823.

Dennis L. Hoover
Mark F. Bellinger

22 Genitourinary Trauma

Serious injuries of the genitourinary (GU) systems are commonly secondary to vehicular accidents, sledding mishaps, and falls from gymnastic equipment. These accidents occur most commonly in the second decade of life. GU trauma is associated with other system injury in nearly 40% of cases.[1] Although the immediate care of central nervous system, orthopedic, or abdominal injuries may overshadow attention to urologic injury, the impact of significant renal, urethral, or genital trauma can be lifelong, especially if neglected during the initial resuscitation of the patient.

RENAL TRAUMA

Of all trauma to the GU system, renal injuries are most common.[2] The significance of renal trauma lies partly in the fact that the minute volume blood flow to the kidney is 25% of the cardiac output. Thus, renal injury can result in very rapid blood loss. The greater mobility and lesser amount of perinephric fat and the pliability of the surrounding ribs make a child's kidney more susceptible to injury than an adult's. Congenital or acquired renal anomalies, including tumors, also can predispose a child to injury. An ectopic kidney is more vulnerable because of its relatively superficial position. An obstructed collecting system, distended with urine, is at risk of rupture with relatively minimal trauma. Most renal injuries are caused by blunt trauma, frequently associated with motor vehicle accidents. Penetrating renal trauma is much less common.

Clinical Features

The child with multiple trauma must be evaluated carefully for signs of renal injury (Figure 22-1). With the high incidence of central nervous system injuries in multiple trauma, pain, guarding, and other subjective findings may be absent. Physical examination should include direct visualization of the back and flanks for abrasions or contusions. Tenderness in the renal fossa, although often musculoskeletal in nature, should indicate possible renal injury. Urinalysis revealing either gross or microscopic hematuria is significant, and x-ray films showing lower rib fractures or transverse process fractures demand further radiologic investigation of the urinary tract.

Pain or tenderness in the flank or costovertebral angle is the most common symptom associated with renal injury.[1,3] The severity and duration of pain may be extremely variable. Renal pain may result from two processes: capsular distension resulting from acute urinary obstruction or subcapsular hematoma, or colicky pain due to ureteral spasm from the passage of tissue, stone, or clot. The differential diagnosis of flank pain includes musculoskeletal pain, splenic or hepatic injury (although these are

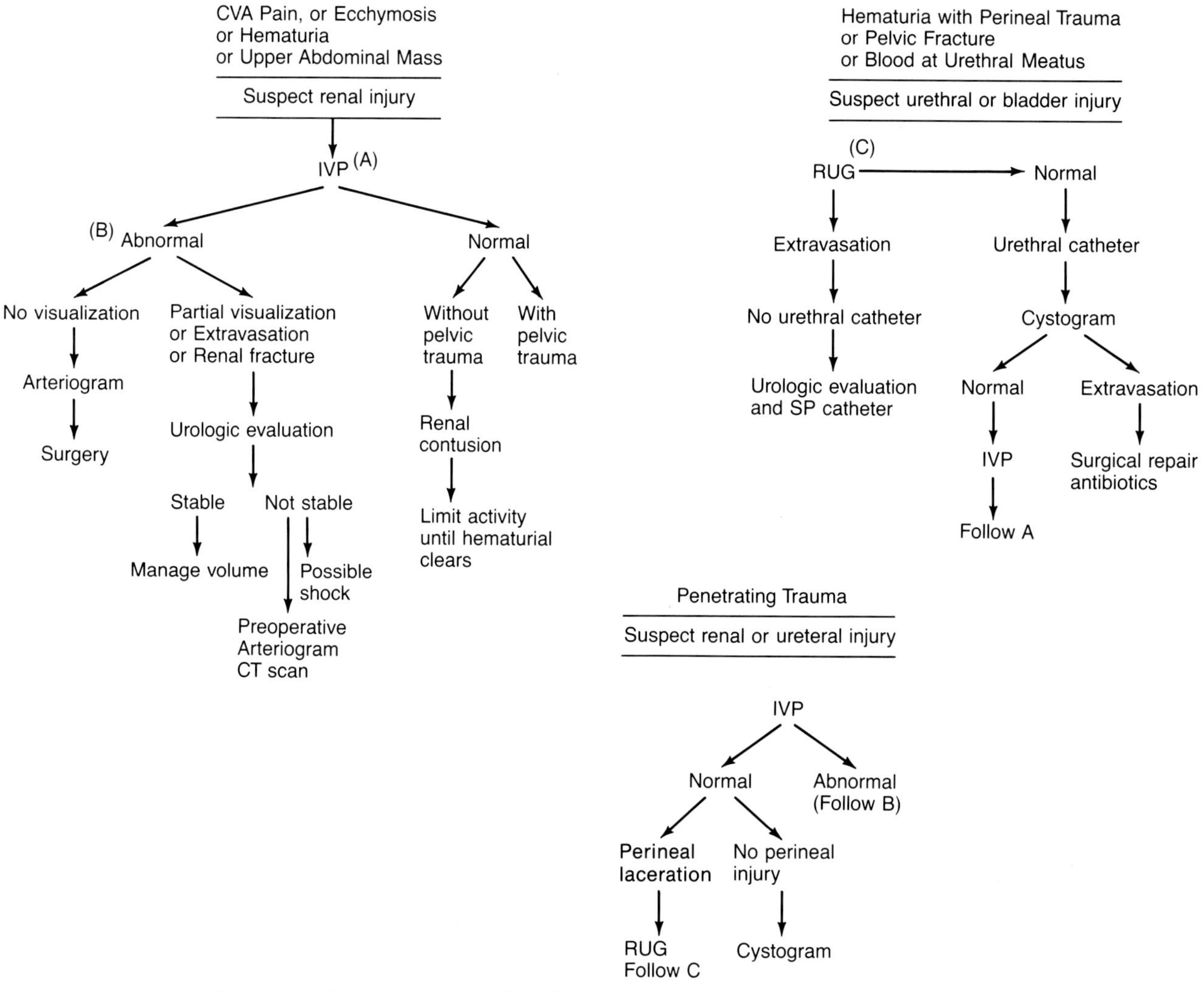

FIGURE 22-1 Evaluation and management of urologic trauma. CT, Computed tomography; IVP, intravenous pyelogram; RUG, retrograde urethrogram; SP, suprapubic.

likely to result in acute abdominal symptoms and peritoneal irritation), and pleuritic pain. Splenic injury has been associated with left renal trauma in up to 25% of pediatric patients, and duodenal and pancreatic trauma are not uncommon. Chest trauma is not infrequently associated with renal injury.[3,4]

Hematuria, whether gross or microscopic, is evidence of injury to the urinary system. Renal injury, being more common, is the most likely source. Although reported series[3,5] indicate that more than 50% of patients with renal trauma have gross hematuria and 20% to 40% have microhematuria, 7% to 20% of pediatric patients with significant renal injuries may have normal urinalysis findings. Therefore, the presence of hematuria is significant, but the absence of blood in the urine does *not* eliminate the possibility of injury to the urinary tract.

A drop of blood at the urethral meatus is pathognomonic of urethral injury. Catheterization of such patients is contraindicated prior to assessment of the urethra, as discussed under "Urethral Injuries."

A flank mass is suggestive of severe renal injury, with extravasation of urine or blood. A flank or upper abdominal mass may be palpable in over 50% of children with renal trauma. Large masses suggest injury to a previously diseased or hydronephrotic kidney.

Diagnosis and Management

The classification of renal injuries proposed by Sargent and Marquardt[6] remains one of the most clinically useful (Figure 22-2):

- type I: a contusion or minor parenchymal fracture with an intact renal capsule
- type II: major parenchymal fracture, possibly extending into the collecting system
- type III: shattered kidneys with multiple fractures or injury to the major renal vessels

Most (80%) are type I, relatively minor renal contusions. Although variable degrees of flank pain or hematuria may be present, an excretory urogram (intravenous pyelogram [IVP]) can confirm a structurally normal kidney and collecting system that is intact. No specific treatment is necessary, although bed rest is recommended until gross hematuria resolves. More serious injuries (type II and type III) also may produce a variable symptom complex. Findings on excretory urogram may include extravasation from a laceration into the collecting system, interruption of the renal contour because of a large parenchymal tear, loss of a portion of the nephrogram because of injury of a segmental vessel, or nonvisualization of the kidney, indicating a shattered kidney or injury to the main renal artery. Patients with these injuries are at greatest risk for missed diagnosis. There are often overshadowing head or gastrointestinal injuries. In an effort to get the patient to the operating room rapidly, an intravenous urogram is sometimes postponed, in which case serious renal injury may not be suspected until an expanding retroperitoneal mass is found at exploration. In that setting the salvage rate of the injured kidney is significantly decreased.[7]

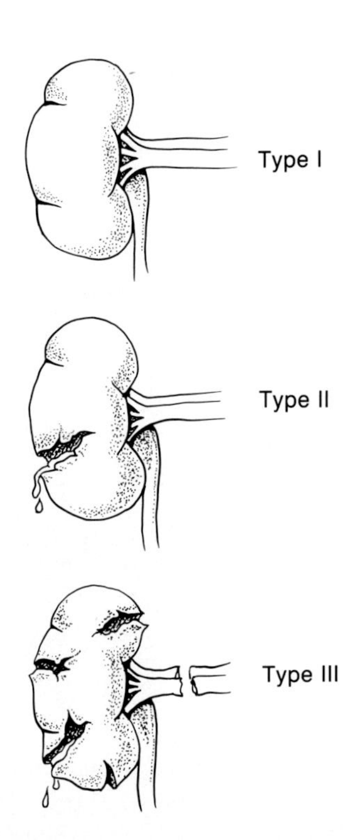

FIGURE 22-2 Classification of renal injuries. Type I, contusion. Capsule and collection system intact. Type II, renal fracture. Possible extension into the collecting system and possible loss of a segmental vessel. Type III, multiple renal fractures or pedicle injury.

Emergency radiologic evaluation is necessary for proper management of the patient with renal trauma. The studies are important not only to delineate the degree of injury and guide treatment but also to confirm the presence of a functioning contralateral kidney. Even for the most critically injured patient, an adequate portable contrast study of the kidneys can be performed in the emergency department. Diatrizoate meglumine (Renografin 60, E.R. Squibb), at a dose of 3 mL/kg (100 mL maximum dose), provides good resolution of renal architecture, even under adverse conditions. A portable abdominal x-ray film can be taken at 1 minute and 10 minutes after injection without interfering with other management efforts. If a type III injury is suspected and the patient's vital signs are stable, further evaluation with renal scan, computed tomography, or arteriography may be helpful. Complete nonfunction on IVP should suggest renal artery avulsion which, although an uncommon injury, occurs in a greater percentage of pediatric trauma cases.[8] In the past, arteriography has been indicated in the preoperative evaluation of patients suspected of having severe renal vascular injury. Since the early 1980s, however, enhanced computed tomography scans have been used effectively to yield nearly as much information, and in some facilities they have supplanted renal arteriography for evaluation of traumatic renal injuries.

In the case of pedicle injury, repair of the renal vessels must be performed within 12 to 18 hours of injury if renal salvage is to be possible. Type II renal injuries resulting from blunt trauma can be managed nonoperatively if the patient remains stable but must be monitored initially in the hospital setting. Penetrating renal trauma requires surgical exploration. Urologic follow-up of the patient who suffers renal trauma includes monitoring with serial urograms and screening for continued hematuria or hypertension as sequelae of the renal injury.

URETERAL INJURIES

Ureteral injuries are rare. They are usually a consequence of penetrating injury and all require surgical intervention. Rarely, the ureter may be dis-

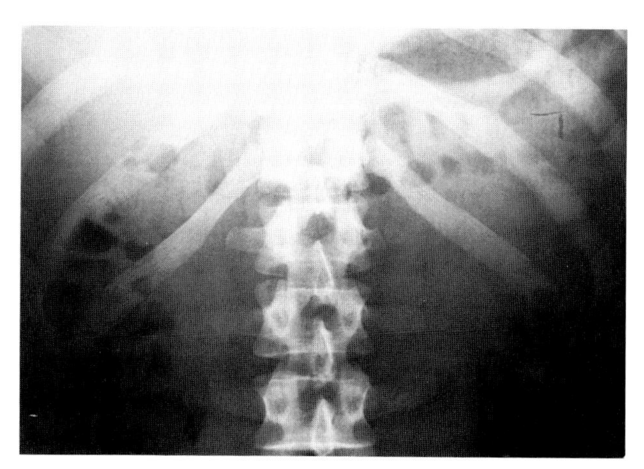

FIGURE 22-3 Fracture of transverse process of first lumbar vertebra. Any child with this injury should have an intravenous urogram to rule out ureteral injury.

rupted from the renal pelvis at the ureteropelvic junction. This consequence of blunt trauma is peculiar to children[9] and is due in part to the increased mobility of the kidney. Because there are no acute signs or symptoms related specifically to ureteral injury, the diagnosis can be easily missed. Avulsion injuries are caused by such a forceful blow that associated fractures of the lumbar transverse processes are commonly noted (Figure 22-3). Therefore, any patient who has such a fracture or who has sustained penetrating trauma near the expected course of a ureter should have an IVP (Figure 22-1). Early diagnosis of ureteral injury affords the best opportunity for surgical repair before infection or devitalization of the ureter has occurred.

BLADDER INJURIES

The bladder is an abdominal organ in the young child. Bladder trauma may be due to penetrating injury or blunt abdominal trauma, but most commonly it is associated with pelvic fracture. Approximately 10% of pelvic fractures are associated with bladder rupture. In the pediatric patient compression of a distended bladder is frequently associated with a peritoneal tear and intraperitoneal leakage of blood and urine.[10] Although hematuria and a lower abdominal mass are common signs, they are not necessarily present, and the diagnosis depends on a high index of suspicion. Every child with a pelvic fracture must have an IVP and cystogram (Figure 21-1). A cystogram is performed by retrograde instillation of a water-soluble (intravenous) contrast agent via a urethral catheter. It is imperative that a retrograde urethrogram be performed prior to catheter insertion if urethral trauma is suspected (see "Urethral Injuries"). During filling, the injured bladder may take on a teardrop configuration because of extrinsic compression by a pelvic hematoma. Intraperitoneal rupture becomes evident as the contrast outlines loops of bowel in the lower abdomen (Figure 22-4). Because extraperitoneal rupture may not be apparent until the bladder is emptied and extravasated contrast is seen in the perivesical space, postdrainage films are very important. Bladder irrigation alone is not a reliable test to rule out bladder rupture since complete return of irrigant may occur even in the presence of a large bladder rent that is transiently plugged with bowel or omentum. Initially, these injuries are adequately managed with urethral catheter drainage but, ultimately, surgical repair is required for all but small extraperitoneal injuries.

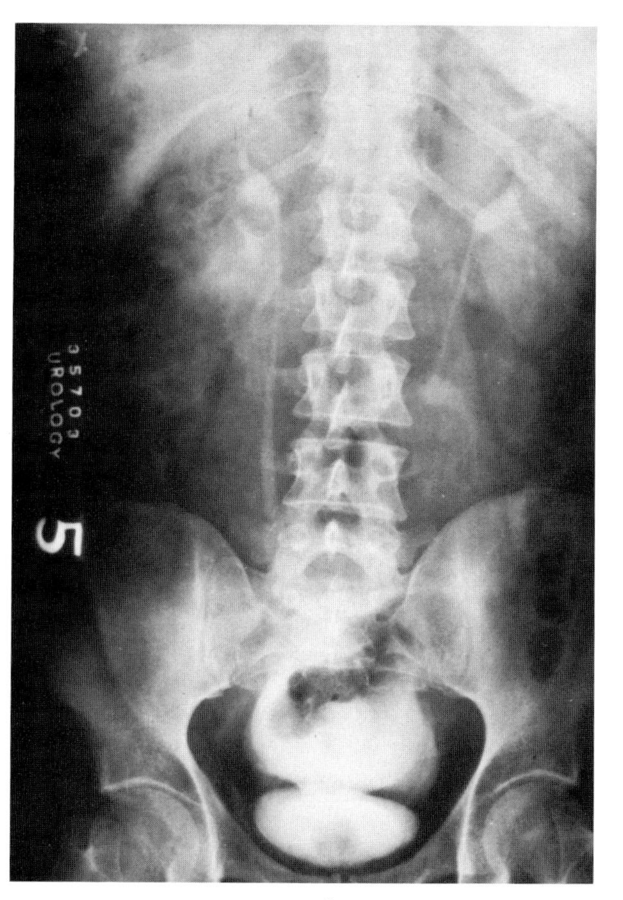

FIGURE 22-4 Cystogram after an intravenous urogram demonstrates rupture of the bladder with intraperitoneal extravasation of contrast medium. The scalloped appearance is caused by contrast medium outlining loops of small bowel.

URETHRAL INJURIES

The length and course of the male urethra make it more liable to injury than the female urethra (Figure 22-5). Complete or partial disruption of the bulbous urethra may occur as an isolated event and should be suspected in all patients with straddle injury or penetrating penile, scrotal, or perineal trauma. Most membranous urethral injuries result from severe trauma and are associated with multiple injuries including pelvic fractures. Blood at the urethral meatus is pathognomonic of urethral injury but is not always present. Other findings may include irregularity of the pubis because of fracture and distended bladder because of retention. Ecchymosis of the perineum in a butterfly pattern can result from blood extravasating along fascial planes. A high-riding prostate and bogginess in the prostatic fossa on rectal examination of the postpubertal male suggests elevation of the bladder, which is possible only with complete urethral disruption. Recognition of urethral injury before attempted catheterization is extremely important. A partially torn urethra does not require as extensive a surgical repair as does a complete disruption.[11] Unwitting damage from urethral catheterization attempted during initial evaluation can easily transform a partial injury into a complete one, with greater risks of impotence, incontinence, and stricture.[11]

If urethral injury is suspected, a gentle retrograde urethral contrast study should be performed in the emergency department or radiology suite prior to catheterization. The tip of a number 5 or number 8 French feeding tube (or simply a blunt-tipped adapter and syringe) is inserted into the urethral meatus, which is then occluded while 10 to 15 mL of water-soluble contrast is injected without force. An oblique x-ray film of the pelvis taken during injection demonstrates the extent of urethral injury (Figure 22-6). (If a Foley catheter has already been inserted and the question of urethral injury is raised, the study should be performed alongside the catheter.) If injury is demonstrated, urinary diversion will be necessary, and immediate referral is mandatory.

It is appropriate here to discuss the trocar cystostomy, which can serve as an excellent form of temporary diversion when surgical or urologic consultation is not immediately available and which is preferable to urethral catheterization when urethral injuries are present. Percutaneous cystostomy catheters are available in most hospitals (Figure 22-7). A perfectly functional alternative may be a long (10-12 cm or greater), 12- or 14-gauge intravenous catheter.

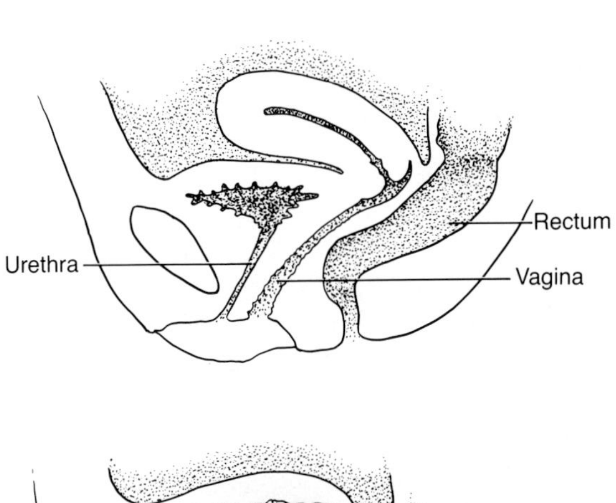

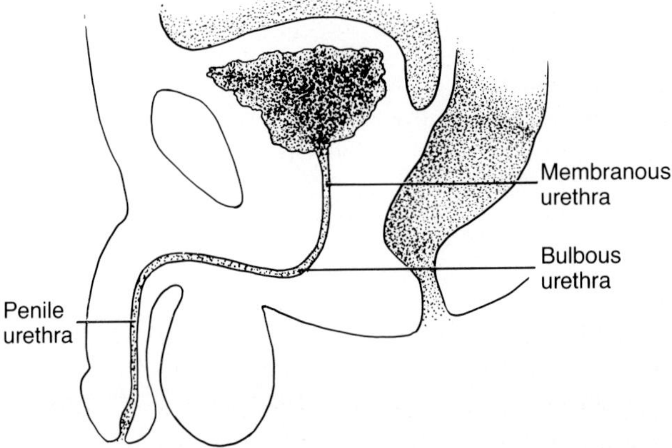

FIGURE 22-5 Anatomy of the urethra. The female urethra is shorter and less vulnerable than that of the male, which is susceptible to injury at the penile urethra, the bulbous urethra, or the membranous urethra.

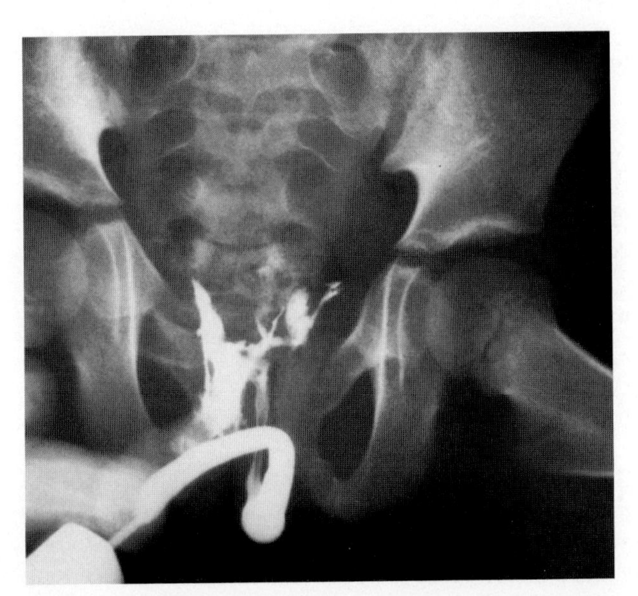

FIGURE 22-6 Retrograde urethrogram demonstrates extravasation of contrast medium from the point of urethral injury. No contrast medium enters the bladder because of complete disruption of the membranous urethra.

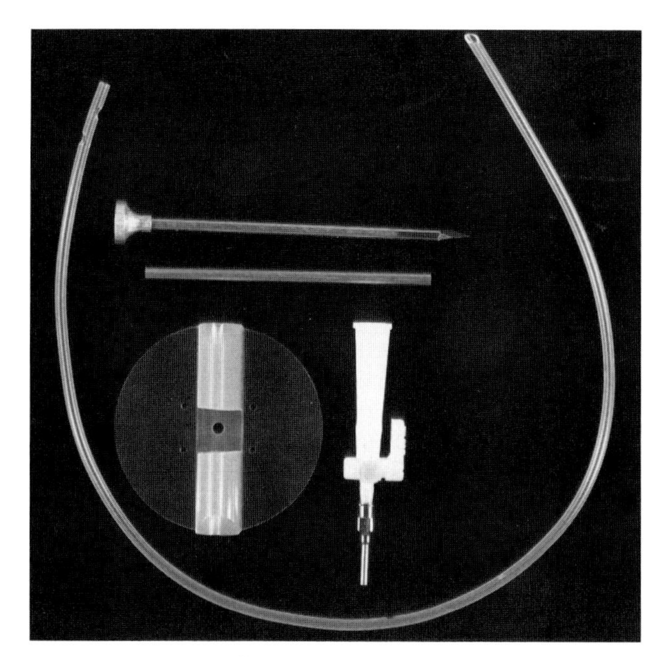

FIGURE 22-7 One type of commercially available trocar for percutaneous placement of a suprapubic tube for cystostomy.

Short lengths should not be used because they may be inadequate to reach the decompressed bladder.

Insertion of the trocar for cystostomy (Figure 22-8) should be in the midline, 2 to 4 cm above the pubic symphysis; the bladder must be fully distended and palpable to ensure that peritoneal contents are pushed cephalad. A probing needle that can be used to inject a local anesthetic should also be used to aspirate urine prior to trocar insertion and thus confirm the location of the bladder.

Insertion of the trocar should be done by those with experience. The inability of the child to cooperate may limit its use. Hazards of bleeding, infection, visceral perforation, and pelvic hematoma are risked by blind insertion, yet in cases of urinary retention due to perineal trauma, urethral stricture, or genital injury, gratifying temporary urinary diversion may be accomplished quickly.

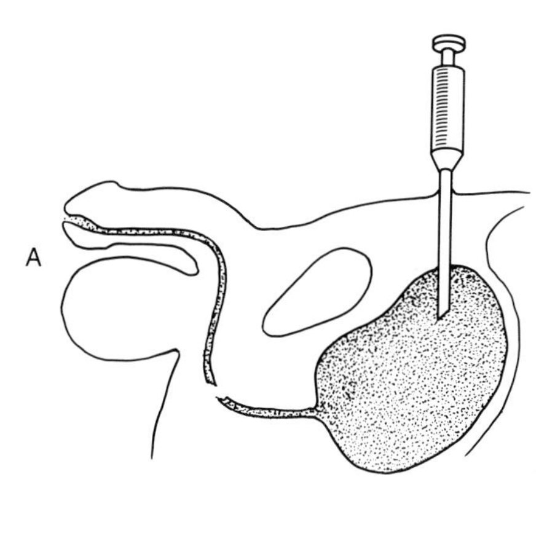

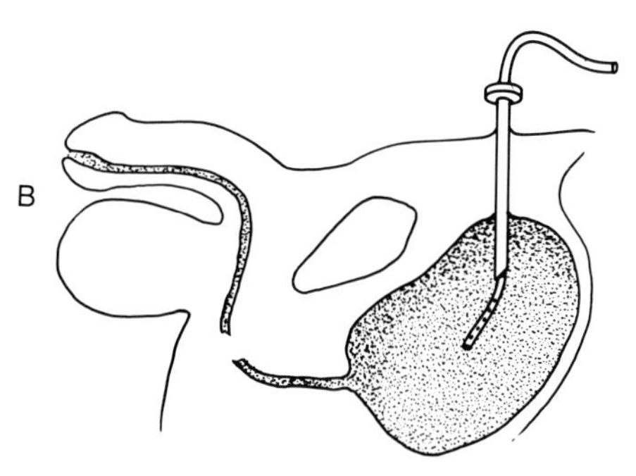

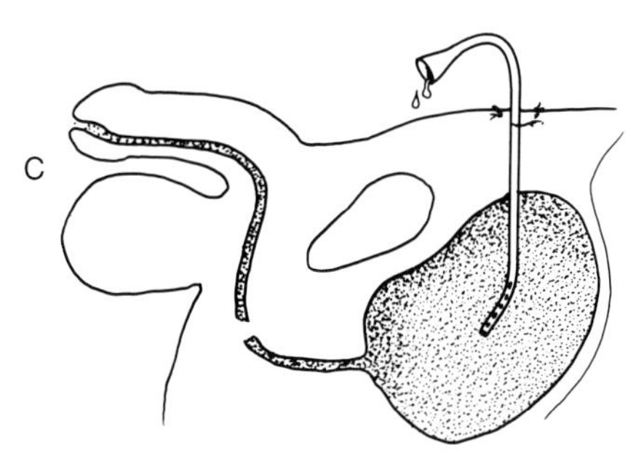

FIGURE 22-8 Placement of a percutaneous suprapubic tube. A, Place the needle in the midline, 2 to 4 cm above the pubis, and confirm the location of the bladder by aspiration. B, Make a 0.5-cm incision in the skin at the site of injection, and insert the trocar with the obturator. C, Remove the trocar sheath, secure the catheter with the face plate, and attach the adapter to a drainage bag.

GENITAL INJURY

The consideration of sexual abuse should not be dismissed during the initial evaluation of the child who has a genital injury. Straddle injuries commonly cause external genital trauma in children, although machinery trauma (wringer injury) and penetrating injuries can occur.

The male genitalia are particularly susceptible to minor injuries such as zipper entrapment and direct trauma from a falling toilet seat (a very common injury). These children usually have mild distal penile swelling and dysuria. If gross hematuria or severe hematoma develops, the patient should be evaluated for urethral trauma. Paraphimosis is a common source of concern in the uncircumcised child. Mothers washing their children, or physicians forcefully retracting the foreskin, may cause it to be trapped proximal to the glans, with resulting severe glanular edema. Generally, gentle and gradual manual compression of the glans decreases edema enough to allow the foreskin to be reduced. If this cannot be easily done, surgical consultation is necessary. Similar tourniquet injuries of the penis may be caused by a hair becoming entrapped, usually at the corona, or by foreign bodies around the penis. Any unexplained distal penile edema should be referred to the urologist immediately, as urethral fistulas or distal penile loss can occur. Similar injuries can damage the clitoris. Testicular trauma is rare, but penetrating scrotal injury or severe crush injury with hematoscrotum may require surgical exploration.

Female perineal trauma, usually associated with straddle injury, may cause vulvar or periurethral ecchymosis, and urinary retention may result. Penetrating vaginal injury has been known to cause peritoneal perforation with little evidence of external injury.

CONCLUSION

Trauma to the GU system is a frequent occurrence in the pediatric age group. Any child who has blunt abdominal trauma or who has sustained forceable blows to the flank or the thoracoabdominal area should be suspected of having sustained significant GU injury until proven otherwise. A high index of suspicion, careful observation, and appropriate radiologic evaluation are essential to successful identification, treatment, and triage of this problem.

References

1. Morse TS: Renal injuries. *Pediatr Clin North Am* 1975;22:379.
2. Malek RS: Genitourinary trauma, in Kelalis PP, King LR (eds): *Clinical Pediatric Urology*. Philadelphia, WB Saunders Co, 1976.
3. Mertz JHO, Wishard WM Jr, Nourse MH, et al: Injury of the kidney in children. *JAMA* 1963;183:730.
4. Cass AS: Renal trauma in the multiple injured patient. *J Urol* 1975;114:495.
5. Javadapour N, Guinan P, Bush IM: Renal trauma in children. *Surg Gynecol Obstet* 1973:136:237.
6. Sargent JC, Marquardt CR: Renal injuries. *J Urol* 1950;63.
7. Thompson IM, LaTourette H, Montie JE, et al: Results of non-operative management of blunt renal trauma. *J Urol* 1977;118:522.
8. Clark DE, Georgitis JW, Ray FS: Renal arterial injuries caused by blunt trauma. *Surgery* 1981;90:87.
9. Beckley DE, Waters EA: Avulsion of the pelvi-ureteric junction: A rare consequence of non-penetrating trauma. *Br J Radiol* 1972;45:423.
10. Brereton RJ, Philip N, Buyukpamukcu: Rupture of the urinary bladder in children. *Br J Urol* 1980;52:15.
11. Mitchell JP: Injuries to the urethra. *Br J Urol* 1968; 40:649.

Dennis L. Hoover
Mark F. Bellinger

23 Nontraumatic Genitourinary Emergencies

Symptoms referable to the genital and urinary systems not infrequently bring children to the care of the emergency physician. Although many of these symptoms reflect problems of an urgent rather than emergent nature, many signify the presence of anatomic abnormalities that will require urologic evaluation. Such symptoms are painless hematuria, incontinence, and urinary infection. True emergency situations may be associated with genital or urinary trauma (frequently associated with multiple trauma), acute scrotal pain, urinary sepsis, or urinary retention. Unrecognized or untreated genitourinary problems can result in deterioration of renal function, infertility, or even death. Consequently, the postemergent evaluation and care of these patients is often as important as the immediate treatment. It is also understandable that parental and (depending on the age of the child) patient concern over genital problems may be inflated out of proportion to the degree of injury.

The history and physical examination of the patient with urologic symptoms should remain the keystone of differential diagnosis (Figure 23-1). Pertinent questioning concerning a past history of hematuria, urinary infection and urologic investigations or surgery; a family history of urogenital disorders, voiding difficulties, or incontinence; and any information about neurologic or perinatal problems should be used to focus on potential areas of concern. The history and physical findings should be augmented by laboratory data and appropriate radiologic investigation. Radiologic studies frequently are pivotal steps in urologic diagnosis and must be logically directed on the basis of history and physical findings.

RENAL PAIN

Pain is a common indication of genitourinary pathology. Historical data concerning the onset, duration, nature, and distribution of the pain are important in formulating a differential diagnosis and deciding whether prompt radiologic and urologic evaluation is essential. Pain originates in the urinary tract primarily because of distension. Gradually progressive or chronic distension caused by low-grade obstruction may result in dull aching but very commonly is completely painless. This is not infrequently seen in children with massive hydronephrosis of a congenital nature. Acute distension of the urinary tract, however, causes severe paroxysmal pain. This colic is known to be one of the most severe pains experienced by man.

Renal pain is secondary to capsular distension. This, in turn, may be the result of ureteral or renal pelvic obstruction or of acute parenchymal distension from pyelonephritis. The latter is associated with fever. Because of the embryologic development of the kidney and its innervation, renal pain

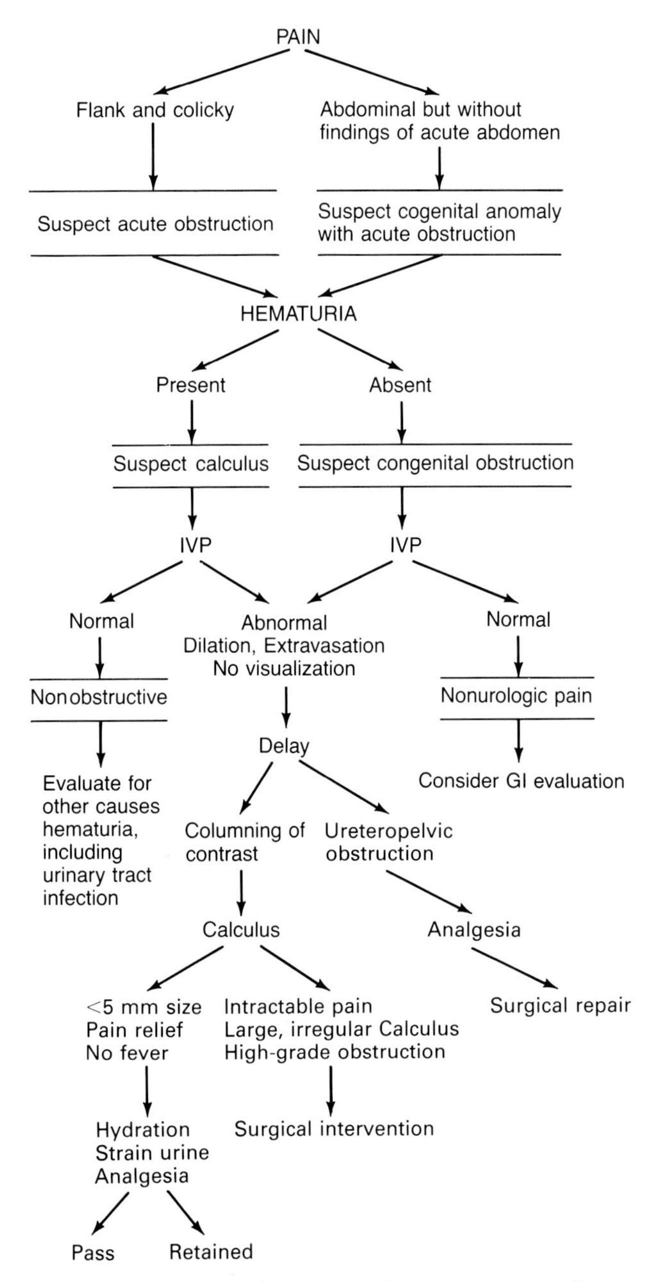

FIGURE 23-1 Evaluation and management of pain caused by obstruction. GI, Gastrointestinal.

may radiate to the ipsilateral gonad, scrotum, or labia. Renal inflammation, in addition to causing localized flank or upper quadrant tenderness, can cause irritation of the overlying posterior peritoneum, resulting in an "acute abdomen" or ileus. Thus, the urine sediment should be examined in all children with acute abdominal pain.

Clinical Features

Acute ureteral colic results from obstruction and distension that causes intense, paroxysmal ureteral spasm. This pain, most commonly precipitated by passage of calculi or a blood clot, is severe, and the intensity of the colic may have no relation to the size of calculus being passed. The child with ureteral colic classically is severely agitated, writhing about in a futile effort to find a comfortable position. The intensity of pain or ileus associated with peritoneal irritation may result in nausea and vomiting. The location of pain associated with ureteral colic is usually segmental, with upper ureteral pain in the upper abdomen and lower ureteral pain in the lower quadrants. Right lower ureteral stones not uncommonly are mistaken for appendicitis, and again x-ray examination and urinalysis are very important here. Stones or a clot passing through the bladder wall are also irritating, usually initiating urinary frequency and dysuria. Thus history alone may allow localization of the point of obstruction.

Although renal colic is usually associated with obstructing calculi, it may also be caused by obstruction of the ureteropelvic junction as a result of congenital abnormality. Sudden diuresis after large fluid intake may trigger acute renal pelvic distension, which subsides slowly as the pelvis drains. The older child may give a history of hydration-induced colic, whereas such a pain history is rare in the young child, whose ureteropelvic junction obstruction is more commonly diagnosed upon evaluation of a urinary-tract infection.

Once obstructive uropathy is suspected, urinalysis should be performed and intravenous urography should be undertaken to determine the degree and level of obstruction. Delayed films are extremely important in these situations because the functioning, obstructed renal unit excretes contrast material that eventually (perhaps as long as 24 hours later) reaches the site of obstruction.

As noted, urinary calculi are capable of causing severe ureteral colic, which may be associated with gross hematuria, microscopic hematuria, or normal urinalysis findings. Stones may be formed secondary to infection, metabolic disorders, or for unknown reasons (idiopathic). The relative frequency is variously reported and depends a great deal on the geographic distribution. Metabolic stones are more common in children of less industrialized countries and more frequently arise in the bladder. In the United States calcium oxalate renal calculi are more common at all ages, particularly along the Atlantic coast. Reports indicate that children nationwide most frequently form stones as the result of infection or obstruction.[1] Such calculi are composed of magnesium ammonium phosphate (struvite). Metabolic calculi that form as the result of an inborn error of metabolism are also seen in children. Cystine calculi and nephrocalcinosis secondary to renal tubular acidosis are examples. Immobilization elevates urinary calcium excretion significantly, so children immobilized by hospitalization, particularly by orthopedic surgery with application of traction or casts, may be prone to develop calculi. Many theories of stone formation have been advanced. Suffice it to say that calculus formation depends on a number of factors, including concentration of solute in the urine, inhibitory factors such as citrate and pyrophosphates, urine pH, and urinary stasis. The incidence reported is variable but ranges from one case per year to one case per 60 new pediatric urologic patients.[1,2]

In evaluation of the patient with renal colic, the history is particularly important because calculi tend to recur and there may be a history of prior episodes. Since some disorders causing renal calculi are inherited, a family history should be obtained.

Ureteral colic is a common manifestation for the child with upper tract calculi. Again, the pain pattern may suggest the level of obstruction. Calcium-containing, struvite, and, to a lesser degree, cystine calculi are radiopaque and can be visualized on a plain film of the abdomen. A word of caution, however: even densely calcified calculi can be missed on a plain film because of bony structures, overlying stool, or bowel gas. Furthermore, many densities within the gut lumen or mesentery of the bowel can appear very similar to a ureteral or renal calculus. Confirmation of the presence of a calculus and delineation of the level and degree of obstruction hinge on the intravenous urogram. In the presence of obstruction, delayed films are usually required (Figure 23-2) to localize the point of obstruction. Dilatation may be minimal after acute obstruction, and there may be extravasation of contrast medium outside the collecting system because of sudden increased pressure and the resultant tear of a calyceal fornix. The duration of delay in "columnating" of contrast material to the site of obstruction is a more accurate indication of the degree of obstruction than the amount of dilatation seen. In the presence of a marked or high-grade obstruction, the collecting system may not be visualized until the 12- or 24-hour delayed film. It is thus imperative for the physician to look at each film and determine whether further follow-up films are necessary. Failure to do so may result in a nondiagnostic intravenous pyelogram.

Management

Relief of the pain requires narcotic analgesia, and usually morphine is more effective than meperidine. Ample oral fluids must be encouraged to maintain good hydration. Activity should not be limited. The urine must be strained with each voiding to recover the calculus when passed. Hospitalization in the older age group is required when (1) nausea and vomiting preclude adequate oral hydration, (2) parenteral analgesics are required for adequate pain relief, (3) significant obstruction is noted

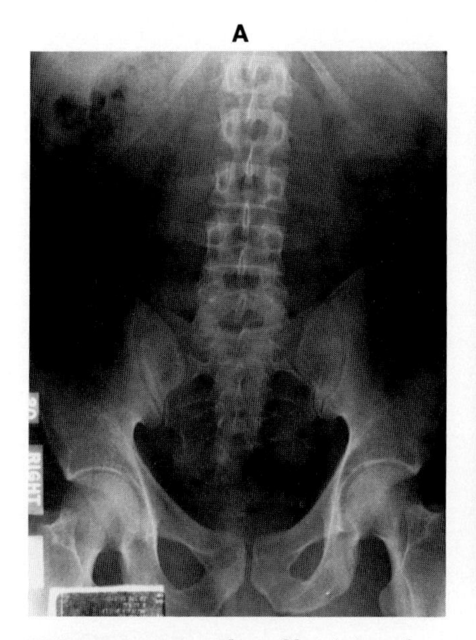

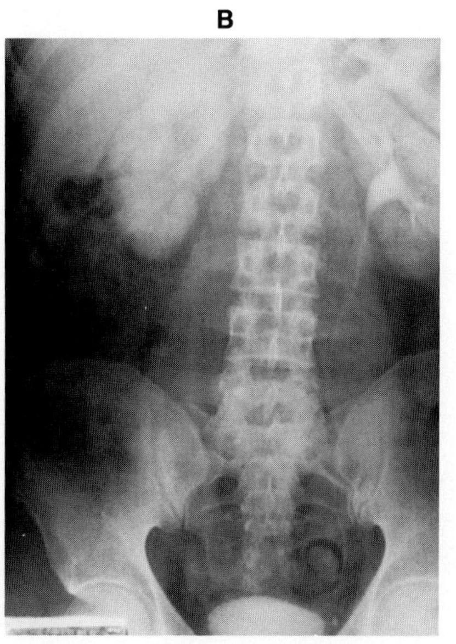

FIGURE 23-2 Plain film (A) and x-ray film taken 10 minutes after intravenous contrast (B). Note columning of contrast medium in the ureter to the point of obstruction.

on intravenous pyelogram, or (4) infected urine behind a calculus results in fever or sepsis. In young children hospitalization is more likely to be necessary to ensure pain relief and proper hydration.

A small calculus may pass if the patient follows the conservative management outlined. Calculi that do not pass or are associated with sepsis may require emergency surgical intervention, and patient disposition appropriate to that possibility must be initiated.

URINARY RETENTION

Urinary retention is uncommon in children. It may occur as the result of a neurologic disorder, neoplasm, calculus, infection, acute pelvic or perineal trauma, or gynecologic lesion. The abdominal location of the child's bladder may even cause such distension to be misinterpreted as an abdominal mass. Except in the case of pelvic fracture with urethral disruption or pelvic mass involving the urethra or severe perineal trauma, insertion of a urethral catheter temporarily relieves the problem. The volume of urine drained must be recorded and would be expected to exceed normal capacity if the diagnosis of true retention is to be confirmed.

Urinary retention can be secondary to congenital anomalies. These chronic conditions may result in urinary infection and an overdistended lower urinary tract but do not usually cause the signs and symptoms associated with sudden acute obstruction. Imperforate hymen with marked hydrocolpos is a possible cause of obstruction in the female infant. The male infant may have obstruction caused by posterior urethral valves (Figure 23-3). These are abnormal leaflets of tissue in the proximal portion of the urethra. Valves are embryologic abnormalities, although the exact cause is debated. The key feature is that they cause occlusion of the urethra with voiding. Despite antegrade obstruction, a catheter generally passes easily. The diagnosis must be made by a voiding cystourethrogram. Drainage by means of an indwelling catheter is adequate interim therapy while awaiting surgical ablation of the valves.

A common cause of urinary retention in the child who is toilet trained is urinary infection. Dysuria resulting from cystitis (or urethritis in the male) may cause a child to retain urine on a voluntary basis. A child who experiences dysuria may very effectively disallow micturition by voluntarily contracting the external urinary sphincter. Treatment of the infection may not resolve the irritative symptoms for a day or more. Phenazopyridine (Pyridium) is cleared into the bladder urine within hours and acts as a topical mucosal anesthetic to reduce dysuria. This can be helpful for the child who is able to swallow a small tablet. Relief of discomfort frequently can be obtained by placing the child in a warm bath and allowing the child to urinate in the warm water. If efforts at local relief fail, a pediatric enema may force the child to relax the perineal musculature and urogenital diaphragm enough to allow micturition.

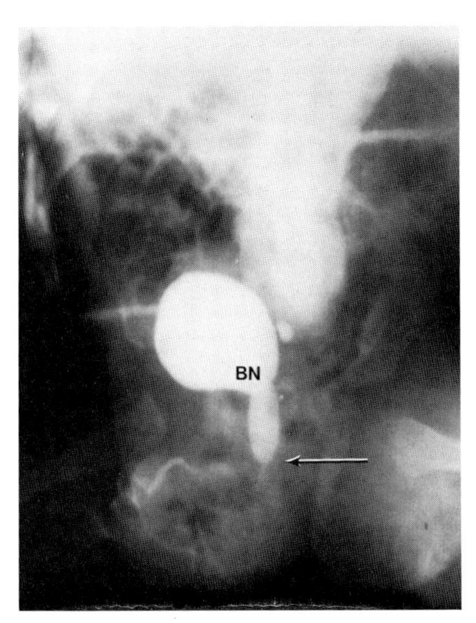

FIGURE 23-3 Voiding urethrogram demonstrates the abnormally dilated posterior urethra above the obstructing posterior urethral valve (*arrow*). The bladder neck (BN) is normal.

ACUTE SCROTAL PAIN AND SWELLING

Acute scrotal pain and swelling ("acute scrotum") is probably the most widely recognized pediatric urologic emergency. It is also one of the most challenging areas of differential diagnosis (Table 23-1). The child who has acute scrotal pain, enlargement, and erythema raises a diagnostic question that sometimes can be resolved only by surgical exploration. Torsion of the spermatic cord eliminates all blood flow to the testis. Irreversible damage occurs in a matter of hours. The expediency with which such a problem is recognized and managed in the emergency department may well make the difference between salvage or irreplaceable loss of the testicle. On the other hand, a nontender mass in the scrotum may (albeit rarely) represent a testicular tumor.

TABLE 23-1 Differential Diagnosis of the Acute Scrotum*

	Age	Pain	Other Symptoms	Swelling	Vascular Flow	Anatomy
Painful Swelling						
Torsion of spermatic cord	Prepubertal	Acute; vague distribution	Nausea and vomiting	Diffuse	None by Doppler scan	Poorly defined
Torsion of testicular appendage	Prepubertal	Acute; well localized	Nausea possible	Localized if early	Intact by Doppler scan	Discrete if early; blue dot
Epididymitis	Postpubertal	Usually gradual; vague distribution	Fever possible	Diffuse	Intact by Doppler scan	Discrete if early; poorly defined later. Suspect urologic anomaly
Incarcerated hernia	Any	Pain and course variable	Fever likely	Extends into groin	Intact	
Painless swelling						
Hydrocele	Infant and prepubertal	None	None	Waxes and wanes		Cystic; transilluminates
Tumor	Infant and postpubertal	Minimal	Unlikely	Persistent		Hard mass; does not transilluminate

* Testicular torsion and neoplasm enter into the differential diagnosis of any scrotal swelling. If both cannot be eliminated as possible diagnoses, surgical scrotal exploration is indicated.

Avoiding delay in diagnosis and referral will no doubt make a difference in long-term survival. A scrotal examination performed with knowledge of testicular anatomy, congenital anomalies that predispose to intrascrotal pathology, and signs and symptoms, helps to differentiate the emergent from the less urgent scrotal malady.

Anatomy

The testicle develops from gonadal tissue in the midsection of the developing embryo near the internal inguinal ring. Late in development the testicle descends into the scrotum, accompanied by an evagination of peritoneum (processus vaginalis). Testicular vessels originate at the aorta, vena cava, and left renal vein and follow the course of the testicle into the scrotum. In a sense the testicle hangs on this vascular pedicle (Figure 23-4). The consequence is that injury or constriction of the pedicle can result in complete loss of blood supply to the testicle. Twisting of the spermatic cord, similar to twisting the neck of a plastic bag, would interrupt the entire blood supply to the gonad. Fortunately, the normal testicle is not at risk for such an event because of attachments of the testicle to the scrotal wall. The congenital anomaly that results in extension of the processus vaginalis (called the tunica vaginalis in the scrotum) around the entire testicle prohibits these normal attachments (Figure 23-5). The result is a testicle that hangs freely on the vascular pedicle, much like a ball on a chain that can be

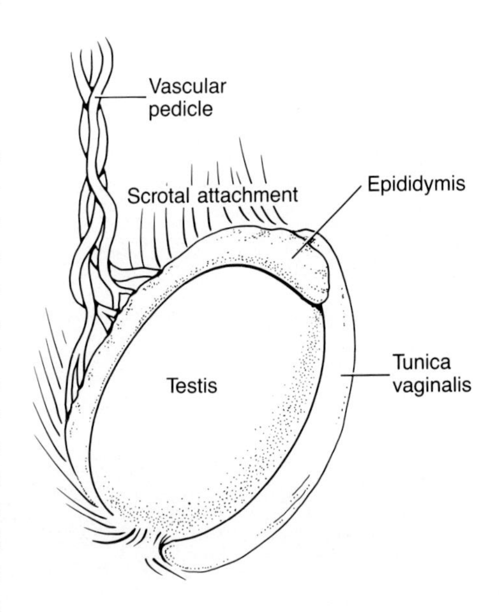

FIGURE 23-4 Anatomy of the normal testicle.

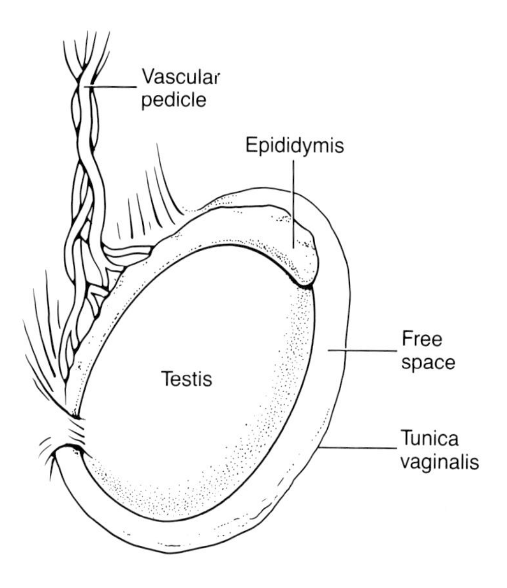

FIGURE 23-5 Bell-and-clapper deformity.

freely rotated. This "bell-and-clapper" configuration occurs as a bilateral phenomenon and predisposes the child to torsion of either or both testicles.

Vestiges of fetal wolffian and müllerian ducts persist in association with the testicle. These remnants of incompletely regressed fetal structures persist as appendages of the testis or epididymis (Figure 23-6) in 90% of males.[3] They have a discrete vascular supply traversing the tiny pedunculated structures. These appendages are freely mobile and

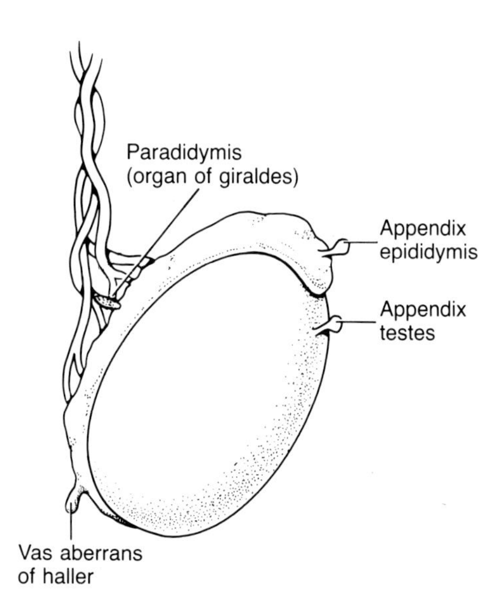

FIGURE 23-6 Testicular appendages.

may rotate, compromising vascularity and resulting in very impressive pain and scrotal swelling. Findings may be so severe as to closely mimic torsion of the entire spermatic cord.

The epididymis is a broad, cordlike structure that represents the proximal end of the male genital duct system. It communicates with the testicle via tiny ductules. Its formation from the wolffian duct, which also gives rise to the ureteral buds, can result in bizarre patterns of abnormal ureteral insertion (ectopic ureters). Although this is a rare phenomenon, epididymal infection or swelling in the prepubertal boy is so uncommon that such an anomaly must be suspected. More frequently, although also uncommon in young boys, inflammation of the epididymis occurs as a result of reflux of infected or sterile urine into the distal ends of the ductal structures (ejaculatory ducts). Therefore, epididymitis in the very young boy suggests predisposing structural anomalies, urinary infection, or a degree of outlet obstruction. Urologic evaluation is indicated.

The patency of the projection of peritoneum that accompanies the testicle in its descent, the processus vaginalis, is obliterated at about the time of birth in full-term pregnancies. Eighty to ninety percent of premature infants are born with a patent processus that closes spontaneously in the subsequent weeks. When patent, this structure allows peritoneal fluid to enter the scrotum on an intermittent basis. This scrotal swelling, which represents a communicating hydrocele, is more marked when the child is active or crying and decreases when the child is resting. If the opening is large enough, omentum or bowel may enter the scrotum, resulting in a true hernia.

Clinical Features

The acute scrotum implies sudden, painful swelling. The differential diagnosis includes torsion of the spermatic cord, torsion of a testicular appendage, trauma, and epididymitis (Table 23-1). Trauma is evident from the history as an insult significant enough to cause noticeable scrotal swelling and pain, whether from testicular fracture and bleeding or from reactive swelling (hydrocele). The history may not be so helpful in the case of epididymitis except that the incidence is greater in adolescence. If associated with urinary infection, there may be preceding irritative symptoms of dysuria, urinary frequency, or incontinence. The pain pattern is extremely variable but often more gradual in onset than that associated with a scrotal vascular accident. Pain is usually quite severe and may radiate to the groin or be associated with nausea and vomiting.

Fever is occasionally present. The involved hemiscrotum is swollen, erythematous, and extremely tender to touch, which makes differentiation of intrascrotal structures difficult. If the child is examined within the first few hours of onset, it may be possible to distinguish a normal testis from a very tender, swollen epididymis on the posterior aspect of the testicle. The spermatic cord may be tender but not enlarged. The testicle typically is in a low, normal scrotal position. Because the pain is, in part, secondary to the weight of the testicle pulling on tender cord structures, gentle elevation of the testicle sometimes relieves the pain (Prehn's sign). Generally, the patient seeks help only after several hours or days of gradually increasing pain. Examination then may only reveal a diffusely swollen, painful testicle with reactive edema and hydrocele, making differentiation of intrascrotal structures impossible. Cord structures also may be quite swollen. At this point pyuria on microscopic urinalysis may be the most helpful finding.

Although epididymitis is invariably included in the differential diagnosis of the acute scrotum in the prepubertal boy, emphasis must be placed on the more likely torsion of an intrascrotal appendage or torsion of the spermatic cord. Pain resulting from intrascrotal torsion is fairly sudden in onset and unrelenting in severity. It is often stated that torsion is associated with activity or mild trauma, but in actual practice there is just as frequently no history of increased activity, and the child may awaken with pain.[4] Initially, the pain is commonly in the inguinal region and may be associated with nausea and vomiting. Interestingly, torsion of an appendiceal structure can result in as much pain, but it is initially localized to the infarcted structure[5] so that, if old enough to cooperate, the child can localize the pain with an index finger. Soon after torsion, intrascrotal structures are definable if only an appendage is involved. The testis is normal, although perhaps with referred tenderness. The epididymis may be somewhat edematous in reaction to the closely associated ischemic process. The twisted appendix testis or appendix epididymis is often palpable as a hard "knot" at the upper pole of the testicle and coincides with the "index finger" localization of pain. At this same point the infarcted appendage may be evident as a black or blue dot visible through the scrotal skin stretched taut over the testicle. If the patient with an appendiceal torsion is seen later in the course, marked reaction and hydrocele accumulation may make differentiation of intrascrotal anatomy impossible. Thus it is indistinguishable on physical examination from the more serious torsion of the spermatic cord. A testicle that is riding high in the scrotum (because of twisting and thus shortening of the spermatic cord) suggests testicular torsion. The cord structures may even be palpably thickened and "knotted." Because of the severe pain in the involved hemiscrotum, examination of the contralateral testicle may provide better clues. Since the bell-and-clapper deformity is a bilateral anomaly, the uninvolved testicle typically has a transverse position in the scrotum and may be more mobile than normal. The epididymis may actually lie anteriorly during examination. A small contralateral testicle would suggest a previous infarction.

Studies

Abnormal findings on urinalysis make epididymitis suspect, but no possibility can be eliminated on the basis of urinalysis alone. The physical examination becomes the most important and expedient means of making the diagnosis. Other studies, which can be helpful if readily available, may better determine the vascular status of the testicle. The Doppler monitoring has been useful in assessing arterial flow to the acutely involved testis.[6] Flow in the testicular artery can be heard by placing the Doppler transmitter directly over the hilus of the testicle on the posterior aspect. If the flow is of similar magnitude to that detected in the uninvolved organ, torsion is less likely. The reliability of Doppler examination has been documented in clinical series. However, caution must be exercised since false-positive results have been obtained in cases of partial torsion and late in the event when inflammation has resulted in increased vascular flow to skin and subcutaneous scrotal tissues.[7] Imaging of the testicle with radionuclide scanning techniques and B-mode ultrasonography has been helpful in differential diagnosis.[8] Testicular scanning is most reliable in establishing the presence of arterial flow to the testicle.[9] Unfortunately, technical problems resulting from the child's inability to cooperate because of severe pain or young age often make this study impractical, even if the facilities are available on an emergency basis.

Management

Time is of the essence whenever testicular torsion is suspected. Although experimental evidence has established that as little as 4 hours of complete arterial occlusion results in total infarction, a history of pain that extends beyond 4 hours does not portend a hopeless situation. Torsion can occur intermittently or may be partial rather than complete. If either is the case, salvage may be possible, even after several hours.[10] Diagnosis and management must be pursued as if there is not a moment to spare. As soon as the diagnosis is suspected, the child is restricted to nothing by mouth. While awaiting evaluation by the urologist or surgeon, the emergency physician can attempt manual detorsion of the testicle. As a general principle, a gonad tends to twist inward. This may be related to orientation of the cremasteric muscle fibers. Detorsion is first attempted by rotating the testicle outward, as if opening the pages of a book. As the examiner faces the child, the child's left testicle is turned clockwise and the right, counterclockwise. If this is unsuccessful, detorsion in the opposite direction should be attempted. Successful detorsion is characterized by a sudden and dramatic relief of pain; when it is unsuccessful, surgical exploration and detorsion must be performed. At that time each testicle is fixed in place with sutures into the tissues of the scrotum to prevent a recurrence. Even when manual detorsion is successful, surgical exploration and suture fixation is necessary but less urgent.

If an unequivocal diagnosis of appendix torsion can be made by the urologist, the testis itself having been palpably identified as normal, the child may be managed without surgical intervention. The appendage eventually completely infarcts and thromboses with no further implications or threat to health or fertility. The usual course is of pain that peaks at 24 to 48 hours and gradually resolves over the ensuing 5 to 7 days.[5] Surgical intervention is used if the diagnosis is in doubt or if pain is severe. In this case the minor procedure of excising the appendage significantly decreases the duration of discomfort and can even be performed under local anesthesia in the older child.

Painless Scrotal Mass

Not infrequently a child with a painless scrotal swelling is brought to the emergency department for evaluation. The most common cause of painless scrotal swelling in a child is the hydrocele. Although the communication allowing for the intermittent hydrocele is present from birth, the swelling may only suddenly be recognized after an episode of crying or activity. The scrotal skin is nonerythematous, although taut skin over a large hydrocele may take on a pinkish hue. If the hydrocele is tense, the testicle may not be palpable, but transillumination demonstrates that the major portion of the scrotal mass is fluid filled. If the hydrocele is large or waxes and wanes, elective surgical repair is warranted.

Although idiopathic scrotal edema is not totally painless, usually a child with this condition is brought to the emergency department for evaluation of the scrotal enlargement. Edema often involves the entire scrotum, but it is localized in the scrotal wall and therefore does not involve the testicle itself; the testicle may not be palpable, depending on the amount of edema. A Doppler flow test or radionuclide scan can confirm that the blood supply of the testicles is intact. If the swelling is clearly demonstrated to be in the scrotal wall, no further diagnostic studies are necessary, but if the testicle cannot be palpated through a markedly swollen hemiscrotum, torsion cannot be ruled out. Some of these children undergo scrotal exploration before the diagnosis is made. The cause of this problem is not clear, but some feel it is an allergic phenomenon. Treatment with diphenhydramine may shorten the clinical course and seems to make the child more comfortable. If no treatment is instituted, the edema resolves in a matter of days.[11]

Finally, a painless swelling in the scrotum may indicate a testicular tumor. Although not a true emergency, the expediency with which such a finding is diagnosed and treated carries obvious significance. A painless testicular mass is often first noticed while the child is being bathed or upon inspection of the genitalia following trauma to the perineum. Testicular tumors represent only about 1% of all childhood cancers. Most appear in boys past the age of 15 years, but there is a prepubertal peak incidence at 1 to 2 years.[12] Physical examination confirms that the scrotal mass is firm, nontender, smooth or irregular, and inseparable from the testicle. Paratesticular tumors arise from the cord structures and are also firm, solid masses. Any mass in the scrotum that is inseparable from the cord structures or testicle and does not transilluminate must be considered a testicular or paratesticular tumor until proven otherwise. Scrotal scan or B-mode ultrasonography may be helpful in demonstrating a nonfunctioning solid mass, but the answer ultimately is obtained at exploration of the scrotal contents performed via an inguinal incision.

FEMALE PERINEAL MASSES

Just as the sudden finding of a painless intrascrotal mass often precipitates a visit to the emergency department, so does the previously unnoticed bulge on the female perineum. The proximity of the vagina and urethra in the pediatric patient often makes evaluation of a sizable perineal mass somewhat challenging. Mucosa protruding from the ure-

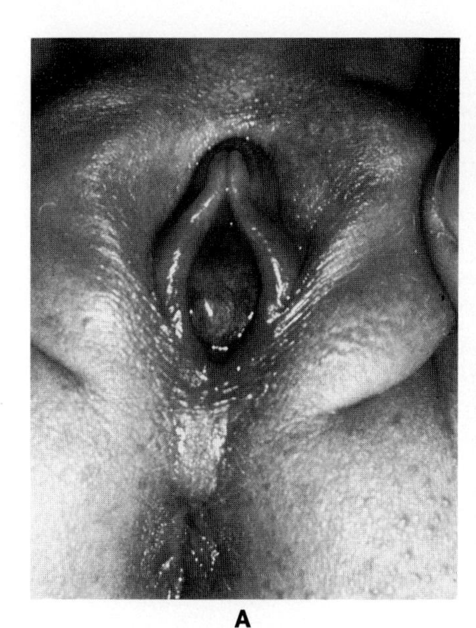

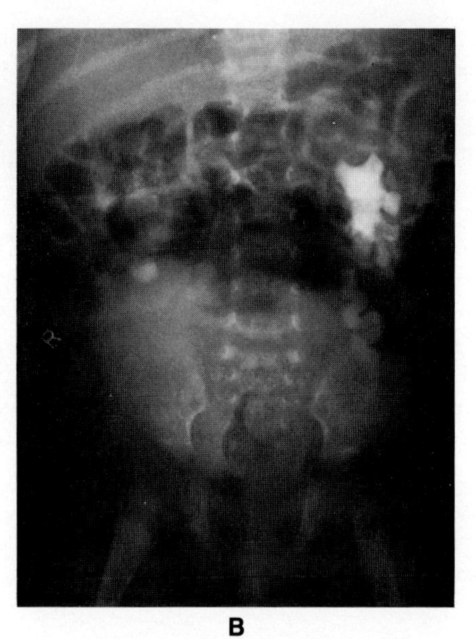

FIGURE 23-7 Imperforate hymen (A) bulging from the perineum. The intravenous urogram (B) shows bilateral hydroureteronephrosis attributable to obstruction of the outlet. The contrast medium is diluted in an overdistended bladder.

thra may be a prolapsing ureterocele (dilated distal portion of an abnormally developed ureter) or a prolapse of the urethra. The former is more likely to occur in infants whereas the latter is more common in the prepubertal girl.[13] Either may become apparent when blood spotting is noticed on diapers or underclothing as a result of excoriation of the involved mucous membranes. The ectopic ureterocele is best diagnosed by renal ultrasound or intravenous urography since it is associated with a duplication of the collecting system and hydroureteronephrosis. The prolapsed urethra is not associated with any other anomaly. The prolapsed mucosa emanates from the urethra circumferentially, and a urethral catheter easily passes through the protruding tissue. Treatment consists of simple excision of the prolapsed mucosa and placement of hemostatic sutures. This requires general anesthesia in most children. Estrogen cream and catheter placement have also resulted in successful resolution in some patients.

Masses protruding from the vagina may be large enough to make determination of the source difficult. A catheter passed via the urethra may help to clarify the anatomy. An infant or newborn who has a lower abdominal mass and a midline bluish bulge on the perineum probably has a hydrocolpos. The abdominal mass is the vagina, dilated with secretions under the influence of maternal estrogens and trapped by an imperforate hymen. The vagina may be so distended as to cause obstruction of the urinary tract (Figure 23-7). Treatment may simply involve excision of the membrane.

Dilated Skene's glands or Gartner's duct cysts may also occur in the infant as the result of maternal estrogen influence. They appear as discrete masses on the perineum very near the vaginal introitus. They are not midline but, if large, can be easily confused with an ectopic ureterocele or imperforate hymen. They resolve spontaneously, although drainage or excision may be appropriate to shorten the clinical course. Cysts or abscesses of Bartholin's gland may enlarge the labia in older children, and the possibility of inguinal hernia should not be discounted in girls who have labial swelling.

OTHER UROLOGIC EMERGENCIES

Both urinary tract infection and abdominal masses are common in children with urologic disorders, and either may prompt a visit to the emergency department. All children with an abdominal mass or documented infection require radiologic evaluation of the urinary tract. Evaluation and treatment of these children is discussed in Chapter 21.

Hematuria not infrequently brings children to the emergency department and should always be considered important. Both gross and microscopic hematuria require radiologic and urologic or nephrologic evaluation (see Chapter 21).

References

1. Walther PC, Lamm D, Kaplan GW: Pediatric urolithiasis: A ten year review. *Pediatrics* 1980;65:1068.
2. Bass HN, Emmanuel B: Nephrolithiasis in childhood. *Clin Pediatr* 1966;5:79.

3. Rolnick D, Kawanoue S, Szanto P, et al: Anatomic incidence of testicular appendages. *J Urol* 1968; 100:755.
4. Allen TD: Disorders of the male genitalia, in Kelalis PP, King LR (eds): *Clinical Pediatric Urology*. Philadelphia, WB Saunders Co, 1976.
5. Skoglund RW, McRoberts JW, Ragde H: Torsion of testicular appendages: Presentation of 43 new cases and a collective review. *J Urol* 1970;104:598.
6. Levy BJ: The diagnosis of torsion of the testicle using Doppler ultrasonic stethoscope. *J Urol* 1975;113:63.
7. Nasrallah PF, Manzone D, King LR: Falsely negative Doppler examinations in testicular torsion. *J Urol* 1977;118:194.
8. Leopold GR, Woo VL, Scheible FW, et al: High resolution ultrasound of scrotal pathology. *Radiology* 1979;131:719.
9. Falkowski WS, Firlit CF: Testicular torsion: The role of radioisotope scanning. *J Urol* 1980;124: 886.
10. Kaplan GW, King LR: Acute scrotal swelling in children. *J Urol* 1970;104:219.
11. Kaplan GW: Acute idiopathic scrotal edema. *J Pediatr Surg* 1977;12:647.
12. The management of testicular tumors in children. *J Urol* 1978;120:96.
13. Klaus H, Stein RT: Urethral prolapse in young girls. *Pediatrics* 1973;52:645.

Catherine DeAngelis

24 Gynecologic Disorders and Sexually Transmitted Diseases

Emergency physicians are occasionally confronted with pediatric gynecologic problems. To discuss in detail the entire realm of these problems is quite beyond the scope of this chapter. For example, dysfunctional bleeding and ovarian cysts and tumors have been omitted. The focus is centered instead on the more common gynecologic problems that can be managed relatively easily.

PHYSICAL EXAMINATION

The basic gynecologic physical evaluation of a child or teenager consists of breast, abdominal, and pelvic-rectal examinations.[1] Since these examinations may provoke anxiety, time should be spent preparing the adolescent or child first.

Breast Examination

Breasts should be examined for stage of development, presence of masses, and discharges.[2] In older girls and adolescents, they should be observed for abnormalities while the girl is sitting with her arms relaxed at the side, with her hands on her hips, and with her hands pressed together over her head. Exhibit 24-1 gives a list of items to check.

Pelvic Examination

It is frequently necessary to perform a pelvic examination when problems such as vaginal discharge or acute abdominal pain are the chief complaint.[3] Every physician who cares for adolescents should be proficient in performing pelvic examinations.

Since this examination may provoke anxiety, time should be spent preparing the young woman or child for it. Also, the gynecologic examination of a youngster involves the parents and their attitudes about this procedure. It is important to remember that there are many taboos concerning the genitalia, especially those of a young child. In most instances discussing the purposes of the various procedures suffices to relieve anxiety. We have found it helpful to assist the teenager in watching the procedure with a mirror and to explain each step of the examination to her. This also provides an excellent opportunity for health education.

COMMON GYNECOLOGIC PROBLEMS

Breast Lesions

Transient breast enlargement is found in most infants of both sexes born after 32 weeks of gestation.[4] By the second week of life, gentle palpation of the breast nodules can result in release of milk similar to the first milk secreted by mothers. This enlargement and milk production is probably a physiologic response to passive hormone stimulation from the mother. Its absence in premature infants may reflect imperfect formation of the breast bud or some other

Exhibit 24-1 Breast Examination

Symmetry: The breasts should look the same except that one may be slightly larger than the other.

Color: Redness, especially with warmth and tenderness, may indicate infection.

Dimpling: An indentation in any part of the breast should be considered serious, as it may indicate fat necrosis from trauma, infection, or cancer.

"Orange peel": The orange peel appearance of the breast may be an indication of cancer and should be further evaluated by a specialist.

Nipples: The nipples should be observed for discharge. Darkening of the nipples and areola occurs during pregnancy and may remain afterward. Inverted nipples are usually normal, especially if they have been inverted since birth. Supernumerary nipples are a normal variant and occur in 1% to 2% of healthy patients. Extra nipples, which may appear like warts or moles, may be found along the nipple line or in the axillary region.

important factor of the intrauterine environment. Milk production has been shown to continue as long as 8 weeks, and the nodules persist into the second half of the first year.

Premature thelarche, a relatively common finding, occurs in girls usually between 1 and 3 years of age. Precocious breast development by itself can occur at any time prior to puberty. One or both breasts may be involved. The hypertrophy may disappear or regress spontaneously, but it may remain even until the normal onset of puberty. There is no history of accelerated growth, no cornification of the vaginal epithelium, and bone age is normal. Urinary excretion of gonadotropins and 17-ketosteroids is normal or only minimally increased for age. Continued observation is all that is necessary in this condition.

Breast Masses

Most breast masses in adolescents are probably the result of fibrocystic disease.[5] Typically, these cordlike nodules are diffuse and thick, and they become larger and tender just prior to the onset of each menses. These masses usually change from month to month.

A fibroadenoma, on the other hand, is rubbery and firm and tends to become enlarged or remain unchanged.[5] The premenstrual changes found in fibrocystic disease are usually not present. Therefore, an adolescent with a breast mass and no discharge or lymphadenopathy should be reexamined right after her menses. If the mass is still present or if any doubt exists, she should be referred to a specialist for further diagnostic management.

Breast abscesses are very uncommon except in lactating women and newborns.[4,5] They have a sudden onset with a red area that is warm and tender to touch. If untreated, the inflammation progresses to an abscess, usually in the subareolar area. Staphylococci are the most commonly found pathogens. Treatment consists of systemic antibiotics and incision and drainage.

Masses caused by fat necrosis or scar tissue resulting from breast trauma may also be found in children and adolescents. Careful evaluation is necessary because often a breast mass unrelated to the trauma is first discovered on examination after an injury.

Cancer of the breast in children and adolescents accounts for less than 1% of all reported cases.[5] However, any of the problems mentioned must include cancer in their differential diagnosis.

Dysmenorrhea

Dysmenorrhea is one of the most common gynecologic complaints of adolescents. It is usually manifested as abdominal or back pain, cramps, breast tenderness, a feeling of bloating, and mild to moderate swelling of the hands and legs as a result of fluid retention. It accounts for a good deal of school absenteeism. Most frequently the problem is primary and no significant pathologic changes are found in the history or physical examination. Occasionally, an adolescent has secondary dysmenorrhea, and conditions such as endometriosis or pelvic inflammatory disease are found.

Dysmenorrhea probably results from prostaglandins, released during the breakdown of endometrial tissue during menses, stimulating contraction of the myometrium, which may have been sensitized by falling progesterone levels.[6] Primary dysmenorrhea does not occur until cyclic ovulation has begun, approximately 12 to 24 months after the onset of menses in most women.

Evaluation includes a thorough menstrual history, including types of therapy attempted, and pelvic examination. Any pathologic finding requires further evaluation. First-line treatment for primary dysmenorrhea includes analgesics such as aspirin or acetaminophen and supportive methods such as local heat. If these do not provide relief, prostaglandin synthetase inhibitors may be used. These include ibuprofen, 400 mg four times daily; naproxyn, 550 mg initially and 275 mg every 6 to 9 hours, as required; mefenamic acid, 500 mg initially and 250 mg every 6 to 8 hours, as required. Some physicians prefer to use combination oral contraceptives that block ovulation and have a reported success rate of up to 90%.[1]

Labial Adhesions or Agglutinations

The labia minora can adhere to each other in the midline, leaving only a small opening dorsal to the clitoris through which urine is passed. A thin, transparent line lies between the fused labia. It rarely occurs in girls over 8 years of age and is not encountered in those who are postmenarchal. This condition is frequently mistaken for congenital absence of the vagina or an imperforate hymen. In both of these conditions, the labia are separate and neither have the vivid line of agglutination extending vertically down the center of the membrane. Another condition to be considered in the differential diagnosis is the relatively rare case of intersexuality, in which other signs such as an enlarged phallus, a thickened perineum, or an atypical location of the urethra are present.

Labial adhesions usually result from an irritation or inflammation of the labia minora that may be accompanied by an underlying vulvovaginitis. It is a self-limited problem and disappears as puberty approaches and estrogen levels rise. However, it probably should be treated to avoid the primary amenorrhea and dysuria that may be caused by labial fusion and to assure parents that the child has normal female genitalia.

The local application of an estrogenic cream, such as Premarin, nightly for 2 weeks induces cornification of the epithelium, causing the adherent labia to open. Occasionally, a second course of therapy is indicated. Care should be taken not to overuse the medication because the estrogen can be absorbed by the vaginal mucosa, causing secondary effects such as tender breasts. The adhesion should not be forcefully torn because it is very traumatic to the child and may, in fact, result in reagglutination of the damaged edges of tissue.

Prepubertal Vulvovaginitis

Vulvovaginitis is a very common problem in premenarchal children. Often the complaints of pruritis, dysuria, or discharge are misleading. The close proximity of the vagina to the anus and the thin atrophic vaginal mucosa make the child especially susceptible to vulvovaginal infections. The parent usually has stopped supervising the toilet practices of the child, who may be wiping from the anus over the vulva towards the urethra. Bubble baths, harsh soaps, tight-fitting underclothing, nylon underpants, perfumed toilet tissues, and sliding or sitting in the dirt can cause irritation. The child then scratches with dirty fingers and finger nails, causing infection. Pinworm infestations are common, and the child may scratch the anus and then the vulva, also causing infection. The child also may cause vaginal irritation during normal exploratory activity.

Dysuria can occur when urine flows over the inflamed vulvar mucosa. The leukocytes found in the voided urine are from the vulva, not the urinary tract, but physicians may make an erroneous diagnosis unless they examine the child.

The discharge material may be sparse or copious, mucoid, purulent, or bloody. A thin, mucoid discharge with irritation may be found during illnesses such as measles, chickenpox, diphtheria, and scarlet fever. The presence of a malodorous, bloody discharge usually indicates a foreign body. Children insert a variety of items into the vagina, and perhaps the item most commonly found is toilet paper.

A physical examination of the genitalia, with the child in the knee-chest position, should be performed. If a copious discharge is present or if there is any reason to suspect sexual abuse, specimens for gonococcal cultures should be taken with sterile cotton applicators or a plastic eyedropper. A wet preparation should be examined for *Trichomonas* or fungal infections, although these are rare in the prepubertal child.

Most cultures that are not positive for gonococcus reveal a mixed flora, including *Escherichia coli*, *Gardnerella vaginalis* (formally known as *Haemophilus vaginalis*), staphylococci, streptococci, *Proteus*, and *Pseudomonas*. These cultures are expensive and are not helpful in deciding on therapy.

The treatment for nonspecific vulvovaginitis involves good perineal hygiene, including wiping front to back after defecation, frequent changing of white cotton underpants, and avoiding bubble bath, harsh soaps, and perfumed toilet tissue. In addition, the child should have sitz baths in plain water 2 to 3 times daily for a week or so, followed by patting the area dry. If possible the child should lie with her knees apart and wearing no underpants for as long as possible after the bath.

A soothing lotion or cream such as calamine or zinc oxide can be used in conjunction with the baths. If pruritis and inflammation are extreme, a mild steroid cream such as 1% hydrocortisone may be helpful. Occasionally, a systemic antipruritic agent such as diphenhydramine can be used.

The treatment of specific vaginitis is discussed later. Fortunately, such infections occur much less frequently in young children than in adolescents.

Vaginal Foreign Bodies

If a foreign body is suspected, it may be palpated on rectal examination. Care must be taken because sharp objects may be impaled in the mucosa. Direct visualization using a speculum and a good light source may be necessary. Small or soft foreign bodies may not be palpable, and the vaginal canal should be flushed using a large syringe, filled with tepid water, to which a soft rubber catheter is attached. The flushing is best performed with the child in a supine position. She and her mother should be told in detail what is to be done, and a small amount of the water can be squirted over the vulva to show the child that it will not hurt.

SEXUALLY TRANSMITTED DISEASES

Postpubertal Vaginitis

The evaluation of the adolescent with suspected vulvovaginitis is different from that of the prepubertal child.[1,3,7] This is not only true of the pathogenesis but also includes the psychosocial and psychosexual responses to the problem. The emerging adolescent is characterized by a rather dramatic increase in self-consciousness and need for privacy. Although most of the causative agents associated with vulvovaginitis in this age group are relatively noninvasive, infections of this nature may create significant discomfort, embarrassment, and concern.

The first pelvic examination may occur in conjunction with an evaluation for vulvovaginitis. It should not be a traumatic experience. Appropriate diagnostic and therapeutic intervention must take this into account if compliance and follow-up are expected.

The five most common agents responsible for vulvovaginitis are *Candida albicans, G. vaginalis* (*H. vaginalis*), herpes simplex, *Neisseria gonorrhoeae,* and *Trichomonas vaginalis* (Table 24-1). Microscopic examination of fresh smears immersed in (1) a drop or two of saline, (2) a potassium hydroxide (KOH) preparation, (3) a Gram stain, and (4) a Wright stain of the material will usually be diagnostic. Cultures may be necessary to make the diagnosis, especially if gonorrhea is suspected.[8]

If douching is done prior to the examination or if the menstrual period has started, the diagnosis may be delayed. Identification and concurrent treatment of an infected sexual partner are essential because treatment failures are usually the result of reinfection. All adolescents with a sexually transmitted vulvovaginitis should be screened for gonorrhea.

Candida Infections

C. albicans (monilial) infection of the vagina and vulva has replaced trichomoniasis as the most common cause of vaginitis. Clinically, the individual is seen with mild itching and dysuria in the week prior to menstruation. The vulva may appear to be wet or dry, erythematous, edematous, and excoriated. The inguinal region, when involved, may appear to be erythematous, with satellite lesions typical of the monilial diaper rash of infancy. Vaginal infection alone may be asymptomatic except for the presence of odor and a curdlike discharge.

Diagnostic Tests Diagnosis must be based on both a suggestive clinical picture and demonstration of the organism. A 10% KOH preparation lyses other cellular elements, thereby enhancing the micro-

TABLE 24-1 Organisms and Characteristics of Vulvovaginitis

	Candida	*Gardnerella*	Herpesvirus	*Trichomonas*
Discharge	Usually absent, curdlike if present	Milky white, somewhat frothy	Scanty	Profuse; yellowish, frothy
Timing	Usually 1 wk prior to onset of menses; during pregnancy	Anytime	Anytime	Anytime
Odor	Rare	Fishy	Rare	Foul
Pruritis	++++	+	++	++ to +++
Other symptoms	Dysuria and dyspareunia	Not usual	Dyspareunia, inguinal lymphadenopathy	Frequency, dysuria, dyspareunia
Diagnosis	KOH, wet smear, Gram's stain	Saline wet mount, "clue cell," Gram's stain	Smear of scrapings from vesicular lesions, viral culture	Saline wet mount, motile organisms on fresh specimen
Treatment of choice	Miconazole (Monistat)	Ampicillin	1% Betadine solution	Metronidazole (Flagyl)

Source: Adapted with permission from DeAngelis, C: *Pediatric Primary Care,* ed 3. Boston, Little Brown & Co, 1984, p 508. Copyright © 1984 Little Brown & Co.

scopic demonstration of the fungi. A Gram stain further increases diagnostic accuracy. Budding yeast cells are from 2 to 5 mm in axis and appear as dense, Gram-positive tubes with a diameter about the same size as that of the yeast form. Many asymptomatic patients have scattered budding cells and pseudohyphae on routine KOH preparation or Gram's stain. In general, culture techniques are too sensitive and not very useful.

Treatment Management involves eradication of the fungus and, if present, treatment of the secondary infection related to the excoriations. Excellent local hygiene is essential. Douching, sprays, and suppositories often make matters worse. Sitz baths with baking soda help to relieve the itching. One percent hydrocortisone cream may be applied locally after the bath. If the vulva and inguinal region are involved, a nystatin preparation may be applied. The current intravaginal agents of choice are miconazole cream or nystatin vaginal suppositories twice daily for 14 days. Candicidin (Candeptin or Vanobid) vaginal tablets, inserted twice daily for a minimum of 14 days, are excellent alternatives. Miconazole cream is more expensive than other medications, but it has been associated with higher cure rates than nystatin.

Gardnerella Vaginalis Infections

Gardnerella vaginalis, otherwise known as *Haemophilus vaginalis,* is a small, pleomorphic Gram-variable, but predominantly Gram-negative, nonmotile rod. Like *N. gonorrhoeae, G. vaginalis* is a fastidious organism, growing best in a reduced oxygen atmosphere.

The vaginal discharge may begin at any time during the menstrual cycle, is milky white in appearance, and has a characteristic "fishy" odor. Pruritis is a frequent complaint. Mild abdominal discomfort is occasionally present.

Diagnostic Tests Diagnosis is made by the microscopic examination of a saline wet mount or a Gram stain. The involved vaginal epithelial cells will have lost their angulated appearance and many will be in a process of degeneration; these cells are called "clue cells" and are specific for this disorder.

Treatment The treatment of choice is ampicillin, 500 mg orally 4 times a day for a week. Tetracycline in the same dosage is also effective for individuals who are allergic to penicillin. Some physicians prefer metronidazole, one tablet three times a day for a week. Simultaneous treatment of sexual partners is recommended because urethral colonization with the bacterium has been found in the vast majority of male partners.

Genital Herpes

Herpes simplex virus, otherwise known as herpesvirus, can be differentiated serologically into two types. Type 1 has been recognized primarily as the virus responsible for cold sores or fever blisters on the oral mucous membranes, lips, and face. Type 2 primarily involves the genital tract. Both types of viruses are known to cross-infect, often in association with orogenital sexual practices. Thus type 2 may cause oral mucosal fever blisters, and type 1 may cause genital lesions.

The patient may have dysuria of such degree that voiding is practically impossible. There are complaints of local pain, itching, and inguinal adenopathy. When the lesions are diffuse, fever, headaches, and malaise are commonly found. The disease starts as a group of vesicles that rupture within 1 to 2 days. They leave crusts, blisters, or ulcers. The ulcers are shallow, small, and round, with bright red bases. Discharge is scanty. The usual duration of primary genital herpes is 10 to 14 days, but it may last for 3 to 4 weeks. Hospitalization in severe cases may be necessary. Complications range from disseminated herpes to local infections involving the eye or meninges.

Diagnostic Tests The laboratory diagnosis can be made by conventional tissue culture methods within 1 to 3 days. Scrapings taken from herpetic lesions and stained with Wright's stain reveal multinucleated giant cells with eosinophilic intranuclear inclusions, often surrounded by a prominent halo. These giant cells are recognized by their dark purplish color and abundant cytoplasm.

Treatment Treatment is primarily symptomatic. The adolescent should be advised to tell his or her partner about any past or present history of herpes, to avoid sexual contacts when any active herpes lesions are present, and to be aware that there is no guarantee that a condom will prevent the spread of infection.

Genital care should be aimed at decreasing pain and the chance of secondary infection. Warm compresses or sitz baths several times daily for 15 to 20 minutes with gentle removal of adherent crusts or discharge are helpful. If the patient is not allergic to iodine, 1% povidone iodine (Betadine) solution may be applied with a cotton swab. This is an antiseptic drying agent that helps to prevent secondary infection.

Application of cold compresses with a modified

Burrow's solution (Domeboro or Blue Boro) helps to reduce pain, itching, and local edema. Affected individuals often need to receive stronger analgesics than aspirin during the acute phase. Increasing the fluid intake decreases local irritation with urination. Urinating while sitting in water, sleeping with pajama bottoms off and legs apart, and wearing absorbent white cotton underwear and a skirt during the day also minimize local irritation.

Trichomoniasis

Clinically, the patient with trichomoniasis complains of urinary frequency and dysuria, pruritus of the labia and introitus, intravaginal and vague pelvic discomfort, and a malodorous vaginal discharge. Physical examination may reveal inflamed, excoriated, and edematous labia and introitus. The vaginal walls and cervix have a similar appearance, and small, punctate hemorrhages may also be present. The malodorous vaginal discharge is often profuse, yellowish, and frothy.

Diagnostic Tests To confirm the diagnosis, a cotton swab is saturated with discharge from the posterovaginal pool and mixed on a slide with a drop of tepid saline. A cover slip is then applied, and scanning under the high-dry objective with reduced lighting often reveals the flagella and undulating membranes of viable parasites. After death the organisms become round and are difficult to differentiate from leukocytes.

Treatment In children up to 50 kg in body weight, metronidazole (Flagyl), 5 mg/kg/dose three times daily, is used. For patients over 50 kg, 250 mg orally three times daily for 7 days, or 500 mg orally twice a day for 5 days, may be prescribed.

TABLE 24-2 Sexually Transmitted Diseases

Agent	Clinical Disorder
Spirochete	
Treponema pallidum	Syphilis
Bacteria	
N. gonorrhoeae	Urethritis, cervicitis, perihepatitis, pelvic inflammatory disease, disseminated infection
Haemophilus ducreyi	Chancroid
Calymmatobacterium granulomatis	Granuloma inguinale
G. vaginalis	Vaginitis, urethritis
Viruses	
Herpesvirus type 2 and type 1	Vaginitis, cervicitis, urethritis, cystitis, ? cervical cancer
Cytomegalovirus	Endometritis, ? cervicitis, urethritis
Molluscum contagiosum	Wartlike lesions
Papilloma virus	Condylomata acuminata
Hepatitis virus (hepatitis-associated antigen positive)	Hepatitis
Protozoan	
T. vaginalis	Vaginitis, cervicitis, urethritis
Insect	
Pthirus pubis	Pediculosis (crabs), acute dermatitis
Mite	
Sarcoptes scabiei, variety *hominis*	Acute dermatitis
Other	
Chlamydia trachomatis	Urethritis, cystitis, cervicitis, nonsuppurative polyarthritis, anterior uveitis, salpingitis
Chlamydia-type agent	Lymphogranuloma venereum
Ureaplasma urealyticum (*T-mycoplasma*)	Urethritis

Source: Adapted with permission from DeAngelis, C: *Pediatric Primary Care*, ed 3. Boston, Little Brown & Co, 1984, p 512. Copyright © 1984 Little Brown & Co.

Venereal Diseases

Classically, gonorrhea and syphilis have been identified as the two major venereal diseases, and chancroid, lymphogranuloma venereum, and granuloma inguinale have been called the minor venereal diseases. In addition, a variety of other infections can be transmitted by sexual contact. All of these are included in Table 24-2. Gonorrhea, syphilis, *Chlamydia* infections, and condyloma are discussed in this section. Pediculosis and scabies are discussed in Chapter 29.

The adolescent who has one of these disorders is a prime candidate for sex education and counseling. Having a sexually transmitted disease has little or no correlation with knowledge regarding the disease or contraception. Often, the adolescent masks a sense of apprehension with an air of indifference or pseudosophistication. The physician must look beyond this facade and provide education.

Gonococcal Infections

Gonorrhea is the number one reported infectious disease and potentially one of the most devastating illnesses in the adolescent age group.[8,9] It is estimated that up to 40% of males and 90% of females with gonococcal infections are asymptomatic.[8] The symptomatic male with gonococcal urethritis usually has a history of urethral discharge and pain on urination and ejaculation. The discharge usually becomes purulent within 2 to 7 days after a contact, but it may take as long as a month. If contiguous spread has occurred, fever may be present. Pain in the perineal, suprapubic, or inguinal areas may indicate prostatic and seminal vesicle involvement. What appears to be testicular torsion or orchitis may actually be gonococcal epididymitis. A careful examination, frank, nonjudgmental questioning, and a high index of suspicion are essential because repeated episodes can lead to sterility.

Rectal and pharyngeal gonorrhea are occurring with increasing frequency in homosexual adolescent males and in heterosexually active females. The physician must be prepared to include questions about sexual practices in the history because standard treatment for uncomplicated gonococcal urethritis may not be consistently effective in eradicating gonorrhea from these other sites.[9]

Accurate and early diagnosis of gonorrhea infection in the adolescent girl is extremely difficult. Clinically, minimal and transient dysuria may be the only symptom present. The vaginal discharge may be profuse, purulent, and yellowish green in the acute stage of the infection. However, in most instances the discharge is scant and not purulent.

Pelvic Inflammatory Disease Pelvic inflammatory disease is usually caused by the gonococcus. Nongonococcal organisms include anaerobes and aerobes. Acute gonococcal salpingitis is manifested by fever, chills, and abdominal pain. The onset typically coincides with menstruation, and the patient may have a bent-over, shuffling gait. Examination usually reveals bilateral adnexal pain that is readily elicited by cervical traction. The Gram stain and cervical culture are usually positive for *N. gonorrhoeae,* the leukocyte count is elevated with a pronounced left shift, and the erythrocyte sedimentation rate is elevated. Pelvic inflammatory disease must be differentiated from appendicitis, pyelonephritis, ruptured ovarian cyst, ectopic pregnancy, and septic abortion.

Pharyngeal Infections Pharyngeal infections appear to be important as a reservoir of *N. gonorrhoeae,* as a potential source of gonococcemia, and as a possible cause of symptomatic pharyngitis. Gonorrhea of the pharynx is usually asymptomatic. On physical examination, the infected pharynx appears to be normal.

Anorectal Infections Clinical symptoms include copious, purulent anal discharge, burning or stinging rectal pain, blood or mucus in the stools, and tenesmus. Milder cases are characterized by perianal itching or burning, some purulent staining of the underwear, and mucus or pus in the stools; however, two thirds of the proven cases were asymptomatic in one study.

Physical examination may reveal a perianal area that is moist or stained with creamy pus. Condylomata acuminata may also be present. Proctoscopic abnormalities are limited to the anal canal and rectum. In severe cases the mucosa is reddened, edematous, and bathed in pus. A perirectal abscess may be present.

Disseminated infections, such as septic arthritis and septicemia, may arise from the infected anorectal area, even in the absence of local symptoms.

Gonococcal Ophthalmia The high incidence of gonorrhea among adolescents is matched by their current pregnancy rates and is also reflected by the rising rate of neonatal gonococcal ophthalmia.[9,10] The disease begins with a conjunctival discharge that progresses from watery to purulent within 2 days. Untreated, the cornea rapidly opacifies, ulcerates, and ruptures. Diagnosis is made by culturing the exudate.

Gonococcal Perihepatitis (Fitz-Hugh-Curtis Syndrome) The diagnosis of gonococcal perihepatitis is a presumptive one based on the presence of pain in the right upper quadrant and the recovery of *N. gonorrhoeae* from the endocervix. *N. gonorrhoeae* has never been recovered by culture from an intraabdominal specimen obtained from a woman with this syndrome. Occasionally, abnormal liver function tests and a perihepatic friction rub are present. Evidence of salpingitis of variable severity is usually present, and other signs of generalized peritonitis may also be found.

Symptoms range from those of pelvic peritonitis or generalized peritonitis to the occasional patient with predominantly perihepatic findings that may be confused with cholecystitis. Because cholecystitis is unusual in the adolescent girl and gonorrhea is increasingly common, a high index of suspicion should exist for making an early diagnosis in adolescents with this disorder. Clinical improvement associated with antibiotic therapy is a further aid in establishing the diagnosis.

Disseminated Gonorrhea Disseminated gonococcal infections involve women more commonly than men, and occur as a result of hematogenous extension of the gonococcus from the site of entry. Dissemination follows asymptomatic, more than symptomatic, genital infection, and it often results from gonococcal pharyngitis and anorectal gonorrhea. Septicemia with arthritis and dermatitis is the most frequent extragenital manifestation, occurring in 1% to 3% of all cases of gonorrhea.[9,10] Endocarditis, meningitis, and pericarditis rarely occur.

The clinical symptoms of systemic gonococcal spread include fever, chills, malaise, migratory polyarthritis, tenosynovitis, and painful, acral skin lesions, including vesiculopustular, hemorrhagic bullous, and urticarial eruptions.

The diagnostic procedure with the highest yield is culturing samples on modified Thayer-Martin medium; specimens are obtained from the cervix, rectum, urethra, and pharynx, as indicated. Blood samples obtained from septic skin lesions and joint aspirates should be cultured on chocolate agar immediately upon suspicion of gonococcal septicemia. Occasionally, smears of specimens from the genitourinary tract, scrapings of involved skin, or aspirates of affected tendon sheaths or joint fluid can prove helpful.

Definitive therapy should be instituted when the diagnosis appears probable and when other diagnoses have been reasonably excluded. The dramatic response to specific therapy may be helpful in the diagnosis.

Diagnostic Tests The improved modified Thayer-Martin culture medium is the foundation of modern gonorrhea detection. In adolescent boys with untreated urethral discharge, demonstration on a stained smear of typical, Gram-negative diplococci within polymorphonuclear leukocytes is sufficient for diagnosis. Immediate treatment is indicated in these cases; however, a negative Gram stain does not exclude gonorrhea, and a culture of the discharge should be performed before nongonococcal urethritis is assumed. Culture, rather than smear, is required as a test of cure after antibiotic therapy.

Gram-stained smears of the urethral or cervical exudates are not as reliable in girls. False-negative smears are common because large numbers of organisms and cellular debris usually obscure the presence of *Neisseria* and interfere with the staining process.

In adolescent girls specimens taken from deep inside the vagina are a good substitute for cervical specimens when the adolescent is unwilling to have a speculum introduced into the vagina. Menstruation is not a contraindication to performing diagnostic studies.

Treatment There are two treatments of choice for uncomplicated gonococcal infections in patients over 50 kg in weight: (1) simultaneous administration of ampicillin, 3.5 g, plus probenecid, 1 g, both given orally; or (2) aqueous procaine penicillin G, 4.8 million U IM divided into at least two doses and injected at two different sites at one visit. One gram of oral probenecid should be given just before the injection.[10]

Individuals who are allergic to either penicillin or probenecid can be treated with tetracycline or erythromycin, each at doses of 1.5 g initially, followed by 0.5 g by mouth four times a day for 4 days. Spectinomycin, 2 mg IM, should be reserved for individuals who are infected with penicillinase-producing organisms, their recent sexual partners, and those with positive follow-up cultures despite initial treatment with the other recommended antibiotics. Tetracycline and probably spectinomycin should not be used in pregnant women.

Adolescents who have had known, recent exposure to gonorrhea should be treated as if they have gonorrhea. Follow-up cultures should be obtained 7 to 14 days after the completion of therapy. All patients with gonorrhea should have a serologic test for syphilis performed at the time of diagnosis.

For patients weighing less than 50 kg, the doses of these medications are based on body weight (see Chapter 3).

Syphilis

Primary Syphilis After an incubation period of 10 to 90 days, initial lesions appear, usually on the genitalia. These lesions vary from slight erosions to deep ulcers, generally accompanied by painless bilateral inguinal lymphadenopathy. Approximately 60% of men and 90% of women do not recall the initial lesions because they are painless and inconspicuous.

Secondary Syphilis This stage is heralded by a generalized macular or maculopapular eruption that is rarely nodular or pustular. The palms and soles are sometimes affected, and oral and anogenital lesions may also be present. The rash may be accompanied by slight fever and sore throat.

Tertiary Syphilis Fifteen to twenty years after the latency period, about one quarter of all affected individuals develop late, multisystem complications. This phase is tertiary syphilis. Discussion of this aspect is beyond the scope of this text, and tertiary syphilis does not usually involve individuals in the pediatric or adolescent age group.

Diagnostic Tests Diagnostic tests for syphilis can be divided into two types based on the antigen used. The Venereal Disease Resource Laboratory (VDRL) and rapid plasma reagin (RPR) are nontreponemal tests and detect a nonspecific antibody-like substance called reagin. The fluorescent treponemal antibody-absorbed (FTA-ABS) test detects the specific antibody to *Treponema pallidum*. The FTA-ABS test should be performed on patients with positive RPR or VDRL tests to decrease false-positive results.

Treatment Treatment is either benzathine penicillin G, 2.4 million U IM at one visit, or procaine penicillin G, 600,000 U IM daily for 8 days. Patients who are allergic to penicillin may be treated with tetracycline or erythromycin, 500 mg orally four times a day for 15 days. Medication for younger patients should be based on the patient's weight (Chapter 3).

Chlamydia Trachomatis Infections

C. trachomatis can cause urethritis and epididymitis in the male and cystitis, cervicitis, and salpingitis in the female. The infection may be manifested by a mucopurulent vaginal discharge in girls or by dysuria and urinary frequency in both sexes. *Chlamydia* should be considered in anyone with these symptoms when usual cultures are negative. It is important to remember that women with gonorrhea vaginitis can also have chlamydial infection and that up to 70% of postgonococcal urethritis is due to *Chlamydia*.[11] Untreated *Chlamydia* infections persist and may lead to salpingitis.

Diagnostic Tests The specific laboratory diagnosis of chlamydial infection requires special tissue culture facilities and the recovery of living cells when a culture is taken. Consequently, the physician may be required to treat on presumptive diagnosis in some cases. Serologic evidence of infection may be obtained by complement-fixation testing, showing a rising titer of immunofluorescent antibodies.

Treatment Adolescents with chlamydial infections can be treated with doxycycline, 100 mg orally twice daily for 7 to 10 days. Girlfriends of boys with urethritis should be treated simultaneously because up to 70% of them harbor the organism in the cervix. Alternative antibiotics include tetracycline, erythromycin, and sulfamethizole.

Condylomata Acuminata

Genital warts are thought to be caused by the papova-papilloma virus. Their spread is primarily by close physical or sexual contact with an infected individual and by autoinoculation. The incubation period ranges from less than 1 month to as long as 20 months. The rapid spread and variable response to therapy can create a discouraging clinical situation.

The warts appear on mucous membranes and the genitalia. Rarely, they can be found on the vocal cords of infants who have been infected at birth. They are grayish white, filiform, coneshaped or cauliflower-like papules, from 3 to 10 mm in diameter. When the warts are adjacent to the urethral meatus or anus, more complete examination of the urethra and rectum is necessary because of frequent contiguous spread. The warts are often associated with vaginitis and intravaginal vegetations, and the irritating vaginal discharge may provoke their growth. The lesions may disappear with successful treatment of the vaginitis.

Diagnostic Tests All patients should have a VDRL test performed because the condyloma latum of secondary syphilis may not be readily distinguishable clinically.

Treatment Treatment consists of the application of 20% podophyllum in tincture of benzoin applied weekly until the lesions are gone. The solution should be rinsed off thoroughly with water in 4 to 6 hours. Petroleum jelly should not be applied at the base of the lesion to protect the skin. This practice may prevent the medication from reaching the base of the lesions. Podophyllum should not be used in pregnant women, and its use in young children is controversial because of absorption and toxicity.

Podophyllum should be applied intravaginally only under the direct vision of a speculum examination, and it need not be removed by douching. Local irritation secondary to local toxic and allergic response can be quite severe. Adolescents should not be allowed to self-medicate.

The eradication of coexisting vaginitis and the treatment of current sexual partners, if indicated, significantly diminishes recurrence and chronicity. Oral mucous membrane involvement may also be a source of reinfection, depending on sexual habits. Frequently, electrodesiccation or surgical excision is necessary. Immunotherapy may be the treatment of choice in extensive, persistent, or recurrent disease.

CONTRACEPTION AND PREGNANCY

Providing family planning, contraceptive advice, and general realistic and pertinent sexual education should be a major function of all physicians who care for adolescents. Basically contraception involves eight categories of methods or devices. These methods and their risks of pregnancy, advantages, and disadvantages are listed in Table 24-3. Risks are expressed in terms of pregnancies per 100

TABLE 24-3 Contraception Methods

Method	Risk of Pregnancy (per 100 woman-yr)	Advantages	Disadvantages
No contraception	75–100		
Withdrawal	20–35	Essentially no side effects, no mechanical intervention necessary	Not usually effective with adolescents because control is necessary
Douching	20–30	No serious side effects, relatively cheap	Inconvenient; by the time douching occurs, most sperm are already well into the canal
Rhythm	14–25	No side effects, religious sanction	Requires sophisticated knowledge of menstrual cycle; requires fairly regular menstrual cycle, therefore not usually effective for adolescents
Foams, jellies, creams, and suppositories	8–20	Essentially no side effects	Interferes with spontaneity, may be too expensive for adolescents, only effective for 60 min. after insertion
Condoms	10–15	No side effects, inexpensive venereal disease protection	Interferes with spontaneity
Diaphragm plus jellies (diaphragms should never be used alone)	6–15	Few side effects	Requires fitting by a physician, interferes with spontaneity, may be too expensive for adolescents
Intrauterine devices (IUDs)	2–4	Few side effects	Requires insertion by physician, breakthrough bleeding, high expulsion rate in nulliparous adolescents
Oral contraceptives		Spontaneity preserved, very effective	Weight gain, nausea, fluid retention, spotting, headaches, change in libido, vertigo, hypertension, thromboembolic disease, requires daily pill ingestion, expensive, requires prescription, good follow-up essential
Sequential	1.0		
Combined	0.5		

Source: Reprinted with permission from Page S, Villee C, Villee J: *Human Reproduction*. Philadelphia, WB Saunders Co, 1972, p 84.

woman-years.[12] A woman-year is based on 13 menstrual cycles; therefore, 100 woman-years represents the risk of pregnancy using a specific method per 1300 menstrual cycles. Although this is the generally accepted method for expressing risk, the actual risk of pregnancy for each woman is not as high as these figures indicate because obviously no woman has 1300 menstrual cycles in a lifetime.

Many adolescents have misconceptions about birth control devices that should be addressed. For example, soda pop douches and using plastic wrap (e.g., Saran wrap) for condoms are not very effective and may be hazardous.

Spermatocides immobilize and kill sperm. In general, foams such as Emko, Delfen, and Conceptrol are more effective than creams, jellies, and suppositories that do not disperse well. The spermatocide should be inserted into the vagina within 1 hour prior to each act of coitus.

Generally, condoms are made of the collagenous lining of sheep intestines and should always be used with a spermatocidal agent. They should not be stored for long periods of time especially in wallets and glove compartments.

Diaphragms, which also should be used with spermatocidal agents, act as barriers to the cervical orifice and hold the spermatocide in place against the cervix. They are relatively easy to fit, and the pediatrician can learn the techniques in one short session with a knowledgeable physician. The diaphragm may be inserted up to 2 hours prior to intercourse, and it should be left in for at least 6 hours after coitus.

After the initial fitting, the diaphragm should be rechecked after 1 week. It should then be rechecked annually to assure proper fitting and sooner if the young woman has been pregnant, has had a pelvic operation, or has lost or gained significant weight.

Oral contraceptive pills prevent ovulation by inhibiting release of the pituitary gonadotropin's follicle-stimulating hormone and luteinizing hormone.

They also cause a decrease in secretion and an increase in viscosity of cervical mucus, thereby inhibiting sperm motility and penetration.

The combination oral contraceptives contain synthetic progestin and estrogen in each pill. In the 28-pill package, at least 7 pills are placebos. The first 14 pills contain estrogen only and the following 7 contain estrogen and progestin.

No matter what contraceptive method is used, constant reassurance and encouragement are necessary for the adolescent to remain motivated to continue use. It is not enough to write a prescription for pills or fit a diaphragm. The role of the physician as confidante and motivator cannot be overemphasized. Because it is very evident that premarital sexual activity is a basic fact of many people's lives, it should be practiced in a manner that will not produce the added problems of pregnancy.

Sterilization has no place in contraception for adolescents. Their lives and ideas will probably change dramatically as they mature. They should not be burdened with a possible undesired infertility based on a decision made before full maturity has been reached.

No matter how much energy is expended in the area of birth control for teenagers, it seems that pregnancies in this age group continue to occur for a variety of reasons. A few teenagers actually plan a pregnancy, but most of them seem to have other factors involved such as ambivalence about birth control and pregnancy.

Before becoming involved with pregnant teenagers or those who desire birth control, an examination and awareness of the practitioner's own feelings are important. If the physician does not feel comfortable in this area, a referral to another qualified professional must be made.

When the pregnant teenager comes for care, it is essential to determine how far she has advanced into the pregnancy, how she and the father feel about it, and, if possible, why it occurred. Was it a planned pregnancy, a birth control failure, or was there denial that pregnancy could occur? An evaluation of the young woman's support system and current living situation is valuable in determining where she might receive assistance. If the father is known, he should be included in the decisions and counseling if it is at all feasible.

The teenage parents' physical and emotional welfare and their rights of privacy and confidentiality must be preserved. Their own parents should take an active part in the overall situation if at all possible. If the teenagers do not have a good relationship with their parents, they may be able to find support from sources such as their brothers, sisters, close friends, or clergy. Ideally, the parents or others might be able to provide the reassurance and assistance necessary to assist the teenagers through the pregnancy. They might also be willing to help care for the infant, providing the necessary emotional and possibly economic support. In all cases the adolescent parents should be encouraged to continue and complete their educations as soon as feasible. Currently, over two thirds of teenage mothers do not complete high school. The practitioner should advise the young parents about local agencies that may provide assistance and help to arrange for the initial contact with the proper agency if assistance is needed.

After an assessment of the resources available to the teenager, the alternatives should be discussed. Basically, there are three options: (1) the mother can keep the baby as a single parent or get married and keep the baby; (2) she can give the baby up for adoption; or (3) she can have an abortion. Before discussing each alternative in detail, it is helpful to determine the teenage parents' reaction to these choices.

If the teenagers feel that they may want to keep the baby, it is important to discuss how a pregnancy will change or influence their lives and future goals. Many adolescents have unrealistic expectations and ideas about child rearing. Some young women feel that it is an act of emancipation to have a child or perhaps they view the baby as someone who will love them unconditionally. It is often valuable to explore the adolescents' goals regarding child rearing and how they plan to meet them. Teenagers are frequently unaware of their needs and available resources in the areas of finances, housing, and emotional support. It is valuable to discuss this with them in a realistic and supportive way.

The options of adoption and abortion should also be discussed in detail, and the feelings of the prospective grandparents about each alternative should be explored. If the teenagers know some individuals who have experienced adoption or abortion, they may wish to speak to them about the decision. The teenagers may have strong moral feelings about abortion or may be influenced by the values of friends and family. Although some adolescents can intellectually see some rationale for an abortion, they often have much difficulty with this concept emotionally. Common concerns regarding abortion include the effect it will have on future children, the possibility of sterility, pain, complications, and the financial cost. The abortion procedure and possible complications should be explained.

Abortion should never be used to replace adequate preventive measures. Sex education and contraception should be provided to the potentially sexually active teenager long before abortion becomes an alternative.

The total care of the teenage parents and their child requires all the resources of the pediatric health team, obstetrician, and local social service agencies. Even with this multidisciplinary approach, the long-range outlook for the teenage mother, father, and child is replete with possible physical and emotional problems. It is much better to have prevented the pregnancy.

RAPE

Rape in this context means the act of having sexual intercourse with a child or an older individual without consent or using threats or force to achieve consent. In children, the attempt itself is generally considered to be sexual assault.

Rape is the fastest growing violent crime in the United States, and sexual abuse of children and adolescents occurs at an estimated rate of 100,000 to 500,000 cases annually.[13] Many, if not most, cases involving children and adolescents are not reported because of psychologic reactions to the incident, fear of reprisals, guilt, and other factors. The assailants can be anyone, including parents, siblings, relatives, baby-sitters, and strangers.

The physician should remember that rape, per se, is a legal term and that the physician's involvement requires careful history taking, performing a thorough physical examination, collecting appropriate specimens in accordance with local protocol, and treating the patient for physical and emotional problems. Informed consent should be obtained for the entire evaluation, including taking pictures, collecting specimens, and releasing information to legal authorities.[14]

Depending on the nature of the incident and the age of the patient, the following specimens should be obtained and transferred according to local legal standards: vaginal, cervical, rectal, pharyngeal, blood, pubic hair, and dried, ultraviolet light-positive specimens on clothing. Evidence of recent coitus includes motile sperm, a vaginal aspirate containing 50 or more King-Armstrong units per milliliter of acid phosphatase, or the presence of acid phosphatase on dried material.[15]

Treatment includes the following as appropriate for the incident: management of physical trauma, antiseptic douching, oral analgesics, prophylaxis for sexually transmitted diseases, and follow-up for evaluation of possible pregnancy, sexually transmitted diseases, and emotional reactions. Many cities or medical centers have rape-crisis teams that are specially trained in managing victims of sexual assault. Physicians should be sure that they or other appropriate health professionals attend to the psychologic needs of the victim and assure protection from recurrence.

References

1. Cowell C (ed): Pediatric and adolescent gynecology. *Pediatr Clin North Am* 1981;28:247–530.
2. Greenwald P, Nasca P, Lawrence C, et al: Estimated effect of breast self-examination and routine physician examinations on breast-cancer mortality. *N Engl J Med* 1978;299:271–273.
3. Emans S, Goldstein D: *Pediatric and Adolescent Gynecology*. Boston, Little Brown & Co, 1977.
4. McKiernan J, Hull D: Breast development in the newborn. *Arch Dis Child* 1981;56:525–529.
5. Foster S, Lang SL, Constanza M, et al: Breast self-examination practices and breast cancer stage. *N Engl J Med* 1978;299:265–270.
6. Pickles V, Hall W: Prostaglandins in endometrium and menstrual flow from normal and dysmenorrheic subjects. *J Obstet Gynaecol Br Commonwealth* 1975; 72:185–188.
7. Hein K, Schreiber K, Cohen M, et al: Cervical cytology: The need for routine screening in the sexually active adolescent. *J Pediatr* 1977;91:123–126.
8. Litt I, Edberg S, Finberg L: Gonorrhea in children and adolescents: A current review. *J Pediatr* 1974; 85:595–607.
9. Kraus S: Complications of gonococcal infections. *Med Clin North Am* 1972;56:1115–1125.
10. Abramowicz M (ed): Treatment of syphilis and gonorrhea. *Med Lett Drugs Ther* 1977;19:26.
11. Schachter J: Chlamydial infections. *N Engl J Med* 1978;298:428–435, 540–549.
12. Dickey R: *Managing Contraceptive Pill Patients*, ed 2. Minneapolis, Creative Informatics Inc, 1980.
13. Summit R, Kryso J: Sexual abuse of children: A clinical spectrum. *Am J Orthopsychiatry* 1978;48:237–255.
14. Hicks DJ: Rape: Sexual assault. *Am J Obstet Gynecol* 1980;137:931–933.
15. Tilelli J, Turek D, Jaffe A: Sexual abuse of children: Clinical findings and implications for management. *N Engl J Med* 1980;302:319–323.

Part VII

Musculoskeletal Disorders

Edward M. Sills

25

Musculoskeletal Disorders

Young people represent a group particularly vulnerable to development of problems of limb movement or locomotion. Traumatic episodes, developmental processes, infections, or specific disease syndromes must be considered when disorders of the musculoskeletal system are encountered.

LIMB DYSFUNCTION

Spasticity

Fixed motor disabilities resulting from central nervous system damage may be the basis of limb dysfunction. In children spastic cerebral palsy should be considered. The usual clinical feature is that of persistent toe walking, flexed or limp arm posture, marked clumsiness, or mild hemiatrophy. Unilateral cerebral palsy usually affects an upper limb, with flexion of the elbow, wrist, and fingers. When a leg is involved, the foot rests on the toes with the heel off the floor and the leg circumducting. An unworn shoe heel with a very worn toe is a good clue. Bilateral spastic cerebral palsy affects all extremities and a quadriplegia results. All children with a spastic form of cerebral palsy have increased muscle tone, are hyperreflexic, and demonstrate a positive Babinski sign. Those with the athetoid form of cerebral palsy have peculiar writhing movements in the distal extremities, have poor speech development, are slow in developing motor milestones, and have compromised hand dexterity. These children often have normal intelligence.

Congenital Torticollis

Congenital torticollis is usually seen in infants after a difficult breech extraction and is caused by shortening of the sternocleidomastoid muscle on one side. Palpation reveals a firm mass in the body of the muscle. If the condition is left untreated, the muscle fibroses and shortens, causing head and face asymmetry. The head is tilted toward the affected side and the mouth is pulled downward. Cervical spine x-ray films should be taken to exclude fractures, dislocations, or Klippel-Feil syndrome. Simple muscle stretching exercises are usually sufficient to correct this problem.

Muscle Weakness

Muscle weakness may be the basis of a child's manifestation of limb dysfunction. Careful distinction between generalized and isolated proximal weakness aids in establishment of the correct diagnosis.

Generalized muscle weakness may result from upper or lower motor neuron lesions. The upper neuron lesions cause, in addition to muscle weakness, some degree of spastic paralysis of the extremities. Sudden appearance of hemiparesis suggests blood vessel disease, whereas gradual weakness suggests a degenerative disorder or tumor. Lower neuron disease usually is manifest as a flaccid weakness and involves anterior horn cells (as in poliomyelitis or Werdnig-Hoffmann disease), peripheral nerve (as in polyneuritis), or muscle (as in muscular dystrophy). Atrophy usually occurs, and there is a negative Babinski sign and diminished or absent deep tendon reflexes. Polyneuritis and poliomyelitis are the most common causes of distal muscle weakness. Lower extremities are more affected than upper extremities. Sensory abnormalities are absent.

Most of the primary muscle diseases carry a prognosis of a relatively normal life span with adequate function. These various disorders can only be distinguished and defined by skeletal muscle biopsy and electron microscopic examination.

Infantile Hypotonia

Infantile hypotonia is detected by history and during ventral suspension. Diseases of the central nervous system, spine, or muscles can cause infants to be floppy. Birth trauma with intraventricular hemorrhage, spinal cord injury, or anoxia can cause flaccidity and poor tone. Inherited metabolic diseases, such as the gangliosidoses, type 2 glycogen storage disease, Niemann-Pick disease, and hyper-β-alaninemia, may all present with generalized hypotonia. In most of these the hypotonia changes to spasticity in later stages of the disorder.

Werdnig-Hoffmann Syndrome

The hypotonic infant might have infantile spinal muscular atrophy (Werdnig-Hoffmann syndrome), secondary to atrophy of the anterior horn cells in the spinal cord and of the brainstem motor nuclei. This disease is transmitted as an autosomal recessive trait. The onset is usually in utero but can appear at any point in the first 2 years of life, with weakness and hypotonia of the intercostal, distal, and proximal limb and tongue muscles. An alert facial expression is maintained. Deep tendon reflexes are absent, and electromyogram findings show denervation with fibrillations and fasciculations. These are easily demonstrated in the tongue. Intelligence is normal. The disease is progressive, and death usually occurs secondary to respiratory failure. Hypotonia, associated with normal deep tendon reflexes and mental alertness, is usually benign, and gradual improvement can be expected.

Myasthenia Gravis

Transient neonatal myasthenia gravis, lasting weeks to months, can occur in infants born to mothers with myasthenia gravis. This disorder of neuromuscular transmission responds rapidly to administration of anticholinesterase drugs.

Congenital Hypertrophic Muscular Dystrophy

Congenital hypertrophic muscular dystrophy (Duchenne's muscular dystrophy) is a rare autosomal recessive disorder in which symptoms rarely appear until 2 to 3 years of age. These youngsters frequently have difficulty climbing stairs or assuming a standing position and often have a waddling gait. Serum muscle enzymes, especially creatine phosphokinase, are elevated in these disorders.

Upper Extremity Paresis

Paresis of the upper extremities can result from nerve damage or clavicular fracture.

Brachial Plexus Injury

Brachial plexus injury can occur in early infancy, often as a result of a traumatic delivery. The roots of C5 and C6 may be injured, causing proximal upper extremity weakness (Erb's palsy), or there may be distal weakness, especially involving hand muscles, when the roots of C7 and C8 are injured (Klumpke's paralysis). These injuries are usually associated with forceful lateral traction and hyperabduction being applied to the infant during delivery.

In Erb's palsy the infant cannot abduct the arm and shoulder, rotate the arm externally, or supinate the forearm. The infant maintains a position of internal rotation and adduction of the upper arm and pronation of the forearm. Hand grasp is preserved. This injury usually involves edema and hemorrhage about nerve fibers; laceration does not usually occur. Unless laceration of the nerve has taken place, function usually returns within a few months. Should laceration have occurred, permanent damage with atrophy of the deltoid muscle and dropping of the shoulder will ensue.

In rarer Klumpke's paralysis, T1 roots are occasionally involved such that ipsilateral miosis and ptosis can be seen in association with a paralyzed hand. If paralysis persists in either condition for more than 6 months, tendon transfer or neuroplasty becomes necessary. Splinting and passive range-of-motion maneuvers of affected joints must be carefully performed to keep the joints sufficiently supple and functionally positioned, so as to maintain range of movement and prevent pulling of antagonistic nonparalyzed muscles.

Clavicular Fracture

During difficult delivery of a shoulder in vertex presentations and during delivery of extended arms in breech presentations, the clavicle can be fractured, causing obliteration of the suprasternal depression, spasm of the sternocleidomastoid muscle, bone irregularity and crepitance, and lack of free movement of the affected arm. As opposed to the problems of brachial plexus palsy, arm immobility due to a fractured clavicle is benign and rapidly resolves. Immobilization with the shoulders and arms held backward for a week or so is all that is indicated.

Limp

Limp associated with hip pathology may be accompanied by hip pain that can be referred to the thigh or knee. The hip is usually externally rotated, and the gait is outtoed. Legg-Calvé-Perthe's disease and slipped capital femoral epiphysis, important entities to be considered in a patient with a limp, are discussed in Chapter 27.

Congenital Hip Dislocation

Congenital hip dislocation has an incidence of 1 to 1.5 per 1000 live births in the general population, with a substantial increase in risk among siblings (40 per 1000) and among identical twins (350 per 1000). Female infants are more commonly affected than are males. Abnormal capsule and ligament laxity secondary to estrogen metabolism and excretion by the mother are believed to play a role in fetal development of this disorder. The condition occurs on the left side more frequently than it does on the right, while bilateral involvement occurs in 25% of cases. First pregnancies are more frequently involved than are any subsequent pregnancies.

Breech extractions increase the incidence of congenital dislocation of the hip. In breech malposition the hips are flexed and the knees are extended. Extension of the hips during breech delivery is a common maneuver. Thus, breech extraction, especially in first-born female infants, is associated with a substantial risk of hip dislocation. In this circumstance the femoral head and acetabulum are of normal configuration, but the angle of anteversion of the proximal femur is 10° to 15° greater than normal.

The majority of hip dislocations are associated with an acetabulum of normal length, depth, and angulation. About 15% of hip dislocations, however, are associated with small, dysplastic acetabula in which the acetabulum faces lateral to its normal position, is foreshortened, and is considerably narrowed. In this condition the femur is displaced superior, lateral, and posterior to its normal positioning. This three-plane displacement accounts for the various clinical and roentgenographic findings.

A dislocatable, unstable hip is detected by Barlow's test, which dislocates the femoral head across the posterior lip of the acetabulum and then allows the femoral head to slip back into the acetabular socket. Ortolani's sign demonstrates frank dislocation by the presence of a palpable click in and out as the hip is reduced by abduction and dislocated by adduction.

Immediate therapy is the prevention of hip adduction and extension, with the femoral head centered in the acetabulum. The effectiveness of simple harness and splinting devices in correcting this disorder diminishes with increased age. Beyond infancy, initial treatment must usually include adductor and psoas muscle releases, surgical reduction, and cast immobilization. Clearly, early diagnosis and management in the neonate are preferable.

Localized Bone or Joint Tenderness

Inflammatory, noninfectious disorders causing bone or joint pain with attendant limb dysfunction have onset more frequently in the preschool-age patient than in any other age group. The most common ultimate diagnosis is juvenile chronic arthritis, most commonly of the pauciarticular type (four or fewer joints involved), often monarticular. Other disorders to be considered and that are discussed later include:

1. postinfective phenomena such as rheumatic fever and Reiter's syndrome
2. allergic disorders such as anaphylactoid purpura and hypersensitivity disorders; these usually cause periarticular rather than discrete articular disease
3. other connective tissue diseases such as psoriatic arthritis, systemic lupus erythematosus, diffuse fasciitis with eosinophilia, scleroderma, mixed connective tissue disease, dermatomyositis, and periarteritis nodosa
4. arthropathy associated with inflammatory bowel diseases such as Crohn's disease and ulcerative colitis
5. inflammatory deficiencies, associated with immunoglobulin deficiencies, especially immunoglobulin A (IgA)

Infiltrative processes may appear initially as bone or joint pain and dysfunction. Juxta-articular epiphyseal involvement resulting from leukemia, neuroblastoma, and histiocytosis is of significance in this group. Direct synovial involvement is also frequently encountered with Lesch-Nyhan syndrome, Farber's syndrome, hypercholesterolemia, and mucopolysaccharidoses.

The inflammatory, infectious disorders of osteomyelitis, septic arthritis, and diskitis, as well as toxic synovitis are covered in Chapter 27. Gonococcal arthritis and Lyme arthritis are discussed later in this chapter.

Bowleg Deformity

Infants normally have leg bowing until 18 months of age, by which time the legs have straightened and even progress to a minimal knock knee (genu valgum). However, progressive bowing of the legs should be evaluated. The initial study is an x-ray taken with the child in a standing position, to evaluate for the presence of tibia vara (Blount's disease) or for renal or nutritional rickets.

Blount's Disease

In Blount's disease there is an irregular medial tibial metaphysis, and distorted tibial epiphyseal center "beaking" occurs at the medial aspect of the proximal tibia as a result of this irregularity. Osteotomy procedures are required to correct this abnormality.

Rickets

In rickets there is suppression of normal calcification and growth of epiphyseal cartilage. An irregular, disrupted epiphyseal line at the end of the shaft results. Inadequate mineralization and the deposition of uncalcified osteoid produces a rachitic metaphysis, characterized by a nonrigid, irregular, frayed, and widened zone. This is easily compressed, causing flaring of the ends of the bones. The earliest radiologic findings of rickets occur in the wrists, although bowlegs are the most frequent limb abnormalities that alert the physician to the possibility of rickets. Appropriate treatment with vitamin D results in radiologic evidence of healing within 4 weeks. The daily requirement of vitamin D to prevent rickets is 400 IU. As much as 5000 IU daily are required to induce healing of rickets, however.

Intoed Gait

The internally rotated foot seen in infants is usually due to metatarsus adductus (varus); when seen in toddlers, it is usually due to internal tibial torsion. Intoed gait seen at age 3 to 4 years is usually the result of the excessive anteversion syndrome or internal femoral torsion.

If metatarsus adductus persists past 6 months of age, it may require treatment with one of various methods: casting, reverse-last shoes and an external rotation splint, or reverse-last shoes with heels tied to each other. It should be noted that metatarsus adductus is often associated with internal tibial torsion, which often persists after the foot deformity is corrected.

The most common cause of intoeing, often noted at the onset of independent walking, is internal tibial torsion. Treatment is directed to prevent the child from sleeping with the feet internally rotated. This is best accomplished by using any of the devices used for treatment of metatarsus adductus.

In internal femoral torsion, femoral neck anteversion, which is normal in the newborn, fails to decrease in the growing child. It usually is first noted at the age of 3 years, most commonly in females, and is usually bilateral. The child has an intoed gait with patellae internally rotated. It usually causes no functional problems in the infant or young child, but if it does not spontaneously improve, it may cause functional or cosmetic disabilities in the older child or adolescent. No devices are effective in treating this disorder. Operative derotational osteotomy gives excellent results but should be reserved for severely disabled youngsters.

Outtoed Gait

Normal infants have externally rotated hips secondary to their intrauterine position. When the infant stands, the feet externally rotate. This spontaneously resolves over the first 3 years and requires no treatment. An outtoed gait, however, should be of concern if it persists beyond 3 years of age or if it is acquired at any time because serious hip pathology may underlie this gait abnormality.

Other causes of out-toed gait include external tibial torsion and a valgus foot. If external tibial torsion presents severe functional and cosmetic difficulties, and does not regress or progresses over time, it is treatable only by tibial derotation osteotomy, as nonoperative treatment is ineffective. Outtoeing caused by an everted valgus flatfoot occurs in children with cerebral palsy or in normal children with hypermobile joints. In most instances of this disorder, no treatment is indicated, although in some situations inner shoe appliances can be useful.

Clubfoot

Congenital foot deformities are referred to as "talipes" because, if untreated, the child will walk on the talus (ankle). Talipes equinovarus (equino-plantar flexion, varus-forefoot adducted, heel and forefoot inverted) is the most severe clubfoot deformity. Talipes calcaneovarus (heel and forefoot are dorsiflexed with toes higher than heel) is the other common form. In utero positioning can cause the newborn foot to develop functional, self-correcting positions that mimic these conditions. If the deformed foot cannot be brought to a neutral or corrected position, a pathologic deformity is present and immediate orthopedic care is indicated. Metatarsus varus deformities (forefoot adduction) occur fairly frequently and may sometimes be mimicked by talipes varus and by metatarsus adductus. These are truly fixed deformities that require splint or cast treatment.

Infantile Cortical Hyperostosis

Infantile cortical hyperostosis is hyperplasia of subperiosteal bone with associated soft tissue edema and discoloration. The cause is unknown. It is abrupt in onset, occurring usually before 5 or 6 months of age, and is associated with hyperirritability and fever. The swollen parts are firm and indurated and are deeply fixed to underlying bones. It may be unifocal, multifocal, or migratory. On rare occasions, recrudescences of swelling and tenderness continue for prolonged periods. The disorder is painful and invariably resolves without treatment, although clinical activity can persist for 9 or 10 months. The mandible and clavicles are most often involved, but long bones in extremities, ribs, and metatarsals have been affected. This disorder is diagnosed by radiologic examination. It was first described by Caffey and Silverman in 1945 and is often referred to as Caffey's disease. Acute osteomyelitis and acute trauma (child abuse) are the major differential diagnoses to consider.

Osteogenesis Imperfecta

Brittle bone disease or osteogenesis imperfecta is seen in two forms. The severe, congenital form is an autosomal recessive disorder usually manifest at birth and characterized by skeletal deformities resulting from intrauterine fractures that healed in abnormal positions and fractures that occurred at the time of delivery. Skull fractures, intracranial bleeding, and progressive hydrocephalus occur. The infants have blue sclerae, deafness with otosclerosis, and teeth that emerge discolored and misshapened. Many succumb to the intracranial insults. Those who survive require many restorative orthopedic procedures. The tarda form of osteogenesis imperfecta is autosomal dominant, less severe, and the more common form of this disorder. Lower limb fractures occur after the first year. Blue sclerae, otosclerosis, and hypoplastic, discolored teeth occur in this form as well.

Painful Knees

Disease in the hip may be referred to the knee, and an examination of the hip should be part of any examination of a knee complaint.

Chondromalacia of the Patella

Patellar chondromalacia is an internal derangement of the knee joint caused by stressful forces on the patella, producing degeneration of the cartilage. A common cause is the excessive anteversion syndrome, which produces an intoed gait with internal rotation of the patellae. It occurs most commonly in adolescent girls. The patella is painful, and there is intermittent effusion and subpatellar crepitus associated with lateral movement of the patella when the knee is being extended. Avoidance of strain by limiting stair climbing, squatting, or prolonged sitting in a flexed position is helpful, as are simple quadriceps-setting exercises. Patellectomy is indicated in only the most severely pained patients.

Osgood-Schlatter Disease

Tenderness and pain in the tibial tuberosity in a young teenager should provoke suspicion of Osgood-Schlatter's disease. It is a sequela of avulsion of the patellar ligament with attached cartilaginous or bony fragments from the tibial tuberosity. The disorder is more frequent in boys than in girls. Knee pain is the initial complaint, with most of the pain at the end of active extension or flexion of the knee. The best x-ray film is taken with the knee rotated inward, giving a tangential view of the affected tibial tuberosity. Soft tissue swelling, an opaque patellar ligament, and a fragmented tuberosity are seen. Relief is provided by rest. In girls the onset is usually between the ages of 10 and 14 years; in boys, between the ages of 12 and 15 years.

Painful Feet

The painful foot is a frequent complaint of the older child or adolescent. The disorders involved are most frequently seen in the obese youngster or in a child undergoing a growth spurt.

Flatfoot

Persistence of foot pronation because of laxity of ligaments supporting the foot causes a wide-based stance that places the weight on the medial aspect of the foot. The strain of continued attempts to shift weight bearing laterally toward the center of the foot results in foot and ankle aching, calf cramping at night, and easy fatigue. Relief is brought with support to the medial longitudinal arch.

Tarsal Coalition

Tarsal coalition is a synostosis between two or more tarsal bones, causing a rigid flatfoot that is often associated with osteochondral inflammatory synovitis. The peroneal or posterior tibial tendon is often sprained, and the subtalar joint is restricted in motion. The inflammation responds to cast immobilization and anti-inflammatory agents. With time the x-ray film shows joint space narrowing with hyperostosis of the talonavicular joint and an irregular talar head. Subtalar motion becomes restricted, and a reactive bone spur forms dorsolaterally on the talar head. Persistence of symptoms despite casting and medications necessitates excision of the coalition. In the older teenager arthrodesis may be required to relieve the pain.

Köhler's Disease

Köhler's disease is an osteochondrosis of the tarsal navicular bone that causes moderate pain at the inner aspect of the midtarsal part of the foot. The patient (usually a boy) walks either on the outer side of the foot or flat-footedly and exhibits some local warmth. There is aseptic necrosis of the ossification center of the tarsal navicular bone; which usually heals spontaneously. The peak age of onset is between 3 and 7 years.

Freiberg's Disease

Freiberg's disease, an osteochondrosis of a metatarsal head (usually the second metatarsal bone), occurs in girls four times more frequently than in boys and is most commonly seen between the ages of 12 and 14 years. There is pain on walking, referred to the region of the affected metatarsal. Plantar pressure elicits tenderness, as does abrupt release of this pressure. Dorsal swelling in the area of the implicated metatarsophalangeal joint ensues, with limitation of plantar function and flattening of the transverse arch of the affected foot. Callus develops on the plantar surface of the foot in the region of the diseased metatarsal head. A deformed, flattened metatarsal head is seen on x-ray. Discontinuation of wearing high heels, avoidance of long walks until the symptoms subside, and symptomatic use of anti-inflammatory agents are recommended treatments.

Back Pain

Spondylolysis and Spondylolisthesis

Spondylolysis, a defect in the continuity of the pars interarticularis of the posterior portion of L4 or L5, may result in forward slippage of the vertebral body, known as spondylolisthesis. The horizontal slippage most commonly involves the fifth lumbar vertebral body moving anteriorly in relationship to S1. This deformity can occur anywhere in the vertebral column, however. Spondylolysis often causes back pain before the spondylolisthesis develops. On physical examination one notes flattening of the normal lumbar lordosis with posterior tilting of the pelvis. Trauma, causing disruption of the pars interarticularis, is believed to be the cause of spondylolysis. Genetic factors are believed to be prominent. The propensity for spondylolysis to become spondylolisthesis with forward slippage is exaggerated during the growth spurts. An oblique x-ray film demonstrates the effect of the pars interarticularis on spondylolysis, and a standing lateral x-ray film demonstrates spondylolisthesis. Activities causing hyperextension of the lumbar spine should be avoided, and exercises to reduce lumbar lordosis can relieve the pain of spondylolysis. Once slippage occurs, spinal fusion by surgery is a necessity.

Scoliosis and Kyphosis

Lateral deviation of the spine is termed scoliosis, and excessive posterior curvature of the thoracic spine is termed kyphosis. Scoliosis can be nonstructural (corrects with side bending) or structural (no improvement with position change). Nonstructural scoliosis is secondary to posture, leg length inequality, muscle spasm, or hysteria. Structural disease is congenital (e.g., absent or fused spinal segments), metabolic (e.g., juvenile osteoporosis), neuromuscular, or idiopathic in origin. The most common is idiopathic scoliosis in the adolescent, seen more commonly in girls than in boys. When the patient bends forward, prominence of one scapula, one side of the rib cage, or lumbar paraspinous muscles can indicate the site and direction of the scoliosis. Pulmonary restriction, significant back pain, and cosmetic deformity are the sequelae of unrecognized and untreated disease. Curves of less than 15° do not require immediate care. Curves of greater than 20° require immediate orthopedic intervention with bracing, and those in excess of 40° require surgical fusion.

Scheuermann's Disease

Scheuermann's disease, a cause of kyphosis, is an osteochondrosis that involves anterior wedging of vertebral bodies. The abnormality is usually in the lower thoracic spine, causing thoracic kyphosis. This can be disablingly painful. Exercises, casting, and bracing are indicated; in rare instances spinal fusion is necessary. The peak age of onset of this disorder is between 14 and 19 years.

Bone Tumors

Malignant Tumors

Occult malignancy is always a possibility in a child with unexplained musculoskeletal pain, joint swelling, or fever. Leukemia often involves large joints with a pauciarticular (four or fewer joints) involvement. Initially, it is frequently mistaken for rheumatoid arthritis. Severe, excruciating pain, unusual in rheumatologic disease, is seen more often in leukemia and should arouse suspicion. Bone tumors occur most commonly in adolescence and usually appear at the end of growth peaks. They can be osteogenic, chondrogenic, collagenic, or myelogenic in origin and are demonstrable radiologically.

Osteogenic sarcoma involves long bones at the metaphyseal ends and often metastasizes before a primary lesion is found. Its peak age of appearance is 10 to 15 years. The most frequent initial findings are pain at the site of the tumor and signs and symptoms associated with pulmonary metastases, such as dyspnea and pneumothorax. Amputation and chemotherapy are indicated.

Chondrosarcoma is less frequently seen. It is usually a disorder of adolescence. Its most frequent sites of origin are the pelvis and shoulder. It metastasizes by local extension. This is a radioresistant tumor requiring amputation and chemotherapy.

Fibrosarcomas are the major collagen-producing bone malignancies. They occur in long bones throughout childhood. They grow slowly and recur locally, rather than by metastatic spread. Surgical excision is indicated.

Of the marrow tumors in childhood, Ewing's sarcoma and reticulum cell sarcoma are the most common other than the leukemias and lymphomas (including Hodgkin's disease). Pain and swelling at the tumor site herald its presence. The pelvis and femur are the most frequent sites of involvement. The x-ray film characteristically demonstrates a bone lesion with a surrounding soft tissue mass. Calcification of periosteum lifted away from the bone causes a characteristic "sunburst" appearance. High-dose irradiation and chemotherapy are indicated.

Benign Tumors

Nonmalignant bone lesions can be arranged by tissue of origin in a manner similar to that of neoplasms. Of the osteogenic group, osteoid osteoma, osteoblastoma, osteoma, and osteochondroma are the major lesions. Both osteoid osteoma and osteoblastoma are reparative rather than infiltrative. Osteoid osteoma occurs in long bones and the posterior portion of the vertebrae, and osteoblastoma occurs in neural arches of the vertebral column. Pain is the usual complaint, especially at night, and is quickly relieved by aspirin. On x-ray film one sees a hyperostotic lesion surrounding a nidus of sclerotic bone separated by a radiolucent zone. Surgical excision is curative. Osteomas arise in the periosteum of the cranium and are best left untreated. Osteochondroma is the most commonly seen lesion in this group. This tumor arises from the epiphyses and grows toward metaphyses, and can cause secondary adjacent joint deformity. These tumors have malignant potential and should be excised as soon as noted.

Of the chondrogenic group, chondroblastomas arising in epiphyses of long bones, causing chronic joint pain and lytic lesions on x-ray films, occur in teenagers. The two metaphyseal tumors in this group are enchondroma and chondromyxoid fibroma. Enchondromata are common in the hands and feet, whereas chondromyxoid fibromata occur in long bones. If painful, they should be excised or curetted.

The collagenic group of benign bone tumors should be curetted if they cause structural bone fragility and the potential for fracture. This category includes periosteal desmoids (distal femur), distal cortical defects (distal femur and tibia), ossifying fibromata (long bone), and fibrous dysplasia (ribs).

Of the marrow tumors, lipomas are best left untreated unless they cause pain by bone expansion. Histiocytosis X (eosinophilic granuloma), which can involve the skull, mandible, ribs, humerus, and proximal femur in metaphyseal areas, should be curetted and treated with radiation.

CONSTITUTIONAL SYNDROMES WITH MAJOR MUSCULOSKELETAL MANIFESTATIONS

Acute Rheumatic Fever

Acute rheumatic fever is closely related to and must follow a streptococcal respiratory tract infection and occurs most commonly between 5 and 10 years of age. The peak incidence of first attacks of rheumatic fever is between the ages of 6 and 10 years, most often in winter and spring months. About 3% of children with untreated streptococcal respiratory tract infections develop acute rheumatic fever. A latent period between subsidence of the streptococcal infection and the first symptoms of rheumatic fever, usually arthritis and fever, is typical and may last from 1 to 5 weeks. The arthritis characteristically is migratory and involves large peripheral joints. Fingers, toes, hips, and spine are rarely, if ever, involved. The pain is intense and diffuse over the entire involved joint. Arthralgia may occur in a few joints and true arthritis in others. Tachycardia, holosystolic and middiastolic murmurs, cardiomegaly, and pericarditis all herald the onset of the serious rheumatic carditis. Distinctive erythema marginatum is rare and transient, and subcutaneous nodules appear late in the disease. The major criteria (modified Jones criteria) must be met and solid supporting evidence of antecedent streptococcal infection must exist before this diagnosis can be made. The arthritis is exquisitely responsive to aspirin. Once the diagnosis is made firmly, lifelong continuous prophylaxis with penicillin (or erythromycin in penicillin-sensitive patients) is indicated to prevent the severe cardiac damage associated with subsequent attacks. Even those patients who did not experience carditis in an initial episode warrant prophylaxis.

Juvenile Chronic Rheumatoid Arthritis Syndromes

This group of disorders, often referred to as JRA, is characterized by chronic synovitis, fever, and subsequent extra-articular manifestations. There are major subgroups based on clinical manifestations at onset. Three of the groups occur primarily in girls, and two occur primarily in boys. The onset is either pauciarticular (four or fewer joints involved), or polyarticular (five or more joints involved). Ninety percent or more of all forms are negative for rheumatoid factor. The presence of rheumatoid factor implies "adult type" disease with erosive dysfunctional changes. Fewer than 1% of young children and fewer than 10% of adolescent girls are positive for rheumatoid factor. Of the seronegative groupings, the polyarticular group is the largest and girls predominate. Any joint can be involved, and severe, deforming arthritis occurs in about 30% of cases. Of the two pauciarticular groups, type I occurs mainly in young girls, has a high risk for iridocyclitis and a very low risk for deforming arthritis. Type II, seen mainly in boys, involves large joints and carries a high risk for development of spondyloarthropathy; many of these youngsters are HLA-B-27 positive. The final subgroup, seen mainly in boys, has a systemic onset with fever, rash, pericarditis, and pleuritis; about 20% of these youngsters have severe arthritis sequelae.

The major concern in children with JRA is the differential diagnosis of other disorders, including malignancy (mainly leukemia) and infective processes. Often, the diagnosis cannot be made with confidence early in the disease, and one can make the diagnosis only after observing chronic arthropathy without other evidence of associated systemic manifestations of other disorders. Maintenance of full activity, preservation of normal epiphyseal growth, and careful ophthalmologic surveillance are the major challenges of the physician caring for youngsters with JRA.

There are several clinical findings that strongly suggest the diagnosis of JRA: narrowing and/or erosion of posterior zygapophyseal joints of the cervical spine, even without clinical complaints in the neck; fusiform swelling of proximal interphalangeal joints; iridocyclitis with peripheral arthritis; and evidence for a chronic course, such as flexion contractures, osteoporosis, and cartilage articular cysts. However, their absence does not exclude the diagnosis.

The treatment includes nonsteroidal anti-inflammatory medication (e.g., aspirin), physical therapy to restore normal function, and twice yearly slit lamp surveillance.

Arthritis with Inflammatory Bowel Disease

Inflammatory bowel disease often becomes manifest in children with a pauciarticular arthritis involving large joints. The majority of children have only the peripheral arthritis, which is nondestructive and essentially coincides with the activity of the bowel disease. Treatment of the bowel disease suppresses this form of the arthritis. Many children develop ankylosing spondylitis, which is independent of bowel activity. In these instances nonsteroidal anti-inflammatory drugs are necessary. The associated disorders usually seen in this setting are ulcerative colitis and Crohn's disease, although there are some patients who develop a transient arthropathy associated with *Shigella*, *Salmonella*, or *Yersinia* gastrointestinal disease. HLA-B-27 positivity is seen with very high frequency in this group.

Psoriatic Arthritis

This disorder is the basis of chronic arthropathy in 15% of the actively arthritic youngsters evaluated in the Rheumatology Clinic of The Johns Hopkins Hospital. The arthritis is asymmetric and characteristically involves distal interphalangeal joints. Either the psoriasis or the arthritis can be manifested first, with a very low incidence of concurrent onset.

Sacroiliitis and ankylosing spondylitis appear frequently. Physical therapy to the joints and the use of nonsteroidal anti-inflammatory drugs are indicated. The skin disease, especially nail involvement, should be treated cautiously and conservatively. Slit lamp surveillance for uveal tract inflammation is indicated at twice yearly intervals. There is frequently a very strong family history for psoriasis in youngsters with this disorder.

Spondylitis Arthritis Syndromes

All of these disorders are associated with an increased incidence of HLA-B-27 positivity. The most frequently seen is the pauciarticular form of JRA with ankylosing spondylitis, which was discussed in an earlier section. All of these conditions are associated with seronegativity for rheumatoid factor.

Reiter's Disease

Reiter's disease includes sterile urethritis, ocular inflammation, and arthritis with skin rash and occasional gastroenteritis. The arthritis is pauciarticular, affecting large joints; heel pain and Achilles tendonitis are common. Sacroiliitis is seen with great frequency and should be sought even in the absence of flagrant symptoms. Treatment is with physical therapy and the use of nonsteroidal anti-inflammatory agents, including aspirin.

Systemic Lupus Erythematosus

This disorder mimics many rheumatologic disorders and, when seen in children, often is manifested by fever, rash, and arthropathy. The presence of renal disease and the form of glomerular involvement, if renal disease is present, determines to a great extent the long-term prognosis. The arthropathy usually presents as arthralgia and joint stiffness, and only rarely is there warmth and swelling. Deforming arthritis is almost never seen, and the only major long-term disabilities of the musculoskeletal system are those secondary to aseptic necrosis, usually of the femur, secondary vasculitis or the use of corticosteroids. Acute musculoskeletal distress may be associated with inflammatory myositis or tenosynovitis. Nonsteroidal treatment is appropriate unless there is one or more of the following: renal disease, seizures and other manifestations of central nervous system disease, platelet antibodies, or circulating anticoagulant. In these instances, steroid therapy is indicated. The American Rheumatism Association has published a listing of definite weighted criteria for the diagnosis of this disorder. In order that the diagnosis be made with certainty, five or more of the criteria must be present. However, if a high-titer antinuclear antibody is present, four criteria are sufficient, and if specific antinative DNA antibody is present in high titer, the diagnosis is firm. The criteria include

1. facial erythema or butterfly eruption
2. discoid lupus
3. Raynaud's phenomenon
4. alopecia
5. photosensitivity
6. oral or nasopharyngeal lesions
7. nondeforming arthritis
8. lupus erythematosus cells
9. chronic false-positive serologic test for syphilis
10. profuse proteinuria (greater than 3.5 g/d)
11. cellular casts in urine sediment
12. pleuritis or pericarditis
13. psychosis of seizures
14. hemolytic anemia, marked leukopenia, or marked thrombocytopenia

High circulating titers of anti-DNA antibodies and marked hypocomplemententemia are important laboratory markers of disease activity.

Myositis

Following viral respiratory epidemics, especially influenza, patients are sometimes seen with a transient inflammatory myositis involving major proximal muscles. A skin rash is absent. Muscle biopsy findings are similar to those of dermatomyositis. In this setting, short-term corticosteroid therapy is indicated unless there is rapid, spontaneous improvement.

Dermatomyositis

This systemic angiopathy of childhood mainly involves skin and striated muscle, but vessels in any organ can be affected. The usual clinical complaints are fatigue and weakness, with the proximal muscles of the thigh, upper arms, and neck involved initially. A characteristic violaceous rash involves the periorbital tissues and a heliotropic and atrophic, scaly, erythematous, edematous rash occurs over surfaces of joints (Gottron's rash). The pediatric patient always has dermatologic abnormalities in the chronic form of this disorder. Serum muscle enzymes (creatine phosphokinase, aldolase) and the erythrocyte sedimentation rate are elevated. Characteristic inflammatory myopathic patterns are seen on electromyography, and muscle biopsy shows perivascular mononuclear infiltrates and fiber size variation. The gastrointestinal tract is frequently involved, with loss of esophageal peristalsis and vasculitic changes in the proximal small bowel. Aggressive early and prolonged use of steroids plus muscle-strengthening physical therapy is indicated. In approximately 20% of cases, healing of the lesion is associated with calcium phosphate deposition in previously inflamed areas. The sheathlike deposits often erode through skin and present major infectious and cosmetic difficulties.

Mixed Connective Tissue Disease

This rheumatic disorder usually has the clinical features of polyarthritis, Raynaud's phenomenon, rash, myositis, lymphadenopathy, autoimmune thyroiditis, and parotiditis. The major musculoskeletal complaints are related to muscle pain and weakness and joint tenderness (usually hands and wrists). The invariable presence of high-titer, speckled antinuclear antibodies, composed mainly of antibody to ribonucleoprotein-extractable nuclear antigen, sets this disorder apart. The patients often have esophageal as well as interstitial pulmonary abnormalities. The acute syndrome usually responds promptly to systemic steroids, although the sclerodermatous component is resistant and ultimately becomes the major clinical challenge. Membranous nephritis is a rare but severe complication.

Scleroderma

This chronic inflammatory disturbance of the epidermis and dermis may sometimes involve the gastrointestinal tract, lung, kidneys, and heart. In children the usual manifestations are focal areas of cutaneous involvement occurring in a linear pattern, usually unilateral. This is known as morphea, and the lesions usually begin as painful, thickened, erythematous patches or areas of atrophy along an extremity. Involved joints are "stiff," and flexion contractures are common concomitants. Progressive systemic sclerosis is characterized by a symmetrical pattern and involvement of hands, feet, distal extremities, and face with induration binding the skin to underlying structures, plus Raynaud's phenomenon, cutaneous ulcers, and synovitis of small joints. This severe form usually includes esophageal dysfunction and intestinal, renal, pulmonary, and cardiac disease. The prognosis for life is excellent in morphea and dismal in progressive systemic disease. No medical therapy has been useful, but substantial benefits accrue from early aggressive physical therapy to prevent or ameliorate crippling contractures.

Shulman's Diffuse Eosinophilic Fasciitis

This recently described disorder is histologically and clinically distinct from the scleroderma group of disorders. The patient frequently has a history of unusual physical exertion antedating the appearance of thickened, rivuleted (orange peel) skin on one or more extremities, associated with stiffened joints and tenderness. The peripheral blood shows a striking eosinophilia and immunoglobulins are elevated. A through-and-through biopsy reveals normal epidermal and dermal structures with a marked thickened fibrosis and perivascular inflammation of the deep fascia. Systemic steroids provide prompt relief.

Vasculitis Syndromes

Vasculitis syndromes appear in the pediatric population in various ways but usually include musculoskeletal complaints. Henoch-Schönlein syndrome is a frequently encountered example. When muscular arteries are involved in an inflammatory process, the disease is a polyarteritis that can be manifested as Kawasaki disease, infantile periarteritis, or Wegener's granulomatosis.

Henoch-Schönlein Syndrome

Henoch-Schönlein syndrome, or anaphylactoid purpura, is a nonnecrotizing capillary inflammatory vasculitis that may involve multiple systems. Schönlein described the combination of purpuric rash, periarticular arthritis, and nephritis; Henoch added the description of colicky abdominal pain and bloody diarrhea to the syndrome. Manifestations of the syndrome may occur sequentially over several weeks or, with acute onset, they may appear simultaneously. In the majority of instances, swelling of large joints (knees and ankles), tenderness, and painful motion are present. Occasionally, there is true serous effusion, although in the majority of instances, periarticular swelling is the finding. Edematous, hemorrhagic bowel wall inflammation causes the abdominal pain and bloody diarrhea, and intussusception can result. The focal nephritis is usually benign, although in a very small percentage of cases, it may progress to chronic renal disease. The course is variable and intermittent and may recur over several months. In the absence of severe renal disease, prognosis is superb for a full recovery.

Kawasaki Disease

Kawasaki disease is a mucocutaneous lymph node syndrome; it is diagnosed on clinical grounds, based on at least 5 days of prolonged high fever with associated conjunctivitis, stomatitis, palm and sole erythema with desquamation of the terminal digits, lymphadenopathy, and the rash of erythema multiforme. The digits initially are diffusely swollen and usually quite tender, with specific interphalangeal joint arthralgia. In most cases there is complete recovery, although coronary artery vasculitis can cause death in about 3% of patients. Laboratory studies show an elevated erythrocyte sedimentation rate and profound thrombocytosis. Aspirin is useful for symptomatic relief and for reducing platelet adhesiveness. Early intervention with IV administration of unsplit gamma globulin reduces likelihood of coronary vessel disease.

Periarteritis Nodosa

Periarteritis nodosa involves small arteries and usually is manifested by arthritis, myositis, erythematous and purpuric rashes, cutaneous ulcers, and edema. The diagnosis is made by arteriography or kidney biopsy. Positive laboratory studies may include an elevated erythrocyte sedimentation rate, eosinophilia, and anemia. Steroids are useful in suppressing the inflammatory phenomena.

Wegener's Granulomatosis

Wegener's granulomatosis is a systemic necrotizing vasculitis involving primarily the upper respiratory tract, lungs, and kidneys. Although arthritis and myositis are present in some cases, destructive granulomatous lesions associated with this systemic vasculitis are most prominent in the lungs and kidney. Cytotoxic agents are mandatory to achieve clinical remission.

Gonococcal Arthritis Syndrome

Gonococcal arthritis is usually associated with gonococcal infection of the urethra or other portions of the genitourinary tract. When wrists and ankle joints are involved, there is often an associated tenosynovitis, which is very characteristic of this syndrome. Skin lesions, which are hemorrhagic and contain necrotic centers, are often found on extremities, clustered around joints. It is not unusual for adolescent girls to report premenstrual polyarthralgia for several cycles prior to the onset of the full-blown syndrome. In the systemic form of the syndrome, with fever, chills, skin lesions, and positive blood cultures, multiple large and small joints are involved. In the more common localized form, blood cultures are negative, there are minimal systemic symptoms, and a monarticular arthritis is seen; the organism may be recovered from the synovial fluid. Thayer-Martin medium, a specially prepared chocolate agar to which antibiotics have been added, inhibits growth of organisms other than *Neisseria* and should be used to cultivate suspect specimens. Disseminated infection requires the use of aqueous, crystalline penicillin G in bactericidal doses for 10 days.

Lyme Arthritis

First described in 1975, this tick-transmitted, multiple system, immune-mediated inflammatory disorder usually occurs in the summer months in the areas of distribution of two tick species, *Ixodes dammini* and *I. pacificus,* in individuals with alloantigen DRW 2. It begins with an annular skin lesion, erythema chronicum migrans, that appears similar to erythema multiforme but does not involve mucous membranes, palms, or soles. In small numbers of patients, a fluctuating meningoencephalitis or myocarditis with heart block can occur weeks after onset of the rash. Frank arthritis occurs in half of those with the rash; its onset can occur months after erythema chronicum migrans and appears as brief recurrent attacks in large joints, occasionally in a migratory pattern. Occasionally, knee involvement can become chronic, with cartilage erosion and pannus. When a patient with rash is found to have high IgM levels and cryoglobulins containing IgM, one can confidently expect the arthritis to appear weeks to months later. The rash should be treated with penicillin, and the arthritis, with high levels of aspirin. Steroids have been found useful in meningoencephalitis and heart block.

Hemoglobin Disorders

Bone infarction, as observed in the various hemoglobinopathies, including sickle cell disease, results from occlusion of small local blood vessels by thrombi of abnormal red cells. These sites of ischemic bone necrosis can occur in tubular bones or in vertebral bodies. In young children the shafts of the phalanges and the metacarpal and metatarsal bones become infarcted, causing pain and dysfunction, sometimes with associated adjacent synovial effusion. On x-rays films there is evidence of repair, with periosteal new bone formation, patches of radiolucency, and areas of radiopacity. In older children and teenagers, the long tubular bones are sites of ischemia; the proximal portion of the femurs is most commonly involved, often with necrosis of the capital femoral epiphysis. In this group of disorders, hematogenous infection of one or more bones or joints can occur, usually as a result of *Salmonella* bacteremia, which often follows a hematologic crisis, with the osteomyelitis developing at the site of a bone infarct. *Salmonella* osteomyelitis is a less acute and less destructive process than that seen with staphylococcal disease.

β-Thalassemia major can be associated with brief episodes of joint pain, swelling, and stiffness in which there is widening of the medullary spaces, osteoporosis, thin cortices, and microfractures. These patients have characteristic "mongoloid" facial features because of the thickening of cranial bones and the nasal recession.

Hemophilias

The manifestations of factor VIII deficiency (hemophilia) and factor IX deficiency (Christmas disease), both seen in males, include repeated intra-articular hemorrhage leading to destructive changes, with associated hypertrophy and hypervascularity of the synovium. (Partial factor VIII deficiency—Von Willebrand's disease—is seen in both sexes and rarely produces joint bleeding.) Any joint can be involved, although the knees are most frequently affected, with elbows and ankles next in frequency. In some instances a single joint is involved repeatedly; in other cases various joints are involved from time to time. Pain is the initial complaint, which is then followed by joint distension. The initial bleeding is primarily intracapsular if it is spontaneous, with extracapsular hemorrhage occurring only if direct trauma has taken place. The first attack is usually followed by a return to normal joint appearance and function within a few weeks. After multiple attacks, chronic arthritis occurs with synovial membrane thickening. The joint remains enlarged, painful, and contracted, with adjacent muscle atrophy and weakness.

Treatment includes replacement of the deficient factor and immobilization of the joint. Aspiration is rarely indicated. Once pain and spasm have subsided, remobilization of the joint and rehabilitation of adjacent muscles should begin. In those instances in which chronic arthritis and bony overgrowth have occurred, nonaspirin, nonsteroidal anti-inflammatory agents can be useful, and tendon releases or arthroplasties may be necessary.

Endocrine Diseases

Several metabolic disorders related to thyroid, adrenal, and parathyroid dysfunction can cause myopathic disorders that are reversible after correction of the myopathy. It should be noted that because most primary muscle disorders present with proximal limb weakness, one must be careful to exclude hip or shoulder pathology, fracture, infection, or inflammation as a primary phenomenon, with the muscle weakness being secondary.

Metabolic Disorders

Limited joint mobility involving small or large joints, predominantly the hand, have been seen and associated with juvenile onset diabetes mellitus. This is believed to be closely associated with generalized microvascular phenomena that affect the soft tissues adjacent to the affected joints. Those patients with diabetes who develop this phenomenon are at high risk for retinal and renal microvascular disease.

Farber's Lipogranulomatosis

Farber's lipogranulomatosis, or foam cell granulomata, results from a deficiency of acid ceramidase and produces synovial plaques and associated arthropathy, which is painful and deforming. Joint function can be improved with anti-inflammatory agents and physical therapy. Chlorambucil has been effective in several case reports.

Nodular Panniculitis

In relapsing nodular panniculitis, subcutaneous nodules appear on the extremities, with adjacent pain, redness, and warmth. When these are recurrent, systemic steroid therapy is found to be useful.

Pancreatitis and Pancreatic Pseudocysts

Acute and chronic pancreatitis and pancreatic pseudocysts cause disseminated fat necrosis associated with tender, erythematous nodules and soft tissue swelling over digits. Measurement of serum amylase and lipase leads to the underlying disorder.

Hypervitaminosis A

Chronic ingestion of large doses of vitamin A causes cortical hyperostosis of the ulna, tibia, clavicles, and metatarsals and associated periosteal elevation and epiphyseal destruction, with tender swelling of soft tissues adjacent to the involved bony area. Children with this condition are irritable, apathetic, alopecic, polydipsic, and complain of limb pain. Hypervitaminosis A has been seen with increased frequency in children whose families subscribe to megavitamin panaceas. Successful treatment can occur by removing the noxious dosages.

Lymphedemas

Diffuse, permanent, pitting edema due to obstruction of lymph drainage can occur secondary to acquired obliteration of lymph nodes or lymphatics. It can also be seen as part of Milroy's disease or as part of the syndrome of gonadal dysgenesis (Turner's syndrome). Congenital lymphedema is often associated with extra eyelashes, yellow nails, and recurrent cholestasis. The marginally adequate or obliterated lymphatics, which are evident in the acquired form, usually appear in teenage girls and are secondary to infection caused by staphylococci or streptococci, cat scratch antigen, filiarisis, fibrosis, immune responses, or malignant infiltration. If a primary cause is not uncovered, symptomatic decrease of swelling can be achieved with local compression garments.

Functional Limb Pain

The most frequently seen rheumatic complaint is that of "growing pains," described as aching or heaviness, predominately in the lower limbs and nonarticular. The pain typically occurs late in the day or at night and is eased by gentle rubbing. The child is well and has had normal growth and development. There is no tenderness, erythema, or swelling of the pained extremity. The erythrocyte sedimentation rate, white blood cell count, and hemoglobin level are normal. Emotional disturbances associated with tension states are common in this group of children and in their families. Pubertal girls who have generalized joint laxity and who are otherwise normal tend to have discomfort after exercise, especially in the lower extremities. True hysteria, whether it be conversion hysteria or hysterical prolongation of symptoms of an organic disease, usually involves one limb or one joint. The child cannot move the limb or straighten the joint, but on examination the part is normal. The disability is disproportional to any objective evidence of muscle weakness or joint deformity. Underlying precipitating psychologic stresses at home or in school should be sought and addressed.

Bibliography

Arnold W: Hemophilic arthropathy. *J Bone Joint Surg [Am]* 1977;59:287.

Bohan A: Medical progress—polymyositis and dermatomyositis. *N Engl J Med* 1975;292:344, 403.

Boone J: Juvenile rheumatoid arthritis. *Pediatr Clin North Am* 1974;21:885.

Caffey J, Silverman WA: Infantile cortical hyperostoses; preliminary report on a new syndrome. *Am J Roentgenol* 1945;54:1.

Dubowitz V: *Muscle Disorders in Childhood.* (ed.) WB Saunders, Co., Philadelphia, 1978.

Espinoza L: Joint manifestations of sickle cell disease. *Medicine* 1974;53:295.

Jaffe H: *Metabolic, Degenerative and Inflammatory Diseases of Bones and Joints.* Philadelphia, Lea & Febiger, 1972.

Kempe C: Pediatric implications of the battered baby syndrome. *Arch Dis Child* 1971;46:28.

Markowitz M: *Rheumatic Fever,* ed 2. Philadelphia, WB Saunders Co, 1972.

Meislin AG and Rothfield N: System lupus erythematosus in childhood: Analysis of 42 cases, with comparative data on 200 adult cases followed concurrently. *Pediatrics* 1968;42:37–49.

Morrey B: Septic arthritis in children. *Orthop Clin North Am* 1975;6:923.

Oetgen WJ, Boice JA, and Lawless OJ: Mixed connective tissue disease in children and adolescents. *Pediatrics* 1981;67:333–337.

Sills E: Psoriatic arthritis in childhood. *J Hopkins Med J* 1980;146:49.

Sills E: Diffuse fasciitis with Eosinophilia in childhood. *J Hopkins Med J* 1982;151:203–207.

Staheli L: Torsional deformities in children. *Journal of Continuing Education in Pediatrics* 1978;20:11.

Steere AC, Grodzicki RL, Kornblatt AN, et al: The spirochetal etiology of Lyme disease. *New Eng J Med* 1983;308:733–742.

Taft LT: Cerebral palsy. *Pediatric Annals,* (December) 1973;2:5–91.

William Herndon

Musculoskeletal Trauma

26

Trauma is now the leading cause of death in children. Extremity injuries in children represent a significant proportion of injuries seen in an emergency department setting. Musculoskeletal injuries often are present in the multiply injured patient, even though injuries to other organ systems frequently take precedence. Attention to the airway and vital signs goes without saying; intrathoracic and intra-abdominal injuries may be life-threatening and need to be delineated and stabilized before attention is directed to the extremity injury. Emergency management of musculoskeletal trauma in multiply injured children is outlined in Figure 26-1.

INITIAL EVALUATION

Examination of an injured child can be time consuming and frustrating, but must be carefully performed. The examiner should look for obvious deformity, malalignment, or swelling. Wounds should be sought; the presence of abrasions or contusions may suggest the mechanism of injury. Fractures are tender. This may seem obvious, but frequently an orthopedist is asked to see a patient with a questionable roentgenographic abnormality in an area that is clinically totally asymptomatic! Stability of injured joints must be carefully and gently checked. Torn ligaments are uncommon in children and adolescents, and what seems to be an unstable joint caused by ligamentous instability may in reality be a fracture through an open growth plate. This is most common in the distal femur of adolescent males. Ligamentous disruption is rarely encountered and stress x-ray films are necessary to make the diagnosis (Figure 26-2). As in adults, complete disruption usually requires surgical repair. Dislocations are unusual and are often accompanied by a fracture.

The circulatory status of any injured extremity must be rapidly assessed. Examination begins with the general color and temperature of the limb, comparing it to the uninjured side. It is important to remember that cool, clammy extremities can signify shock; the distal extremity should be assessed for good capillary refill. The peripheral pulses must be checked carefully. A Doppler ultrasonic monitor may indicate their presence or a change in their status. Absence of a pulse does not guarantee that the vascular status is compromised nor does the presence of a pulse assure adequate circulation. Severe pain in the forearm or calf, pain with passive stretch of the fingers or toes, or sensory deficit in the distal extremity are more important indicators and, if present, imply ischemia of the extremity. Ischemia may be secondary to arterial injury or to a compartment syndrome in which increased tissue pressure within a muscular compartment leads to compromise of blood flow in the arterioles and cap-

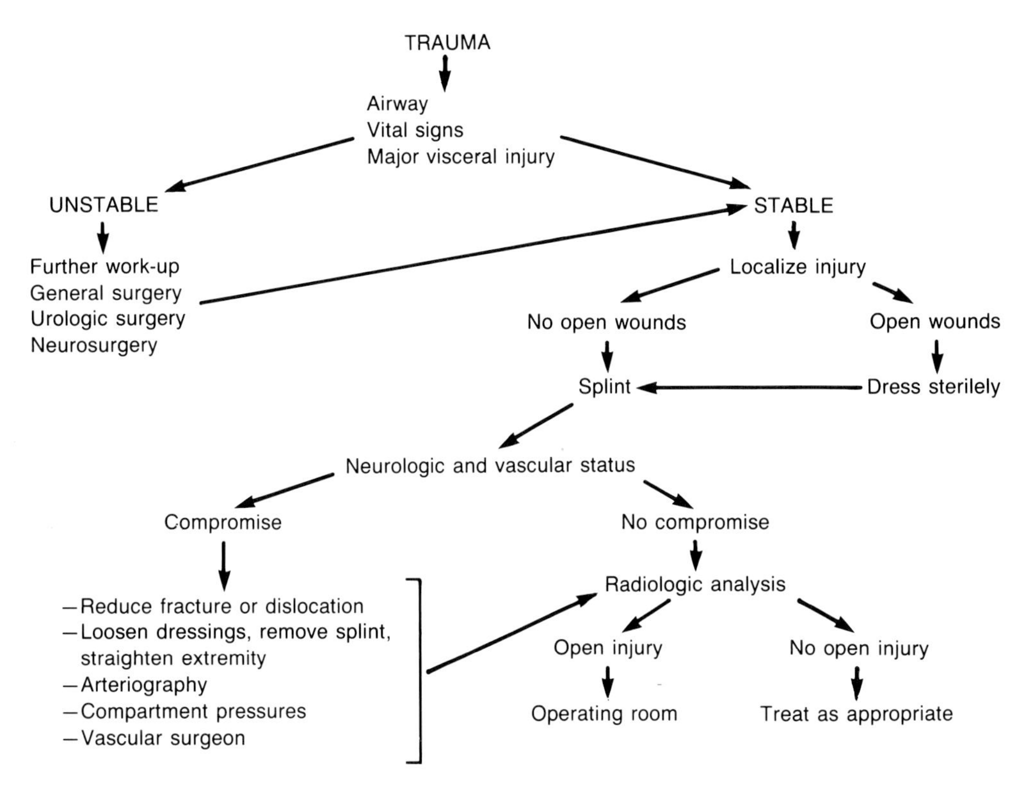

FIGURE 26-1 Flow chart for management of musculoskeletal trauma in multiply injured children.

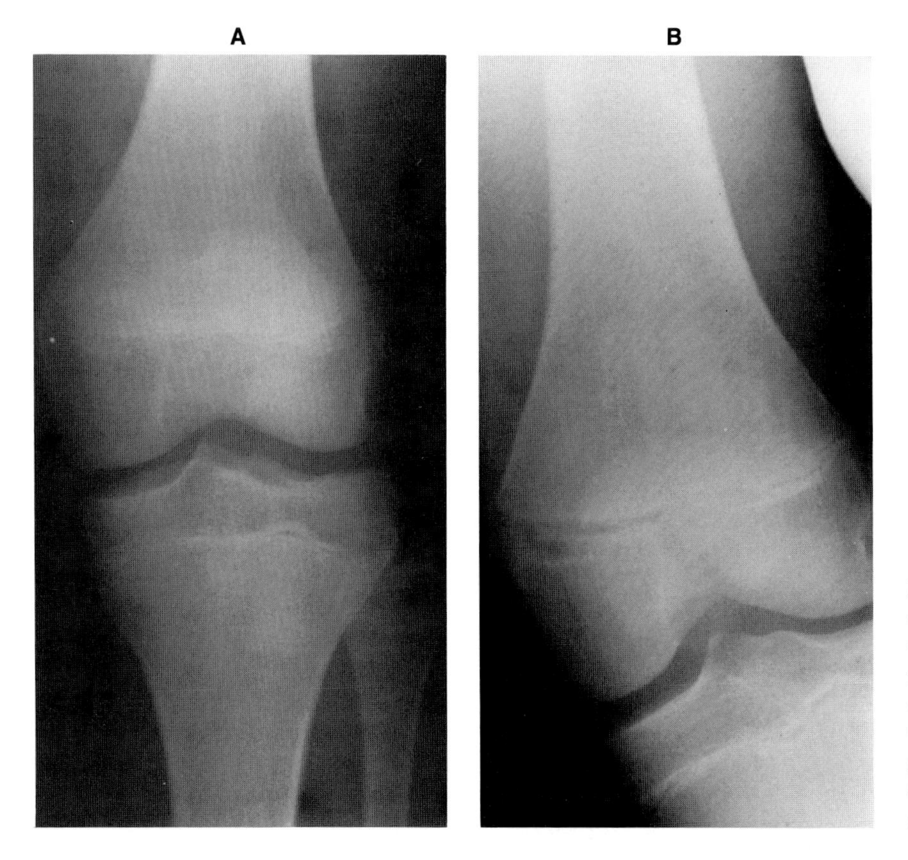

FIGURE 26-2 A, Plain x-ray film of left knee of a 15-year-old boy who sustained an injury playing football. Clinically there was medial instability of the knee. B, Stress view demonstrating opening of the growth plate. This represents a fracture through the growth plate rather than ligamentous instability.

illaries. If differentiation is difficult, measurement of intracompartmental pressures is usually helpful.[1] Since compartment syndromes are most common in the forearm and leg distal to the knee, a high index of suspicion should be maintained with injuries about the elbow, forearm, and lower leg. Arteriography may be required if a major vessel injury is suspected.

An accurate neurologic examination should follow the circulatory assessment. Nerves may be contused or lacerated by fracture fragments or penetrating wounds. Motor and sensory examinations should be quickly and carefully performed. Deep tendon reflexes are usually difficult to assess in a traumatized limb. Sensory changes may represent early ischemia. The sensory assessment is often not reliable in children and the motor examination is usually more accurate in the uncooperative, frightened child. An accurate baseline neurologic examination is mandatory, as a change following application of a splint or after reduction of a fracture usually indicates a need for change in treatment. The examiner must not assume that the child cannot move the extremity on the basis of pain alone since that is usually not the case.

The primary responsibility of those initially taking care of fractures is to prevent the development of neurocirculatory compromise and further contamination of open fractures, and to ensure that definitive treatment is undertaken as soon as possible. Following stabilization of the patient, stabilization of the fracture should be undertaken.

All fractures should be splinted in the emergency department. Splinting lessens discomfort, decreases further blood loss and swelling, prevents additional injury to soft tissue and further displacement of fragments, and makes radiologic examination easier.

Most lower leg and forearm fractures can be easily immobilized by commercially available low-pressure air splints. Care must be taken that the splint is not overinflated. Air splints are not usually satisfactory for shoulder, upper arm, hip, and thigh injuries and at times may cause difficulty by straightening an extremity and causing more pain or neurovascular deficit. Femur and hip fractures can be temporarily stabilized with a Hare-traction splint. When severe deformity is present and the neurologic and circulatory status is stable, it is often appropriate to splint the extremity in that position since attempts at straightening it may endanger the neurovascular status of the extremity. Splints made from eight to ten thicknesses of 3- to 4-inch plaster of Paris, backed by Webril and held on by a loose elastic bandage, are ideal for this purpose.

If any degree of neurovascular injury is present, immediate consultation with an orthopedic surgeon is mandatory. In the meantime a bandage or splint should be totally loosened or removed. Neurologic or vascular compromise in a markedly deformed extremity may respond to reduction of the fracture. If appropriate consultation is not available in a short period of time, simple longitudinal traction usually straightens the extremity. If there is no response, continued vascular compromise usually requires surgical exploration.

Prevention of infection in open fractures is of utmost importance. A break in the skin that leads to the fracture site means that the fracture is open. Whether the wound was produced from outside in or inside out is not important. Even the smallest puncture wound can produce serious sequelae if not recognized and handled properly. Proper management consists of gentle wound cleansing and application of a sterile dressing, followed by splinting of the limb. The emergency physician *should not* push the bones into the skin or attempt to reduce the fracture unless the extremity is in danger from acute circulatory embarrassment. A set of wound cultures should be obtained in the emergency department. Open fractures require thorough, meticulous debridement and irrigation under proper anesthesia, usually in the operating room. Every attempt should be made to accomplish this within 6 to 8 hours after injury. Broad-spectrum intravenous antibiotic therapy should commence in the emergency department as soon as cultures are obtained.

GENERAL PRINCIPLES OF FRACTURES IN CHILDREN

A fracture or dislocation is initially described as open or closed. It can occur through the epiphysis, metaphysis, or diaphysis (Figure 26-3). Diaphyseal fractures can be further described by dividing the bone into thirds, e.g., fracture of the proximal, middle, and distal thirds of the femur. A fracture may extend completely through the bone or be incomplete. A linear fracture has two main fracture fragments, whereas a comminuted fracture consists of multiple fracture fragments (Figure 26-4D). Comminuted fractures are rare in children. In complete fractures the fracture line may be transverse (Figure 26-4A), spiral (Figure 26-4B), or oblique. The fracture may be displaced, i.e., named according to the direction the distal fragment takes with respect to the proximal, or angulated, i.e., named according to the direction the apex is pointing (Figure 26-4C).

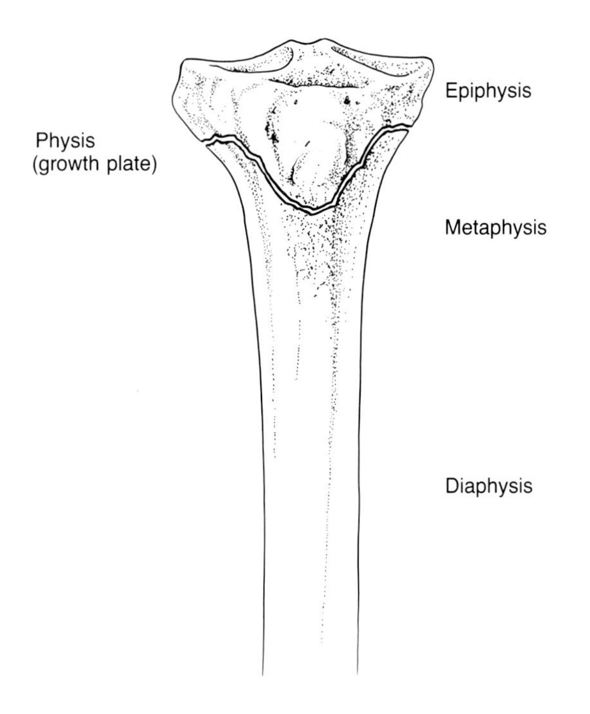

FIGURE 26-3 Anatomy of a long bone.

The biomechanical properties of children's bones are responsible for several unique incomplete fracture patterns. One cortex may fail in compression and result in a torus or buckle fracture (Figure 26-5A). If one cortex fails in tension, a so-called greenstick fracture results (Figure 26-5B). In addition, children's bones may actually bend and remain in a permanently deformed position. Injuries to the growth plate, differences in healing rate, overgrowth, and potential for remodeling are factors unique to children's fractures.

With very rare exceptions, nonunion is not a problem in children, and healing takes place rapidly. This reduces the decision-making time, and definitive treatment needs to be carried out expeditiously.

Fractures of the long bones in children between the ages of 2 and 10 years often result in overgrowth of the corresponding extremity. The mechanism is unknown, but it is felt to be related to growth plate stimulation caused by the hyperemia that occurs with fracture healing. For that reason overriding may be intentionally allowed in certain fractures, notably those of the femur.

Fractures that are imperfectly reduced often remodel to give an acceptable result in children with at least 2 years of growth left. As a rule, mild angulation in the plane of motion of a joint remodels satisfactorily and fractures near the joint remodel better than midshaft fractures. Rotation usually does not remodel nor do significant angular deformities near the midshaft of a bone. The surest way to achieve good final alignment is with an adequate initial reduction. Too much reliance must not be placed on remodeling potential in severely malaligned fractures.

As many as one third of children's fractures involve the growth plate. The prognosis following injury to the growth plate depends on the type of injury to the plate and quality of reduction. The most commonly used system of classification is one devised by Salter and Harris.[2] Growth plate injuries are divided into five types, as follows (Figure 26-6):

- Type I: the epiphysis separates from the metaphysis.
- Type II: the epiphysis separates as in type I, but the fracture traverses a portion of the metaphysis.
- Type III: the fracture runs through part of the growth plate and exits through the epiphysis into the joint.
- Type IV: the fracture runs from the joint surface, across the epiphysis and growth plate, and exits through the metaphysis.
- Type V: a crushing injury to the growth plate that is usually discovered retrospectively because the initial x-ray films appeared normal. The existence of this fracture is somewhat controversial because the mechanism of growth plate damage is difficult to prove.

Type I and II injuries usually are benign and heal with minimal sequelae, although certain type II fractures, notably of the distal femur, can cause serious growth disturbances.[3,4] Type III injuries involve the joint surface and, if displaced, require open reduction and anatomic alignment. Type IV injuries involve the joint surface also and, if not anatomically reduced, lead to growth arrest when a bony bridge forms between the epiphysis and metaphysis. Displaced type IV fractures require open reduction and anatomic alignment. Growth arrest in any of these injuries may be partial or complete and lead to serious angular deformity or shortening. In addition, type III and IV injuries are intra-articular and, if not anatomically reduced, lead to joint incongruity and possible early degenerative arthritis.

The growth plate is fragile and reduction must be gentle. These injuries heal very rapidly, and reduction should be performed early. The parents should understand that growth arrest is a potential complication from the time treatment is begun.

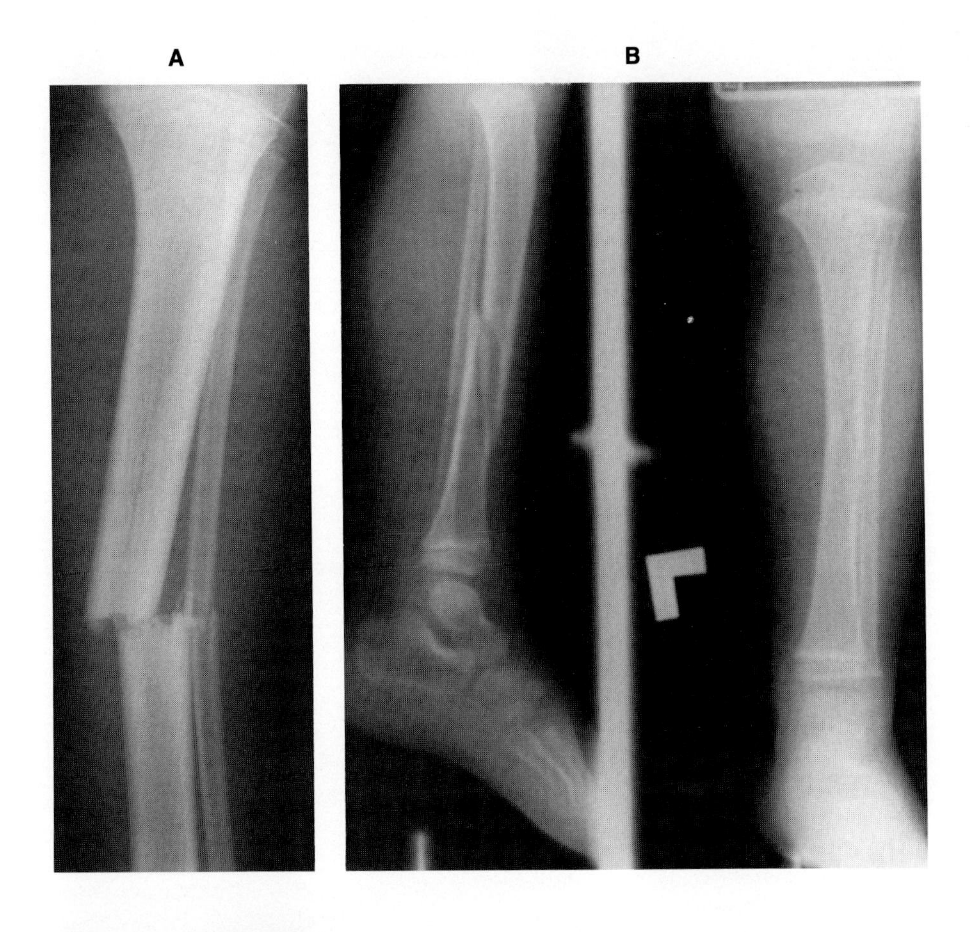

FIGURE 26-4 A, Transverse fracture of the tibia. B, Spiral fracture of the tibia. C, Volar angulation of a fracture of both bones of the forearm. D, A comminuted fracture of the proximal ulna.

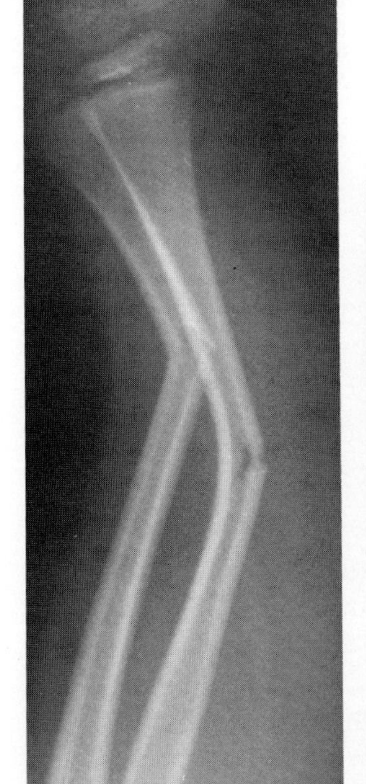

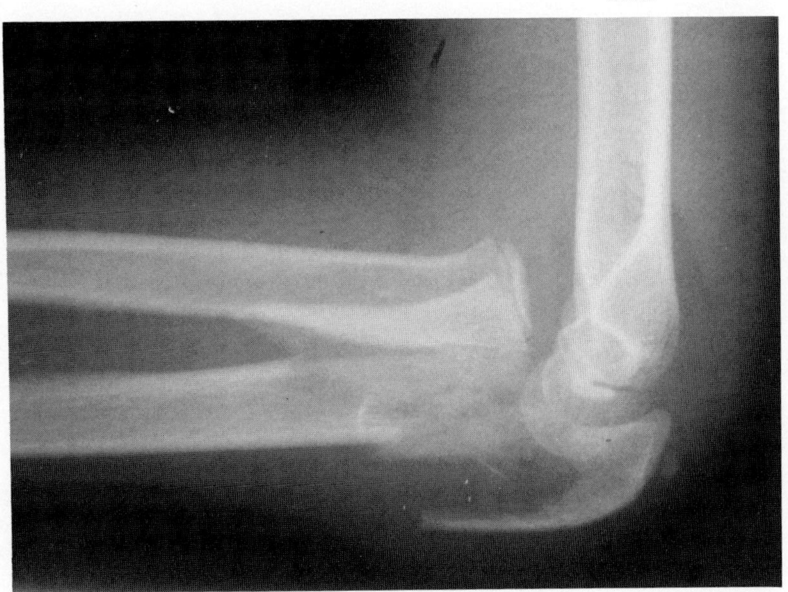

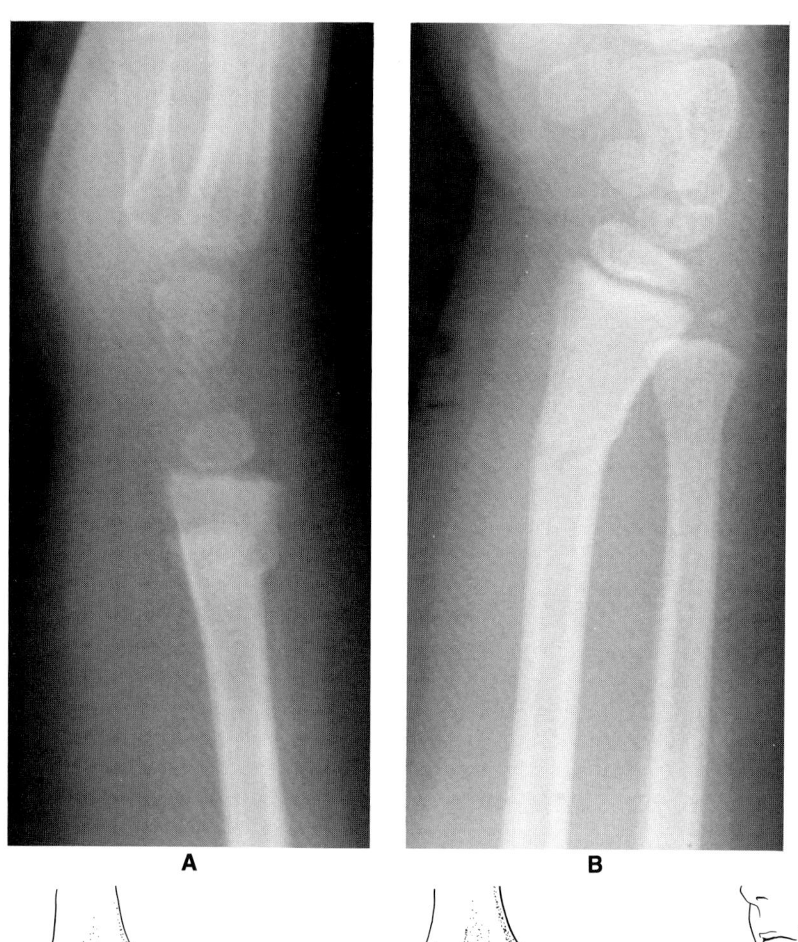

FIGURE 26-5 A, Torus fracture of the distal radius. B, Greenstick fracture of the distal radius. There is volar angulation.

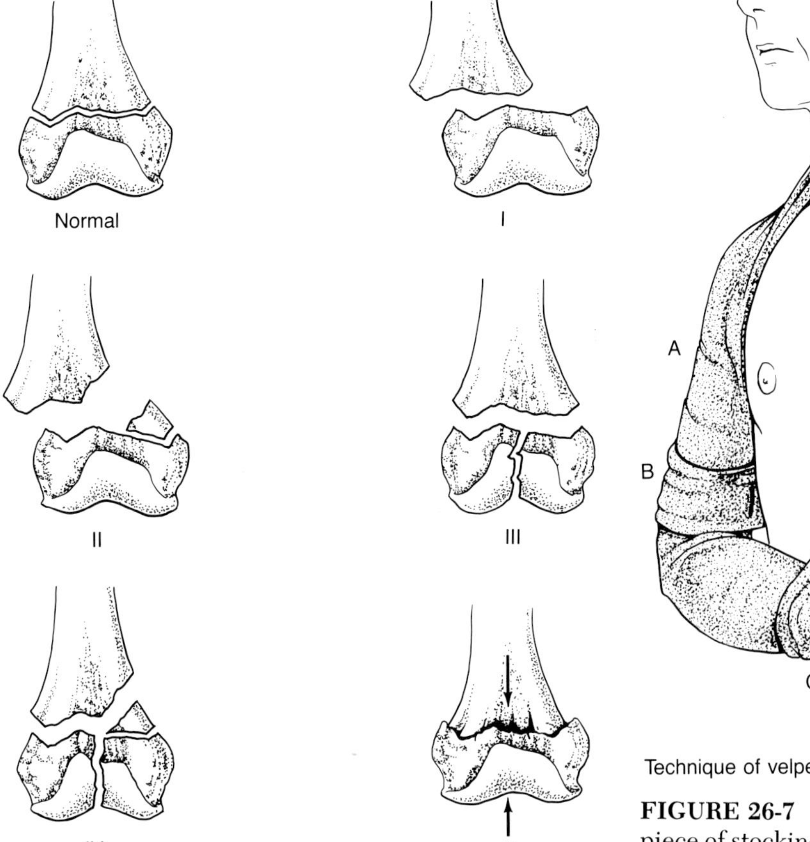

FIGURE 26-6 Patterns of growth plate fractures as described by Salter and Harris.

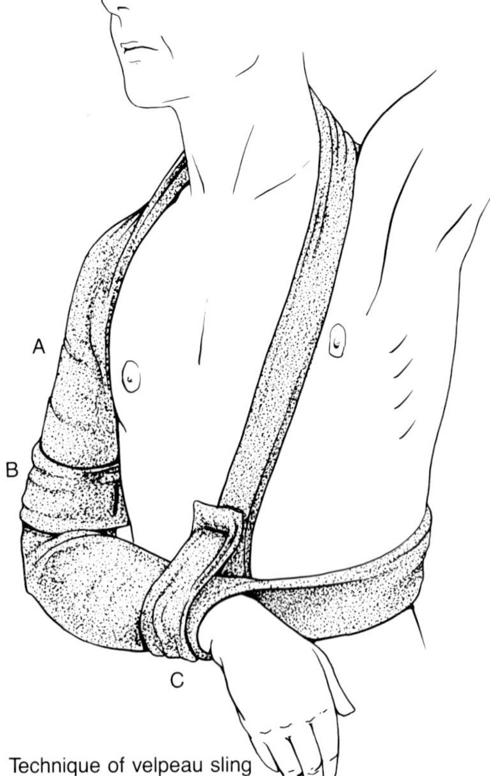

FIGURE 26-7 Technique of the Velpeau sling. A, One piece of stockinette is drawn over the arm, with a hole cut for the wrist. B, The axillary end is brought over the shoulder and pinned around the wrist. C, The hand end is brought around the waist and is pinned around the arm above the elbow.

SPECIFIC FRACTURES

Clavicle

Fracture of the clavicle represents the most common broken bone in children. Although fracture may occur in any part of the bone, it is usually in the midshaft. Neurovascular compromise is unusual but the possibility should not be overlooked. Reduction is generally not required, and treatment consists of a simple figure-of-eight clavicle splint for 3 to 4 weeks.

Humerus

Fractures of the proximal end of the humerus occur most commonly in adolescents and are usually Salter-Harris type II epiphyseal fractures. Closed treatment is almost always successful and rarely requires more than a Velpeau or sling-and-swathe bandage for 3 to 4 weeks (Figure 26-7).

Fractures of the humeral shaft are usually successfully treated with plaster coaptation splints and a sling-and-swathe bandage. They are fairly uncommon in children.

Elbow

Elbow fractures can present difficult diagnostic and management problems. The presence of multiple ossification centers and growth plates can be confusing, but the judicious use of comparison views of the normal extremity usually solves the problem. A positive "fat pad" sign indicates an elbow fracture, although a radiographic fracture line may not be seen (Figure 26-8).

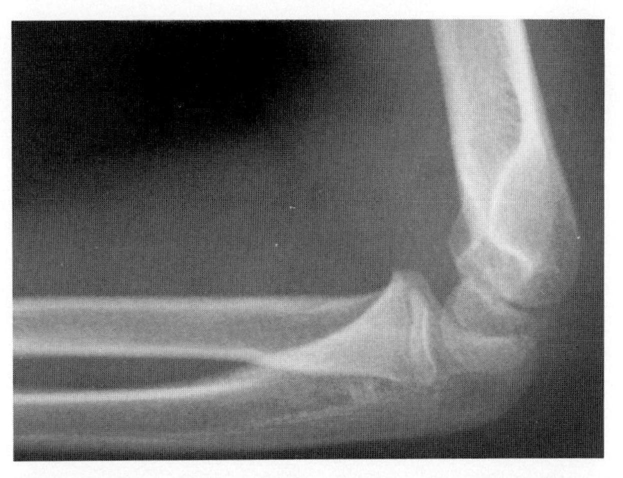

FIGURE 26-8 The radiolucent area adjacent to the posterior aspect of the distal humerus represents a positive fat pad sign and suggests the presence of a fracture, although none can be seen on the radiograph. The radiolucent area adjacent to the anterior distal humerus is a normal finding.

Supracondylar fractures represent the most common children's elbow fracture (Figure 26-9). Displaced fractures are treated at our institution by closed reduction and percutaneous pinning,[5–7] although closed reduction and traction[7,8] and open reduction and internal fixation[9] are widely used. These fractures can be difficult to reduce but perhaps are more well known for their significant risk of neurovascular compromise. Injury to the radial, ulnar, or median nerve is not uncommon, although function usually returns spontaneously after reduction. A nerve that loses function during reduction may have been lacerated, contused, or even trapped in the fracture and usually requires operative exploration. The most dangerous sequela of this fracture is ischemic necrosis of the muscles of the forearm, so-called Volkmann's ischemic contracture. This may occur from vascular damage at the time of fracture, from swelling about the elbow, or from tight, constricting bandages.

Prior to reduction the elbow should be splinted in extension and the arm should be elevated, followed by rapid reduction if vascular compromise is apparent. Careful observation for at least 12 hours after reduction is absolutely mandatory. At the first sign of vascular compromise following reduction, the elbow should again be straightened and all bandages should be split. If no improvement is seen promptly, surgical exploration and fasciotomy should be performed.

Once ischemia is present, there is little place for preoperative angiography because it only delays surgical relief of ischemia. Occasionally, arteriography may be helpful either intraoperatively or in the patient with persistent absence of pulses in a nonischemic limb. The presence of ischemia is a surgical emergency. Absence of circulation for more than 12 hours can lead to irreversible changes. Ischemic contracture of muscles is a preventable complication with adequately evaluated, promptly treated children's elbow fractures.

Lateral condyle fractures represent a Salter-Harris type IV epiphyseal injury (Figure 26-10) and require open reduction and internal fixation in most instances. These fractures often appear innocuous, but if they are improperly treated, the result may be nonunion or malunion initially, with angular deformity and ulnar nerve palsy as late findings.[10]

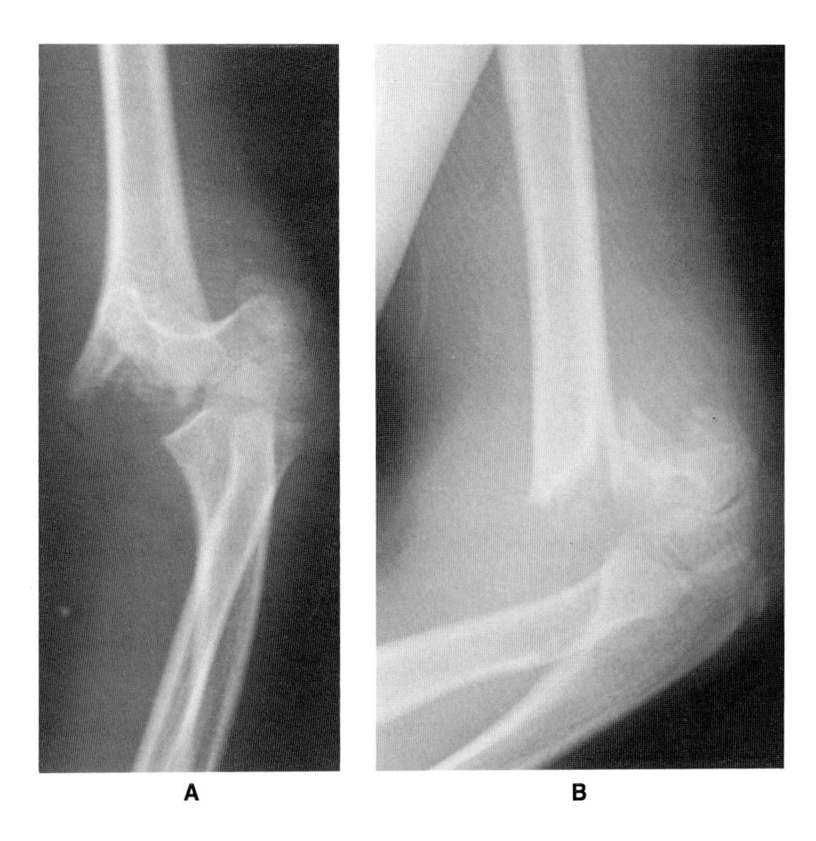

FIGURE 26-9 A, Anteroposterior view of supracondylar fracture of the distal humerus. B, Lateral view of same fracture.

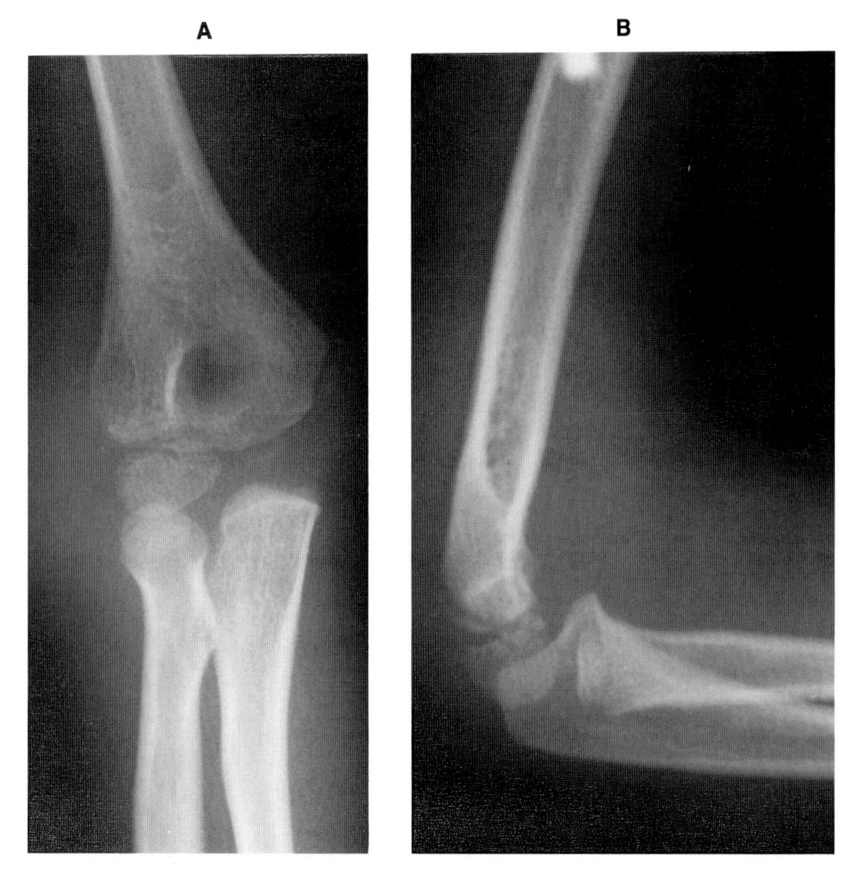

FIGURE 26-10 A, Minimally displaced lateral condyle fracture of the distal humerus. The fracture can barely be seen through the lateral cortex of the distal humerus just proximal to the normal growth plate. B, Lateral view of the same fracture. The fracture is much more easily seen extending through the posterior cortex of the distal humerus.

A

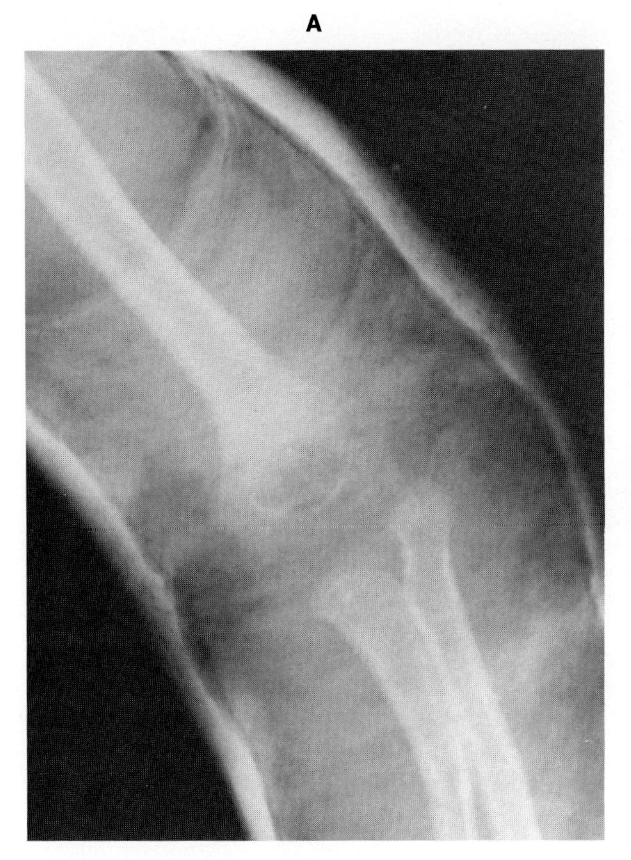

B

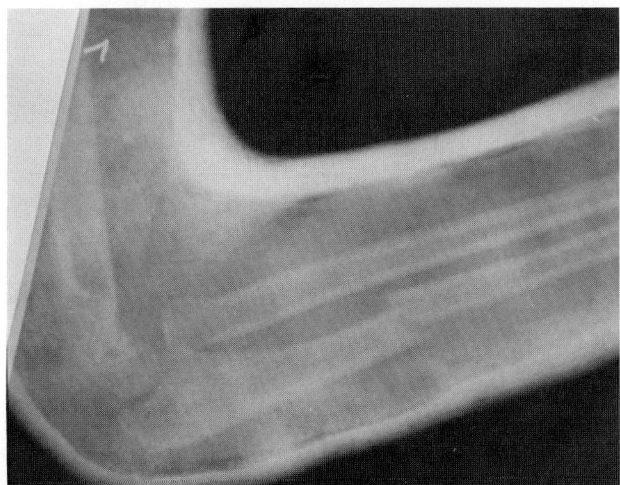

FIGURE 26-11 A, Alleged fracture of the ulna that has been reduced and casted. Close examination reveals a dislocation of the radial head, a so-called Monteggia fracture. Compare this anteroposterior view with Figure 26-9A. The radial head points lateral to the capitellum in this view. B, Lateral view of the same Monteggia fracture. Compare this to the position of the radial head in Figure 26-9B. The radial head points proximal to the capitellum in this view. This injury did nicely following reduction and immobilization.

Fractures of the radial neck may be markedly angulated and, if irreducible, require open reduction.

The association of an ulnar fracture and a dislocation of the ipsilateral radial head is known as a Monteggia fracture. It is a common injury, and films of the elbow should be carefully evaluated in forearm fractures. It is important to note that the radial head points to the capitellum in all radiographic views of the elbow, and absence of this relationship indicates dislocation of the radial head (Figure 26-11).

The so-called nursemaid's elbow results from a pull on the outstretched arm of a child between 1 and 5 years old. The child does not use the arm, and any attempt to move it causes the child to cry out. The elbow is held slightly flexed with the forearm pronated. This injury is probably due to a tear of the annular ligament, which partially displaces into the joint between the radius and capitellum. After x-ray films to rule out a more serious injury, the arm should be mildly flexed and the forearm should be supinated fully. A slight click is usually felt, and the child will begin to use the arm. It is important that the parents understand the mechanism of injury so that it does not recur. A sling and follow-up by an orthopedist are required.

Pelvis

Pelvic fractures usually occur in children who have sustained significant trauma, and associated injuries are common. The pelvic injury itself is usually not a problem, but injuries to abdominal or genitourinary viscera as well as vascular and neural structures must be carefully sought and often require further urologic, vascular, or general surgical work-up. Massive bleeding may occur. The orthopedic injury is often the least of the worries in the care of these children.

Hip and Femur

Fractures of the growth plate of the proximal femur or through the femoral neck usually require operative treatment (Figure 26-12). Unfortunately, avascular necrosis, early growth plate closure, and nonunion may occur,[10] even with the best treatment, and are responsible for a large number of unsatisfactory results in these fractures. Intertrochanteric fractures can usually be treated by closed means involving traction and casting.

Dislocation of the hip does occur in children and, in fact, is more common than femoral neck fractures

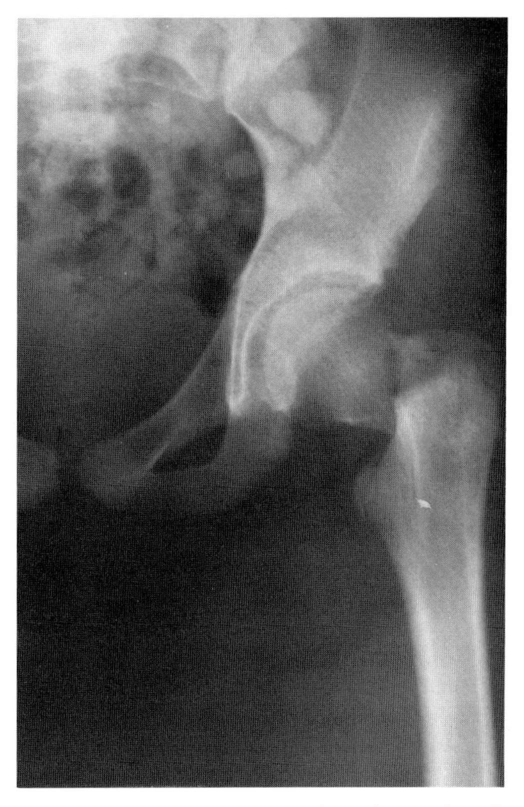

FIGURE 26-12 Fracture of the femoral neck in an 11-year-old girl. This injury required open reduction and internal fixation.

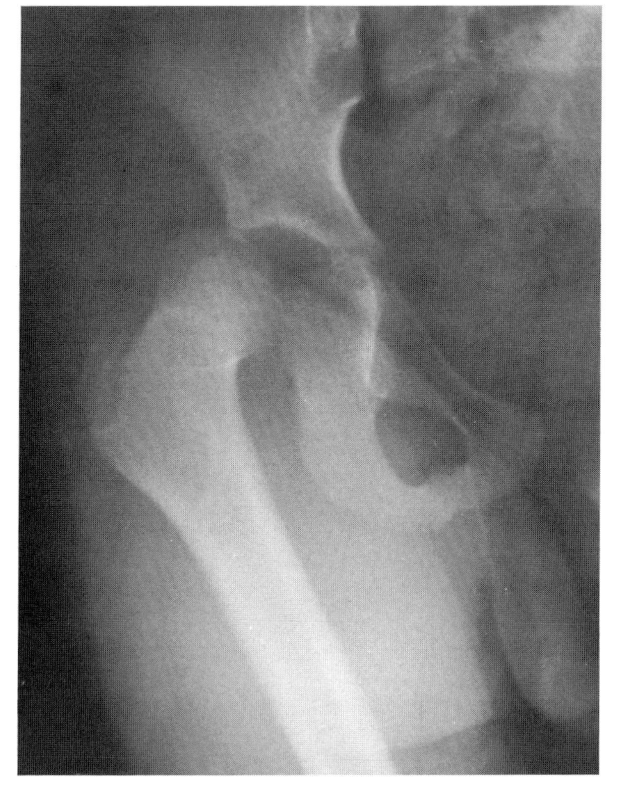

FIGURE 26-13 Posterior dislocation of the right hip in a 9-year-old boy who fell out of a tree.

(Figure 26-13). With posterior dislocation the leg is held in a flexed, adducted, internally rotated position. Early, gentle reduction is absolutely essential to prevent avascular necrosis.

Fractures of the femoral shaft are usually treated closed. Blood loss can be significant. Initial management consists of splinting and accurate neurocirculatory examination. X-ray films of the hip must be included so that an associated hip dislocation is not neglected. Overgrowth is most common in these fractures.

Knee

Because of the relative strength of joint ligaments compared to the incompletely calcified growing bones of a child, epiphyseal fractures of the distal femur may initially be misinterpreted as knee ligament disruption (Figure 26-14). This may not be apparent on the initial plain films, and stress views are necessary to make the diagnosis.

The injury that tears the anterior cruciate ligament in adults usually fractures the tibial spine in children (Figure 26-15). The diagnosis is made from

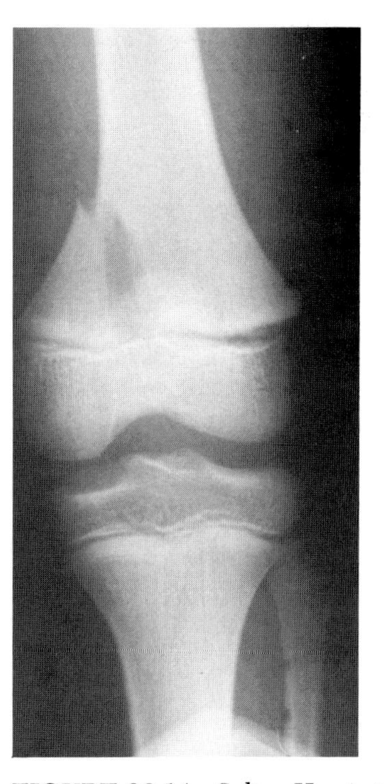

FIGURE 26-14 Salter-Harris type II fracture of the distal femur. This was treated by closed reduction and casting and did nicely. Unfortunately, growth plate arrest can occur after this injury.

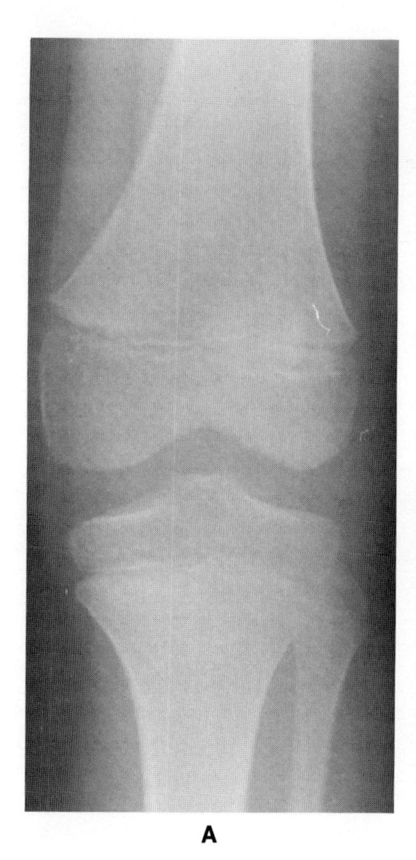

A

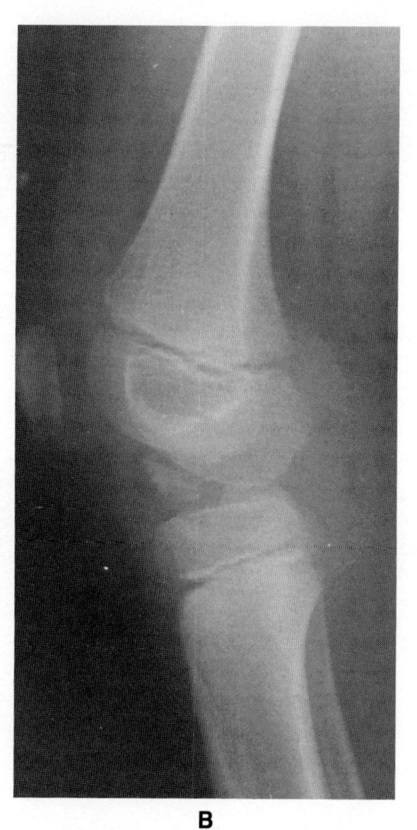

B

FIGURE 26-15 A, X-ray film of a painful swollen knee in an 11-year-old boy injured playing football. The injury is difficult to delineate on the anteroposterior view. B, An avulsion of the tibial spine is easily seen on the lateral view. Open reduction and internal fixation were performed.

plain films, and displaced fractures usually require open reduction.

Tibia

Tibial shaft fractures are much easier to treat in children than in adults. Closed reduction and casting for a period of time, depending of the age of the patient, are all that is necessary.

Epiphyseal fractures of the distal tibia need to be carefully delineated. Type III and IV injuries require open reduction if displaced.

CONCLUSION

The injured child who sustains any type of fracture must be evaluated thoroughly and expeditiously. Associated injuries must be assessed, the possibility of contamination should be considered, and appropriate splinting to prevent further damage must be provided. Prompt referral to an orthopedic surgeon experienced in the care of children's injuries should then be done.

References

1. Matsen FA, Winquist RA, Krugmire RB: Diagnosis and management of compartmental syndromes. *J Bone Joint Surg* [*Am*] 1980;62:286–291.
2. Salter RB, Harris WR: Injuries involving the epiphyseal plate. *J Bone Joint Surg* [*Am*] 1963;45:587.
3. Lombardo SJ, Harvey JP: Fractures of the distal femoral epiphysis. *J Bone Joint Surg* [*Am*] 1977;59:742–751.
4. Stephens DC, Louis DS: Traumatic separation of the distal femoral epiphyseal cartilage plate. *J Bone Joint Surg* [*Am*] 1974;56:1383–1390.
5. Arino VC, Lluch EE, Ramirez AM, et al: Percutaneous fixation of supracondylar fractures of the humerus in children. *J Bone Joint Surg* [*Am*] 1977;59:914–916.
6. Flynn J, Mathews JG, Benoit RL: Blind pinning of displaced supracondylar fractures of the humerus in children. *J Bone Joint Surg* [*Am*] 1974;56:263.
7. Prietto CA: Supracondylar fractures of the humerus. *J Bone Joint Surg* [*Am*] 1979;61:425–428.
8. Dodge HS: Displaced supracondylar fractures of the humerus in children—treatment by Dunlop's traction. *J Bone Joint Surg* [*Am*] 1972;54:1408.
9. Weiland AJ, Meyer S, Tolo VT, et al: Surgical treatment of displaced supracondylar fractures of the humerus in children. *J Bone Joint Surg* [*Am*] 1978;60:657–661.
10. Tachdjian MO: *Pediatric Orthopaedics.* Philadelphia, WB Saunders Co, 1972.

William Herndon

27 Nontraumatic Musculoskeletal Emergencies

The majority of musculoskeletal problems seen in the emergency department are the result of trauma and consist of contusions, lacerations, fractures, and other injuries that are readily diagnosed.[1] However, an occasional patient is seen with no history of trauma and a limp, refusal to bear weight, or refusal to use an extremity. Common entities, such as bone and joint infection, discitis, Legg-Calvé-Perthes disease, slipped capital femoral epiphysis, and toxic synovitis, are discussed in this chapter, but less common diseases such as juvenile rheumatoid arthritis or neoplasm must not be overlooked.

INITIAL EVALUATION

As with any other medical examination, a detailed history should first be obtained.[1,2] Usually, the parents are the primary historians, but it is important to listen to the child. Where is the discomfort? How long has it been present and what brought it on? Has there been trauma and who observed it? The examiner must remember that children fall every day, and a presumed etiology of trauma may be misleading. Does the child use the involved extremity or bear weight on it? Did the child awaken with the problem or did it begin at play? Has there been a recent febrile illness or is there a history of an underlying disease, such as sickle cell anemia or osteogenesis imperfecta? Has another member of the family been ill or is there a family history of a similar complaint? Injuries in multiple stages of healing and obvious trauma with poor explanations should alert the physician to the possibility of child abuse.

The physical examination should be systematic and careful. The child should be unclothed and handled gently; above all, the examiner must be patient. Does the child walk or use the involved extremity? Is there an apparent deformity? Does the child appear ill or have a fever? Is there swelling, warmth, erythema, or decreased motion of involved joints?

Adequate x-ray films are important. Generally, views taken at right angles (anteroposterior and lateral) to one another of the involved, injured, or symptomatic area are appropriate.[1,2] The opposite normal extremity provides comparison views when necessary. It must be remembered that pain in the thigh or knee may be referred from a lesion about the hip.

This chapter emphasizes diagnosis and early management. Most of the following situations require orthopedic consultation, but early diagnosis and appropriate early management may often mean the difference between success and failure.

ACUTE SEPTIC ARTHRITIS

Septic arthritis in children is an emergency.[1] Delayed treatment can result in disaster, with a destroyed joint and growth arrest. The inflammatory response yields proteolytic enzymes that irreversibly destroy articular cartilage.

Bacteria usually enter the joint in one of two ways. Septic arthritis may occur by hematogenous bacterial seeding of the synovium or by direct extension from a preexisting osteomyelitis (Figure 27-1). The latter occurs in joints where the metaphysis is intra-articular, most often the hip. Differential diagnosis includes osteomyelitis, juvenile rheumatoid arthritis, and rheumatic fever. Legg-Calvé-Perthes disease and toxic synovitis also must be considered when the hip joint is involved.

The history may include previous trauma or a previous site of infection elsewhere in the body. The child is irritable, febrile, and refuses to use the extremity. The hip joint is most frequently involved and is held in a position of flexion, abduction, and external rotation. Any attempted motion of the involved joint is met with resistance. More superficial joints such as the knee, elbow, or ankle are swollen, red, warm, and tender.

The white blood cell count is usually elevated, although it may be normal. The erythrocyte sedimentation rate may be quite high. Roentgenograms usually show surrounding soft tissue swelling and capsular distension. Later, joint subluxation or even dislocation may be present. The most important diagnostic finding is the presence of pus upon aspiration of the involved joint. Patients with suspected or possible pyogenic arthritis must be referred as soon as possible to an orthopedic surgeon since aspiration of the involved joint may be required. Any fluid obtained should be Gram stained and cultured, and the number of cells should be counted. Pyogenic arthritis has a white cell count in the range of 50,000–200,000/μL, with a marked predominance of polymorphonuclear leukocytes. If enough fluid is aspirated, it should be sent for measurement of glucose; blood samples for determination of the serum glucose level also should be obtained and sent to the laboratory at the same time. A difference of 50 mg/dL or greater is virtually diagnostic of pyogenic arthritis.

The most common organism in children 6 to 24 months old is *Haemophilus influenzae,* whereas *Staphylococcus aureus* is the common organism in older children.[3] Septic joints secondary to hematogenous osteomyelitis are usually due to *S. aureus.*

As in osteomyelitis, treatment of septic arthritis is directed at getting the appropriate antibiotic to the involved area in an adequate concentration. In the hip joint open drainage is required. Although some physicians feel that other joints may be handled by repeated aspiration, I prefer to surgically incise all septic joints. Choice of antibiotics depends upon the age of the child. In younger children a combination of semisynthetic penicillin and chloramphenicol is appropriate since a significant percentage of *H. influenzae* is resistant to ampicillin. Older children usually receive a semisynthetic penicillin or one of the cephalosporins. When culture results are available, the antibiotic is changed if necessary. There is controversy over the appropriate time of treatment, but antibiotics must be used a minimum of 2 to 3 weeks. Because these antibiotics readily cross the synovial membrane, there is no need for intra-articular instillation.

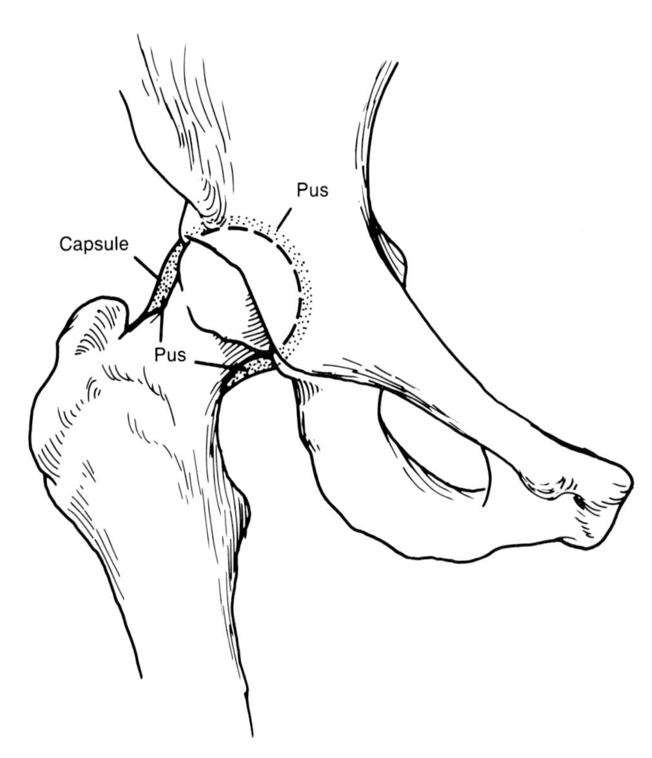

FIGURE 27-1 The mechanism of septic arthritis occurring by direct extension from a preexisting osteomyelitis of the metaphyseal region.

ACUTE HEMATOGENOUS OSTEOMYELITIS

Osteomyelitis in children is usually hematogenous, the primary source often being a previous upper respiratory tract infection. Although any bone may be involved, it is most commonly the metaphyseal region of the long bones. Bacteria lodge in the vascular channels of the metaphysis and an inflammatory response ensues. *S. aureus* is the offending organism in up to 90% of cases.[1,4]

Osteomyelitis is a clinical diagnosis. An ill child with pain in a limb, fever, and tenderness, swelling, and erythema over the metaphyseal region of a long bone should be presumed to have osteomyelitis until proven otherwise. The adjacent joint can usually be placed through a nearly normal range of motion. This is an important finding when trying to differentiate osteomyelitis from a septic joint.

The erythrocyte sedimentation rate and white blood cell count are usually elevated. Blood cultures may be positive. Early roentgenographic changes consist of blurring and swelling of the soft tissues. Bone involvement does not usually become apparent on x-ray films for 10 to 14 days. The earliest bony abnormalities are lytic changes in the metaphyseal region. Shortly thereafter, a thin line of periosteal reaction forms about the metaphysis. Bone imaging has proved useful,[1] usually demonstrating increased uptake in the involved area, although it may not be reliable in children less than 6 months old. A "cold" bone scan in acute osteomyelitis has recently been described.[5]

Treatment depends on delivering adequate doses of the appropriate antibiotic to the site of infection. Currently, we start with a parenteral semisynthetic penicillin or cephalosporin and switch to the appropriate drug when an organism is identified. *Salmonella* may be the offending organism in children with sickle cell anemia, and initial coverage should include the appropriate antibiotic in those children. If treatment is begun within 48 hours of the onset of symptoms, antibiotic therapy alone for 3 to 6 weeks may be sufficient. Later in the course the inflammatory response has progressed, and pressure within the bone has cut off the local capillary flow. Pus then moves through the cortex and becomes subperiosteal. When this occurs, adequate surgical drainage is required in addition to antibiotics. The length of treatment is arbitrary, and recent studies have shown that a short period of intravenous antibiotics followed by oral antibiotics can be successful.

DISCITIS

Discitis, the symptomatic narrowing of the disk space, may manifest itself in several ways.[2,6,7] Younger children (less than 3 years old) usually will not stand or walk, whereas older children usually have various degrees of abdominal or back pain. Frequently, a history of a preceding viral illness or trauma is present. Physical examination may show an abnormal posture, refusal to stand or walk, limited back motion, or hamstring tightness. The patient is usually mildly febrile and has an elevated sedimentation rate. The white blood cell count may be normal or mildly elevated. Blood cultures are frequently positive.

Early in the course of the disease, roentgenograms of the spine may be normal; 2 to 4 weeks later, disk space narrowing becomes apparent. The earliest changes appear on bone scan, and any child with fever, refusal to bear weight, and abdominal or back pain in whom a diagnosis is not readily apparent should have a bone scan (Figure 27-2).

The etiology appears to be inflammatory, proba-

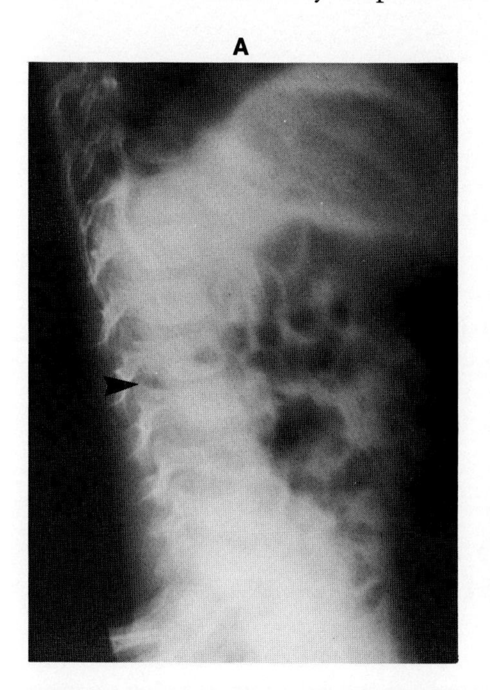

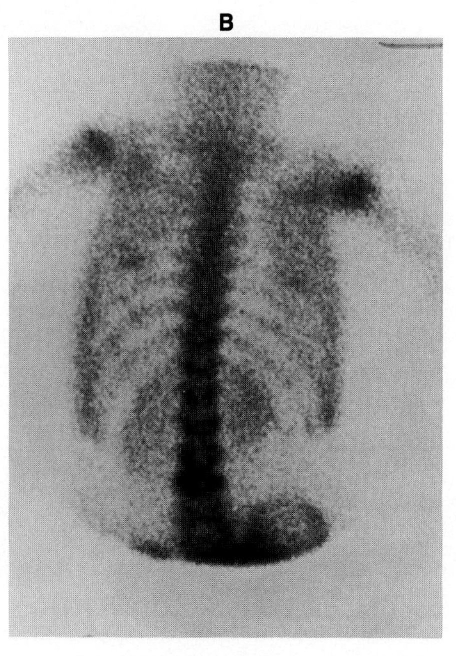

FIGURE 27-2 A, A lateral view of the spine in a 3-year-old girl with a 3-week history of refusal to walk. Note the narrowing of the L2-L3 disk space (*arrow*). B, A bone scan that demonstrates increased uptake within the body of L3. This child had a discitis that responded to a course of antibiotics and immobilization.

bly an *S. aureus* infection in most cases. It is still not clear whether this represents a primary infection of the disk space or an infection secondary to a primary vertebral osteomyelitis. Treatment consists of rest and spine immobilization. The use of antibiotics is controversial.

LEGG-CALVÉ-PERTHES DISEASE

Legg-Calvé-Perthes disease is an abnormality of the hip joint in children, usually between the ages of 4 and 10 years. It is much more common in boys and is bilateral in about 15% of cases. The etiology is unknown, and although the pathogenesis has not been defined, most orthopedists believe that the process results from a disturbance of the vascular supply to the femoral head, producing avascular necrosis.[1,2]

The child usually has a limp that was initially sporadic but became more constant. Initially, the limp may have been painless. When pain is present, it may be experienced in the region of the groin or medial thigh but, as with other hip disturbances in children, may be referred to the medial aspect of the distal thigh or the knee region. Physical examination usually reveals limitation of internal rotation and abduction of the hip. There may be a mild hip flexion contracture. The child is afebrile, and the white blood cell count and sedimentation rate are normal.

Roentgenograms show sequential changes, depending on the length of time the process has been present. Proper films to evaluate hip pathology are a standing anteroposterior and supine frog lateral view of both hips. The earliest change is slight decrease in the size of the capital femoral epiphysis, followed by an increased density of a portion or all of the femoral head. On the frog lateral view, a so-called crescent sign may be visible as a thin area of lucency just below the subchondral bone in the anterolateral portion of the head. With time, fragmentation occurs, followed by gradual reconstitution that results in a widened, enlarged, and sometimes flattened or irregular femoral head (Figure 27-3).

Early differential diagnosis includes infection, juvenile rheumatoid arthritis, and toxic synovitis. Hypothyroidism and multiple epiphyseal dysplasia may give a radiologic appearance much like that of bilateral Legg-Calvé-Perthes disease in the fragmentation stage.

Preventing deformity of the femoral head is the main goal of therapy. Treatment usually consists of bedrest and traction to restore range of motion to the hip, followed by containment of the hip joint either by a brace or surgical measures. Prognosis depends primarily on the age of the patient at onset of the disease and the degree of involvement of the femoral head. As a rule, younger patients have a better result.

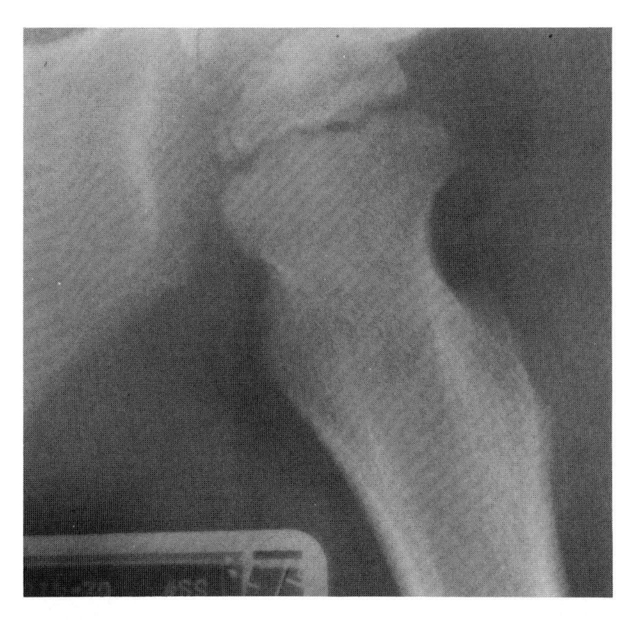

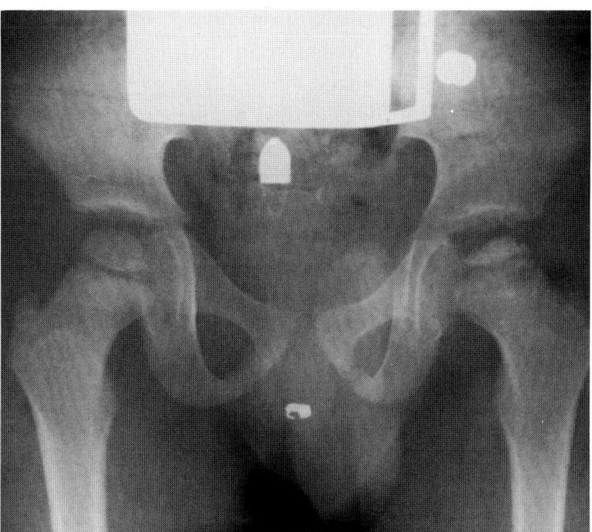

FIGURE 27-3 A, The crescent sign demonstrated on the frog lateral view of a patient with Legg-Calvé-Perthes disease. B, Changes of the necrotic stage in another patient with Legg-Calvé-Perthes disease. Note the increase in density and decrease in size of the left capital femoral epiphysis.

SLIPPED CAPITAL FEMORAL EPIPHYSIS

Slipped capital femoral epiphysis affects the hip joint of adolescents. Boys are affected twice as often as girls and usually about 2 years earlier. Blacks are more frequently affected than whites. The process may be bilateral in up to 30% of cases.

The etiology is unknown, but most investigators believe that a combination of endocrine and mechanical factors is responsible.[1,2] Affected boys are very often overweight with poor gonadal development, although tall, thin individuals may also be seen. It is postulated that the former group has a low level of sex hormone whereas the latter group has excessive growth hormone. Experimental evidence has shown that the perichondrium about the femoral neck gives the epiphysis its primary support. During adolescence, thinning of the perichondrium occurs and the bone-cartilage junction of the growth plate is thereby weakened.[2,8]

Clinically, patients are affected in one of three ways. Acute slippage may occur following trauma. Chronic slippage may occur in a patient who has had symptoms for weeks or months. The third possibility is an acute slippage occurring in a patient who has already had this condition on a chronic basis.

Acute slippage after trauma is usually too painful for weight bearing. Patients with chronic slippage complain of pain localized to the groin or medial thigh or referred to the knee region. Examination reveals a characteristic limp with the leg externally rotated. There is marked limitation of internal rotation; as the thigh is flexed, the leg rolls into external rotation. The earliest radiologic change is widening of the growth plate. The slippage may be difficult to see on the anteroposterior view and is best observed on the frog lateral view, where the capital femoral epiphysis is shifted posteriorly (Figure 27-4).

Treatment is directed at preventing further slippage and achieving fusion of the growth plate. This most often involves surgical pinning in situ for chronic conditions. Acute slippage usually requires gentle reduction with traction, followed by pinning.

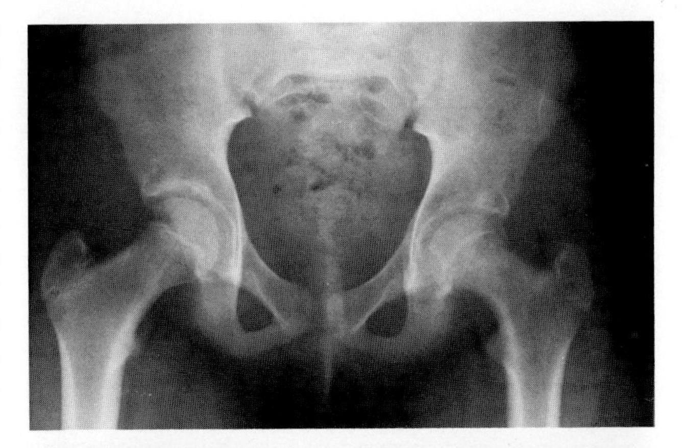

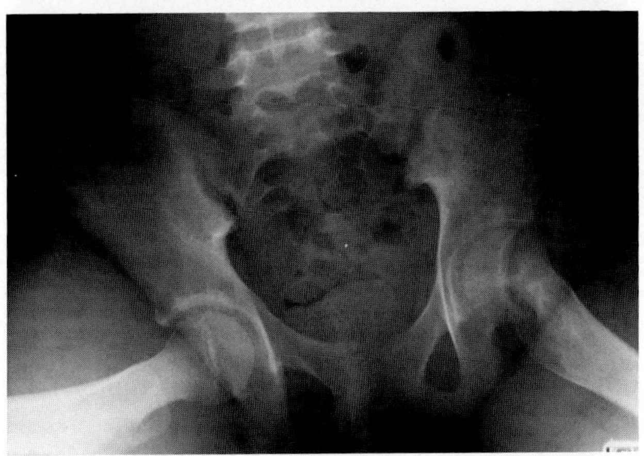

FIGURE 27-4 A, Anteroposterior view of the pelvis in an 11-year-old girl with a 6-week history of a painful limp. There is irregularity in the region of the growth plate on the left side when compared with the normal right proximal femur. B, The diagnosis is readily made on the frog lateral view where the left slipped capital femoral epiphysis can easily be seen. This patient underwent traction, followed by pinning in situ.

TOXIC SYNOVITIS

Toxic synovitis, also known as transient synovitis or observation hip, is a self-limiting hip disorder in children of the same age group vulnerable to Legg-Calvé-Perthes disease. It is unilateral and there is minimal difference in sex preponderance.

Physical findings are similar to those of Legg-Calvé-Perthes disease: a limp and limited internal rotation and abduction of the involved hip. The child is afebrile, and laboratory studies usually reveal a normal white blood cell count and erythrocyte sedimentation rate, although these may be minimally elevated.

The etiology is unclear. Trauma, infection, and allergic hypersensitivity all have been implicated. Differential diagnosis includes infection, juvenile rheumatoid arthritis, and Legg-Calvé-Perthes disease.

Roentgenograms are usually normal, although mild widening of the joint space may be visible. If symptoms are severe and infection is felt to be a possibility, aspiration of the hip joint is mandatory.

Treatment consists of relief from weight bearing. Traction is often helpful. The symptoms may recur, but chronic prolonged symptoms should lead to a search for another cause.

INTRASPINAL TUMORS

Intraspinal tumors are extremely rare and are mentioned for the sake of completeness. Although the initial complaints are usually musculoskeletal, this is a neurosurgical problem. The most common complaint is pain in the neck, back, or extremities.[9] The parents may note the slow onset of a limp or obvious difficulty climbing stairs or running. A change in bowel or bladder function may be noted.

The most common physical finding is weakness that may be spastic or flaccid, depending on the level of the lesion. Foot deformities or scoliosis may be present. Painful scoliosis in a child should be attributed to a tumor until proven otherwise. Often paraspinal muscle spasm and spinal rigidity are seen.

Proper diagnosis requires a high index of suspicion. Plain roentgenograms may demonstrate widening of the spinal canal or bony erosion. Diagnosis is confirmed by lumbar puncture and myelography. Treatment is usually neurosurgical.

CONCLUSION

Any child with a painful joint represents a potential orthopedic emergency. Inaccurate assessment or injudicious disposition may allow a severe inflammatory process to go untreated long enough to cause major destruction to the involved joint. Awareness of this possibility, compulsive examination, and thorough assessment are the best means of avoiding this potential catastrophe.

References

1. Lovell WW, Winter RB: *Pediatric Orthopaedics*. Philadelphia, JB Lippincott Co, 1978.
2. Tachdjian MO: *Pediatric Orthopaedics*. Philadelphia, WB Saunders Co, 1972.
3. Griffin PP: Septic arthritis. Read before the American Orthopaedic Symposium on Common Hip Disorders in Children. AI duPont Institute, Oct, 1980.
4. Morrey BF, Peterson HA: Hematogenous pyogenic osteomyelitis in children. *Orthop Clin North Am* 1975;6:935–951.
5. Jones DC, Cady RB: "Cold" bone scans in acute osteomyelitis. *J Bone Joint Surg* [*Br*] 1981;63:376–378.
6. Boston HC Jr, Bianco AJ Jr, Rhodes KH: Disk space infections in children. *Orthop Clin North Am* 1975;6:953–964.
7. Wenger DR, Bobechko WP, Gilday DL: The spectrum of intervertebral disc-space infection in children. *J Bone Joint Surg* [*Am*] 1978;60:100–108.
8. Chung SMK, Batterman SC, Brighton CT: Shear strength of the human capital epiphyseal plate. *J Bone Joint Surg* [*Am*] 1976;58:94–103.
9. Tachdjian MO, Matson DD: Orthopaedic aspects of intraspinal tumors in infants and children. *J Bone Joint Surg* [*Am*] 1965;47:223–248.

Theodore E. DuPuy
Pat L. Aulicino

28 Hand Injuries

Hand injuries in children occur frequently. As the physician treating a child's hand, it is imperative to be knowledgeable of all of the structures that may be injured—skin, nerve, joint, bone, tendon, and vessel—and their anatomic relationships. One should keep in mind the old adage, "You see only what you look for and recognize only what you know."

ANATOMIC CONSIDERATIONS

The skin covering the volar aspect of the palm and fingers is relatively thick compared to the dorsal skin. The volar finger skin creases have a paucity of subcutaneous tissue covering the tendon sheath. A superficial laceration or puncture in this area is more likely to damage the tendon or cause infection (Figure 28-1).

The proper digital nerves and arteries lie volar to the midaxial line of the finger. The nerve is volar to the artery. Therefore, digital arterial bleeding usually means that the nerve is transected (Figure 28-2).

Three nerves innervate the muscles that move the wrist and fingers. The radial nerve supinates the hand and extends the wrist, fingers, and thumb (Figure 28-3). The ulnar nerve spreads and approximates the fingers and adducts the thumb (Figure 28-4). The median nerve flexes the wrist and fingers and opposes the thumb to the fingers (Figure 28-5).

The median and ulnar nerves are the "eyes" of the hand, providing the sensibility that is so important for function and protection. Classically, the median nerve innervates the volar aspect of the radial three and a half digits, and the ulnar nerve innervates the ulnar one and a half digits (Figure 28-6).

On the volar aspect of the wrist, there are 12 flexor tendons: 2 to each finger, 1 to the thumb, and 3 to the wrist (Figure 28-7). The flexor digitorum profundi flex the distal phalanx and are deep to the superficialis in the palm. The flexor digitorum superficialis flexes the middle phalanx. It is superficial to the profundus in the palm and splits in the proximal finger, allowing the profundus to continue to its insertion in the distal phalanx (Figure 28-8).

The extensor tendons of the fingers, thumb, and wrist are also 12 in number (Figure 28-9). There are 4 common extensor tendons, which extend the index, middle, ring, and little fingers. The extensor indicis proprius and extensor digiti quinti provide independent extension of the index and fifth digits, respectively. The extensor pollicis longus extends the distal phalanx of the thumb, and the extensor pollicis brevis extends the proximal phalanx of the thumb. The abductor pollicis longus abducts the thumb metacarpal. The extensor carpi radialis longus and brevis and the extensor carpi ulnaris ex-

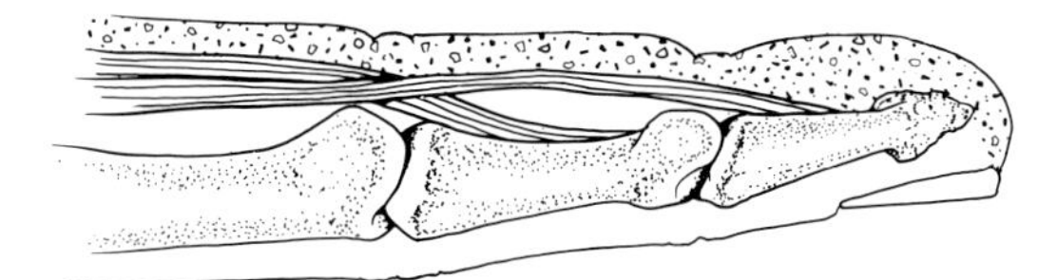

FIGURE 28-1 Longitudinal cross section of a finger. Note the paucity of fat between the skin and tendons at the level of the flexion creases.

tend and deviate the wrist in radial and ulnar directions, respectively.

The joints of the fingers are hinge type, with the exception of the metacarpal-phalangeal (MP) joints. The MP joints are cam shaped and have some lateral motion in full extension because of the eccentricity of the metacarpal head. The collateral ligaments of the MP joints are lax in extension and are tightened in flexion (Figure 28-10).

ROENTGENOGRAMS

Suspected fractures of the fingers must always be examined roentgenographically with a lateral and an anteroposterior view of both the injured and the noninjured hand for comparison. The injured phalanx should be placed against the film cassette in order to get true anteroposterior and lateral views. Roentgenograms are a necessary part of the hand examination and should not be eliminated for any reason. Fractured fingers are able to function even though they may be painful.

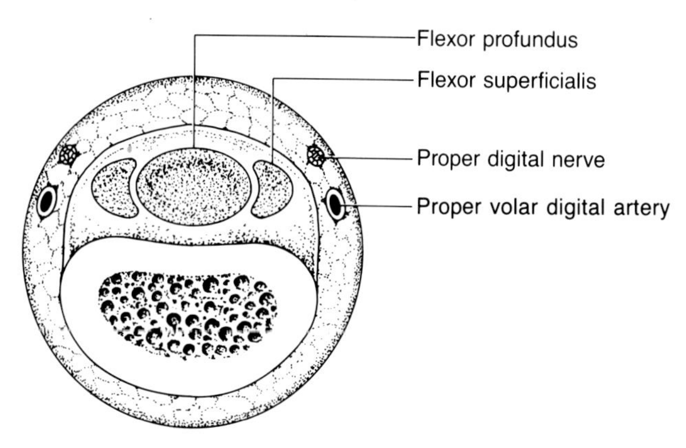

FIGURE 28-2 Cross section of the midproximal phalanx. Note the superficial location of the neurovascular bundle and the volar relationship of the nerve to the artery.

HAND EXAMINATION FOR INJURY

Observation of the position of the hand can reveal significant pathology. Starting from the index finger, each finger flexes more than the adjacent one when

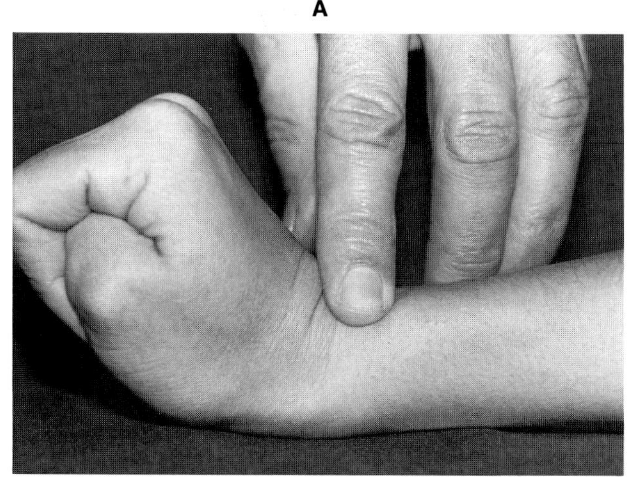

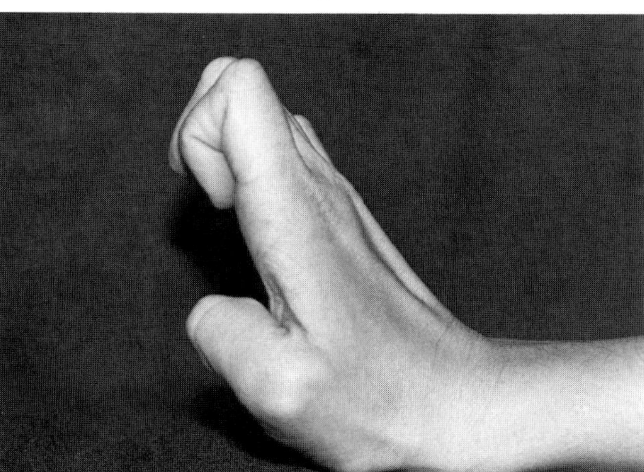

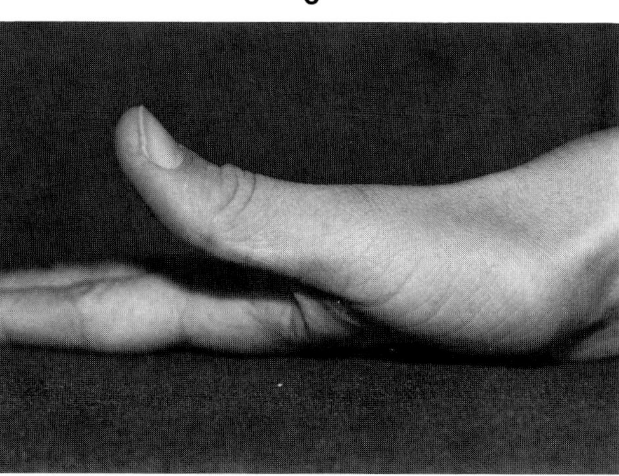

FIGURE 28-3 The radial nerve extends the wrist (A), metacarpophalangeal joints (B), and the thumb (C).

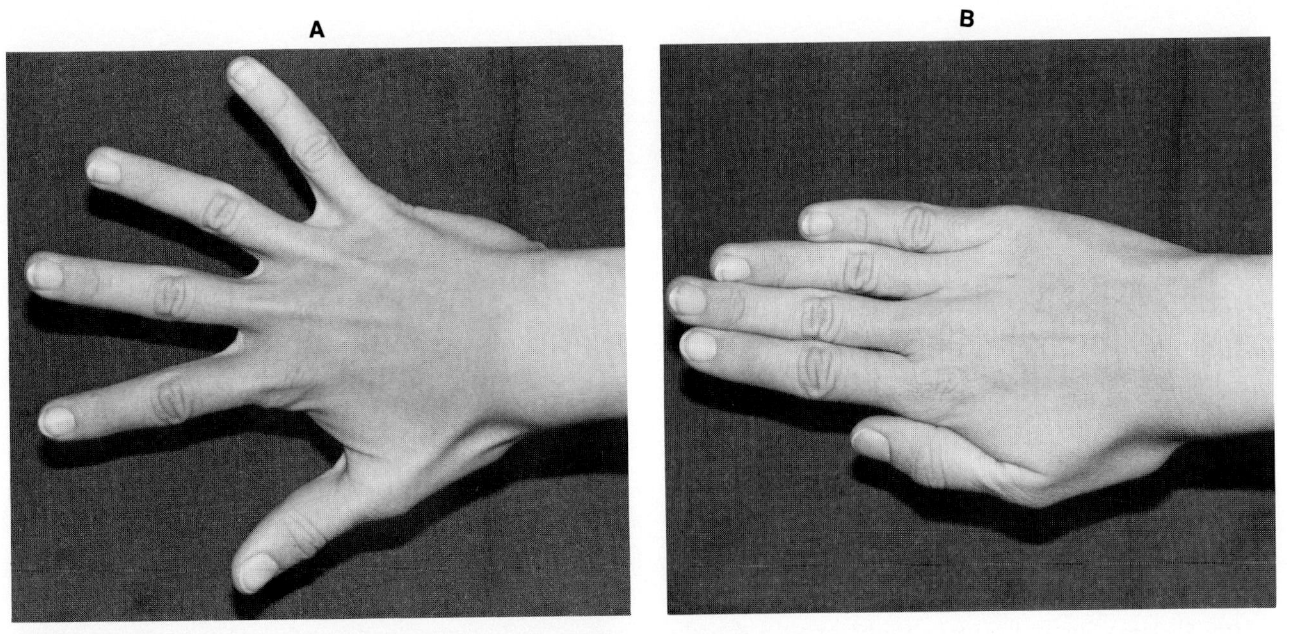

FIGURE 28-4 The ulnar nerve abducts (A) and adducts (B) the fingers.

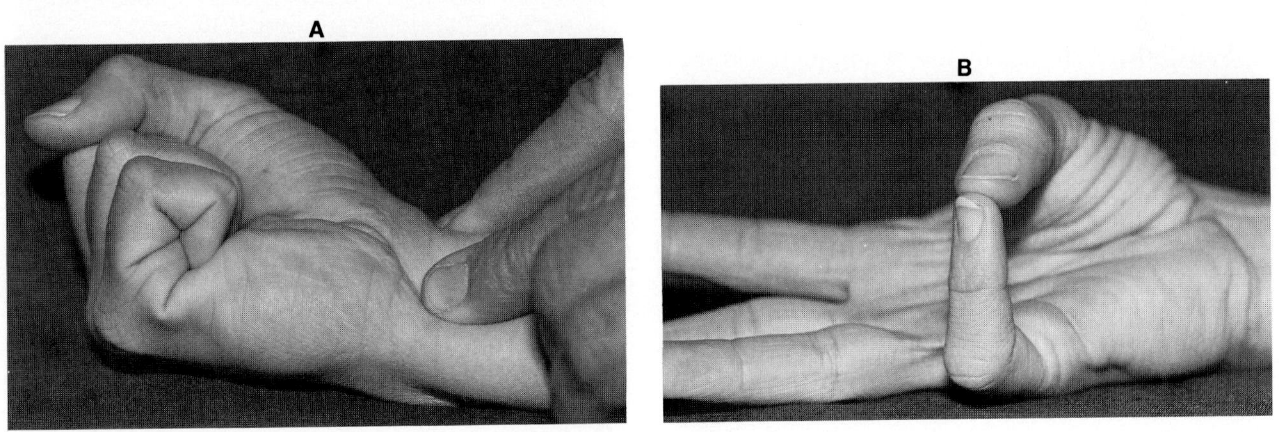

FIGURE 28-5 The median nerve flexes the fingers (A) and opposes the thumb to the little finger (B).

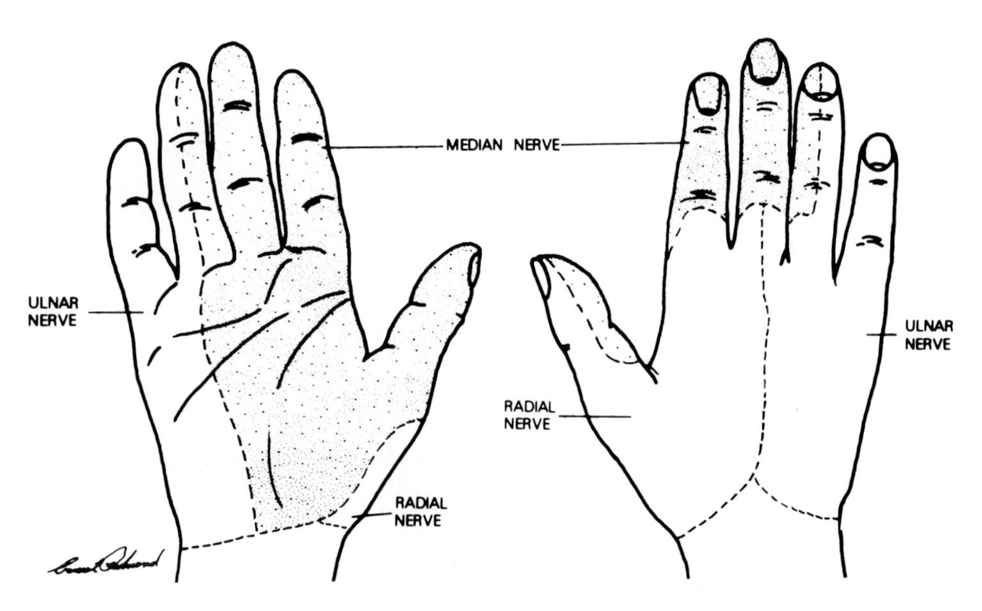

FIGURE 28-6 Cutaneous innervation of the hand.

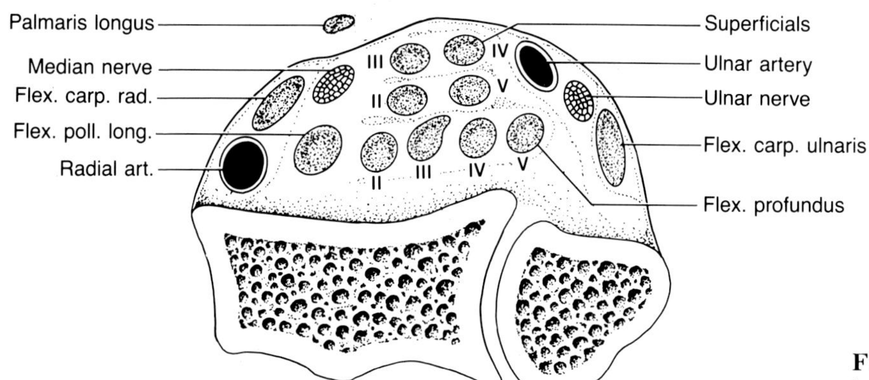

FIGURE 28-7 Cross section of the left wrist.

at rest (Figure 28-11). If one finger is out of place, a tendon injury is likely (Figure 28-12). The tenodesis effect of the tendons with passive wrist motion is an aid in determining whether tendons are in continuity. Passive wrist flexion should extend the fingers and passive wrist extension should flex the fingers (Figure 28-13).

Sensibility is tested by the two-point discrimination test using the blunt points of a paper clip. The normal range is 3 to 5 mm at the fingertip (Figure 28-14). A sharp pin stuck into a fingertip gives much pain and little information. The ophthalmoscope can be used to visualize the lack of sudomotor function distal to a nerve laceration. In children a high index of suspicion for a lacerated nerve is enough to warrant surgical exploration.

The flexor superficialis tendons are tested individually by holding the uninvolved fingers in extension to inhibit profundus action and allowing flexion at the proximal interphalangeal joint (Figure 28-15). The profundi are tested either in full extension or flexion (Figure 28-16). The inability to flex the distal interphalangeal joint indicates an injury to the profundus tendon.

The extensor digitorum communis tendons extend all the MP joints (Figure 28-17A), and the extensor indicis proprius and extensor digiti quinti extend the MP joints of the index and the little finger independently (Figure 28-17B).

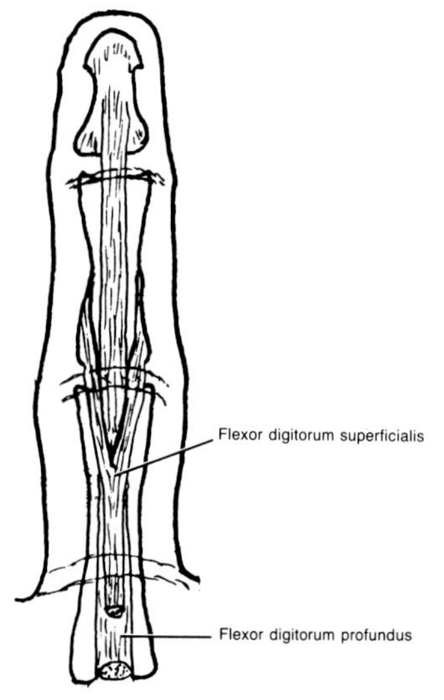

FIGURE 28-8 Flexor digitorum profundus inserting onto the base of distal phalanx, and the flexor digitorum superficialis splitting and inserting onto the proximal half of the middle phalanx.

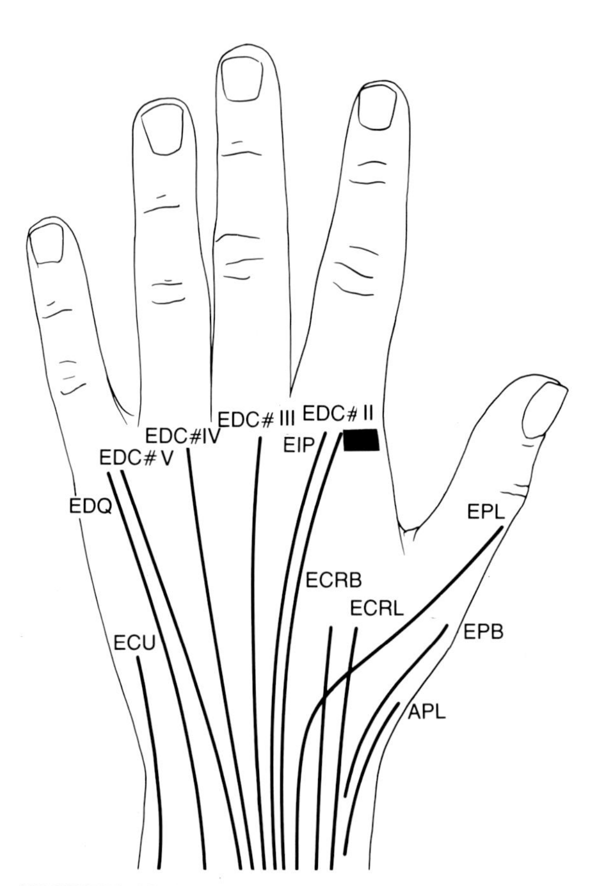

FIGURE 28-9 Extensors of the hand: ECU, extensor carpi ulnaris; EDQ, extensor digiti quinti; EDC, II–V, extensor digitorum communis of II–V; EIP, extensor indicis proprius; ECRB and ECRL, extensor carpi radialis brevis and longus; EPL, extensor pollicis longus; EPB, extensor pollicis brevis; APL, abductor pollicis longus.

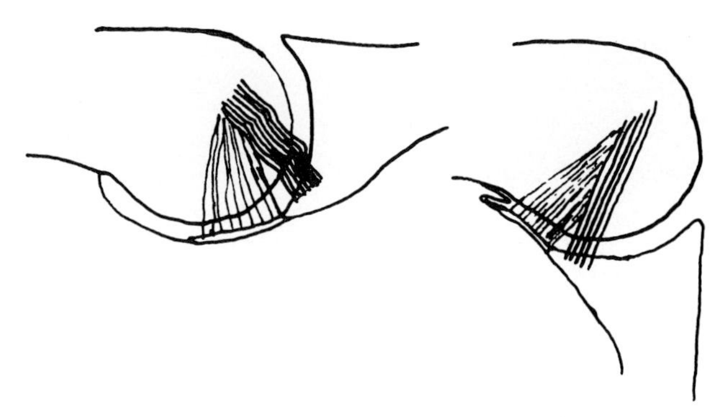

FIGURE 28-10 The collateral ligaments of the MP joint are lax in extension and tight in flexion due to the cam-shaped metacarpal head.

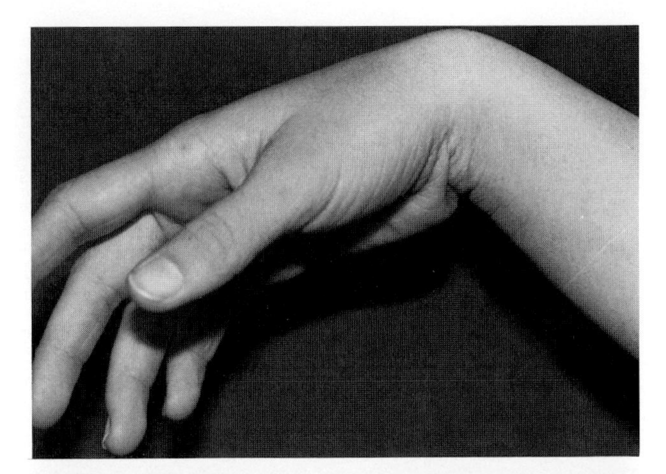

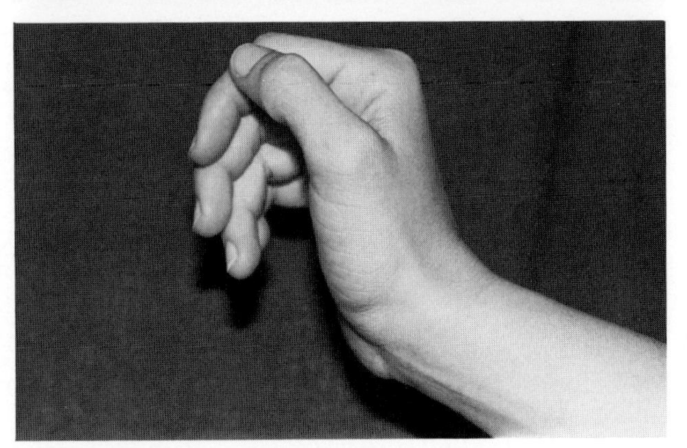

FIGURE 28-13 Tenodesis effect. Passive flexion of the wrist causes finger extension (A). Passive extension of the wrist causes finger flexion (B).

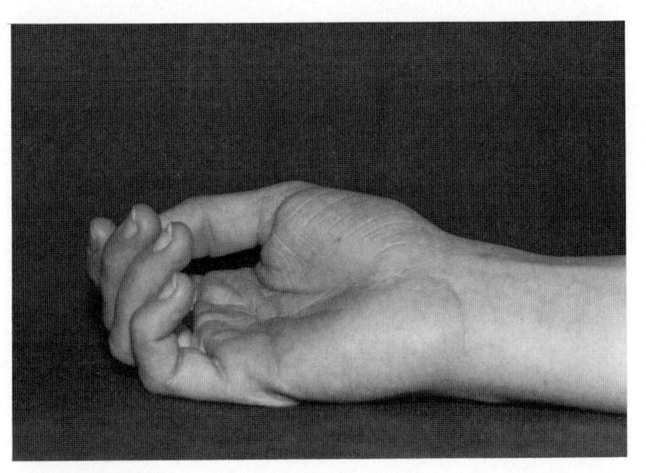

FIGURE 28-11 Position of the hand at rest. Note progressive flexion of the digits from index to fifth finger.

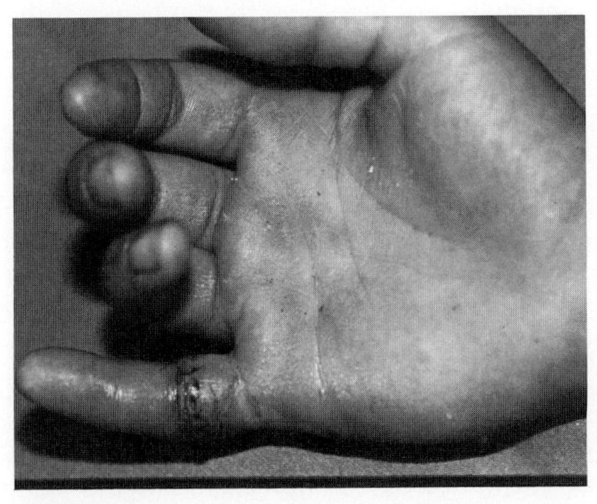

FIGURE 28-12 Right fifth digit lacks its normal position of flexion because of a tendon laceration.

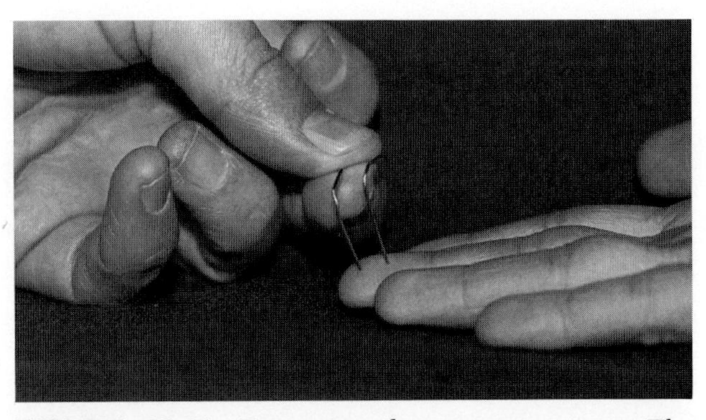

FIGURE 28-14 Two-point discrimination test. The blunt tipped paper clip is applied to the skin in the distribution of a digital nerve. The pressure should be light and barely cause blanching of the skin. Normally, one can discern two distinct points of the paper clip when they are 3 to 5 mm apart.

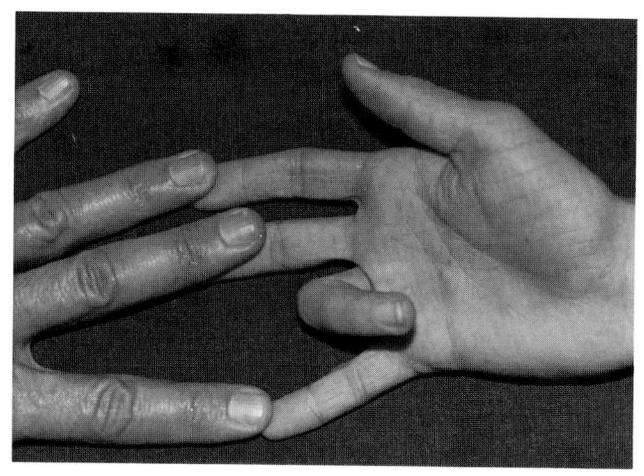

FIGURE 28-15 The superficialis test. The adjacent fingers are held in extension while testing superficialis function of the involved finger. Ability to flex the proximal interphalangeal joint indicates normal function.

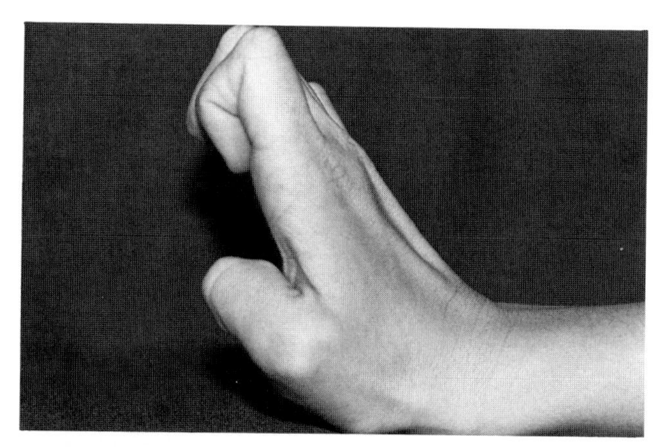

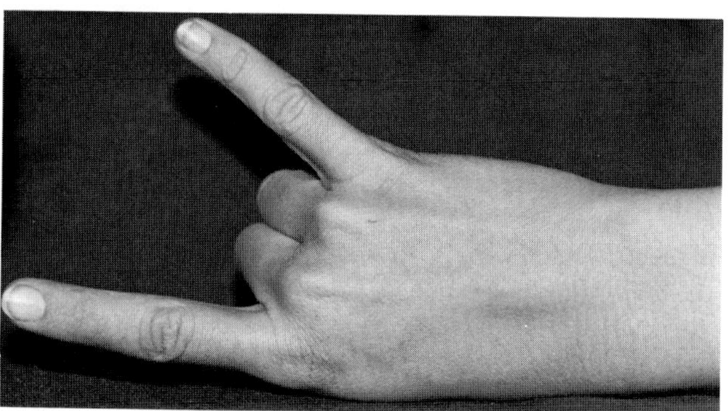

FIGURE 28-17 The extensor digitorum communis tendons extend the MP joints of all of the fingers (A). Independent extension of the index and fifth digits is provided by the extensor indicis proprius and extensor digiti quinti, respectively (B).

ANESTHESIA

Although adequate anesthesia of the hand can be achieved in many ways, there are two absolute principles that must be considered in every case: (1) no anesthetic is placed into the finger proper, as this increases intradigital pressure enough to jeopardize the blood supply; and (2) epinephrine-containing anesthetics are absolutely contraindicated. Because of the end-arterial blood supply of the digit, the vasoconstrictive action of epinephrine may jeopardize the viability of the injured finger (Figure 28-18).

A finger block can be accomplished with 1.5 to 3 mL of 1% lidocaine. Via a 26-gauge needle, 0.5 to 1.0 mL is injected through the finger webs on each side of the finger to block the proper digital nerves. Dorsally, the base of the finger over the head of the metacarpal is injected subcutaneously with 0.5 to 1.0 mL to block the dorsal nerves (Figure 28-19).

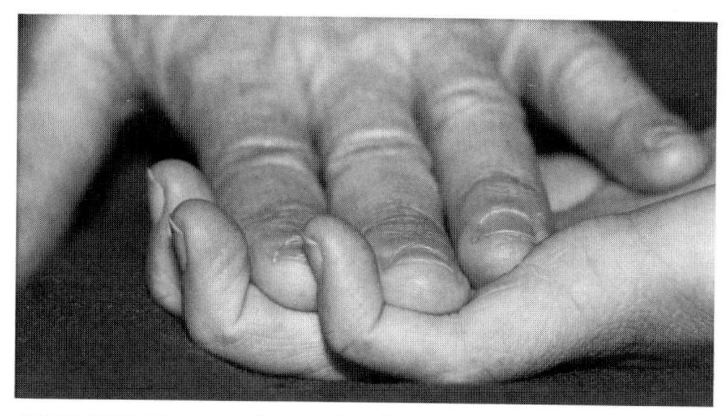

FIGURE 28-16 The profundus test. The profundus tendon is tested by having the patient flex the distal interphalangeal joint. Inability to do so indicates an injury to the profundus tendon.

FINGERTIP INJURIES

Crushed Fingertip

This common injury is frequently the result of the child versus a door. The tip has jagged lacerations.

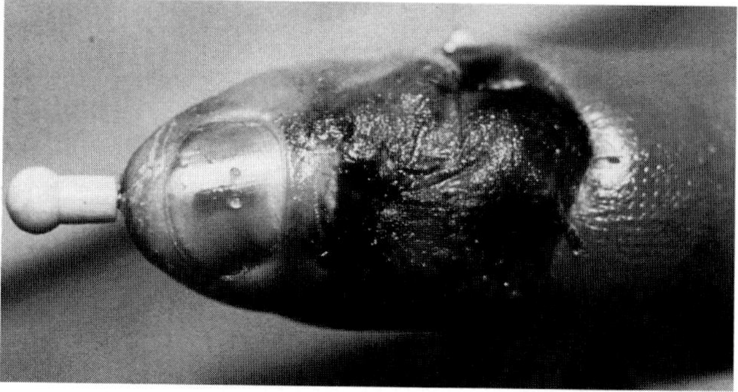

FIGURE 28-18 Necrosis of the thumb distal to interphalangeal joint secondary to a "ring block" with anesthetic containing epinephrine.

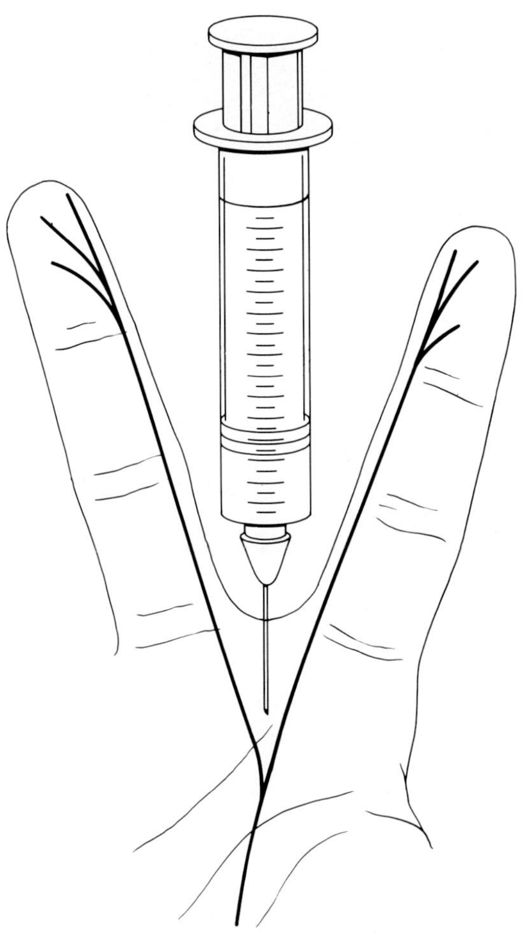

FIGURE 28-19 One percent lidocaine without epinephrine is injected with a 26-gauge syringe in the web space, toward the bifurcation of the digital nerves. The anesthetic is injected proximal to the web space just distal to the distal palmar crease.

The nail is avulsed proximally, the nail bed may be torn, and the distal phalanx may be fractured (Figure 28-20).

The wound is cleansed with copious amounts of saline after the rest of the hand is washed with a mild antiseptic soap solution. There may be very little nonviable tissue to debride other than the proximal portion of the nail, which may be lifted from the nail bed. If the nail bed has been torn, it is repaired with 5-0 or 6-0 absorbable suture (plain catgut) to prevent nail distortion. A torn nail bed may indicate an open fracture of the distal phalanx, which is relatively stable. The edges of the fingertip laceration are approximated with Steri-strips, molding the tip back in shape without encircling the finger, which may jeopardize the blood supply because of swelling (Figure 28-21). All of the above may be done without anesthesia, with the exception of suturing the nail bed.

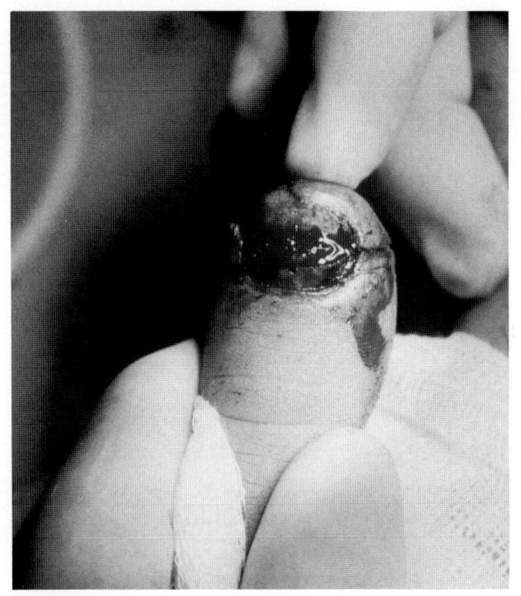

FIGURE 28-20 Fingertip crush injury.

Lacerated Fingertips

Lacerated fingertips usually cause little or no problem. However, the fingertip injury that has more than 1 cm^2 of skin loss or loss of the volar fat pad is of major concern (Figure 28-22C).

The child less than 5 years old has remarkable recuperative powers. If the fingertip is injured (as in Figure 28-22, A and B), there are two approaches to treatment: closed or open.

To close the fingertip of an injury as shown in Figure 28-22, A or B, a V-Y-plasty may be performed (Figures 28-23 and 28-24).[1] A large triangular flap is outlined on the volar surface of the tip. The proximal apex of the triangle should not cross the distal volar flexion crease. The skin is incised through to

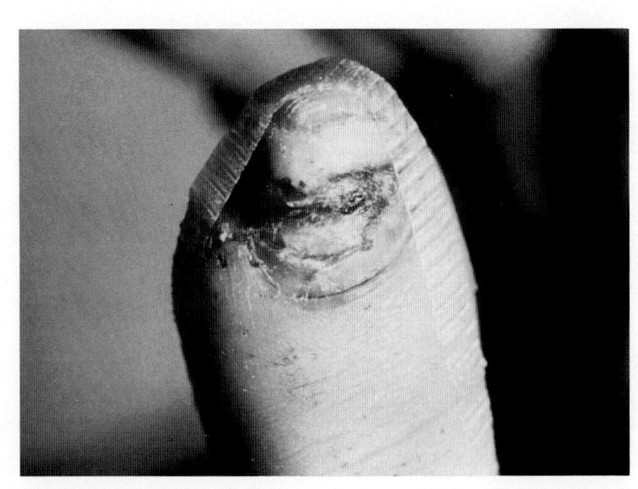

FIGURE 28-21 Steri-strips help mold the fingertip back into normal shape.

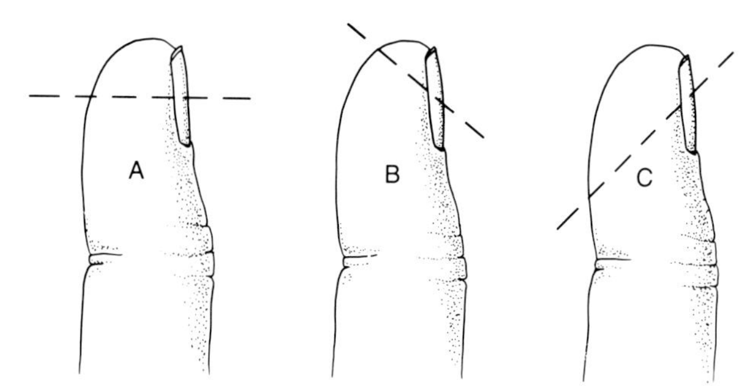

FIGURE 28-22 Fingertip amputation levels.

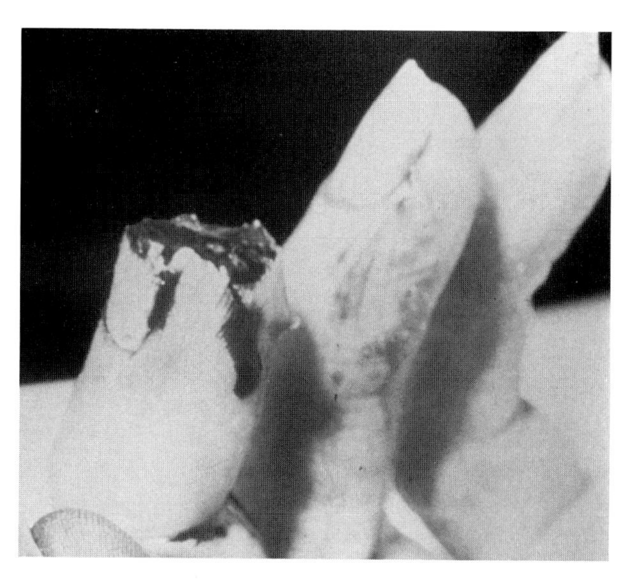

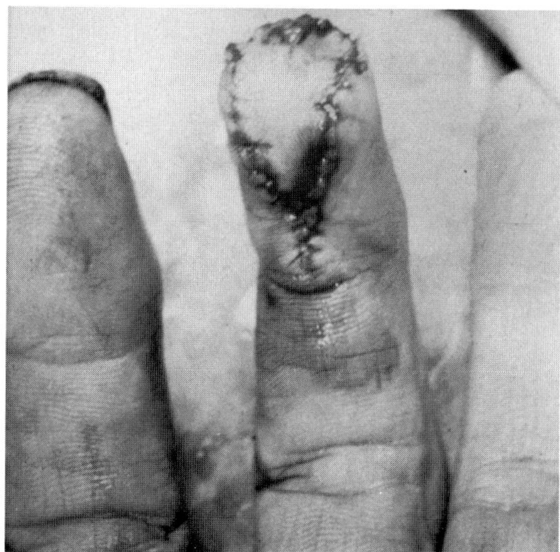

FIGURE 28-24 A and B, V-Y-plasty performed on a young girl.

the subcutaneous fat. The subcutaneous tissue is spread gently away from the bone with sharp pointed scissors, and the triangular flap, including all its subcutaneous tissue, is pulled distalward. The fibrous septal attachment at the proximal apex of the triangular flap must be transected to advance this flap over the bone to the tip. The base of the triangle is sutured to the nail and the V is converted to a Y.

Open treatment consists of cleansing the wound and placing a piece of tape or Steri-strip from the volar skin surface over the wound to the dorsal finger surface. This eventually heals within 4 to 8 weeks with little or no problem as long as the bone is covered with viable soft tissue. Usually there is no problem with infection.

Loss of the pulp (Figure 28-22C) is a difficult problem as there is no local flap able to cover the defect without shortening the bone. A split-thickness skin graft is unsatisfactory because there is no soft tissue covering the bone. A cross-finger flap will cover the defect and retain length, but sensibility will be lacking. This problem should be relegated to the experienced hand surgeon for definitive care.

Dislocations

Understanding and treating finger joint dislocations requires adequate knowledge of the anatomy of the joint.[2] The structures surrounding the joint can be compared to a chair with arms. The back of the chair is analogous to the base of the middle phalanx; the arms, to the collateral ligament complex; and the seat, to the volar plate (Figure 28-25).

The common "jammed finger" injury usually involves a dislocation of the proximal interphalangeal joint. The dorsal dislocation of the proximal interphalangeal joint avulses the volar plate from the middle phalangeal base and tears the accessory collateral ligaments (Figure 28-26), leaving the main collateral ligaments intact and thus resulting in excellent lateral stability when reduced. There are other combinations of tears and avulsions of these structures that lead to instability.

A dorsal dislocation that has only soft tissue damage need not be repaired surgically. An open dislo-

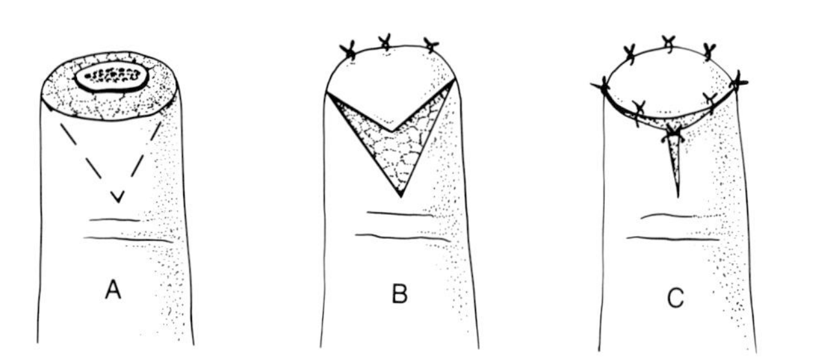

FIGURE 28-23 Diagramatic illustration of V-Y-plasty for fingertip amputation.

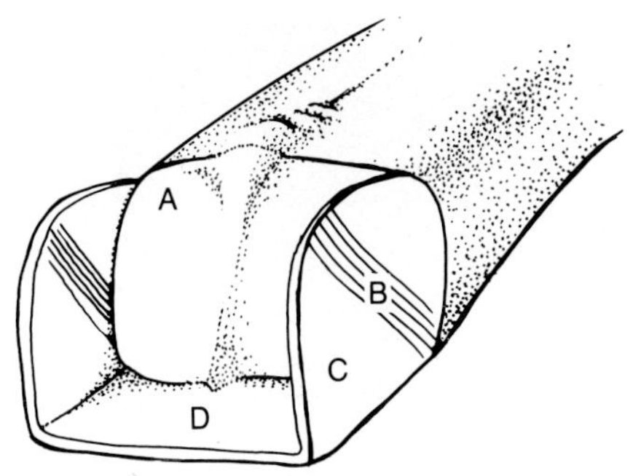

FIGURE 28-25 View of a disarticulated proximal interphalangeal joint. The proximal phalanx has been removed. A, Base of the middle phalanx; B, main collateral ligament; C, accessory collateral ligament; D, volar plate. A dislocation of the proximal interphalangeal joint cannot occur without tearing at least two of the ligamentous structures.

cation, where the flexor tendons dislocate lateral to the proximal phalangeal head, needs surgical intervention to cleanse and relocate the flexor tendons and repair the volar plate (Figure 28-27).

Treatment of the closed dorsal dislocation begins with adequate finger anesthesia after which the MP joint is flexed to relax the flexor and intrinsic tendon forces on the middle phalanx. Traction is applied to the middle phalanx in the direction of the dislocation. Reduction is accomplished by flexing and applying pressure to the base of the middle phalanx. Once reduced, the joint range of motion is tested actively to see if the joint dislocates when fully extended. The finger joint is also passively tested for lateral stability. A dorsal extension block splint is applied to the finger, allowing active flexion and preventing full extension. The splint is worn for approximately 3 weeks, and then the finger is "buddy taped" to the normal adjacent digit for the next 3 weeks.

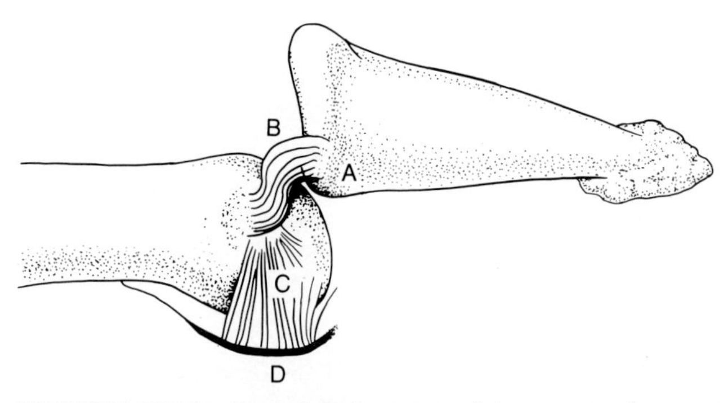

FIGURE 28-26 Dorsal dislocation of the proximal interphalangeal joint. Note that the volar plate (D) is avulsed from the base of the middle phalanx (A). The accessory collateral ligaments (C) are also torn. B, collateral ligament.

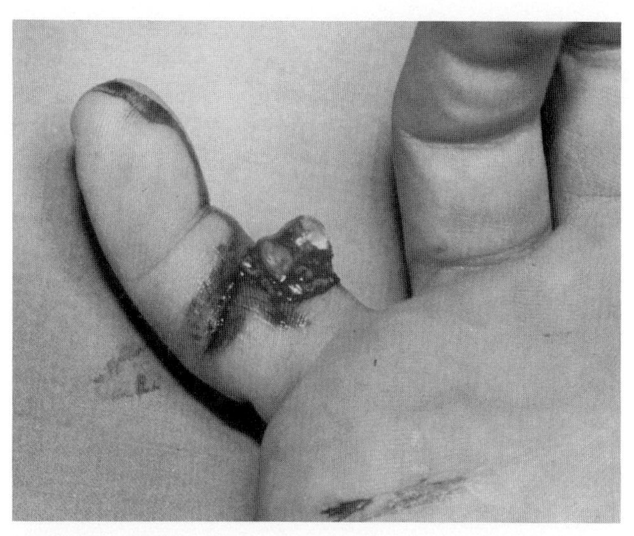

FIGURE 28-27 Open proximal interphalangeal joint dislocation. This should be treated with surgical debridement, relocation of the flexor tendon, and repair of the volar plate.

Dorsal dislocations of the MP and distal interphalangeal joints may be handled in a similar manner. Irreducible, "complex" dislocations of the MP joints can occur. Interposition of the volar plate between the metacarpal head and the proximal phalanx is the obstacle that blocks closed reduction. Open reduction is usually necessary (Figure 28-28).[3]

A volar proximal interphalangeal joint dislocation is a more severe injury. The extensor mechanism of the middle phalanx is avulsed and both col-

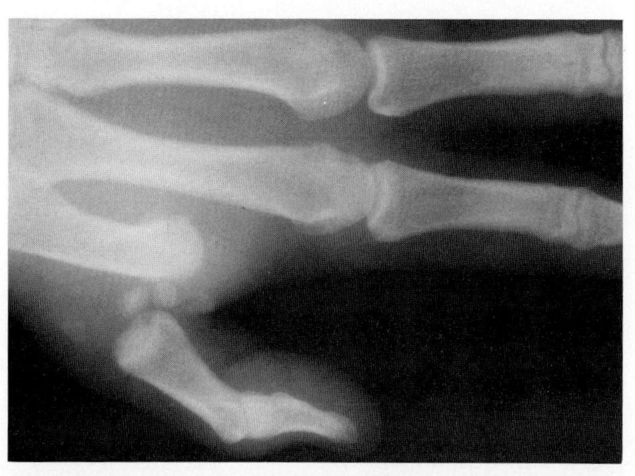

FIGURE 28-28 Complex dislocation of the thumb MP joint. The volar plate is blocking reduction of this dislocation. The sesamoids of the thumb, which are located in the volar plate, can be visualized dorsal to the first metacarpal.

lateral ligaments are torn. Open reduction and internal fixation are required.

FRACTURES

The difference between a child's and an adult's bone is the growth plate (physis) found in children. It is located near the joint and is responsible for the longitudinal growth of bone. The physis is weaker than the bone and ligaments. When the digit is subjected to tensile and shearing forces, physeal type injuries occur. As the child matures and the growth plates close, ligament injuries occur instead of physeal fractures.

In 1963 Salter and Harris[4] classified epiphyseal plate (physeal) injuries into five types and gave a prognosis for each (see Chapter 26, Figure 26-6).

Type I is a complete shearing through the physis not involving bone. A closed reduction accomplished early will be stable and have an excellent result.

Type II is a partial shear through the physis and out through the metaphysis. The treatment and result are the same as for type I. This is the most common type of fracture in children.

Type III is an intra-articular fracture, which is a partial shear through the physis and out through the epiphysis. It is an uncommon type of fracture that may require open reduction to obtain congruity of the joint and good results.

Type IV is an intra-articular fracture through the epiphysis, physis, and metaphysis. It is an unstable fracture that requires anatomic reduction, usually open, to provide a good result.

Type V is a crush of the physis, which may alter or stop growth. This is an uncommon injury with a very poor prognosis.

The potential complications of physeal fractures in regard to possible growth abnormalities should always be explained to the parents.

Fractures of the Distal Phalanx

The fractured distal phalanx is usually the result of a crush from a door. The fracture can be simple or comminuted and is quite stable unless it is open.

The closed fracture of the distal phalanx in children heals in approximately 3 to 4 weeks, although the fracture lines may be seen radiographically for many months. If there is no tenderness at the fracture site, the finger should be considered healed.

A subungual hematoma may occur with this fracture. The finger pulp can become distended and tender from bone bleeding (Figure 28-29A). Theoretically, the increased pressure from this bleeding may compromise the blood supply and necrose the pulp. This is easily avoided by applying a red-hot paper clip to the nail gently with no pressure, allowing it to burn a hole and decompressing the subungual hematoma (Figure 28-29B). This not only relieves the pressure on the pulp, but also dramatically decreases the patient's discomfort.

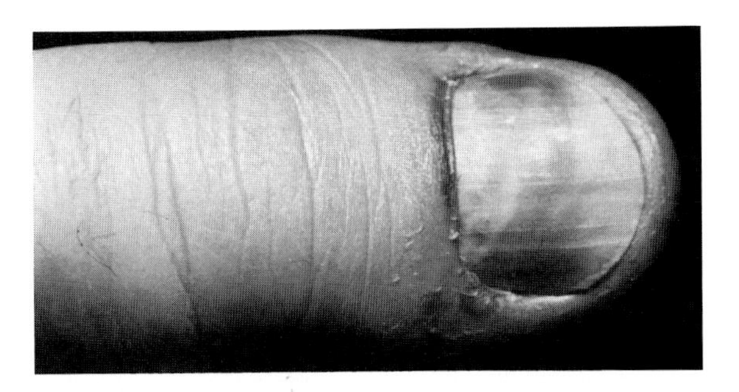

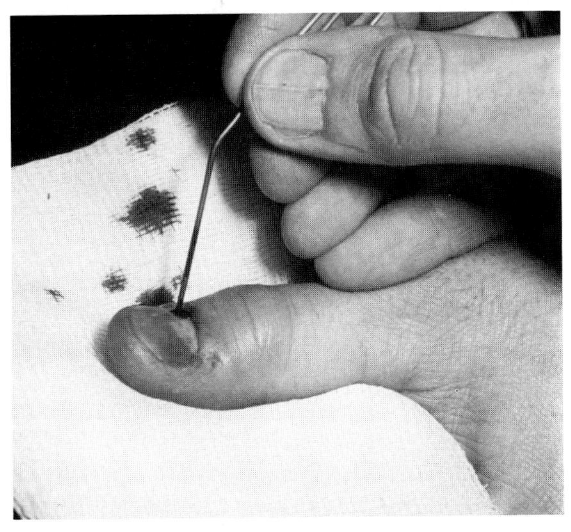

FIGURE 28-29 Subungual hematoma (A) being drained with a hot paper clip (B). The red hot clip requires very little pressure to burn through the nail. Burning the nail is not painful; pressure is painful.

Intra-articular fractures of the distal phalanx with a closed physis may be avulsion fractures of either the terminal extensor slip, i.e., "mallet finger," or an avulsion of the flexor profundus tendon, i.e., "football jersey injury" (Figure 28-30). The latter avulsion fracture needs to be repaired surgically to return flexion to the distal phalanx and strength to the finger.

Mallet Finger

Baseball or mallet finger is the inability of the distal joint of the finger to be fully extended. This malady is secondary to the lack of extensor power, which

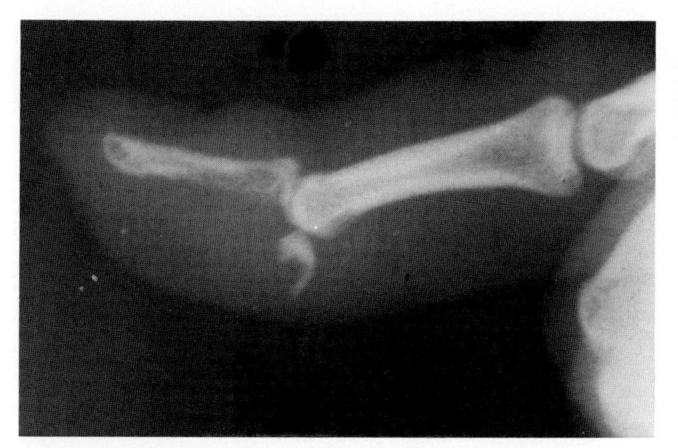

FIGURE 28-30 Intra-articular fracture of the distal phalanx. The flexor digitorum profundus tendon is attached to this fragment of bone. Early open reduction and internal fixation are mandatory. This injury usually affects the ring finger and occurs when a player is grabbing an opponent's football jersey while attempting to tackle him.

may be the result of a terminal slip rupture, laceration, or avulsion fracture (Figure 28-31).

Treatment is tailored to the severity of the injury. A ruptured terminal slip with or without avulsion of bone and a stable unsubluxed joint is treated with a splint. The distal joint is held in extension and the proximal interphalangeal joint is held in 30° of flexion, which advances the terminal slip. This position is held for 3 weeks to allow soft tissue healing, after which just the distal interphalangeal joint is held in full extension for 4 to 5 weeks more. A large bone fragment, more than one third of the joint surface, and a subluxed or dislocated joint need to be reduced with internal fixation (Figure 28-32).

The soft tissue mallet finger, if not treated, will lack approximately 45° or less of full extension with a minimal amount of functional loss.

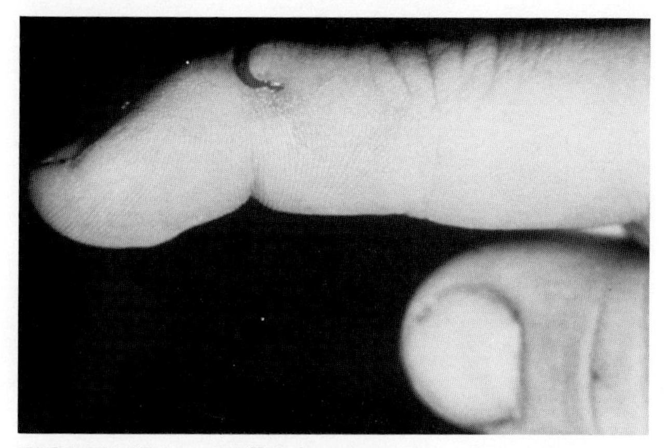

FIGURE 28-31 Mallet finger resulting from a laceration of the terminal slip. This requires surgical repair and a transarticular wire for 6 weeks.

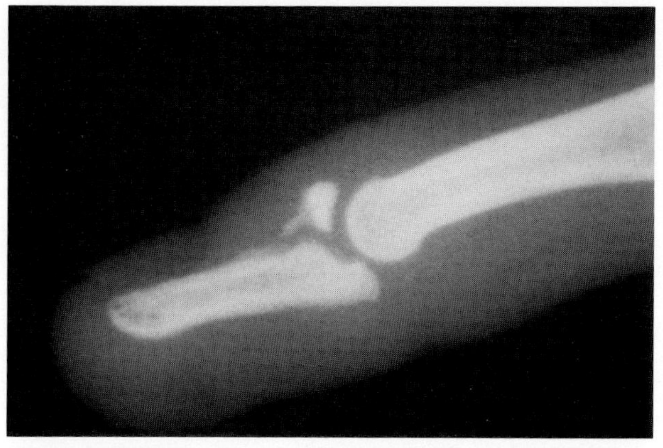

FIGURE 28-32 Bony mallet finger. Note that there is a large intra-articular component. The distal phalanx is subluxed volarly because of the pull of the profundus tendon. This injury must be treated surgically.

An open Salter-Harris type I or II fracture of the distal phalanx can mimic a mallet finger (Figure 28-33). This is usually associated with an avulsion of the base of the nail. Treatment does not require removal of the whole nail. Instead, a V-shaped notch is cut at the base of the nail, and the fracture is irrigated, if open, and reduced. If torn, the nail bed is closed with 6-0 plain catgut. The nail is resewn into its fold, and the distal phalanx is held in full extension rather than hyperextension in a splint for 3 weeks. Internal fixation with K-wires may be unwarranted because of the complication of infection.

Intra-Articular Fractures

Intra-articular fractures of the proximal interphalangeal joint are common in the older child. A baseball strikes the end of the finger and transmits the force proximally, fracturing the volar base of the middle phalanx and dislocating it dorsally (Figure 28-34, A and B). The middle phalangeal joint fragment may

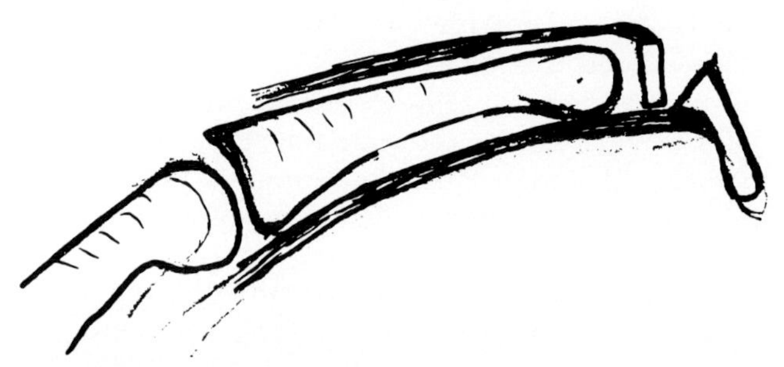

FIGURE 28-33 Diagramatic representation of a Salter-Harris type I fracture of the distal phalanx. This is often an open fracture and requires irrigation, debridement, antibiotics, and reduction. All mallet fingers should be radiologically examined.

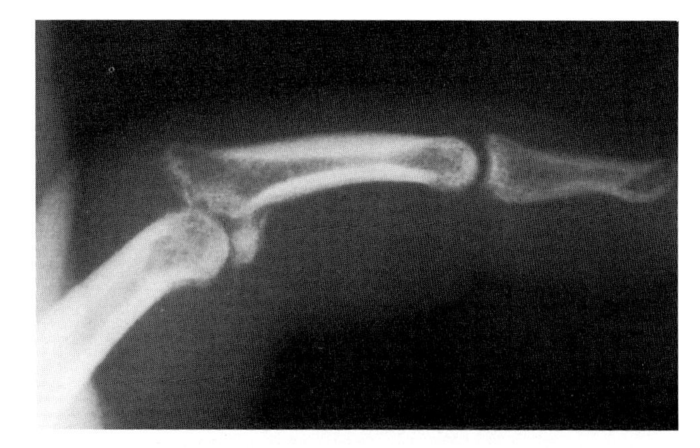

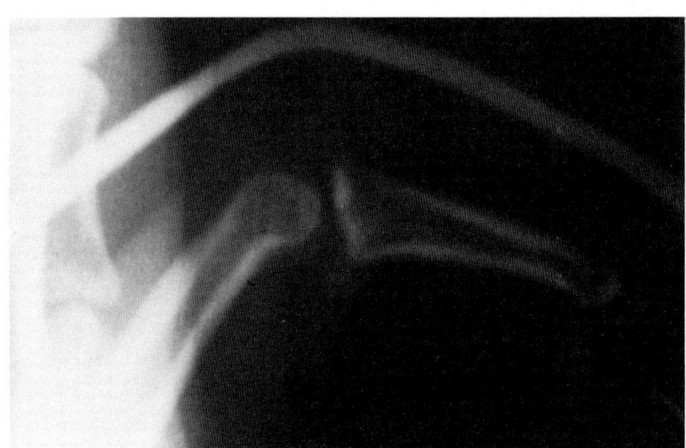

FIGURE 28-34 Dorsal fracture-dislocation of the proximal interphalangeal joint (A). Satisfactory closed reduction was obtained, and the patient was placed in a dorsal extension block splint. He was allowed to flex in the splint but not extend beyond the point of instability for approximately 3 weeks (B).

range in size from a small fleck to the entire joint surface. The lack of integrity of the joint may cause dorsal subluxation or dislocation.

If a closed reduction is attempted, the proximal interphalangeal joint must be distracted and flexed enough to obtain opposition of the fracture fragments. An avulsion fracture of the volar plate can be reduced and treated as a dorsal dislocation. It may be necessary to flex the proximal interphalangeal joint to 90° to reduce the large fragment and prevent dorsal subluxation. This would require immobilization for 3 weeks, after which range-of-motion exercises should be started.

Failure to attain a good intra-articular reduction will lead to traumatic degenerative joint disease. Therefore, an open procedure may be indicated. Experience has shown that this particular type of fracture is most difficult to treat and obtain good results.[1] Any injury to the proximal interphalangeal joint of the finger causes a great amount of disability. Swelling may last a year or more. It is a gross understatement to say "it is just a sprained joint."

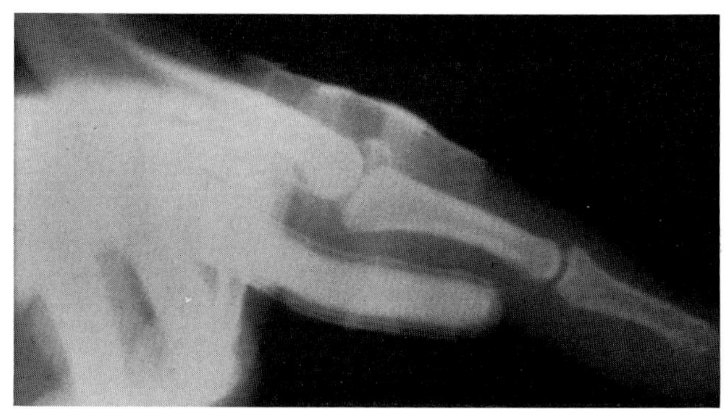

FIGURE 28-35 Postreduction x-ray film of a volar dislocation of the proximal interphalangeal joint. The fragment of bone on the midphalanx has been avulsed by the central slip. This fracture should be internally fixed for optimum results.

A volar fracture-dislocation of the proximal interphalangeal joint is relatively uncommon. A roentgenogram revealing bone avulsed by the central slip from the dorsal middle phalangeal base (Figure 28-35), with or without subluxation of the joint volarly, suggests the diagnosis. The joint may be quite unstable and must be relocated and pinned. The fragment with the central slip is replaced anatomically to attain congruity of the joint and extensor power of the middle phalanx.

Avulsion fractures of the base of the proximal phalanx of the MP joints (Figure 28-36) are usually stable injuries. If minimally displaced, they will heal and have a good prognosis. Fractures with joint

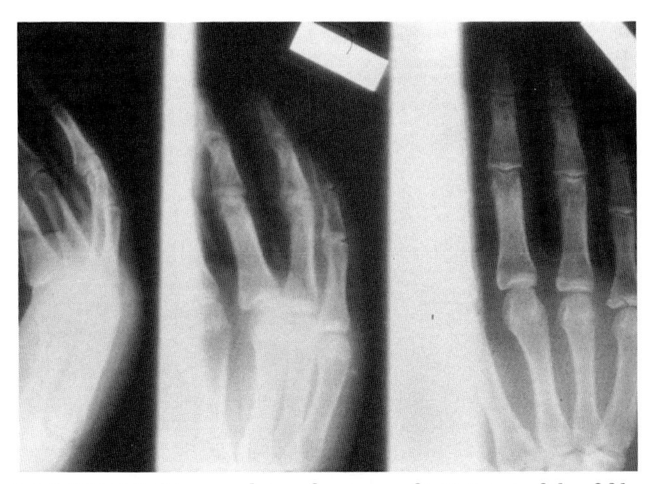

FIGURE 28-36 Avulsion fracture of MP joint of the fifth digit. There is a nondisplaced Salter-Harris type III fracture of the proximal phalanx of the fifth digit. This is stable and can be treated closed.

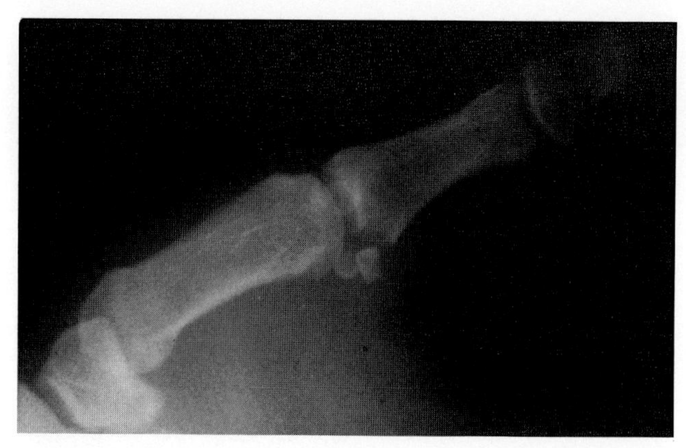

FIGURE 28-37 Bony gamekeeper's thumb. This portion of bone is avulsed with the ulnar collateral ligament. Open reduction and internal fixation are required for optimum results.

incongruity need to be opened, reduced, and internally fixed.

The "gamekeeper's thumb" or "skier's thumb," which is an avulsed ulnar collateral ligament, with or without a bony fragment from the base of the proximal phalanx, is a common entity (Figure 28-37). This injury is a major insult to hand function, as the stability of the thumb is lost in grasp and pinch. When both thumbs are examined in full extension, a definite stop is felt with an intact ulnar collateral ligament; but a springy sensation is present if the ulnar collateral ligament complex is avulsed. Roentgenograms may reveal a displaced avulsion fracture, but in either case the pathology is the same, i.e., loss of ulnar stability. Treatment of the torn ulnar collateral ligament complex, with or without an avulsion fracture, requires operative repair by a knowledgeable surgeon. The results of immediate repair are far more favorable than those of later reconstruction for chronic instability.

Diaphyseal Fractures

Nondisplaced fractures of the diaphysis of the phalanx in children are relatively stable. The thick periosteal sleeve holds the fragments in place. The shaft fracture can usually be reduced with traction and held with a splint. If adequate reduction cannot be maintained despite repeated attempts at balancing all the displacing forces, then open reduction and internal fixation are indicated.

Treating shaft fractures of the hand requires knowledge of anatomy and dynamic forces.[5] Transverse fractures are stable longitudinally but angulate readily (Figure 28-38). The force of the interosseous muscles angulates the fracture of the

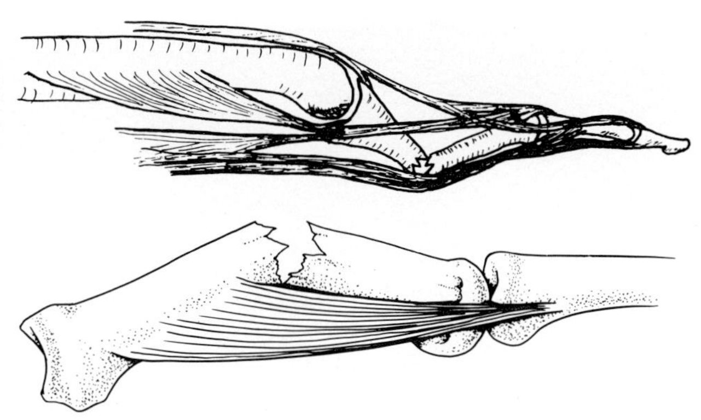

FIGURE 28-38 Diaphyseal fractures of the proximal phalanx angulate volarly (A), whereas fractures of the metacarpal angulate dorsally (B).

metacarpal shaft dorsally and the fracture of the proximal phalangeal shaft volarly when the MP joint is in full extension. Flexing the MP joint to approximately 60° diminishes the angulatory force, allowing reduction to be achieved and held. Finger alignment is important. Each finger, when flexed individually, points to the tubercle of the scaphoid (Figure 28-39). This is an excellent check for malrotation of the metacarpal and proximal phalangeal fracture. The fractured finger should be splinted pointing toward the scaphoid tubercle.

The shortening that occurs with an unstable oblique fracture of the phalangeal shaft can only be tolerated in the distal phalanx and, at times, the metacarpal. The middle and proximal phalangeal shafts are unable to tolerate much shortening because of the fine balance of the flexor and extensor

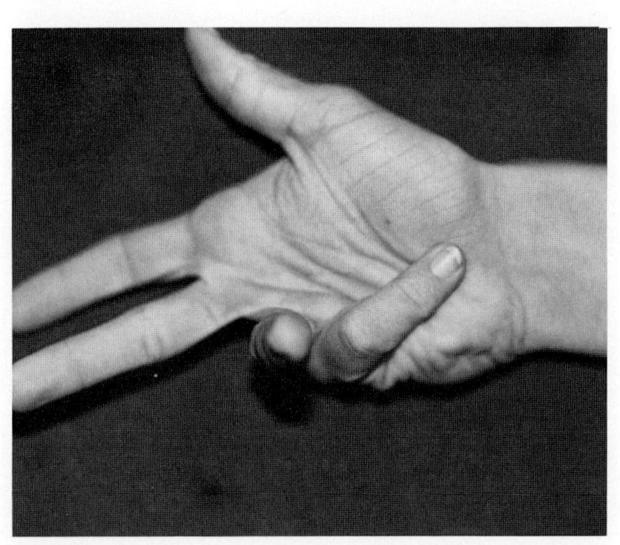

FIGURE 28-39 Each finger when individually flexed will point toward the tubercle of the scaphoid. This alignment should always be checked after fracture reduction.

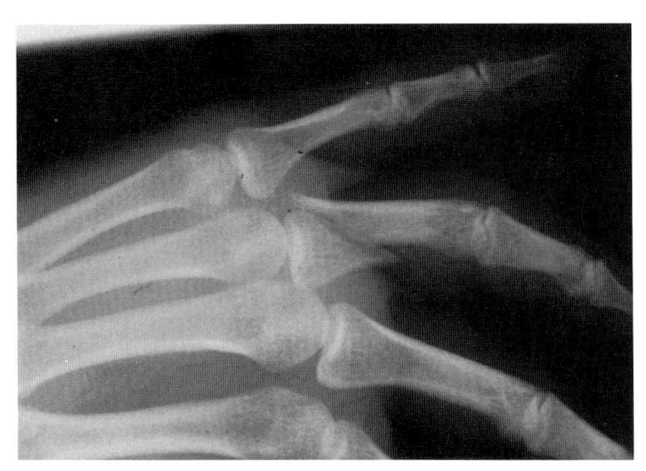

FIGURE 28-40 Oblique proximal phalanx fracture. Open reduction and internal fixation are necessary for optimum results.

forces. Therefore, unstable oblique, transverse, or comminuted fractures of the proximal and middle phalangeal shaft that are not amenable to closed reduction should be opened and internally fixed (Figure 28-40).

The key to hand function is the wrist. Every splint applied to hold the fingers needs to incorporate the wrist. If the wrist moves, the fingers also will move by the tenodesis effect.

Metaphyseal fractures (i.e., Salter-Harris type II fractures) of the proximal phalanx are common. Reduction is accomplished by (1) flexing the proximal phalanx to 90°, which tightens the collateral ligaments; (2) holding the base of the proximal phalanx rigidly to the metacarpal head; and (3) sharply manipulating the finger into the anatomic position (Figure 28-41). A relatively stable metaphyseal fracture, one that will stay reduced after manipulation, can be buddy-taped to the adjacent finger and moved.

Metacarpal Fractures

The most common fracture of the hand is the "boxer's fracture," which is a fracture at the neck of the fifth metacarpal (Figure 28-42).[6] This is usually secondary to striking a hard object, e.g., a wall or jaw. Flexing the MP joint and pushing up the metacarpal head volarly help decrease the dorsal angulation. Anatomic reduction is usually not accomplished and 45° of dorsal angulation is acceptable. A rotational deformity, however, is not acceptable. Once reduction is performed, the hand is immobilized by a short arm cast with an outrigger to both the ring and little fingers to control rotation.

Most fractures of the metacarpal shaft can be treated in a short-arm plaster cast with the wrist in dorsiflexion and the fingers splinted in flexion at the MP joint to eliminate the deforming forces of the interosseous muscles and to correct malrotation. In 3 weeks, fractures are usually healed enough that the hand can be used. If the patient still has tenderness over the fracture site, immobilization is continued for an additional week.

Fractures of the metacarpal base need to be aligned by traction and manipulation and are relatively stable. They are treated in a short-arm cast for 3 weeks.

Bennett's Fracture

This intra-articular fracture of the base of the first metacarpal is unstable and requires reduction and

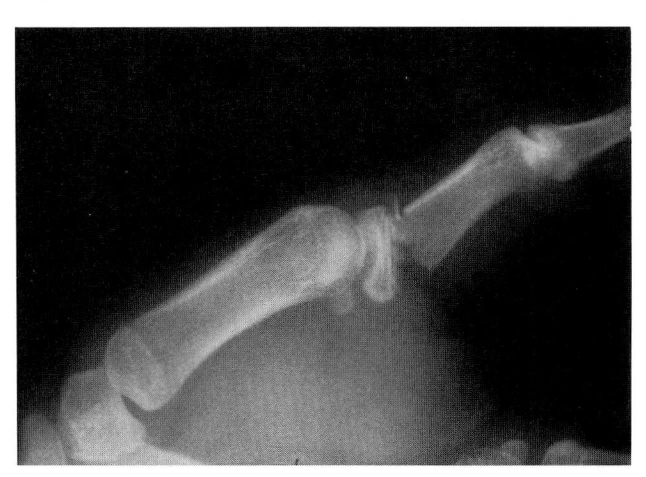

FIGURE 28-41 Salter-Harris type II fracture of the proximal phalanx of the thumb. The thumb must be flexed and forcibly adducted to achieve reduction.

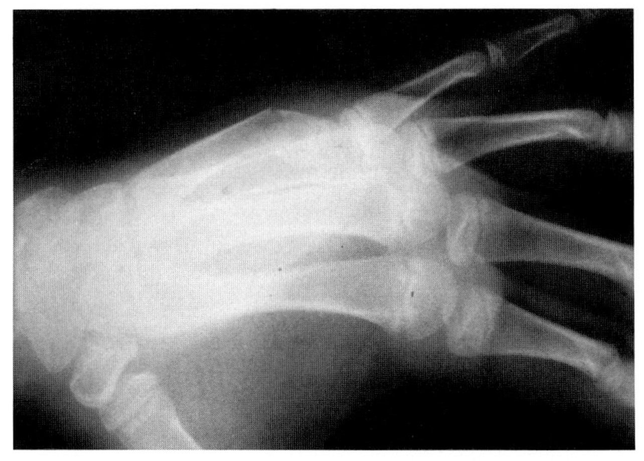

FIGURE 28-42 Boxer's fracture of the fifth metacarpal neck. Forty-five degrees of dorsal angulation is acceptable and compatible with normal function.

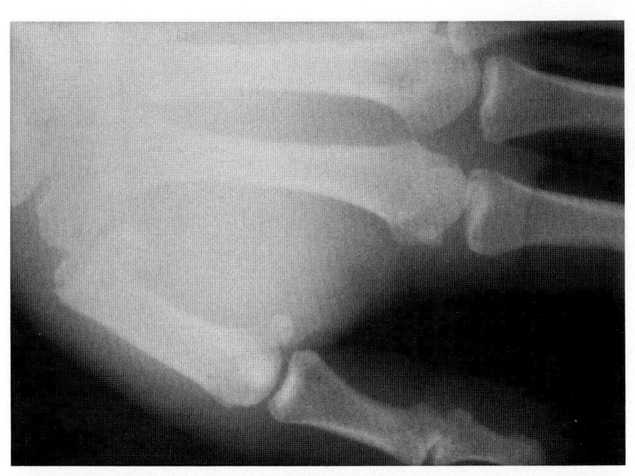

FIGURE 28-43 Bennett's fracture of the first metacarpal. This is an unstable intra-articular fracture-dislocation. Either closed reduction with percutaneous pinning or open reduction and internal fixation are required.

anatomic percutaneous pinning within 12 to 24 hours. Open reduction and internal fixation are required if closed reduction is not possible or if there has been a delay in treatment. The thumb is the most important digit of the hand, for without it grasp is not possible (Figure 28-43).

Carpal Bone Fractures

The history of a fall on the outstretched arm and pain in the anatomical snuff box should alert the examiner to the possibility of a scaphoid fracture. Roentgenograms may reveal the nondisplaced fracture initially. However, if a fracture is not visualized on the initial film, the patient should be immobilized in a thumb spica cast for 2 to 3 weeks and then x-ray films should be repeated. After the cast is removed, if the hand is nontender and the repeat film shows no fracture, the patient's "sprained wrist" has been treated ideally. If, on the other hand, the patient has a fracture of the scaphoid, the short-arm thumb spica cast is continued until the fracture is healed. Since the fractured scaphoid is frequently missed, all wrist injuries should be treated as a fractured scaphoid until proven otherwise (Figure 28-44).

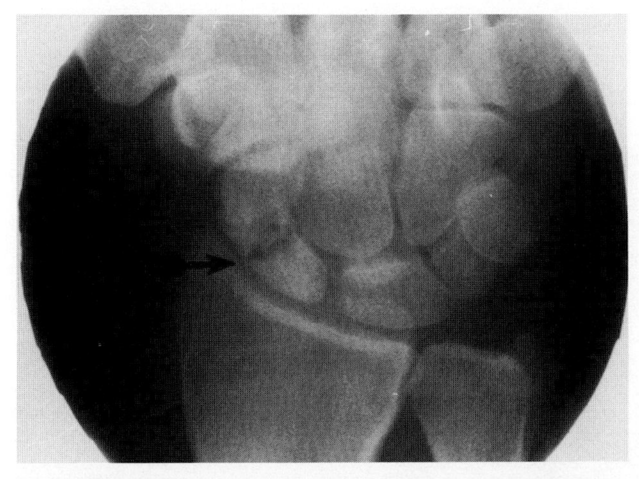

FIGURE 28-44 Fracture of the scaphoid. This fracture is often missed and has a very high incidence of nonunion if left untreated.

HAND WOUND EVALUATION

Hand injuries should be evaluated thoroughly by the emergency physician. If there is profuse arterial bleeding, direct pressure and elevation are all that is necessary to control it. Hemostats can cause more problems than they solve: they not only crush an artery that may need repair, but they often damage nerves permanently.

Adequate anatomic knowledge and a detailed physical examination of all the structures distal to the wound make for a straightforward diagnosis.

Soft tissue injuries that have not violated any important structures and are not contaminated can be cleansed and closed primarily. The use of a pneumatic tourniquet placed high on the arm and inflated to 50 mmHg above systolic blood pressure allows excellent visualization of the wound depths and the important structures during debridement. Exsanguination of the extremity prior to tourniquet inflation is obtained by elevation of the limb higher than the heart for 3 minutes. Without axillary block anesthesia the tourniquet may be tolerated only 10 to 20 minutes and usually no longer than 45 minutes. After the wound has been debrided, irrigated copiously ("the solution to pollution is dilution"), and appears completely clean, the tourniquet is deflated and removed. Pressure is applied to the wound site for approximately 10 to 15 minutes to allow for tissue equilibrium and blood clotting after tourniquet removal.

In young children the use of interrupted absorbable 5-0 plain catgut sutures to approximate skin is recommended. In older children a similar sized nonabsorbable monofilament suture is recommended for skin closure.

A contaminated wound should never be closed, even if flexor tendons and neurovascular bundles are exposed. The incidence of severe infections complicating closed contaminated wounds is unacceptably high. Open treatment with or without antibiotics is the safest course whenever the status of the wound is in question. Most wounds that parallel the normal skin creases heal with minimal scarring when allowed to heal by secondary intention.

TENDON INJURIES

Flexor Tendons

Careful observation and examination will detect a flexor tendon laceration (see Figure 28-12). Flexor tendon and nerve repair should be carried out by an experienced surgeon who is able to provide the appropriate rehabilitation and care for the complications that may ensue.[3]

Extensor Tendons

Extrinsic extensor tendons of the fingers extend both the MP and the proximal interphalangeal joints. The interossei and lumbricales flex the MP joint and extend the proximal interphalangeal joint and the distal interphalangeal joints.

Extrinsic extensor tendon lacerations (Figures 28-45, A and B) are repaired by approximating the ends of the tendons with one or two 4-0 nonabsorbable sutures. The wrist is splinted in 35° of extension and the fingers are splinted in full extension for 4 weeks.

Intrinsic extensor mechanism or dorsal apparatus lacerations need to be repaired and splinted in the same manner as above for 4 weeks and then are moved gently.

Splinting the MP joint in full extension relaxes the collateral ligament (see Figure 28-10). In adults, if this position is held for more than 3 weeks, shortening of these ligaments will occur, causing inability of the joint to fully flex. However, splinting children's hands 4 to 5 weeks in this position presents minimal difficulty in regaining flexion.

INFECTION

A closed-space infection, if not treated correctly, can severely and permanently damage a child's hand. Large open wounds are readily noticed, treated promptly, and usually heal without infection. It is usually the small puncture or scratch that goes unnoticed until an infection has become established. Antibiotics have reduced the number of significant hand infections; however, knowledge of the course and treatment is necessary to prevent disastrous complications.

Paronychia

Local redness, swelling, and pain in the paronychium at the side of the nail are the signs and symptoms of a paronychial infection (Figure 28-46, A and B). Drainage of purulence by a small incision in the depth of the sulcus is usually curative. If the infection is left untreated, pus dissects around the base of the nail under the eponychium and nail plate. Treatment at this stage is removal of the base of the nail plate, using sharp pointed scissors and gently placing a doubled piece of xeroform gauze in the sulcus of the nail base. In 5 to 7 days, the finger is relatively asymptomatic, and in 10 to 14 days the wound is healed.

Felon

A felon is an infection of the fingertip pulp space, which becomes distended with pus. If this pressure is not released, the blood supply of the pulp and the

A

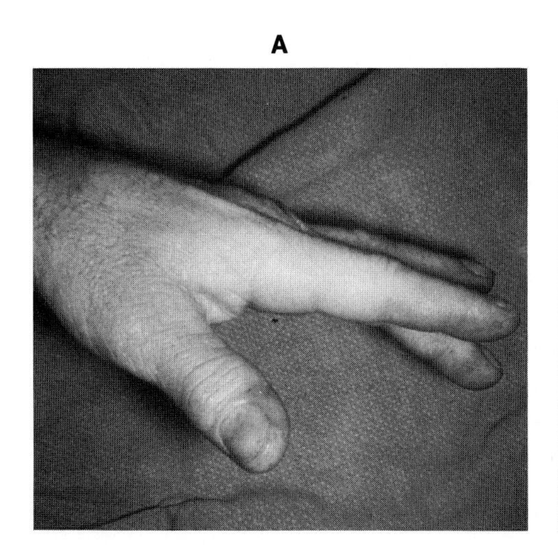

B

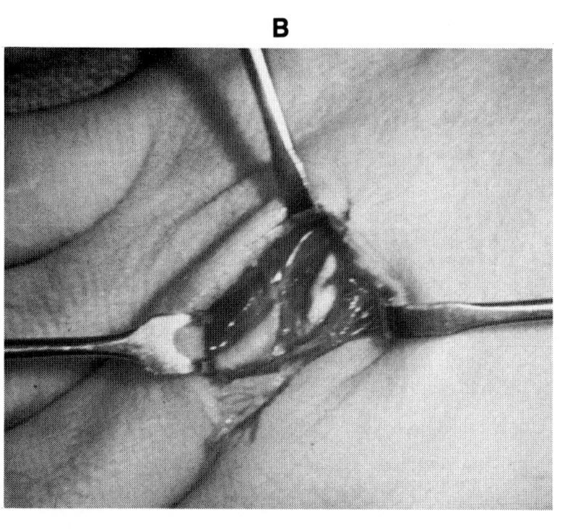

FIGURE 28-45 Long finger lacks 30° of extension (A) as a result of an extensor communis tendon laceration (B).

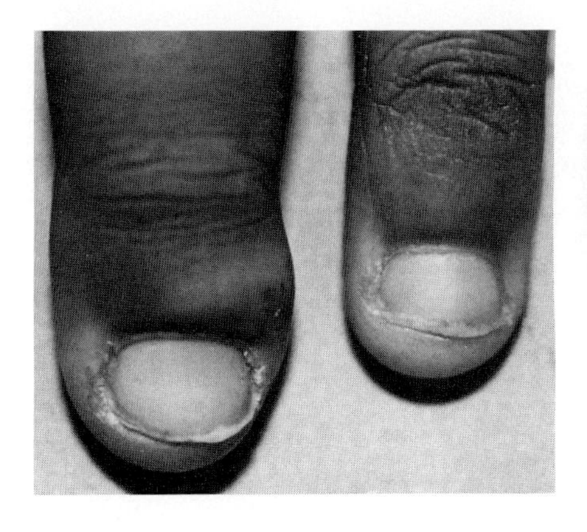

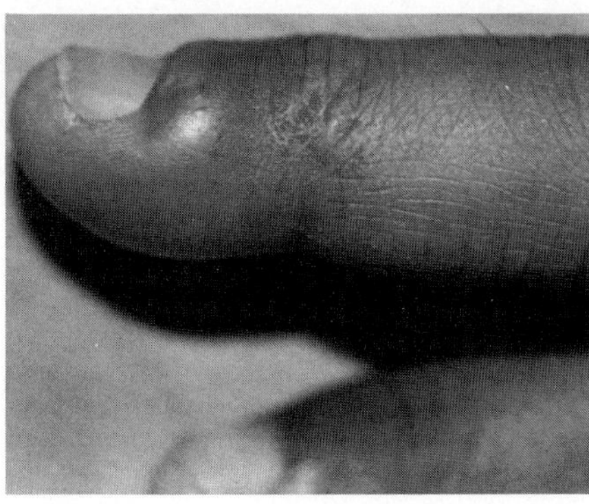

FIGURE 28-46 Paronychia, dorsal view (A) and lateral view (B). These infections can be drained where they point. However, the nail matrix must not be incised or a deformed nail will result.

diaphysis of the distal phalanx is jeopardized, causing necrosis. A patient complaining of a severe throbbing pain and a markedly distended finger pulp that is exquisitely tender to touch is a candidate for prompt treatment (Figure 28-47).

Treatment consists of draining the pulp where the abscess is pointing. While keeping in mind the innervation of the fingertip, a longitudinal incision is made through the skin. A pair of sharp, pointed scissors is used to spread the subcutaneous tissue in the same longitudinal direction. The tendon sheath should not be violated. If the felon is not pointing or more adequate drainage is required, a longitudinal lateral incision with a number 11 blade is made just volar to the dorsum of the distal phalanx. The incision proceeds to, but not through, the skin on the opposite side of the tip of the finger. A small Silastic or rubber Penrose drain can be used, but if the incision has been adequate, often no drain is needed. A fish-mouth incision is not necessary and may lead to retraction of the pulp.[1]

Purulent Flexor Tenosynovitis

Septic tenosynovitis is a true surgical emergency and calls for immediate attention. Kanaval's four cardinal symptoms of acute septic tenosynovitis are: (1) a painful finger held rigid in a semiflexed position; (2) pain with passive extension of the finger; (3) fusiform swelling; and (4) marked tenderness on palpation along the entire tendon sheath, with maximal pain over the metacarpal head (Figure 28-48).[3]

The course is rapid in onset. In 6 to 12 hours, the patient is usually complaining bitterly of a painful, throbbing finger. The pain is secondary to the distended synovial sheath, which compromises the blood supply to the tendon. The infection may rupture into a fascial space with marked decrease of pain, fooling both the physician and the patient into thinking the finger is better, while the infection is actually spreading.

Although very early treatment with antibiotics can abort tendon sheath infections, the treatment of choice is prompt drainage of the infected sheath through an incision at the midaxial line. This procedure should be performed by one who is familiar with the course of infection and all of the structures of the finger. The treatment of most infections in the hand calls for excellent anesthesia, tourniquet, adequate light, and good help. The operating suite of the hospital usually has all of these.

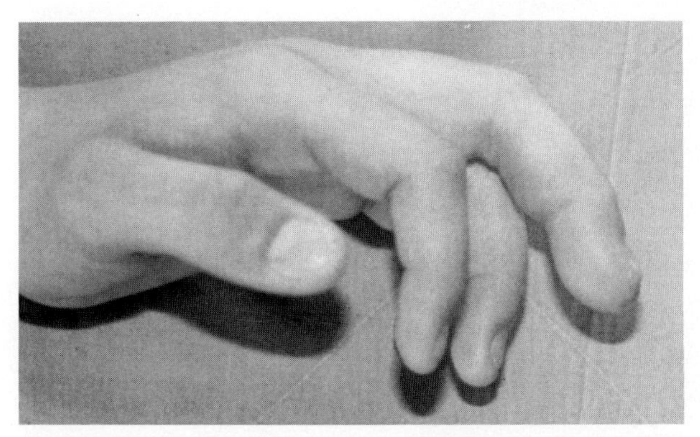

FIGURE 28-47 Felon of the middle finger. Note the red, swollen, tense fingertip.

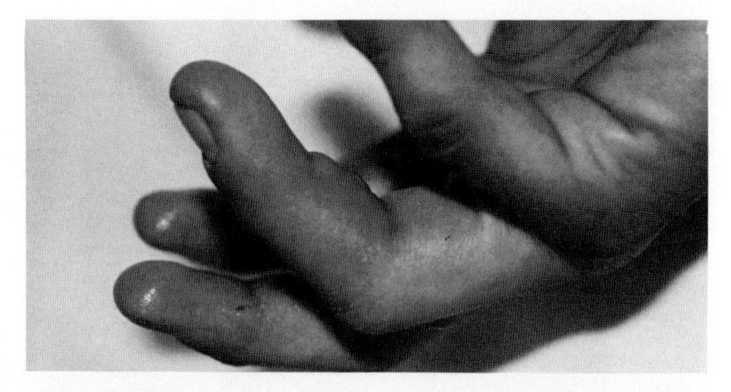

FIGURE 28-48 Flexor tenosynovitis. Note the fusiform swelling and the semiflexed position. This is a true surgical emergency and demands prompt incision and drainage.

HUMAN AND ANIMAL BITES

There is very little difference in the treatment of these types of wounds, with the exception of those caused by an animal that may be rabid. All wounds should be cleansed thoroughly and left open. The majority of human bites are inflicted in the MP joint area when the clenched fist strikes the teeth. The tooth lacerates the skin, dorsal apparatus, joint capsule, and metacarpal head with the proximal phalanx in full flexion. When the laceration is explored, one should place the hand in the same position as when struck. This "clenched-fist position" gives you a better idea as to the depth of the wound and the structures injured. If the joint has been violated by a "fight bite," it needs to be opened adequately and irrigated copiously. No repair of the damaged structures should be attempted primarily because of the potential danger of infection. This is the time for hospitalization, tetanus toxoid, prophylactic systemic antibiotics, elevation, and immobilization. At 5 to 6 days, once the danger of infection has passed, tendon repair and skin closure may be accomplished (Figure 28-49, A and B).

REPLANTATION

Microsurgical techniques have made it possible to replant digits, hands, and even arms. Proper care begins in the emergency department with resuscitation, tetanus prophylaxis, initiation of treatment with broad-spectrum antibiotics, and preparation for surgery. The possibility of replantation should be discussed, informing the patient and parents that not all amputations can or should be replanted. Roentgenograms of the limb and amputated part should be taken and sent with the patient if time permits.

The wound should be cleansed with sterile saline and dressed. Wash the part gently, wrap in a sterile saline moist sponge, put in a plastic bag, and place on ice. The part should not directly touch the ice nor should dry ice be used. If the amputation is partial, treat it the same way, as cooling lengthens the survivability of the part. The warm ischemia time should be recorded.

The next step is to notify the replantation center. The following information is required: age of the patient; dominant vs nondominant extremity; level of the amputation, such as thumb at the MP joint; mechanism of injury, such as crush or clean cut; time of the injury; and time of cooling. The decision to replant an amputated part must be made by the microvascular surgeon in the operating room.

CONCLUSION

Although emergency department physicians must have a broad base of knowledge, they are not expected to treat all emergencies definitively. A quali-

A

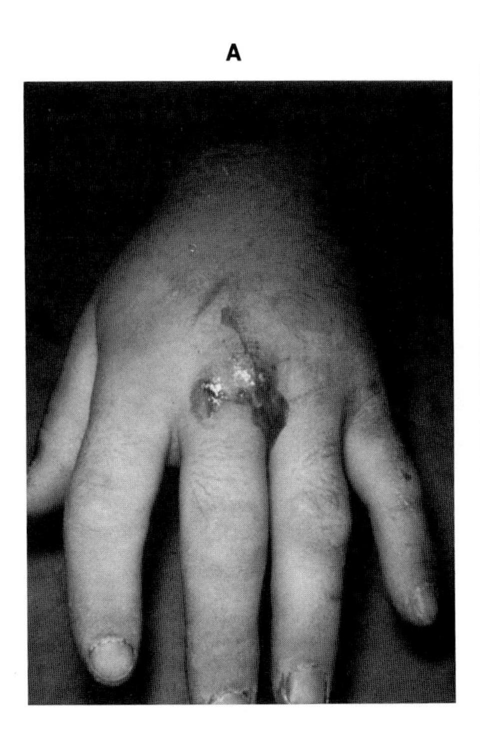

B

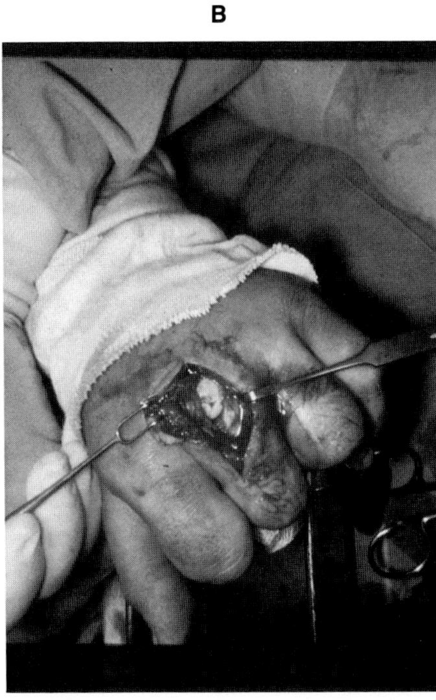

FIGURE 28-49 Fight bite wound over the middle MP joint (A). When the wound is debrided in the clenched-fist position, the laceration of the tendon and the tooth indentation in the metacarpal head are visualized (B).

fied hand surgeon is a good source of advice and should be consulted frequently, both for unusual problems and definitive follow-up.

References

1. Green DP: *Operative Hand Surgery.* New York, Churchill Livingstone, 1982.
2. Aryian S: *The Hand Book.* Baltimore, Williams & Wilkins, 1978.
3. Flynn JE: *Hand Surgery.* Baltimore, Williams & Wilkins, 1982.
4. Salter RB, Harris WR: Injuries involving the epiphyseal plate. *J Bone Joint Surg* [*Am*] 1963;45:587.
5. Semple C: *The Primary Management of Hand Injuries.* Chicago, Yearbook Medical Publishers Inc, 1979.
6. Weeks PM, Wray RC: *Management of Acute Hand Injuries.* St. Louis, CV Mosby Co, 1973.

Part VIII

Dermatologic Disorders

Nancy K. Barnett
Antoinette F. Hood

29

Dermatologic Disorders

To facilitate rapid diagnosis and treatment in an emergency department setting, the diseases discussed in this chapter are organized by their morphologic appearance (e.g., macules, papules, pustules). Optimal utilization of this chapter requires the use of standardized terminology for the description of cutaneous lesions. Figure 29-1 provides an illustrated diagramatic vocabulary for individual skin lesions. Because the morphology of skin lesions may change or evolve during the course of an illness and because a common etiology may produce a variety of lesions, some of the disorders described in this chapter are found in more than one section. Finally, since certain pediatric dermatologic emergencies are more common at different times in a child's life, at the beginning of each section there is a table that organizes the diseases according to age of presentation: neonate, infant or child, and adolescent.

DIFFUSE AND LOCALIZED MACULAR ERYTHEMA

Macular (flat or nonelevated) erythema is usually caused by dilatation of the superficial blood vessels in the skin. Light pressure applied to erythematous skin pushes the blood out of the engorged vessels and produces a transient blanching effect. This simple maneuver can be used to differentiate erythema associated with vasodilation from erythema associated with hemorrhage (see "Nonpalpable Purpura"). Macular erythema, which may vary in intensity from faint pink to bright red, can be difficult to detect in individuals with dark skin.

Diffuse, generalized macular erythema is usually associated with a systemic disease process. In contrast, localized macular erythema is usually associated with an exogenous cause such as thermal or ultraviolet light-induced injury. The most common causes of localized and diffuse blanchable macular erythema in various pediatric age groups are given in Table 29-1.

Staphylococcal Scalded Skin Syndrome

Clinical Picture

The patient has generalized *tender* macular erythema. Pressure on the skin produces erosions (Nikolsky's sign). Flaccid blisters filled with clear fluid are occasionally present. Large sheets of superficial epidermis may peel off, leaving a raw, shiny red surface.

Fever and malaise frequently accompany the eruption but vary considerably in severity. Conjunctivitis, pharyngitis, and mucous membrane erosions may be present.

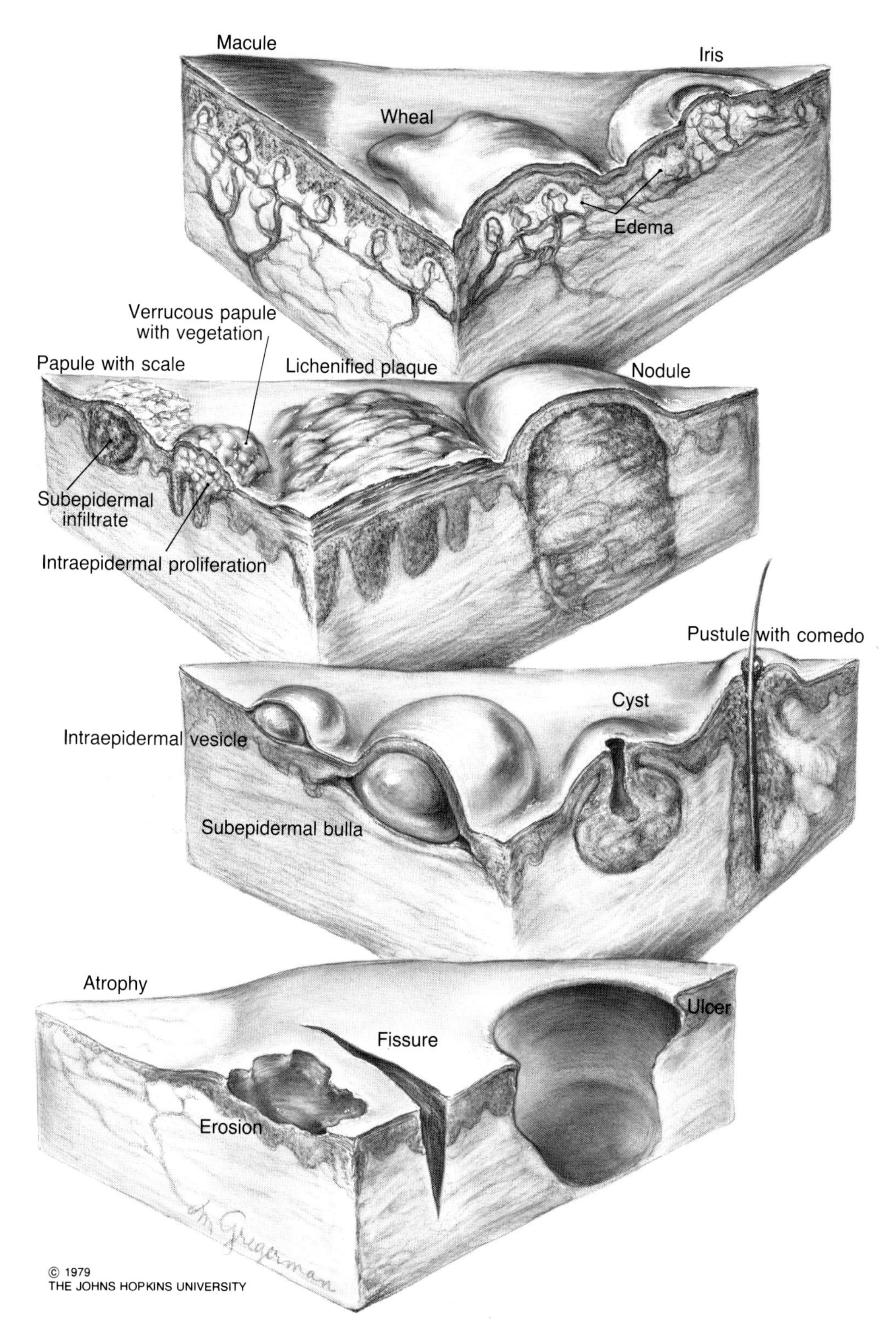

FIGURE 29-1 Various lesions of the skin. (© 1979 The Johns Hopkins University. Reprinted with permission.)

TABLE 29-1 Diffuse and Localized Macular Erythema

Neonate	Infant and Child	Adolescent
Staphylococcal scalded skin (SSS) syndrome	SSS syndrome	Toxic shock syndrome
	Toxic epidermal necrolysis (TEN)	TEN
	Mucocutaneous lymph node syndrome (Kawasaki disease)	
	Sunburn	Sunburn
	Phototoxic reaction	Phototoxic reaction

Etiology
The causative agent is *Staphylococcus aureus*, phage group II.

Diagnostic Studies
The causative organism may be cultured from any pyogenic focus on the skin (e.g., the umbilical stump) or from the conjunctiva, nasopharynx, or stool. Blood cultures and cultures from intact blisters are usually sterile. A skin biopsy may be helpful in diagnosing a difficult or atypical case. In staphylococcal scalded skin syndrome a characteristic split is observed in the granular or upper malpighian layers of the epidermis. A rapid diagnosis may be obtained by histologically examining a frozen section or a sheet of peeling skin and determining the level of the split within the epidermis.

Differential Diagnosis
The following conditions must be considered: drug-induced toxic epidermal necrolysis, severe epidermolysis bullosa, boric acid poisoning, and second-degree burns.

Treatment
The patient should be hospitalized and treated with penicillinase-resistant antistaphylococcal antibiotics. Body temperature and fluid and electrolyte balance should be carefully monitored. The patient is isolated from other susceptible patients until cultures are negative. Excessive or traumatic handling is avoided, and the skin is kept moist with saline compresses. (See Chapter 36, "Infectious Diseases," for additional discussion.)

Toxic Epidermal Necrolysis

Clinical Picture
The initial clinical picture is similar to that described for staphylococcal scalded skin syndrome, with widespread, tender macular erythema. Subsequently, scattered tense blisters appear, which rupture and produce moist ulcerations. Stomatitis may be severe. This clinical picture may be preceded by target lesions of erythema multiforme.

Etiology
Ingestion of drugs, most commonly sulfonamides, penicillin, barbiturates, diphenylhydantoin, or salicylates, is responsible for toxic epidermal necrolysis.

Diagnostic Studies
The diagnosis is confirmed with a skin biopsy or the examination of a frozen section of denuded skin. In drug-induced toxic epidermal necrolysis there is loss of the entire epidermis (as opposed to only the upper layers in staphylococcal scalded skin syndrome). Skin and blood cultures should be obtained while awaiting the biopsy report.

Differential Diagnosis
Staphylococcal scalded skin syndrome, second-degree burns, and erythema multiforme major (Stevens-Johnson syndrome) must be ruled out.

Treatment
If denudation is extensive, admission to a burn unit may be warranted. Penicillinase-resistant antistaphylococcal antibiotics are administered until cultures have been reported. Temperature and fluids should be carefully monitored. Although conclusive data supporting the use of corticosteroids are not available, most physicians recommend administration of high-dose corticosteroids (prednisone, 1 mg/kg/d) or the equivalent. (See Chapter 36, "Infectious Diseases," for further discussion.)

Mucocutaneous Lymph Node Syndrome (Kawasaki Disease)

Clinical Picture
Discrete and confluent polymorphous (morbilliform, scarlatiniform, erythema multiforme-like, urticarial) macular and papular erythema appears on the palms and soles and subsequently progresses over the trunk. Significant edema of the hands and feet may occur with desquamation 2 to 3 weeks later. The diagnosis of Kawasaki disease requires at least *5 days of fever without an obvious detectable*

source, plus four of the following five criteria: (1) exanthem, as described; (2) bilateral conjunctival injection; (3) acral edema with desquamation, as noted; (4) cervical lymphadenopathy; and (5) pharyngeal injection, strawberry tongue or dry lips.

Etiology
The cause is unknown.

Diagnostic Studies
A platelet count can be helpful since thrombocytosis occurs in almost all cases 3 to 5 weeks after onset of illness.

Differential Diagnosis
The following disorders should be ruled out: scarlet fever, toxic epidermal necrolysis, drug eruption, viral exanthem, erythema multiforme, toxic shock syndrome, staphylococcal scalded skin syndrome, infectious mononucleosis, acrodynia.

Treatment
Supportive care is provided. Early in the course gamma globulin may be given and aspirin can be administered at 80 to 100 mg/kg/d, with a decrease to 20 to 30 mg/kg/d when the patient is afebrile. (See Chapter 36, "Infectious Diseases," for additional discussion.)

Sunburn

Clinical Picture
In areas exposed to the sun, a diffuse, tender macular erythema appears 4 to 8 hours after exposure to ultraviolet light. The erythema may be accompanied by edema, blister formation, pain, and fever if the intensity of radiation was great or if the duration of exposure was prolonged.

Etiology
Burning is produced by ultraviolet light (290 to 320-nm wavelength).

Diagnostic Studies
The diagnosis is facilitated by obtaining a history of sun exposure and by observing normal skin in unexposed areas.

Differential Diagnosis
Phototoxic reaction and thermal burn must be considered in the differential diagnosis.

Treatment
Cool saline compresses and bland emollients are applied to the involved skin. Systemic analgesics may be necessary if the sunburn involves a large area of skin. Preparations containing topical analgesics (e.g., diphenhydramine or the "caines") are to be avoided because of their potential for sensitization. The patient should be encouraged to use available sunscreen preparations prior to future exposures.

Phototoxic Reaction

Clinical Picture
The morphology of the lesions is similar to that described for sunburn. Phototoxic reactions secondary to topical preparations are usually limited to the area to which the chemical was applied.

Etiology
With phototoxic reactions an exaggerated response to ultraviolet light is induced either by topical preparations (tars, dyes, and photosensitizing plant oils incorporated into colognes and skin products) or by systemic drugs (sulfonamides, phenothiazine, demeclocycline, and methotrexate).

Diagnostic Studies
No diagnostic studies are needed.

Differential Diagnosis
Sunburn must be ruled out.

Treatment
Cool compresses and bland emollients are applied to affected skin. Systemic analgesics may be necessary if the area of involvement is extensive.

Toxic Shock Syndrome

Clinical Picture
Diffuse, tender macular erythema is particularly prominent in a "bathing suit" distribution. Desquamation of palms and soles may occur. Fever, vomiting, diarrhea, myalgias, hypotension, disorientation, and alterations in consciousness may be accompanying signs and symptoms.

Etiology
S. aureus, phage group I or III, is the causative agent. This entity has been described in young (menstruating) women and is associated with the use of tampons or contraceptive devices. It should be noted, however, that toxic shock syndrome was initially recognized in children and that there have been case reports of toxic shock syndrome occurring in both sexes with staphylococcal infections.[1,2]

Diagnostic Tests
Cultures should be obtained from all orifices and the blood.

Differential Diagnosis
Scarlet fever, staphylococcal scalded skin syndrome, toxic epidermal necrolysis, and drug eruption must be considered.

Treatment
The patient should be admitted to the hospital and receive β-lactam-resistant antibiotics. Fluid and electrolyte balance and blood pressure must be monitored carefully. (See Chapter 36, "Infectious Diseases," for further discussion.)

MACULES AND PAPULES

Blanchable macular erythema with discrete or confluent papules is a common presentation for viral exanthems and drug eruptions. The adjective "morbilliform," or measles-like, has been applied to these eruptions, but with the widespread administration of measles vaccine, this term may have lost much of its meaning, especially for younger physicians. The morphology of these eruptions may be clinically indistinguishable, and a differential diagnosis is often based on the pattern and evolution of the rash, the accompanying signs and symptoms, and an adequate drug history. The common causes of macular and papular erythematous eruptions in the various pediatric age groups are listed in Table 29-2.

TABLE 29-2 Macules and Papules

Neonate	Infant and Child	Adolescent
Drug eruption	Drug eruption	Drug eruption
	Scarlet fever	
	Roseola	
	Erythema infectiosum	Erythema infectiosum
	Infectious mononucleosis	Infectious mononucleosis
	Echovirus 16 (Boston exanthem)	
		Hepatitis
Rubella	Rubella	Rubella
Cytomegalovirus		
	Measles	Atypical measles
Graft-versus-host reaction	Graft-versus-host reaction	Graft-versus-host reaction

Drug Eruption

Clinical Picture
There is a widespread, bright red macular and papular eruption that often involves the palms and soles. Pruritus may be intense. Fever is variably present.

Etiology
The most common causative agents are penicillin and penicillin derivatives such as ampicillin, trimethoprim, and sulfamethoxazole. Barbiturates, salicylic acid, isoniazid, phenothiazine, and thiazides can also produce drug eruptions.

Diagnostic Studies
Blood studies may show leukocytosis with eosinophilia. The diagnosis is facilitated by a history of drug ingestion within the preceding 2 weeks.

Differential Diagnosis
Viral exanthem must be ruled out.

Treatment
The suspected drug should be discontinued. Antihistamines can be administered for symptomatic relief of severe pruritus (Table 29-3).

Rubella

Clinical Picture
Pink lesions appear first on the face, spreading to the trunk and then the extremities. The eruption fades in a similar progression. The total duration of the rash is 48 to 72 hours. The rash is usually accompanied by fever, palatal petechiae, and postauricular and suboccipital lymphadenopathy. A monarticular arthritis may occur but is more common in older children and adolescents.

Etiology
Rubella virus is the causative agent.

TABLE 29-3 Antipruritic Agents

Agent (Trade Name)	Dosage (mg/kg/d)*
Chlorpheniramine maleate (Chlor-Trimeton)	0.35
Diphenhydramine hydrochloride (Benadryl)	5.00
Hydroxyzine hydrochloride (Atarax, Vistaril)	2.00–4.00

* Given in divided doses q4–6h.

Diagnostic Studies
A fourfold increase in convalescent-stage antibody titer compared with the acute-phase antibody titer is considered indicative of a recent infection.

Differential Diagnosis
Other viral exanthems should be considered (see Table 29-2).

Treatment
Treatment is symptomatic. (See Chapter 36, "Infectious Diseases," for further discussion.)

Cytomegalovirus

Clinical Picture
An erythematous, occasionally petechial, macular and papular eruption may occur in infants or children who are immunosuppressed by disease or drugs. Pharyngitis, jaundice, and hepatosplenomegaly may accompany the rash.

Etiology
Cytomegalovirus is the causative agent.

Diagnostic Studies
Viral cultures and serologic tests should be arranged. A skin biopsy may reveal characteristic intranuclear inclusion bodies within dermal endothelial cells.

Differential Diagnosis
Drug eruption, hepatitis, and other viral exanthems must be part of the differential diagnosis.

Treatment
No specific treatment is available.

Graft-versus-Host Reaction

Clinical Picture
Transient, erythematous, blanchable macular and papular eruption appears on the trunk, face, and extremities. This eruption appears in children who are immunosuppressed and have received blood transfusion products or bone marrow transplants.

Etiology
Immunocompetent donor lymphoid cells recognize the recipient as "foreign" and attempt to immunologically reject certain host organs such as the skin, liver, and intestinal tract.

Diagnostic Studies
Liver function tests may be abnormally elevated. The skin biopsy may demonstrate basal vacuolization, epidermal dyskeratosis, and a mild superficial perivascular mononuclear cell infiltrate.

Differential Diagnosis
Viral exanthem and drug eruption must be excluded.

Treatment
Most cases are mild and require no treatment. Severe graft-versus-host reaction may require high-dose systemic corticosteroids.

Scarlet Fever

Clinical Picture
Scarlet fever is characterized by a diffusely erythematous eruption with numerous punctuate papules, which produce a rough "sandpaper" skin texture. The rash begins on the neck and spreads to the trunk and extremities. A characteristic accentuation of the eruption in the groin, axillae, and antecubital fossae may be accompanied by petechiae. Facial erythema is macular and diffuse with circumoral pallor commonly present. After 4 to 5 days, the erythema fades and desquamation occurs. Pharyngitis and a white or red "strawberry tongue" are present early in the course of the disease.

Etiology
The eruption is caused by an erythrogenic toxin produced by group A β-hemolytic streptococci.

Diagnostic Studies
Pharnygeal cultures should be obtained.

Differential Diagnosis
Scarlatiniform eruptions associated with *S. aureus*, Kawasaki disease, rubella, infectious mononucleosis, and certain drug eruptions must all be ruled out.

Treatment
Penicillin is administered for scarlet fever. If the patient is penicillin sensitive, erythromycin is given instead.

Erythema Infectiosum (Fifth Disease)

Clinical Picture
Confluent macular erythema appears on both cheeks ("slapped cheeks") and is followed in 1 or 2 days by a nonpruritic reticulated eruption on the

trunk and proximal extremities. The lesions may come and go for several weeks.

Etiology
Although presumed to be a viral exanthem, no agent has been isolated in this disease.

Diagnostic Studies
No diagnostic studies are needed, although blood tests may indicate eosinophilia and lymphocytosis.

Differential Diagnosis
The clinical appearance is usually characteristic and diagnostic.

Treatment
No treatment is necessary.

Infectious Mononucleosis

Clinical Picture
A macular and occasionally papular erythematous eruption involves the trunk and extremities. Eyelid edema may occur. An enanthem consisting of pharyngitis and petechiae at the junction of the soft and hard palate is commonly seen. Cervical adenopathy is characteristic, and lymphadenopathy and splenomegaly may be present.

Etiology
Epstein-Barr virus is the responsible agent. Patients receiving ampicillin or allopurinol have a higher incidence of skin lesions.

Diagnostic Studies
The following studies should be obtained: mononucleosis spot test, heterophile antibody titers, and a complete blood count (CBC) with a smear to show atypical lymphocytes.

Differential Diagnosis
Viral exanthem and drug eruption should be considered in the differential diagnosis.

Treatment
Treatment is symptomatic. (See Chapter 36, "Infectious Diseases," for additional discussion.)

Echovirus 16 (Boston Exanthem)

Clinical Picture
Red macules and/or papules are scattered over the head, trunk, and occasionally the extremities. Vesicles are occasionally observed. Shallow ulcerations may be seen on the soft palate and tonsils. Cervical, suboccipital, and postauricular lymphadenopathy are often present.

Etiology
Echovirus 16 is the causative agent.

Diagnostic Studies
Serologic tests should be arranged.

Differential Diagnosis
Other viral exanthems must be ruled out.

Treatment
No treatment is needed.

Roseola Infantum (Exanthem Subitum)

Clinical Picture
The rash is preceded by 3 to 5 days of high fever occasionally accompanied by convulsions. Discrete small pink macules and papules appear on the neck and trunk as the fever resolves. The distal extremities and face are usually spared. Periorbital edema is occasionally present. Postoccipital lymphadenopathy may appear during the febrile period and persist during the rash.

Etiology
The causative agent has not been isolated.

Diagnostic Studies
No diagnostic studies are available. A CBC may reveal leukopenia.

Differential Diagnosis
Other viral exanthems should be excluded.

Treatment
Treatment is symptomatic. (See Chapter 36, "Infectious Diseases," for further discussion.)

Measles

Clinical Picture
A macular and/or papular erythematous eruption appears first on the anterior scalp, spreads rapidly over the face, and then extends to the trunk and extremities. The eruption is accompanied by a fever and is preceded by conjunctivitis, rhinitis, cough, and white Koplik's spots on the buccal mucosa.

Etiology
Measles virus is the causative agent.

Diagnostic Studies
Serologic studies should be obtained.

Differential Diagnosis
Viral exanthem and drug reaction must be considered in the differential diagnosis.

Treatment
Treatment is symptomatic. (See Chapter 36, "Infectious Diseases," for additional discussion.)

Atypical Measles

Clinical Picture
Pruritic macules, papules, and/or vesicopustules begin acrally and extend centripetally 2 to 3 days after the onset of fever, myalgias, and abdominal pain. Most individuals with atypical measles develop pneumonia. Pedal edema is common.

Etiology
This variant is the result of exposure to natural measles virus in an individual vaccinated with killed vaccine or ineffective live vaccine.

Diagnostic Studies
Serologic studies should be obtained.

Differential Diagnosis
Rocky Mountain spotted fever, meningococcemia, and other viral exanthems should be excluded.

Treatment
Treatment is symptomatic. (See Chapter 36, "Infectious Diseases," for additional discussion.)

Hepatitis

Clinical Picture
A generalized erythematous macular and papular, or occasionally urticarial, eruption is usually accompanied by malaise, posterior cervical adenopathy, anorexia, and polyarthritis. The eruption may precede jaundice by 10 days.

Etiology
Hepatitis B virus is the causative agent.

Diagnostic Studies
Studies should be arranged to measure liver function and hepatitis B surface antigen.

Differential Diagnosis
Viral exanthem and drug eruption must be ruled out.

Treatment
Treatment is symptomatic. (See Chapter 14, "Gastroenterologic Disorders," for further discussion.)

PAPULES AND PLAQUES WITH SCALE OR CRUST

A number of dermatologic disorders are morphologically characterized by discrete individual papules 1 to 3 mm in size or by larger plaques. These lesions may be flesh colored, erythematous, or hyperpigmented and often have an overlying white scale or yellowish crust. The differential diagnosis for scaly papules and plaques is given in Table 29-4.

Seborrheic Dermatitis

Clinical Picture
Scaly, greasy, often well demarcated erythematous plaques may be seen on the scalp (cradle cap, seborrhea), face, diaper area, or midchest. Rarely, seborrheic dermatitis may become widespread. Severe, persistent infantile seborrheic dermatitis associated with diarrhea and failure to thrive is known as Leiner's disease.

Etiology
The cause is unknown.

Diagnostic Studies
The appearance of the lesions is usually quite characteristic. Occasionally, a biopsy may be necessary to differentiate this entity from other similar-appearing lesions.

Differential Diagnosis
Psoriasis, atopic eczema, and histiocytosis must be excluded.

TABLE 29-4 Papules and Plaques with Scale or Crust

Neonate	Infant and Child	Adolescent
Seborrheic dermatitis	Atopic eczema	Atopic eczema
	Seborrheic dermatitis	Seborrheic dermatitis
		Guttate psoriasis
	Impetigo	
Diaper dermatitis		Pityriasis rosea
		Secondary syphilis
	Tinea corporis and versicolor	Tinea corporis and versicolor

Treatment
For scalp manifestations a medicated shampoo containing sulfur or salicylic acid, used two to three times per week, is usually sufficient to control scaling. If the scales are very thick and adherent, apply mineral oil to the scalp. Severe erythema should be treated with an application of hydrocortisone cream or lotion once or twice a day.

Localized and generalized disease is treated with 1% hydrocortisone lotion or cream, applied twice a day. The patient should be followed closely to avoid prolonged injudicious use of corticosteroid medication.

Diaper Dermatitis

Clinical Picture
Erythema involving the buttocks, genitalia, lower abdomen, and upper thighs may be accompanied by scaling or erosion. The flexural folds may be spared.

Etiology
Maceration, dampness, and chemical irritation with or without bacterial and yeast (*Candida*) superinfection combine to produce this problem.

Diagnostic Studies
Microscopic examination of a KOH preparation of scale may show the budding yeast forms that are characteristic of *Candida albicans*.

Differential Diagnosis
Seborrheic dermatitis, psoriasis, histiocytosis, and atopic dermatitis should be ruled out.

Treatment
Avoidance of an occlusive environment is paramount in the treatment of diaper dermatitis. Diapers must be changed frequently, and the area should be rinsed with tepid tap water. Application of a nonfluorinated corticosteroid cream or 1% hydrocortisone cream three times daily will reduce inflammation. If *Candida* organisms are present, also apply an appropriate antimicrobial cream (nystatin or any preparation listed in Table 29-5).

TABLE 29-5 Antifungal Agents

Agent (Trade Name)	Sizes Available	
	Cream (g)	(Solution (mL)
Clotrimazole (Lotrimin)	15, 30, 45, 90	10, 30
Haloprogin (Halotex)	15, 30	10, 30
Miconazole (Micatin)	15, 30	3.5-oz spray liquid

Impetigo

Clinical Picture
The small vesicles that appear rupture easily and form superficial erosions with a "honey-colored" crust. Lesions may be anywhere but are most commonly seen on the face, around the mouth, and on the extremities.

Etiology
Streptococci and/or *S. aureus*, phage group II, are the responsible organisms.

Diagnostic Studies
A Gram stain of a smear taken from beneath the crust shows numerous (Gram-positive) cocci in pairs and clusters. The culture is usually positive for streptococci and/or staphylococci.

Differential Diagnosis
Disorders to be considered in the differential diagnosis are listed on Table 29-4.

Treatment
Penicillin VK, Ampicillin, or Amoxicillin is administered orally for 10 days, or benzathine penicillin is given intramuscularly in doses appropriate for weight or age. If lesions do not begin to resolve in a few days or cultures show heavy growth of staphylococci, dicloxacillin, cloxacillin, cefaclor, or erythromycin should be administered. (See Chapter 36, "Infectious Diseases," for further discussion.)

Atopic Eczema

Clinical Picture
Atopic eczema appears as ill-defined, erythematous, minimally elevated lesions with variable microvesiculation, excoriation, crust, scale, and lichenification (accentuation of skin markings secondary to rubbing). The lesions are intensely pruritic. The distribution of eruption varies with the age of the patient:

- infant: head (cheeks and scalp), neck, trunk, diaper area, and extensor surfaces of arms and legs
- child: antecubital and popliteal fossae, neck, and feet
- adolescent: hands, feet, and flexural surfaces

Etiology
Atopic eczema is a hereditary disorder commonly seen in association with a personal or family history of hay fever and asthma.

Diagnostic Studies

Diagnostic tests are not routinely obtained. Allergy testing (scratch, intradermal, or patch) is generally time consuming, expensive, and unrewarding. If secondary infection is clinically suspected, a skin culture and tests for antibiotic sensitivities should be arranged.

Differential Diagnosis

Disorders to be considered in the differential diagnosis are shown in Table 29-4.

Treatment

Aggravating stimuli, such as wool and other "itchy" materials, should be removed, and excessive soap and other drying agents should be avoided. Pruritus can be reduced with systemic antipruritic agents (Table 29-3). Dryness can be relieved with emollients (Eucerin cream, hydrated petrolatum), and inflammation can be treated with a topical corticosteroid cream or ointment such as 0.1% triamcinolone.

Tinea Corporis

Clinical Picture

Tinea corporis appears as one or more slightly elevated, mildly erythematous, scaly lesions. These lesions often have a well-defined, papular border and some central clearing. Superficial pustules are occasionally present. The trunk and proximal extremities are the most commonly involved areas.

Etiology

Trichophyton rubrum, *Trichophyton mentagrophytes*, and *Microsporum canis* are the primary causative agents.

Diagnostic Studies

A scraping of scale prepared with KOH and examined microscopically demonstrates long, thin, branching, septate hyphae. A culture may be helpful if the scraping is negative.

Differential Diagnosis

Granuloma annulare and the herald patch of pityriasis rosea must be ruled out.

Treatment

For mild to moderate localized involvement, antifungal cream (Table 29-5) is applied three times per day and continued for 10 days after the lesions have completely cleared. For extensive or very inflammatory disease, griseofulvin is administered orally for 2 to 3 weeks.

Tinea Versicolor

Clinical Picture

There are numerous round to oval and flat to slightly elevated lesions that are flesh colored, pink, hyper- or hypopigmented (hence the name versicolor), with fine scale. They are scattered on the trunk, neck, and proximal extremities.

Etiology

This infection is produced by a yeastlike organism known as *Malassezia furfur* or *Pityrosporum orbiculare*.

Diagnostic Studies

Microscopic examination of a KOH preparation of a scale demonstrates short hyphae and spores (so-called spaghetti and meatballs).

Differential Diagnosis

Other disorders to be excluded are tinea corporis, vitiligo, and seborrheic dermatitis.

Treatment

Selenium sulfide (Selsun) shampoo is applied liberally for 20 minutes, lathered up, and washed off for 14 consecutive days. An overnight application once a month helps prevent recurrence. The topical preparations listed in Table 29-5, applied twice a day for 2 to 3 weeks, are an effective but expensive alternative therapy.

Guttate Psoriasis

Clinical Picture

Guttate psoriasis appears as multiple discrete erythematous papules and small plaques covered with silvery scale. The lesions are scattered over the trunk and proximal extremities. When the onset is abrupt, there may be a history of a sore throat 2 to 3 weeks previously. Pruritus is variable.

Etiology

Psoriasis is transmitted by a polygenic inheritance and is subject to environmental or infectious influences.

Diagnostic Studies

An antistreptolysin O titer and a throat culture should be obtained to rule out a streptococcal infection which may precipitate guttate psoriasis.

Differential Diagnosis

Pityriasis rosea, secondary syphilis, and viral exanthem should be considered in the differential diagnosis.

Treatment
Treatment includes topical application of fluorinated corticosteroid creams, three times per day for 2 to 3 weeks; emollients; and ultraviolet light therapy.

Pityriasis Rosea

Clinical Picture
Multiple round to oval, pink to fawn colored, slightly elevated, scaly grouped papules or plaques, 5 to 10 mm in diameter, are present on the neck, trunk and proximal extremities. Lesions on the trunk follow skin lines, giving a "Christmas tree" appearance on the back and a chevron pattern on the chest. Typically, pityriasis rosea spares the face, palms, and soles. A single larger lesion called a "herald patch" may precede the generalized eruption by days to weeks. Pruritus is variable.

Etiology
The cause is unknown.

Diagnostic Studies
A serologic test for secondary syphilis should be obtained.

Differential Diagnosis
Secondary syphilis, tinea corporis, and guttate psoriasis must be considered in the differential diagnosis.

Treatment
The disease is self-limiting. Reassurance and symptomatic therapy with oral antipruritic agents and emollients are usually the only treatment necessary. Exposure to sunlight may reduce the duration of the eruption. A short course of tapering oral corticosteroids may "shut off" severe inflammatory disease and prevent excessive postinflammatory hyperpigmentation in dark-skinned individuals.

Secondary Syphilis

Clinical Picture
The lesions appear as numerous, well-demarcated, erythematous to tan papules and annular plaques with variable scale. The lesions can occur anywhere but are commonly present on the palms and soles, where they may be macular and hyperpigmented ("copper pennies"). Warty genital or oral lesions and patchy alopecia are often seen. The primary chancre is occasionally still visible, especially if patient is seen during the early stage of the generalized eruption.

Etiology
Treponema pallidum is the responsible organism.

Diagnostic Studies
Dark-field microscopic examination of samples from genital or palmar lesions may show spirochetes. The serologic test for syphilis is always positive.

Differential Diagnosis
Because secondary syphilis can have a varied appearance, the differential diagnosis is extensive but includes viral exanthem, pityriasis rosea, psoriasis, and atypic exzema.

Treatment
Treatment consists of benzathine penicillin G, 2.4 million U IM, repeated in 7 days. Erythromycin or tetracycline, 500 mg four times per day for 15 days, may be given to penicillin-sensitive individuals. (See Chapter 24, "Gynecologic Disorders and Sexually Transmitted Diseases," for additional discussion.)

VESICLES AND PUSTULES

Clear, fluid-filled vesicles and turbid pustules may arise on normal-appearing skin or may occur in association with erythema, papules, or plaques. Since many vesiculopustular lesions have an infectious etiology, diagnostic testing performed at the time of examination is often important. Material from the vesicles and pustules can be smeared on a glass slide and examined for bacteria (Gram's stain), fungi (KOH preparation), and evidence of viral infection (Tzanck test). Examining the cellular content of the lesion for the presence of neutrophils, eosinophils, or monocytes (Wright's stain) may also provide important diagnostic information. Table 29-6 provides a differential diagnosis for most of the common vesiculopustular disorders seen in pediatrics.

Herpes Simplex

Clinical Picture
Grouped (umbilicated) vesicles on an erythematous base are the classic lesions seen in all herpes simplex infections. The appearance and extent of the eruption may vary according to the age of the infected individual, the presence of underlying dis-

TABLE 29-6 Vesicles and Pustules

Neonate	Infant and Child	Adolescent
Herpes simplex neonatal	Herpes simplex Gingivostomatitis Labialis Whitlow Kaposi's varicelliform eruption Herpes varicella-zoster	Herpes simplex Progenitalis Labialis Whitlow Kaposi's varicelliform eruption Herpes varicella-zoster
Erythema toxicum neonatorum		
Transient neonatal pustular melanosis	Hand-foot-and-mouth disease	Hand-foot-and-mouth disease
Incontinentia pigmenti		
Miliaria	Miliaria	Miliaria
Candidiasis	Candidiasis	Dermatophytosis
Impetigo*	Impetigo Contact dermatitis	Impetigo Contact dermatitis
Septicemia†	Septicemia Scabies‡ Erythema multiforme	Septicemia Erythema multiforme

* See "Papules and Plaques with Scale or Crust."
† See "Palpable Purpura."
‡ See "Papules and Nodules."

ease, the location of lesions, and whether the lesions represent a primary infection or a reactivation (recurrence).

Neonatal Herpes Simplex Occurring in a small percentage of infants born to parents with active herpes progenitalis, neonatal herpes simplex is a potentially life-threatening infection that appears within 7 days of birth with scattered vesicular lesions. Although the disease may be primarily localized to the skin, systemic involvement occurs commonly and may result in neurologic impairment or even death.

Herpes Gingivostomatitis Vesicles occurring on mucous membranes are rarely seen because they are easily ruptured and rapidly evolve to become erosions and ulcerations. Gingivostomatitis is the most common symptomatic presentation for primary infection with herpes simplex in infants and young children. Characterized by extensive erosions on the tongue and buccal mucosa, herpes gingivostomatitis is accompanied by general irritability, difficulty in eating, and fever. Lesions may persist for as long as 14 days. Intraoral recurrences are rare.

Herpes Labialis Recurrent infections most commonly occur on the vermillion (red) surface of the lip or adjacent skin. They tend to be localized, last 5 to 7 days, and recur at the same site.

Herpes Progenitalis Genital herpes occurs almost exclusively in adolescents and older individuals. The primary infection, which lasts 7 to 14 days, may be widespread and debilitating. Recurrences are localized and of shorter duration. (See also Chapter 24, "Gynecologic Disorders and Sexually Transmitted Diseases.")

Kaposi's Varicelliform Eruption (Eczema Herpeticum) Kaposi's varicelliform eruption occurs in individuals with a defective skin barrier (e.g., atopic eczema, burn), which may permit cutaneous dissemination of virus from a localized herpes lesion. Systemic involvement may result in death.

Herpes Simplex in Immunocompromised Individuals Infections with herpes simplex may appear in unusual locations; produce blisters or deep, scarring, ulcerations; and persist longer than normal or disseminate.

Herpetic Whitlow Deep-seated pustular lesions on the finger caused by primary viral inoculation with herpes simplex may be confused with bacterial abscesses or cellulitis.

Etiology

Herpes simplex, type I or II, is the causative agent in all these disorders.

Diagnostic Studies

The Tzanck preparation is a quick and easy test to confirm the diagnosis of herpes virus infection. A relatively fresh lesion is wiped with alcohol. The roof of a vesicle or blister is gently removed with a scalpel blade. The base of the blister is then scraped with the scalpel blade, and the material is smeared on a clean glass microscope slide. The preparation is air dried and then is fixed in methanol, stained with Giemsa's or Wright's stain, and examined under the microscope. The presence of multinucleate giant epithelial cells confirms the diagnosis of herpes (simplex or varicella-zoster) infection.

A viral culture permits differentiation between herpes simplex and herpes varicella-zoster.

Differential Diagnosis
Impetigo, herpes zoster, and contact dermatitis must be ruled out.

Treatment
Gingivostomatitis Symptomatic relief of pain can be provided with topical or systemic analgesics. Hydration should be maintained. There is no effective topical treatment that erradicates recurrences.

Herpes Labialis and Progenitalis Application of 5% benzoyl peroxide may help lesions dry faster.

Herpes Simplex Neonatorum and Kaposi's Varicelliform Eruption Systemic acyclovir is effective in preventing progression of the eruption.

Herpes Varicella-Zoster

Clinical Picture
The classic picture is that of scattered or grouped umbilicated vesicles.

Varicella "Teardrop" vesicles resting on an erythematous base appear in crops on the trunk and face. The vesicles evolve into pustules and then into crusted erosions. Pruritus is common. Constitutional symptoms are usually present including fever, malaise, and headache.

Zoster Umbilicated vesicles and pustules are grouped in a unilateral dermatomal distribution. The eruption may be preceded or accompanied by pruritus, tenderness, or pain. Regional lymphadenopathy, fever, and malaise also may be present.

Etiology
The cause is infection with herpes varicella-zoster virus, either primary (varicella) or recurrent (zoster).

Diagnostic Studies
A Tzanck preparation confirms the diagnosis of herpes infection (see "Herpes Simplex" for technique). A viral culture permits the differentiation between herpes simplex and herpes varicella-zoster.

Differential Diagnosis
Impetigo must be excluded.

Treatment
Symptomatic treatment is usually sufficient for the varicella form; however, aspirin should be avoided because of its association with Reye's syndrome. (See Chapter 36, "Infectious Diseases," for further discussion.) Zoster infections can be treated with saline or Burow's solution, followed by a topical antibiotic ointment to prevent secondary bacterial infection.

Erythema Toxicum Neonatorum

Clinical Picture
The eruption is characterized by ill-defined (splotchy) macular erythema with minute vesicles scattered over the face, trunk, and extremities. Lesions usually appear during the second and third day of life; occasionally, the onset may be delayed to as late as the fourth or fifth day after birth.

Etiology
The cause is unknown.

Diagnostic Studies
A Wright's stain of a smear from a vesicle shows a predominance of eosinophils.

Differential Diagnosis
Herpes simplex infection, miliaria, folliculitis, and transient neonatal pustular melanosis must be part of the differential diagnosis.

Treatment
No treatment is required. The lesions stop appearing by about one month of age.

Transient Neonatal Pustular Melanosis

Clinical Picture
Pigmented macules and vesiculopustules appear on narrow erythematous bases, which frequently have a superficial collarette of desquamating scale. These lesions are present at birth and are more numerous about the face and neck. Vesicles may occur on scalp, palms, and soles. Macules may persist for months.

Etiology
The cause is unknown.

Diagnostic Studies
Pustules are sterile and smears show numerous neutrophils when examined with a Wright's stain. A skin biopsy shows a thickened stratum corneum with intra- and subcorneal collections of neutrophils and rare eosinophils; the macules have focal areas of basilar and occasionally suprabasilar melanin increase.

Differential Diagnosis
Erythema toxicum neonatorum, staphylococcal pustulosis, herpes infection, and miliaria must be excluded.

Treatment
No treatment is required. Vesiculopustules disappear in 24 to 48 hours, while pigmented macules may fade in 3 weeks to 3 months.

Incontinentia Pigmenti

Clinical Picture
During infancy there is a gradual onset of tense vesicles arising on slightly erythematous skin and arranged in a distinctive linear and whorled ("marble cake") pattern. The majority of affected individuals are girls.

Etiology
The cause is unknown.

Diagnostic Studies
A skin biopsy reveals intraepidermal vesicles containing eosinophils.

Differential Diagnosis
The distribution of lesions is characteristic.

Treatment
No treatment is required. A whorled pattern of hyperpigmentation persists indefinitely.

Miliaria

Clinical Picture
Miliaria is characterized by nonfollicular lesions, 1 to 4 mm in diameter, with variable morphology:

- miliaria crystallina: superficial clear vesicles on a nonerythematous base
- miliaria rubra ("prickly heat"): papules and papulovesicles on an erythematous base
- miliaria pustulosa: pustules on an erythematous base
- miliaria profunda: firm erythematous papulopustules

These eruptions occur in areas of sweating subject to occlusion.

Etiology
Miliaria is a result of blockage of sweat ducts, with rupture into the stratum corneum (miliaria crystallina), the epidermis (miliaria rubra and miliaria pustulosa), or the dermis (miliaria profunda).

Diagnostic Studies
A Gram's stain of miliaria crystallina and miliaria rubra lesions reveals only cellular debris, whereas miliaria pustulosa pustules show neutrophils and cellular debris. No organisms are observed.

Differential Diagnosis
Miliaria crystallina must be distinguished from burns, bullous impetigo, viral eruption (e.g., herpes lesions), and acute eczematous dermatitis. In diagnosing miliaria rubra, folliculitis must be ruled out. The differential diagnosis for miliaria pustulosa must consider erythema toxicum neonatorum, transient neonatal pustular melanosis, and folliculitis.

Treatment
Heat and occlusion of body parts should be avoided. The skin should be kept dry to reduce sweating.

Candidiasis

Clinical Picture
Candidiasis appears as erythematous plaques with peripheral or satellite pustules. These occur most commonly in the anogenital (diaper) area but occasionally may be seen in other warm, moist areas such as the neck and axilla.

Etiology
Candida albicans is the causative agent.

Diagnostic Studies
A smear from a pustule treated with KOH and examined under the microscope reveals nonseptate pseudohyphae and budding yeast. A fungus culture confirms the diagnosis.

Differential Diagnosis
Eczema, psoriasis, and seborrheic dermatitis must be excluded.

Treatment
Clotrimazole or nystatin cream is applied two to three times daily. The area is kept as dry as possible. If the inflammation is severe, 1% hydrocortisone cream should also be applied twice a day for a few days.

Hand-Foot-and-Mouth Disease

Clinical Picture
Painful vesicles and cloudy pustules, some of which may be oval or linear, appear on the hands (palms and dorsal surfaces) and feet. Acral lesions are accompanied by painful oral erosions.

Etiology
Coxsackievirus A16 is the most commonly implicated organism.

Diagnostic Studies
No studies are needed.

Differential Diagnosis
Erythema multiforme and dyshidrotic eczema should be part of the differential diagnosis.

Treatment
Symptomatic relief should be provided for mucosal erosions, along with reassurance that the illness is short lived.

Acute Contact Dermatitis

Clinical Picture
In acute contact dermatitis, tense vesicles and blisters are present on erythematous skin, often associated with red papules and plaques. Oozing and crusting are common sequelae. Pruritus may be intense. The distribution and arrangement of lesions may point to the responsible agent:

- earlobes: nickel sensitivity (earrings)
- linear lesions on arms: poison ivy, oak, and sumac
- dorsum of foot: any one of a number of potentially sensitizing products in shoes
- scalp: hair dyes, permanents, or relaxing solutions

Etiology
Sensitization to contact allergens is responsible for this condition.

Diagnostic Studies
No tests are indicated for a single episode. If the problem persists or recurs, patch testing may be helpful in determining the offending allergen.

Differential Diagnosis
Bullous disease of childhood, dermatitis herpetiformis, and herpes infection must be ruled out.

Treatment
Cool compresses (tap water, saline, or aluminum acetate) are applied for 15 to 30 minutes several times a day to help relieve itching and to remove crusts. Calamine lotion with 0.25% menthol is soothing and drying. Topical preparations containing analgesic agents must be avoided since these are potential sensitizers themselves. Topical corticosteroid creams may be useful once vesiculation has subsided. Oral antipruritic agents (Table 29-3) provide symptomatic relief. If involvement is extensive, oral prednisone is indicated, starting at 1 mg/kg/d and gradually tapering over 12 to 14 days. When prednisone is given for 7 days or less, patients often experience a marked rebound and a recurrence of their eruption.

Erythema Multiforme

Clinical Picture
Elevated, erythematous, urticaria-like round lesions are scattered randomly over the body, including the palms and soles. The pathognomonic lesion resembles a target or "bull's eye," with central erythema surrounded by a pale ring that in turn is surrounded by a red ring. Vesicles and bullae may be present. Mucosal erosions (eyes, mouth, genitalia) differentiate erythema multiforme major (so-called Stevens-Johnson syndrome) from erythema multiforme minor. The condition may recur.

Etiology
Presumably erythema multiforme is a hypersensitivity reaction that may be provoked by a variety of widely diversified agents including drugs (penicillin, sulfonamide, barbiturate) and infectious organisms (*Streptococcus*, *Mycoplasma pneumoniae*, herpes simplex).

Diagnostic Studies
Appropriate cultures or serologic tests should be obtained to rule out suspected infectious agents.

Differential Diagnosis
The presence of a definite target lesion is diagnostic.

Treatment
Symptomatic treatment is usually sufficient for mild cases. In severe cases the administration of systemic prednisone, 1 to 2 mg/kg/d, can shorten the course and reduce discomfort. With significant oral lesions careful monitoring of fluid and electrolyte balance is important. Concomitant infection should be appropriately treated.

Dermatophytosis

Clinical Picture
Dermatophytosis is characterized by erythematous scaly lesions, with or without vesicles. They are more commonly present on the extremities, especially the palms and soles.

Etiology
This condition is caused by dermatophytes of the *Trichophyton* or *Epidermophyton* genera.

Diagnostic Studies
The roof of a vesicle is scraped, KOH is added, and the sample is examined microscopically. The presence of septate branching hyphae confirms the diagnosis of dermatophytosis.

Differential Diagnosis
Acute eczematous dermatitis and contact dermatitis must be ruled out.

Treatment
Oral griseofulvin, 15 mg/kg/d in a single dose with a fatty meal, e.g., milk, is administered if the eruption is extensive or very inflammatory. Topical preparations (Table 29-5) can be used for less severe infections. The cream (or lotion for hairy areas) is applied three times per day, continuing for 10 days after the lesion has disappeared.

BLISTERS

Blisters may be produced by widely diverse causes including heritable disorders, infections, trauma, and allergies. Table 29-7 provides a differential diagnosis for blistering disorders.

Epidermolysis Bullosa

Clinical Picture
Vesicles and blisters occur on normal-appearing skin at sites of trauma, particularly the knees, elbows, hands, and feet. Erosions and crusting with or without scarring are common.

TABLE 29-7 Blisters

Neonate	Infant or Child	Adolescent
Epidermolysis bullosa	Epidermolysis bullosa Contact dermatitis*	Epidermolysis bullosa Contact dermatitis
Friction	Friction Bullous impetigo Insect bites†	Friction Dermatophytosis* Insect bites
Staphylococcal scalded skin syndrome‡	Staphylococcal scalded skin syndrome Toxic epidermal necrolysis‡	 Toxic epidermal necrolysis

* See "Vesicles and Pustules."
† See "Papules and Nodules."
‡ See "Diffuse and Localized Macular Erythema."

Etiology
Minimal trauma produces separation of epidermis from dermis in individuals with this genetic disorder.

Diagnostic Studies
The clinical appearance of the dystrophic form and the junctional form of epidermolysis bullosa may be quite similar early in the course of the disease. Electron microscopic examination of the edge of a blister to determine the exact location of the epidermal-dermal split is usually necessary to differentiate the two entities.

Differential Diagnosis
Friction blisters, burns, and bullous impetigo must be considered in the differential diagnosis.

Treatment
Neonates and infants who develop blistering in pressure areas should be hospitalized for evaluation and diagnosis, as well as to control pain and infection.

Bullous Impetigo

Clinical Picture
In bullous impetigo, flaccid blisters containing cloudy fluid arise on a slightly erythematous base. Older lesions may show denudation of epidermis and an oozing, honey-colored crust. Lesions can occur anywhere but are most commonly seen on the face, especially around the nose and mouth.

Etiology
S. aureus is the causative organism.

Diagnostic Studies
A Gram's stain of a smear from the base of the blister shows numerous Gram-positive cocci in clusters. A culture confirms the diagnosis.

Differential Diagnosis
The differential diagnosis includes friction blisters, burns, bullous erythema multiforme, dermatitis herpetiformis, bullous pemphigoid, and bullous dermatosis of childhood.

Treatment
A semisynthetic penicillinase-resistant penicillin should be administered. Erythromycin may be used

as an alternative drug for patients allergic to penicillin. (See Chapter 36, "Infectious Diseases," for additional discussion.)

PAPULES AND NODULES

Papules are small (less than 1 cm) lesions that are elevated above the surface of the skin and may have a rough, smooth, or ulcerated surface. They may be solitary or multiple, isolated or confluent. Papules may be produced by epidermal or dermal proliferation, dermal inflammation, or by metabolic depositions in the dermis. Nodules, which are palpable elevated lesions larger and deeper than papules, may be due to epidermal, dermal, or subcutaneous proliferation, metastatic infiltrates, metabolic depositions, or inflammatory processes in the dermis or fat. A differential diagnosis for papules and nodules in children and adolescents is given in Table 29-8.

Neuroblastoma

Clinical Picture

Neuroblastomas are multiple, nontender, flesh-colored to bluish subcutaneous nodules that are randomly scattered over the body.

Etiology

The lesions are metastases from a primary sympathetic nervous system tumor, which is most commonly found in the adrenal gland.

TABLE 29-8 Papules and Nodules

Neonate	Infant and Child	Adolescent
	Molluscum contagiosum	Molluscum contagiosum
	Warts	Warts
	Common wart	
	Flat wart	
	Genital wart	
	Insect bites	Insect bites
Neuroblastoma	Scabies	Scabies
	Urticaria pigmentosa	Urticaria pigmentosa
	Pyogenic granuloma	Pyogenic granuloma
Leukemia cutis*	Leukemia cutis	Leukemia cutis
	Cold panniculitis	Cold panniculitis
	Erythema nodosum	Erythema nodosum
	Primary syphilis	Primary syphilis

* See "Palpable Purpura."

Diagnostic Studies

Characteristic tumor cells are visualized on microscopic examination of a biopsy from one of these nodules.

Differential Diagnosis

The differential diagnosis should include leukemia cutis and "TORCH" syndrome (toxoplasmosis, rubella, cytomegalovirus and herpesvirus infections).

Treatment

Treatment is aimed against the primary tumor.

Molluscum Contagiosum

Clinical Picture

Flesh-colored, smooth, dome-shaped pearly papules, 1 to 10 mm in diameter with a central dell (umbilication), may be surrounded by a rim of erythema. The most common site is the face, but lesions may occur anywhere.

Etiology

Molluscum contagiosum is caused by cutaneous infection with an intracytoplasmic DNA poxvirus.

Diagnostic Studies

A shave biopsy confirms the diagnosis in doubtful cases by revealing characteristic eosinophilic intracytoplasmic inclusions.

Differential Diagnosis

Comedones, warts, and nevi must be excluded.

Treatment

The treatment depends on the number of lesions and age of patient. Effective therapies include curettage, liquid nitrogen, podophyllin, and cantharidin.

Warts

Clinical Picture

The clinical presentation of a wart varies with its type and location.

Common Wart (Verruca Vulgaris) Common warts appear as flesh-colored to pink papules or plaques with an irregular, sometimes scaly surface. Removing excess scale reveals pinpoint bleeding sites. Common warts may be located anywhere but more often are seen on the fingers and hands, soles of the feet, lips, and genital area.

Flat Wart (Verruca Plana) Flat warts are multiple, small (2 to 5 mm), flesh-colored papules with a slightly irregular surface. They are most commonly found on the face and dorsal surface of the hand. They may be arranged in a linear configuration.

Genital Wart (Condyloma Acuminatum) Genital warts are flesh-colored, erythematous, or white papules with a moist verrucous surface. They are dispersed singly or in clusters in the anogenital region.

Etiology
Human papilloma virus infects human epidermal cells to produce characteristic lesions. The different kinds of warts are caused by different subtypes of human papilloma virus.

Diagnostic Studies
A serologic test for syphilis should be obtained from persons with genital warts since (1) condyloma latum occasionally resembles condyloma acuminatum, and (2) viral and spirochetal infections may occur concomitantly.

Treatment
Therapy depends to a great extent on the number, location, and type of lesions present. All patients require outpatient follow-up.

Common Warts Effective therapies include dessication and curettage, liquid nitrogen, cantharidin, or salicylic acid and lactic acid in a flexible collodion (Duofilm). Plantar warts may respond to the repetitive application of salicylic acid plasters, followed by gentle paring of the surrounding callus.

Flat Warts Salicylic acid and lactic acid in a flexible collodion (Duofilm), applied once a day for several days, may be helpful, as may be cautious application of cantharidin. Topical vitamin A cream can be tried also.

Genital Warts Podophyllin in benzoin should be applied carefully to each individual lesion, left on the lesion for 4 to 6 hours, and then washed off with soap and water. Additional applications are usually necessary at 5 to 7-day intervals.

Insect Bites

Clinical Picture
Reactions to bites from insects are characterized by the acute onset of multiple pruritic red papules, most frequently occurring on exposed surfaces such as the distal extremities. Sometimes a central punctum is visible, but more commonly the lesions are excoriated or impetiginized. Occasionally, insect bites are grouped in threes ("breakfast, lunch, and dinner"), and vesicles or even blisters may be present. (For a detailed discussion of venomous bites and stings, see Chapter 33, "Animal and Insect Bites.")

Etiology
"Hungry" insects such as mites and fleas are usually responsible.

Diagnostic Studies
In persistent lesions or doubtful cases, a skin biopsy may be helpful. An insect bite reaction is histologically characterized by a superficial and deep perivascular lymphohistiocytic and eosinophilic infiltrate.

Differential Diagnosis
Viral exanthem and drug eruption must be excluded.

Treatment
Antibiotics should be given if the bites are secondarily infected. Topical steroids or systemic antihistamines may help reduce pruritus.

Scabies

Clinical Picture
Intensely pruritic erythematous papules and vesicles are seen most prominently between the fingers, on the wrists, around the areolae and umbilicus, in the axillary folds, and on the genitalia. The face and scalp are almost always spared. Threadlike sepiginous lesions are occasionally visible. Excoriations are common. Infants may have flesh-colored or hyperpigmented nodules in the axillary and groin folds and a vesicular eruption on the palms and soles.

Etiology
Sarcoptes scabiei is the causative organism.

Diagnostic Studies
A carefully obtained scraping from a lesion may reveal diagnostic organisms, ova, or feces. After the skin is cleansed with alcohol, a drop of immersion or mineral oil is placed on a papule. The papule is then scraped vigorously with a scalpel blade, and the scraping is placed on a clean glass microscope slide. This procedure is repeated on multiple lesions. A coverslip is then applied, and the slide is examined microscopically. The presence of intact organisms, organism parts, ova, or feces confirms the diagnosis.

Differential Diagnosis
Scabies infestation can be so varied in its appearance that it is called the "great imposter." The differential diagnosis includes atopic dermatitis, contact dermatitis, impetigo, dermatitis herpetiformis, and lichen planus.

Treatment
All family members and any other individuals in close contact with the infected individual, such as playmates or babysitters, should receive treatment. After the patient is bathed, a thin coat of gamma-benzene hexachloride lotion is applied to the entire skin surface from the chin to the toes. The preparation is left on for 12 hours, after which time another bath or shower is taken. Clothing, towels, and bed linen used before or during therapy should be washed or dry cleaned before reusing. Pruritus may continue for as long as 2 to 3 weeks after treatment and may require antihistamines or systemic corticosteroids for control. Because a small percentage of individuals fail to respond to a single application of medicine, patients should be reexamined in 1 to 2 weeks, and if signs and symptoms persist, they should undergo a second course of therapy.

Urticaria Pigmentosa

Clinical Picture
Red-brown macules, papules, plaques, or nodules may be present as solitary or multiple lesions. When stroked, individual lesions urticate (Darier's sign) and/or occasionally vesiculate. Pruritus is variable. Multiple macular lesions are rarely associated with systemic mastocytosis.

Etiology
The lesions are caused by a perivascular or diffuse dermal mast cell infiltrate.

Diagnostic Studies
A skin biopsy reveals the characteristic mast cell infiltrate in the dermis.

Differential Diagnosis
Juvenile xanthogranuloma, spindle and epithelioid cell nevus, and xanthomata must be considered in the differential diagnosis.

Treatment
Lesions usually spontaneously resolve, leaving residual hypopigmentation or hyperpigmentation. When lesions are multiple, avoidance of certain stimulators of mast cell histamine release is suggested to prevent systemic symptoms (flushing, tachycardia, pruritus). Thus patients should be warned to avoid hot baths, vigorous rubbing of lesions, and ingestion of opiates (codeine, morphine, meperidine), aspirin, polymyxin B, and alcohol. Antihistamines may relieve itching and prevent flushing.

Pyogenic Granuloma

Clinical Picture
A pyogenic granuloma appears as a papule or nodule that is pink to red, with an oozing, crusted, or even slightly scaly surface; it bleeds easily. There is usually a solitary lesion on the face or hand, but lesions may occur elsewhere. A pyogenic granuloma occasionally appears as a large central lesion surrounded by multiple smaller "satellite" lesions.

Etiology
Pyogenic granuloma is thought to be an overexuberant reaction to trauma or a foreign body.

Diagnostic Studies
The clinical impression may be confirmed by a shave biopsy, which shows thin epithelium overlying an edematous dermis that contains a proliferation of small blood vessels and a variable amount of inflammation.

Differential Diagnosis
Hemangioma, spindle and epithelioid cell nevus (Spitz nevus), and traumatized nevocellular nevus must be excluded.

Treatment
Depending on its location and size, the lesion may be excised or it may be shaved off, with the base cauterized. The specimen should be submitted to the pathology department for microscopic examination.

Cold Panniculitis

Clinical Picture
Firm, tender, slightly erythematous subcutaneous nodules may appear at sites of direct cold injury. "Popsicle panniculitis" is a term used to describe circumoral lesions that occur after sucking on a Popsicle.

Etiology
Cold panniculitis is produced by direct exposure of involved tissue to cold.

Differential Diagnosis
Trauma and neoplasia must be ruled out.

Diagnostic Studies
The diagnosis is usually made on the basis of a history of cold exposure and the appearance of the characteristic lesions. In difficult or confusing cases, a skin biopsy may be helpful. Characteristic histologic features include lymphocytic infiltration and necrosis of the panniculus.

Treatment
Observation is usually sufficient; the natural history is that of gradual resolution over a 2- to 3-week period.

Erythema Nodosum

Clinical Picture
One or more tender, red to slightly bluish nodules, 1 to 3 cm in diameter, appear most commonly on the anterior surface of the legs. The lesions are often bilateral in distribution.

Etiology
Erythema nodosum is a panniculitis with a characteristic histology and is associated with a great variety of disorders, including infections (streptococcal pharyngitis, herpes simplex infection, and tuberculosis) and drug reactions.

Diagnostic Studies
Appropriate tests should be ordered to search for an underlying precipitating cause.

Differential Diagnosis
Trauma and thrombophlebitis must be considered in the differential diagnosis.

Treatment
Bed rest (with leg elevation) plus anti-inflammatory agents such as aspirin are often sufficient for symptomatic relief. For chronic or debilitating recurrent disease, short courses of saturated solution of potassium iodide, 5 to 10 drops three times per day, or prednisone, 1 mg/kg/d, may be helpful.

Primary Syphilis (Chancre)

Clinical Picture
A chancre is a flesh-colored, ulcerated papule or nodule that is usually solitary and nontender. Although a chancre may occur anywhere, it is most commonly present in the genital or perirectal area. Oral chancres may appear as erosions.

Etiology
T. pallidum is the causative organism.

Diagnostic Studies
A dark-field microscopic examination usually confirms the diagnosis. False-negative findings may occur if an antibacterial cream or ointment has been applied to the lesion. If the dark-field examination of a suspected lesion is negative, serologic testing should be done at weekly intervals for 1 month. Dark-field examinations are not reliable for oral lesions since other nonpathogenic spirochetes normally reside in the mouth.

Differential Diagnosis
Herpes simplex, chancroid, pyoderma, and trauma must be ruled out.

Treatment
Benzathine penicillin G, 2.4 million U IM, is the treatment of choice. Erythromycin or tetracycline, 500 mg four times per day for 15 days, may be given to penicillin-sensitive patients. (See Chapter 24, "Gynecologic Disorders and Sexually Transmitted Diseases," for additional discussion.)

NONPALPABLE PURPURA

The extravasation of erythrocytes into the dermis results in a reddish to reddish brown discoloration that is called petechia, purpura, or ecchymosis, depending upon the extent of the hemorrhage and size of the lesion. Extravasation of blood unaccompanied by inflammation produces flat, nonpalpable lesions. The differential diagnosis of nonpalpable purpura is given in Table 29-9.

TABLE 29-9 Nonpalpable Purpura

Neonate	Infant and Child	Adolescent
Platelet disorders	Platelet disorders	Platelet disorders
	Idiopathic thrombocytopenic purpura	
	Drug induced	Progressive pigmented purpura
	Associated with malignancy	
	Viral and bacterial infections	
	Collagen vascular diseases	
	Physical exertion (coughing, vomiting)	Physical exertion
	Trauma	Trauma
		Maculae caeruleae (pediculosis)

Platelet Disorders

Clinical Picture

Platelet disorders produce scattered macular purpuric lesions (petechiae or ecchymoses) that can occur anywhere on the body, including the mucous membranes, but are often more prominent on the distal extremities. The palms and soles may be involved. The patient may manifest systemic symptoms.

Etiology

Quantitative or qualitative alterations in platelets result in focal dermal hemorrhage. Causes include drug reactions, infections (bacterial and viral), collagen vascular diseases, malignancy, and idiopathic thrombocytopenic purpura.

Diagnostic Studies

Laboratory work should include a platelet count, prothrombin time, partial thromboplastin time, and bleeding time, plus other specific studies as needed to identify the cause.

Differential Diagnosis

Progressive pigmented purpura and maculae caeruleae must be ruled out.

Treatment

The underlying disease must be treated. (See Chapter 34, "Hematologic and Oncologic Emergencies.")

Progressive Pigmented Purpura

Clinical Picture

Individual or grouped red to brown-colored nonblanchable macules, 1 to 3 mm in diameter, are scattered over the distal lower extremities bilaterally. The soles are not involved. The lesions are usually asymptomatic but may be pruritic. There are no associated systemic symptoms.

Etiology

The cause is unknown.

Diagnostic Studies

Platelet studies are all normal. A skin biopsy reveals a perivenular mononuclear cell infiltrate and hemorrhage.

Differential Diagnosis

This purpura must be distinguished from petechiae produced by platelet disorders. The gradual onset, localization to lower legs, and general well-being of the patient are features that help distinguish progressive pigmented purpura from other entities.

Treatment

The eruption may persist from months to years. Some authors report that resolution may be hastened by using fluorinated corticosteroid cream under an occlusive wrap.

Maculae Caeruleae (Pediculosis)

Clinical Picture

Maculae caeruleae is characterized by several macular gray-blue purpuric lesions on the chest, abdomen, thighs, and upper arms. Although the lesions themselves are asymptomatic, the patient usually complains of pruritus involving the pubis or axillae.

Etiology

Pthirus pubis is the causative organism.

Diagnostic Studies

Discovery of an adult organism on the skin or nits (deposited eggs) on the hair confirms the diagnosis.

Differential Diagnosis

Platelet disorders and trauma must be ruled out.

Treatment

This condition is treated with 1% gamma-benzene hexachloride shampoo or lotion. Rid is a satisfactory alternative.

PALPABLE PURPURA

Purpuric lesions that are elevated and palpable are usually associated with inflammation and/or vessel thrombosis. Patients with palpable purpura are often acutely ill and require an extensive and rapid evaluation to determine the underlying cause for their eruption. The most common causes for palpable purpura are listed in Table 29-10.

Disseminated Intravascular Coagulopathy

Clinical Picture

The patient has multiple large, flat to slightly raised purpuric lesions with sharply demarcated, often red borders. Blisters are common. The patient is always toxic, with fever, hypotension, lethargy, or coma.

Etiology

Rapid consumption of coagulation factors including platelets, Factors V and VII, prothrombin, and fi-

TABLE 29-10 Palpable Purpura

Neonate	Infant and Child	Adolescent
Infections	Disseminated intravascular coagulopathy	Disseminated intravascular coagulopathy
Enterovirus		
Syphilis		
TORCH syndrome		
Toxoplasmosis		
Rubella		
Cytomegalovirus	Rocky Mountain spotted fever	Rocky Mountain spotted fever
Herpes		
Neuroblastoma*		
Leukemia cutis	Leukemia cutis	Leukemia cutis
	Bacterial endocarditis	Bacterial endocarditis
	Septicemia	Septicemia
	Staphylococcus	*Staphylococcus*
	Candida	*Candida*
	Meningococcus	Meningococcus
		Gonococcus
	Atypical measles†	Atypical measles
	Leukocytoclastic vasculitis	Leukocytoclastic vasculitis
	Henoch-Schönlein purpura	Henoch-Schönlein purpura
	Drug induced	Drug induced
	Idiopathic	Idiopathic
		Collagen vascular disease

* See "Papules and Nodules."
† See "Macules and Papules."

brinogen results in noncoagulation. Disseminated intravascular coagulopathy may be triggered by infections (bacterial, viral, and fungal), surgery, and transfusion reactions.

Diagnostic Studies

The following studies should be obtained: platelet count, prothrombin time, partial thromboplastin time, circulating split products of fibrin, and blood cultures. A skin biopsy also may be helpful in establishing the cause of the eruption.

Differential Diagnosis

Early in the evolution of the eruption, individual lesions may resemble vasculitis, sepsis, or a viral exanthem. With time the lesions develop their characteristic appearance and the diagnosis is established.

Treatment

The patient should be hospitalized and treated for the underlying disease. Heparin should be administered. (For additional discussion of disseminated vascular coagulopathy, see Chapter 34, "Hematologic and Oncologic Emergencies.")

Rocky Mountain Spotted Fever

Clinical Picture

Rocky Mountain spotted fever begins with erythematous macules that progress to form purpuric papules. The lesions often appear first on the wrists and ankles and then spread centrifugally. Fever, headache, photophobia, and myalgias are common. This classic manifestation may be altered if medication (antibiotics) is administered early in the course of the disease.

Etiology

Rickettsia rickettsii, the causative organism, is transmitted by the bite of a tick (*Dermacentor*). Endemic areas include the Rocky Mountain states, Maryland, Virginia, North Carolina, and Massachusetts.

Diagnostic Studies

Organisms are occasionally observed on skin biopsy. Confirmation of diagnosis is by specific complement-fixation test and a positive Weil-Felix reaction to OX-2 and OX-19 strains of *Proteus vulgaris*.

Differential Diagnosis

Viral exanthem (coxsackievirus A5 or B3), atypical measles, and cutaneous vasculitis must be ruled out.

Treatment

If the disease is clinically suspected, an appropriate dose of tetracycline or chloramphenicol should be administered as soon as diagnostic studies are obtained. Hospitalization should be considered to observe and monitor the patient. (See Chapter 36, "Infectious Diseases," for further discussion.)

Leukemia Cutis

Clinical Picture

One or more flesh-colored to purpuric nontender dermal or subcutaneous nodules are scattered randomly over the body.

Etiology

This condition is produced by proliferation of malignant hematopoietic cells in the skin.

Diagnostic Studies

A skin biopsy confirms the presence of abnormal cells in the dermis. A peripheral smear or bone marrow aspirate establishes the cell of origin.

Differential Diagnosis

TORCH syndrome, and neuroblastoma should be considered in the differential diagnosis.

Treatment

Treatment is directed at the underlying disease. (See Chapter 34, "Hematologic and Oncologic Emergencies," for additional discussion.)

Bacterial Endocarditis

Clinical Picture

Bacterial endocarditis can be associated with a countable number of small (1 to 3 mm) purpuric papules that are scattered over fingers, toes, and, occasionally, conjunctival mucosa. Splinter hemorrhages are often present under the nails. The patient usually appears quite toxic, with fever, lethargy, malaise, arthralgias, and cardiac murmurs.

Etiology

Streptococcus viridans and *S. aureus* are causative agents.

Diagnostic Studies

Blood cultures confirm the diagnosis. A skin biopsy may be helpful.

Differential Diagnosis

Cutaneous vasculitis and collagen vascular disease must be excluded.

Treatment

Appropriate antibiotic therapy is administered. (See Chapter 10, "Cardiovascular Disorders," for further discussion.)

Septicemia

Clinical Picture

Septicemia is manifested as a variable number of purpuric papules, up to several centimeters in size, that are usually acrally distributed. Pustules, hemorrhagic blisters, necrotic lesions, and ulcerations may occur. Systemic symptoms are variable, depending on the causative agent.

Etiology

Neisseria gonorrhoeae A sparse number of lesions are usually present on the fingers or toes. The lesions range from erythematous papules to hemorrhagic pustules. Fever, pharyngitis, tenosynovitis, arthritis, vaginitis, urethritis, and lower abdominal pain may be accompanying symptoms.

Neisseria meningitidis Small purpuric lesions may enlarge to form larger areas with sharp borders and central necrosis. Fever, headache, lethargy, meningism, nausea, vomiting, pharyngitis, and polyarthritis are common.

Staphylococcus aureus Pustular and hemorrhagic acral lesions are accompanied by fever and variable systemic symptoms.

Pseudomonas* and *Candida albicans Lesions are indistinguishable from those caused by other bacteria.

Diagnostic Studies

Blood cultures should be obtained. A Gram's stain of a sample from a pustule, blister, or infarcted lesion may demonstrate the causative organism. A skin biopsy also may be helpful in demonstrating the causative organism.

Differential Diagnosis

Vasculitis and endocarditis should be considered in the differential diagnosis.

Treatment

The patient should be admitted to the hospital and receive the appropriate antibiotics. (See Chapter 36, "Infectious Diseases," for further discussion.)

Leukocytoclastic Vasculitis

Clinical Picture

Numerous purpuric papules ranging in size from 2 to 10 mm may be present anywhere on the body; however, the heaviest concentration is usually seen on the arms, legs, and buttocks. Hemorrhagic vesicles, blisters, and necrotic lesions may occasionally occur. Accompanying systemic symptoms are variable but may include fever, malaise, headache, arthralgias or arthritis, and abdominal pain.

Etiology

Henoch-Schönlein Purpura Occasionally, vasculitis follows streptococcal infection or upper respiratory tract infection. Purpura often appears in crops; urticarial lesions and localized edema of scalp, face, hands, and feet also may be present.

Drug-Induced Vasculitis Antibiotics and diuretics are the most frequently implicated medications.

Collagen Vascular Disease Vaculitis may accompany rheumatoid arthritis and systemic lupus erythematosus, but it is rarely the presenting symptom.

In addition to the aforementioned causes, there is also an idiopathic manifestation of leukocytoclastic vasculitis.

Diagnostic Studies

The following studies should be performed: CBC, platelet count, stool guaiac test, urinalysis, testing for antinuclear antibodies and rheumatoid factor (if symptoms suggest collagen vascular disease), and skin biopsy.

Differential Diagnosis

Sepsis and endocarditis must be ruled out.

Treatment

Treatment is usually directed against the underlying cause.

MISCELLANEOUS

Pediculosis

Clinical Picture

The patient usually complains of pruritus of the scalp, axillae, or pubis. Careful examination reveals adult lice on the skin (these may be brown from engorged blood) and 1 to 2-mm white or opalescent nits (egg cases) on the hair shafts. Lice and nits occasionally may be seen on the eyelashes of young children. Excoriations and lymphadenopathy are often present.

Etiology

The causative organisms are *Pediculus humanus* var. *capitis* (head louse) and *Pthirus pubis* (pubic "crab" louse). Organisms can be transferred person-to-person or via personal items such as clothing, bedding, and hair brushes.

Diagnostic Studies

No diagnostic studies are needed.

Differential Diagnosis

The clinical picture is sufficiently characteristic to be diagnostic.

Treatment

Pediculosis Capitis The hair should be washed with 1% gamma-benzene hexachloride shampoo, which is left on for 5 to 10 minutes and then is rinsed off. The treatment is repeated after 24 hours.

Pediculosis Pubis One percent gamma-benzene hexachloride lotion is applied to the pubic area and left on overnight.

Eyelash Involvement An ointment of 0.25% physostigmine (Eserine) is applied daily with a cotton-tipped swab until the infestation is eliminated.

Objects in contact with the infested skin, such as bedding, underwear, and hats, should be washed with detergent in hot water.

Bibliography

Arndt KA: *Manual of Dermatologic Therapeutics*, ed 2. Boston, Little Brown & Co, 1978.

Fitzpatrick TB, et al. (eds): *Dermatology in General Medicine*, ed 2. New York, McGraw-Hill Book Co, 1979.

Hurwitz S: *Clinical Pediatric Dermatology*. Philadelphia, WB Saunders Co, 1981.

Lazarus GS, Goldsmith LA, Tharp MD: *Diagnosis of Skin Diseases*. Philadelphia, FA Davis Co, 1980.

Rippon JW: *Medical Mycology. The Pathogenic Fungi and the Pathogenic Actinomyces*. Philadelphia, WB Saunders Co, 1974.

Rook A, Wilkinson DS, Ebling FJG (eds): *Textbook of Dermatology*, ed 3. London, Blackwell Scientific Publications, 1979.

Solomon LM, Esterly WB: *Neonatal Dermatology*. Philadelphia, WB Saunders Co, 1973.

Weston WL: *Practical Pediatric Dermatology*. Boston, Little Brown & Co, 1979.

Thomas R. Weber
Dennis W. Vane
Jay L. Grosfeld

30 Skin and Subcutaneous Injuries

Children with skin and soft tissue injuries make up a large portion of pediatric cases seen in the emergency department. Usually these injuries are relatively minor and can be treated adequately with a minimum of medical attention; however, each wound must be thoroughly investigated as to its cause and extent of injury to avoid potentially serious complications. An apparently superficial laceration may involve deep tissues, and, similarly, a small bruise on the arm may in fact be a wringer injury. Pediatric patients are frequently frightened of physicians and the unfamiliar hospital emergency department. In addition, the injury may be the result of an act of disobedience, increasing the child's anxiety.[1] For these reasons it is often helpful to enlist the aid of a parent or friend in compiling the history and to interview the child privately.

ASSESSING THE WOUND

Examination of the wound and assessment of the extent of injury are the prime objectives of the emergency physician. Determination of the general condition of the child and identification of associated injuries are critical in any pediatric trauma case. In a child for whom the history is incomplete, a thorough physical examination must be undertaken. Only after other life-threatening injuries have been ruled out should the care of the obvious soft tissue injury be addressed.

A soft tissue injury should always be explored with aseptic technique. Ideally, the examining physician should scrub, glove, and don a cap and mask. Open wounds should be covered with a temporary sterile dressing to prevent hospital flora from infecting the wound.

Thorough examination of the injury obviously requires a cooperative patient. In general, older children can usually understand and cooperate adequately after the parents have been excused to the waiting area. For infants and young children, sedation is usually necessary, especially when examination involves tender areas. Meperidine (1.0 mg/kg) combined with promethazine (0.5 mg/kg) and chlorpromazine (0.5 mg/kg) administered intramuscularly allows detailed examination of a wound with relative comfort for the child.[1] Prior to administration of the medication, vital signs should be normal and all systemic injuries must be ruled out. Restraining the child with a commercially available device is often valuable in both assessment and treatment of injuries (Figure 30-1).

Assessing the injury requires answers to several important questions. First, identification of the mechanism of injury is critical. Lacerations resulting from falls may involve a retained foreign body. Circumferential bruising of an extremity should suggest a wringer-type injury with the possibility of

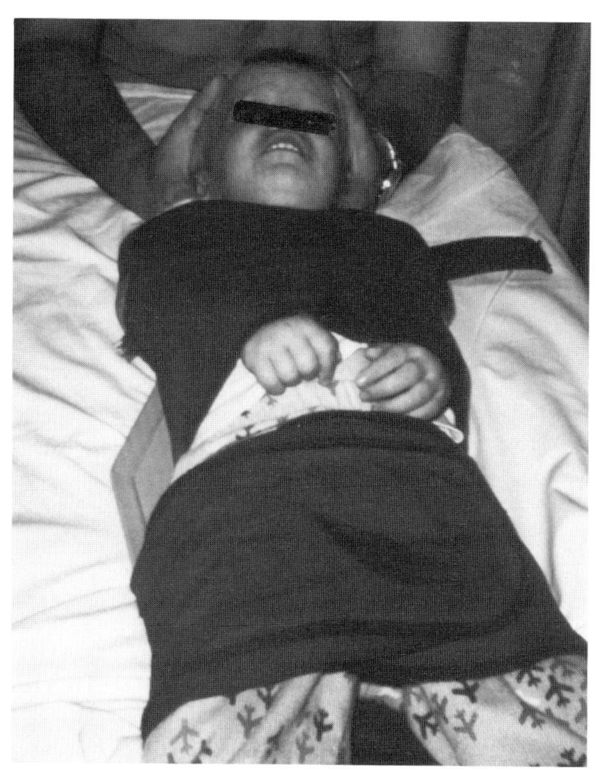

FIGURE 30-1 A commercially available device for restraining the chlid.

a compartment syndrome. A complete neurovascular examination of the extremity distal to an injury is mandatory. Missile wounds cause considerable soft tissue damage in areas surrounding entry and exit wounds. Abrasions and irregular lacerations caused by falls may contain contaminating objects such as soil, glass, pebbles, and sand. Some of these foreign materials are radiopaque, but frequently only careful inspection and debridement of the wound itself lead to their discovery.

Second, the location of the injury is important. Lacerations or soft tissue loss near major vessels or nerve trunks must be carefully examined to ensure no underlying injury to vital structures. A thorough familiarity with extremity anatomy as well as facial nerves is essential to avoid unnecessary complications.

Finally, the specific circumstances at the time the wound occurred should be investigated, especially with regard to the possibility of child abuse. It is the responsibility of the emergency department staff to recognize and bring suspicious cases of trauma to the attention of a child abuse team for follow-up. Failure to do so may result in repetitive inflicted injuries that are potentially life-threatening. In many states medical personnel are legally responsible to report any suspect case. (See Chapter 39, "Child Abuse and Neglect.")

LOCAL ANESTHESIA

Local anesthesia is usually administered with a 25- to 27-gauge needle directly under the skin edges of the wound. Preparation of the skin for injection should not be extensive to limit the child's discomfort as much as possible. It is helpful to tell the child that a small "sting" will accompany the injection, since this makes the child more trustful when told that subsequent suturing will be painless. In general, 0.5% to 1.0% lidocaine without epinephrine is used, after allergy to the drug has been ruled out by questioning the parents. Epinephrine 1 : 100,000 can be used with the lidocaine in selective cases and is helpful in the suturing of wounds in highly vascular areas such as the face.[2] Local anesthetics containing epinephrine should never be used in extremity wounds because this may lead to vasoconstriction with digital necrosis of toes or fingers. Administration should not exceed 3 mg/kg with plain lidocaine or 5 mg/kg when lidocaine with epinephrine is used.[1]

CLEANSING THE WOUND

One of the most important aspects of treating soft tissue trauma is adequate cleansing of the wound. In general, totally different sets of instruments should be used for cleansing and repairing the wound. Any antiseptic the physician or hospital feels comfortable with can be used.[2] We generally prefer an iodine-based antiseptic for preparation, although this has the minor disadvantage of staining the tissue. Peroxide 1.0% is also useful, especially in wounds with considerable capillary hemorrhage, since it provides a hemostatic component. Gentle scrubbing is important in all wounds to provide adequate antisepsis.

Irrigation should be employed, using normal (physiologic) saline (0.9% NaCl) in large volumes, to adequately remove foreign bodies and to provide a diluent effect on microorganisms. In this regard a syringe with a 20- or 21-gauge needle is useful as it provides good hydrostatic pressure for removal of foreign bodies and debridement of devascularized tissue. Extremely dirty wounds can be irrigated by intravenous tubing connected to a 1-L bottle of saline, elevated high on a pole to provide a vigorous flow of the solution. It is not uncommon to use 4 to 6 L of solution to completely cleanse an extremely dirty laceration. Cleansing action is dependent on both the volume and velocity of the irrigation. Commercially available irrigation sets can also be employed.

HEMOSTASIS

To avoid complications, hemostasis should be established before attempting wound repair. This allows visualization of all of the damaged tissue and prevents the development of a postclosure hematoma, which is an excellent growth medium for subsequent wound infection. In most instances adequate hemostasis can be obtained with direct pressure on the wound. If the wound is bleeding profusely and hemostasis cannot be achieved with pressure, this often indicates a major vessel injury and suggests that wound exploration and vessel repair should be undertaken in the operating room under more controlled conditions than exist in most emergency departments. Hemostats should never be applied blindly to the child, especially in instances of extremity or facial injury. Nerves and arteries can be extremely small in children and are often anatomically located in proximity (e.g., neurovascular bundle), and serious injury may be created by haphazard clamping. Similarly, chemical hemostatic agents have little place in the emergency department, except possibly in the case of a large abrasion with considerable bleeding. In this instance the use of topical thrombin gently rubbed with the glove directly on the blotted surface of such an injury aids both in hemostasis as well as reduction of pain in the area.

WOUND DEBRIDEMENT

Mechanical debridement of the wound should be undertaken just prior to closure, if at all possible. In most cases mechanical debridement is accomplished simultaneously with irrigation and cleansing of the wound. When the wound is fully debrided, it is essential that recontamination does not occur.

The basis for debriding a wound is that devitalized tissue with compromised blood flow does not heal properly and may increase the risk of infection.[3] All questionable tissue in a traumatic wound must be excised prior to closure. Any devascularized tissue left in the closed laceration, no matter how sterile, will probably become infected. Similarly, all foreign bodies should be removed from the wound. Dirt and gravel embedded securely in tissue may require removal of the tissue itself to ensure adequate removal of the foreign body. However, if the removal of foreign bodies requires damaging essential structures, then their removal should be completed in the operating room. In addition, the so-called tattoo injuries of the face caused by gravel or carbonaceous materials may require later dermabrasion that should not be attempted in the emergency setting.

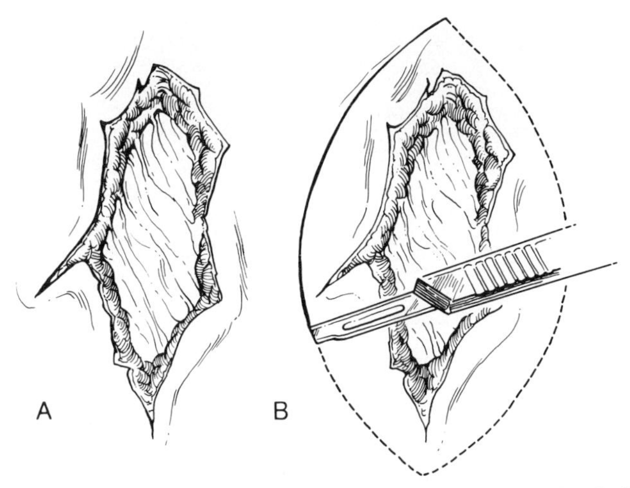

FIGURE 30-2 Irregular lacerations should be debrided to assure clean, viable wound edges before closure is attempted.

Irregular and beveled skin edges should be carefully debrided to obtain satisfactory closure (Figure 30-2). A linear wound is not essential, provided the edges are viable, and even L-shaped wounds are acceptable if they are closed properly. Excessive tissue loss is undesirable in wound debridement, especially when it results in excessive tension on the wound edges for approximation, lengthening of a facial scar, or extension of wounds over moving joints. If tissue loss is necessary, then the wound should be designed so that scar will result in a minimum of deformity and loss of mobility. This may require the assistance of a plastic surgeon if the laceration is on the face or over a joint.

WOUND CLOSURE

Wound closure in most traumatic wounds is straightforward and uncomplicated if certain principles are followed.[3] Wounds must be closed without tension and without a "dead space" in the deep tissues, if possible (Figure 30-3). If a wound is deep, several deep-layer sutures may be required. Commonly, this deep closure is done with an absorbable suture material. Closure is accomplished with a tapered needle and suture material 4-0 or smaller. Deep closure requiring larger sutures may have to be done in the operating room, particularly if special techniques of relaxing wound edges are necessary. Closure of the deep layer must be done ana-

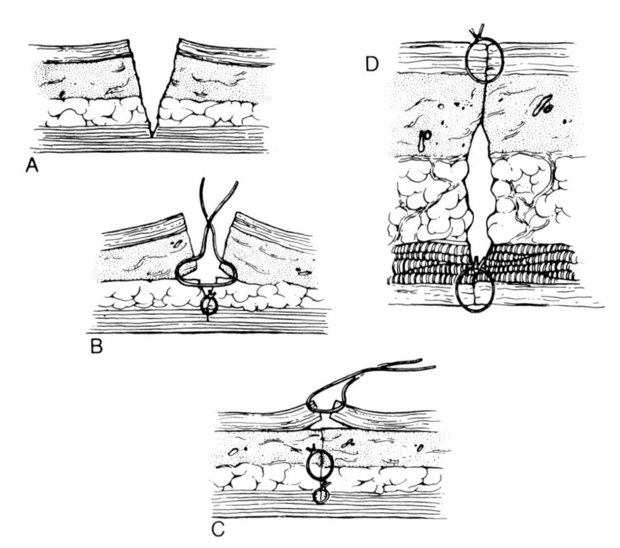

FIGURE 30-3 Deep wounds should be closed in layers (A, B, and C) to prevent tension on wound edges and eliminate dead space. A poorly closed deep wound with dead space present (D) can lead to wound infection with infected hematoma or serum.

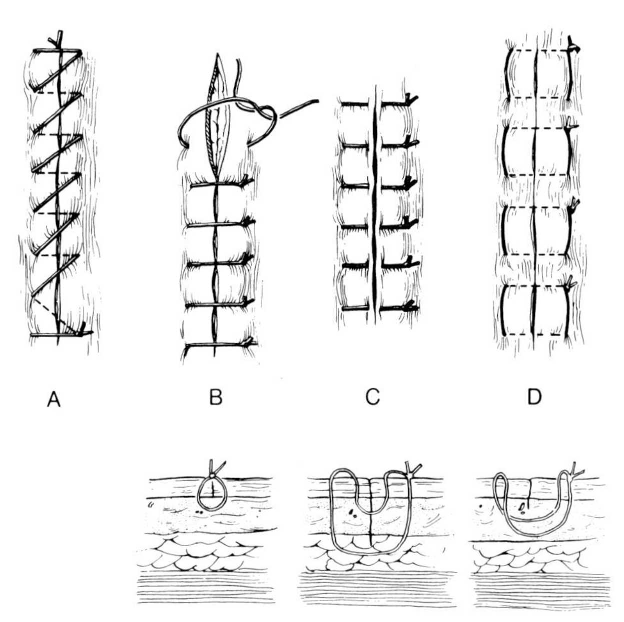

FIGURE 30-4 Commonly employed suture techniques. A, Simple running suture is well suited for straight, superficial lacerations. B, Simple, interrupted sutures are also used in superficial wounds. C, Vertical mattress sutures allow deep and superficial approximation without skin tension. D, Horizontal mattress technique is valuable in areas of thickened skin to maintain skin eversion.

tomically to prevent an overlying irregular skin closure.

Closure of the skin can be accomplished by a variety of operative techniques.[3] We usually prefer a fine nonabsorbable monofilament suture placed in interrupted fashion, especially since many traumatic wounds are contaminated. Nylon and polypropylene are well suited, with 4-0 or 5-0 suture most commonly employed on the trunk and extremities and 6-0 used for fascial closures. A fine cutting needle is used for skin closure. The specific technique of suture placement depends on the preference of the particular physician involved; however, several types of suturing techniques can be used with specific wound problems (Figure 30-4). In clean, straight wounds a running suture is quite acceptable. In irregular, superficial lacerations or in deep wounds with the deep layers closed, simple interrupted sutures suffice. In wounds with a slight amount of tension or when the skin is thick or subject to considerable motion, horizontal mattress sutures may prove useful. In moderately deep wounds, when deep layers are not closed, vertical mattress sutures can be used. This last technique gives good approximation of the skin and deeper layers and eliminates dead space and skin-edge tension. Many physicians currently prefer subcuticular sutures, where both absorbable and nonabsorbable material can be used. If absorbable sutures are used, subsequent removal is unnecessary. In general, these sutures should be used only in relatively straight wounds that are considered clean. Close follow-up is necessary to avoid a wound infection promoted by the foreign body effect of the subcuticular suture.

Numerous cutaneous tape closure materials are commercially available. These are highly acceptable for small, superficial wounds where the skin does not undergo much motion, and therefore they should not be used near or on joints. It is essential that the skin be defatted and completely dry before the strips are applied. Tincture of benzoin is very helpful in obtaining a good "stick" for the strips (Figure 30-5A). Care must be taken to obtain a good closure, and the rules of good skin approximation must be followed (Figure 30-5B).

Anatomic apposition of the skin layers is extremely important (Figure 30-6). Skin edges must be approximated until they just touch and are slightly everted. Inverted skin edges or overlapping edges result in poor healing or a "step-off" wound. Similarly, closing the wound too tightly results in strangulation of the wound edge and subsequent tissue necrosis. In extremely long wounds or wounds associated with some tissue loss, it is helpful to identify landmarks such as direction of hair

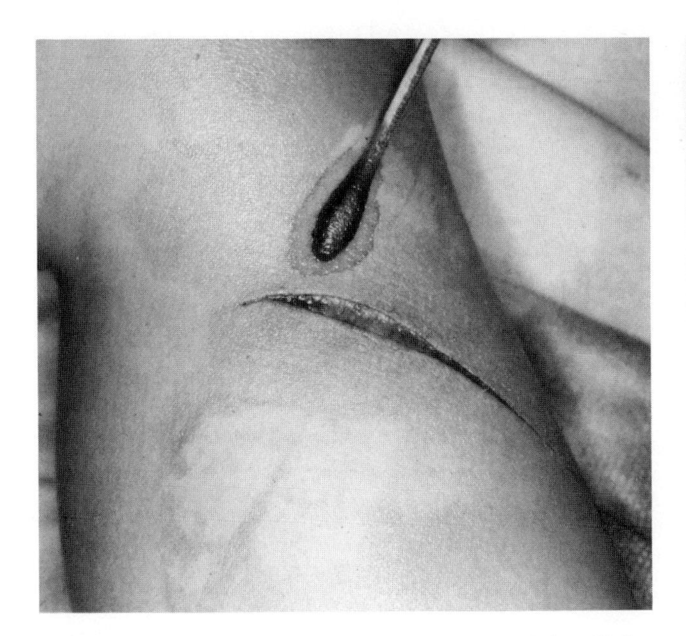

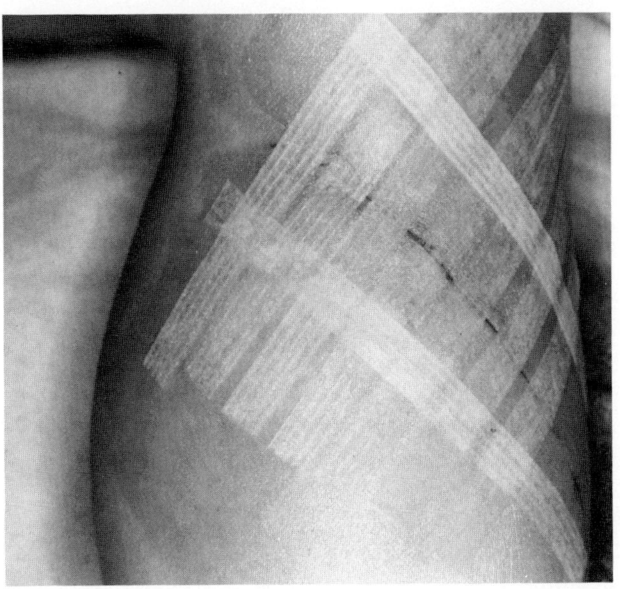

FIGURE 30-5 Benzoin (**A**) and Steristrips (**B**) will frequently produce excellent cosmetic results.

lines, moles or freckles, scratches, or even old scars to aid in reapproximation of skin edges.

DRESSINGS

Dressings must be functional for the child, provide sterile protection for the new wound, and protect the wound from the stresses of excessive movement. It is often helpful to use aids such as crutches for lower extremity wounds or splints and sling for upper extremity wounds to assist in adequate wound immobilization. A brief period (48 hours) of immobilization aids considerably in healing.

Simple Lacerations

For simple lacerations an occlusive gauze dressing is applied. Tape is used to cover the area entirely to provide a sterile barrier. A sterile ointment is helpful in preventing adherence of the dressing to the normally formed protein eschar. Considerable evidence has shown that the simple wound is sealed in a period of 24 to 48 hours; therefore, if the dressing remains clean and intact, it should be left for 48 hours, and afterwards no further external dressing should be necessary.[3] In general, areas around wounds can be washed at this time. Regular skin care can be resumed when the sutures or Steristrips are removed, usually within 10 days to 2

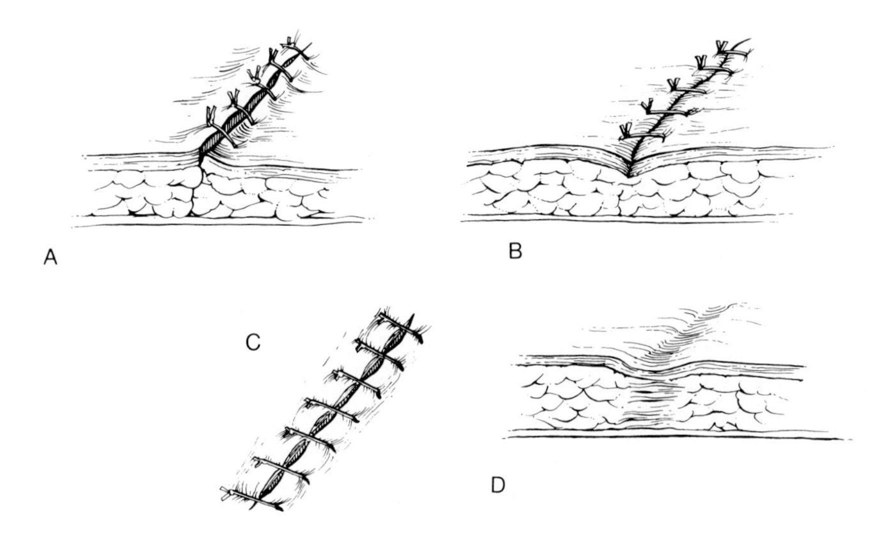

FIGURE 30-6 Common errors in wound closure. A, Unequal length of suture placement results in a "step-off" wound. B, Inversion of wound edges leads to poor healing and may result in wound separation when the sutures are removed. C, Sutures placed too far apart or tied too tightly may create an unsightly scar. D, Wounds healing by secondary intention frequently leave a broad, depressed scar.

weeks (3 to 4 days on the face), depending on the area involved.

Abrasions

Abrasion injury, if it is severe, should be treated similar to a burn. Appropriate therapy is to cover the area with an occlusive dressing. Petroleum-impregnated gauze and nitrofurazone or silver sulfadiazine creams have been used as dressings. Also, plastic skin coverings (Op-Site) have become available. Any of these techniques are useful if appropriate follow-up is available. It is essential that these dressings remain intact to provide maximum benefit. If a break in sterile technique occurs, the wound must be cleaned and the dressing should be reapplied. Effective treatment of these wounds must include keeping them clean and free of cellular debris to allow complete reepithelization. They must be followed closely to prevent infection; to prevent pain, they should be kept covered for approximately 48 hours or until a superficial eschar forms.

SUTURE REMOVAL

Suture removal is an important part of wound care and should be done under the supervision of a physician. Sutures are removed on a varying schedule, depending upon their location. Sutures in the face should be removed in 3 to 5 days, with few exceptions, and be replaced with tape strips, which are left in place for 1 week. Sutures on the head within the hairline can be left in place 1 week, whereas sutures on the extremities and back should remain 10 to 14 days, depending on the degree of tension, vascularity of the original wound, and its location (e.g., over moveable joints).

TETANUS IMMUNIZATION

Guidelines for tetanus immunization are shown in Table 30-1. (See also Chapter 36, "Infectious Diseases," for treatment of tetanus.)

ANTIBIOTIC USAGE

In general, most traumatic wounds do not require antibiotics if treated appropriately. Exceptions may include puncture wounds, human and other bites, and extremely dirty wounds of the hand, face, or feet. Questionable wounds should be left open, with either delayed primary closure or healing by secondary intention. Cosmetically poor results from these latter techniques can be revised at a later date.

GROSSLY INFECTED WOUNDS

Even with the most careful and thorough preparation and closure, a small percentage of wounds become infected.[4] In addition, lacerations treated without physician attention frequently become infected and are seen at the emergency department several days after the initial injury. These infections must be treated promptly to prevent systemic complications. If the infection is well localized to the area of the wound, with neither signs of systemic infection (elevated white cell count and temperature) nor cellulitis or lymphangitis (red "streaks" radiating away from the wound), removal of sutures and opening the wound are usually adequate treatment. The wound is cultured and can then be treated with irrigation or "wet-to-dry" dressings on

TABLE 30-1 Tetanus Immunization*

Patient Status	Nontetanus-Prone Wounds	Tetanus-Prone Wounds
Child adequately immunized		
Previously fully immunized and last dose given within the last 10 yr	No booster needed	If 5 yr since last dose, 0.5 mL adsorbed toxoid IM; if excessive prior toxoid injections, can omit this booster
Two or more prior injections of toxoid and the last dose given more than 10 yr previously	0.5 mL adsorbed toxoid	0.5 mL adsorbed toxoid IM
Child not adequately immunized		
Only 1 or no prior injection of toxoid or immunization history unknown	0.5 mL adsorbed toxoid IM, followed by two injections at 60-d intervals	0.5 mL adsorbed toxoid IM and subsequent boosters; 250 U (or more) of human TIG† IM Consider giving antibiotics

* Based on recommendations of the Committee on Trauma of the American College of Physicians.
† Tetanus immune globulin.

an outpatient basis, with healing by secondary intention. Other local care includes warm soaks to the area and elevation of an extremity, if it is involved. If any signs of systemic toxic effects, lymphangitis, or cellulitis are present, the child should be admitted to the hospital and given broad-spectrum antibiotics intravenously. The antibiotic can eventually be changed when specific cultures are available. After improvement antibiotic therapy then can be changed to an oral regimen, and the child can be treated as an outpatient, with frequent follow-up visits.

L-shaped Lacerations

Although L-shaped lacerations often appear to have significant skin loss, in most situations this is not the case. Approximation of the deep layer of the corner of an L-shaped laceration usually allows for adequate closure of the wound in straight lines (Figure 30-7).

Dirty Lacerations

Children's wounds are frequently contaminated with soil, gravel, or organic materials. If the wound can be cleaned and debrided adequately, it can be closed, and the child is followed closely for infection. If there is a question of follow-up or if the wound is grossly contaminated and areas of questionable tissue viability are present, the wound should be left open and saline "wet-to-dry" dressings should be applied.[1]

Puncture Wounds

Puncture wounds should virtually never be closed. In general, treatment is local with elevation and warm soaks. In cases of contaminated wounds, a broad-spectrum antibiotic may be helpful, especially in wounds of the feet.

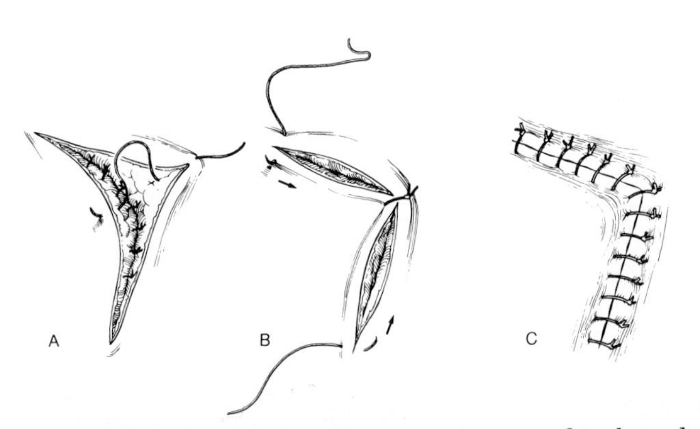

FIGURE 30-7 The curvilinear appearance of L-shaped lacerations (A) frequently appears to represent skin loss, but this can usually be repaired primarily. The center of the wound is reapproximated first (B); each limb of the laceration is then closed individually (C).

Retained Foreign Body Punctures

Treatment of puncture wounds with a retained foreign body (e.g., splinters, needles) should be similar to simple puncture wounds. If the foreign body is clearly visible, it can be removed. However, if it is not visible, exploration should not be carried out in the emergency department. Documentation of the presence of foreign bodies frequently requires radiologic procedures (Figures 30-8 through 30-12). The wounds usually remain asymptomatic until the foreign body extrudes itself to the skin, and at this time the object can be removed with local anesthesia. Exploration of the wound in the emergency department is tempting but often extremely frustrating. Deep foreign bodies are almost never found, and a simple puncture wound can be converted to a larger, often contaminated, laceration. Symptomatic foreign bodies should be treated by formal operative exploration, often under fluoroscopic control.

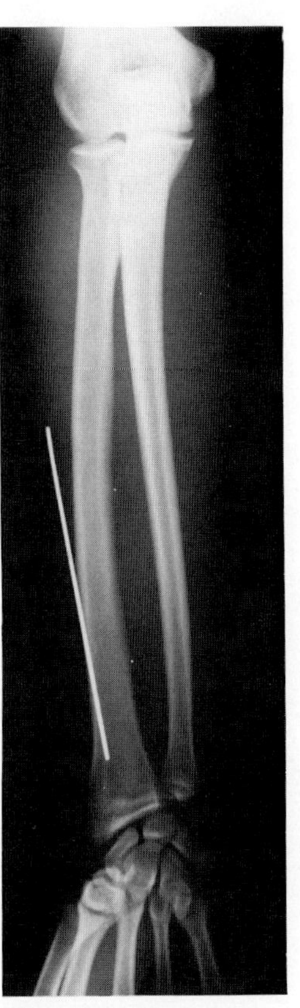

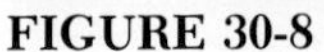

FIGURE 30-8

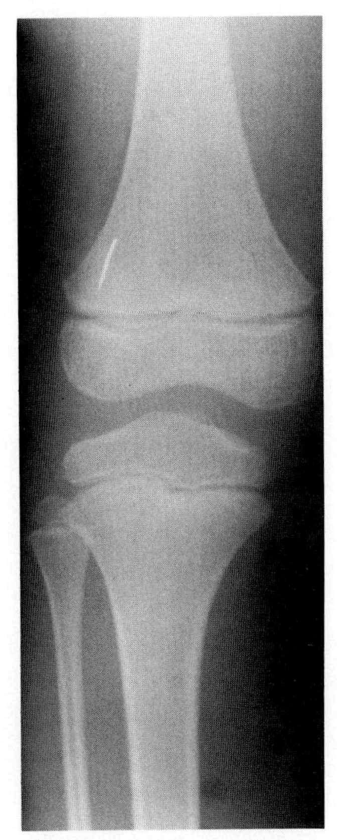

FIGURE 30-9

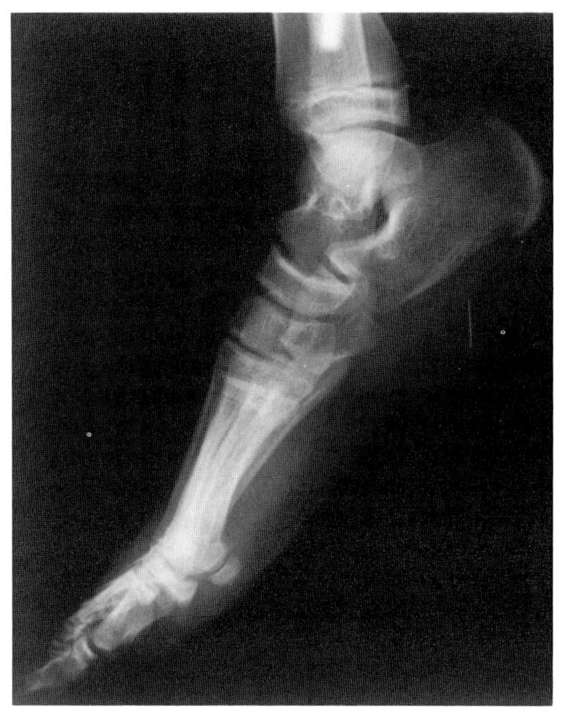

FIGURE 30-10

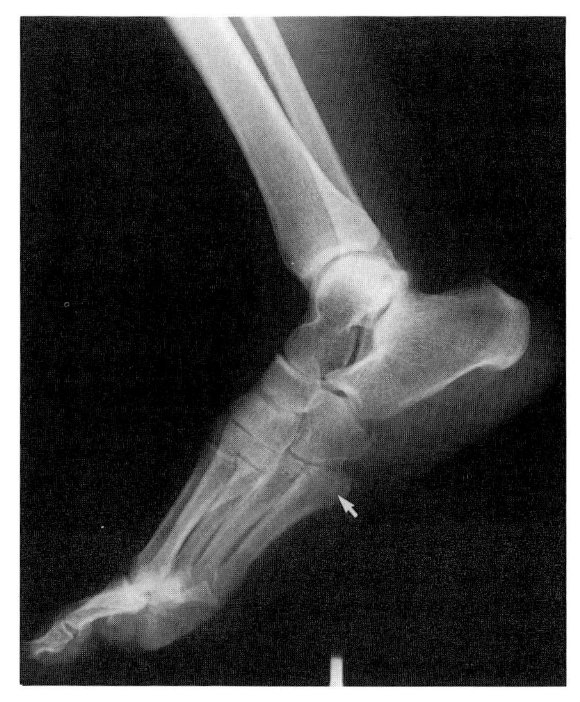

FIGURE 30-12

AVULSION INJURIES

Wringer Injuries

Wringer injuries are becoming less common in children because of the modernization of washing machines; however, these injuries continue to be seen in large emergency departments. Wringer injuries often have two components: the skin and superficial injury, and the deep and often more serious underlying crush injury. Avulsions of the skin can range from a slight skin abrasion to a severe skin loss (Figure 30-13). The skin lesion is treated like an abrasion, with the appropriate dressing. If significant skin loss occurs, the child may require a skin graft. The deep injury often appears later (4 to 8 hours) and occasionally results in a compartment syndrome with accompanying neurovascular compromise; thus all children with suspected or proven wringer injury must be admitted for a 24-hour close observation and elevation of the limb (Figure 30-14). Neurovascular checks of the affected extremity every few hours are mandatory to prevent possible catastrophy. Fasciotomy may be required if compartment compression develops.

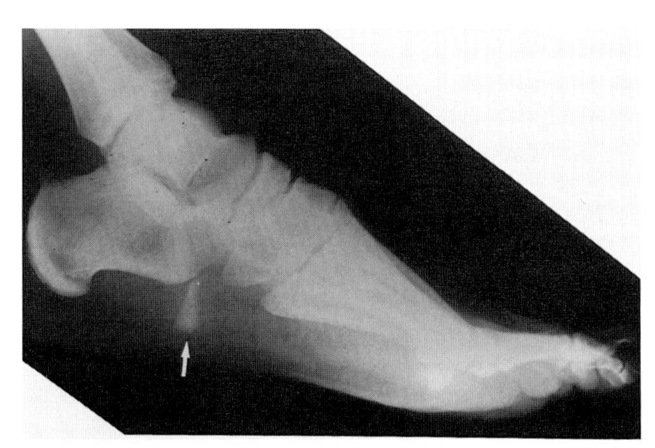

FIGURE 30-11

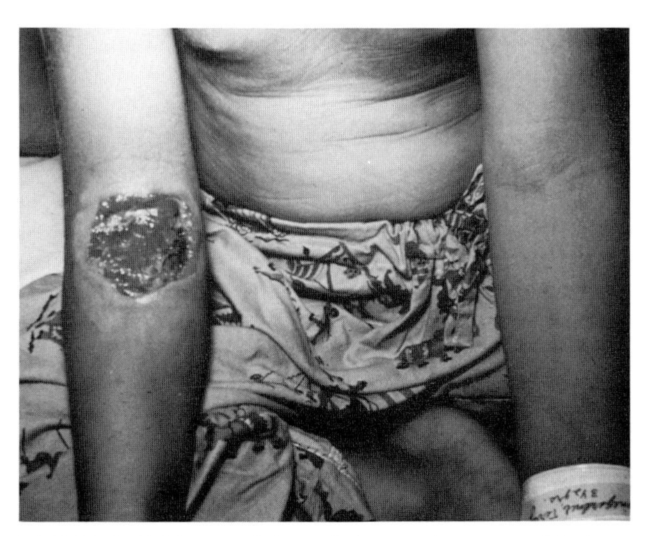

FIGURE 30-13 Avulsion of skin with severe skin loss.

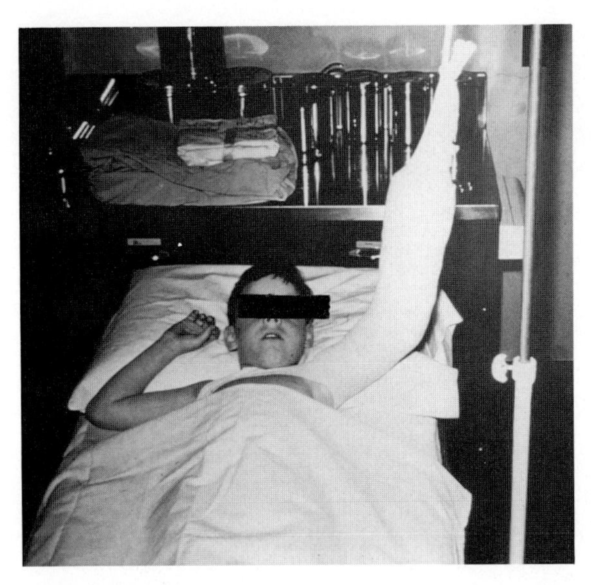

FIGURE 30-14 Elevation of limb with suspected or proven wringer injury.

Bicycle Spoke Injuries

This injury occurs as the bicycle rider's foot is caught between the frame and wheel spoke. If extensive skin loss is present, grafting may be required (Figures 30-15 and 30-16), but often simple local care is enough. Treatment consists of sterile dressings and extremity elevation. Depending on the extent of injury, hospital admission may be required. If the skin injury results in a flap, simple closure usually can be performed. Occasionally, the flap may require removal if vascularity is compromised, but it can then be reapplied as a skin graft after cleansing and defatting of the wound. This usually requires the technical expertise of a surgeon

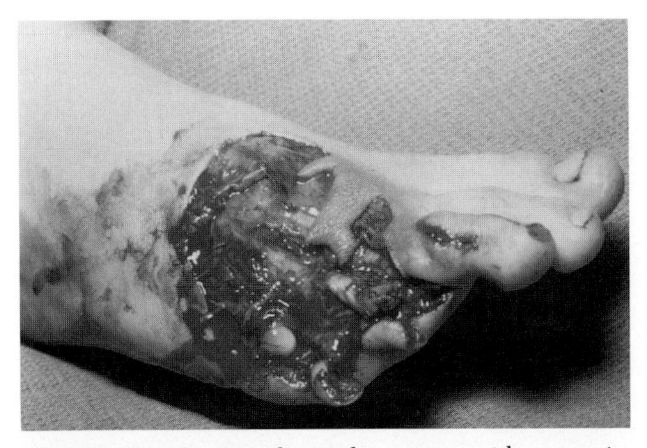

FIGURE 30-15 Bicycle spoke injury with extensive skin loss.

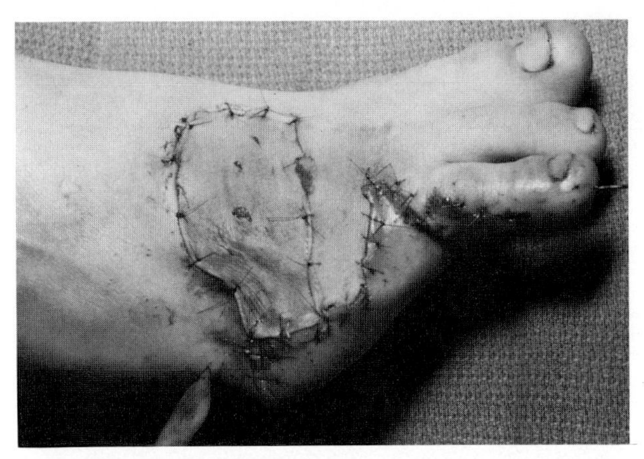

FIGURE 30-16 Bicycle spoke injury with extensive skin loss requiring skin grafts.

and generally should not be attempted in the emergency department.

Severe Scrape Abrasions

Dragging an extremity from a moving object, (swing, cart, bicycle) often results in severe abrasions. These may be treated with sterile dressings, but if tendon or fascia is exposed, grafting or pedicle flaps may be required.[2]

Degloving Injuries

Degloving injuries are usually more extensive than first impression would indicate. The laceration and degree of underlying soft tissue damage are often not immediately apparent, and joint spaces or deep structure such as nerves, tendons, and vessels may be involved. These injuries mandate x-ray films, and extensive exploration is the rule. They cannot be treated with local care, and all require expert surgical consultation to prevent loss of function in the involved area.[3]

References

1. Paletta FX: *Pediatric Plastic Surgery.* St. Louis, CV Mosby Co, 1967.
2. Schultz RC: *Facial Injuries.* Chicago, Year Book Medical Publishers, 1977.
3. Grabb WC, Smith JW (eds): *Plastic Surgery: A Concise Guide to Clinical Practice.* Boston, Little Brown & Co, 1973.
4. Irby WB: *Facial Trauma and Concomitant Problems.* St. Louis, CV Mosby Co, 1974.

William Carl Bailey

31 Burns

Burns represent a significant portion of injuries in children, ranking only behind automobile accidents, drownings, and falls as a cause of death. Approximately 2 to 3 million people in the United States are burned annually; of these 95% are treated on an ambulatory or outpatient basis. An estimated 100,000 to 300,000 of burn patients require hospitalization, 20,000 of them in burn centers. It is estimated that 5% to 10% of these burn victims die as a direct result of their burn injuries.

Approximately 30% of burn victims are children. The majority are under the age of 3 years, and the burn is usually caused by hot liquids. Such burns usually occur in the kitchen or bathroom and most are considered preventable. By reaching up on a stove or becoming entangled in an electrical cord, small children may pull down a container of hot liquid that drenches the head, upper body, and arms producing a classic injury. Another common injury occurs when children climb into a tub of hot water or are placed there carelessly or deliberately by an adult. Sometimes the victim or another child turns on the hot water tap and causes a scald. The importance of hot tap water as a source of scald injuries has been more keenly appreciated in recent years. Several years ago Moritz and Henriques showed that adult skin sustained a full-thickness injury in 1 second at a temperature of 159 °F, in 6 seconds at 140 °F, and in 15 seconds at 133 °F.[1] Feldman et al found that 80% of homes surveyed in Seattle had a tap water temperature greater than 130 °F.[2] Many scald injuries produce a superficial partial-thickness burn that heals well in about 2 weeks when properly treated. Because children's skin is thinner than that of adults, however, a surprising number of scald injuries in children are deep partial-thickness or full-thickness injuries that can result in serious morbidity, contractures, and long-term complications.

In children older than 3 years, flame burns are more common than scalds. These are caused by circumstances such as house or mobile home fires, space heaters, kitchen stoves, playing with matches, and trash fires. Furthermore, children frequently have access to gasoline. Flame burns often involve flammable clothing, are most often full thickness, and account for the majority of fatal burns. Interestingly, the number of child arsonists appears to be increasing dramatically.

Feller et al found that burn deaths are related to many factors including age, sex, and the extent of the burn.[3] The most favorable survival rate was found in the 5–34 year age group in which a 70% survival rate was achieved with a burn size of 55% body surface area burned (BSAB). The same survival rate was achieved only in burns of 42% BSAB in children age 0–4 years (see Figure 31-1). Thus younger children, who are less able to cope mentally and physically with the hazards of their environment, are not only more likely to be burned but

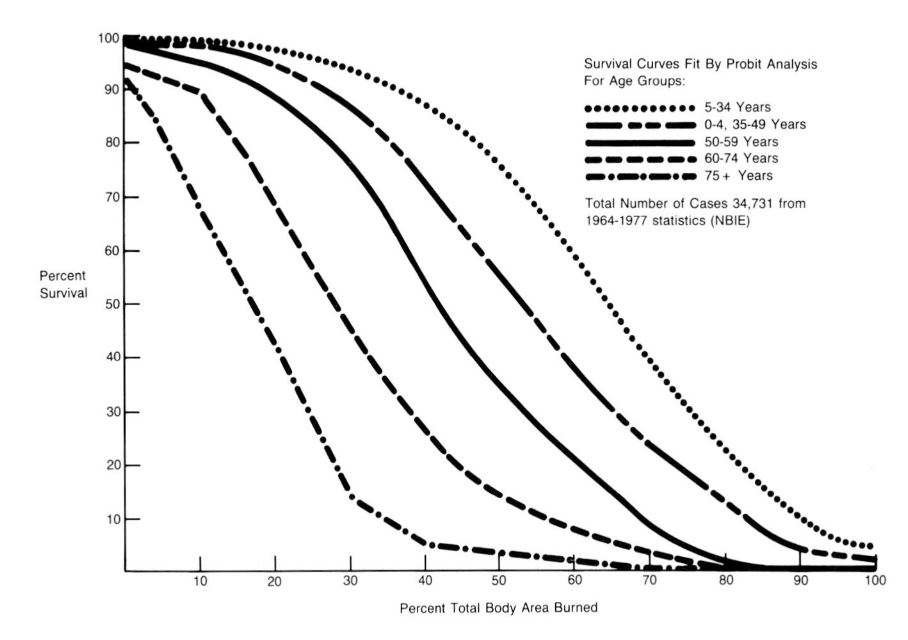

FIGURE 31-1 Survival curves for age groups. Reprinted with permission from Feller I, Crane K, Flanders S: Baseline data on the mortality of burn patients. Reprinted with permission from *Quality Review Bulletin,* July 1979, p 4. Copyright Joint Commission on Accreditation of Hospitals, July 1979.

also appear subject to higher mortality. Carvajal and Parks have suggested, however, that the difference in mortality between younger and older children may not be substantial when care is administered according to modern pediatric burn care standards.[4]

PATHOPHYSIOLOGY

A detailed discussion of the myriad derangements of physiology that follow burn injury is beyond the purview of this discussion; however, a few which have particular significance in the acute period are mentioned briefly.

Cell and Tissue Damage

Thermal energy applied to tissue initially destroys normal enzyme systems, damages cells, and may destroy them by coagulation necrosis, depending on the temperature and the duration applied. Marked elevation of tissue osmolality, with an initial rapid increase in extravascular volume and lymphatic flow, produces local edema. Destruction of blood vessels and red cells disrupts the microcirculation. Vasoconstrictive activity and aggregation of formed elements, such as platelets and red cells, augments the plugging of lymphatic vessels secondary to coagulation of extravasated protein, thereby increasing edema.

Certain active substances, which are currently the subject of much research, are released at the site of a burn with remote as well as local effects. One of the most well-known effects is increased capillary permeability, which permits fluid containing sodium and plasma protein to pour into the extravascular space. In burns greater than 25% BSAB, increased capillary permeability is noted in unburned tissue as well as at the burn site. This capillary leakage appears to follow a biphasic curve with an early peak 15 to 30 minutes after the injury and a second higher peak at about 3 hours after injury.[5] The effect appears to decline toward normal after this time and largely disappears 12 to 24 hours after the injury, although this is variable and traces of the effect may remain for several days.

Fluid Requirements

In addition to capillary leakage, large burns have been shown to produce increased fluid requirements because of the movement of sodium and water into the cells of unburned tissue, particularly skeletal muscle. Baxter has measured transmembrane potentials and performed simultaneous serial muscle biopsies showing that the depression of transmembrane potential was more persistent and the interstitial distribution of sodium significantly different in burns larger than 40% BSAB. This indicates a greater increase in cell permeability to sodium in large burns.[6]

The loss of varying amounts of fluid from the circulating blood volume into interstitial fluid and cells may culminate in classic burn shock. The magnitude of these changes is illustrated by the fact that an adequately resuscitated patient with a major burn may gain over 15% in total body weight as sequestered fluid. Following restoration of near normal capillary integrity, the patient usually enters a diuretic phase 24 to 48 hours after burn with a significant initial loss of tissue edema, a process that continues over the next several days.

Cardiac Output

Cardiac output after large burns may be depressed to as low as 30% of preburn values within 30 minutes of the injury, slowly returning to normal and then supranormal until the wound is closed. Initial work suggested the presence of a myocardial depressant factor, but more recent opinion suggests that depression of cardiac output is more likely a reflection of the combined effect of decreased plasma volume and increased peripheral resistance.[7] With adequate fluid resuscitation, cardiac output returns to normal values within 18 to 24 hours, at the same time that plasma volumes are still decreasing somewhat, and is associated with a reciprocal decline in peripheral vascular resistance. Cardiac output thus appears to be a more reliable indicator of adequate resuscitation than intravascular volume change. In the immediate postburn period, both peripheral and pulmonary vascular resistance rise. The rise in pulmonary vascular resistance persists longer and has been related to diminution of blood volume, embolization of platelet aggregates, or release of substances such as histamines and prostaglandins.

Renal Effects

Decreased cardiac output and increased peripheral resistance results in decreased glomerular filtration rate and renal plasma flow that may produce oliguria. Acute renal failure is rare in adequately resuscitated patients but may occur in those with high levels of circulating hemoglobin or myoglobin resulting from high-voltage electrical injury, crush injury, burned muscle, or in some immersion scald burns. Plasma renin levels are elevated in proportion to burn size, and elevation of angiotensin, adrenocorticotropin, cortisol, and aldosterone also occur.

Hematologic Effects

Following major burn injury, a number of hematologic effects appear. An increase in the hematocrit occurs routinely, concomitant with a rise in blood viscosity. In extensive burns, an initial loss of up to 10% or even 15% of red cell mass may be experienced as a direct result of the injury, and a daily loss by hemolysis of about 8% of the total red cell mass per day may be seen for a few days following injury.[8] This appears to be related to high levels of circulating free fatty acids.[9] Platelets and fibrinogen levels show a significant drop immediately after burn injury and rise later to elevated levels with concomitant increases in factors I and VIII. Elevated levels of fibrin split products are noted immediately after injury and may persist for 8 to 10 days. Platelets exhibit increased adhesiveness in the postburn period.

CLASSIFICATION OF BURNS

Burns may be classified by mode, depth, and extent of injury. All of these factors are important in establishing the prognosis and treatment.

Mode of Injury

There are four modes of energy transmission to tissue that result in damage:

1. thermal: scald, contact, flame, or flash
2. electrical
3. chemical
4. radiation

Depth of Injury

The depth of burn injury has been classified as first degree, second degree, and third degree. It is more descriptive and less confusing to designate partial-thickness or full-thickness injury. Burns described as first degree are superficial injuries characterized by erythema but with little other discernible evidence of thermal effect. A classic example is sunburn, which may be quite painful initially but heals rapidly with no residual scarring.

What has been described as a second-degree burn is partial-thickness injury. A mild to moderate partial-thickness burn exhibits blister formation and devitalization of the superficial levels of epidermis, which are readily stripped away revealing a red, wet, hypersensitive, and blanching surface that is edematous and slightly raised above the surrounding tissue. Unless exposed to excessive drying or infection, these burns heal spontaneously in 1 to 2 weeks, leaving little obvious effect. Deep partial-thickness burns are characterized by a waxy appearance of the underlying tissue when the devitalized epidermis is removed. The wound is soft, dry, and not initially edematous or raised. It is relatively insensitive to pinprick, but perception of deep pressure remains intact. Because some elements of the skin and its appendages remain, these burns can heal spontaneously in 3 to 4 weeks, but usually with a significant amount of hypertrophic scarring.

Full-thickness, or third-degree burns, are characterized by hard, leathery, inelastic eschar, which may be charred or yellow-brown and translucent, and exhibit thrombosed vessels in the deeper tissues. Certain full-thickness scalding injuries may be deceptive, however, because they appear red due to hemoglobin fixed in the tissues which may lead the unwary observer to misread the injury as a partial-thickness burn. Since in a full-thickness burn all elements of skin have been lost, these injuries cannot heal spontaneously and are especially vulnerable to infection. They form granulation tissue, which results in a thick, hypertrophied scar.[10]

The depth of burn injury is a function of temperature, time of exposure, and thickness of the skin which varies from area to area of the body. The skin of children is generally thinner than that of adults, and a given thermal insult may produce a deeper injury in the child than in an adult.

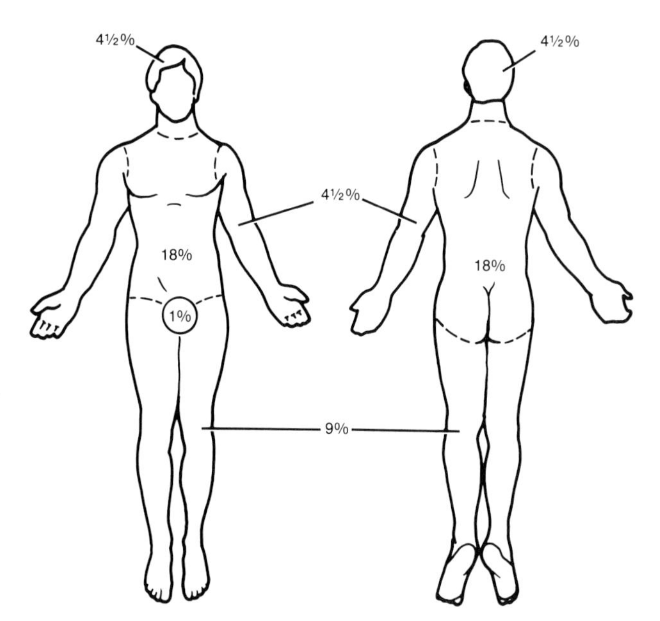

FIGURE 31-2 Rule of nines for adults. (Reprinted with permission from Parks DH, Carvahal HF, Larson DL: Management of burns. *Surg Clin North Am* 1977;57(5): 877. Copyright © 1977 WB Saunders Co.)

Extent of Injury

A third classification of burn injury considers the extent or body surface area burned (BSAB). Calculation of the burn surface area is somewhat inaccurate even by skilled observers, but it is essential in estimating the severity of injury and in determining fluid requirements. The simplest formula for estimating BSAB of adults and older children uses the "rule of nines," in which a value of 9% of the total body surface area (TBSA) is given to the head and neck, 18% to the anterior surface area of the trunk, 18% to the posterior surface, 9% to each upper extremity, 18% to each lower extremity, and the remaining 1% to the perineum (Figure 31–2). Because the head of a child is relatively larger and the lower extremities are correspondingly smaller in proportion to the remainder of the body, the rule of nines must be modified for children (Figure 31–3). For each year of age under 10, 1% is added to the value for the head and neck, and 0.5% is subtracted from each of the two lower extremities. Thus the head and neck of a 5 year old would be calculated as 9% plus 5% for a total of 14%. Each lower extremity would be calculated as 18% minus 2.5% for a value of 15.5% for each lower extremity. Above the age of 10 years, the adult formula can be used. It is also important to note that not only the body proportions of children are different from those of adults, but also the surface area is relatively larger compared to the body mass. This is of importance in metabolic functions, including thermal and water balance.

A chart such as that devised by Lund and Browder[11] is a more accurate method of calculating percent of BSAB and is quite simple to use (Exhibit 31–1). Charts of this type are readily obtained and should be kept on hand in any medical facility required to care for burns.

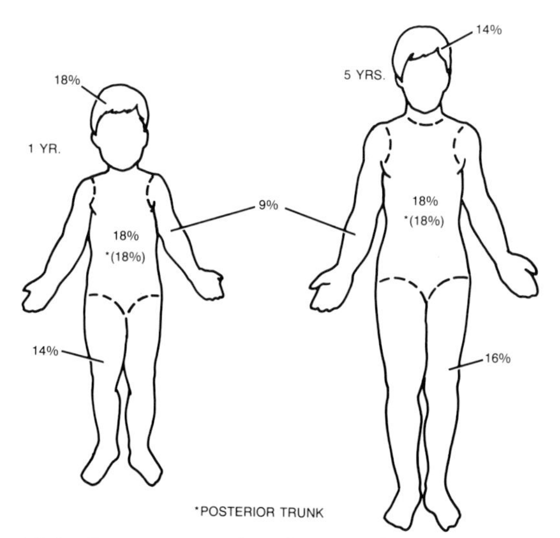

FIGURE 31-3 Rule of nines for children. (Reprinted with permission from Parks DH, Carvahal HF, Larson DL: Management of burns. *Surg Clin North Am* 1977; 57(5):878. Copyright © 1977 WB Saunders Co.)

NATIONAL BURN INFORMATION EXCHANGE
UNIVERSITY OF MICHIGAN BURN CENTER
ST. JOSEPH MERCY HOSPITAL BURN UNIT
I. Feller, M.D., Director

Name:
Hospital:
Date:
Form completed by: ____________

Estimation of Size of Burn by Percent

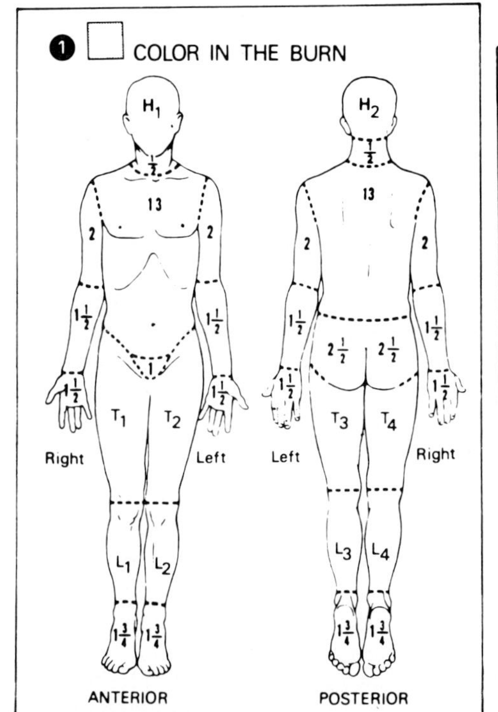

3 CALCULATE EXTENT BURN

	ANTERIOR	POSTERIOR
Head	H1 ____	H2 ____
Neck	____	____
Rt. Arm	____	____
Rt. Forearm	____	____
Rt. Hand	____	____
Lt. Arm	____	____
Lt. Forearm	____	____
Lt. Hand	____	____
Trunk	____	____
Buttock		____
Perineum	____	
Rt. Thigh	T1 ____	T4 ____
Rt. Leg	L1 ____	L4 ____
Rt Foot	____	____
Lt. Thigh	T2 ____	T3 ____
Lt. Leg	L2 ____	L3 ____
Lt. Foot	____	____
SUB TOTAL	____	____
% TOTAL AREA BURNED		____ %

2 CIRCLE AGE FACTOR

PERCENT OF AREAS AFFECTED BY GROWTH

	AGE 0	1	5	10	15	Adult
H(1 or 2) = ½ of the Head	9½	8½	6½	5½	4½	3½
T(1,2,3 or 4) = ½ of a Thigh	2¾	3¼	4	4¼	4½	4¾
L(1,2,3 or 4) = ½ of a Leg	2½	2½	2¾	3	3¼	3½

(see instructions on back)

Exhibit 31-1 Chart for Calculating the Extent of a Burn. (Reprinted with permission from Feller I, National Burn Information Exchange, Ann Arbor, MI.)

The extent or volume of damaged tissue correlates with the degree of pathophysiologic changes that occur. Thus, calculating the surface area of a burn injury (length × width) correlates well with the magnitude of injury because of the relatively shallow depth of the typical burn injury, which usually extends only through the dermis. However, the same relationship does not exist for electrical injury or in very deep burns and consequently the third dimension is indeterminate. Calculation of surface area is of little or no help in defining the extent of these injuries and thus in determining fluid resuscitation.

Utilizing the three methods of burn classification, the American Burn Association has identified 3 treatment categories for burned patients (Exhibit 31-2). In general, minor burns can be treated on an ambulatory or outpatient basis. Most moderate injuries, particularly in children, require hospitalization. All major burns require hospitalization, preferably in a specialized burn treatment facility.[12] Guidelines for hospitalization are given in Exhibit 31–3. Evidence of child abuse is an absolute indication for hospitalization.

First Aid

Emergency measures at the scene of a burning accident are summarized in Exhibit 31-4. The first step

Exhibit 31-2 ABA Treatment Categories

- Minor
  - Partial-thickness burns
    - <10% TBSA in children
    - <15% TBSA in adults
  - Full-thickness burns
    - <2% TBSA
  - Exclusions
    - Electrical injury
    - Inhalation injury
    - Burns of the hands, feet, or perineum
    - Poor-risk patients
- Moderate
  - Partial-thickness burns
    - 10%–20% TBSA in children
    - 15%–20% TBSA in adults
  - Full-thickness burns
    - 10% TBSA
  - Exclusions: Same as for minor burns
- Major
  - Partial-thickness burns
    - >20% TBSA in children
    - >25% TBSA in adults
  - Full-thickness burns
    - >10% TBSA
  - Exclusions: None

Source: American Burn Association: Total Care for Burn Patients, a guide to hospital resources, in *Bulletin American College of Surgeons*, Oct 1977, p. 8.

is to stop the burning. Burning clothing can be extinguished by applying water, wrapping the patient in heavy materials, such as a coat, blanket, or rug, or slowly rolling the victim on the ground. In scald injuries, clothing that is soaked in hot liquid should be removed immediately or dashed with cold water to stop the burning process. Hot, viscous fluids such as tar are better treated by rapid cooling with cold water than by attempting removal in the field.

Chemical burns in most cases should be treated by immediate copious and protracted (minimum 15 minutes) irrigation with tap water. Time should not be wasted searching for specific neutralizing agents. Some neutralizing materials applied to a strong acid or alkali may actually make the injury worse by producing an exothermic reaction.

Exhibit 31-3 Guidelines for Admission to the Hospital

- Adults with mixed second-degree and third-degree burns >15% TBSA
- Children with mixed second-degree and third-degree burns >10% TBSA
- Full-thickness burns
- Burns of the face
- Burns of the perineum
- Burns of the hands or feet
- Inhalation injuries
- Electrical injuries
- Complicated burns, e.g., associated injury or disease
- High-risk patients, e.g., infants or the elderly
- Nonaccidental trauma, i.e., child abuse

Exhibit 31-4 First Aid

1. Stop the burning.
   a. Extinguish flames.
   b. Remove hot clothing.
   c. Cool viscous hot liquids.
   d. Irrigate chemical burns.
2. Apply cold water to limited burns.
3. Dress the wounds with dry, sterile (or clean) dressings.
4. Check the airway; use oxygen if needed.
5. Treat shock.
6. Treat associated injuries.
7. Keep records.
8. Transport the victims.

The immediate application of cold to small burns, particularly partial-thickness burns, has been advocated for many years. Cold applications may dramatically reduce pain, particularly if applied within moments of the injury, and are alleged to decrease edema, lower the infection rate, shorten the recovery period, and lessen the need for grafting. There is evidence that very cold water applied within 30 minutes of the burn and continued up to 1 hour afterward may suppress conversion of arachidonic acid to detrimental metabolites which affect microcirculation.[13] Ice should never be applied directly to the burn, and the cooling technique should be reserved for small burns. In particular, children with large burns are susceptible to hypothermia, and body temperature may drop precipitously while the patient is being transported to a medical facility. Hypothermia may cause fibrillation and death from cardiac arrest.

Care of the burn wound in the field should be simple. Grease or ointments should not be applied, because they will have to be removed on arrival at the care facility. Instead, a clean sheet or dry dressings should be used to cover the wounds during transport.

The airway should be checked immediately for obstruction, and appropriate measures should be taken to clear it. Any patient with a history of unconsciousness, suspected smoke inhalation, or carbon monoxide should receive 100% oxygen at once. if the patient is unconscious, ventilation should be provided with a snug-fitting face mask or endotracheal tube, utilizing an Ambu bag or respirator.

If shock is present or imminent or if a significantly long transport time is anticipated, a large-bore intravenous access route should be established preferably through unburned skin, and appropriate intravenous fluid resuscitation should be initiated en route. Concomitant injuries, lacerations, fractures, and the like should be identified and appropriate first-aid measures should be applied.

The patient should be closely monitored and simple, accurate records should be kept. It must be emphasized that treatment in the field should be limited to the essentials, and the patient should be transported as quickly as possible to a medical facility that has the capabilities appropriate for the degree and complexity of the injury.

INITIAL TREATMENT

Upon arrival in the emergency department, most burn-injured patients can be assessed quickly by an experienced observer. Virtually all minor injuries, and even some moderate ones, may be treated on an ambulatory basis or by brief hospitalization for stabilization followed by outpatient care. Most moderate and all major burns, however, require the same care as is given to other forms of major trauma. Exhibit 31-5 presents an outline for the initial management of these burns. The patient must be stabilized in preparation for hospitalization or transport to a burn center. If transport seems likely, the burn center should be contacted to coordinate resuscitation and smooth transfer. The treatment of a seriously burned patient requires that many things be done, often simultaneously, and priorities may be difficult to establish. Clearly, maintenance of ventilation and treatment of shock are the most urgent early considerations.

Exhibit 31-5 Initial Management of Moderate to Large Burns

1. Cessation of Burning
   a. Extinguish smoldering clothing.
   b. Remove or immediately cool adherent hot substances.
   c. Irrigate chemical burns with large volumes of water.
   d. Apply cold water (4° C) to small burns (if seen within 30–60 min).
2. Ensuring an Airway
   a. Clear obstructions from the airway.
   b. Supply oxygen therapy immediately to any patient who is unconscious or who has been hypoxic or exposed to carbon monoxide or smoke.
   c. Be prepared to intubate a patient who has smoke inhalation injury.
3. Management of Shock
   a. Install a large-bore (16- to 18-gauge) IV line, preferably through unburned skin.
   b. Administer lactated Ringer's or normal saline solution according to formula and clinical state.
4. Physical Examination
   a. Remove all clothing; avoid hypothermia.
   b. Assess the location, extent, and depth of the burn.
   c. Perform laryngotracheobronchoscopy if required.
   d. Evaluate the patient for hemorrhage and concomitant injuries, e.g., fractures, head injury, internal injuries.
   e. Determine the patient's height, weight, and surface area.
   f. Assess the patient's physical status as for any serious illness.
5. History
   a. Determine the time the burn occurred.
   b. Determine the circumstance of the burning.
   c. Determine the mode of burning: thermal, electrical, chemical, radiation.
   d. Determine if there is a past history of disease or disability.
   e. Obtain a record of immunizations.
   f. Determine if the patient has been exposed to any infectious agent, e.g., *Streptococcus*, chickenpox.
6. Accurate Record Keeping
   a. Keep accurate records from the moment of arrival.
   b. Pay special attention to vital signs, intake and output, drugs, and fluid administration.
7. Laboratory Studies
   a. Obtain blood samples for the following:
      (1) Complete blood count
      (2) Blood urea nitrogen, creatinine, and serum electrolytes
      (3) Blood gases
      (4) Carboxyhemoglobin
      (5) Typing and cross-matching
   b. Obtain urine for a urinalysis, especially for the following:
      (1) Specific gravity
      (2) Glucose
      (3) Protein
      (4) Myoglobin and hemoglobin
   c. Obtain samples from the nose and throat for culture.
8. Foley or Indwelling Straight Catheterization
9. Nasogastric Intubation
10. Tetanus Prophylaxis
11. Antibiotics (optional)
12. Analgesia
    a. Give as indicated in the text.
    b. Use the IV route only.
13. Wound Care
    a. Avoid hypothermia.
    b. For immediate transport, wrap the patient in sterile or clean sheets or dressings.
    c. For delayed transport or definitive therapy:
       (1) Wash wounds carefully with bland soap or povidone-iodine detergent and water.
       (2) Remove loose skin, gross debris, grease, and dirt.
       (3) Apply a topical antibacterial agent such as silver sulfadiazine, mafenide, or 0.5% aqueous silver nitrate.
       (4) Perform escharotomy, if required, for circumferential burns of the trunk or extremities.
       (5) Consider fasciotomy in electrical and crush injuries.

Ventilation and Control of Shock

The airway must be quickly assessed for evidence of obstruction, and any debris or obstruction should be removed. If upper airway compromise secondary to smoke inhalation is suspected, preparations must be made to intubate the patient quickly before the obstruction becomes complete. Warm, humidified oxygen should be administered in suspected cases of carbon monoxide poisoning or smoke inhalation. If the patient is unconscious or ventilating poorly, ventilatory assistance may be required. With large burns, shock may develop quickly, and intravenous fluid therapy must be started immediately, as described at Fluid Replacement.

Physical Examination

After life-threatening conditions are controlled, all of the patient's clothing and jewelry, should be removed, and the patient should be carefully examined. Other injuries, such as lacerations, fractures, intra-abdominal or intrathoracic injuries, and hemorrhage, must be identified. The patient's height and weight should be recorded, and total body surface area (TBSA) in square meters should be calculated by a standard nomogram (Figures 31-4 and 31-5). The depth, anatomic location, and extent of

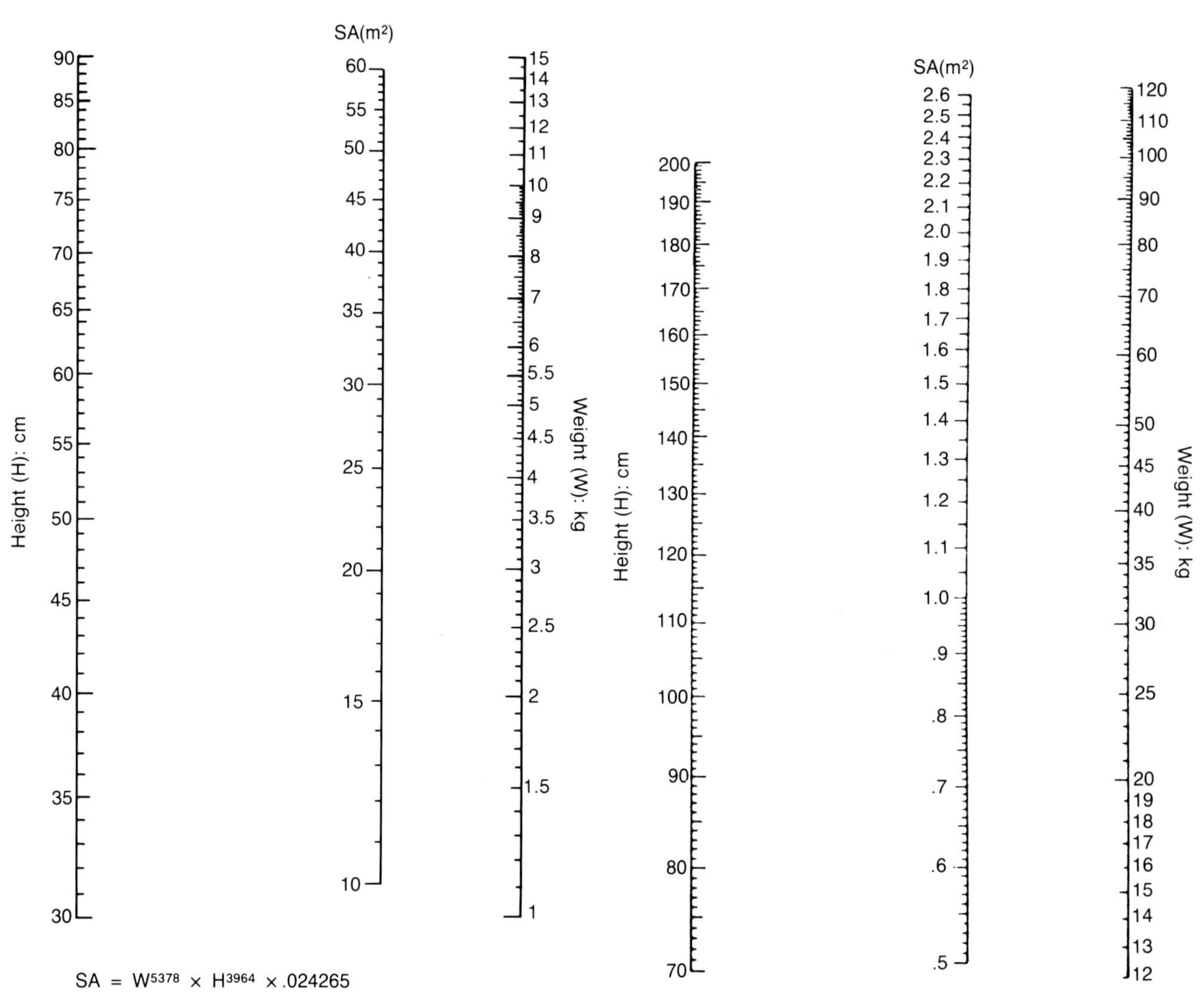

FIGURE 31-4 Nomogram for calculating the surface area (SA) of infants and young children. (Reprinted with permission from Haycock GB, Schwartz GJ, Wisotsky DH: Geometric method for measuring body surface area: A height, weight formula validated in infants, children and adults. *J Pediatr* 1978;93(1):65. Copyright © 1978 CV Mosby Co.)

SA = W^{5378} x H^{3964} x .024265

FIGURE 31-5 Nomogram for calculating the surface area (SA) of children and adults. (Reprinted with permission from Haycock GB, Schwartz GJ, Wisotsky DH: Geometric method for measuring body surface area: A height, weight formula validated in infants, children, and adults. *J Pediatr* 1978;93(1):64. Copyright © 1978 CV Mosby Co.)

the burn can be estimated using a standard Lund and Browder or similar diagram (see Exhibit 31-1).

History

A good history should be obtained, including the time of injury, mode of burning, and the circumstances. These data are of great importance in assessment, treatment, and for legal purposes. Routine past medical history should include the status of immunizations, recent exposure to infectious disease (e.g., *Streptococcus*, chickenpox), bleeding disorders, allergy or sensitivity to medications, and any medications that the patient may be currently receiving.

Record Keeping

It is essential to establish precisely what drugs, topical applications, intravenous fluids, or other therapy have been administered prior to the patient's arrival at the receiving unit and if the patient has voided. The importance of continued close charting is self-evident.

Laboratory Studies

Routine laboratory data should be obtained as for any serious injury: complete blood count, blood glucose, blood urea nitrogen, creatinine, serum electrolytes, arterial blood gases, and pH. A carboxyhemoglobin level is indicated when smoke inhalation is suspected. If acute blood loss has occurred, typing and crossmatching for transfusion may be indicated. Urine should be studied for specific gravity, glucose, protein, sediment, and free hemoglobin. Bacterial cultures of the throat and any infected skin lesions should be obtained routinely.

Urinary Catheterization

An indwelling urinary catheter should be installed in children whose burns exceed 15% to 20% BSAB to monitor quality and quantity of urine on an hourly basis. A Foley catheter is most often used, but care must be taken not to damage a very small urethra by forcibly inserting the catheter. In these cases a small plastic feeding tube may be more safely inserted and taped in place.

Nasogastric Intubation

A nasogastric tube should be inserted in children with significant burns because gastric dilatation and ileus commonly occur. Acute gastric dilatation may impair resuscitation and, on occasion, can be life-threatening. This problem is compounded significantly in air-transported burn victims, as intestinal gases expand with increasing altitude and lowered atmospheric pressure. Furthermore, children even more than adults are liable to develop an acute peptic ulcer (Curlings's ulcer) as a complication of burns. Gastroduodenal erosions may develop within 5 hours after an acute burn and then progress to frank ulceration within 72 hours. The use of a nasogastric tube may help ameliorate this tendency, but it should be continuously and effectively aspirated. Later the tube may be used for the hourly instillation of antacids and milk. The largest tube that comfortably fits the nasal passage should be selected.

Tetanus Prophylaxis

Tetanus prophylaxis should be provided for all burn victims regardless of the size of the burn. A tetanus toxoid booster dose should be administered as active immunization for any patient who has not had one for 5 years or when an accurate history of immunization is not available. Any patient who has not been immunized or has not received the complete course of immunizations should receive human tetanus immunoglobulin (Hypertet) in one extremity and the first of a series of active immunization injections with tetanus toxoid in another. The series should be completed as per schedule.

Antibiotics

The use of prophylactic antibiotics in burn therapy has been largely discontinued because of concern about the development of resistant organisms. Within the first 5 days after a burn, the most common infecting organisms are Gram-positive cocci, of which the group A β-hemolytic streptococci are the most serious. Infection can rapidly convert a partial-thickness burn into a full-thickness burn within a short period. However, infection with these organisms can usually be detected when the patient is under close surveillance by the presence of erythema surrounding the burn and other stigmata. The prophylactic use of penicillin for brief periods while awaiting the results of a throat culture may be indicated in patients at high risk, who live in an area where the streptococcus is endemic or have an obvious pharyngitis or preexisting infected skin lesions.

Analgesia

Analgesia should be provided as appropriate for the patient's degree of pain and level of consciousness. The pain of superficial burns may be intense, while that of a deep partial-thickness or full-thickness burn may be minimal. The average pediatric burn patient can tolerate intramuscular doses of meperidine up to 1.5 mg/kg body weight and of morphine sulfate up to 0.2 mg/kg body weight. As a general principle, however, narcotics should never be administered to a patient with an acute major burn except by the intravenous route. Intramuscular administration in the vasoconstricted and hypoperfused patient is poorly absorbed. Also, they may cause an overdose when blood volume has been restored and normal perfusion returns. For intravenous use, approximately one fourth to one half of the intramuscular dose may be administered cautiously and repeated at intervals of 15 to 30 minutes, titrating the dose until the desired effect is achieved. The respiratory center of very young infants is sensitive to narcotics, and appropriate caution should be exercised. A mild tranquilizer, such as diazepam (5 mg/m^2/dose), may also be useful.

Children with minor to moderate burn injury who are not experiencing perfusion difficulties may be premedicated for debridement and wound dressing with a single intramuscular injection of meperidine (1 mg/kg body weight), promethazine (0.5 mg/kg body weight), and chlorpromazine (0.5–1.0 mg/kg body weight) as advocated by Shuck.[14]

FLUID REPLACEMENT

Loss of fluid and changes in fluid distribution occur in all injuries as a pattern of tissue response. The translocation of fluid from the intravascular space to the interstitial and intracellular spaces in burns occurs rapidly and may lead to shock in a relatively short time.

In major burns it is essential to establish intravenous access as quickly as possible. A single large-bore cannula (16 to 18 gauge) may be inserted into the veins of even small children, particularly if done prior to the development of hypovolemia and attendant venous constriction. Insertion through unburned skin is desirable, but vessels under freshly burned and uninfected skin may be used temporarily. Although not ideal, cutdowns on the greater saphenous vein anterior to the medial malleolus provide quick access to a large vessel. Central venous pressure recordings are sometimes helpful, and rarely a Swan-Ganz catheter may be required. However, central line sites are best preserved for use later in the course of treatment.

The fluid loss from the intravascular space closely resembles plasma, and the amount lost appears to be related to the size of the burn. Sodium loss has been calculated at 0.52 mEq/%BSAB/kg body weight/24 h; plasma loss, at 0.3 to 0.5 mL/%BSAB/kg body weight/24 h.[15] Because both sodium and plasma proteins are lost, it may seem desirable that both be replaced. However, because of the loss of capillary integrity, which permits protein molecules as large as 150,000 to 350,000 molecular weight to escape, many investigators have questioned the value of colloid infusion when administered earlier than 24 hours after burn. They argue that in the "leak" phase, colloid does nothing that cannot be accomplished by crystalloid alone.

Crystalloids

The most well-known method of "crystalloid only" use is that of Baxter (Parkland formula).[16] During the first three 8-hour periods, an isotonic crystalloid solution is the only fluid given. It is administered parenterally and nothing is given by mouth. Lactated Ringer's solution is used because it is readily available and is a balanced salt solution, with a ratio of lactate (as bicarbonate) to chloride of 27:103 mEq/L. Since the sodium concentration is 130 mEq/L, it furnishes between 60 to 80 mL of free water per liter and, therefore, free water is not given during the first 24 hours. This formula is intended to meet maintenance as well as burn requirements.

Calculation of the burn surface includes only second-degree and third-degree areas and is not limited to maximum 50% BSAB as in some other formulas. Half of the calculated amount is administered in the first 8 hours after injury, and the remaining half is given over the next two 8-hour periods. During the fourth 8-hour period, plasma equivalent is given in the amount of 0.5 mL/%BSAB/kg body weight. Enough free water should be given to maintain adequate urinary output. Baxter points out that the reestablishment of the capillary membrane may occur somewhat earlier than 24 hours in some patients, permitting earlier effective plasma restoration. Perhaps even more important, in some extensive burns the capillary seal may not occur until after 24 to 32 hours, making administration of additional plasma necessary. Sufficient amounts of 5% or 10% glucose in water or oral fluids are then administered to provide for adequate urine production and to compensate for increased evaporative water loss, which may be 4 to 13 times greater through burned than unburned skin.[17]

A similar formula has been advocated by the U.S. Army Institute of Surgical Research, based on studies of their case material.[18] These researchers found that fluid requirements are somewhat less than those given in the Parkland formula. They achieved satisfactory fluid replacement in adults with 2 mL and in children with 3.0 to 3.75 mL/%BSAB/kg body weight in the first 24 hours.

Colloids

While acknowledging the importance of sodium and the utility of these formulas, a number of investigators feel that, particularly in children, resuscitation is more effective when colloid is combined with crystalloid.[19–21] They contend that with the combination of crystalloid and colloid, resuscitation is accomplished more quickly, cardiac output is better, and there is less pulmonary vascular resistance, less lung water, and better arterial oxygenation. Carvajal believes that colloid leakage is a short-lived phenomenon, lasting only 12 hours after injury, and is of importance for only 3 to 6 hours postinjury. He and his coworkers advocate a composite solution for resuscitation, consisting of lactated Ringer's solution in 5% Dextrose containing 12.5 g of albumin per liter. This is administered on the basis of surface area rather than body weight, at the rate of 5,000 mL/m^2 BSAB/24 h to meet "burn requirements" and 2,000 mL/m^2 TBSA/24 h for maintenance. The solution is given at a constant rate, half in the first 8 hours and the remainder in the next 16 hours.

Because albumin and globulin are lost in equal measure from the blood, some practitioners prefer to use plasma rather than albumin for fluid replacement. They argue that fresh or fresh-frozen plasma provides coagulation factors and opsonic proteins that may be of value.[19,22] Stored plasma or plasma protein fraction (Plasmanate) does not contain these factors but minimizes the risk of hepatitis. Others, however, claim that, after processing, albumin represents almost a foreign protein and is rapidly metabolized by the liver, thus having only a transient effect on plasma volume.[19]

Hypertonic Solutions

A discussion of replacement fluids must include hypertonic solutions. These solutions contain 250 mEq/L of sodium, 100 mEq/L of chloride per liter of solution. Monafo and Robinson,[23] Caldwell and Bowser,[24] and others have used this solution safely in children as well as adults by closely monitoring serum electrolytes and osmolality.[23,24] They claim that the required salt load can be administered with one third of the usual water load resulting in less edema. As a result burns are softer and more pliable, and there is less need for tracheostomy and escharotomy, less ileus, and better production of urine under the condition of maximal antidiuresis that exists in the burn patient. However, critics suggest that administration may be difficult, particularly for the inexperienced, and there have been reports of sudden death, renal failure, severe hypokalemia, and extreme hypernatremia (greater than 160 mEq/dL).[25]

The major objection to the use of hypertonic solutions is that water must be extracted from the intracellular space to maintain near normal physiologic ranges of sodium concentration. This results in intracellular dehydration, which can be tolerated up to a level of 15% before structural damage occurs. Burns increase cell permeability to sodium ion, however, which in turn promotes the movement of potassium out of cells. Therefore, raising the sodium in interstitial fluid markedly favors the gain of intracellular sodium and the loss of intracellular potassium.[25]

Signs of Adequate Replacement

One of the most commonly accepted signs of satisfactory fluid replacement is adequate urinary output. This is generally considered to be 50 to 70 mL/hr in adults, 25 to 35 mL/hr in adults over the age of 60 years, and 1 to 1.5 mL/kg body weight/hr (45 mL/m^2 TBSA/h) in children. Urine should be evaluated for specific gravity, sodium, osmolality, and sediment. Hyperglycemia is common following a major burn injury, and the rapid infusion of large volumes of 5% to 10% glucose may produce an osmotic diuresis. In this situation, solutions containing dextrose should be withheld while glucosuria persists. Insulin may be required. If hemoglobin or myoglobin is detected in the urine, indicating the threat of acute renal failure, fluid administration should be increased and osmotic diuretics and bicarbonate are indicated.

An adequately resuscitated patient is responsive, lucid, alert, and has a clear sensorium. Return of a normal core body temperature indicates good resuscitation, but subnormal temperatures are common because of diminished heat production associated with the burn injury, cool environment, and the administration of cool fluids. Blood pressure should be normal or high as a result of peripheral vasoconstriction. The pulse rate is usually high, but rates above 140 beats per minute suggest volume depletion. In children, changes in pulse rate may be a more sensitive indication of volume status than blood pressure.

Serum electrolytes, blood urea nitrogen, creatinine, protein, glucose, and osmolality should be monitored routinely. Return of blood pH, carbon dioxide pressure, and bicarbonate to normal reflects complete correction of metabolic acidosis. The hemoglobin level and hematocrit are of limited value until about 24 hours after a burn because of the hemoconcentration that is common in the early hours. Serum albumin should not be allowed to fall below 2 g/dL. The most valuable laboratory aids for determining physiologic resuscitation are cardiac output and oxygen consumption. Cardiac output returns to normal between 6 and 12 hours after burn and increases proportionately to twice normal by 32 to 36 hours. Oxygen consumption remains low until shock is completely alleviated and increases to normal or supranormal levels during or before the first 32 hours.

Choice of Formulas

The controversies that surround burn resuscitation formulas make the choice of formulas difficult and confusing, particularly for the physician who treats burns infrequently. The best advice is to choose a single method and then to follow it in detail. At the same time, formulas must be regarded as guidelines only and must never be pursued blindly. Individual differences of response, coexisting injury or disease, age of the patient, and other factors require the exercise of good clinical judgment and appropriate modification of therapy.

The fact that "adequate" replacement of fluids can be achieved by several methods that appear to differ significantly is an eloquent testimonial to the innate physiologic resiliency of the average healthy young burn patient. Burn formulas have in common the use of water, sodium, and plasma protein, and are based on a calculation of the percentage of body surface burned multiplied either by the mass or surface area of the body. The "sheet anchor" of burn fluid management is clearly the sodium ion. Formulas differ not so much in the amount of sodium supplied but in its concentration, or more accurately the amount of water supplied either in the solution or by mouth. Virtually all formulas utilize plasma protein at some point in the resuscitation of major burns. The main difference appears to be whether colloid is indeed indicated in a given patient and the perception of the point after a burn that capillary leakage has sealed sufficiently to permit colloid to be retained to a useful degree. Nevertheless, it is often useful to introduce colloid 6 to 12 hours postinjury, rather than after 24 hours as recommended in some formulas.

It has been noted that young children require relatively larger amounts of fluid for adequate resuscitation.[18,24] The young child's total body water and intravascular and extracellular fluid compartments are relatively larger than those of an adult. Since a number of metabolic functions, including water metabolism, appear to correlate more closely with surface area than body weight, a formula based on surface area has an advantage, especially in smaller children. In small children, 4 mg/kg/%BSAB/24 hr may fail to provide adequate fluids, which leads to a preference for the Galveston formula.

When the patient fails to respond to resuscitative efforts, other causes such as acute gastric dilatation, hypoxia secondary to airway obstruction, or ventilatory insufficiency should be investigated. Common causes of error in the use of formulas include failure to correct the entire early deficit, miscalculation of the burn size, and failure to recognize those injuries that are known to require additional fluids (eg, electrical burns, smoke inhalation, associated trauma, and burns greater than 60% of BSAB).[25]

WOUND CARE

The goal of therapy in all surgical wounds is the prevention of infection, preservation of tissue, maintenance of function, and timely closure.[26] MacMillan[27] pointed out that the burn wound differs from other surgical wounds in several important respects:

- The cutaneous barrier to infection is lost.
- There are large amounts of devitalized tissue, which provide a rich medium for the growth of the pathogens with which it is often colonized.
- Large quantities of water, serum, and blood are exuded.
- The wound may remain open for long periods of time.
- Tissue frequently must be mobilized for permanent wound closure.

The care of a burn wound requires isolation of the wound from sources of contamination, rapid removal of nonviable tissue, removal of purulent and enzymatic secretions, prevention of wound desiccation, maintenance of an environment conducive to wound healing, keeping the wound at rest, and preventing further damage.

In minor injuries local wound care is undertaken immediately but in moderate or major burns, such care is deferred until resuscitation is well underway and the patient is relatively stable and comfortable. During this time in which the patient is exposed, great care must be taken to avoid hypothermia by the appropriate use of warm solutions, heated blankets, and overhead heating lamps. If possible, the room temperature should be approximately 88 °F.

Cleansing and Debridement

Wounds may be washed initially with mild soap or povidone-iodine detergent and water. Washing should be done as gently as possible to avoid further injury to tissues yet still remove all gross dirt, grease, and debris. In patients who are sufficiently stable, the Hubbard or a similar tank may be useful, either immersing the patient in a 1:60 or 1:120 Chlorox solution or suspending the patient on a slanted plinth over the tank and gently irrigating the wounds with warm water. Hair should be shaved for a distance of 3 to 4 cm immediately around the burns. Remaining hair may be cut to a shorter length, and a shampoo and body bath with povidone-iodine detergent should be administered to minimize endogenous sources of wound contamination. Blisters should be completely debrided and dressed carefully to prevent desiccation of underlying viable tissue.

Escharotomy and Fasciotomy

Circumferential burns of the extremities require careful monitoring to guard against impaired distal circulation. The extravasated plasma in the subcutaneous tissue under a tight, unyielding eschar may cause tissue pressure to exceed that of capillaries and to approach arterial pressures. This results in marked impairment of blood flow to the affected extremity with ischemia and ultimate necrosis of deep tissues. These effects may be relieved by escharotomy, (ie, incising the eschar to permit the underlying tissues to expand). This can be done at the bedside with minimal pain and blood loss, since the full-thickness burn is insensate and essentially bloodless. Elevation of upper extremities to 90 degrees and lower extremities to 45 degrees, with active exercise carried out for 5 minutes of each hour, may help to eliminate the need for escharotomy.

Swelling and coolness to touch in the distal, unburned skin of an involved extremity is not unusual; however, cyanosis of unburned skin, delayed capillary refilling, progressive neurologic disturbance, especially paresthesias, and deep tissue pain suggest impaired circulation. Neurologic changes are the most reliable clinical indicators, but clinical signs are relatively inaccurate.[28] Plethysmography and the Doppler flow meter are more accurate monitors of the need to incise the eschar. Blood flow in the distal palmar arch of the hand or the posterior tibial artery of the leg should be monitored hourly for the first 48 hours after the burn.

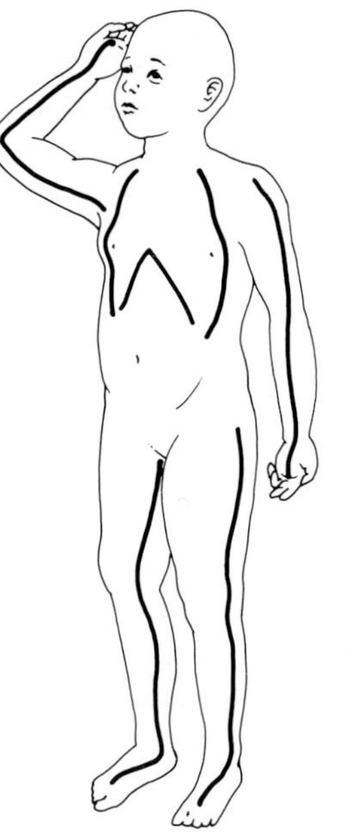

FIGURE 31-6 Recommended locations of incisions for escharotomy and fasciotomy. (Reprinted with permission from Artz CP, Moncrief JA, Pruitt PA Jr (eds): *Burns: A Team Approach.* Philadelphia, WB Saunders Co, 1979. Copyright © 1979 WB Saunders Co.)

The escharotomy incision should be placed in the long axis in the midlateral or mid-medial aspects of the involved limb or digits and should cross the joints (Figure 31-6). Care should be taken at the elbow to pass anteriorly to the medial epicondyle to avoid injury to the nerve. A circumferential burn of the thorax may produce an escharotic cuirass, severely restricting respiratory excursion exchange. The respiratory status of such a patient may be dramatically improved by escharotomies incising through the eschar and the anterior axillary lines bilaterally, extending to the abdomen if necessary. Transverse escharotomies should be made inferior and parallel to the subcostal margin, particularly if the burn extends under the abdomen. Other incisions, such as on the dorsum of the hand, sides of the fingers, long access of the penis, or the neck may be made as required.

Fasciotomy is necessary both to prevent pressure necrosis and to permit debridement of devitalized tissue. After escharotomy or fasciotomy the open wounds must be protected from contamination by the application of a topical chemotherapeutic agent and a biological or synthetic dressing.

Dressings

Burn wounds may be treated by closed technique or by the open method. The closed technique traditionally employs a nonadherent petrolatum gauze dressing with overlying layers of absorbent materials. Sometimes an antibacterial agent is also used. These dressings are particularly useful for burns of extremities and for children to prevent picking or scratching at the burn. Such dressings may be changed in 1 to 5 days but experience has shown that careful monitoring for infection may require changes daily or twice a day. In the hospital setting, dressings are soaked in 0.5% silver nitrate or 5% mafenide acetate.

In recent years, synthetic materials such as Biobrane® have appeared which are in effect occlusive or semiocclusive dressings. Biobrane is a bilaminate product consisting of a thin perforated layer of silicone rubber and a nylon fabric that has been impregnated with collagen. Biobrane adheres to the wound when applied to cleanly debrided, viable tissue, providing protection and an environment conducive to regeneration of underlying tissue. Similar qualities are claimed for Opsite®, Epilock®, and other materials. Such products reduce the frequency of dressing changes, although wounds must still be monitored for the development of infection. The materials have a long shelf life and do not transmit disease.

Biological dressings, such as commercially prepared pigskin, have been used for the past several years. They are beneficial when properly used and may be helpful in the debridement of wounds. Wounds must be monitored closely and the dressings changed as necessary until a tendency to "take" is noted which often indicates that the burn bed is ready to receive an autologous graft. However, biological dressings have the disadvantage of a relatively short shelf life.

The open method of burn wound management usually involves the direct application or "buttering" of topical antibacterial creams or ointments on the wounds. These applications are usually reinforced with a thin layer of fine mesh gauze.

Topical Antibacterial Agents

The advent of topical antibiotics, beginning with silver nitrate, has been one of the great breakthroughs in burn therapy. Burn mortality rates have been markedly improved due to the control of wound infection and sepsis. While invasive sepsis is seldom a problem in burns less than 30% BSAB, infection may convert a partial-thickness injury to a full-thickness injury with significant morbidity. Three agents are commonly used, and the choice often depends on whether the patient is to be treated on an inpatient or ambulatory basis.

Silver nitrate soaks have proved effective and are used in the hospital setting. Silver nitrate 0.5% has a broad spectrum of antibacterial activities and is nontoxic and nonpainful on application, is associated with no hypersensitive reaction, and reduces the evaporative loss of the wound. However, the dressings must be kept moist by the application of fresh solution to prevent the silver nitrate from reaching toxic levels, and the bulk of exclusive dressings impairs joint mobility. Silver nitrate is precipitated immediately by contact with proteinaceous material and thus has little ability to penetrate eschar. In addition, because silver nitrate soaks leach quantities of sodium, potassium, calcium, and chloride from the burn wound, careful management of the patient's electrolyte status is required. Fluid balance also must be closely monitored because absorption of the aqueous medium can produce water overloading. A further although minor disadvantage is the discoloration of the unburned skin, bed linens, and anything that the substance touches. Rare cases of methemoglobinemia have been reported in wounds colonized by nitrate-reducing bacteria, which results in the absorption of nitrites.

Silver sulfadiazine is the most popular agent and lends well to outpatient management. It is used as a 1% suspension in a water-soluble base, but because it is only slightly soluble in water it has a limited penetration of eschar. The antibacterial properties of the drug derive both from its sulfa and silver components. It has the advantages of being painless on application and not causing electrolyte and acid-based disturbances. It is applied easily by buttering it on the wounds; a layer of impregnated gauze may be placed over the basic application. It is removed once or twice daily at bathing or debridement and is reapplied as it rubs or washes off. Because it is not used with dressings, mobility of involved joints may be maintained. The disadvantages of silver sulfadiazine are rare hypersensitivity, neutropenia, and ineffectiveness against *Enterobacter cloacae*. Both silver sulfadiazine and silver nitrate solutions are best used on fresh burns to prevent colonization of the burn wound surface.

Sulfamylon cream is a 11.1% suspension of mafenide acetate in a water base. While it has little effectiveness against staphylococci it has a broad range of effectiveness against Gram-negative organisms and provides better control of *Candida* species than does silver sulfadiazine. Its main advantage is its superior ability to penetrate eschar and establish an effective antibacterial concentration at the viable-nonviable skin interface. The disadvantages are pain and discomfort lasting 20 to 30 minutes when it is applied to partial-thickness burns and carbonic anhydrase inhibition. This reduces bicarbonate absorption in renal tubules lowering bicarbonate. The drug should be avoided in the presence of pulmonary or renal impairment. Hypersensitivity reactions occur in about 7% of patients but are often responsive to antihistamine. Mafenide is used with an open technique in much the same fashion as silver sulfadiazine and should not be used under dressings. Because of its ability to diffuse into eschar and its effectiveness in Gram-negative organisms, mafenide is indicated in treatment of burns with thick eschar and older burns with specific applications, such as burns of the ear where penetration may help prevent the development of perichondritis.

SMOKE INHALATION AND PULMONARY COMPLICATIONS

Smoke inhalation is the leading cause of death by fire. Many victims are not burned, as in recent hotel fires and airplane crashes. Among burn victims, pulmonary complications are the leading cause of death exceeding that from burn shock and sepsis.

Three categories of respiratory injury are seen: (1) smoke inhalation alone; (2) burns without concomitant smoke inhalation; and (3) the combination of burns plus smoke inhalation. With expert care, morbidity and mortality in the first two categories is low. However, mortality in the third category is very high.[29] For example, Thompson et al. found inhalation injury to be present in 88 of 1,018 patients studied, an overall incidence of 8.6%. The mortality rate of burned individuals with inhalation injury was 56%. Burn patients without inhalation injury had a mortality of only 4.1%.[30] The authors conclude that inhalation injury is the most important determinant of mortality in patients with thermal injury, exceeding that of age or BSAB.

Pulmonary restrictive disease caused by circumferential eschar of the thorax and abdomen should be treated promptly by appropriate escharotomy.

Apart from smoke inhalation, burn injury alone is attended by airway and pulmonary complications. Upper airway obstruction from edema, hyperventilation, atelectasis, and pulmonary edema may occur in the early stages of acute burn injury. These effects may be minimized by avoiding fluid overload, gastric dilatation, and by providing adequate perfusion and ventilatory assistance.

Mechanism of Injury

Heat may injure the upper airway, but because of the heat sink effect, direct thermal injury virtually never occurs in the lower airway except when live steam is inhaled.

The initial injury from smoke inhalation is described as the asphyxiaobtundation syndrome.[31] Oxygen deprivation occurs when ambient oxygen in a closed-space fire drops to 10% or less, as the fire consumes atmospheric oxygen. The inhalation of carbon dioxide and carbon monoxide aggravates the situation. Hemoglobin has an affinity of 200 times, and myoglobin 50 times greater for carbon monoxide than for oxygen. In the presence of large amounts of carboxyhemoglobin, the oxygen dissociation curve is moved to the left, further decreasing tissue oxygenation. The primary targets of carbon monoxide poisoning are the brain and heart. Mild cases may exhibit cardiac arrhythmias, headaches, dizziness, visual disturbances, and confusion. Severe poisoning may result in coma, demyelinization, and long-term neuropsychiatric effects.

In addition to carbon monoxide, pyrolysis or combustion of wood, cotton, wool, paint, lacquer, and various synthetic materials such as plastic produces many noxious substances, including oxides of nitrogen, lead, and sulfur; hydrocholoric acid; phosgene; ammonia; chlorine; fluorine; and aldehydes, acrylics, cyanide, and particles of carbon. In the second phase of inhalation injury, direct damage to respiratory epithelium causes edema and mucous membrane irritation, producing upper airway obstructive disease. Adherence of acid compounds to carbon particles prolongs this irritation. Injury to tracheobronchial mucosa can produce mucosal slough 24 to 36 hours post-injury leading to obstruction of small airways and distal infection with the risk of superinfection. A later, third phase has been called the hypoxemia-hypoventilation syndrome.[31]

Burned patients without smoke inhalation may experience respiratory failure both from upper airway injury and edema in the early phase and atelectasis and pneumonitis later. The mechanism by which the lethal effects of the combination of the burned skin and inhalation injury is enhanced is not well understood. The occurrence of cutaneous burn with intravascular complement activation triggers the release of a cascade of effects which affect the lung in various ways, including increased pulmonary vascular resistance, loss of capillary integrity, fibrin emboli, and entrapment of leukocytes in the pulmonary capillaries by increased endothelial adhesiveness. Leukocytes under these conditions may produce prodigious amounts of oxygen metabolites, including superoxide anions, hydrogen peroxide, and extremely unstable oxygen free radicals which are thought to result in the histopathologic changes of hyaline membrane disease and acute respiratory distress syndrome.[32]

Diagnosis

The presence of burns of the anterior chest, neck, and face; singed nasal vibrissae, sooty sputum, and burned clothing; a history of exposure to fire in a closed space or to petroleum fires are indicators of probable smoke inhalation. The historical value of these data, however, is perhaps less than 50%. The history of unconsciousness and the persistence of carbonaceous sputum are perhaps the most valuable predictors of inhalation injury. Direct examination of the airway with a fiberoptic bronchoscope is useful in suspected inhalation injury. Using this method in unselected burn patients, Moylan found that about one third had evidence of inhalation injury.[33] The criteria indicating inhalation injury are chemical burn of the airway, mucosal erythema, edema, ulceration, hemorrhage, and the presence of carbonaceous material in the airways. If any of these stigmata are present in the larynx and vocal cords, the fiberoptic bronchoscope should be passed into the tracheobronchial tree. Moylan found that among patients with inhalation injury, damage was confined to the upper airway in 60% and extended to the major airways in 35%. Only 5% of these patients had a true gas exchange problem as the primary presenting complication.

Intravenous xenon scanning has been used with accuracy and reliability in the diagnosis of inhalation injury involving the major airways or parenchymal injuries. Ten microcuries of 133 xenon injected into a peripheral vein should be completely cleared from the lung by ventilation in 90 seconds. Delayed clearance or inequality of the clearing pattern from segments of lung noted on the scintigram indicates injury. Because the technique relies on the presence of edema to produce entrapment of the isotope in the lung, it may not be positive in the first hours post-injury.

Routine blood gas and electrolyte measurements are required to monitor patients with inhalation injury and pulmonary complication, although the initial arterial blood gases are almost routinely within normal limits. Determination of alveolar to arterial oxygen gradient may be helpful in following patients.

Carboxyhemoglobin determinations are indicated if carbon monoxide poisoning is suspected. Arterial blood gas measurements in CO poisoning may show normal oxygen pressures since the dissolved oxygen is at normal tension, although the absolute amount of oxygen available is markedly reduced. Since the chemoreceptor mechanism responds to the tension of dissolved oxygen and not that combined with hemoglobin, these patients may show no respiratory changes.[34] The classic "cherry-red" skin color of CO poisoning is unreliable.

Pulmonary function studies may be valuable, particularly flow volume curve analysis that may help to distinguish between obstructive and restrictive deficits.

Chest roentgenograms are also valuable but may be expected to be within normal limits in an early examination. It may take as long as 24 to 96 hours to show significant changes.

Treatment

Warm humidified oxygen should be administered immediately when smoke inhalation or carbon monoxide poisoning is suspected. The carboxyhemoglobin level of patients breathing room air will be lowered by 50% in about two hours. This can be shortened to 20 to 30 minutes by administering 100% oxygen with a nonrebreathing face mask. Assisted ventilation may be required.[34] There clearly is a place for the use of hyperbaric oxygen in the treatment of acute CO poisoning and its subacute sequelae.[35]

All patients with smoke inhalation should be very carefully monitored for upper airway obstruction. Hoarseness and stridor indicate impending airway obstruction which may not be fully evident until it occurs. Attempts at airway control at the time of occlusion may be extremely difficult, and many practitioners favor early endotracheal intubation. However, since the endotracheal tube may be needed for less than four to six days, tracheostomy, which is poorly tolerated by burn patients, may be avoided. Warm moist oxygen and vigorous pulmonary physical therapy are essential. Endotracheal suction and bronchoscopy may be needed frequently to remove thick secretions and sloughing mucosa that cause small airway obstruction and atelectasis. Mild upper airway edema may be treated by nebulized epinephrine (0.5 mL diluted to 2 mL) every four hours together with large doses of Decadron every four to six hours.[8] It should be remembered that in the small diameter airway of the child, edema produces a much greater proportionate loss of airway than the same amount of edema in an adult (cross-section area of airway = πr^2). Such patients require exceedingly close monitoring in the early hours post-injury.

Bronchorrhea, bronchospasm, and wheezing may be severe and occasionally lethal. Systemic or nebulized bronchodilators may be used. Intravenous aminophylline and large doses of corticosteroids may be necessary for severe continuing bronchospasm. Ventilatory support requiring large tidal volumes of 10 to 15 mL/kg may be necessary to treat respiratory insufficiency resulting from pulmonary edema, severe bronchospasm, or superimposed edema. Positive end-expiratory pressure may be valuable in overcoming the effects of decreased lung compliance, increased airway resistance, and the increased work of breathing.

Controversy exists regarding the use of corticosteroids in respiratory injury. Many advocate the use of single or short-term large doses, but there has been evidence that steroids may have no therapeutic benefit and may increase the infection rate and salt retention.[33,36]

Prophylactic antibiotics are not recommended in smoke inhalation injury because of the possible development of infection with resistant organisms. Serial cultures should be performed and specific antibiotics used for demonstrated infection.

ELECTRICAL INJURIES

Electrical injuries account for 3% to 4% of burn center admissions, and there are an estimated 1,100 deaths per year, with 2 to 4 times that number of nonfatal injuries.[37–39]

Pathophysiology

The factors that affect the severity of electrical injury include the characteristics of the current (voltage, amperage, and type of circuit); the duration of current flow; and the resistance of body tissues and pathway through the body.[38]

Voltage

Electrical current that causes injury is classified as high voltage (greater than 1,000 V) or low voltage (less than 1,000 V). Both may cause death by cardiac and respiratory arrest, but high-voltage injuries are much more likely to be associated with extensive thermal damage.[39] The relationship between voltage and amperage is illustrated by Ohm's law (voltage = amperage × resistance). Amperage is a better measure of electrical injury, but it is less easily determined than voltage. While ionic and structural changes in tissue may be induced by electrical current, heat production accounts for most of the tissue damage. Joule's law (heat = amperages^2 × resistance × time) is used to calculate the thermal effect.

Resistance

Electrical resistances, measured in ohms, vary from one tissue to the next. Heat production is directly related to electrical resistance and duration of current flow. Resistance is greatest in bone and becomes progressively less in fat, tendon, skin, muscle, blood vessels, and nerves. The greatest portion of current applied to a limb is transported by muscle, fat, skin, and tendon.[37] Bone passes little current because of its high resistance, but generates considerable heat. Blood vessels and nerves conduct relatively little current in spite of their high-current density, because of their minimal cross-sectional area.

When an electrical potential is contacted, the skin is the primary resistor and its resistance varies according to the thickness, wetness, and cleanness of the skin. A thickly calloused palm may have a resistance of 1,000,000 Ω/cm^2, contrasted with 5,000 Ω/cm^2 for normal dry skin, and only 1,000 Ω/cm^2 for wet skin.[40] Skin resistances also change with current flow. Hunt et al showed three phases of electrical injury in an animal model.[41] In the first phase, a slow rise in current occurred with a parallel decrease in skin resistance. The second phase was characterized by an abrupt and rapid rise in amperage as skin resistance completely broke down allowing unimpeded flow of current through the animal's body. In this phase, the animal's body behaved as a volume conductor. In the third phase, current arcing occurred. This produced temperatures of 2,500 °C–3,000 °C that resulted in explosive volatilization of tissue and fluids, desiccation, and carbonization, thereby producing a sudden increase in tissue resistance. At this point, tissue in contact with the power source ceased to be a conductor and became an insulator with cessation of current flow and tissue damage. Burning and charring occurred at the contact site and severity of damage decreased as distance from the current pathway increased.

If body tissues function as a volume conductor, two important considerations emerge. First, when current enters a portion of a limb with a small cross-sectional area, current density, and therefore heat production, is high. Conversely, in portions with a larger cross-sectional area, current density and associated heat production are lower. Second, in a volume conductor, the rate of temperature increase depends on both heat capacity and the rate at which heat escapes by radiation, convection, and conduction. The differences in rate of heat loss from superficial and deep tissues may explain the common clinical observation of nonviable periosseous tissue underlying viable more superficial muscle from which heat is more readily lost. The pattern of deep tissue necrosis in such an injury is variable and necrotic tissue is found distributed in a patchy fashion. Severe edema develops beneath fascia requiring immediate fasciotomy to reduce the pressure in the muscle compartments and to prevent further necrosis from ischemia.

Type of Current

Direct current (DC) produces a single muscle contraction that tends to repel the victim from the power source, particularly if a fall is produced. By contrast, alternating current (AC) with its rapidly depolarizing effects produces a cycle of tetanic muscular contraction and relaxation such that the hand grasping the power source is unable to let go. Thus, AC is particularly treacherous and produces three times as much damage as DC.

The frequency of AC is also critical since low-frequency currents in the range of 10 to 120 cycles per second (c/s) have a specific cardiorespiratory effect that can produce ventricular fibrillation and apnea. The clinical importance of this resides in the fact that commercial current in the United States is 60 c/s, which explains the relatively high incidence of death from low-voltage household current.

Pathways

The pathway taken by the electrical current as it passes through the body determines the structures which are damaged. The course of the current does not necessarily follow a predicted line from the external points of entry to exit, and damage at distant sites may occur.

Types of Electrical Injuries

Burn Injury

Electrical injuries are usually accompanied by burns. An exception may be found in the bathtub or sink accident in which an electrical appliance fell into the water transmitting the current to the victim. Because of low skin resistance, no burn is suffered, yet fatal cardiac arrest may occur. Burns are caused by direct contact, flame, flash, and current arcs. Often all of these occur in the same accident. Direct contact at one or more sites of entry and one or more sites of exit produces severe destruction of skin, and charring is evident. The most common entry sites are located on the head or hands, and exit sites on the heel.[38] Secondary thermal burns occur from contact with ignited clothing or hot metal, such as jewelry, which the patient may be wearing. Electrical explosions produce flash burns which are generally fairly superficial. Arc burns may occur not only at entry and exit points, but between flexor skin surfaces as the joint contracts due to muscle stimulation induced by the current.

Oral Burns

The most common electrical injury experienced by children occurs in the mouth.[42] The victims are usually under the age 4 years, most commonly 1½ to 2 years. Boys outnumber girls by two to one. The injury occurs when a toddler sucks on the live end of an extension cord, the junction between two cords, chews through an electrical wire, comes in contact with exposed live wires, or sucks on a wall or floor socket. The flow of saliva completes the circuit and the resultant electric arc produces a severe burn of the lips, labial commissures, gums, teeth, and tongue. It is estimated that there is an associated cardiorespiratory arrest in 5% of victims.

Neurological

Damage to the brain, brainstem, spinal cord, peripheral nerves, and sympathetic nervous system may occur producing brainstem damage, seizures, paralysis, intracranial hemorrhage, and death. Devastating spinal cord injuries have been reported after latent periods of 2 to 3 years.

Cardiopulmonary

Conduction defects, arrhythmias, posterior wall ischemia, and acute myocardial infarction have all been reported following electrical injury. Cardiac arrest may present in either ventricular fibrillation or asystole. Respiratory arrest is common.

Eye

Cataracts occur from electrical injury, usually as a late development.

Genitourinary

Renal failure is the most serious complication of electrical injury. It occurs because of the large quantities of circulating hemoglobin and myoglobin that are released from massive destruction of muscle and blood components. Late urinary tract complications include lithiasis and impotence.

Gastrointestinal

Curling's ulcer is not uncommon in electrical injury, and prolonged ileus, damage to the liver, pancreas, and gallbladder also may occur. Mesenteric thrombosis and injury to the small and large bowel are also seen.[40,43]

Blood Vessels

Pronounced vasculitis, primarily arteritis with necrosis of the vascular wall occurs, sometimes resulting in delayed hemorrhage. Large and medium-sized vessels are commonly thrombosed and may affect any organ.

Associated Injuries

Blunt trauma and fractures of the skull, ribs, and long bones are common concomitant injuries that result from intense muscular contractions produced by electrical current and falls. Primary head injury, rather than electrical damage, should be suspected in the event of decreasing consciousness.[38]

Infection

Infection, including clostridial myositis, is a very serious potential complication in electrical injury, because of the large volume of necrotic tissue that may be produced and the difficulties of adequate debridement. When sepsis occurs in the victim of electrical injury, the site is usually necrotic muscle.

Treatment

Cardiorespiratory

Cardiac and respiratory arrest are the most common causes of death in electrical injuries and cardiopulmonary resuscitation is often required in the field. Endotracheal intubation, administration of 100% oxygen, and ventilatory assistance may be required. Electroshock therapy may convert a lethal ventricular fibrillation into a supraventricular tachycardia or ectopic-focus arrhythmia that can be pharmacologically changed to a normal rhythm.[40] Patients should be monitored post-injury with serial electrocardiograms and cardiac isoenzyme determinations.

Fluid Resuscitation

The volume of tissue damaged in a conduction burn may be very large and the visible burns of the skin may be only the tip of the iceberg. Formulas for fluid resuscitation based on BSAB are essentially of no value. Large volumes of lactated Ringer's solution without glucose must be administered until adequate urinary flow is established and the criteria for adequate resuscitation, described previously, have been met.

Myoglobinuria

Urine and serum should be monitored for the presence of hemoglobin and myoglobin. When coupled with hypovolemia and acidosis, these substances may produce acute tubular necrosis and renal failure. The administration of large volumes of fluid not only helps prevent shock but also helps the renal glomeruli and tubules to filter myoglobin and hemoglobin. An osmotic diuretic in the form of mannitol should be administered. Furosemide has also been advocated to increase renal flow. It should be noted that the use of diuretics makes urinary flow an unreliable measure of resuscitation. Acidosis frequently accompanies myoglobinuria and should be treated with enough sodium bicarbonate to maintain serum pH above 7.35.

Wound Management

Escharotomy and particularly fasciotomy are an essential part of therapy in electrical injury. Early and deep exploration of all muscle compartments in an involved extremity should be carried out to relieve pressure, restore circulation, and debride devitalized tissue to reduce hyperkalemia, myoglobin load, and the risk of infection. Muscle damage is often spotty and necrotic periosseous muscle may be covered by viable muscle.

Carpal tunnel release and fasciotomy of the intrinsic muscles of the hands and feet may be beneficial. Adequacy of circulation should be monitored by the Doppler technique and occasionally by arteriogram. Early amputation may be lifesaving. Abdominal injuries should be explored promptly. When possible, salvage of exposed major blood vessels, nerves, and tendons should be attempted by covering them with viable skin and muscle flaps.

Burns of the skin are treated in the conventional manner. Arc burns should be excised. Topical antibodies may be applied as appropriate, and open areas following debridement should be protected with biological or synthetic dressings.

Oral burns in children may require hospitalization, depending on severity and ability of the family to care for the patient at home. Such burns produce profuse delayed hemorrhage, and if a child is to be treated as an outpatient, parents need to be instructed on emergency digital compression of the labial artery until the vessel can be ligated. Treatment may be by: (1) early excision and reconstruction; (2) healing by secondary intention with subsequent restoration; (3) early and continuous oral splinting; or (4) no reconstruction. Tetanus prophylaxis should be administered, and antibiotics are usually given. These injuries may heal relatively well when minor, but often have serious cosmetic and functional sequelae.[42]

Gastrointestinal Injuries

Antacids and cimetidine should be administered early to prevent Curling's ulcer. Prolonged ileus requires nasogastric intubation. Peritoneal tap or abdominal exploration may be indicated in appropriate circumstances.

Associated Injuries

Blunt trauma, fractures, and closed head injuries should be sought and treated in the usual way. Skeletal traction should be used for reduction and stabilization of fractures in the presence of burn injuries rather than internal fixation and plaster casting to prevent infection and to provide easy access to the wounds.

Tetanus

Routine prophylaxis for tetanus should always be administered in electrical wounds.

LIGHTNING INJURIES

Lightning kills about 300 to 600 persons annually in the United States, more than any other natural disaster.[44] Several thousand more people experience lightning injury but survive. Twenty to thirty percent of seriously injured victims die and up to 74% of the survivors have serious sequelae.[45]

Lightning is a direct current which may reach energies of 100 million V and peak currents of 2000,000 A. Temperatures of 15,000 °F to 60,000 °F may be generated. "Cold" lightning lasts only 1/1000 second, but "hot" lightning may last up to 1/10 second, enough to cause ignition of flammable materials.

Lightning injuries occur in four ways: (1) direct strike; (2) side flash or splash; (3) ground current; and (4) blunt injury.[28] Direct strike needs no explanation. Side flash occurs when the current splashes from the primary conductor, such as a tree or other object or person, to the victim. Ground current produced by a ground strike near the victim may produce a current through the victim when the feet are placed far enough apart to create a difference of potential (ie, "stride potential"). Injury to the body may occur at points distant from the presumed direct path of the current through the legs and trunk and may be as dangerous as a direct strike. The cylindrical shock waves surrounding a lightning bolt (thunder) may cause blunt injury similar to that seen in an explosion. Blunt injuries may also occur when the victim is thrown by a violent propulsive muscular contraction. Electric current normally flows over the outside of a metal conductor. In a similar way, most of the lightning energy flows around the outside of the victim's body producing the "flashover" phenomenon in which relatively less energy flows through the victim's body.

Types of Lightning Injuries

Burns

Burns in lightning injury are usually superficial because of the flashover phenomenon, even though clothing may be burned or blown away. The burns are characteristically dendriform, streaked, and feather-like. Minimal treatment is often adequate.

Cardiopulmonary

A lightning strike is often accompanied by cardiac and respiratory arrest because part of the current flows internally. The effect on the heart is that of a massive DC countershock that produces asystole. After an interval, the heart tends to resume normal rhythmic contractures spontaneously. Unfortunately, the concomitant respiratory arrest usually lasts longer than the cardiac standstill. Unless the victim receives immediate ventilatory assistance, anoxia supervenes and a second and usually fatal cardiac arrest occurs. Cardiac arrhythmias, ischemia, and elevation of cardiac isoenzymes occur.

Neurological Injury

Direct damage to the central nervous system is common with cerebral edema, unconsciousness, coma, retrograde amnesia, disorientation, seizures, and neurological sequelae. Lightning paralysis or keraunoparalysis is the most common immediate neurological sequela. This consists of a flaccid paralysis of legs and lower trunk, usually associated with extreme vasoconstriction, loss of pulsations, blue livid discoloration and extreme coolness, and loss of sensation. It is frequently the result of stride potential, is relatively transient, seldom requires extensive treatment, and has a generally good prognosis.[46]

Eye and Ear Injury

Multiple types of eye injuries result from lightning including retinal hemorrhage and optic atrophy. Cataracts occur more commonly than in electrical injury. There are reports of spontaneous absorption of lightning-induced cataracts.

Neurosensory deafness and vestibular abnormalities occur, but the most common cause of deafness is rupture of the tympanic membrane.[38]

Treatment

Treatment focuses on cardiac arrest. A lightning victim who has no pulse or respiration—who appears dead—may in fact survive if ventilation or cardiopulmonary resuscitation is administered quickly enough to avoid secondary cardiac arrest from anoxia.[47,48] Cases are reported of victims who remained comatose on a ventilator for weeks following lightning injury and finally recovered without significant neurological deficit. The large volumes of salt solution required in the resuscitation electrical injury victims are seldom needed. Fluid resuscitation is usually carried out with glucose and water solutions, avoiding fluid overload in comatose patients. Fasciotomies, escharotomies, and extensive burn treatment are rarely needed. Patients who have been struck by lightning should receive an electrocardiogram and cardiac isoenzyme determinations and should be monitored for 24 hours to rule out cardiac injury.

CHILD ABUSE INJURIES

Burning as a manifestation of child abuse is being increasingly recognized by those who care for pediatric trauma victims. Recognition depends in part upon the alertness and sophistication of the physician and other health care providers.[49] Exhibit 31–6 lists criteria that indicate the possibility of child abuse. Burns are estimated to occur in about 10% of child abuse victims. Evidence of child abuse or overt neglect is found in approximately 20% of our hospitalized burn patients.

Patterns of Inflicted Burns

Lenoski and Hunter have defined specific patterns of inflicted burn injury.[50]

Exhibit 31-6 Conditions Suggesting the Possibility of Child Abuse

- Multiple hematomas or scars in various stages of healing.
- Concurrent injuries or evidence of neglect such as malnutrition or failure to thrive.
- History of prior hospitalizations for "accidental" trauma.
- An unexplained delay between the time of injury and the first attempt to obtain medical attention.
- Burns that appear older than they are alleged to be.
- Account of the accident is not compatible with the age and ability of the child.
- Responsible adults allege that the child was merely "discovered" to be burned.
- Relatives bring the injured child to the hospital.
- Burn is attributed to the action of a sibling or another child (which does in fact occur).
- Injured child is excessively withdrawn, passive, submissive, or overly polite or does not cry during painful procedures.
- Child has scalded hands or feet, and the appearance of the injury—often symmetrical and full-thickness burns—suggests that the extremities were forcibly immersed or held in hot liquid.
- The child has isolated burns of the buttocks that in children would hardly have been produced by accidental means.
- The child has fractures or internal or central nervous system injuries.

Source: Stone NH, Rinaldo L, Humphrey CR, et al: Child abuse by burning. *Surg Clin North Am* 1970; 50:1419

Immersion Burns

Immersion in hot tap water or other fluid produces a uniform burn in all areas exposed to the hot liquid. A distinct line separates the burned from the unburned areas. These lines may be made parallel by positioning of the body and body members of the patient and indicate the position of the child at the time of immersion. Forced immersion into hot liquid held in an unheated container (e.g., hot water run into a bathtub) produces a doughnut-shaped injury in which a central portion of the injury areas is spared, representing the part of the body pressed against the side or bottom of the cooler container (Figure 31–7A and B).

Splash Burns

Splash burns occur when hot liquid is poured or thrown on the victim. They are usually less deep, less uniform, and more irregular in pattern, as would be expected from splashing. As the hot liquid runs off the skin it may leave a cascade or "arrowhead" configuration, permitting an analysis of the

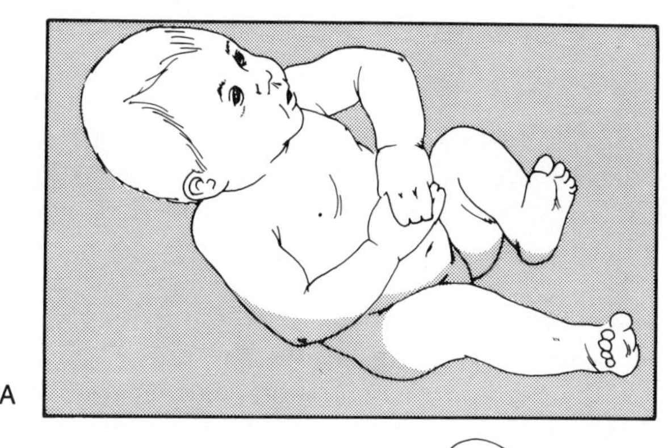

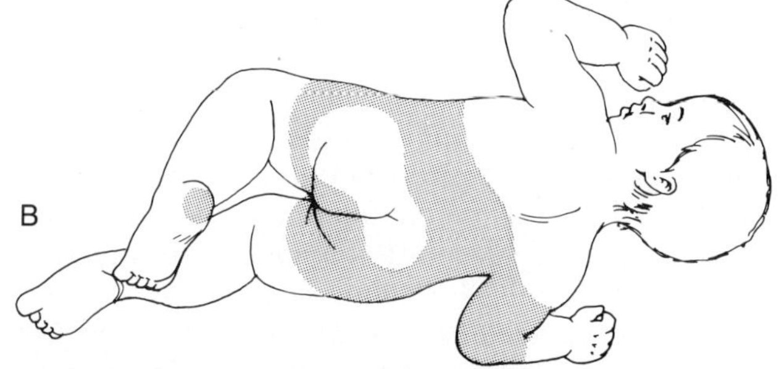

FIGURE 31-7 A, View of patient from right side. Note flexed extremities, which protected skin surfaces in apposition. Note left heel dipped into water because of left knee flexion. B, Pattern of burn inflicted by forced immersion depicted in Figure 31-7A. Note the doughnut area of spared skin on buttocks, which were pressed against tub surface, which is at lower temperature than the hot water. (Reprinted with permission from Lenoski EF, Hunter KA: Specific pattern of inflicted burn injuries. *J Trauma* 1977; 17(11):843, 844. Copyright © 1977 Williams & Wilkins Co.)

position of the child's body relative to the direction from which the burning fluid came.

Flexion Burns

A victim upon threatened by immersion or splashing with hot liquid assumes a fetus-like posture with marked flexion of all extremities. A burn suffered in this position frequently spares flexion creases at the axillae, antecubital, popliteal, hip flexion, and neck areas.

Contact Burns

Contact burns are the easiest to identify, and, like a brand on livestock, reproduce the shape of whatever hot object was used to inflict them (eg, a cigarette, hot wire, or grill).

Family Characteristics

The families of abused children often are severely stressed, highly mobile, economically insecure, and prone to violent behavior. As in many burns in which child abuse is not implicated, there is often a history of psychiatric illness in the patient or the family. Often the abusing parent is found to have been abused as a child. Many times the perpetrator of the burn alleges that it was only an attempt to impose discipline and frequently fails to appreciate the destructiveness of hot tap water. It is striking that many of such injuries revolve around the issue of toilet training.

Obligations of Health Care Providers

The physician and other health care providers who suspect child abuse have a moral and legal obligation to report cases to appropriate authorities. The first responsibility is to the patient, and such patients should always be admitted to the hospital pending appropriate disposition. The help of a child advocacy team with special investigation skills may spare the physician from simultaneously having to fulfill the conflicting roles of care provider and investigator. A high degree of skill and professionalism is required of the investigator to prevent overlooked child abuse on the one hand, and the separation of wrongfully accused parents from their child on the other. (For an in-depth discussion of child abuse and neglect, see Chapter 39, "Child Abuse and Neglect.")

CONCLUSION

The physician who cares for a burned child must recognize the essential differences that separate the pediatric from the adult patient and must modify therapy appropriately. The child with a severe burn, whose body and personality are still growing and developing, is uniquely vulnerable. The cost of such injuries in human and economic terms to the patient, the patient's family, and society are incalculable.

References

1. Moritz AR, Henriques FC: Studies of thermal injury: The relative importance of time and surface temperature in the causation of cutaneous burns. *Am J Pathol* 1947;23:695.
2. Feldman KW, Schaller RT, Feldman JA, et al: Tap water scald burns in children. *Pediatrics* 1978;62:1–7.
3. Feller I, Crane K, Flanders S: Baseline data on the mortality of burn patients. *QRB* 1979.
4. Carvajal H, Parks DH: Survival statistics in burned children. *JBCR* 1982;3:81–84.
5. Moncrief J: *Burns: A Team Approach.* Philadelphia, WB Saunders Co, 1979, p 29.
6. Baxter CR: Guidelines for fluid resuscitation. *J Trauma* 1981;21(suppl): 687–689.
7. Pruitt BA Jr: Fluid resuscitation for extensively burned patients. *J Trauma* 1981;21:690–692.
8. Pruitt BA Jr: The burn patient: I. Initial care. *Curr Prob Surg* 1979;16:25.
9. Baxter CR: Guidelines for fluid resuscitation. *J Trauma* 1981;21:689.
10. Moncrief JA: Burns: I. Assessment. *JAMA* 1979; 242:72.
11. Lund CL, Browder JC: The estimation of areas of burns. *Surg Gynec Obstet* 1944;79:352.
12. Total care of burn patients: A guide to hospital resources. Compiled by the American Burn Association: *ACS Bulletin,* October 1977, p 8.
13. Raine TJ, Heggers JP, Robson MC, et al: Cooling the burn wound to maintain microcirculation. *J Trauma* 1981;21:394–397.
14. Shuck LW, Shuck JM: The outpatient burn. *Current Concepts in Trauma Care,* Spring 1982, p 15–21.
15. Baxter CR: Fluid resuscitation, burn percentage and physiologic age. *J Trauma* 1979;19(suppl):864–865.
16. Baxter CR: Guidelines for fluid resuscitation. *J Trauma* 1981;21(suppl):687–689.
17. Baxter CR: Controversies in the resuscitation of burn shock. *Current Concepts in Trauma Care,* Spring 1982, p 6.
18. Pruitt BA Jr: The effectiveness of fluid resuscitation. Proceedings of the NIH consensus development conference in supportive therapy in burn care. *J Trauma* 1979;19(suppl):868.
19. Burke JF, Quinby WC Jr, Behringer GD, Bondoc CC: 1981—Approach to burn therapy. *Surg Annu* 1981.
20. Carvajal HF: A physiologic approach to fluid therapy

in severely burned children. *Surg Gynec Obstet* 1980;150:379.
21. Recinos PR, Hartford CA, Ziffren, SE: Fluid resuscitation of burn patients comparing a crystalloid with a colloid containing solution: A prospective study. *J Iowa Med Soc* 1975;65:426–432.
22. Alexander JW, Ogle CK, Stinnett JD, et al: Fresh frozen plasma vs. plasma derivatives as adjunctive therapy for patients with massive burns. *J Trauma* 1979;19:502.
23. Monafo WW, Robinson HN: The treatment of burned children. *Clin Plast Surg* 1977;4:537.
24. Caldwell FT, Bowser BH: Critical evaluation of hypertonic and hypotonic solutions to resuscitate severely burned children. A prospective study. *Ann Surg* 1979;189:546.
25. Baxter CR: Controversies in the resuscitation of burn shock. *Current Concepts in Trauma Care,* Spring, 1982, p 11.
26. Pruitt BA Jr: The burn patient: II. *Curr Probl Surg* 1979;16 (no. 5).
27. MacMillan BG: Burns. *A Team Approach.* WB Saunders Co, Philadelphia, 1979, p 195.
28. Pruitt BA Jr: The burn patient: I. Initial care. *Curr Probl Surg* 1979;16(no. 4):28.
29. Bartlett RH: Types of respiratory injury. Proceedings of the NIH consensus development conference in supportive therapy in burn care. *J Trauma* 1979;19(suppl):918.
30. Thompson PB, Herndon DN, Traber DL, et al: Effect on mortality of inhalation injury. *J Trauma* 1986;26:163.
31. Horowitz JW: Abnormalities caused by smoke inhalation. Proceedings of the NIH consensus development conference in supportive therapy in burn care. *J Trauma* 1979;19(suppl):915.
32. Ward PA: The role of the complement system in smoke inhalation. Second conference on supportive therapy in burn care. *J. Trauma* 1981;21(suppl):722.
33. Moylan JA: Inhalation injury. Second conference on supportive therapy in burn care. *J Trauma* 1981;21(suppl):720.
34. Gilman JI: Pediatric burns, in *Yearbook Medical Publishers.* Chicago, London, 1979.
35. Meyers RA, Snyder SK, Emhoff TA: Subacute sequelae of carbon monoxide poisoning. *Ann Emerg Med* 1985;14:1163.
36. Moylan JA: Inhalation injury. Proceedings of the NIH consensus development conference in supportive therapy in burn care. *J Trauma* 1979; 19(suppl):917.
37. Sances A Jr, Myklebust JB, Larson SJ, et al: Experimental electrical injury studies. *J. Trauma* 1981;21:589.
38. Cooper MA: Electrical and lightning injuries. *Emerg Med Clin North Am* 1984;2:489.
39. Parshley PF, Kilgore J, Pulito JF, et al: Aggressive approach to the extremity damaged by electrical current. *Am J Surg* 1985;150:78.
40. Bingham H: Electrical burns. *Clin Plast Surg* 1986;13:75.
41. Hunt JL, Mason AD, Masterson TS, et al: The pathophysiology of acute electric injuries. *J Trauma* 1976;16:335.
42. Leake JE, Curtin JW: Electrical burns of the mouth in children. *Clin Plast Surg* 1984;11:669.
43. Baxter CR: Present concepts in the management of major electrical injury. *Surgical Clin North Am* 1970;50:1401.
44. Craig SR: When lightning strikes. *Postgrad Med* 1966;79:109.
45. Cooper MA: Lightning injuries: Prognostic signs for death. *Ann Emerg Med* 1980;9:134.
46. TenDuis HJ, Klasen HJ: Keraunoparalysis, a "specific" lightning injury. *Burns* 1985;12:54.
47. Ravitch MM, Lane R, Safar, P: Lightning stroke. *N Engl J Med* 1961;264:36.
48. Taussig HB: "Death" from lightning—and the possibility of living again. *Am Intern Med* 1968;68:1345.
49. Stone NH, Rinaldo L, Humphrey CR, et al: Child abuse by burning. *Surg Clin North Am* 1970;50:1419–1424.
50. Lenoski EF, Hunter KA: Specific patterns of inflicted burn injury. *J Trauma* 1977;17:842.

Moritz M. Ziegler

32

Skin and Subcutaneous Lesions

Skin and subcutaneous lesions of childhood form a major part of pediatric outpatient and pediatric surgical practices. Prompt recognition, correct differential diagnosis, appropriate triage, and judicious emergency management of such masses form a large part of the medical care of the child. To facilitate an orderly discussion of differential diagnosis and treatment, this chapter is organized according to anatomic sites and clearly states when emergency department therapy is indicated as opposed to primary emergency triage with subsequent elective treatment.

FACE AND SCALP

Cysts

Cysts located about the face and scalp most commonly are inclusion or dermoid cysts. They may be located either in the midline of the face, in the scalp, or over the lateral aspect of the eyebrow. Such lesions are subcutaneous, vary from several millimeters to more than a centimeter in diameter, and are mobile and nontender. Dermoid cysts require surgical excision to establish a diagnosis or prevent erosion of the underlying outer table of the skull. Such benign lesions are not characterized by recurrence. Their potential cranial penetration contraindicates removal in an emergency department.

Sebaceous cysts are related to the hair follicle and the glandular oily sebaceous secretions from such follicular glands. Sebaceous cysts most often appear as subcutaneous nodules in a hair-bearing area. Since they are prone to infection, such lesions are best treated by elective surgical excision. Acute abscess formation requires incision and drainage in the emergency department.

Preauricular Lesions

Preauricular lesions may be classified as a simple pit with a cutaneous orifice, a sinus tract with an associated subcutaneous cyst or tract extending to the auditory canal or to the base of the skull, or a cutaneous tag with or without a cartilaginous component. They may be unilateral or bilateral and are quite common in the population at large, but in only a few circumstances do they require operative intervention. Surgery for cutaneous tags is optional, usually for cosmetic purposes; however, it is the best treatment for sinus tracts and cysts if there is a previous history of infection or if there is a palpable cystic component in the subcutaneous tissue lying below the sinus. Because of the deep extension of these lesions, emergency department procedures should be limited to only the incision and drainage of an acutely infected cyst.

Tongue and Oral Cavity Lesions

Tongue-tie is a condition in which the ventral frenulum of the tongue binds the tongue tip to the floor of the mouth. The difficulty of patient selection for frenotomy, the potential tissue vascularity, and the nonurgent nature of this problem mitigate against surgery in the emergency department.

An enlarged tongue, or macroglossia, may indicate a lingual thyroid gland or a lymphangioma involving the tongue, with the associated abnormal lymphatic cysts being prone to secondary infection. These infections are best managed by outpatient antibiotics, and only in the face of potential airway compromise is urgent hospital admission indicated.

The most common lesions in the mouth include gingival papillomas (abnormal papillary protrusions) and gingival mucoceles (collections of mucus beneath the gingival mucosa). A bulge in the floor of the mouth beneath the mucosa suggests a ranula, an aberrant remnant of the salivary secretory glands. None of these problems requires urgent surgical intervention, and all should be referred to appropriate surgical specialists when identified.

An acute, painful swelling about the base of a tooth may suggest a periodontal abscess. Whether an emergency department drainage procedure in addition to antibiotics is indicated should be decided only after emergency dental consultation.

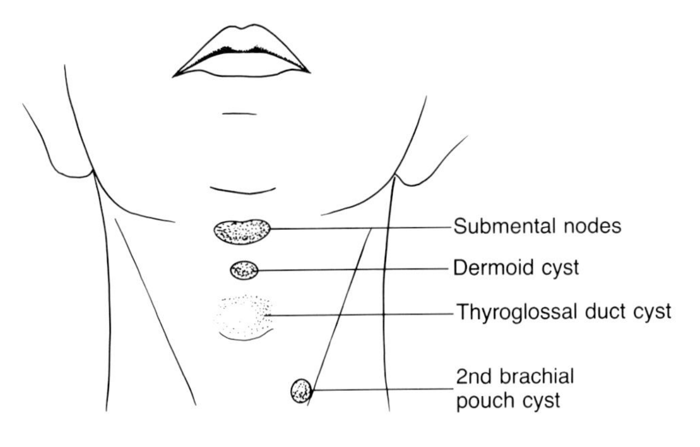

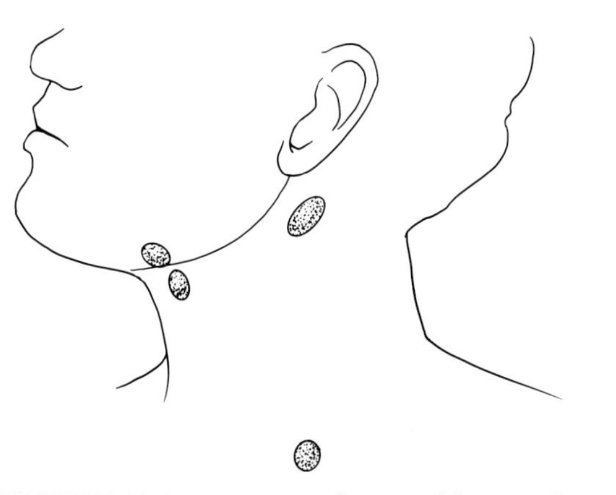

FIGURE 32-1 Location of cervical lesions that manifest themselves as masses or spots.

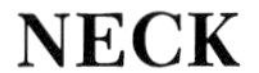

NECK

Midline Lesions

Midline neck lesions (Figure 32-1) include submental lymph nodes in the upper midline of the neck. These nodes are normally present but become enlarged following an infection in the floor of the mouth or the perioral area.

Dermoid cysts may be located anywhere within the midline of the neck, from the mandible to the supraclavicular fossa. These small (0.5 to 1.0 cm) lesions most commonly are nontender, mobile, and located in the subcutaneous tissue. They commonly are high in the midline of the neck, above the area of a classic thyroglossal duct cyst.

A thyroglossal duct cyst (Figure 32-2) represents an aberrant cystic remnant from the normal descent of the thyroid gland and may occur anywhere along the tract, from the foramen cecum of the tongue down to the midline of the neck just above the thyroid cartilage. Such lesions are characterized by a painless midline neck mass, which moves with swallowing and protrusion of the tongue. If children with such lesions come to the emergency department because of the discovery of an undiagnosed but asymptomatic mass, then triage for elective surgical consultation is appropriate. If treatment is sought because of tenderness and redness, then outpatient antibiotic therapy is indicated. For an acute abscess a limited incision and drainage are appropriate, but subsequent definitive excision after cessation of infection is then required to remove the tract of the thyroglossal duct cyst and its attached central portion of the hyoid bone.

Lateral Lesions

The most common neck lesion in childhood is cervical lymphadenitis, which is usually due to a suppurative bacterial process. Acute suppurative lymphadenitis is characterized by the onset of swelling and tenderness in the neck, with heat and redness overlying the area. It frequently follows an episode of pharyngitis or otitis. Initially such lymph nodes may be rubbery hard, and when children have such a mass in a known location of a nodal group, a course of outpatient antibiotic therapy effective against staphylococcal organisms is indicated. With progression and suppuration the inflamed nodes develop central softening as abscess formation occurs. Such suppurative lymphadenitis is best treated by drainage along with antistaphylococcal antibiotics. To facilitate the proper selection of antibiotic treatment, drainage may be accomplished by needle aspiration and culture of the aspirate prior to the initiation of antibiotic therapy. Aspiration plus antibiotics is often the only treatment necessary for controlling suppurative lymphadenitis, but if repeated aspiration is necessary or if signs of toxemia exist, then formal surgical drainage is the preferred method of management, combined with hospital admission and parenteral administration of antibiotics.

Tuberculous lymphadenitis (scrofula) is characterized by a more chronic lymphadenopathy with tenderness and enlargement, suggesting an inflammatory process. Initial evaluation is best accompanied by a diagnostic chest x-ray film and a tuberculin skin test. The rubbery, woody lymph nodes require elective surgical excision (with culture and histology). Needle aspiration or simple drainage are not appropriate because of the high incidence of chronic cervicocutaneous fistula formation. The offending organism in these tuberculous lesions is often an atypical mycobacterium (Figure 32-3). (For further discussion of infectious lymphadenitis, see Chapter 36, "Infectious Diseases.")

Lymphadenopathy also may be due to neoplasm, which in children is usually a primary lymphoid tumor of the lymphoma type. Both posterior and

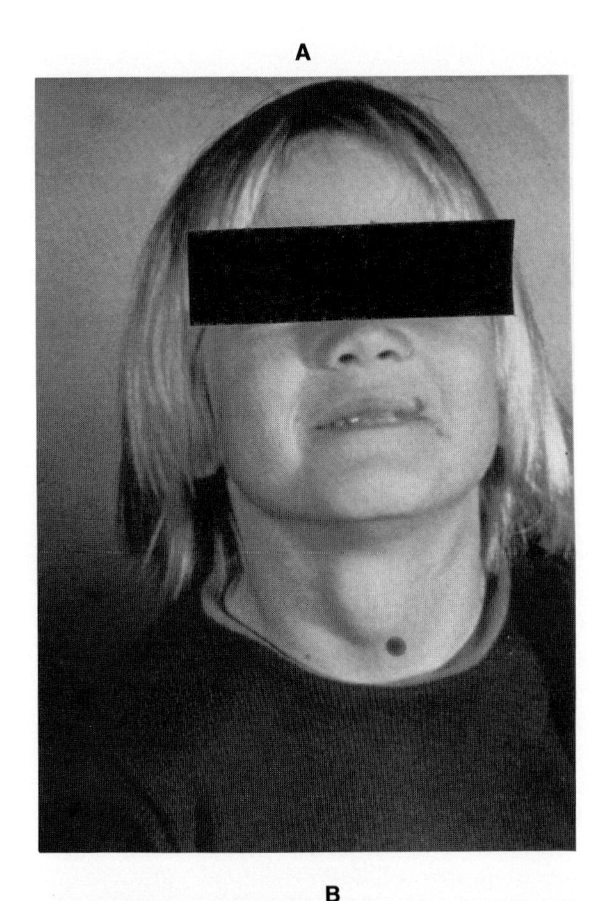

FIGURE 32-2 Anterior (A) and lateral (B) views of a child with a thyroglossal duct cyst. (Courtesy of J.J. Tepas, M.D.)

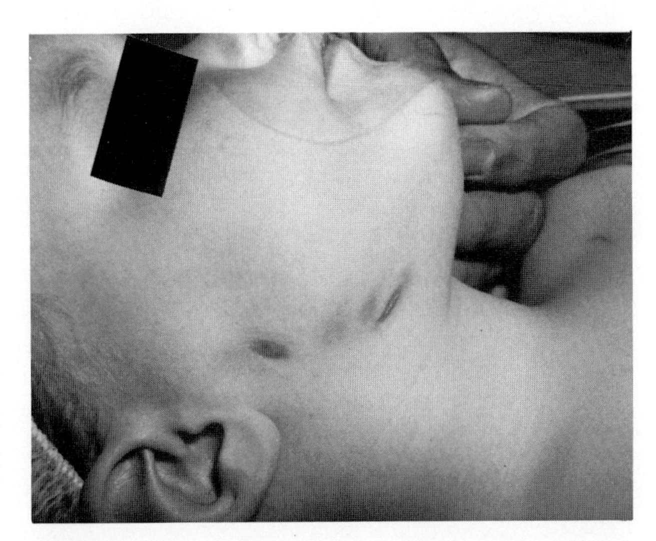

FIGURE 32-3 Child with a nonhealing, chronic lymphadenitis secondary to an infection caused by an atypical mycobacterium. (Courtesy of J.J. Tepas, M.D.)

anterior cervical nodes may be involved in these processes. Prompt surgical referral is especially indicated whenever there is no evidence of acute inflammation. Other malignant neoplasms, specifically neuroblastoma, may metastasize to cervical lymph nodes. Definitive histologic diagnosis of neoplastic involvement of cervical nodes requires a gentle excisional biopsy; proper specimen handling for touch preparation, lymphocyte markers, and microscopic histology; and proper processing for staining and culture of bacterial, fungal, and acid-fast organisms. Only needle aspiration or limited incision is safely in the realm of the emergency department physician. More extensive excisional biopsies and drainage procedures require operating room care.

Salivary gland pathology in the lateral neck includes sialadenitis of the submandibular or parotid gland, with or without secondary abscess formation. These infectious processes are unusual, result in systemic symptoms of infection and sepsis, and require prompt antibiotic therapy and operative drainage after surgical consultation.

Salivary glands are more commonly involved by such vascular lesions as hemangioendotheliomas (Figure 32-4). Rarely, they may be involved by tumors. These painless, progressive salivary gland swellings all require nonemergent surgical evaluation.

Branchial cleft cysts and sinus tracts in the lateral neck occur either along the anterior border of the sternocleidomastoid muscle from the upper to the lower neck (branchial pouch type II, cysts and sinus tracts), or they occur in the submandibular triangle up onto the anterior face (branchial pouch type I, cleft deformities). Such lesions vary and may consist of a pore in the skin, a subcutaneous cyst associated with that pore, and a proximally ascending sinus tract. There also may be only a subcutaneous cystic component or a subcutaneous soft tissue component, which includes cartilaginous remnants (Figure 32-5). If the type II branchial pouch persists as a proximally extending sinus tract, it courses between the external and internal carotid artery and ends in the pharyngeal tonsillar fossa. In the type I branchial pouch deformity, such tracts extend to the external auditory canal.

Suspected branchial cleft lesions should be referred for surgical excision to establish the histologic diagnosis of a subcutaneous nodule, to remove skin-communicating cystic mass prone to infectious problems, and to prevent the statistically increased likelihood of an in situ carcinoma forming in the branchial cleft remnant. Urgent emergency department treatment of these lesions is restricted to needle aspiration or limited incision and drainage of the acutely infected cyst or sinus.

Torticollis or wry neck is most commonly associated with breech presentation and a traumatic extraction of the head from the vaginal canal, inducing a contusion of the sternocleidomastoid muscle. The local hemorrhage is followed by an inflammatory healing response characterized by fibrosis and thickening of the muscle itself, which limits its motion, twists the head and neck, and produces a palpable nodule within the muscle. Such children are usually seen within the first few weeks of life with impaired mobility of their head and neck, but they also may be seen later in life with hypoplastic development of the neck and face. The differential diagnosis of wry neck includes neurologic syndromes, Sandifer's syndrome secondary to gastro-

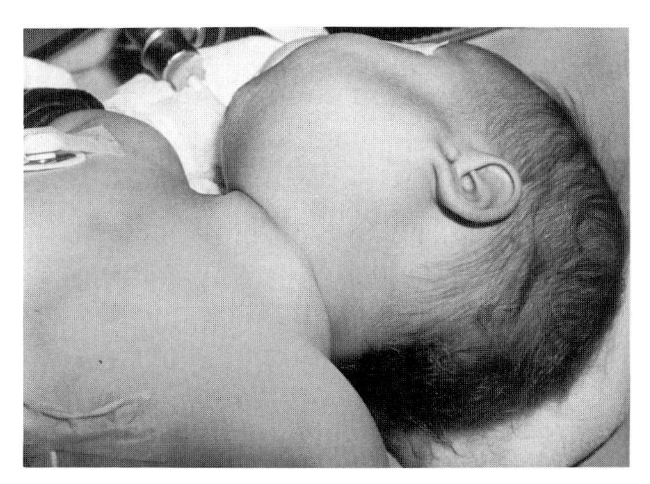

FIGURE 32-4 Infant with a large, soft cervical lesion that was a hemangioendothelioma of the parotid gland. Note also preauricular skin tag (Courtesy of J.J. Tepas, M.D.)

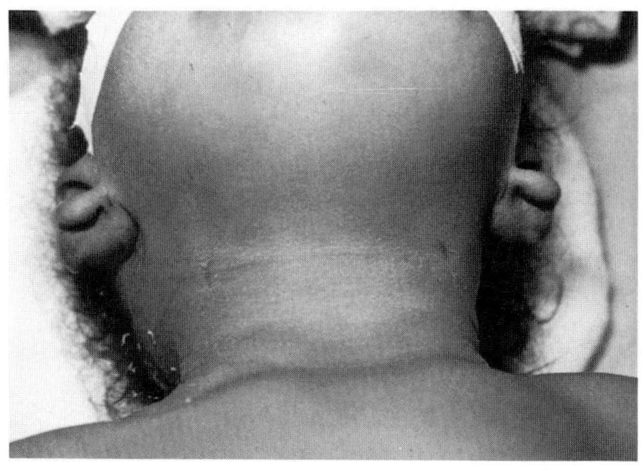

FIGURE 32-5 Bilateral branchial cleft remnants (pouch type II). Both lesions chronically drained a mucoid discharge. (Courtesy of J.J. Tepas, M.D.)

esophageal reflux, a primary muscle tumor, or even lymphadenitis. Torticollis is best treated by aggressive, active range-of-motion exercises: the child is placed in the supine position on a flat surface, and, with the shoulders held flat, the head is actively turned through a full 180° range of motion to slowly stretch the tightened sternocleidomastoid muscle. It is appropriate to teach the parents this exercise in the emergency department and then refer the child for surgical follow-up and evaluation in several weeks, since the nonresponders may require operative intervention.

Lymphangiomas are congenital aberrant lymphatic system tumors consisting of a "cluster of grapes" or multiple cystic lesions resulting from an abnormal continuity in or dilatation of lymphatic channels. Such lymphangiomas or cystic hygromas are most commonly located in the neck, although they can be found throughout a child's body, especially on the chest wall, axillae, and the extremities. These soft tissue tumors are variable in size, spongy, and filled with clear yellow or hemorrhagic fluid. Aspiration of fluid from the mass frequently confirms the diagnosis. Lymphangiomas per se are not characterized by spontaneous regression, but they do demonstrate a gradual coalescence, with restriction of their boundaries and better definition of their margins. They frequently have a history of recurrent lymphangitis with its associated acute swelling, tenderness, and occasional erythema of the overlying skin. These are the lesions that require emergent institution of broad-spectrum antibiotic therapy. Hospital admission is indicated if the acute inflammatory swelling might potentially compromise the airway or if there is evidence of a proximal lymphangitis or systemic infection. Surgical referral is indicated electively or urgently, depending on the clinical manifestations.

Vascular malformations of the head and neck are common. These lesions can be located over the nape of the neck as the classic "stork bite" of the neonate, or they can be located anywhere on the face or neck margin itself. At one end of the spectrum of hemangiomatous lesions are port-wine stains, in which there is a purplish discoloration of the skin by a lesion located beneath the skin surface. These port-wine stains are best treated by nonoperative means such as cosmetic coverage (Covermark), although possibly the future application of laser surgery will offer even better control.

Capillary hemangiomas are characterized by a raised reddish lesion, which makes them not only visible but palpable (Figure 32-6A). Such capillary or strawberry hemangiomas spontaneously regress after an initial growth phase, the peak of the aggressive period being 2.5 to 3 years of age. This "apparent growth" in size is, in reality, the opening of more vascular channels. As the lesion begins to regress, the central portion begins to undergo an ischemic change, with formation of a whitish skin

A

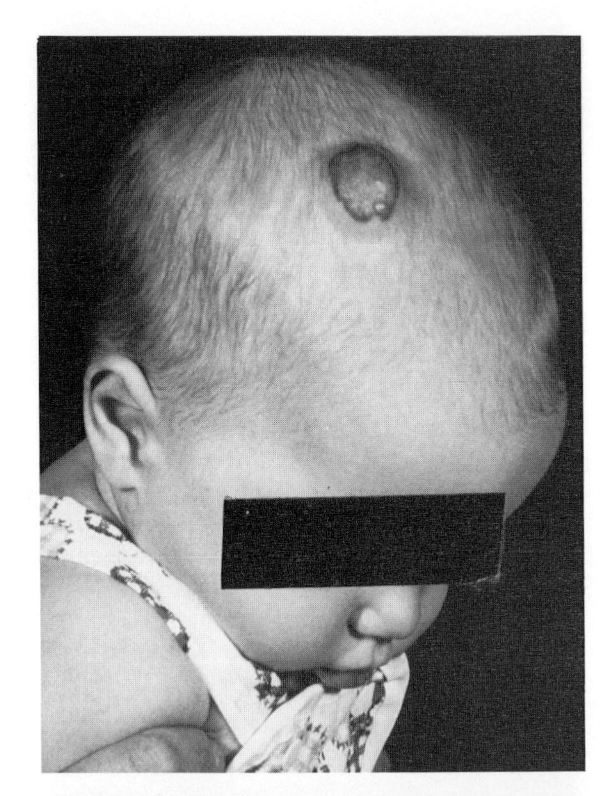

B

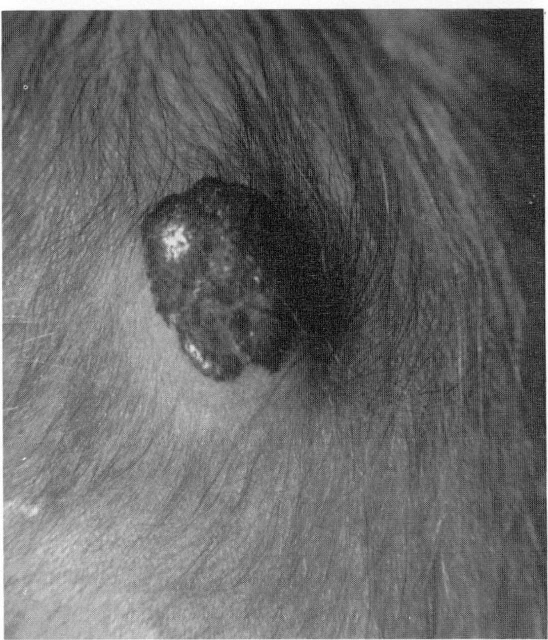

FIGURE 32-6 A, Capillary hemangioma on the scalp of an 8-month-old infant. Note the raised appearance. B, Close-up shows white, shiny skin replacing the lesion as regression occurs. (Courtesy of J.J. Tepas, M.D.)

sheen followed by occasional frank ulceration and crust formation (Figure 32-6B). Although such infarcting lesions are prone to bleeding and irritation, it is these characteristics that suggest regression and possible complete spontaneous remission. When such bleeding does occur, simple direct pressure for several minutes effectively controls the problem.

Hemangioendotheliomas are characterized by discolored skin associated commonly with a soft tissue swelling beneath the surface. Such lesions likewise undergo spontaneous regression of their capillary elements, although stromal residua may persist (Figure 32-7). Their natural history is similar to that of a standard capillary hemangioma, and preferred management is also a conservative wait for spontaneous regression. These lesions may occasionally cause platelet trapping, with a bleeding diathesis or cardiac failure (Figure 32-8). Such potential problems should be considered in the emergency department assessment.

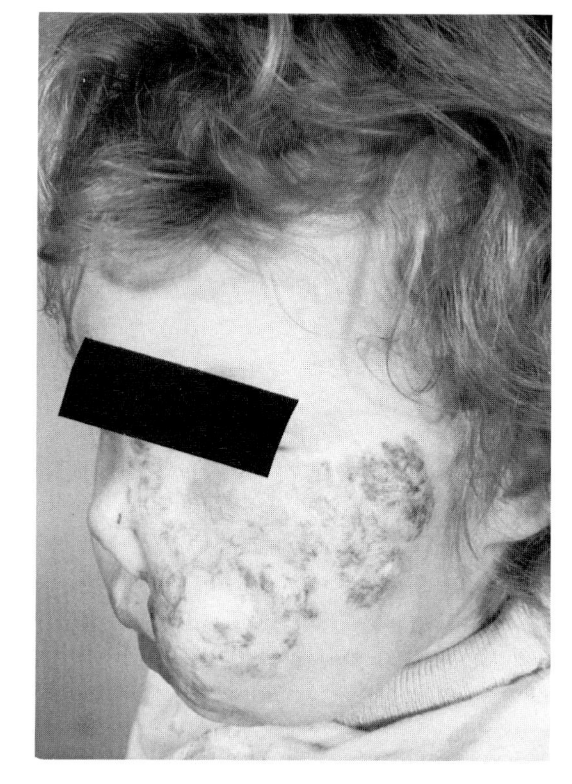

A

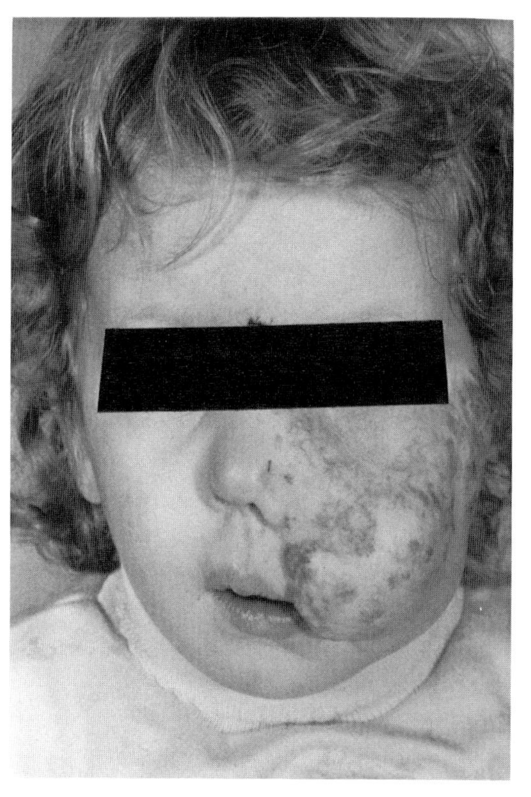

B

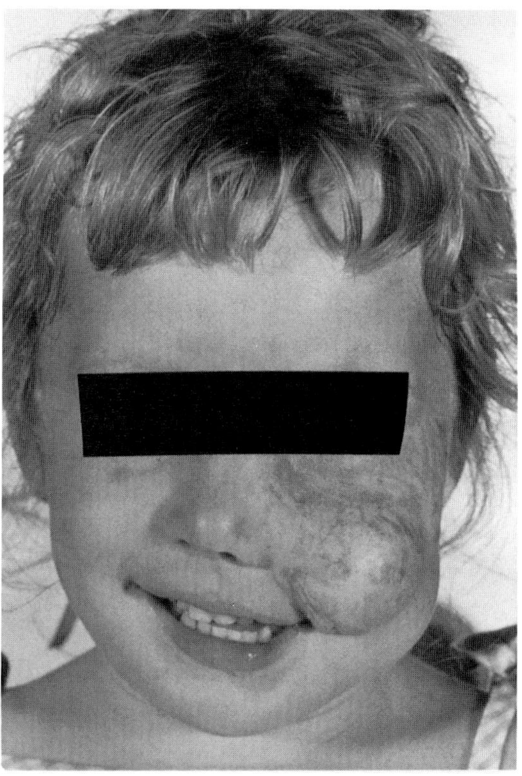

C

FIGURE 32-7 Anterior (A) and lateral (B) views of a 13-month-old girl with a large facial hemangioendothelioma. Note displacement of the nares, corner of the mouth, and medial anthus of the left eye. Views of the same child 6 months later (C and D) show regression of the lesion. Same type of lesion on the shoulder of a child (E) shows the white areas of regression. (Courtesy of J.J. Tepas, M.D.)

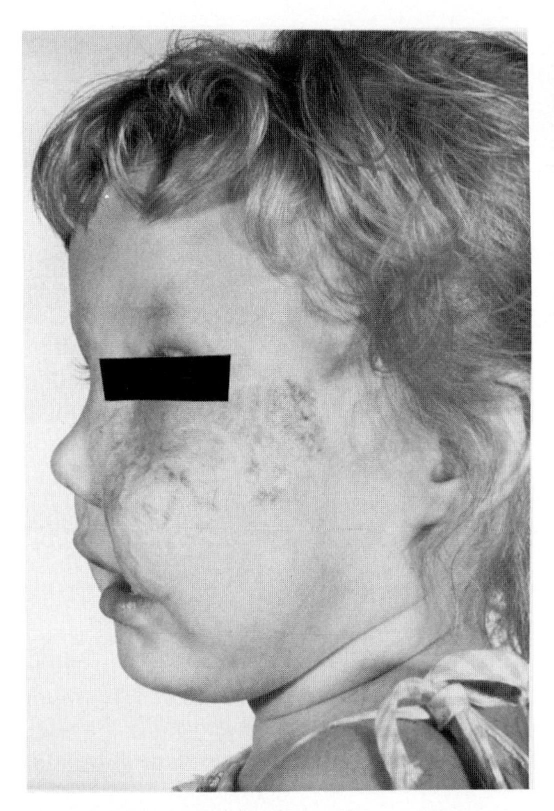

D

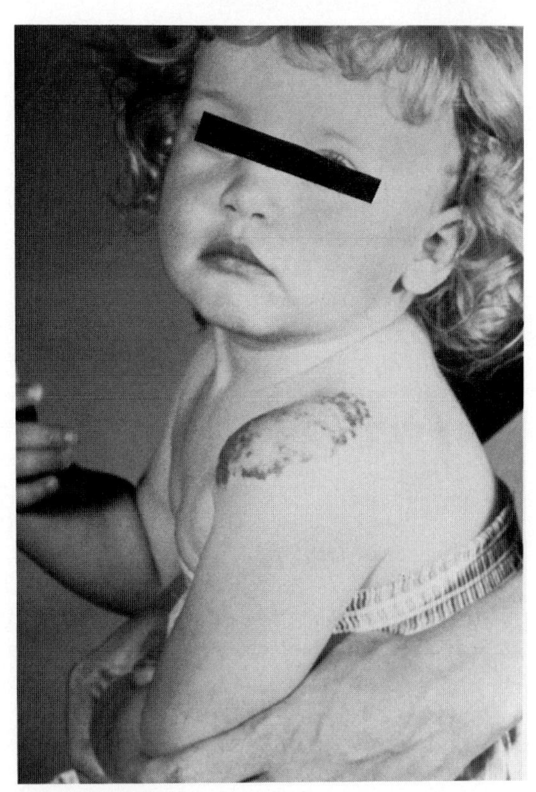

E

FIGURE 32-7 (*continued*)

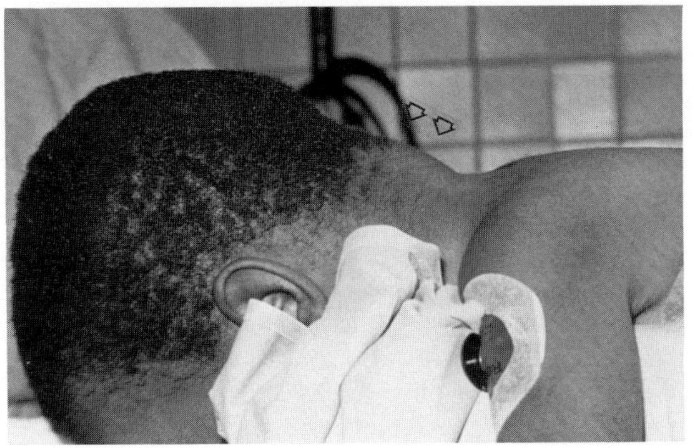

FIGURE 32-8 Six-year-old boy with a small hemangioma in the suboccipital area (*arrows*) that required excision because of severe thrombocytopenia caused by platelet trapping. (Courtesy of J.J. Tepas, M.D.)

Cavernous hemangiomas consist of large "lakes" of vascular channels and are not characterized by spontaneous regression. Many lesions are true mixed hemangiomas with capillary, port-wine, and cavernous components, and their treatment needs to be individualized.

Arteriovenous fistulas represent still another form of vascular malformation, but such congenital fistulas are characterized by multiple connecting channels rather than the single isolated channel that occurs after vascular trauma and is amenable to surgical division. The diagnosis can be suspected from the presence of increased blood flow (warmth, erythema, overgrowth, bruit) to a part.

Venous lakes may occur in the head and neck, especially in the supraclavicular area. When such patients perform the Valsalva maneuver, increasing their intrathoracic pressure, a bulge becomes visible anterior to the sternocleidomastoid muscle or in the supraclavicular space, representing a venous lake of the jugular system. Angiography is a necessity to define this pathology.

THORAX

Breast Lesions

Breast lesions requiring emergency disposition are those that are infectious. These include a neonatal breast abscess or a breast abscess in an older child. Although the former is usually secondary to infection with staphylococcal organisms, the proper treatment to prevent damage to the breast bud is prompt surgical referral followed by incision and drainage, culture of the drained material, and appropriate systemic antibiotic selection.

Additional nonemergent breast pathology in the newborn child includes the extra or supernumerary nipples of polythelia and newborn breast hypertrophy secondary to the transplacental passage of maternal hormones. Premature thelarche may include drainage of secretions from the nipple, commonly occurs in the first several months of life, and is characterized by a prominent breast bud and spontaneous disappearance. Virginal hypertrophy usually occurs in adolescence, although it may precede puberty and be unilateral or bilateral. Precocious puberty may also produce breast enlargement in a premature fashion; such children point out the need for genital examination in all children with abnormal breast development.

Gynecomastia, or breast enlargement in boys, may be unilateral or bilateral and frequently appears as a tender breast enlargement and/or a subareolar nodule. These lesions usually regress spontaneously and do not require surgical excision. However, surgical excision is occasionally indicated for a very large or very tender lesion, or for one that persists unchanged for over a year.

Childhood breast tumors are usually benign. Carcinoma of the breast in a young girl is very rare. Most breast tumors in adolescent girls are fibroadenomas characterized by a discrete, firm, nontender, moveable nodule. These lesions may change with menstruation and are sensitive to hormonal growth stimulation, especially in the adolescent using contraceptive pills. A breast tumor associated with a nipple discharge most commonly is an intraductal papilloma, but it is also possible that breast lesions are secondary to true fibrocystic disease.

In the young adolescent a dominant breast nodule is ideally managed by serial examinations over one or two menstrual periods to confirm its presence and persistence. Breast biopsy under any circumstance is rarely indicated in children younger than 5 years of age. In this age group an inappropriately done biopsy may damage the breast bud and severely limit subsequent breast development.

ABDOMEN

Abdominal wall defects may occur in the midline, the lateral abdominal wall, and in the inguinoscrotal region.

Midline Abdominal Wall Lesions

Midline abdominal lesions can be localized to the area around the umbilicus or above and below that region. A weeping umbilicus may be due to either a granuloma at the site of the previous umbilical cord attachment, a patent urachus secondary to persistence of the urachal remnant at the dome of the bladder, or a patent omphalomesenteric duct connecting an epithelialized remnant extending from the antemesenteric border of the distal ileum to the umbilicus. A granuloma is best treated by outpatient excision and/or cautery using silver nitrate; usually no further difficulties occur. A patent urachus requires operative intervention after study for the presence of bladder neck or posterior urethral valve obstruction. A patent omphalomesenteric duct represents an extension of the area of the ileum from a Meckel's diverticulum and requires formal laparotomy with excision of the sinus.

Umbilical hernias are an extremely common developmental anomaly. Such hernias represent a failure of closure of the abdominal wall at the body stalk or umbilical cord. Umbilical hernias are characterized by a fascial defect through which bulges a true peritoneal sac, thereby exposing the patient to the risk of incarceration, strangulation, or even evisceration with rupture of the sac and overlying skin. All of these events require emergent surgical care and are quite rare. The more common course of a neonatal umbilical hernia is gradual contracture of the fascial ring, with spontaneous closure of the defect after several years. Elective operative intervention is deferred in boys until 4 or 5 years of age and in girls until the age of 2 or 3 years. Supraumbilical hernias, fascial defects located just above the umbilicus, with associated protrusion of intra-abdominal contents, are not characterized by spontaneous regression, and the detection of a supraumbilical hernia is an indication for elective operative repair.

A midline fascial defect extending from the umbilicus to the xiphoid process of the sternum, with prominent rectus muscle margins on either side, is a normal anatomic variant termed diastasis recti. This finding is best demonstrated by a Valsalva maneuver or by having the patient lie supine with subsequent lifting of the head to tense the abdominal wall musculature.

A midline 1.0- to 1.5-cm abdominal wall nodule between the xiphoid and umbilicus most likely represents an epiplocele. An epiplocele, in contrast to a true ventral hernia, is a protrusion of preperitoneal fat through a small midline fascial defect. Epiploceles may mimic an "acute abdomen" because of incarceration and strangulation of the fat; in such circumstances they require prompt surgical evaluation. More often they appear as an undiagnosed soft tissue nodule and should be referred for elective operative excision with closure of the fascial defect.

Lateral Abdominal Wall Lesions

Lateral abdominal wall protrusions include the very rare lumbar hernia, located in the posterior lateral lumbar triangle. A spigelian hernia is similarly rare and occurs along the lateral border of the rectus muscle where it interdigitates with the oblique musculature. Both lumbar and spigelian hernias may require elective or, rarely, urgent operative repair of the fascial weakness, but their major interest is their very infrequent occurrence and peculiar presentation inconsistent with the more classic hernias.

The inguinal hernia represents a failure of the congenital obliteration of the processus vaginalis, which normally occurs in the last trimester of pregnancy (Figure 32-9). Patency of the processus vaginalis may result in (1) a physiologic hydrocele, in which case the proximal processus has been obliterated, but fluid has been trapped in the distal scrotum; (2) a hydrocele of the spermatic cord, in which there is loculation of fluid in the midprocessus vaginalis with a proximal patency; or (3) a frank communicating or hernia-hydrocele, in which the entire processus is patent and is filled either with fluid from the abdominal cavity or with other intra-abdominal contents, depending on the diameter of the neck of the hernia sac. A physiologic hydrocele is characterized by mild scrotal swelling, present since birth, with no history of suprapubic bulging or scrotal size change. A hydrocele of the cord is represented by a swelling confined to the midinguinal canal, with an empty space in the area of the deep inguinal ring. It is at times impossible to make a distinction between this lesion and an incarcerated inguinal hernia, in which case prompt surgical referral for operative exploration is indicated. A communicating hydrocele may also be noted during the newborn period and demonstrates intermittent scrotal size change. It is more appropriately designated an indirect inguinal hernia whenever the diameter of the neck of the processus vaginalis is large enough to accommodate any of the intra-abdominal contents. Inguinal hernias are more common in the premature child, on the right side, in boys, and in children with a previous family history of such hernias.

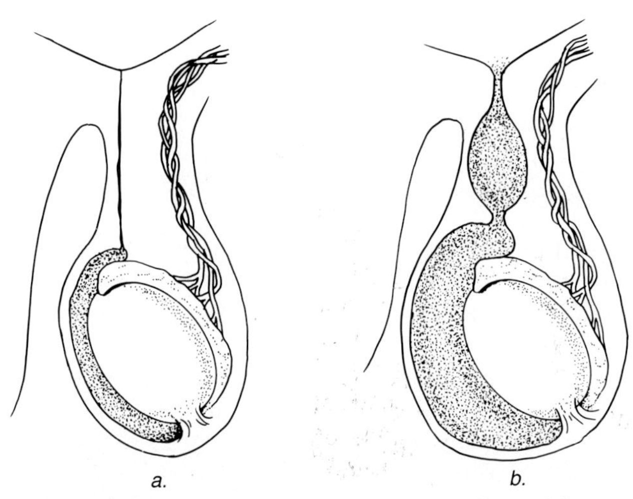

FIGURE 32-9 Lesions related to incomplete obliteration of processus vaginalis. A, Normal obligation of processus vaginalis; B, communicating hydrocele or hernia-hydrocele.

Once an inguinal hernia is diagnosed, it should be electively repaired to prevent the potential complications of incarceration and strangulation. Although this complication occurs in only 5% to 10% of children, it is nevertheless a devastating event that complicates greatly the operative repair of an inguinal hernia.

The differential diagnosis of an inguinal canal swelling in the presence of a normally placed scrotal testis includes an inguinal hernia, a hydrocele of the spermatic cord, or ilioinguinal lymphadenopathy, the last being suggested especially in the presence of an infected distal extremity lesion. If the swelling is sudden in onset, the child seems irritable with signs and symptoms of a partial bowel obstruction, and the mass is tubular in nature, extending out of the area of the deep inguinal ring, then an incarcerated inguinal hernia is the likely diagnosis.

Emergency department hernia reduction is best accomplished by V-shaped distal traction of the examiner's upper hand at the area of the deep inguinal ring while simultaneously performing a distal-to-proximal transcrotal compression of the hernial contents by the lower hand. After reduction of such an incarcerated hernia, hospital admission may be needed and an early elective operative repair is indicated; but if the hernia cannot be reduced, then prompt inguinal exploration is required to avoid hernia strangulation.

PERINEUM

Scrotal Lesions

The undescended testis may arrest in descent anywhere within the abdomen, the inguinal canal, the medial to lateral thigh, or, its most common site, the suprapubic pouch. It is also possible that the empty scrotum represents an agenesis of the testis. The diagnosis of the undescended testicle necessitates a clear understanding of its embryological development and requires a relaxed child examined in a comfortable and warm environment. An undescended testicle most commonly needs to be differentiated from a retractile testis, which can be identified, grasped, and pulled to the bottom of the scrotum. The child who has pain and an acutely tender mass in the right or left side of the groin with the absence of a palpable testis in the scrotum on that side should be suspected of having either incarceration of a hernia associated with that undescended testis or torsion of the undescended testis. Testicular torsion itself is an uncommon event, but torsion of an undescended testis is statistically more likely. Such a diagnosis represents a true surgical emergency, and testicular salvage is possible only by rapid operative intervention.

Testicular torsion may also occur in the intrascrotal testis when it is twisted either extra- or intravaginally and the twisted and foreshortened spermatic cord pulls the testis to the top of the scrotum. These suddenly tender scrotal masses oftentimes are associated with pain, nausea, and vomiting, and they are absolute surgical emergencies requiring rapid differential diagnosis by physical examination, urinalysis, ultrasound, or nuclear medicine scan to evaluate testicular blood flow.

The differential diagnosis of a painful scrotal mass includes an incarcerated hernia, testicular torsion, acute epididymitis, and torsion of the appendix testis. The last is diagnosed by localizing a discrete tender spot on the spermatic cord-testis surface in a patient whose scrotal pain is not severe. Epididymitis may produce abnormal urinalysis results and is manifest by increased testicular vascularity, as shown by either ultrasound or scanning techniques. Still another cause of the acutely tender scrotum is acute hemorrhage into a testicular tumor.

Anorectal Lesions

Anal fissures may occur secondary to local anal canal trauma, often resulting from constipation. Fissures are the most common cause of bright red rectal bleeding in childhood and are best diagnosed by either direct physical inspection or limited proctoscopy with either a proctoscope or a glass test tube. Acute fissures are best treated by stool softeners, sitz baths, and rectal lubricants such as glycerine suppositories. Chronic fissures require elective surgical referral.

Perianal abscesses require drainage and adequate decompression, a procedure best done formally in the operating room, although emergency department drainage of a tiny abscess in an infant is not inappropriate. Sitz baths help treat the acute inflammatory response and keep the area cleansed.

A late-appearing anal fistula extending from the crypts of the rectal glands through perianal soft tissue to the skin requires elective surgical follow-up.

Rectal prolapse may be without apparent cause or it may herald underlying chronic constipation or cystic fibrosis. Gentle compression usually reduces the prolapsed rectum, after which surgical referral should be obtained as soon as possible. In the interim, efforts should be made to soften the stool and limit the time a child spends on the toilet.

Pilonidal dimples are common congenital variations in children. Such dimples may appear only as a skin lesion over the sacrococcygeal area, or they may be associated with a subcutaneous sinus leading to a cyst beneath the skin. The acute pilonidal abscess following a secondary infection requires incision and drainage. Subsequent elective operative removal of the chronically infected lesion is then indicated. Prophylactic surgical excision is not required for the shallow, broad-based, noninfected dimple.

EXTREMITIES

Cysts

Cystic lesions of the extremities include ganglia, which represent synovial sheath cysts. These are usually located on the dorsum of the wrist, although they can be located in any joint or tendon synovial sheath area. These soft, spongy subcutaneous masses may produce discomfort and are best treated by splinting and joint rest. A Baker's cyst represents a ganglion-type synovial sheath cyst located in the popliteal space. This lesion may produce a mass as well as discomfort, and elective surgical referral is indicated.

Infections

Infections of the extremities require a categorization of severity with a logical treatment plan. Most skin infections are discussed in Chapters 28 and 29.

Lymphangitis represents infection in the lymphatic channels and may extend proximally from a paronychia, felon, an infected abrasion, or some other infectious source. It is recognized by a red streaking up an arm or leg. If it progresses to the point of proximal lymphadenitis in the axilla or inguinal area, the possibility of bacteremia or sepsis mandates immediate referral for admission and systemic antibiotic therapy.

Foreign Bodies

Metallic, glass, or wooden foreign bodies should be suspected as a cause for any chronically draining extremity wound. Radiologic analysis in the emergency department is helpful to confirm the presence of radiopaque materials. Only the most superficial foreign bodies should be removed in the emergency department. Deeper materials should be referred for elective removal in a controlled operating room environment. (For additional discussion, see Chapter 30, "Skin and Subcutaneous Injuries.")

Nevi

Nevi are classified as raised or flat, pigmented or nonpigmented, and hair bearing or hair free. Spider nevi or spider angiomas represent true vascular hamartomas and are not true nevi. Congenital nevi do have a documented increased incidence of malignant degeneration, and such patients should be referred for surgical evaluation. The presence of irritation and erythema, bleeding, growth, or darkening are all warning signs that biopsy and surgical excision should be considered. The location of a nevus on the plantar surface of the foot, the palm of the hand, or the genitalia does not per se indicate considering operative intervention.

Bibliography

Koop CE: *Visible and Palpable Lesions in Children.* New York, Grune & Stratton, 1976.

Dennis J. Hoelzer
Bruce D. Taylor

33 Animal, Insect, and Snake Bites

ANIMAL AND HUMAN BITES

Domestic Animals

Approximately 85% of the reported animal bites in the United States are inflicted by dogs, and it is estimated that there are one million people bitten each year.[1–3] The incidence of dog bites is increasing and is felt to be due to the greater number of canines and the growing use of trained guard dogs for private and commercial security.

The typical dog bite victim is a male under 20 years of age who is bitten by his own pet or some other familiar dog. Injuries most frequently occur between 1 and 9 P.M. and during the summer months. Injuries to the upper and lower extremities account for 74% of reported cases, with head and neck involvement in 10% to 15%.[4] Facial wounds are more common in young children and teenagers.

Therapy in the emergency department includes washing of the wound with soap and water, debridement of devitalized tissue under local anesthesia, and copious, forceful irrigation with sterile saline solution.[5,6] (The last can be effectively accomplished by irrigating the wound with saline delivered through a 19-gauge needle and a 20-mL syringe.) In general, wounds of the face can be excised, debrided, irrigated, and closed primarily, but surgical consultation is strongly recommended.[7] Wounds elsewhere on the body are best allowed to heal by secondary intention. Bites near bones and joints are at risk for joint space infections and osteomyelitis, and baseline x-ray films should be considered.

Adequate tetanus prophylaxis is mandatory as the possibility of infection and intoxication from *Clostridium tetani*, while remote, is real. Tetanus toxoids should be given on the basis of the patient's immunization status (see Chapter 30, Table 30-1).

The prophylactic use of antibiotics for dog bite wounds is controversial.[8,9] Some experts recommend culturing samples from all wounds as well as administering antibiotics. Even with good wound care and prophylactic antibiotics, approximately 5% to 15% of patients develop secondary wound infections with *Pasteurella multocida, Streptococcus viridans,* and other aerobic and anaerobic bacteria.[10] We recommend the use of penicillin V or ampicillin prophylacticly for a 3- to 5-day period. For children with penicillin allergies, erythromycin can be substituted.

The bites of cats and other animals may be handled in a similar fashion. Injuries from farm animals often result in greater tissue damage and frequently necessitate surgical intervention. A summary of animal bite management is provided in Exhibit 33-1.

Human Bites

Human bites, because of the quantity and quality of the bacterial flora of the human mouth, need to be

Exhibit 33-1 Management of Animal and Human Bites

Animal Bites
1. Wash the wound with soap and water.
2. Debride devitalized tissue after administering local anesthesia.
3. Irrigate the wound forcefully with a copious quantity of sterile saline.
4. Give penicillin V, 40 mg/kg/24 h po, q6h for 3–5 d.*
5. Provide tetanus prophylaxis.
6. Consider primary closure and surgical consultation for facial wounds.
7. Take x-ray films of wounds near bones or joints.

Human Bites
1. Take samples from the wound for culturing.
2. Wash the wound with soap and water.
3. Debride devitalized tissue after administering local anesthesia.
4. Irrigate the wound forcefully with a copious quantity of sterile saline.
5. Consider hospitalization for all but the most trivial injuries.
6. For minimal wounds give penicillin V, 40 mg/kg/24 h po, q6h for 3–5 d.*

* If the patient is allergic to penicillin, give erythromycin, 50 mg/kg/24 h po, q6h for 3–5 d.

treated aggressively. All but the most trivial human bites require hospitalization for operative debridement, intravenous antibiotics, and immobilization of the affected part.[11,12] Bites of the head and neck, in most cases, can be closed primarily after adequate wound preparation. Many authorities feel strongly that samples for culturing should be taken from the depth of the wound before treatment, with changes made in antibiotic administration as culture results become available. Human bites to the hand may damage nerve, tendon, and neurovascular structures, and the risk of soft tissue infection and subsequent loss of function must be remembered. Management of human bites is summarized in Exhibit 33-1.

Rabies

Human rabies is fortunately a rare occurrence in the United States. In 1981 there were only two cases reported to the Center for Disease Control. Still, approximately 30,000 individuals are vaccinated yearly for rabies prophylaxis.[13]

Table 33-1 depicts the relative risk of rabies transmission by different animal species. Wild animals are the major reservoir for rabies and transmit the virus to humans, pets, and livestock. In the United States and Canada, foxes, skunks, raccoons, and bats are the major vectors. State health departments survey both wild and domestic animals and can help define the degree of risk of rabies virus transmission by animal species.

TABLE 33-1 Risk of Rabies Transmission by Animal Species

Degree of Risk	Animal
High	Bats, skunks, bobcats, badgers, wolves, coyotes, weasels, racoons, foxes
Moderate	Stray dogs and cats; pet skunks and mongooses; abnormally behaving dogs, cats, farm animals
Low	Normal pet dogs, cats, farm animals
Negligible	Rats, mice, squirrels, gerbils, chipmunks, guinea pigs, hamsters, rabbits

Domestic animals are rarely rabid because of widespread vaccination programs. Dogs and cats, both capable of transmitting rabies, do so only when the virus appears in their saliva.[14] Those animals who remain asymptomatic during a 10-day period of observation after the bite are not considered infectious, and, in general, the risk of rabies from an immunized pet is negligible. On the other hand, the unprovoked bite of a stray dog or cat must be seriously considered as a potential source of rabies, especially if local wild animals are known to be rabid.

The initiation of antirabies therapy must be based upon the type of animal that has inflicted the bite as well as other determining factors: the severity of the bite, its location (on the head, neck, or hands), the type of virus in the animal's saliva and the virulence of that viral strain, the immune status of the biting animal, and the adequacy of wound management and vaccination.[15] Once it has been determined that there was a chance of rabies transmission, additional therapy is necessary (Exhibit 33-2).

Treatment is passive immunotherapy with rabies immune globulin at a dose of 20 IU/kg. Half of this

Exhibit 33-2 Initiation of Antirabies Therapy*

Bites from Animals of Low or Negligible Risk
1. Report the injury to local authorities.
2. Observe the animal for 10 d. If it remains asymptomatic, no antirabies therapy is required. If the animal becomes symptomatic (purposeless movements, drooling, spasms of neck, vocal cord paralysis), submit it for pathologic examination and initiate antirabies therapy.

Bites from Animals of High or Moderate Risk
1. Report the injury to the local or state health department.
2. If possible, capture the animal and deliver it to the appropriate authorities for confinement, observation, or examination of brain tissues (microscopic examination with Seller's stain or fluorescent antibody test).
3. Begin antirabies therapy.

* Your state health departments can estimate the degree of risk of rabies transmission and recommend the appropriateness of antirabies treatment.

dose is injected into the tissues adjacent to the wound, when feasible, and the other half is administered intramuscularly. Immunotherapeutic vaccination with human diploid cell rabies vaccine is given on days 0, 3, 7, 14, and 28. Adequate follow-up for the vaccination program must be established before the patient is discharged from the emergency department.

INSECT BITES

Millions of people are bitten by insects each year. For the most part these injuries can be managed conservatively and will result in no serious sequelae. Approximately 25,000 people per year suffer hypersensitivity reactions, and 40 to 50 people die each year as the result of insect stings or bites.[16,17] These deaths are attributed almost exclusively to anaphylactic reactions and not to the direct effect of the insect's venom. Table 33-2 and Exhibit 33-3 summarize the characteristics and management of anaphylactic reactions.

Insect bites may be divided into two groups: (1) those of biting and piercing arthropods that inject their venom with an apparatus located anteriorly or associated with their mouth parts (black widow spider, brown recluse spider, tarantula, centipede, and kissing bug) and (2) those of stinging arthropods who inject their venom by a stinger located posteriorly (ants, bees, wasps, hornets, yellow jackets, and scorpions).

It is estimated that eight people per thousand are allergic to insect bites and that four of these individuals are severely sensitive. Part of the treatment of these individuals should include patient education about desensitization programs; the availability of emergency kits; the risk of serum sickness, which may occur from 1 to 2 weeks after a systemic reaction to an insect bite; and the advisability of wearing or carrying identification that describes the allergy.

TABLE 33-2 Characteristics of an Anaphylactic Reaction

Effects	Characteristics
Local	Pain and swelling at the site of injury
Systemic	Pruritus, urticaria, flushing of the skin, dyspnea, weakness, anxiety, nausea, abdominal cramps, loss of consciousness
Respiratory	Dyspnea, rhinitis, sneezing, cough, bronchospasm, wheezing, angioedema, respiratory arrest
Gastrointestinal	Abdominal cramps, diarrhea, sudden involuntary defecation, nausea and vomiting
Cardiovascular	Vasodilation with hypotension, cardiac arrhythmias, syncope, circulatory collapse
Late	Urinary incontinence, uterine contractions, serum sickness

Exhibit 33-3 Management of Anaphylaxis

Mild: Itching and Urticaria

1. Epinephrine (1 : 1000): 0.1–0.3 mL SC
2. Tourniquet, placed proximal to the site of injury
3. Remove stinger if still present

Anaphylactic Shock

1. Epinephrine (1 : 1000): 0.1–0.3 mL SC
2. Epinephrine (1 : 1000): 0.1–0.3 mL injected into the site of injury (to decrease absorption of the insect venom)
3. Epinephrine (1 : 10,000): 1–2 mL IV for severe hypotension
4. Epinephrine may be repeated at 10- to 20-min intervals
5. Tourniquet, placed proximal to the site of injury
6. Ensure an adequate airway (endotracheal intubation, tracheotomy)
7. Supplemental O_2
8. Urticaria: administer diphenhydramine, 2 mg/kg IV or 5 mg/kg/24 h po
9. Intravenous fluids: saline or plasma expanders to treat hypotension
10. Hydrocortisone: 7 mg/kg IV, then 7 mg/kg/24 h IV
11. Bronchospasm: aminophylline, 7 mg/kg diluted in 2 equal volumes of saline, given IV over a 5- to 10-min period
12. Persistent hypotension: metaraminol, 0.4 mg/kg IV, or norepinephrine bitartrate, 4 mL in 1000-mL infusion—titrate effect by minidrip infusion
13. Warm patient: Trendelenburg position
14. Empty gastric contents

Stinging Arthropods

The major offenders of the order of stinging arthropods are the yellow jacket, wasp, hornet, and honeybee. Although the yellow jacket bite is the most likely to produce anaphylaxis, there is cross-sensitivity to the antigens of these insects, and one insect's bite can trigger an allergic response to any of the others. The yellow jacket, wasp, and hornet have stingers usually contaminated with bacteria whereas the honeybee is seldom colonized. Only the female members can sting because the stinging apparatus is a modification of their ovipositor. The honeybee is unable to remove her stinger after introduction, and subsequently, as the bee exits, a portion of her abdomen and venom sac remain in contact with the victim.

Reactions to these injuries depends on several factors: amount of venom, site of sting, number of

Exhibit 33-4 Management of Local Reactions to Stings from Bees, Wasps, Hornets, Yellow Jackets, and Ants

1. *Scrape* the bee stinger out of the site of injury.
2. Wash the site with soap and water.
3. For itching give diphenhydramine, 5 mg/kg/24 h po in 4 doses.
4. For pain use topical application of cold compresses, calamine lotion, corticosteroid cream or lotion, or aerosol spray of benzocaine.

stings, and degree of sensitivity of the individual. Therapy is summarized in Exhibit 33-4.

Black Widow Spiders

Black widow spiders are identified by their shiny, coal black, button-shaped bodies. The female is much larger than the male and is the one that induces injury. She has a red hourglass marking on her underside and is approximately one-half inch long with a leg span of about two inches. Her normal habitat is around rocks, debris, basements, garages, and privies. She weaves a characteristically tangled web that leads into a dark corner. The species is prevalent in the south, the Ohio valley, and the west coast but can be found in all states except Alaska.[18]

Her bite is characterized by a pinprick sensation, redness, and fang marks. A dull, numbing pain develops in the affected extremity after several hours and may persist for several days. A bite of the lower extremity may cause abdominal pain whereas a bite of the upper extremity can cause shoulder, back, and chest pain with associated rigidity, fasciculation, and weakness of large muscle groups. Nausea, vomiting, headache, sweating, and abdominal pain are frequent findings.[19] Severe reactions include convulsions, paralysis, shock, cyanosis, and respiratory and cardiac collapse. Death occurs in 4% to 5% of untreated cases.

These patients require hospitalization. The area of the bite should be cleansed with soap and water and ice packs should be applied. Antivenin is the mainstay of treatment and should be administered as soon as possible (2.5 mL IM or IV following a negative skin test for horse serum sensitivity).[20] Symptoms usually subside within 3 to 5 hours, but a second dose of antivenin may be required. Calcium gluconate, 500 mg/kg/d IV, and methocarbamol, 60 mg/kg/d, in four to six divided IV doses, are useful for relieving muscle spasm.[21] Treatment is summarized in Exhibit 33-5.

Exhibit 33-5 Management of Spider Bites

Black Widow Spider Bite

1. Wash the wound with soap and water.
2. Apply an ice pack.
3. Admit the victim to the hospital.
4. Give antivenin (after negative skin test for horse serum sensitivity).
   a. Lyovac antivenin (Merck Sharp & Dohme), 2.5 mL IM or IV for victims with severe symptoms or children less than 12 yr of age
   b. Calcium gluconate, 500 mg/kg/24 h IV in 4 to 6 divided doses
   c. Methocarbamol, 60 mg/kg/24 h IV q6h
5. Do not give narcotics (potentiates effects of venom).

Brown Recluse Spider Bite

1. Wash the wound with soap and water.
2. Give antihistamines for itching.
3. Admit symptomatic victims to the hospital.
4. Administer parenteral corticosteroids.
5. Perform an early total excision if the lesion is greater than 1 cm.
6. Give analgesics and antibiotics as indicated.
7. Order baseline laboratory coagulation tests.

Brown Recluse Spiders

Both the male and the female brown recluse spider are venomous. They have a tan to brown body and are approximately one-half inch in length with a leg span of two inches. A distinct, dark, violin-shaped marking appears at the top of the spider's cephalothorax and has accounted for its nickname of the "fiddle back" spider. This venomous spider is found most commonly in the south central United States and is a nocturnal hunter that often bites its victims while they are in bed or dressing.

The initial symptom of a bite is a mild sting. Pain becomes prevalent within 2 to 8 hours after injury, with erythema and blister formation. Within 3 to 4 days, the central area of the wound turns dark violet in color, becomes firm, ulcerates, and forms a black eschar. This eschar separates after several weeks and the wound heals by secondary epithelialization. Systemic symptoms occur within 24 to 48 hours; they are not related to the degree of local reaction and can even precede significant local findings. Symptoms and signs are headache, fever, chills, nausea, vomiting, drowsiness, joint pain, morbilliform rash, cyanosis, hypotension, convulsions, hemolysis, disseminated intravascular coagulation, and, rarely, death.

Medical management (Exhibit 33-5) includes antihistamines to control itching, corticosteroids for systemic symptoms, and early total excision of the bite area if it measures greater than 1 cm in width.[22] These patients require hospitalization.

Other Arthropods

Tarantula bites have an unearned sinister reputation in the United States. Fortunately, the tarantulas of Central America, which are poisonous, are not common in the United States. The clinical picture includes local pain, edema, and erythema. Symptomatic treatment with antibiotics and analgesics for pain relief is all that is necessary.

Centipede, kissing bug, and tick bites are treated conservatively with antihistamines, local wound care, and analgesics. (For a discussion of tick bites and Rocky Mountain spotted fever, see Chapter 29, "Dermatologic Disorders," and Chapter 36, "Infectious Diseases.")

SNAKE BITES

Annually, it is estimated that there are 45,000 snake bites of which 8,000 are poisonous.[23] Only about 15 people die each year as a result of these injuries, but local tissue involvement often leads to permanent deformity or amputation. The treatment of poisonous snake bites is controversial, and various treatment recommendations are often diametrically opposed, but it is clear that the low mortality is due to early and aggressive medical management.

Because snakes hibernate, 90% of all snake bites occur between April and October.[24] The majority of bites are to males; about half of the victims are children and young adults. Ninety percent of the bites are to the extremities, with the majority to the legs.

There are two families of poisonous snakes native to the United States. The *Crotalidae* or pit vipers include the rattlesnake, the cottonmouth or water moccasin, and the copperhead. They are identified by facial pits located between the nostril and eye on each side of the head, vertical elliptical pupils, a triangular head, prominent maxillary fangs, and a single row of subcaudal plates on the tail. Rattlesnakes have interlocking horny segments on the distal tail.

The *Elapidae* family is represented by the coral snake. It has a characteristic tricolor pattern of red, yellow or white, and black circular bands. Coral snakes are fairly shy reptiles and do not lunge or immediately inject their venom like the pit vipers. Instead, they must chew on their victim in order to envenomate. Unlike pit vipers, their bites may demonstrate little local reaction but have severe systemic involvement.

About 20% of the bites of poisonous snakes do not involve envenomation (even higher with the coral snake).[25] Russell[23] feels that many "cures" described in the literature are attributable simply to the lack of envenomation.

Following envenomation by a pit viper, there is immediate swelling around the area of bite, often within 5 minutes. Within an hour edema may involve the entire extremity. Immediate pain is common, especially with rattlesnake bites. Ecchymosis occurs within hours, followed by vesiculations with thrombosis of the superficial vessels and sloughing of injured tissues. Untreated bites may compromise the neurovascular bundle with necrosis and gangrene.

Exhibit 33-6 Management of Snake Bites

First Aid

1. Discontinue contact with the snake to prevent further bites.
2. Identify the snake. If possible, kill the snake and transport it with the child for definitive identification. If this cannot be accomplished, note important body characteristics, e.g., configuration of eyes, coloring, length.
3. Keep the child calm.
4. Apply tourniquets above and below the wound tight enough to occlude only venous and lymphatic drainage. If edema increases, place new tourniquets before releasing the initial ones.
5. Use incision and suction for bites of moderate to great severity. If this cannot be done immediately, it should be omitted.
6. Do not give the child anything by mouth.
7. Maintain the injured body part at the level of the victim's heart in a normal physiologic position.
8. Do not apply ice packs to the area of the wound.
9. Transport the patient safely and quickly to the nearest emergency center capable of delivering therapy.

Treatment in the Emergency Department

1. Contact appropriate personnel for definitive care.
2. Confirm envenomation. If it occurred, admit the child to the hospital.
3. Obtain a thorough but rapid history that includes the child's age, weight, allergies, and health status. Identify the snake and determine its size. Elicit an interval history, including a description of first aid measures taken.
4. Perform a physical examination to evaluate the child's cardiopulmonary status; pay careful attention to the airway and perfusion. Perform a neurologic examination that includes the patient's ability to handle secretions and diaphragmatic strength. Carefully note the quality of pulses, motor function, sensation, and amount of swelling in the affected extremity.
5. Start a large-bore IV (5% lactated Ringer's solution).
6. Order laboratory tests: complete blood count, clotting time, prothrombin time, partial thromboplastin time, fibrinogen level, fibrin split products, platelet count, serum creatine phosphokinase level, serum electrolytes, typing and cross-matching for blood products.
7. Do not release the tourniquets until the appropriate antivenin and tests for sensitivity to horse serum are available and until medical personnel are in attendance.

Systemic symptoms include nausea, fatigue, sweating, muscle fasciculations, salivation, melena, and hematemesis. Alterations in renal function include decreased glomerular filtration, hematuria, hemoglobinuria, glycosuria, and proteinuria. Disseminated intravascular coagulopathy, manifested by decreased platelets, thrombocytopenia, prolonged prothrombin time, low fibrinogen, and elevated fibrin split products, is an ominous sign. Coral snake envenomation classically results in neurologic involvement, but cardiopulmonary collapse can also occur. Bulbar paralysis may cause respiratory failure; marked salivation is also a problem. Durand[25] found that if death occurs, it is usually within 24 hours.

The management of poisonous snake bites is indeed a true medical emergency. Because of the complexity of successful management, children with snake bites should be admitted to the hospital, and their care should be provided by personnel familiar and ready to handle the spectrum of problems that may occur. Exhibit 33-6 is a brief outline of first aid and emergency center care.

References

1. Newman EC: Animal bites as a public health disease. *Tex Med,* November 1977, pp 49–52.
2. *Veterinary Public Health Notes,* US Dept of Health, Education and Welfare publication, Atlanta, Center for Disease Control, November 1975.
3. Moore RM Jr, Zehmer RB, Moulthrop JI, et al: Surveillance of animal-bite cases in the United States, 1971–1972. *Arch Environ Health* 1977;32:267–270.
4. Harris D, Imperato PJ, Oken B: Dog bites—an unrecognized epidemic. *Bull NY Acad Med* 1974;50:981–1000.
5. Dean DJ, Baer GM, Thompson WR: Studies on the local treatment of rabies-infected wounds. *Bull WHO* 1963;28:477–486.
6. Callaham ML: Treatment of common dog bites: Infection risk factors. *JACEP* 1978;7:83–87.
7. Graham WP III, Calabretta AM, Miller SH: Dog bites. *Am Fam Physician,* January 1977, pp 132–137.
8. Callaham ML: Prophylactic antibiotics in common dog bite wounds: A controlled study. *Ann Emerg Med* 1980;9:410–414.
9. Elenbaas RM, McNabney WK, Robinson WA: Prophylactic antibiotics and dog bite wounds. *JAMA* 1981;246:833–834.
10. Saphir DA, Carter GR: Gingival flora of the dog with special reference to bacteria associated with bites. *J Clin Microbiol* 1976;3:344–349.
11. Tomasetti BJ, Walker L, Gormley MB, et al: Human bites of the face. *J Oral Surg* 1979;37:565–568.
12. Brandt FA: Human bites of the ear. *Plast Reconstr Surg* 1969;43:130–134.
13. Rabies prevention. *MMWR* 1980;29:265–280.
14. Cat rabies exposure in Iowa—1981. *MMWR* 1982;31:67–73.
15. Johnson HN: Rabies virus, in Horsfall FL, Tamm I (eds): *Viral and Rickettsial Infections of Man,* ed 4. Philadelphia, JB Lippincott Co, 1965, pp 814–840.
16. Frazier CA: Insect stings—a medical emergency. *JAMA* 1976;235:2410–2411.
17. Light WC, Reisman RE: Stinging insect allergy: Changing concepts. *Postgrad Med,* April 1976, pp 153–157.
18. Baerg WJ: The black widow and five other venomous spiders in the United States. *Ark Agr Exp Sta Bull* 1959;608:1–43.
19. James JA, Sellars WA, Austin OM, et al: Reactions following suspected spider bite: A form of loxoscelism? *Am J Dis Child* 1961;102:395–398.
20. Schmaus JW: Bites of spiders and other arthropods, in Conn HF (ed): *Current Therapy, 1970.* Philadelphia, WB Saunders Co, 1970, pp 883–884.
21. Russell FE: Venomous animal injuries. *Curr Probl Pediatr,* July 1973, pp 1–48.
22. Auer AI, Hershey FB: Surgery for necrotic bites of the brown spider. *Arch Surg* 1974;108:612–618.
23. Russell FE, Carlson RW, Wainschel J, et al: Snake venom poisoning in the United States: Experiences with 550 cases. *JAMA* 1975;233:341–344.
24. Parrish HM: Incidence of treated snakebites in the United States. *Public Health Rep* 1966;81:269–276.
25. Durand LS, Hiebert JM, Rodeheaver GT, et al: Snake venom poisoning. *Compr Ther,* May 1981, pp 51–62.

Part IX

Hematologic, Endocrine, and Metabolic Disorders

Thomas H. Howard
William H. Meyer

34 Hematologic and Oncologic Emergencies

HEMATOLOGIC EMERGENCIES

The emergencies that occur with hematologic diseases are primarily due to the development of severe anemia, bleeding, and infection. Initial management of these emergencies requires a rapid, definitive diagnosis. Management often involves transfusion with blood products or use of antibiotics. The diagnosis of the disorder must be accurate since it often determines whether infusion of blood products is necessary and which products should be used.

Severe Anemia

Anemia is defined by the patient's hematocrit and hemoglobin level. Age-related values for the mean and lower limit of normal hemoglobin levels and hematocrit are shown in Table 34-1. Coulter counter values that fall below the lower limits for hemoglobin and hematocrit constitute anemia. For the purposes of this discussion, hemoglobin values less than 8.5 g/dL define severe anemia, and those greater than 8.5 g/dL define mild and moderate degrees of anemia.

Severe anemia can occur in association with any congenital or acquired anemia, and any patient with hemolysis or blood loss can rapidly make the transition from a mild or moderate to a severe degree of anemia in less than 24 hours. Although the office approach to mild degrees of anemia is variable, many of these patients receive trials of iron with limited diagnostic evaluation. Ideally, any patient with anemia should be evaluated by determination of a Coulter blood count (CBC), a platelet count, differential white cell count, reticulocyte count, and review of the peripheral smear. In a patient with a hemoglobin value less than 8.5 g/dL, such a diagnostic evaluation and, *at least,* close outpatient follow-up are imperative. Hospital admission for evaluation of severe anemia should be considered for the patient with

1. an uncertain diagnosis and previously normal hemoglobin levels
2. active bleeding
3. a documented rapidly decreasing hematocrit
4. reticulocytopenia
5. a clinically ill appearance

Transfusion is necessary in a minority of patients with severe anemia; however, blood typing and cross-matching should be instituted for any patient whose hemoglobin values or clinical status is deteriorating or could potentially deteriorate. Transfusion should be administered to severely anemic patients who have (1) active hemorrhage and hypotension, (2) altered sensorium, or (3) signs of congestive heart failure. A hemoglobin level less

TABLE 34-1 Red Blood Cell Values at Various Ages: Mean and Lower Limit of Normal (−2 SD)*

	Hemoglobin (g/dL)		Hematocrit (%)		Red Cell Count (10^{12}/L)		MCV† (fL)		MCH (pg)		MCHC (g/dL)	
Age	Mean	−2 SD	Mean	−2 SD	Mean	−2 SD	Mean	−2 SD	Mean	−2 SD	Mean	−2 SD
Birth (cord blood)	16.5	13.5	51	42	4.7	3.9	108	98	34	31	33	30
1–3 d (capillary)	18.5	14.5	56	45	5.3	4.0	108	95	34	31	33	29
1 wk	17.5	13.5	54	42	5.1	3.9	107	88	34	28	33	28
2 wk	16.5	12.5	51	39	4.9	3.6	105	86	34	28	33	28
1 mo	14.0	10.0	43	31	4.2	3.0	104	85	34	28	33	29
2 mo	11.5	9.0	35	28	3.8	2.7	96	77	30	26	33	29
3–6 mo	11.5	9.5	35	29	3.8	3.1	91	74	30	25	33	30
0.5–2 yr	12.0	10.5	36	33	4.5	3.7	78	70	27	23	33	30
2–6 yr	12.5	11.5	37	34	4.6	3.9	81	75	27	24	34	31
6–12 yr	13.5	11.5	40	35	4.6	4.0	86	77	29	25	34	31
12–18 yr												
Female	14.0	12.0	41	36	4.6	4.1	90	78	30	25	34	31
Male	14.5	13.0	43	37	4.9	4.5	88	78	30	25	34	31
18–49 hr												
Female	14.0	12.0	41	36	4.6	4.0	90	80	30	26	34	31
Male	15.5	13.5	47	41	5.2	4.5	90	80	30	26	34	31

* These data have been compiled from several sources. Emphasis is given to recent studies employing electronic counters and to the selection of populations that are likely to exclude individuals with iron deficiency. The mean ±2 SD can be expected to include 95% of the observations in a normal population.
† Abbreviations: MCV, mean corpuscular volume; MCH, mean corpuscular hemoglobin; MCHC, mean corpuscular hemoglobin concentration.
Source: Adapted with permission from Dallman PR: Blood and blood-forming tissues, in Rudolph AM, Barnett HL, Einhorn AH (eds): *Pediatrics*, ed 16. New York, Appleton-Century-Crofts, 1977, p 1111. Copyright © 1977 Appleton-Century-Crofts Inc.

than 4.5 g/dL combined with reticulocytopenia is an indication for transfusion unless the diagnostic evaluation identifies a specific therapeutic intervention that will rapidly reverse the anemia. In general, children tolerate uncomplicated anemia with hemoglobin levels of 4.5 to 6.0 g/dL with remarkable ease, and the necessity for transfusion often depends upon the specific cause of the anemia and the potential for its abrupt reversal. Transfusion is only a temporary, lifesaving solution for severe anemia and should not preempt a thorough diagnostic evaluation. Toward that end, every effort should be made to establish the cause of anemia prior to transfusion, since subsequent management of the patient depends upon that specific cause. If the patient requires transfusion, several blood samples should be stored in tubes with EDTA* anticoagulant and refrigerated. This allows specific diagnostic testing without the confusing presence of transfused, normal red cells.

A diagnostic approach to the patient with severe anemia is presented in Exhibit 34-1. This schema is constructed from the basic laboratory parameters of the CBC (hemoglobin level, hematocrit, indices, white blood count [WBC]), smear, differential WBC, platelet count, and reticulocyte count. The purpose of this approach is to channel the diagnostic efforts of the physician in general directions and ultimately to arrive at a diagnosis that a specific test can confirm.

All of the core laboratory parameters of anemia are doubtless familiar to all physicians, with the exception of the peripheral smear. The peripheral smear is a window on the causes of anemia in that recognition of specific cellular forms, e.g., ovalocytes, spherocytes, and abnormal leukocytes or platelets, may allow one to suspect a specific diagnosis almost instantly. Although the initial steps in the diagnostic approach presented here are based upon the CBC, platelet count, and reticulocyte count, the steps toward a specific diagnosis usually require information from the peripheral smear. No one is blessed with an innate ability to interpret the smear; however, failure to review the peripheral smear ignores important information and assures a continued inability to make maximum use of this simple tool.

Anemia with Acute Blood Loss

In the emergency department or the primary care setting where one may encounter patients with traumatic injuries, such as those from sledding accidents or bicycle falls, acute blood loss should come to mind in an anemic patient with no prior history of

* Ethylenediaminetetraacetic acid.

Exhibit 34-1 A Diagnostic Approach to Anemia

Step 1: Hemoglobin reveals anemia.

Step 2: Determine the following:
Hb,* Hct, indices, reticulocyte count
WBC, differential WBC
Platelet count

Step 3: Consider blood loss. Note active bleeding; test stool for occult blood.

Step 4: Consider WBC, platelet count, and WBC morphology. If numbers are decreased or morphology is abnormal, obtain a bone marrow aspirate.
- A. Bone marrow abnormal
  - 1. Infiltrated with malignant cells
    - a. Leukemia
    - b. Lymphoma
    - c. Neuroblastoma
  - 2. Aplastic or fibrotic
    - a. Aplastic anemia
      - 1) Constitutional: Fanconi's anemia, dyskeratosis congenita, Schwachman-Diamond syndrome
      - 2) Acquired: chemically related or postinfectious
    - b. Fibrotic: myelofibrosis
- B. Bone marrow normal
  - 1. Microangiopathic anemia
    - a. Disseminated intravascular coagulation
    - b. Hemolytic-uremic syndrome
    - c. Kasabach-Merritt syndrome
  - 2. Hypersplenism
    - a. Secondary to chronic hepatic disease
    - b. Secondary to vascular abnormality
    - c. Secondary to metabolic disorder, e.g., lipid storage disease or mucopolysaccharidosis
  - 3. Autoimmune disorders

Step 5: Consider the reticulocyte count. An elevated reticulocyte count suggests that anemia is due to blood loss or hemolysis.
- A. Anemia with acute blood loss
- B. Acquired causes of hemolysis
  - 1. Antibodies
    - a. Idiopathic
    - b. With autoimmune disease
    - c. With immunodeficiency
    - d. With malignancy, e.g., Hodgkin's disease
  - 2. Drug exposures
    - a. G6PD deficiency
    - b. Unstable hemoglobins
  - 3. Infectious illnesses
  - 4. Mechanical injury to red cells
- C. Congenital causes of hemolysis
  - 1. Abnormal hemoglobins, e.g., SS, SC, Sβ^o thalassemia
  - 2. Abnormal membranes, e.g., HS, HE
  - 3. Enzyme deficiencies, e.g., G6PD, pyruvate kinase

Step 6: Consider the reticulocyte count and the MCV. If reticulocyte count is low (<2.5%):
- A. With decreased MCV:
  - 1. Iron deficiency
  - 2. β-Thalassemia
  - 3. α-Thalassemia
  - 4. Lead poisoning
  - 5. Anemia of chronic disease (ACD)
- B. With normal MCV:
  - 1. Transient erythroblastopenia of childhood
  - 2. ACD
  - 3. Aplastic crisis with a hemolytic process
- C. With increased MCV:
  - 1. Diamond-Blackfan anemia
  - 2. Folate deficiency
  - 3. B_{12} deficiency

* Abbreviations: Hb, hemoglobin; Hct, hematocrit; WBC, white blood count; HS, hereditary spherocytosis; HE, hereditary elliptocytosis; G6PD, glucose-6-phosphate dehydrogenase; MCV, mean corpuscular volume.

anemia. In the absence of obvious external blood loss, anemia, especially when coupled with abdominal pain, orthostatic hypotension, or gross hematuria, should suggest injury to internal organs, such as liver laceration, splenic rupture, or renal damage. The pediatric patient may also have melena, hematochezia, or hematemesis as a result of acute gastrointestinal (GI) bleeding. Acute GI bleeding in the pediatric patient can result from peptic ulceration or varices; in patients less than 2 years of age, GI bleeding may be due to such "nonadult" entities as intussusception, malrotation with gut infarction, or Meckel's diverticulum. A careful history and stool guaiac test are important in establishing blood loss as the cause of anemia. If the blood loss is acute, the red cells are normochromic and normocytic on smear, with normal indices. The reticulocyte and platelet counts are usually increased. Initial therapy of anemia caused by hemorrhage requires transfusion with whole blood, packed red cells, and fresh frozen plasma (FFP), depending upon the site of bleeding and the blood pressure. Definitive therapy depends upon the specific cause of blood loss.

Anemia with Abnormal Leukocytes or Platelets

Once acute blood loss is excluded as the cause of anemia, the next important diagnostic question is whether anemia is the sole hematologic abnormality or is combined with abnormal leukocytes or platelets. Review of the WBC, differential WBC, and platelet count should quickly answer this question. Leukopenia, neutropenia, or thrombocytopenia alone or in combination usually occurs with anemia in disease states associated with (1) generalized marrow failure (e.g., aplastic anemia, leukemia, myelofibrosis, osteopetrosis, Schwachman-Diamond syndrome), or (2) destruction of more than one peripheral blood element (e.g., systemic lupus erythematosus, hemolytic-uremic syndrome [HUS], disseminated intravascular coagulation [DIC]).

Any patient with an anemia associated with decreased or abnormal leukocytes or platelets should undergo bone marrow aspiration. The marrow may be diagnostic and reveal a myelophthistic process such as replacement of marrow with the malignant cells of lymphoma, leukemia, or neuroblastoma, or the marrow may show a significant decrease in all marrow elements and be diagnostic of an aplastic process. The bone marrow is usually normal in disorders associated with destruction of peripheral blood elements.

Leukemia and Lymphoma. The clinical picture of leukemia is varied. Usually fever, lymphadenopathy, hepatosplenomegaly, petechiae, and purpura predominate. Alternatively, some patients may have chronic bone pain, orthopedic problems such as hip pain, or arthritic pain and fever suggestive of juvenile rheumatoid arthritis. Essential laboratory abnormalities may include an elevated WBC; however, one third or more of patients with leukemia have normal or decreased leukocyte counts. Thrombocytopenia and neutropenia are common in leukemia. The anemia is often severe, and the peripheral smear may exhibit nucleated red cells and teardrop forms. Identification of immature leukocytes (blasts) on the peripheral smear should lead one to suspect leukemia. The diagnosis is clinched by finding that the bone marrow is replaced with immature blasts. Essential steps in the immediate management of the patient with leukemia are addressed in "Oncologic Emergencies."

Aplastic Anemia. Like the patient with leukemia, the patient with aplastic anemia usually has pallor, nosebleeds, petechiae and purpura, and often fever from an acute infection. However, unlike those with leukemia, patients with aplastic anemia usually do not have hepatosplenomegaly, lymphadenopathy, or bone and joint complaints. Aplastic anemia may be constitutional or acquired following exposure to toxins (e.g., benzene, insecticides), infectious agents (e.g., hepatitis B), or drugs, (e.g., chloramphenicol). People with constitutional aplastic anemia (e.g., Fanconi's anemia, dyskeratosis congenita, Schwachman-Diamond syndrome) may exhibit a variety of clinical, physical, or roentgenographic findings of a congenital nature: skin hyperpigmentation, absent thumbs or radii, microcephaly, mental retardation, renal anomalies, abnormal genitalia, short stature, and dystrophic fingernails. The peripheral smear in aplastic anemia (acquired and congenital) usually contains macrocytes and sometimes ovals and teardrops. The mean corpuscular volume (MCV) is usually normal or elevated, and the reticulocyte count is usually low and inappropriate for the degree of anemia. The diagnostic finding in aplastic anemia is marked decrease or absence of myeloid elements, erythroid elements, and megakaryocytes in the bone marrow. Bone marrow biopsy is often required to assess marrow cellularity. Differentiation of acquired from congenital forms of aplastic anemia depends upon identifying dysmorphic or constitutional abnormalities in a patient with this condition. The diagnosis of Fanconi's anemia is confirmed in the laboratory by finding increased numbers of breaks in the chromosomes of a patient with congenital abnormalities such as absent thumbs, renal anomalies, short stature, and hyperpigmentation.

Appropriate initial management of the patient with aplastic anemia is essential to maintain maximum opportunity for cure. For patients with severe aplastic anemia (platelets $\leq$ 20,000/μL, absolute granulocytes $<$ 500/μL, reticulocytes $\leq$ 1.0% corrected for hematocrit, and marrow cellularity $<$ 30% of normal), the primary treatment, if possible, should be HLA-matched bone marrow transplantation. Primary objectives in the management of aplastic anemia are (1) to determine whether an HLA-identical sibling exists, and (2) if an HLA match exists, where possible, to avoid transfusion of any blood products and to transfer the patient to a center capable of doing marrow transplants. In many instances transfusion with platelets or red cells cannot be avoided. If transfusion is required, the blood should be from a random donor, *not* a family member. This minimizes sensitization to the cells of potential bone marrow donors. Equally important is the need to treat potential sepsis, manifested by fever and neutropenia (see "Oncologic Emergencies").

Long-term treatment, in the absence of an HLA match, involves androgen therapy, supportive therapy, antibiotic coverage of febrile episodes, and transfusion with platelets and red cells.

Microangiopathic Anemia with Decreased Platelet Count

Microangiopathic anemias are hemolytic anemias resulting from mechanical fragmentation of red cells as they flow across vascular irregularities such as intravascular fibrin deposits. The hallmark of microangiopathic hemolysis is fragmented erythrocytes or schistocytes on the peripheral smear. Thrombocytopenia accompanies the microangiopathic hemolysis associated with several disease entities in the pediatric age group. The bone marrow is normal in these disorders. HUS, Kasabach-Merritt syndrome, and DIC, which may be induced by a variety of insults, are associated with hemolysis and decreased numbers of platelets.

Hemolytic-Uremic Syndrome. HUS is a disease of acute onset. It usually occurs in children less than 6 years of age in whom a mild viral illness with GI or respiratory symptoms is followed by the development of pallor, jaundice, and oliguria. Clinically, patients usually have icteric sclerae, hypertension, and petechiae and purpura; occasionally, the spleen is palpable. Laboratory values should show an elevated reticulocyte count, peripheral smear with fragmented red cells, decreased platelet count, and, usually, leukocytosis. The prothrombin time (PT) and partial thromboplastin time (PTT) are normal or mildly prolonged, and the direct Coombs' test is negative. Initially, the hemolytic anemia may dominate the clinical picture; subsequently, clinical and laboratory evidence of renal failure dominates as the hemolysis abates. Urinary sediment is remarkable for red cells, red cell casts, and proteinuria early in the illness.

Short-term management of anemia in HUS is supportive. Since the cause of hemolysis is extrinsic to the red cell, both transfused and indigenous cells are lysed. In some instances repeated transfusions are necessary. Blood loss can also contribute significantly to anemia, and patients may require transfusion with packed red cells. Platelet transfusions are indicated if severe thrombocytopenia (platelets $\leq 20,000/\mu L$) and hypertension are present. Long-term treatment of HUS requires management of the variable degrees of residual renal failure that occur. Hemolysis does not persist.

Kasabach-Merritt Syndrome. Patients with Kasabach-Merritt syndrome have giant cavernous hemangiomata, thrombocytopenia, and, sometimes, chronic hemolysis. Usually, bleeding attributable to thrombocytopenia alone or in combination with DIC dominates the clinical picture. During acute episodes of increased bleeding or hemolysis, management includes transfusion support with packed red cells, FFP, or platelets. No definitive therapy is available; surgery often carries significant morbidity and is of limited benefit. Trials of radiation and corticosteroids have met with variable success.

Hypersplenism. Hypersplenism is defined as anemia, leukopenia, and thrombocytopenia in a patient with a massively enlarged spleen and a bone marrow that is cellular and free of malignant cells. The anemia of hypersplenism is usually mild to moderate, and thrombocytopenia is usually the most severe abnormality. If the cause of splenomegaly is portal hypertension and varices are present, the anemia can rapidly become severe when acute variceal bleeding occurs. The causes of hypersplenism include portal hypertension secondary to primary chronic liver disease (e.g., chronic active hepatitis, α-1-antitrypsin deficiency, Wilson's disease, and a variety of metabolic disorders), vascular obstruction of splenic drainage (Banti's syndrome), and enlargement resulting from accumulation of lipid, as occurs with Gaucher's or Niemann-Pick disease. Erythrocytes on the peripheral smear are normochromic and normocytic; however, if the hypersplenism is complicated by chronic blood loss, the red cells appear hypochromic and microcytic. Thrombocytopenia, often of mild to moderate degree, is a constant finding. The reticulocyte count may be minimally elevated.

The diagnosis of anemia with hypersplenism is always a presumptive one. Bone marrow aspiration must be done. The marrow should not contain malignant cells; however, lipid-laden storage cells may be present and diagnostic of a lipid storage disorder, such as Gaucher's or Niemann-Pick disease.

The success of therapy for hypersplenism depends upon the underlying cause of the splenomegaly. Bleeding and anemia associated with primary liver disease may not improve after splenectomy, whereas that associated with lipid storage disease usually resolves following splenectomy.

Autoimmune Disease. Many autoimmune diseases or immunodeficiencies are associated with anemia combined with leukopenia or thrombocytopenia. In these disorders the anemia may result from antibody-mediated destruction of red cells (see "Autoimmune Hemolytic Anemia") or from chronic inflammation. If thrombocytopenia or leukopenia accompany the anemia, a bone marrow aspirate should be obtained to exclude malignancy as a cause of the cytopenias.

Anemia with Elevated Reticulocyte Count

If the leukocyte count, differential WBC, and platelet count are normal, then the reticulocyte count is the next major aid in differential diagnosis of severe anemia. Severe anemias with elevated reticulocyte counts are usually caused by hemolysis, congenital or acquired, or blood loss.

Acquired anemia caused by acute blood loss is discussed earlier in this chapter. Briefly, the patient usually has bleeding evidenced by history, guaiac test, or predisposing disease. The smear is normochromic and normocytic, and usually the reticulocyte count and platelet count are elevated.

Acquired hemolytic anemia may be the result of

antibodies, infections, drug exposures, or mechanical damage to red cells.

Autoimmune Hemolytic Anemia. Autoimmune hemolytic anemia (AIHA) is an antibody-mediated hemolytic anemia. AIHA can occur as an isolated episode following a viral infection or as a manifestation of an underlying or preexisting autoimmune disease such as systemic lupus erythematosus. In childhood the onset may be abrupt, with fever, vomiting, lassitude, pallor, hemoglobinuria, and jaundice. Typically, the liver and spleen are enlarged, and the hemoglobin is often low enough to necessitate transfusion. However, not all patients with AIHA have such an explosive manifestation. Equally common is the gradual development of pallor, fatigue, and light-headedness, with darkening of the urine and modest degrees of scleral icterus. Physically, such patients manifest splenomegaly, and if an underlying autoimmune disorder exists, they may manifest other physical findings consistent with that disorder. The blood smear in AIHA is remarkable for spherocytes, marked polychromasia, and nucleated red cells. The reticulocyte count may be sharply elevated (up 20% to 50% in some instances). Concurrent with significant reticulocytosis, the MCV may be elevated, which reflects the presence of large reticulocytes and is not due to megaloblastic anemia. In general, the MCV increases 1 μm^3/cell for each 1% increase in reticulocyte count. In patients with collagen vascular disorders such as systemic lupus erythematosus, antibody-mediated thrombocytopenia or leukopenia may accompany the hemolytic anemia. In those cases with thrombocytopenia, a bone marrow aspirate should be obtained to exclude malignancy as a cause of decreased peripheral blood counts.

A positive direct Coombs' test in an anemic patient with reticulocytosis establishes the diagnosis of AIHA. The direct Coombs' test utilizes an antibody to human globulin to detect globulins attached to the red cell of the patient. The globulin on the red cell may be immunoglobulin G (IgG), IgM, or complement. Every patient with a positive direct Coombs' test and hemolysis has an AIHA; however, not every patient with a positive Coombs' test manifests hemolysis.

Management of AIHA with anemia and active hemolysis includes prednisone, 2 mg/kg, and in some instances transfusion with packed red cells. Transfusion is often required in children with an explosive onset of hemolysis and rapidly declining hematocrit. One special problem in the short-term management of AIHA is the inability to cross-match red cells for transfusion. This problem arises because many of the antibodies in AIHA are panagglutinins (i.e., they react with any red cell regardless of the antigenic profile of the cell). The following are suggestions for planning transfusions in AIHA:

1. If the antibody is not a panagglutinin but has specificity, transfuse with any unit that cross-matches.
2. If the antibody is a panagglutinin and a compatible cross-match is not possible, transfuse with major blood group-compatible red cells despite their incompatibility.
3. If the antibody prevents typing of the patient's red cells, infuse washed O-negative red cells.

Since management of AIHA sometimes requires transfusion with incompatible red cells, it must be remembered that the transfused red cells, like the indigenous cells, will be destroyed. For this reason patients with AIHA often require frequent transfusions and may consume large volumes of red cells. If AIHA coexists with bleeding resulting from thrombocytopenia or reticulocytopenia, then the hemoglobin level should be monitored every 4 to 6 hours and maintained above 7 g/dL. Such measures avoid development of life-threatening anemia until hemolysis abates or reticulocyte levels return to normal.

Long-term management of AIHA includes two important areas: (1) tapering of steroids and (2) determining the predisposing factors that led to development of autoimmune hemolysis. A careful history should include a listing of drugs taken by the patient. Drug-induced, antibody-mediated hemolysis is infrequent in children. However, it has been associated with a large number of commonly used drugs including penicillin (in high doses), sulfa drugs, and α-methyldopa.

It is essential to determine whether AIHA is a manifestation of an underlying autoimmune disorder. It can also be a manifestation of disease states associated with alterations of the immune system (e.g., immunodeficiencies, systemic lupus erythematosus, Hodgkin's disease). AIHA associated with these underlying disorders is sometimes chronic and often corticosteroid dependent. The laboratory evaluation of the patient with AIHA should include testing for antinuclear antibody, examination of urinary sediment, and quantitative assessment of immunoglobulins. If the history or physical examination is suggestive, an extended immunologic evaluation is indicated. If AIHA is acute and not a manifestation of an underlying disorder, corticosteroids can usually be tapered rapidly. Chronic forms of the disorder may require more intensive immunosuppressive therapy with cyclophosphamide (Cytoxan) or azathioprine (Imuran), or splenectomy. In children with underlying immunodeficiency, splenectomy should be reserved as an absolute last resort.

Drug-Induced Hemolytic Anemia. Some individuals develop explosive hemolysis and prompt decrease of the hematocrit to life-threatening levels during infectious illnesses or following exposure to oxidant chemicals. Patients with glucose-6-phosphate dehydrogenase (G6PD) deficiency (10% of black males) and rarer individuals with unstable hemoglobins are genetically predisposed to oxidant-induced hemolysis. G6PD deficiency is X-linked, and the unstable hemoglobins are inherited as autosomal codominant traits. The oxidant chemicals that have been implicated include both drugs and common household items such as mothballs. The infectious processes that induce hemolysis are usually febrile viral illnesses. The patient's history is that of a previously healthy child who has been medicinally or environmentally exposed to an oxidant or has had an infection.

The clinical expression of drug-induced hemolysis with G6PD deficiency is variable. It ranges from a critically ill child with severe anemia, rapidly declining hematocrit, disorientation, lassitude, scleral icterus, and hemoglobinuria to a child with moderate degrees of anemia, mild scleral icterus, and a moderately elevated reticulocyte count. On physical examination splenomegaly is a constant finding; hepatomegaly is more variable. Scleral icterus may be present. In the laboratory the smear contains so-called drug reactor or "bite" cells (Figure 34-1), marked polychromasia, and nucleated red cells; the reticulocyte count is sharply elevated, as is the WBC. Heinz bodies (intraerythrocytic clumps of denatured hemoglobin) may be seen on methyl violet stains of peripheral blood. There may be accompanying renal dysfunction and elevated liver function test results with increased direct and indirect bilirubin. The diagnosis is difficult to make during the acute hemolytic episode because reticulocytes have increased G6PD activity even in G6PD-deficient persons. However, identification of Heinz bodies within peripheral red cells during the acute hemolytic period is suggestive. Usually, it is necessary to allow the patient to return to a steady state before the G6PD activity can be quantified. If the patient received a bona fide oxidant drug, developed hemolysis, and is known to be G6PD deficient, evidence for hemolysis because of G6PD deficiency is adequate, and no rechallenge with drug is necessary.

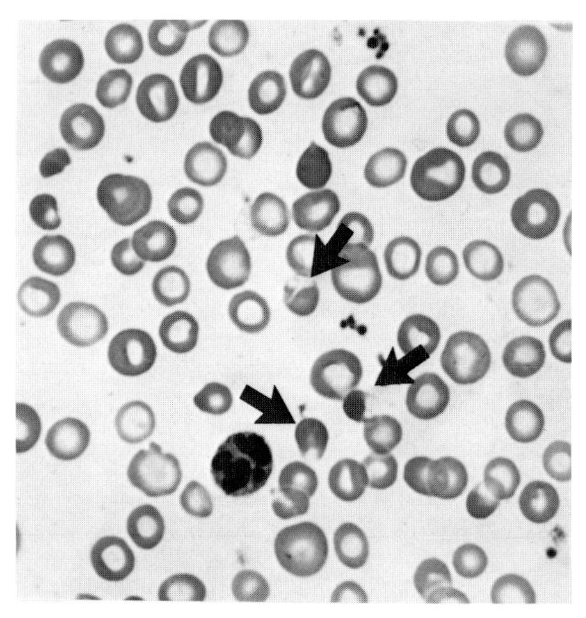

FIGURE 34-1 Blood smear showing "Bite" cells (*arrows*). (Courtesy W.H. Zinkham, M.D.)

The case is strengthened if Heinz bodies were noted during the hemolytic episode.

The diagnosis of hemolysis caused by an unstable hemoglobin that is sensitive to oxidant drugs or denatures during febrile infectious illnesses requires hemoglobin electrophoresis on cellulose acetate and acid agar. If the hemoglobin has abnormal electrophoretic mobility, electrophoresis may be diagnostic; however, many unstable hemoglobins result from neutral amino acid substitutions that do not alter the electrophoretic mobility of the hemoglobin and are not detected by electrophoresis. In this case specialized testing of Heinz body formation in vitro upon exposure to oxidizing stains (brilliant cresyl blue) and hemoglobin precipitation in 30% isopropanol or heat are required to recognize an unstable hemoglobin.

Initial management of patients with hemolysis induced by oxidant drugs depends upon their clinical status. The offending drug should be discontinued. If a severe hemolytic reaction occurs, the patient should be transfused with packed red cells that have normal G6PD activity. However, if the hemolytic reaction is mild and reticulocytosis is adequate, the hemoglobin level and reticulocyte count should return to normal following discontinuation of the oxidant drug.

Long-term management should focus on increasing the patient's and parents' awareness of those drugs that can induce hemolysis and of the clinical signs that indicate hemolysis (Exhibit 34-2).

Exhibit 34-2 Drugs Commonly Associated with Hemolysis in G6PD Deficiency

Antimalarials
- Primaquine
- Quinacrine (Atabrine)

Sulfonamides
- Sulfanilamide
- Salicylazosulfapyridine (Azulfidine)
- Sulfisoxazole (Gantrisin)*

Nitrofurans
- Nitrofurantoin (Furadantin)
- Nitrofurazone (Furacin)

Analgesics
- Acetophenetidin (phenacetin)*

Sulfones
- 4,4′-Diaminodiphenyl sulfone (dapsone)

Miscellaneous
- Dimercaprol (British anti-Lewisite)
- Methylene blue
- Naphthalene (moth balls)
- Vitamin K (water-soluble analogs)*
- Ascorbic acid*

* Hemolysis is infrequent and generally requires a high concentration of the drug.
Source: Reprinted with permission from Sullivan DW, Glader BE: Erythrocyte enzyme disorders in children. *Pediatr Clin North Am* 1980;27:458.

Hemolytic Anemia Associated with Infections. Hemolytic anemia may accompany a variety of infectious illnesses in the absence of G6PD deficiency or an unstable hemoglobin. Such infections include bacterial sepsis attributable to *Streptococcus pyogenes, Haemophilus influenzae,* and *Escherichia coli.* Antibody-mediated red cell destruction manifest as AIHA may also follow mycoplasma or Epstein-Barr virus infections. Acute intravascular hemolysis also can be seen with malaria or be induced by the toxins released from *Clostridium perfringens* infections of gangrenous tissues.

Hemolysis Caused by Mechanical Injury. Hemolytic anemias that result from fragmentation of the red cells as they flow across vascular irregularities and whose hallmark is the schistocyte on smear are usually associated with thrombocytopenia. The "Waring blender syndrome" is an exception; in this disorder an anemia occurs in the absence of thrombocytopenia. This acquired hemolytic anemia results from mechanical damage to red cells as they are forced at high pressure through small openings such as arteriovenous fistulas or fistulas that remain after closure of ventricular septal defects with synthetic materials.

Congenital Hemolytic Anemia. Identification of a new anemia in a person with previously normal hemoglobin levels is the essential clue that the anemia is acquired. Conversely, a history of chronic anemia in a patient suggests that it may be hereditary. Hereditary causes of hemolytic anemia should be suspected in the patient with chronic anemia, splenomegaly, and increased reticulocyte count. The hereditary hemolytic anemias are categorized according to location of the abnormality within the red cell: hemoglobinopathies, membranopathies, and enzymopathies. Specific changes in red cell morphology are often characteristic of specific inherited hemolytic anemias; therefore, the peripheral smear is an essential tool for differential diagnosis of congenital hemolytic anemias. A brief review of the most common disorders follows.

Hemoglobinopathies and Sickle Syndromes. The most common hereditary hemolytic disorders in blacks are the sickle syndromes. The term "sickle syndrome" refers to diseases produced by a gene for hemoglobin S combined with a second gene for either hemoglobin S, C, or D or for β-thalassemia. The resultant disease states, respectively, are sickle cell anemia, SC disease, SD disease, or Sβ-thalassemia. The β-thalassemia genes exist as + and o variants (also known as African and Mediterranean variants, respectively). The "+" and "o" refer respectively to complete or partial suppression of normal β^A-globin production. The major clinical, morphologic, and laboratory findings associated with the most common sickle syndromes are reviewed in Table 34-2.

Patients with sickle cell anemia, Sβ^o thalassemia, SC disease, and SD disease often suffer vasoocclusive episodes that can affect any body organ. Usually children complain of abdominal or bone pain. These painful crises are often manageable with forced fluids and analgesics. However, when (1) crisis is prolonged, (2) oral fluid intake is inadequate, or (3) the nature of the pain requires exclusion of osteomyelitis or an "acute abdomen," these patients require hospitalization, aggressive intravenous hydration, and, if crisis is unrelenting, transfusion. Four life-threatening events can occur in patients with sickle syndrome. Three—cerebrovascular accidents (CVAs), chest syndrome, and sepsis—are unique to sickle syndromes. The other—profound anemia resulting from aplastic crisis—can occur with any chronic hemolytic disorder.

CVAs occur most frequently in patients with sickle cell disease, Sβ^o thalassemia, and SC disease. Patients are usually seen during the first two decades of life with the acute onset of focal neurologic deficits. Occasionally, patients have transient episodes of neurologic abnormalities prior to a CVA. Clinical or laboratory data cannot predict which patients will develop CVAs; however, any patient

TABLE 34-2 Differential Diagnosis of Common Hemoglobinopathies

Diagnosis	Clinical Severity	Mean and Range of Hb* (g/dL)	Mean and Range of Hct (%)	MCV (μm^3)	Mean and Range of Count Reticulocyte	Red Cell Morphology	Hemoglobin Composition† Type	Hemoglobin Composition† %
SS	Moderate–severe	7.5 (6–10)	22 (18–30)	93 Increased or normal	11 (4–30)	Many sickled cells, nucleated red cells	S F A_2	80–90 2–20 <3.6
SC	Mild–moderate	10 (9–14)	30 (26–40)	80 Increased or normal	3 (1.5–6)	Many target cells, rare sickled cells	S C F	45–55 45–55 0.2–8
Sβ^o Thal	Moderate–severe	8.1 (7–12)	25 (20–36)	69 Decreased	8 (3–18)	Marked hypochromia, microcytosis, and target cells; variable sickled cells	S F A_2	50–85 2–30 >3.6
Sβ^+ Thal	Mild–moderate	11 (8–13)	32 (25–40)	76 Decreased	3 (1.5–6)	Mild microcytosis, hypochromia, rare sickled cells	S A F A_2	55–75 15–30 1–20 >3.6
CC	Mild	9–13	28–40	80 Normal	3.2	Target cells, oat cells, microspherocytes		
AS	Asymptomatic carrier	Normal	Normal	Normal	Normal	Normal	S A A_2	38–45 60–55 1–3
AC	Asymptomatic carrier	Normal	Normal	Normal	Normal	Occasional target cells	C A A_2	40–50 50–60 1–3

* Abbreviations: Hb, hemoglobin; Hct, hematocrit; Thal, thalassemia; CC, homozygous C hemoglobin; AS, sickle cell trait; AC, hemoglobin C trait.
† By electrophoresis.

who has a CVA is at increased risk of developing another one. The majority of repeat CVAs develop within 3 years of the initial CVA. A patient with sickle cell disease who develops a CVA should have an emergency partial exchange transfusion with sickle-hemoglobin-negative blood. The purpose of exchange transfusion is to rapidly reduce the number of hemoglobin S-containing red cells to approximately 40% to 50% and to improve oxygenation by increasing the hemoglobin without changing the blood volume or blood pressure. Subsequently, the percentage of hemoglobin S should be maintained at less than 30% by transfusions for at least 1 year. Extensive clinical trials on the value of partial exchange transfusion or chronic transfusion programs have not yet proved the benefit of these interventions. However, the morbidity associated with CVAs in sickle cell disease warrants their use.

Chest syndrome is another complication of sickle cell disease that can be life-threatening if it progresses to generalized pulmonary infarction. Chest syndrome is the term applied to the combination of acute onset of fever, cough, pleuritic pain, tachypnea, and pulmonary infiltrate in a patient with sickle cell disease. It may be caused by pulmonary infarction or infection or a combination of these two processes. Most frequently, children less than 4 years old are affected; however, chest syndrome can occur at any age. When the patient is first seen, it is often impossible to determine whether pulmonary infiltrate is due to infection or infarction. It is important to obtain blood cultures, initiate appropriate antibiotic therapy, administer oxygen, and follow the patient carefully. Any patient with significant respiratory distress combined with decreased arterial oxygen pressure should receive transfusion with packed red cells. Some patients develop rapidly progressive pulmonary disease with severe respiratory distress and decreases in oxygen pressure to less than 65 mmHg, with auscultatory and roentgenographic progression. Presumably, the rapid progression reflects occlusion of pulmonary vessels by red cells that sickle because of hypoxemia. These acute ill patients should receive partial exchange transfusions to improve oxygenation, decrease the number of sickle cells, and interrupt the vicious cycle of hypoxia-sickling-infarction-hypoxia.

High fever in patients with sickle cell disease may be a sign of life-threatening sepsis. Patients with sickle cell disease are immunodeficient, have abnormalities in the alternate pathway of complement, and have functional or anatomic asplenia. Any patient with sickle cell disease who has fever must be evaluated carefully for sepsis. At a minimum those who have temperatures greater than or equal to 39° C without a source should be hospitalized, have blood cultures done, and receive antibiotics until a source is obvious or the cultures are negative. Any ill-appearing patient, regardless of the level of temperature, should be admitted for treatment. Individuals at particular risk of sepsis are children less than 4 years of age or those with a prior history of sepsis. Prophylaxis against sepsis, although not of proven benefit, may be important for patients with sickle cell disease. All children over 2 years of age should receive pneumococcal vaccine (Pneumovax), and all children with sickle cell disease should receive penicillin prophylaxis (250 mg orally twice per day) from the time of diagnosis. Failures of both Pneumovax and prophylactic penicillin are well known. All patients with high fever should be evaluated and hospitalized if no source is found, even if they have received Pneumovax and are on penicillin.

Life-threatening anemia can occur with aplastic crisis in sickle cell disease. Such crises may complicate *any* hemolytic anemia. An aplastic crisis occurs when red cell production ceases in a patient with a hemolytic anemia; this disturbs the balance between production and destruction of red cells, and continued hemolysis causes the development of profound anemia. Aplastic crises usually occur during or after a viral illness. The hemoglobin decreases to levels well below that typically associated with the patient's hemolytic anemia. Reticulocytes, which usually are increased with hemolytic disease, are significantly decreased and may be absent. The total bilirubin also decreases. Treatment of aplastic crisis requires transfusion with packed red cells if anemia is severe (hemoglobin < 4.5 g/dL) or accompanied by clinical symptoms. Patients can spontaneously recover from aplastic crisis. For patients with lesser degrees of anemia, clinical observation with serial (every 6 hours) determinations of hemoglobin may be appropriate. Frequent monitoring is necessary because patients with aplastic crisis can develop profound anemia in less than 24 hours.

Membranopathies. Hereditary spherocytosis is the most common membranopathy. It usually affects whites, and the degree of associated anemia is highly variable. This disorder is usually associated with splenomegaly. The essential diagnostic finding on the peripheral blood smear is spherocytes, and diagnosis requires documentation of increased osmotic fragility of erythrocytes. As with all hemolytic anemias, severe life-threatening anemia occasionally develops during periods when red cell production ceases (aplastic crises). Hereditary spherocytosis exhibits autosomal dominant inheritance, and a positive family history of this disorder is obvious in approximately 70% of cases.

Spherocytes on the smear and increased osmotic fragility of red cells are not exclusively diagnostic of hereditary spherocytosis. These findings also occur with Coombs-positive AIHAs. Therefore, in patients with no family history of hereditary spherocytosis, a direct Coombs' test is necessary to exclude AIHA. Most of the membranopathies cause mild to moderate anemia and mild elevation of the reticulocyte count. Some are morphologic curiosities not associated with anemia. Table 34-3 reviews the clinical presentations, laboratory findings, and specific diagnostic tests associated with some membranopathies.

Enzymopathies. Enzymopathies are relatively rare. They are usually autosomal recessive disorders. The most common are G6PD deficiency, pyruvate kinase deficiency, and 5′-nucleotidase deficiency. G6PD deficiency is discussed in an earlier section. Pyruvate kinase deficiency can be the cause of severe hemolytic anemia. At birth, patients with pyruvate kinase deficiency usually have splenomegaly, indirect hyperbilirubinemia, and severe anemia; in some instances they require splenectomy to avoid chronic transfusion. However, milder forms with moderate degrees of anemia, modest elevations of the reticulocyte count, and mild splenomegaly do exist. The clue to diagnosis is finding spiculated red cells in the peripheral blood of a child who has congenital hemolytic anemia. Quantification of the enzyme activity is necessary for accurate final diagnosis. Emergency treatment of some patients may entail transfusion because of severely depressed hemoglobin levels. Those children who have marked degrees of reticulocytosis are particularly susceptible to aplastic crises. Long-term management may require splenectomy to avoid transfusion dependency.

After G6PD and pyruvate kinase deficiencies, the third most frequent enzymopathy is 5′-nucleotidase deficiency. Although it is relatively common among inherited hemolytic diseases, it is rare in the general population. The patients usually have moderate to severe anemia, a significantly elevated reticulocyte count, and, on peripheral smear, marked basophilic stippling of erythrocytes. The majority of patients have a palpable spleen. The clinical characteristics and morphologic features of this dis-

TABLE 34-3 Clinical and Laboratory Features of Membranopathies

	Occurrence	Manifestations	Physical Findings	Family History	Range of Hb* (g/dL)	Reticulocyte Range (%)	Smear	Diagnostic Tests
Hereditary spherocytosis	Common	Jaundice, splenomegaly, anemia	Palpable spleen, jaundice	Positive in 70%–80% of cases	7.5–11.0	5.0–18	Dense microspherocytes	Osmotic fragility increased; direct Coombs' test negative
Hereditary elliptocytosis	Common	Jaundice, morphologic curiosity, occasionally anemia	Occasional palpable spleen	Usually one parent affected	>9.5 Usually normal	<3.0 Usually normal	Elliptical cells	Peripheral smear shows elliptocytes
Hereditary pyropoikilocytosis	Rare	Jaundice, anemia, splenomegaly	Splenomegaly, jaundice	Parents and siblings normal or have hereditary spherocytosis	7.0–9.0	10–20	Bizarre poikilocytosis	Osmotic fragility increased; RBCs fragment when incubated at 37° C for 6 h

* Abbreviations: Hb, hemoglobin; RBCs, red blood cells.

order and other enzymopathies are summarized in Table 34-4.

Anemia with Low Reticulocyte Count

A decreased or normal reticulocyte count occurs in those anemias with the common feature of deficient production of new erythrocytes. Deficient production of red cells may result from absence of erythroid precursors in the marrow or from deficiency of a factor required for the production of red cells (e.g., iron, vitamin B_{12}, folate). These disorders can be categorized according to red cell size (reflected in the MCV) from the CBC.

Microcytic Anemia. Anemias associated with low reticulocyte count and low MCV include the thalassemias (major or minor), iron deficiency, lead poisoning, anemia of chronic disorders, and sideroblastic anemias. Adult hemoglobin (hemoglobin A) is composed of α- and β-globin chains and is designated $\alpha_2\beta_2$. The thalassemias are inherited deficiencies of globin chain synthesis.

β-Thalassemia. In β-thalassemia, synthesis of β-globin is deficient; in α-thalassemia, α-globin synthesis is deficient. In general, the severity of the clinical disease parallels the degree of deficient globin chain synthesis. Total deficiency of β-globin synthesis (β-thalassemia major) produces a severely anemic infant who, at 2 to 4 months of age, has marked pallor and hepatosplenomegaly and is transfusion dependent for life. Milder deficiency of β-globin synthesis produces mild to moderate anemia in a well child who has no organomegaly and whose anemia mimics iron deficiency anemia. β-Thalassemia syndromes of intermediate severity also exist. They may be associated with severe anemia and organomegaly but do not require chronic transfusion to sustain life.

Patients with β-thalassemia major have noticeably abnormal smears with nucleated red cells, mildly elevated but inadequate reticulocyte counts, microcytosis, and hypochromasia. MCV is decreased, and hemoglobin electrophoresis shows almost 100% fetal hemoglobin. Both parents have laboratory findings consistent with β-thalassemia minor.

β-Thalassemia minor is a disease that occurs in persons who inherit one β-thalassemia gene. The anemia of this disorder is characterized on peripheral smear by microcytosis, ovalocytes, target cells, and basophilic stippling. The degree of anemia is mild to moderate. The reticulocyte count is normal. Hemoglobin electrophoresis reveals a preponderance of hemoglobin A. The quantity of hemoglobin A_2 or F is increased. Serum ferritin and free erythrocyte protoporphyrin are normal and exclude iron deficiency as the cause of anemia. Since β-thalasse-

TABLE 34-4 Clinical and Laboratory Features of Enzymopathies

Deficiency	Occurrence	Hemolysis	Hb* (g/dL)	Reticulocyte Count (%)	RBC Morphology	Inheritance	Diagnostic Tests
G6PD in black Americans	~10% black males	Episodic (exposure to oxidants or infections)	Normal except with exposure to oxidants	Normal except with exposure to oxidants	Normal; with exposure, "bite cells" or drug reactor cells appear	X-linked; carrier-mother has ~50% of normal G6PD activity	Decreased G6PD activity A^- isozyme by electrophoresis
G6PD, chronic hemolytic variants	Rare	Chronic	7.0–10.0	10–20	Variable degrees of abnormality	X-linked; carrier-mother has ~50% of normal G6PD activity	Decreased G6PD activity; characteristic kinetic changes
Pyruvate kinase (PK)	Rare	Chronic	5.0–10.5	Presplenectomy, 10–20; postsplenectomy, >50	Shrunken, spiculated cells	Autosomal recessive; nonanemic parents have ~50% PK activity	Decreased PK activity
Glucose phosphate isomerase (GPI)	Rare	Chronic	7.0–10.0	20–80	Not distinctive	Autosomal recessive; nonanemic parents have ~50% GPI activity	Decreased GPI activity
Pyridine 5′-nucleotidase	Rare	Chronic	7.5–10.0	10–20	Prominent basophilic stippling	Autosomal recessive	Decreased pyridine 5′-nucleotidase activity

* Abbreviations: Hb, hemoglobin; RBC, red blood cell.

mia minor is inherited, one of the parents must be hematologically identical to the child.

α-Thalassemia. Clinically significant α-thalassemia syndromes can be divided into α-thalassemia minor, which causes a mild anemia; hemoglobin H disease, which causes a moderate to severe hemolytic anemia with splenomegaly; and hydrops fetalis resulting from profound anemia. The increasing severity of the syndromes reflects inherited absence of two, three, or all four of the genes that normally produce α-globin. Patients with α-thalassemia minor have mild anemia with decreased MCV, normal hemoglobin electrophoresis, and normal quantities of hemoglobin F and A_2. The anemia mimics iron deficiency; however, unlike children with iron deficiency, these patients have normal ferritins and normal levels of free erythrocyte protoporphyrins, and they do not respond to trials of iron. It is not possible to establish a definitive diagnosis of α-thalassemia minor unless the synthesis of α-globin is measured or the number of α-globin genes is determined. Hence diagnosis usually requires exclusion of other causes of microcytic anemia.

Persons with hemoglobin H disease have a hemolytic anemia with splenomegaly, abnormal peripheral smear, increased reticulocyte count, and elevated amounts of a fast-moving hemoglobin (hemoglobin H = β_4) on electrophoresis. Patients with hemoglobin H disease have only one of four normally occurring α-globin genes.

The α-thalassemia syndromes are not rare diseases in pediatric practice. Studies of blacks show that 23% are nonanemic α-thalassemia carriers, approximately 3% are affected with α-thalassemia minor, and approximately 0.2% have hemoglobin H disease.

Iron Deficiency Anemia. Iron deficiency is the most common cause of microcytic anemia with a low reticulocyte count. Iron deficiency is usually associated with a mild to moderate degree of anemia; however, particularly in the first year of life, if rapid growth is paired with poor diet or blood loss, iron deficiency can result in hemoglobin levels less than 6.5 g/dL. Patients with uncomplicated iron deficiency are pale and irritable and have no other physical abnormality. Children with iron deficiency anemia may have a history of poor diet, prolonged intake of whole cow's milk, or occult GI bleeding. The anemia is associated with low MCV and a peripheral blood smear showing microcytosis and hypochromia. Reticulocyte counts are usually low or normal, and the serum ferritin is decreased. If the patient is mildly anemic, has a decreased MCV, and a smear consistent with iron deficiency, it is appropriate to institute an iron trial (6 mg/kg/d elemental iron). The reticulocyte count should increase in 4 to 5 days, and the hemoglobin level should increase within 7 to 10 days after initiation of therapy. Reticulocytosis or increase in hemoglobin in response to oral iron documents iron deficiency, and iron should be continued for 6 to 8 weeks.

In severely anemic patients (hemoglobin $\leq$ 8.5 g/dL), iron deficiency, if suspected, should be documented by measurement of serum ferritin. GI bleeding should be excluded by a stool guaiac test, and the patient should be followed carefully for reticulocytosis during iron supplementation. Failure of iron trial in patients with microcytic anemia may be due to (1) noncompliance, (2) GI blood loss, or (3) incorrect diagnosis. Patients who fail iron trials should have a stool guaiac test, and thalassemia syndromes should be excluded. Usually, with severe degrees of iron deficiency anemia, even with hemoglobin levels less than 7.0 g/dL, transfusion is not necessary unless there is ongoing GI blood loss. Treatment with oral iron is adequate. If transfusion is clinically indicated, transfuse to a hemoglobin level of approximately 8.5 g/dL and then treat with oral iron. At this level of hemoglobin, documentation of response to oral iron is still possible.

Anemia of Chronic Disease. Iron deficiency must always be differentiated from the anemia of chronic disease (ACD). This anemia occurs in patients with chronic inflammatory disease (e.g., juvenile rheumatoid arthritis, chronic osteomyelitis, or systemic lupus erythematosus). Usually, these patients have a mild to moderate anemia, and the laboratory findings may be similar to those of iron deficiency, except that the total iron-binding capacity is usually low or normal in ACD and high in iron deficiency. The serum ferritin is usually normal or elevated in ACD, and the bone marrow contains stainable iron. The essential point is that this normocytic or microcytic anemia complicates a chronic inflammatory disease. Therapy should be directed primarily at the basic disease process if iron stores are normal.

Lead Poisoning Anemia. Lead poisoning can also cause a mild degree of anemia with low MCV. Even if lead poisoning is documented, the patient should be evaluated for iron deficiency, since both can occur concurrently. The diagnostic tests should measure free erythrocyte protoporphyrin, which is markedly elevated in lead poisoning and mildly elevated in iron deficiency, and determine levels of lead in the blood and ferritin in the serum.

Macrocytic Anemia. The megaloblastic anemias are associated with inadequate production of erythrocytes caused by deficient maturation of erythroid precursors. Anemia with low reticulocyte counts and elevated MCV can be caused by either folate or vitamin B_{12} deficiency. Both disorders are rare. Folate deficiency usually accompanies diseases that cause malabsorption of folate (e.g., celiac disease, blind loop syndrome, chronic diarrhea, poor nutrition, and, rarely, phenytoin therapy for seizures). Vitamin B_{12} deficiency is a rare finding in childhood, except in patients with surgical absence of the terminal ileum. Although rare, pernicious anemia (intrinsic factor deficiency) in children does exist. Severe deficiency of either B_{12} or folate may be associated with leukopenia and thrombocytopenia. The diagnostic test for these diseases is the measurement of serum folate and B_{12} levels. Bone marrow aspirates show characteristically large erythroid percursors with delayed nuclear maturation. There are two areas of caution regarding B_{12} or folate deficiency: (1) MCVs can be increased with marked reticulocytosis and do not always suggest megaloblastic anemia, and (2) large doses of folate can improve the anemia caused by B_{12} deficiency but do not correct the posterior column degeneration of the spinal cord that is associated with B_{12} deficiency.

Another group of anemias, those attributable to inadequate production of red cells, can also result from absence of erythroid precursors in the bone marrow. This situation describes transient erythroblastopenia of childhood (TEC), a transient absence of erythroid precursors in the marrow, and Diamond-Blackfan anemia, a chronic, constitutional absence of erythroid precursors in the marrow. Sometimes it is impossible to differentiate between these two disorders. Both cause anemia and reticulocytopenia. Usually, the anemia is severe and patients may require transfusion. The essential laboratory features that help differentiate these two entities are their clinical course, the MCV, and the levels of hemoglobin F. In both cases erythroid precursors are decreased or absent in the marrow. However, patients with Diamond-Blackfan syndrome usually have increased MCVs and elevated hemoglobin F; they are chronically anemic and sometimes transfusion dependent. In TEC, inability to produce red cells is a transient phenomenon; MCV and hemoglobin F are normal.

Whenever possible, transfusion should be withheld to allow maximum opportunity for the patient's marrow to recover. If transfusion is required, the patient should be transfused to a hemoglobin level of 8.5 to 9 g/dL and followed for evidence of reticulocytosis, which would reflect spontaneous recovery of red cell production. The spontaneous return of red cell production suggests, but does not prove, the diagnosis of TEC. Since aplastic crises in hemolytic disease can mimic episodes of TEC, it is important to exclude an underlying hemolytic disease when the hemoglobin level and reticulocyte count return to a steady state.

Bleeding

The clinical picture of patients with bleeding disorders varies widely. Some patients exhibit clinically obvious signs, such as an acute onset of showers of petechiae or spontaneous hemorrhage into soft tissue and joints, whereas other patients with abnor-

TABLE 34-5 Therapy for Plasma Clotting Factor Deficiencies

	Available Replacement Products	Factor Content	Expected Factor Response	Half-life of Factor	Risks	Clinical Bleeding	Suggested Level of Factor Coverage (%)
VII deficiency	FFP	1 U VII/mL	1% increase/U VIII infused/kg	4–6 h	Hepatitis	Surgery	>25
	Prothrombin complex concentrates	Marked on bottle			DIC with severe liver disease	Surgery Head trauma	>25 >25
VIII deficiency	FFP	1 U VIII/mL	2% increase/U VIII infused/kg	8–12 hr	Allergic reactions	Soft tissue or joint	60
	Cryoprecipitate	80–100 U VIII/bag				Head trauma Tooth extraction	100 60
	Factor VIII concentrate	Marked on bottle			Hepatitis	Stitches	60
von Willebrand's disease	FFP Cryoprecipitate		2% increase/U of VIII infused/kg	Factor VIII variable vWd factor not known		Surgery Stitches Tooth extraction	50–100 VIII 60 VIII 60 VIII
IX deficiency	FFP	1 U IX/mL	1% increase IX/U IX infused/kg	12–18 h	Hepatitis	Soft tissue or joint Head trauma	60 100
	Prothrombin complex concentrates	Marked on bottle			DIC with severe liver disease	Tooth extraction Surgery	60 100
XI deficiency	FFP	1 U XI/mL	2% increase/kg/U XI given	24–48 h		Surgery	100

mal bleeding may escape diagnosis for years, with occasional nosebleeds, slightly heavy menstrual bleeding, or minimally prolonged bleeding following tooth extraction. The manifestations and clinical aspects of a bleeding disorder, although not pathognomonic, are suggestive of the type of abnormality and can help direct evaluation of the patient. Exhibit 34-3 lists some pertinent points to investigate in a bleeding history, and Table 34-5 relates the types of bleeding associated with abnormalities of specific factors in the coagulation pathway. In general, defects in the intrinsic pathway, measured by the PTT, predispose patients to the most severe bleeding abnormalities (e.g., spontaneous or trauma-induced soft tissue and joint hemorrhage). Abnormalities of the extrinsic and common pathway, measured by the PT, are associated with menorrhagia and mucosal bleeding. Petechial lesions are specific for qualitative and quantitative deficiencies of platelets or vasculitis.

Once the clinical findings and history suggest a bleeding disorder, the platelet count, PT, and PTT direct the evaluation of the patient. Figure 34-2 presents a diagnostic approach to the bleeding patient.

Exhibit 34-3 Important Historical and Physical Points that Reveal Abnormal Bleeding

Family history: affected siblings, parents, maternal uncles, grandfather, or nephews
Minor surgery: prolonged umbilical cord bleeding, poor healing and bleeding of stitched lacerations, circumcision bleeding
Prolonged bleeding following tooth loss
Hematomata at immunization sites
Prolonged bleeding with major surgery or child delivery
Poor wound healing

Bleeding with Decreased Platelet Count

The most common cause of bleeding in the pediatric patient is thrombocytopenia. The normal range of platelets is 150,000 to 300,000/μL. Severity of the clinical manifestations of thrombocytopenia (bruises, petechiae, nosebleeds) generally relates to the level of the count. Obvious clinical abnormality may not occur unless platelets are less than 50,000/

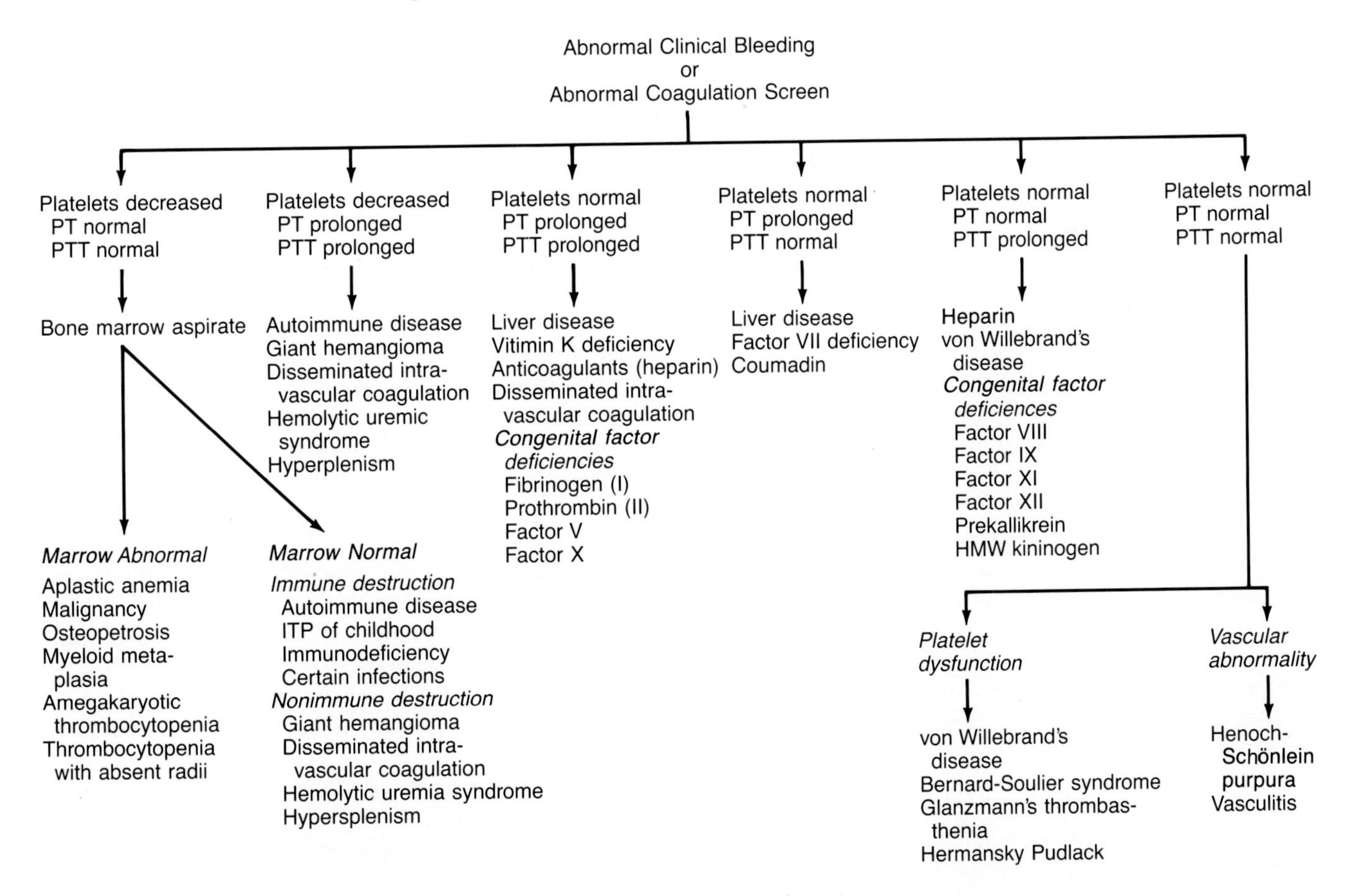

FIGURE 34-2 Differential diagnoses in abnormal clinical bleeding or abnormal coagulation screen. ITP, Idiopathic thrombocytopenic purpura; HMW, high molecular weight.

μL. Minimal decreases in platelet count (100,000 to 150,000) are usually not associated with abnormal bleeding. Regardless of the platelet count or the presence or absence of clinical bleeding, the cause of thrombocytopenia should be determined in any patient in whom it persists.

Thrombocytopenia may occur alone or in combination with either anemia or qualitatively or quantitatively abnormal leukocytes. Regardless, a bone marrow aspirate should be obtained from all patients with thrombocytopenia. Microscopy of marrow aspirates allows assessment of marrow cellularity, determination of megakaryocyte numbers, and diagnosis of disease processes that replace normal marrow, such as leukemia, lymphoma, and neuroblastoma.

A generally hypocellular marrow or isolated absence of megakaryocytes in the marrow of a thrombocytopenic patient indicates that the patient is not making adequate numbers of platelets. Such findings may be diagnostic of aplastic anemia (congenital or acquired), thrombocytopenia-absent radii syndrome, amegakaryocytic thrombocytopenia, osteopetrosis, or myeloid metaplasia, depending upon the complex of associated clinical and laboratory findings. (See "Severe Anemia" for discussion of management of aplastic anemia.) In general, thrombocytopenias resulting from decreased platelet production respond to allogeneic platelet transfusion. Since the life span of infused platelets is short (8 to 11 days total; half life = 4.5 days), frequent repeated transfusions may be required. Usually, a response in platelet count of 10,000 to 12,000/m^2/unit of platelets given can be expected.

The marrow aspirate in the patient with thrombocytopenia may also contain abnormal cellular forms consistent with marrow replacement by malignant cells, such as those of leukemia, lymphoma, or neuroblastoma. Although this is an unusual cause of isolated thrombocytopenia, it can occur and should always be considered in the differential diagnosis of thrombocytopenia.

Thrombocytopenia with normal bone marrow aspirate occurs with disease processes that cause decreased survival of platelets in the peripheral blood. Decreased platelet survival can result from immune-mediated destruction, consumption during disordered intravascular clot formation, or mechanical entrapment.

Immune-Mediated Destruction of Platelets. Acute idiopathic thrombocytopenic purpura (ITP) of childhood occurs as an acute onset of bleeding following a nonspecific viral illness in well-appearing children 2 to 8 years of age, who are otherwise hematologically and physically normal. The diagnosis of acute ITP of childhood requires that other disease processes causing thrombocytopenia be excluded and that the thrombocytopenia resolve, with or without corticosteroids, in a short period of time. All laboratory studies in patients with acute ITP of childhood should be normal, except for the thrombocytopenia and an anemia consistent with any obvious blood loss. Furthermore, the course should be acute and transient, not chronic and relapsing. Thrombocytopenia from immune-mediated destruction of platelets also occurs after specific viral illnesses (e.g., infectious mononucleosis, chickenpox, measles, rubella). In such cases, the clinical and laboratory manifestations include those of the underlying infectious process.

Spontaneous recovery from ITP of childhood is the rule. However, in cases with marked cutaneous hemorrhage, mucosal petechiae, guaiac-positive stools, or hematuria, prednisone therapy (2 mg/kg) should be instituted; after normalization of platelet count, the corticosteroid dosage should be rapidly tapered. Splenectomy can be effective in childhood ITP, but with the initial occurrence of ITP, splenectomy should be reserved for patients with life-threatening GI or central nervous system hemorrhage. In follow-up it should be considered for patients who fail to respond to corticosteroids and continue to bleed or for patients who are corticosteroid responsive but have prohibitive side effects. Since most patients with ITP of childhood remit within weeks of the diagnosis, patients who persist with even minimal thrombocytopenia or who are corticosteroid dependent should have repeat antinuclear antibody, direct Coombs', and urinary sediment tests to detect development of any underlying systemic autoimmune process.

Immune-mediated thrombocytopenia may be the major manifestation or simply occur in the course of an underlying autoimmune disease of immunodeficiency, such as systemic lupus erythematosus, mixed collagen vascular diseases, dysgammaglobulinemias, selective IgA deficiency, systemic combined immunodeficiency disease, and common variable immunodeficiency. In these cases thrombocytopenia usually follows a relapsing or chronic course and is usually associated with other historical, physical, hematologic, or immunologic abnormalities. These abnormalities are often specific and may be diagnostic.

Thrombocytopenia associated with autoimmunity or immunodeficiency usually responds initially to prednisone (2 mg/kg); however, it often subsequently follows a chronic, relapsing course. Because of the chronicity, splenectomy is often considered in these cases. Since postsplenectomy sepsis is a particular threat to patients with immunodeficiency, a thorough immunologic evaluation should precede any decision to splenectomize any patient with chronic thrombocytopenia. If an immunodeficiency is documented, splenectomy should be reserved only for severe, life-threatening bleeding.

Nonimmune Consumption of Platelets. Thrombocytopenia may be caused by nonimmune consumption of platelets in disorders associated with disordered intravascular clot formation. This occurs with the Kasabach-Merritt syndrome, DIC, and HUS. Kasabach-Merritt syndrome is manifest by single or multiple cavernous hemangiomata that occur anywhere in the body. These may cause isolated thrombocytopenia or DIC with thrombocytopenia and microangiopathic hemolytic anemia. The DIC is manifest by elevated fibrin degradation products (FDPs) and/or prolongation of PT and PTT. HUS is manifest by hematuria, proteinuria, acute renal failure, hemolytic anemia, decreased platelets, and variable prolongation of PT and PTT. Similar combinations of coagulation abnormalities are seen with DIC, which may be caused by a variety of severe insults, such as sepsis, hypoxia, and massive head trauma.

There is no specific therapy for any of the disorders associated with nonimmune consumption of platelets. Variable success is claimed for corticosteroid and radiation treatment in the Kasabach-Merritt syndrome; however, reported results are conflicting. Careful management of renal failure in HUS is the primary focus in that disorder. Transfusion with platelets and FFP to replace deficient clotting factors has been done with variable success in patients with bleeding manifestations and HUS. The bleeding associated with DIC is highly variable, even though evidence of laboratory abnormality may be obvious. The primary focus of DIC therapy is to treat the predisposing condition by use of oxygen, ventilation, or antibiotics if hypoxia or sepsis is the underlying condition. Should hemorrhage become life-threatening, support of the patient with platelet transfusion and FFP may be helpful.

Mechanical Entrapment of Platelets. A spleen that is massively enlarged because of either portal hypertension or intrinsic splenic abnormality, such as lysosomal storage disease, often traps platelets and induces thrombocytopenia. The resulting condition is called hypersplenism. The complete clinical picture consists of a patient with marked splenic enlargement, thrombocytopenia, leukopenia, mild anemia, and normal bone marrow. The therapeutic approach to patients with hypersplenism and hemorrhage depends on the source of the enlarged spleen. If enlargement is due to an abnormality extrinsic to the spleen (e.g., chronic liver disease) and the PT or PTT is prolonged, hemorrhage may respond to parenteral vitamin K (1 to 5 mg/dose). If the primary cause of hemorrhage is thrombocytopenia resulting from a process intrinsic to the spleen, splenectomy may be required to treat or prevent hemorrhage. The results of splenectomy are usually most gratifying when splenomegaly is due to intrinsic abnormality, as occurs with storage disorders such as Niemann-Pick and Gaucher's disease or the mucopolysaccharidoses.

Bleeding with Normal Platelet Count, Prolonged PT, and Prolonged PTT

Among bleeding disorders not associated with thrombocytopenia, those in which both the PT and PTT are prolonged are the most common. This combination of laboratory findings may occur with liver disease of any cause, vitamin K deficiency, DIC, and exposure to anticoagulants, or they may indicate a congenital deficiency of specific clotting factors—I, II, V, X

Liver Disease and Disseminated Intravascular Coagulopathy. If the hemorrhagic tendency is due to liver disease, additional physical findings (hepatomegaly, splenomegaly, jaundice) and laboratory abnormalities (elevated total and direct bilirubin and serum transaminases) are usually noted. However, even severe liver disease can be subtle in its clinical presentation. The prolonged PT and PTT associated with liver disease often respond to parenteral administration of vitamin K, 3 to 5 mg/dose; if the disease is severe, repeated large doses of vitamin K may be required.

Although DIC is typically associated with prolonged PT and PTT and a decreased platelet count, the first two may be the only laboratory abnormalities in DIC. Because of the similarity of this coagulation profile with that of liver disease, the distinction between DIC and liver disease can be difficult. Usually, with uncomplicated liver disease, FDPs are not elevated, and unless the liver disease is extremely severe, the fibrinogen level is not depressed. In contrast, the FDPs may be elevated and the fibrinogen may be depressed with DIC; hence, quantification of FDP and fibrinogen may differentiate between liver disease and DIC. In addition, quantification of factor VIII can be helpful because it is consumed and decreased in DIC but normal in liver disease.

DIC and severe liver disease can coexist. Presumably, the impaired ability of cirrhotic liver to remove FDPs predisposes to initiation of DIC by insults such as sepsis. Therapy of bleeding accompanying liver failure, with or without DIC, should include platelets, FFP, and vitamin K. Administration of prothrombin complex (Konȳne or Proplex) in the presence of liver failure may induce DIC and thus should be avoided in those patients with bleeding and liver failure.

Vitamin K Deficiency. Vitamin K deficiency is another cause of bleeding with prolonged PT and PTT but normal platelet levels. Vitamin K deficiency as the cause of hemorrhagic disease of the newborn is well known but rare. It also occurs in patients with malabsorption, and the resultant hemorrhagic tendency may be a clinical feature of malabsorption disorders such as cystic fibrosis or celiac disease in the pediatric patient. Prolonged PT and PTT are due to the deficiency of vitamin K-dependent factors II, VII, IX, and X and is readily reversed with parenteral administration of 3 to 5 mg of vitamin K. Unlike patients with severe liver disease, those with malabsorption should show a rapid (within 8 to 12 hours) normalization of PT and PTT after a single injection of vitamin K.

Anticoagulant Exposure. Therapeutic use of the anticoagulants heparin and coumadin is not widespread in pediatric practice. The increasing use of heparin locks for intermittent intravenous infusion may account for the prolongation of PT and PTT seen in many hospitalized patients who are not bleeding. Heparin potentiates the effect of antithrombin III on prothrombin activation and inhibits coagulation. Its primary effect is to prolong the PTT; however, in high doses, both PT and PTT are prolonged. Blood drawn through a heparin lock may contain significant amounts of heparin even if the line is initially cleared. Therefore, the PT and PTT should be determined only on blood samples obtained from a free-flowing venipuncture distant from the heparinized line. In addition, heparin is used intraoperatively on occasion and can be the cause of postoperative bleeding. Sometimes this effect must be differentiated from DIC. Heparin-induced prolongation of PT and PTT can be identified by the protamine titration test or batroxobin (Reptilase) time. Both protamine and Reptilase bypass the heparin effect and normalize clotting times in the absence of deficiencies of clotting factors that occur with DIC.

Congenital Clotting Factor Deficiencies. PT and PTT prolongation can reflect congenital deficiency of specific clotting factors. Only those factors common to both the intrinsic pathway (measured by PTT) and the extrinsic pathway (measured by PT) can cause prolonged PT and PTT. These factors include fibrinogen (I), prothrombin (II), proaccelerin (V), and Stuart factor (X). Characteristically, patients with these disorders suffer mucosal hemorrhage, traumatic bleeding, and bleeding after minor surgery. Diagnosis requires measurement of the activity of the specific factors and documented absence of liver disease or other explanation for the abnormality.

Bleeding with Normal Platelet Count, Normal PTT, and Prolonged PT

Bleeding with prolonged PT but normal PTT and platelet number can be associated with early primary liver disease, early vitamin K deficiency, coumadin therapy, or congenital factor VII deficiency. Differentiation of these disorders requires determination of liver function, direct and total bilirubin, and repeat coagulation tests after administration of parenteral vitamin K. Normal liver function test results and bilirubin level combined with failure of PT to normalize after parenteral vitamin K in a patient who has spontaneous nosebleeds, mucosal hemorrhage, and occasional hemarthroses suggest the diagnosis of congenital factor VII deficiency. Specific diagnosis of factor VII deficiency requires (1) exclusion of other diseases by finding normal factor X levels and (2) documentation of a specific decrease (less than 25%) of factor VII activity. Patients with congenital factor VII deficiency should have normal levels of other factors synthesized by the liver: II, V, IX, and X. The congenital deficiency is inherited as an autosomal recessive trait. Heterozygotes may have a prolonged PT with factor VII activity in the 17% to 40% range. Guidelines for therapy are given in Table 34-5.

Bleeding with Normal Platelet Count, Normal PT, and Prolonged PTT

The majority of inherited coagulopathies are manifest as a hemorrhagic tendency in patients with normal platelet numbers, normal PT, and prolonged PTT. A similar constellation of results with the coagulation screen can occur with therapeutic heparinization; however, exposure to heparin is usually obvious by history. The inherited coagulopathies segregate into two groups: (1) disorders with abnormal bleeding and prolonged PTT (VIII, IX, and XI deficiency and von Willebrand's disease) and (2) disorders with prolonged PTT and no abnormal bleeding (XII and prekallikrein deficiency and high-molecular-weight kininogen deficiency).

Factor VIII and Factor IX Deficiency. Patients with severe (less than 1%) factor VIII or IX deficiency typically suffer spontaneous bleeding into joints and soft tissues or bleeding at sites of minimal trauma. Factor levels of greater than 5% activity occur in milder variants of VIII and IX deficiency. Mildly deficient patients can experience spontaneous bleeding; however, bleeding typically follows trauma, lacerations, tooth extractions, or surgery. Usually, patients have a family history of abnormal bleeding or documented factor VIII or IX deficiency, which is sex-linked (i.e., occurring in maternal uncles, nephews, or grandfather). Therapy for factor VIII or IX deficiency consists of replacement with plasma products. Available products, expected responses, and suggested replacement for common problems are outlined briefly in Table 34-5. Dose calculation is reviewed in Exhibit 34-4. Three other important problems that may face primary physicians include closed head trauma, minor lacerations, and mouth injuries in hemophiliacs.

Closed head trauma, even of insignificant severity by normal standards, can result in intracranial hemorrhage in hemophiliacs. This can be acutely life-threatening and chronically debilitating. A patient with factor VIII or IX deficiency exposed to closed head trauma must be evaluated immediately; without regard to the presence or absence of neurologic abnormality or history of loss of consciousness, vomiting, or headache, immediate coverage with factor VIII at a level of 100% is indicated. Following initiation of treatment, extensive radiologic and neurologic evaluations are appropriate. Computed tomography of the head may be particularly helpful; however, a negative scan does not exclude the possibility of significant intracranial hemorrhage. Admission to the hospital and continued factor replacement for 3 to 5 days are indicated in any hemophiliac with a history of closed head trauma.

Exhibit 34-4 Calculation for Replacement in Factor VIII and Factor IX Deficiencies

Formula:

Total quantity (units of activity) to be infused = weight (kg) × desired level of factor (%) × [1/expected factor response (% increase in factor/unit factor given/kg)].

For example:

To raise factor VIII in a severely deficient patient (<1% VIII baseline) who weighs 20 kg to a 60% level would require

20 kg × 60% × 1/2 = 600 U factor VIII.

In contrast, to raise factor IX in a severely deficient patient (<1% IX baseline) who weighs 20 kg to a 60% level would require

20 kg × 60% × 1/1 = 1200 U factor IX.

Minor lacerations in hemophiliacs can be problematic. A laceration that requires sutures should be covered initially at 40% to 50% levels of activity until sutures are removed. Otherwise, chronic oozing and hematoma formation can lead to wound dehiscence, infection, and retarded healing. Small, seemingly inconsequential lacerations of the oral mucosa in infants up to 18 months of age can present a difficult management problem. Small tears or cuts of the frenulum may result from the trauma of gnawing during teething or from hard plastic nipple mounts of formula bottles. The repetitive nature of such trauma can result in repeated small hemorrhages, formation of highly vascular granulation tissue at the site, and then continuous bleeding. Interruption of this cycle and healing often requires daily factor replacement for 2 to 3 days, and aminocaproic acid (Amicar), 50 mg/kg/dose every 6 hours for 3 to 5 days. Significant drops in hematocrit can occur with such minor cuts.

Factor XI Deficiency. The hemorrhagic manifestations of factor XI deficiency are generally less severe than those of factor VIII and IX deficiency. Although some patients experience spontaneous soft tissue or joint bleeds and occasional mucous membrane bleeding, the majority of patients with factor XI deficiency bleed only after surgery. The disease is inherited as an autosomal recessive trait. Diagnosis is made by specific factor assay. Replacement therapy requires FFP, and guidelines are given in Table 34-5.

Von Willebrand's Disease. Von Willebrand's disease is considered here as a disorder characterized by abnormal clinical bleeding *and* abnormal PTT. In fact, neither, both, or either characteristic may be noted. Both the bleeding tendency and abnormalities of coagulation screens vary from kindred to kindred, individual to individual, and in a single patient over time. This variability probably reflects molecular and genetic heterogeneity within the clinical disease. Patients exhibit mucosal and GI hemorrhage and often bleed after surgery or tooth extractions. Unlike hemophiliacs, patients with von Willebrand's disease do not have spontaneous hemorrhage, and inheritance is autosomal dominant.

In laboratory tests patients with von Willebrand's

disease usually show mild to moderate reductions of factor VIII activity (20% to 50%). The PTT is not prolonged in patients with factor VIII activity greater than 30%. Patients with von Willebrand's disease are differentiated from mild hemophiliacs by their prolonged bleeding time, their one-to-one ratio of factor VIII coagulant activity and factor VIII antigen (hemophiliacs have gross excess of antigen to coagulant), and failure of ristocetin to induce platelet aggregation. Therapy for von Willebrand's disease consists of infusion with FFP or cryoprecipitate. (See Table 34-5 for therapeutic guidelines.)

Deficiencies with Prolonged PTT and No Abnormal Bleeding. The remainder of the inherited abnormalities of coagulation are characterized by a prolonged PTT in the absence of abnormal bleeding. This group includes deficiency of prekallikrein (Fletcher factor), high-molecular-weight kininogen (Fitzgerald factor), and factor XII (Hageman factor). Usually, these disorders are identified during routine preoperative coagulation screening of patients with no previous history of bleeding. Accurate laboratory definition of these disorders is required prior to surgery. Specific diagnosis requires exclusion of abnormalities associated with hemorrhagic tendency (i.e., PT, bleeding time, and levels of factors VIII, IX, and XI must be normal, and deficiency of the specific factor must be documented). In contrast to the other inherited coagulopathies, patients with deficiency of factor XII, prekallikrein, or high-molecular-weight kininogen do not require intra- or postoperative coverage with plasma products to prevent bleeding.

Bleeding Disorders with Normal Coagulation Screens

The coagulation screen (platelet count, PT, PTT) does not recognize all patients who manifest clinically abnormal bleeding. Those not identified include patients with vascular abnormalities, e.g., Henoch-Schönlein purpura, factor XIII deficiency, and diseases of platelet dysfunction (Glanzmann's thrombasthenia, Bernard-Soulier syndrome, von Willebrand's disease, and storage pool disease). Von Willebrand's disease is mentioned because in some individuals with factor VIII activities of greater than 30%, the sole laboratory abnormality may be deficiency of the plasma factor (von Willebrand's factor) that promotes ristocetin-induced aggregation of platelets. If the patient bleeds abnormally and the coagulation screen is normal, these disorders must be considered.

ONCOLOGIC EMERGENCIES

Emergencies occurring in the child with cancer are uncommon. However, the appropriate management of such situations is critical for a satisfactory outcome. For the purposes of this discussion, we have arbitrarily divided emergency situations into those occurring around the time of diagnosis and those occurring during therapy.

Emergencies at Diagnosis

The most important role for the physician when faced with a child who potentially has a malignant disease is to make an accurate and complete diagnosis without delay. This is best accomplished at a major pediatric center with staff experienced in the management of childhood cancer. Making the proper decisions regarding appropriate diagnostic interventions frequently requires modern imaging capabilities, specialized laboratory facilities, and input from a surgeon, pathologist, radiotherapist, and chemotherapist. For the child who is acutely ill, the input of this multidisciplinary team during this phase of illness is all the more critical. Inappropriate surgical interventions, including attempts at biopsy or excision, without the input of such a group of experts may lead to incomplete or inaccurate diagnosis and staging and the inability to plan radiation fields. A second operation may also be required at the cancer center so that appropriate planning for therapy may proceed. Likewise, bone marrow aspirations to diagnose leukemia will need to be repeated at the cancer center so that appropriate material for histochemical stains, marker studies, and other tests can be obtained. Many of the most common pediatric malignancies are highly curable with up-to-date care, and no child should be offered less than the best chance for long-term survival.

This section outlines those interventions that can and should be done when the diagnosis of malignancy is suspected. They are aimed at stabilizing the patient who is critically ill prior to referral to a pediatric cancer center. In addition, there is a brief discussion about what immediate steps are taken at the center when dealing with emergency situations in the child with suspected malignancy.

Anemia

Anemia detected at diagnosis in the child with cancer is usually secondary to either marrow infiltration by tumor or blood loss. Later during the treatment phase, the most frequent cause of anemia is inadequate production of new red cells secondary to chemotherapy-induced marrow suppression.

The history and physical examination may give clues about the existence and cause of anemia secondary to marrow infiltration. Because of the very gradual onset of anemia, the parents may note little change in the child's color, in spite of significant pallor with severe anemia. The child may complain of tiredness, decreasing activity, and increasing fatiguability. Fever, bone pain, easy bruising, and swollen glands may be associated with marrow infiltration. The physical examination may reveal paleness, tachycardia, signs of heart failure, adenopathy, petechiae, and areas of local infection. The hemoglobin level and hematocrit are low. Reticulocytes are absent or present in decreased numbers. The red cells are normochromic and normocytic, although some changes in red cell shape are sometimes seen. Platelets are usually decreased in number. The total WBC may be low, normal, or increased; abnormal blast forms are seen in the peripheral smear and in many cases may be the predominant white blood cell. Occasional nucleated red blood cells are noted.

In the clinical situation in which leukemia is suspected, a bone marrow aspiration is mandatory for diagnosis. As noted earlier, this is best performed at the multidisciplinary cancer center. In addition to sampling of bone marrow for a morphologic diagnosis, extra quantities of marrow should be withdrawn and immediately processed for histochemical staining, detection of membrane antigens, determination of membrane and cytoplasmic immunoglobulin, and other potential studies.

The treatment of moderate to severe anemia in the child with newly diagnosed leukemia is transfusion of packed red blood cells. During the first 2 to 3 weeks of chemotherapy, the bone marrow produces few new red cells; consequently, indications for transfusion are fairly liberal. Children with hemoglobin values less than 7 g/dL are transfused to a level usually greater than 12 g/dL. In the child with suspected malignancy, severe anemia, and incipient or gross heart failure, immediate transfusion prior to referral is indicated. Because a gradual elevation of hemoglobin is desired, the rate of administration of packed red cells should not exceed 2 mL/kg/h. Diuretic agents are a valuable means of decreasing the risk of overt congestive failure.

Hemorrhage

Hemorrhage in the child with suspected malignancy is most frequently due to thrombocytopenia, usually secondary to a productive defect caused by marrow infiltration. Less commonly, thrombocytopenia occurs because of peripheral destruction. Finally, the hemorrhage may be the result of defects in the fluid phase of coagulation, particularly when DIC accompanies the malignancy. This is most commonly seen in promyelocytic leukemia.

Evidence of bleeding, including mucosal hemorrhage, easy bruising, and a fine, red, nonblanching rash (petechiae), is noted in the history. The physical examination may reveal these areas of bleeding and petechiae. The CBC reveals a low platelet count and other abnormalities previously noted. If the fluid phase of coagulation is involved, the PT and PTT are prolonged.

Severe thrombocytopenia secondary to tumor infiltration of marrow is treated by platelet transfusions. Patients with platelet counts greater than 50,000/μL do not have an increased tendency to bleed unless there are other alterations of coagulation. Platelet counts less than 20,000/μL put the patient at an increased risk of hemorrhage, and spontaneous bleeding may occur when platelet counts are less than 5,000/μL. Patients with a platelet count less than 20,000/μL who are actively bleeding should be transfused to levels greater than 50,000/μL. Controversy exists regarding the proper management of the oncology patient who is not bleeding but has a platelet count less than 20,000/μL. We recommend transfusing these patients prophylactically to prevent hemorrhage and, in the patient with circulating leukemic blasts, to prevent possible seeding of leukemia cells secondary to microscopic bleeding into the meninges. This approach, however, cannot be supported by any controlled clinical trials at the present time. Random donor platelet transfusions are the platelet product of choice in newly diagnosed patients.

Excessive Tumor Burden

The child with suspected leukemia or lymphoma who has a markedly elevated WBC, tremendous organomegaly, or a large anterior mediastinal mass is at great risk for a variety of complications prior to and during the initiation of therapy. These complications can be fatal, and prompt, appropriate management must begin at the first physician contact.

Patients with very elevated WBCs at diagnosis (over 100,000/μL) are at risk for leukostasis and secondary hemorrhage in the central nervous system and lungs. These patients most commonly have acute myelocytic leukemia, although this syndrome also occurs in patients with acute lymphoblastic leukemia. The child has signs and symptoms of anemia and thrombocytopenia secondary to marrow replacement by tumor cells. There may be no signs or symptoms directly related to the elevated WBC; however, the patient may have evidence of central nervous system dysfunction (headache, vomiting, cranial nerve palsies, coma, and convulsions) or pulmonary insufficiency (tachypnea, dyspnea, and cyanosis). The risk of fatal brain hemorrhage, occurring in up to 15% of these patients, necessitates prompt intervention. Immediate referral is indicated. At the cancer center, aspiration of bone marrow is performed for diagnosis, and emergency measures aimed at rapid lowering of the WBC are instituted. Hydroxyurea, cytosine arabinoside, other chemotherapeutic agents, and leukophoresis have all been used. Frequently, prophylactic cranial irradiation is also indicated. If for some compelling reason immediate referral to a cancer center is not possible, adequate hydration and alkalinization must be started (see "Metabolic and Renal Complications"), and hydroxyurea (50 to 100 mg/kg as a single oral dose) should be administered.

A large anterior mediastinal mass is a common feature of Hodgkin's disease, non-Hodgkin's lymphoma, and certain subtypes of acute lymphoblastic leukemia. Children with these disorders frequently have cough; less commonly, they may have severe narrowing of the airway and obstruction of the superior vena cava occur. Patients with no or minimal signs of airway or vascular obstruction may quickly develop severe signs and symptoms of obstruction, particularly during general anesthesia induced for biopsy of the lesion. The care of these children must be closely coordinated with the surgeon, chemotherapist, anesthesiologist, and radiotherapist. Other areas of tumor involvement must be investigated, including the bone marrow, so as not to miss more easily accessible sites for diagnosis. If no other areas of suspected tumor are found, biopsy of the anterior mediastinal mass is indicated. The patient must be prepared to begin therapy prior to the induction of anesthesia. The anesthesiologist should be prepared to give high-dose intravenous corticosteroids, and the radiotherapist must be available to give mediastinal irradiation should severe compromise of respiratory status occur. Unless the patient's airway is critically compromised, short pulses of corticosteroids should be avoided prior to biopsy because even relatively small doses may cause enough tumor necrosis so that no definitive histologic diagnosis is possible.

Metabolic and Renal Complications

Many children with acute leukemia (particularly with elevated peripheral blast counts) and lymphoma (notably Burkitt's lymphoma) develop significant metabolic complications prior to and during the induction phase of therapy. These problems should be anticipated; proper management can begin as soon as the diagnosis is suspected and prior to referral to a cancer center.

Uric acid nephropathy may be life-threatening in these children. Lymphomatous malignancies have a high rate of cellular turnover and lyse very quickly when chemotherapy is started. Large quantities of purine analogs are released and metabolized to xanthine, hypoxanthine, and finally uric acid by xanthine oxidase. Consequently, the serum uric acid level should be determined in all patients with suspected lymphoid malignancies. Uric acid may precipitate in the renal tubule when the serum concentration exceeds 7 mg/dL. Xanthine and hypoxanthine are more soluble than uric acid, and all three compounds are more soluble in an alkaline environment. Consequently, the administration of allopurinol (a xanthine oxidase inhibitor) at 10 mg/kg/d orally, hydration with twice maintenance level intravenous fluids (2500 to 3000 mL/m^2/d), and alkalinization of the urine (50 to 75 mEq $NaHCO_3$ per liter in 5% dextrose in water) are recommended. Less commonly, mannitol is used to induce diuresis. If the patient fails to respond to an initial dose of mannitol, it should be discontinued. Acetazolamide (150 mg/m^2/d) is also used to produce urinary alkalinization. However, this drug may aggravate systemic acidosis. The goal is to stop all new uric acid production and to maintain the urine specific gravity at less than 1.010 and urine pH at greater than 7.0. These measures all can be started prior to referral.

In addition to the release of intracellular purines, phosphates and potassium are also liberated as tumor cells lyse. In most instances the increased phosphate and potassium loads are well handled, as long as good renal output continues. In some instances (particularly in children with very large tumor burdens or Burkitt's lymphoma), an elevated serum phosphate concentration results in secondary hypocalcemia. Efforts should be aimed at maintaining good urine output to increase phosphate excretion. Calcium infusions should be avoided, except when *symptomatic* hypocalcemia occurs, because increases in calcium concentration with preexisting elevated serum phosphate levels will increase the calcium-phosphorus product and increase the risk of $CaPO_4$ deposition in the renal tubule. This increased deposition may result in acute renal failure. In these children the urine pH should be maintained at 6.0 to 7.0 to decrease the risk of $CaPO_4$ deposition.

The children at greatest risk for metabolic and renal complications are those with elevated peripheral WBCs, large tumor burdens, renal obstruction, or abnormal renal function prior to therapy. In these high-risk patients many pediatric oncologists begin the induction of chemotherapy with a gradual escalation of drug doses, in hopes of more gradually inducing the initial tumor lysis. In such children we recommend initiating therapy with 25% of the recommended corticosteroid dose, doubling this dose daily, and then administering other indicated chemotherapeutic agents with the third or fourth day of corticosteroids. Even with all of the outlined precautions, a rare child develops acute renal failure during induction. Sometimes radiotherapy (400 rads) to the renal bed improves renal function. The availability of dialysis may be lifesaving if acute renal failure develops. In many instances these children require aggressive chemotherapy in the face of decreased renal function, and artificial mechanisms for the removal of large quantities of toxic cellular metabolites are required.

Fever

Fever is common in the child newly diagnosed with a hematogenous malignancy. Fever may be secondary to the tumor itself when the marrow is replaced with tumor and inadequate numbers of normal granulocytes are present in the peripheral circulation; however, fever should always indicate to the physician the presence of infection. The child with leukemia during initial induction of therapy and at relapse is at the highest risk for severe infection. The management of fever is discussed in "Emergencies during Treatment."

Spinal Cord Involvement

A tumor causing spinal cord dysfunction may be extradural (hematogenous metastatic disease or primary tumor eroding through the vertebrae) or intradural (drop metastases from primary brain tumors). Dysfunction may be present at diagnosis or occur later when widespread metastatic disease exists. Prompt diagnosis and appropriate intervention require a high index of suspicion and may result in a better outcome for the child. It is easier to preserve neurologic function than to reverse significant deficits.

The child frequently complains of local pain in the vertebral column; radicular pain is less common. Weakness, paralysis (usually involving the lower extremities), bowel and bladder dysfunction, and sensory deficits can occur. In the child with a suspected or proven spinal mass lesion and no prior diagnosis of malignancy, an immediate and thorough evaluation for tumor is mandatory. In the child with a proven malignancy who begins to complain of localized back pain, weakness, or sensory changes, the index of suspicion for spinal metastases must be very high so that an early diagnosis can be made.

The emergency therapy of spinal cord involvement is controversial and must be based on sound knowledge of the biology of the tumor and its response to various therapeutic interventions. Immediate laminectomy relieves pressure on the spinal cord, preventing further deterioration of motor and sensory function and has the added advantage of providing tissue for diagnostic tests. However, there is no evidence in children that the preservation of neurologic function with laminectomy is superior to immediate local radiotherapy and/or chemotherapy for those tumors responsive to such therapies. In addition, laminectomy in the young child is associated with significant short-term and long-term morbidity.

In the previously well child with signs and symptoms of spinal cord compression, immediate evaluation by a neurologist or neurosurgeon is indicated. In addition to computed tomography of the head (to evaluate the possibility of intracranial tumor), plain spinal films, radioisotopic bone scans, and myelography to define the presence and extent of the tumor, radiologic evaluation for intrathoracic and intra-abdominal tumors is mandatory, possibly including plain chest films, computed tomography of the chest and abdomen, and abdominal sonography. If the presence of a thoracic or abdominal mass is suggested, urine testing for catecholamines (including vanillylmandelic acid) and a bone marrow aspiration to define neuroblastoma should be done. At this point, if no tumor outside the central nervous system is found, immediate diagnostic surgery and coverage with high-dose dexamethasone (12 to 15 mg/d) should be undertaken. However, if the workup suggests neuroblastoma, therapeutic approaches must be coordinated with the neurosurgeon, radiotherapist, and chemotherapist. Some investigators suggest that these children may be treated with chemotherapy and/or radiotherapy without immediate laminectomy.

In the child with known malignancy and signs and symptoms suggesting spinal cord compression, immediate neurologic evaluation again is imperative. Myelography is performed to define the location and extent of involvement. If the tumor is known to be sensitive to chemotherapy or radiotherapy, these modalities, particularly radiotherapy (along with high-dose dexamethasone), should be immediately started. Surgical intervention should be reserved for spinal instability or compression by bone, for tumors that fail to respond to radiotherapy or are known to be radioresistant, and in patients with previous radiation exposure of the spinal cord.

The prognosis for neurologic outcome in children with spinal cord compression depends on the type and histology of the tumor and its sensitivity to therapy, the stage of disease, the neurologic status prior to intervention, the rate of onset of neurologic deficit, and the intraspinal location of the tumor (anterior compression of the cord creates more technical problems for the neurosurgeon). It must be stressed that it is easier to preserve neurologic function than to reverse severe neurologic deficits; therefore, the work-up and therapy of these children must be completed expeditiously.

Emergencies during Treatment

Infection

Infection continues to be a leading cause of death in the child with cancer, despite the availability of second-generation and third-generation antimicrobial agents. This is likely due to a number of factors, including increasingly intensive multiagent chemotherapy protocols, development of resistant strains of infectious agents, and the limited sensitivity of various culture systems in identifying specific pathogens. Consequently, many of the recommendations for management of infectious complications are empirically based.

Fever (oral temperature† greater than 38.2° C and lasting longer than 2 to 3 hours) in the child with neutropenia (circulating polymorphonuclear leukocytes $< 500/\mu L$) indicates infection unless another specific cause is found. Newly diagnosed and relapsing patients with extensive disseminated malignancies and with marrow replacement by tumor are at the highest risk of developing fatal infections. All patients with fever and neutropenia should be hospitalized for appropriate evaluation and management.

These patients require a complete interval history and a thorough physical examination. Specific areas to cover in the history are episodes of shaking chills; headache; stiff neck; presence of lesions on the skin, in the mouth, and around the anal opening; cough; dyspnea; recent exposure to others with infections; and present medications. (Many patients under active intensive chemotherapy are receiving oral prophylactic antibiotics, most commonly trimethoprim-sulfonamide combinations.) The physical examination should be complete and performed *only* after strict handwashing. Particular attention should be paid to the oral cavity, rectum, and skin, which are colonized by normal bacterial and fungal flora and are frequent sites of infection by opportunistic organisms. Many minor-appearing lesions commonly cause life-threatening bacteremias. With severe neutropenia few signs of inflammation with little or no purulent exudate can accompany severe infection.

The laboratory evaluation of the child with fever and neutropenia should include a CBC and urinalysis. Specimens of the blood and urine and samples taken from any sites of infection noted on physical examination should be cultured for identification of bacterial and possibly fungal organisms. X-ray films of the chest are mandatory, and if the clinical evaluation suggests, sinus films also should be obtained. Culturing of the cerebrospinal fluid is not done routinely except when clinical signs and symptoms suggest central nervous system infection.

Once the appropriate evaluation is completed, the child is placed empirically on broad-spectrum antimicrobial agents. The specific choice of drugs depends on the types of bacterial pathogens common in neutropenic patients at the treating institution and their antimicrobial sensitivities. Pathogens common in these children include *Staphylococcus aureus, Staphylococcus epidermidis,* streptococci, enterococci, *E. coli, Pseudomonas* species. *Klebsiella pneumoniae,* and species of *Serratia, Enterobacter, Candida,* and *Aspergillus.* We are presently using a combination of nafcillin, 50 to 100 mg/kg/d, to cover staphylococci and other Gram-positive organisms; tobramycin, 6 to 7.5 mg/kg/d, for Gram-negative organisms; and ticarcillin, 200 to 300 mg/kg/d, for its additional synergistic action against *Pseudomonas* organisms. Empiric combinations of trimethoprim and sulfonamides plus an aminoglycoside also provide appropriate coverage for these children. We avoid the routine use of combinations of cephalosporins and aminoglycosides because these combinations have not proved superior to the combination of ticarcillin, nafcillin, and tobramycin and are potentially more nephrotoxic. In addition, because of the potential nephrotoxicity of aminoglycosides, this group of drugs should be avoided in a child who has received *cis*-platinum, a nephrotoxic chemotherapeutic agent.

A much more complex problem occurs in those children who have prolonged neutropenia (greater than 2 weeks). These children usually have leukemia in relapse or have received intensive combinations of chemotherapeutic agents. The initial approach is the same as in patients with brief periods of neutropenia. However, continued or recurrent fe-

† Rectal temperatures should be absolutely avoided in children with neutropenia.

ver in these children suggests superinfection, frequently with fungal organisms. Intensive attempts to isolate and identify a specific pathogen are important. Frequently, empiric addition of amphotericin B is recommended; however, the morbidity from this approach must be weighed against the possible benefits.

Pneumonia in the child under active chemotherapy may be caused by common bacterial and viral pathogens. However, both fungi and *Pneumocystis carinii* are important pathogens in these children. Usually, the pneumonia should be treated the same as if occurring in an otherwise well child of similar age. However, if the chest film suggests an unusual organism or if the child is not responding clinically, a lung aspirate or biopsy may be required to determine the appropriate therapy.

Chickenpox (varicella) poses a particular threat to the child undergoing chemotherapy for a malignant disease. In some series, dissemination of varicella to the liver, lung, or brain occurs in almost one third of children receiving anticancer drugs, with up to 7% dying of disseminated varicella infections. Zoster immune globulin (ZIG) or zoster immune plasma (ZIP), when administered within 48 to 72 hours of exposure, prevents the occurrence of clinical varicella in over two thirds of children on chemotherapy and ameliorates the disease in those children contracting clinical varicella. Consequently, all children on active chemotherapy who are exposed to chickenpox (member of household, indoor exposure to a playmate for longer than 1 to 2 hours, or close school exposure, such as a child in the same classroom who has or soon develops clinical varicella) should receive ZIG or ZIP within 48 hours of such an exposure. ZIG and ZIP are presently available through regional Red Cross Blood banks.

Pain

Children with disseminated malignancies, particularly when such cancers reach a terminal state, have chronic, debilitating pain. Many of these children suffer needlessly primarily because of the physician's reluctance to prescribe adequate analgesic relief. The child with severe pain must be evaluated thoroughly in an attempt to define a treatable cause for the pain. The type and magnitude of such an evaluation must be based on the individual clinical circumstances. Frequently, plain X-ray films or radionuclide bone scans reveal a metastatic lesion as a source of pain; this can sometimes be locally irradiated, with good relief from pain. Occasionally, this evaluation also reveals nonmalignant causes for pain that can be readily treated.

Analgesic drugs play a primary role in pain relief. Acetaminophen is effective in controlling mild pain; aspirin is avoided because of its effect on platelet function. Codeine, frequently combined with acetaminophen, is effective in controlling moderate pain and may be preferable to other combination analgesics in the child.

The use of potent narcotics is clearly indicated for the control of pain not responding to adequate doses of codeine and acetaminophen. Morphine (0.1 to 0.2 mg/kg/dose), meperidine (Demerol; 1 mg/kg/dose), hydromorphone (Dilaudid), and others have about the same analgesic effects if given in appropriate doses. The selection of one of these agents can be based primarily on the physician's familiarity with each agent. We have found methadone particularly useful in those children with intractable pain; its long half-life allows less frequent administration. However, the physician must remember to titrate this drug more gradually because of its long half-life. The addition of a phenothiazine occasionally potentiates the narcotic analgesia.

It must be remembered that the key to controlling pain is to give adequate doses of pain relievers at frequent enough intervals, with some children requiring higher than recommended doses. Analgesics given at appropriate intervals on a scheduled basis, rather than a "prn" basis, frequently can prevent severe pain from occurring in these patients. These children may also benefit from consultation with a pain clinic. We have had good success with transcutaneous electrical stimulation, even in very young children.

Toxic Effects of Chemotherapy

Multiagent chemotherapy (along with advances in radiotherapy and surgery) has provided a realistic hope for long-term disease-free survival and cure for many childhood malignancies that only a decade or so ago were rapidly fatal. However, this success is not without both short-term and long-term morbidity. Local referring physicians are frequently called on to help administer various chemotherapeutic agents and treat the side effects of these drugs, in consultation with the cancer center. They must familiarize themselves with the proper mixing, dilution, route and method of administration, and frequent side effects of each drug they give.

Table 34-6 lists the more commonly used chemotherapeutic agents and their side effects. Several points require explanation. All drugs producing vesication can cause severe tissue destruction if infiltrated into the subcutaneous tissues around the vein, leading to tissue necrosis with poor healing

TABLE 34-6 Side Effects of Chemotherapy

Drug	Alopecia	Vesication	Marrow Suppression	Nausea, Vomiting	Pulmonary Effects	Cardiac Effects	Neurologic Effects	Hepatic Effects	Renal Effects	Stomatitis	Route of Administration
Vincristine	+	+	+	0/+	0	0	2+	*	0	0/+	IV
Vinblastine	+	+	2+/3+	0/+	0	0	+	*	0	+	IV
VM-26 (teniposide)†	+	+	2+/3+	+	0	0‡	0	0	0	+	IV
Adriamycin†	+	+	3+	+	0	+	0	*	0	+	IV
Daunomycin†	+	+	3+	+	0	+	0	*	0	+	IV
Actinomycin	+	+	3+	+	0	0	0	+	0	+	IV
Cyclophosphamide†	+	0	2+/3+	+	Rare	Rare	0	Rare	Cystitis	Rare	po/IV
Mustard	Uncommon	+	2+	+	0	0	0	Rare	0	0	IV
Procarbazine	Rare	0	2+	+	Rare	0	+	+	0	+	po
cis-Platinum†	0	0	1+/2+	+	0	Rare	+	Rare	+	0	IV
Bleomycin†	+	0	0	Rare	+	0	0	0	0	0	IV/IM
Nitrosureas	Rare	0	2+/3+	+	Rare	0	+	+	Rare	+	po/IV
Methotrexate	+	0	1+/3+	+	Rare	0	Infrequent	+	+	+	po/IV/IM/IT§
6-Mercaptopurine	0	0	1+/2+	+	0	0	0	+	0	0	po
6-Thioguanine	0	0	1+/2+	+	0	0	0	0	0	0	po
Cytosine arabinoside	+	0	2+/3+	+	0	0	Rare	+	0	0	IV/SC/IT
L-Asparaginase†	0	0	0/+	±	0	0	+	+	0	0	IV/IM

* Drug excreted by liver.
† Hypersensitivity reactions.
‡ Hypotension during too rapid infusion.
§ Intratumor.

and sometimes requiring skin grafting. Care must be exercised so that these drugs are administered directly into the vein. If any questions exists about the location of an intravenous needle or catheter, it is preferable to remove the device and repeat the venipuncture at another site. Once the needle is placed within the vein, a flush of normal saline is first introduced to help assure intravenous injection; then the drug is pushed, followed by a second flush of normal saline ("two-syringe" technique). If any of the chemotherapeutic drug escapes from the vein, it is recommended in many of the drug instructions to instill hydrocortisone and/or apply topical hydrocortisone cream. Recent experimentation in animal models, however, has failed to demonstrate any dramatic decrease in local tissue reaction with the application of local corticosteroids.

Marrow suppression occurs with most chemotherapeutic agents. The degree of suppression depends on the drug, the dose, sometimes the method of administration, and whether the drug is used in combination with other agents. With single-agent therapy, the nadir for peripheral counts usually occurs 10 to 12 days after administration, with recovery in 7 to 10 days. However, combination chemotherapy and some single agents (particularly the nitrosureas) may produce prolonged suppression. The management of chemotherapy-induced marrow suppression is discussed earlier.

Bibliography

Levine A (ed): *Cancer in the Young.* New York, Masson Publishing USA Inc, 1982.

Miller D, Baehner R, MacMillan C: *Blood Diseases of Infancy and Childhood,* ed 5. St. Louis, CV Mosby Co, 1984.

Nathans D, Oski F (eds): *The Hematology of Infancy and Childhood.* WB Saunders Co, Philadelphia, 1981.

Sutow W, Fernbach D, Vietti T (eds): *Clinical Pediatric Oncology,* ed 3. St. Louis, CV Mosby Co, 1984.

Michael S. Kappy
William E. Winter

35 Endocrine and Metabolic Emergencies

Metabolic and endocrine emergencies in children are not uncommon, and can lead to disordered consciousness, seizures, and death.[1] Children who survive may have permanent sequelae. Prompt recognition of the specific disorder or class of disorder (Exhibit 35-1) is therefore imperative for appropriate treatment to prevent irreversible central nervous system (CNS) damage.

This chapter is confined to conditions that occur beyond the newborn period. The emergency physician is unlikely to encounter neonates, and the differential diagnosis of metabolic and endocrine emergencies is enlarged considerably if the newborn group is included.[2] Inherited conditions that are seen in infancy, however, are included in this discussion.

CLINICAL FEATURES

Diminished levels of consciousness and generalized seizures are common signs in most of the endocrine and metabolic emergencies in children. Levels of consciousness can range from drowsiness to total unresponsiveness and are usually related to the severity of the metabolic disturbance. Fulop's classification of level of consciousness[3] is shown in Table 35-1. Seizures are commonly seen when hypoglycemia, hyponatremia, or hypocalcemia are present, and they may be severe. As a rule the seizures are generalized; however, focal seizures also may be seen, and their presence is not evidence against a generalized metabolic disturbance.

There are other signs that may accompany metabolic and endocrine emergencies. Failure to thrive, poor feeding, vomiting, lethargy, and unusual body or urine odor are seen especially in inborn errors of metabolism. Hepatomegaly (in the absence of cardiac failure) can signify glycogen storage disease, galactosemia, or inflammatory liver disease, and its presence in the child with hypoglycemia usually rules out excessive insulin secretion as a cause. Jaundice can accompany galactosemia or inflammatory liver disease, and cataracts also can be associated with galactosemia. As with other emergencies hypertension or hypotension and shock can be present. The specific pertinent historical and physical findings are discussed under each disease entity.

DIAGNOSTIC TESTS

A number of general laboratory tests can be used for short-term evaluation of the child with a suspected endocrine-metabolic emergency (Exhibit 35-2). More specific tests may have to be ordered as the diagnostic possibilities narrow. For this reason ex-

Exhibit 35-1 Metabolic and Endocrine Emergencies in Children and Adolescents

- Metabolic Acidosis
  - Diabetic ketoacidosis
  - Lactic acidosis: primary inborn error of metabolism or secondary to hypoxia
  - Salicylate intoxication
  - Inborn errors of amino acid or organic acid metabolism
  - Some conditions characterized by hypoglycemia (e.g., glycogen storage disease type I, von Gierke's disease, glucose 6-phosphatase deficiency)
  - Renal tubular acidosis
  - Renal failure
  - Congenital adrenal hyperplasia
  - Diarrhea
- Nonketotic Hyperosmolar Coma
- Hypoglycemia
  - Excessive utilization of glucose
    - Oversecretion of insulin
      - Islet (β) cell adenoma
      - Nesidioblastosis
      - β-Cell hyperplasia
      - Leucine sensitive?
      - Ingestion of sulfonylureas
    - Factitious or accidental insulin overdose
    - Fevers*
    - Infections*
    - Tumors
    - Hyperthyroidism
    - Cold stress
    - Vigorous exercise*
  - Deficient production of glucose
    - Fasting or prolonged illness:* ketotic hypoglycemia
    - Defects in glycogenolysis,* usually congenital (e.g., von Gierke's disease, galactosemia)
    - Defects in gluconeogenesis*
      - Hormone defects: panhypopituitarism or isolated deficiency of pituitary hormones (e.g., GH,† ACTH: idiopathic or secondary to tumors), adrenal insufficiency (CAH, Addison's disease, or acute corticosteroid withdrawal)
      - Enzyme defects: fructose-1,6-diphosphatase deficiency, disorders of amino acid and organic acid metabolism
      - Hereditary fructose intolerance
      - Reye's syndrome
    - Intoxications: salicylate, alcohol
- Hypocalcemia and Hypercalcemia
  - Hypocalcemia
    - Parathyroid deficiency
      - Idiopathic or familial
      - DiGeorge's syndrome
      - Postoperative thyroidectomy
      - Hypokalemia
      - Hypomagnesemia
    - Pseudohypoparathyroidism
    - Renal failure or tubule disorders
    - Rickets
      - Vitamin D deficiency
      - Lack of sunshine
      - Liver disease
      - Malabsorption syndromes
      - Low phosphate intake (preemies)
      - 1α-hydroxylase deficiency (vitamin D-dependent rickets)
      - Familial hypophosphatemia
    - Metabolic alkalosis (decreased ionized calcium)
    - Acute pancreatitis
  - Hypercalcemia
    - Hyperparathyroidism: primary hyperplasia or secondary to renal failure
    - Drugs: vitamin D overdose
    - Tumors that secrete calcium-mobilizing peptides
    - Tumors that metastasize to bone
    - Bone immobilization
- Thyroid Disorders
  - Hyperthyroid states (if cardiac output is excessive)
    - Neonatal hyperthyroidism
    - Graves' disease
    - Hashimoto's thyroiditis
    - Accompanying diabetes mellitus type I
    - Excessive ingestion of thyroid hormone
  - Hypothyroidism (rarely a cause of emergencies in children)
    - Congenital
      - Transient, due to maternal propylthiouracil ingestion in last trimester.
      - Defect in biosynthesis of thyroid hormone: goitrous hypothyroidism (goiter rarely may obstruct trachea and require surgical removal)
      - Thyroid remnants (incomplete gland)
    - Autoimmune (e.g., Hashimoto's thyroiditis, late): may accompany diabetes mellitus type I
    - Postoperative thyroidectomy when replacement therapy is insufficient or not taken
    - Hypopituitarism
- Adrenal Disorders
  - Hyperactivity
    - Cushing's syndrome
    - Adrenal tumor
    - Excessive ACTH secretion (pituitary adenoma or extrapituitary source)
    - Pharmacologic corticosteroid hormone ingestion
  - Hypoactivity
    - Adrenal hemorrhage (trauma, meningococcemia)
    - Congenital adrenal hypoplasia
    - CAH
      - Defect in cortisol biosynthesis
      - Defect in aldosterone biosynthesis
    - Other infection: tuberculosis, coccidioidomycosis, blastomycosis, histoplasmosis
    - Congenital unresponsiveness to ACTH (Migeon's syndrome)
    - Autoimmune (Addison's disease): may accompany diabetes mellitus type I or hypoparathyroidism
    - Acute corticosteroid hormone withdrawal
    - Hypopituitarism
- Hyper- and Hyponatremia
  - Hypernatremia
    - Excessive sodium intake: boiled milk, hyperalimentation, excessive IV sodium infusions
    - Excessive water loss
      - Diarrhea (hypertonic or hypernatremic dehydration)
      - Vomiting?
      - Antidiuretic hormone deficiency
        - CNS lesions
        - Idiopathic
        - Hypercalcemia
        - Hypokalemia
      - Nephrogenic diabetes insipidus
    - Decreased sodium loss
      - Excessive steroid hormone intake

Exhibit 35-1 *(continued)*

Cushing's syndrome or adrenal tumor
Hyperaldosteronism
Head injury
Hyponatremia
Excessive water intake (water intoxication)
Hypotonic IV infusions
Diminished water loss
Renal failure
Syndrome of inappropriate antidiuretic hormone secretion
Cirrhosis
Cystic fibrosis, pneumonias
CNS irritations
Increased sodium loss
Diarrhea (hyponatremic dehydration)
Mineralocorticoid deficiency
CAH
Addison's disease
Defects in aldosterone biosynthesis
Renal tubule diseases
Cystic fibrosis
Diuretics
Osmotic diuresis (e.g., in diabetic ketoacidosis)
Apparent hyponatremia: in the presence of hyperglycemia and/or hyperlipidemia (e.g., in diabetes mellitus types I and II)

* Usually associated with ketonuria.
† Abbreviations: GH, growth hormone; ACTH, adrenocorticotropic hormone; CAH, congenital adrenal hyperplasia; CNS, central nervous system.

tra blood (5 to 10 mL) is usually sent to the laboratory, where the plasma or serum is frozen for later use. In each section these tests are discussed under "special tests."

Blood Tests

Glucose

The blood glucose concentration can be estimated quickly from a drop of blood by using one of the readily available test strip methods. Either Chemstrips bG (Bio-Dynamics, Indianapolis, IN), read visually, or Dextrostix (Ames Co., Elkhart, IN), read with a meter, can be used. Routine determination of the blood glucose concentration also should be

TABLE 35-1 Classification of Level of Consciousness

Stage	Condition
1	Awake or mildly drowsy
2	Moderately drowsy but easily aroused and fully oriented
3	Very drowsy but aroused by loud questioning and then partially oriented
4	Stuporous, barely responsive, and then not oriented
5	Comatose

Source: Reprinted with permission from Fulop M, Tannenbaum H, Dreyer N: Ketotic hyperosmolar coma. *Lancet* 1973;2:000.

Exhibit 35-2 Laboratory Evaluation of Children with Suspected Endocrine-Metabolic Emergencies

Blood Tests
Glucose (screen initially with blood test strip [Chemstrip bG])
Electrolytes (Na^+, K^+, Cl^-, CO_2 content) and BUN*
Calculated anion gap: $Na^+ - (Cl^- + CO_2$ content)
Calculated plasma osmolality:
$(2 \times Na^+) + (Glucose/18) + (BUN/3)$
Measured plasma osmolality
Blood pH
Serum ketones (screen with nitroprusside [Acetest] tablet)
Calcium, phosphorus
Ammonia
Special tests (see individual sections)
Urine Tests
Routine urinalysis, including sediment
Toxin screen
Electrocardiogram

* Blood urea nitrogen.

done by the laboratory to ensure greater accuracy and for irreproachable records.

Severe hyperglycemia (>500 mg/dL) suggests diabetic ketoacidosis (DKA) or nonketotic hyperosmolar coma as causes, although many patients with DKA have initial blood glucose concentrations as low as 250 to 350 mg/dL.

Nonendocrine emergencies, such as head injury, severe stress, or infection, also can be accompanied by hyperglycemia, but this is rarely greater than 250 to 350 mg/dL. Acute salicylate intoxication is usually associated with hypo- or normoglycemia, but such patients occasionally have blood glucose concentrations up to 300 mg/dL.

Electrolytes and Osmolality

Measurement of serum electrolytes (Exhibit 35-2) enables the emergency physician to narrow considerably the diagnostic possibilities in the child with an endocrine-metabolic emergency. Hyper- or hyponatremia, hyper- or hypokalemia, and metabolic acidosis can all be diagnosed with a standard electrolyte "package," e.g., sequential mutichannel autoanalyzer (SMA)-6 or a renal profile. In addition, the blood urea nitrogen (BUN) and creatinine concentrations may suggest dehydration or renal disease as contributing factors. Blood pH measurement is important in determining the extent of compromise of the body's defense mechanisms in metabolic acidosis and can be an important guide to therapy.

The calculated anion gap (Exhibit 35-2) can help differentiate the metabolic acidosis that accompanies diabetes or salicylate ingestion (high anion gap) from that accompanying loss of bicarbonate from the body (normal anion gap, hyperchloremic acidosis).

The calculated plasma or serum osmolality is helpful in diagnosing diabetes insipidus (DI) and inappropriate secretion of antidiuretic hormone (ADH) in children. Although familial and idiopathic DI are quite rare, DI may accompany head trauma with intracranial bleeding, central nervous system (CNS) infection, or tumor. In such instances the plasma sodium concentration is high, the calculated plasma osmolality is high (≥300 mosm/kg), and the urine specific gravity is low (<1.008), suggesting a failure of normal ADH secretion in response to plasma hyperosmolality. A similar picture may be seen as a result of relative renal unresponsiveness to ADH if the serum K^+ is decreased or the serum calcium is increased, or in the rare condition of familial nephrogenic DI. In conditions characterized by inappropriate secretion of ADH, plasma sodium can reach dangerously low levels; the plasma osmolality is low (≤260 mosm/kg), yet the osmolality or the specific gravity of the urine is high.

The calculated and measured serum osmolality should agree within 10 mosm/kg. If the measured osmolality is much greater than calculated, the presence of an unmeasured osmole, such as glycerol, ethylene glycol, or mannitol, is suggested. A calculated osmolality greater than measured usually suggests laboratory error.

Ketones

In cases of suspected DKA, serum or plasma can be screened for the presence of "ketone bodies" by using a crushed nitroprusside (Acetest) tablet. Note that this test measures acetoacetate and acetone (to a lesser degree), but not β-hydroxybutyrate, the major ketone body in DKA. Also, if the patient is moderately hypoxic, very little of the total ketone body concentration will be acetoacetate and the Acetest screening test *may be negative*.

Calcium and Phosphorus

Tests for calcium and phosphorus are particularly useful in arriving at a diagnosis in children who have seizures or signs of tetany. The usual finding is a decreased serum calcium concentration (<7.0 mg/dL) coupled with an increased phosphorus concentration (>6.0 mg/dL); however, the latter finding is variable. Hypercalcemia of clinical significance is usually associated with serum calcium concentrations of greater than 11.0 mg/dL.

Ammonia

Measuring ammonia aids in the diagnosis of liver failure, Reye's syndrome, and certain inborn errors of the urea cycle.

Urine Tests

Urine tests are helpful in documenting the glucosuria and ketonuria that are typical of DKA. Ketonuria without glucosuria is often found in hypoglycemia, particularly ketotic hypoglycemia, the most common cause of hypoglycemia in the 1- to 5-year-old age group.

Urine specific gravity should be commensurate with the serum osmolality and should be greater than 1.015 when serum osmolality is greater than 300 mosm/kg. If the urine is more dilute (i.e., ≤1.008) at that point, diminished ADH secretion or diminished renal responsiveness to ADH is suggested. In cases of inappropriate ADH secretion, on the other hand, the urine specific gravity will be high (≤1.015 to 1.020) in the face of reduced serum osmolality (≤ 260 mosm/kg). Documentation of urine osmolality by direct measurement can be helpful in these situations.

Electrocardiogram

A lead II rhythm strip tracing can be helpful in screening for major electrolyte abnormalities or in following the short-term course of change in a particular electrolyte if an abnormality has been de-

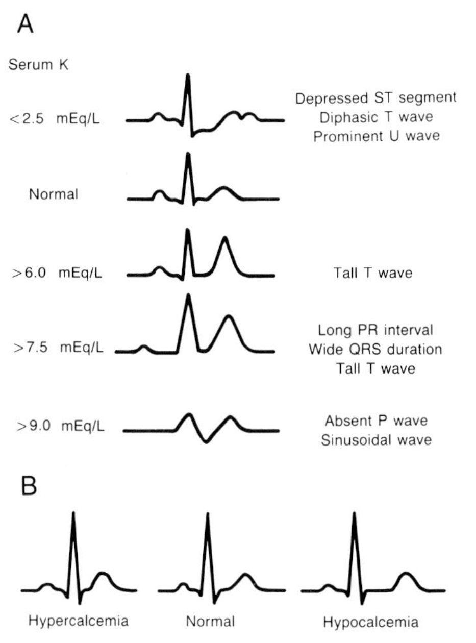

FIGURE 35-1 A, Electrocardiogram findings of hypokalemia and hyperkalemia. B, Electrocardiogram findings of hypercalcemia and hypocalcemia. Hypercalcemia shortens and hypocalcemia lengthens the ST segment. The T wave is not altered. (Adapted with permission from Park MK, Guntheroth WG: *How to Read Pediatric ECG's*, pp 83–84. Copyright © 1981 Year Book Medical Publishers, Inc.)

tected. Figure 35-1 shows the typical changes in the QRS-T complex found in each of several common electrolyte disturbances.

DIABETIC KETOACIDOSIS

DKA is probably the most common endocrine-metabolic disturbance requiring emergency care in children. The cause of DKA in newly diagnosed patients is prolonged insulin deficiency, which may be accompanied by emotional stress or the stress of an infectious disease. Children with established diabetes may omit insulin or develop DKA with the stress of anxiety, illness, or hypoglycemia (rebound). About 20% of established diabetic patients with DKA have no known or identifiable precipitating cause.

Pathophysiology

Before developing ketoacidosis, diabetic patients go through a phase of relative insulin deficiency, either from a gradually exhausted pancreas, as in newly diagnosed diabetes, or from continually missed doses of insulin, as with established patients. Initially, insulin deficiency results in diminished peripheral utilization of glucose and a gradual rise in the plasma glucose concentration. The increase in plasma glucose results in movement of water from the intracellular and interstitial spaces into the plasma space to maintain normal plasma osmolality. Consequently, there is an osmotic dilution of plasma sodium and chloride, resulting in apparent hyponatremia and hypochloremia. As the insulin deficiency is prolonged and plasma glucose concentrations increase further, the renal threshold for glucose reabsorption is finally exceeded and glucose begins to appear in the urine. At this point there is a net loss of water from the body that, at least indirectly, comes from the intracellular space as well as the vascular space. Accompanying this water loss are extracellular electrolytes, primarily sodium and chloride, and true hyponatremia and hypochloremia develop (Figure 35-2).

Signs and symptoms at this point are the result of prolonged hyperglycemia and glycosuria and typically consist of polyuria with polydipsia, hunger, and weight loss. However, children often have anorexia, possibly because of ketosis.

The complete development of DKA depends on the secretion of the so-called counterregulatory hormones: epinephrine, glucagon, growth hormone, and cortisol. These hormones are secreted during times of stress, such as emotional turmoil, infectious disease, surgery, or significant injury, and can precipitate DKA in a patient with relative insulin deficiency. Under the influence of these hormones, the breakdown of glycogen, as well as the synthesis of new glucose from protein stores (gluconeogenesis), proceeds rapidly so that plasma glucose concentrations become considerably elevated. The subsequent urinary loss of fluid and electrolytes becomes critical; dehydration can become so severe that shock is present.

At the same time, the breakdown of lipids from fat stores is stimulated by epinephrine and cortisol, and large amounts of fatty acids are released into the circulation for energy. The increased load of fatty acids exceeds the liver's ability to metabolize them through the Krebs cycle, and they are diverted to the synthesis of ketone bodies (Figure 35-3). The ketone bodies (β-hydroxybutyrate and acetoacetate) are moderately strong acids (i.e., they are ionized) at physiologic pH and release hydrogen ions, which combine with bicarbonate to produce a bicarbonate deficit or metabolic acidosis. The decrease in plasma bicarbonate (or total CO_2 content) is directly proportional to the accumulation of ketone bodies in patients without coexisting pulmonary disease.

The metabolic acidosis causes displacement of both potassium and phosphorus from within cells, and these ions are then lost in the urine as the acidosis progresses. However, during the acute stage of the acidosis, both potassium and phosphorus con-

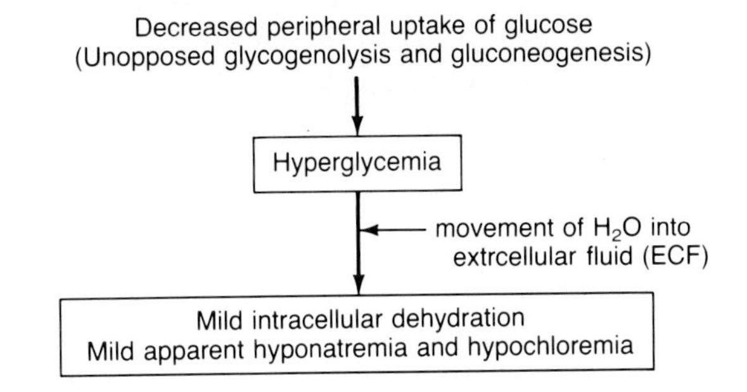

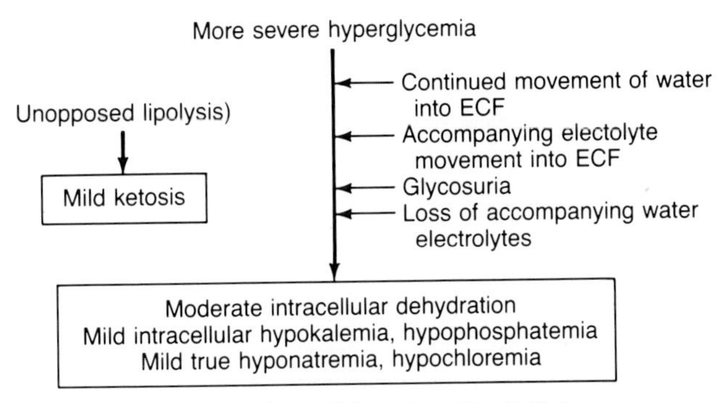

FIGURE 35-2 Early and late insulin deficiency.

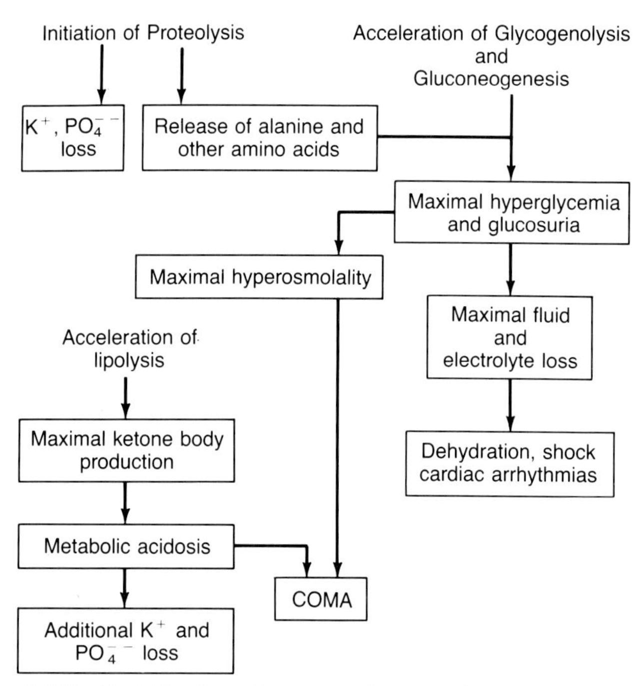

FIGURE 35-3 Development of ketoacidosis.

centrations in the plasma are increased at the expense of intracellular concentrations.

Therefore, the goals of therapy are to halt the continued production of ketone bodies and to correct the hyperglycemia, both of which contribute to the patient's morbidity.

Clinical Features

In patients with new or established diabetes mellitus, there is often a history of recent emotional stress or infection that can be elicited as a precipitating factor in the development of DKA. Surgical procedures and major trauma are also factors that may be identified. Occasionally, a patient admits to skipping one or more doses of insulin. Hypoglycemia with rebound hyperglycemia and ketosis also can be a cause. In many cases no particular precipitating event can be identified.

The physical findings (Table 35-2) reflect the severity of the metabolic disturbance. The dehydration accompanying DKA may be mild, moderate, or severe, but usually it is moderate (about 10% of body weight). If it is more severe, the signs and symptoms of diminished circulation and shock, such as pallor, tachycardia, and hypotension, may be present.

The metabolic ketoacidosis and plasma hyperosmolality combine to affect the level of consciousness so that a patient's state can range from mildly drowsy to comatose at the time of admission. Occasionally, the acidosis has been present for so long that the patient's coma is irreversible. A few patients may require ventilatory assistance for varying periods of time in the treatment of their acidosis, but more commonly, even the most acidotic child demonstrates hyperventilation or Kussmaul breathing.

TABLE 35-2 Signs and Symptoms in DKA

Condition	Signs and Symptoms
Moderate to severe dehydration	Circulatory disturbance, shock, CNS hypoxia, coma
Moderate to severe ketoacidosis	Kussmaul respirations, vomiting, abdominal pain Acetone odor to breath Disordered consciousness, coma Seizures Respiratory depression Death
Hyperosmolality	Disordered consciousness, coma
Hypokalemia	Weakness, cardiac arrhythmias

Vomiting and abdominal pain are also common and are usually nonspecific symptoms of metabolic acidosis. If they have not resolved after the patient is no longer acidotic, then an evaluation of the "acute abdomen" is indicated.

The severity of hypokalemia varies considerably, but where it is evident on electrocardiogram tracings (Figure 35-1), cardiac arrythmias may soon develop.

Differential Diagnosis

Nonketotic Hyperosmolar Coma

In the differential diagnosis of DKA, nonketotic hyperosmolar coma (NKHC) must be considered. By definition this is a condition similar to DKA except that the pH is greater than 7.30. This condition is rarely seen in children who do not have associated retardation (e.g., Down's syndrome). The initial management is similar to that for DKA. A more complete discussion is given in the next section.

Salicylism

Acute salicylism may be accompanied by coma and rapid breathing because of the associated metabolic acidosis (see Chapter 18, "Poisonings and Ingestions"). In contrast to DKA, however, the blood glucose level is rarely above 250 mg/dL, and it is frequently below normal. Furthermore, a screening of the plasma with nitroprusside tablets is rarely positive for ketones in more than trace amounts because of the minimal reactivity of salicylates with the reagent. However, a screen of the urine or plasma with ferric chloride (Phenistix) often gives a positive red result. When the diagnosis is in doubt, the level of salicylate in the serum can be measured (see "Special Tests" in this section).

Head Injury

Head injury is often accompanied by hyperglycemia, but again the plasma glucose concentration is rarely greater than 250 mg/dL. In addition, head injury is rarely accompanied by metabolic acidosis unless hypoventilation is present. The nitroprusside screen is usually negative or trace positive in cases of head injury because the acidosis present is usually due to CO_2 and lactic acid accumulation.

Laboratory Findings

The typical laboratory findings in patients with DKA are a hyperglycemia of between 300 and 1000 mg/dL, hyponatremia and hypochloremia, and normal or elevated plasma potassium and phosphorus concentrations. Plasma and urine osmolalities are increased.

The plasma creatinine concentration may be falsely increased at this time because of the presence of acetoacetate, which reacts with the standard colorimetric procedure for measuring creatinine. Therefore, an increased plasma creatinine level in the absence of a proportionally elevated BUN and abnormal urinary sediment should not be taken as a sign of acute tubular necrosis. If a determination of the true plasma concentration of creatinine is important, most laboratories can measure it by an alternative procedure in which acetoacetate does not interfere.

The plasma total CO_2 is routinely decreased, proportional to the severity of the metabolic acidosis, and is frequently in the range of 3 to 8 mEq/L. This represents a base deficit of approximately 15 to 20 mEq/L. Accordingly, whole blood pH, whether venous or arterial, is in the range of 7.0 to 7.2 in most cases; however, some profoundly acidotic individuals have pH values in the range of 6.85 to 6.95.

The serum amylase concentration may be nonspecifically increased (because of salivary amylase) in the acute course of DKA. This does not represent pancreatitis unless lipase is also elevated and the level of amylase does not return to normal after the acidosis has been corrected.

Special Tests

Special tests include the measurement of salicylate in the serum if the differential diagnosis between acute salicylism and DKA is still difficult. A measured plasma osmolality can be a useful guide to the speed with which replacement fluids are given, although the calculated plasma osmolality in DKA usually reflects the measured value closely.

Direct measurements of β-hydroxybutyrate and acetoacetate are difficult and are rarely necessary in the management of patients with DKA. It is sufficient to assume (in patients without significant respiratory disease) that the difference between the plasma total CO_2 content measured and the normal plasma total CO_2 value of 23 mEq/L represents the concentration of accumulated ketone bodies.

Initial Management

The goals and methods of therapy are given in Table 35-3. The initial management should include an assessment of the need for ventilatory assistance and for catheterization of the bladder in an unconscious patient. It is rarely necessary to aspirate gastric contents, and we have not done so, particularly in the unconscious patient.

An intravenous line is begun quickly after the laboratory tests have been drawn. During the first hour of therapy, the patient receives either normal saline or lactated Ringer's solution at 20 mL/kg of body weight or 360 mL/m^2. This initial phase is essential to reexpand the plasma volume and restore adequate circulation to the kidneys, which helps resolve the metabolic acidosis.

Ongoing Treatment

Ongoing management of DKA depends on replacing fluid and electrolyte deficits over 24 to 48 hours, depending on the patient's initial plasma osmolality, and providing maintenance fluids and electro-

TABLE 35-3 Treatment of DKA

Goals	Therapeutic Measures
Correct hyperglycemia	Insulin
Terminate ketogenesis	Insulin
Correct dehydration and restore adequate circulation and renal function	Maintenance fluids Deficit fluid replacement
Correct metabolic acidosis	Insulin and fluids (bicarbonate rarely)
Correct electrolyte losses	Adequate Na^+, Cl^-, K^+, and PO_4^{--} replacement
Prevent hypoglycemia	IV glucose to keep blood glucose = 250–300 mg/dL
Prevent cerebral edema	Avoid rapid correction of fluid deficits
Prevent hypokalemia	Avoid routine use of bicarbonate Use potassium chloride and phosphate in IV fluids

Exhibit 35-3 Treatment of Fluid and Electrolyte Abnormalities in DKA

1. Maintenance: give evenly over 24 h
   Fluids:
   100 mL/kg × first 10 kg of body weight
   50 mL/kg × next 10 kg
   20 mL/kg × remaining kg
   } or 1500 mL/m²
   Sodium: 2–3 mEq/kg
   Potassium: 1–2 mEq/kg
2. Deficits: Correct evenly over a 24-h period if initial calculated or measured plasma osmolality <320 mosm/kg; over 36 h for osmolalities are 320–340 mosm/kg; over 48 h if osmolality is >340 mosm/kg.
   Estimates for DKA with 10% dehydration
   Fluids: 100 mL/kg
   Sodium: 10 mEq/kg
   Potassium: 6–8 mEq/kg (*use half KCl and half K_2HPO_4*)

Source: Reprinted with permission from Kappy MS, Lightner ES: Low-dose intravenous insulin: Treatment of diabetic ketoacidosis in children (suitability for use in community hospitals). *J Fam Pract* 1977;5:000.

lytes at the same time. Although various schemes are used to determine a fluid and electrolyte treatment regimen, a satisfactory emergency intravenous solution after the first hour is half-normal saline with 40 mEq of potassium (half as potassium chloride and half as potassium phosphate) per liter over the next 8 hours or so. A sample calculation and a listing of approximate deficits in DKA are given in Exhibit 35-3.

Insulin Therapy

Insulin therapy can be initiated during the first hour's plasma expansion. The therapy of choice is the constant low-dose intravenous insulin infusion.[4] The following standard procedure can be used:

1. Administer insulin in an intravenous solution piggybacked into the main intravenous line until the patient's plasma total CO_2 content is greater than 15 mEq/L.
2. Use 1 U of regular insulin per 5 mL of normal saline, e.g., add 50 U regular insulin (1 mL) to 500 mL normal saline; change this solution every 6 hours.
3. Begin with an IV bolus of regular insulin, 0.1 U/kg (maximum, 3 U/kg), and run at 0.1 U/kg/h (maximum of 3 U/h or 15 mL of insulin solution per h) to start.
4. If there is little response in the patient's plasma glucose or bicarbonate (total CO_2 content), increase this rate by 2 or 3 U to approximately 5 U/h.

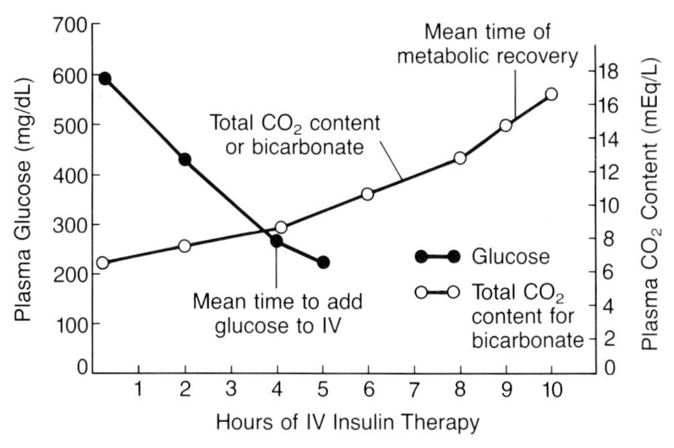

FIGURE 35-4 Results of intravenous insulin regimen in DKA (120 patients).

The *average* rate of fall of plasma glucose concentration using this regimen is 75 mg/dL/h (Figure 35-4), but the range is *35 to 300* mg/dL/h. Therefore, it is *mandatory to monitor plasma glucose HOURLY* (use a blood test strip) for the first 2 to 4 hours after intravenous insulin is begun and then every 2 hours thereafter. *Glucose should be added to the intravenous fluids* when the test strip or laboratory result in approximately 240 mg/dL, to prevent hypoglycemia and the too rapid correction of plasma osmolality, which can predispose the patient to cerebral edema.

A summary of the effectiveness of this mode of therapy is given in Table 35-4. It can be seen that the time to add glucose to the patient's intravenous fluids is approximately 5 hours before the correction of metabolic acidosis (total plasma CO_2 content > 15 mEq/L). Therefore the patient's blood glucose level must be maintained between 250 and 300 mg/dL during this entire period before the intravenous insulin infusion is discontinued. When the patient's total plasma CO_2 content is greater than 15 mEq/L, the intravenous insulin infusion can be discontinued. Then the patient is placed on a standard subcutaneous insulin regimen using regular insulin at a dosage of 0.2 to 0.3 U/kg of body weight every 4 to 6 hours, depending on plasma glucose concentration.

TABLE 35-4 Response to Therapy

	IV Glucose Needed*	Time to Metabolic Recovery†	Insulin Used
Mean ± SEM	3.4 ± 0.6 h	8.4 ± 1.0 h	24 ± 4 U
Range	0.0–8.0 h	2.0–17.0 h	7–46 U
Episodes	100	100	100

* Blood glucose = 250 to 300 mg/dL.
† Bicarbonate >15 mEq/L.

The intravenous fluids are continued until the patient is fully conscious and is eating and drinking without nausea or vomiting.

Special Points

1. *Do not push bicarbonate.* Adequate insulin plus fluid therapy will stop ketogenesis, allow oxidation of ketoacids (an endogenous source of bicarbonate), and restore normal blood flow (thus improving renal tubular excretion of H^+ and increasing bicarbonate production). The use of bicarbonate in DKA is *rarely, if ever,* indicated, for the following reasons:
   - Reduction of ketonemia and the metabolism of β-hydroxybutyrate provide an endogenous source of bicarbonate.
   - There is *no* evidence that the addition of bicarbonate facilitates metabolic recovery (reduction in plasma glucose or ketoacid levels).
   - Bicarbonate treatment can accentuate the tendency of cerebrospinal fluid pH to fall, definitely increases K^+ needs, and can decrease tissue O_2 delivery.

   However, bicarbonate therapy should be considered if there is evidence of the following:

   - Decreased myocardial contractility (*extremely* rare in children without arteriosclerotic or hypertensive cardiac disease): this may be manifested clinically by hypotension unresponsive to appropriate fluid therapy.
   - Severe acidosis ($pH < 7.0$) with depression of the respiratory center: most children with severe ketoacidosis have marked hyperventilation; if this is not present, it suggests that the respiratory center is depressed by the acidosis, and thus correction to a pH of 7.0 to 7.1 with bicarbonate is indicated.

   If bicarbonate therapy is indicated, it should be given as a *diluted,* isotonic solution during the first 2 hours or so of intravenous fluid therapy by continuous infusion; the NaCl is replaced with $NaHCO_3$. Approximately 2 to 3 mEq/kg should be given. Bicarbonate infusion should not be continued if the pH is greater than 7.1.
2. If admission plasma osmolality is greater than 320 mosm/kg, fluid deficits should be corrected over 36 to 48 hours.
3. Continue insulin infusion until plasma total CO_2 content or calculated plasma bicarbonate exceeds 15 mEq/L.
4. *Hypoglycemia must be avoided.* Add glucose (5% to 10%) to intravenous fluids whenever the plasma glucose concentration is 240 mg/dL or less (even if this is the level on admission). After the glucose is added, if the plasma glucose level increases to more than 300 mg/dL, the insulin flow rate can be increased by 1 to 2 U/h. The need to add glucose to the intravenous fluid almost always *precedes* the correction of metabolic acidosis (see Figure 35-4).
5. Urinary or plasma ketones as measured by nitroprusside tablets or test strips (Ketostix) are poor guides to therapy after DKA has been diagnosed since they are predominantly acetoacetate, which does not change much during the first few hours of treatment, and acetone, which is metabolically inert. Also, the useful life of Ketostix (if these are used for urine testing) is short once the bottle is opened.
6. Many patients with *severe* acidosis have relatively low plasma levels of glucose (250 to 300 mg/dL). The acidosis still needs treatment.

OTHER METABOLIC ACIDOSES

Acidosis refers to an abnormal increase in circulating acid with an accompanying decrease in the buffering capacity of the blood, as manifest by a low serum bicarbonate level. Acidosis that ultimately exceeds the body's compensatory buffering mechanisms leads to an increase in extracellular fluid H^+ concentration such that pH is reduced below 7.35. This state is referred to as acidemia. Its presence implies that the patient's compensatory mechanisms have failed to maintain normal extracellular fluid H^+ concentration, and prompt treatment is indicated to prevent severe alterations in extracellular (and then intracellular) pH that might be incompatible with life.

Pathophysiology

To maintain electrical neutrality in the body, the total positively charged cations must always equal the negatively charged anions. A great deal of information can be gathered about the extracellular metabolic state of a patient by interpretation of the commonly ordered serum electrolytes Na^+, K^+, Cl^-, and HCO_3^-.[5] Normally, Na^+ accounts for more than 90% of the extracellular cations, whereas Cl^- and HCO_3^- constitute approximately 85% of the anions. The anion gap, as used clinically, is calculated by subtracting the sum of Cl^- and HCO_3^- from the Na^+ concentration. The normal mean value is 12 mEq/L, with a range of 8 to 16 mEq/L.

Normal Anion Gap

Diarrhea and small-bowel drainage can lead to excessive loss of HCO_3^- (with accompanying Na^+) from the gastrointestinal tract, with the subsequent development of metabolic acidosis. Sodium and HCO_3^- are lost together, but since Cl^- is not usually lost to the same extent, a state of relative hyperchloremia develops, with a normal calculated anion gap. In addition, renal tubular acidosis (proximal type), ureterosigmoidostomy, or carbonic anhydrase inhibitors (acetazolamide, mafenide acetate) interfere with the kidney's ability to resorb filtered bicarbonate, and relative hyperchloremic metabolic acidosis can develop. The calculated anion gap is normal in these situations as well.

Increased Anion Gap

The endogenous production or ingestion of an increased acid load or a failure on the part of the kidneys to excrete sufficient H^+ daily results in metabolic acidosis that may progress to acidemia if the body's compensatory mechanisms are exceeded. This is accompanied by a measurable fall in plasma bicarbonate because of the buffering of H^+, and the calculated anion gap is increased. In the neonatal period, metabolic errors that lead to defective metabolism of amino and organic acids produce a high anion gap metabolic acidosis. In infancy the ingestion of excessive protein or potential nonvolatile acid in commercial infant formulas or cow's milk also can lead to metabolic acidosis, especially in premature infants.

There are several other causes of excess acid in childhood. One is the ingestion of toxins that are acid precursors (e.g., methanol, acetylsalicylic acid). Many of the errors in glycogenolysis and gluconeogenesis that lead to fasting hypoglycemia result in metabolic acidosis because of excessive production of the ketone bodies acetoacetate and β-hydroxybutyrate that are derived from the breakdown of the fat being used as an alternate energy source. Lactic acid also can accumulate in some of these disorders, as well as in primary disorders of lactate metabolism. DKA also leads to an accumulation of ketone bodies (but not usually lactic acid) as a result of the inability to metabolize glucose effectively. Thus when fat is utilized as an energy source, ketone bodies accumulate in the extracellular fluid and urine. Since most of these excessively accumulated anions are not included in the calculation of the anion gap, the gap is increased. Finally, renal failure at any age is also accompanied by a high anion gap acidosis in most instances.

Clinical Features

A history of early infant deaths in the family is compatible with many of the inborn errors of metabolism. Known metabolic disease in the family is, of course, a valuable clue. Symptoms of hypoglycemia during fasting or after specific foods (e.g., fruit) also can be diagnostic of an inborn metabolic error, as is a history of unusual urine ordor.

The general signs that should alert the clinician to the possibility of metabolic acidosis and acidemia include persistent vomiting, tachypnea, and feeding difficulties. Other frequently encountered symptoms include disordered consciousness (lethargy or coma), seizures, or spasticity. These can reflect relatively severe decreases in CNS pH. Over longer periods of time, metabolic acidosis that progresses to acidemia can cause failure to gain weight during infancy or failure to achieve normal stature during childhood. Metabolic acidosis also can accompany diseases associated with mental retardation, ataxia, and hypotonia. In addition, specific physical findings associated with some causes of metabolic acidosis include ambiguous genitalia (congenital adrenal hyperplasia), hepatosplenomegaly (glycogen storage disease), osteoporosis (methylmalonic acidemia), and unusual urine odor (isovaleric acidemia, maple syrup urine disease).

Laboratory Findings

Blood pH and total CO_2 content are reduced in proportion to the degree of metabolic acidosis. The accumulation of organic anions in salicylism and inborn errors of metabolism (lactic acidosis, errors of amino and organic acid metabolism, errors in glycogenolysis and gluconeogenesis) results in a lowering of plasma total CO_2 content primarily, so that the calculated anion gap is greater than 14 to 16 mEq/L. Metabolic acidosis accompanying loss of bicarbonate from the body usually results in a proportionate decrease in sodium but not chloride, so that the anion gap is normal (<14 mEq/L).

Hypoglycemia can accompany inborn errors of glycogenolysis of gluconeogenesis. Urine pH is usually low (<6) unless renal tubular acidosis is present.

Differential Diagnosis

See Exhibit 35-1.

Special Tests

Blood and urine should be sent for determination of amino acid and organic acid concentrations, including those of lactic and pyruvic acid. Blood salicylate concentrations also can be measured, as well as 17-hydroxyprogesterone concentrations in infants with suspected congenital adrenal hyperplasia (ambiguous genitalia in females, occasional large penis in males). Special tests of enzyme activity can be ordered in cases of suspected glycogen storage disease or disorders of gluconeogenesis (hypoglycemic syndromes), but many of these are done in research laboratories only, and consultation from a pediatric geneticist or endocrinologist should be obtained.

Treatment

It should be reemphasized that a blood pH of less than 7.35 suggests failing metabolic compensatory mechanisms, and prompt therapy is indicated.

Except in cases of DKA, in which an endogenous source of bicarbonate (i.e., ketone bodies) is present, bicarbonate therapy may be used to bring the patient's total plasma CO_2 content into the range of 15 to 18 mEq/L. Sodium bicarbonate (1 mEq/mL) can be used in a 1:6 dilution as part of the patient's calculated maintenance and deficit requirements, in a dose as follows:

Dose (mEq) = bicarbonate deficit (mEq/L) × 0.3 × body weight (kg).

This usually is given over 4 to 6 hours and must be accompanied by monitoring of serum potassium, with replacement as needed.

Specific long-term therapy depends on the specific cause of the acidosis and can include dietary or hormonal regimens. Consultation should be obtained.

NONKETOTIC HYPEROSMOLAR COMA

NKHC is only rarely seen in children and either accompanies true insulin-dependent diabetes mellitus or represents a transient response to stress, head injury, or infection.

Laboratory Findings

By definition the plasma glucose concentration is quite high (≥700 mg/dL) and may even reach 1000 to 2000 mg/dL. As a consequence the plasma osmolality is high (>310 mosm/kg), occasionally as high as 400 mosm/kg. The blood pH (venous or arterial) is 7.30 or higher, and the serum ketone body concentration is less than 3 mEq/L.

Treatment

The treatment regimen is similar to that for DKA, i.e., low dosage of regular insulin by intravenous infusion, 0.05 to 0.10 U/kg/h or 2 to 3 U/h, whichever is less.

Plasma K^+ in the form of KCl should be added to the patient's intravenous fluids, 20 mEq/L. The rate of fluid administration should be calculated to repair deficits over at least 48 hours to prevent cerebral edema. Blood glucose concentrations should be monitored hourly. The intravenous infusion may be discontinued when the patient's plasma glucose concentration reaches 200 to 250 mg/dL; however, the plasma glucose should be monitored every 2 hours in case of rebound. When NKHC is due to stress, head injury, or infection, without true diabetes, rebound hyperglycemia should not occur after the other effects have resolved. In a few instances the patient has true insulin-dependent diabetes mellitus, and long-term subcutaneous insulin administration will be necessary. Most of the reported cases of NKHC in children have been associated with problems that might affect spontaneous hydration, such as Down's syndrome with diabetes, or with the use of the hypoglycemic drug diazoxide.

HYPOGLYCEMIA

The cerebral cortex, renal cortex, and mature erythrocyte require a continuous supply of glucose to maintain normal function. Ordinarily, the rate of glucose use is in balance with glucose availability. The glucose comes from the dietary intake of carbohydrates or, in the fasting state, from either the breakdown of glycogen (glycogenolysis) or the synthesis of new glucose (gluconeogenesis) from protein stores (muscle).

Pathophysiology

When glucose uptake exceeds availability, as in starvation, vigorous exercise, or excessive insulin secretion, hypoglycemia can occur.[6] To prevent this, the secretion of the counterregulatory hormones (catecholamines, glucagon, cortisol, and growth hormone) is stimulated. These hormones, acting individually or in concert, stimulate glycogenolysis and gluconeogenesis to restore and maintain normal blood glucose concentration. Deficiencies in the secretion of counterregulatory hormones or in the enzymes involved in glycogenolysis or gluconeogenesis can result in hypoglycemia.

In addition to their effect on carbohydrate metabolism, the counterregulatory hormones promote the breakdown of fat stores (triglycerides) to fatty acids, particularly in the absence of insulin. The fatty acids are then used by most peripheral tissues for energy; however, the excess fatty acids are metabolized to ketone bodies (β-hydroxybutyrate and acetoacetate) and are partly excreted in the urine.

Thus one of the most important laboratory tests in the differential diagnosis of hypoglycemia is the *presence or absence of ketones* in the urine, in addition to the low blood glucose level. Because insulin suppresses fat breakdown, the presence of significant (more than trace) ketonuria is incompatible with excessive insulin secretion as a cause and suggests instead a failure to produce glucose. A plasma glucose concentration less than 40 mg/dL generally signifies hypoglycemia in children.

Clinical Features

Patients may be relatively asymptomatic or may have pallor, tachycardia, and sweating (reflecting the secretion of catecholamines), with varying degrees of weakness and coma. There also may be seizures (generalized or focal). Fatalities are not common but do occur.

The CNS signs in hypoglycemia (seizures, weakness, and coma) reflect the need of the cerebral cortex for glucose to maintain normal function.

Historical points of particular relevance include a positive family history of childhood hypoglycemia, recent introduction of fruit into the diet (hereditary fructose intolerance), antecedent illness with decreased food intake (ketotic hypoglycemia), toxin ingestion (acetylsalicylic acid, ethanol), or known insulin use (diabetes mellitus, type I).

Physical findings of importance, primarily in infancy, include jaundice (liver failure or galactosemia), cataracts (galactosemia), hepatomegaly (galactosemia, glycogen storage diseases), or ambiguous genitalia (congenital adrenal hyperplasia). In childhood or adolescence the presence of a varicella-like rash (Reye's syndrome) or darkening of the skin (Addison's disease) may be helpful in the differential diagnosis.

Laboratory Findings

The initial blood chemistry findings document the emergency as hypoglycemia if an abnormally low glucose concentration is found. In practice it is best to do bedside screening with a blood test strip (Chemstrips) so that treatment can begin before the laboratory results are available.

Except in rare cases of inborn errors of metabolism, including von Gierke's glycogen storage disease, *serum* acetone may not be elevated in patients with hypoglycemia, but profound ketonuria may exist unless insulin excess is present. This should be screened for with nitroprusside tablets.

In the rarer inborn errors of metabolism, profound metabolic acidosis (mixed retention of ketoacids, amino acid precursors or metabolites, and lactic acid) may be present. In these instances the anion gap ($Na^+ - [Cl^- + CO_2$ content]) increases to greater than 14 mEq/L.

Differential Diagnosis

See Table 35-5 and Exhibit 35-1.

Special Tests

Blood should be saved for serum insulin and C-peptide if insulin excess appears likely on the

TABLE 35-5 Major Causes of Hypoglycemia by Age

Age	Cause
Up to 6 mo	Islet cell hyperplasia, adenoma, or nesidioblastosis
	Defects in glycogenolysis* (galactosemia, von Gierke's disease)
	Defects in gluconeogenesis*
	Panhypopituitarism
	Congenital adrenal hyperplasia
	Amino acid disorders
	Fructose-1,6-diphosphatase deficiency
	Hereditary fructose intolerance
	Liver failure (various causes)*
	Fevers,* infections*
>6 mo to 5 yr	Ketotic hypoglycemia (exaggerated starvation)*
	Fevers, infections*
	Intoxications*
	Ethanol
	Aspirin
	Isopropyl alcohol
	Liver failure*
	Viral hepatitis (postinfection)
	Chronic active hepatitis
	Carbon tetrachloride intoxication
5 yr to adolescence	Vigorous exercise*
	Diabetes mellitus (insulin overdosage)
	Reye's syndrome and other causes of liver failure*
	Intoxications*
	Ethanol
	Aspirin
	Withdrawal from corticosteroids*

* Usually accompanied by ketonuria.
Source: Reprinted with permission from Cornblath M, Schwartz R: *Disorders of Carbohydrate Metabolism in Infancy*, ed 2. Copyright © 1976 WB Saunders Co.

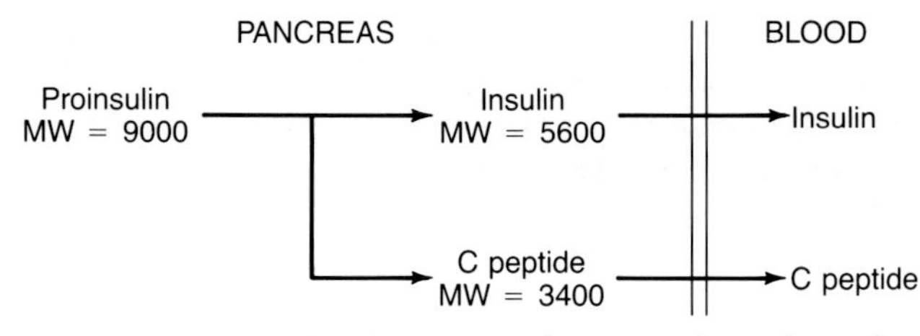

FIGURE 35-5 The formation of C peptide and insulin from proinsulin in the pancreas. MW, Molecular weight.

basis of the remainder of the patient's evaluation or clinical course. *Endogenous* hyperinsulinemia (plasma insulin concentration > 15 μU/mL, with simultaneous plasma glucose < 40 mg/dL), as seen in islet (β) cell adenoma, nesidioblastosis, or β-cell hyperplasia, is usually accompanied by an elevation in plasma C-peptide concentration. This peptide is released into the blood along with insulin when the larger proinsulin molecule is cleaved in the pancreas (Figure 35-5). Hypoglycemic patients who have accidentally or purposely received exogenous insulin will not have increased blood levels of C peptide because it is not contained in commercial insulin preparations.

If there is a history or suspicion of aspirin or ethanol intoxication, samples of gastric contents, blood, and urine should be tested to determine the presence of these substances. Blood ammonia and serum glutamic-oxaloacetic transaminase concentrations are helpful in the diagnosis and management of children with suspected Reye's syndrome and other causes of liver failure that may produce hypoglycemia.

Blood also should be saved for measurement of growth hormone and cortisol to rule out hypopituitarism. In addition, cortisol measurement can be used to rule out congenital adrenal hyperplasia or Addison's disease, in the face of normal growth hormone responses to hypoglycemia.

Various tolerance tests and challenges as well as elimination diets may be necessary to diagnose and treat hypoglycemia over the long term.[6]

Treatment

Short-term management of hypoglycemia consists of rapid administration of glucose, usually by the intravenous route. A dose of 25% glucose at 2 to 4 mL/kg (0.5 to 1.0 mg/kg) is recommended, followed by infusion of a 10% to 15% glucose solution at 6 to 8 mg/kg/min. This may be increased up to 24 mg/kg/min using a 20% to 25% glucose solution if plasma glucose concentrations do not increase and stabilize or if symptoms do not abate. Except in cases of endogenous insulin excess, however, it is rarely necessary to use rates of glucose administration exceeding 10 mg/kg/min.

Initially, a dose of glucagon (0.03 mg/kg IV or IM; maximum, 1 mg) also can be given. The glycemic response may be dramatic, but this is transitory and oral or intravenous carbohydrate must be provided.

Prolonged difficulty in maintaining normal blood glucose concentrations can be alleviated by giving (1) hydrocortisone, 10 mg/kg IV immediately and then 10 mg/kg/d in three divided oral doses, or (2) cortisone acetate, 12 mg/kg/d IM once a day.

Long-range treatment is tailored to the specific cause and may consist of frequent feedings, special drugs (e.g., diazoxide for endogenous insulin excess) and diets, or hormone therapy (e.g., in hypopituitarism or congenital virilizing adrenal hyperplasia). Surgical intervention (partial pancreatectomy) may be necessary in the treatment of unremitting hypoglycemia caused by excessive insulin secretion and unresponsive to medical therapy.

HYPOCALCEMIA

Normal serum calcium concentration is maintained by (1) dietary intake and absorption of calcium and vitamin D and (2) the response of the parathyroid glands to a fall in serum calcium concentration by mobilizing calcium from bone, gut, and kidney into the blood. Deficiencies in calcium or vitamin D, or tissue unresponsiveness to the actions of activated vitamin D or parathyroid hormone (PTH) may lead to hypocalcemia; however, lack of PTH and resistance to its effects are the major causes of severe hypocalcemia.[7]

Pathophysiology

The daily elemental calcium requirement of the young child is approximately 600 to 800 mg/d and that of the adolescent, about 1200 mg/d. This is provided primarily in milk, milk products, and certain green vegetables such as spinach, turnip greens, and collard greens. Although a dietary deficiency of calcium could lead to hypocalcemia, sufficient bone stores of calcium exist so that this would be an unusual cause of hypocalcemia in the child.

Vitamin D may come from endogenous synthesis: natural ultraviolet irradiation from sunlight acts on 7-dehydrocholesterol in the skin to produce cholecalciferol (vitamin D_3). Alternatively, milk and infant formulas are fortified with irradiated ergosterol or ergocalciferol (vitamin D_2) in amounts (400 IU/L) sufficient to ensure normal absorption of calcium (and phosphorus). Vitamins D_3 and D_2 must be further metabolized in the liver and kidney to provide the active forms 1α,25-dihydroxycholecalciferol and 25-hydroxyergocalciferol, respectively, which are necessary to promote maximal absorption of calcium from gut, kidney, and bone.

The conversion of vitamin D_3 or D_2 to its active form is stimulated by PTH. Deficiencies of sunlight or milk products, malabsorption of vitamin D, failure to activate vitamin D, or tissue unresponsiveness to activated vitamin D all can predispose the child to hypocalcemia. However, normal PTH response to hypocalcemia may prevent undue lowering of serum calcium in these instances.

PTH is secreted by the parathyroid glands in response to decreased serum calcium concentrations and is the *primary* defense mechanism against severe (or fatal) hypocalcemia. The actions of PTH are facilitated by active vitamin D and result in mobilization of calcium into the blood from the bones, gut, and kidney. Insufficient secretion of PTH by the parathyroid glands (Exhibit 35-1), severe vitamin D deficiency, or tissue unresponsiveness to PTH (hypernatremia, hypokalemia, hypomagnesemia, pseudohypoparathyroidism) can all lead to severe hypocalcemia and tetany.

Calcium in the blood is either free (ionized; 40%) or transported by albumin (60%). It is the free or ionized form of calcium that is necessary to maintain normal tissue excitability. Thus in hypocalcemia the ionized fraction of serum calcium correlates well with clinical signs, but its measurement is difficult. In practice the total serum calcium concentration is easier to measure and is used as an estimate of the ionized calcium. Hypoalbuminemia or acidosis (metabolic or respiratory) raises the ionized calcium fraction for a given total serum calcium concentration, and metabolic or respiratory alkalosis (as with hyperventilation) lowers it. Total serum calcium concentrations less than or equal to 7.5 mg/dL or ionized serum calcium concentrations less than or equal to 3.0 mg/dL are often associated with the physical signs of hypocalcemia.

Clinical Features

Patients who are on replacement calcium for such conditions as hypoparathyroidism (autoimmune or postthyroidectomy) or pseudohypoparathyroidism are the most likely to have signs of hypocalcemia since they may intentionally or accidentally not take their medicine for days at a time. Other individuals who are prone to significant hypocalcemia are children on vegetarian diets, premature infants, and hysterical children who hyperventilate. The carpopedal spasm that often accompanies hyperventilation may not be due entirely to lowered ionized calcium but also to "hysteria" per se. A precise mechanism for this association is not known, but all symptoms appear to subside with rebreathing therapy.

The signs and symptoms of hypocalcemia are varied. In infants and young children, lethargy, poor feeding, and vomiting may be the only signs present. Congestive heart failure also has been associated with hypocalcemia in the pediatric population. Tetanic contractions of any or all extremities can be present at any age, and generalized seizures are not uncommon. Carpopedal spasm is more or less typical of hypocalcemia, and hyperirritability of the facial musculature (Chvostek's sign) may be demonstrated. If rickets is present, the limbs have a characteristic bowed appearance, and a "rachitic rosary" may be evident along the costochondral junctions on the chest wall.

Laboratory Findings

A lowered concentration of total serum calcium (<7.5 mg/dL) or ionized serum calcium (<3.0 mg/dL) is the rule, with an elevated serum inorganic phosphate concentration (>6.0 mg/dL) as a common and not inadvertent accompaniment. Hypomagnesemia (<1.0 mg/dL) is sometimes present and can make the treatment of hypocalcemia futile unless it is also corrected, since hypomagnesemia reduces peripheral tissue responsiveness to PTH and prevents normal PTH release as well. Hypocalcemia is demonstrated electrocardiographically by lengthening of the ST segment without alteration of the T wave (Figure 35-1). Radiologic findings in cases of rickets include generalized bone demineralization and wide, frayed metaphyseal ends of the long bones, giving a characteristic cupped appearance to the metaphyses.

Differential Diagnosis

There is nothing characteristic about the physical findings that accompany hypocalcemia, except perhaps for carpopedal spasm, which, as noted, can be a nonspecific finding in hysteria. The laboratory results are diagnostic in cases of suspected hypocalcemia.

Special Tests

Blood should be analyzed for magnesium concentration since hypomagnesemia can mimic hypoparathyroidism, and the hypocalcemia may not resolve unless the hypomagnesemia is corrected. Hypernatremia and hypokalemia also reduce peripheral responsiveness to PTH. Serum should be sent for measurement of PTH concentrations so that a distinction can be made between true and pseudohypoparathyroidism (Albright's osteodystrophy).

Treatment

Intravenous administration of a dilute calcium solution is the treatment of choice. The usual solution is 10% calcium gluconate (9 mg *elemental* calcium per milliliter), 1 to 2 mL/kg IV every 6 to 8 hours.

Long-term treatment depends on the cause but usually consists of 1 g *elemental* calcium per day (in older children) as calcium carbonate (10 g/d) or calcium lactate (8 g/d). Infants are treated with either calcium lactate powder in the formula (5 to 6 g/d) or calcium gluconate syrup (Neo-Calglucon Syrup, 90 mg elemental calcium per teaspoon), approximately 6 to 8 tsp/d.

Vitamin D preparations, such as dihydrotachysterol or 1α,25-dihydroxyvitamin D_3 (Rocaltrol) are added in the treatment of hypoparathyroidism, pseudohypoparathyroidism, or vitamin D deficiencies. Coexisting magnesium deficiencies can be treated with magnesium chloride, citrate, or lactate, 24 to 48 mg of magnesium per kilogram per day in divided doses up to a maximum of 1 g *elemental* magnesium per day.

HYPERCALCEMIA

Hypercalcemia is a rare cause of pediatric emergencies.[3] It is often discovered incidentally during evaluation for conditions such as failure to gain weight, short stature, or polyuria.

Pathophysiology

Hypercalcemia can arise because of excessive mobilization of calcium from bone or excessive absorption of calcium from the intestine. Clinically, these can occur as a result of over ingesting vitamin D or its metabolites, primary hyperparathyroidism caused by parathyroid hyperplasia, or secondary hyperparathyroidism accompanying renal failure. Rarely, tumors produce hormones such as PTH-like peptides or invade the bones so that osteoclastic activity occurs and excessive calcium is mobilized. This process is also seen occasionally in children with bone fractures (femur) who must remain relatively immobile for long periods of time.

Clinical Features

The symptoms of hypercalcemia from any cause are nonspecific and include nausea and vomiting, constipation, poor feeding, and polyuria (from peripheral interference with the action of ADH). A history of familial hyperparathyroidism may be elicited from some patients. Patients may be fully alert, but if hypercalcemia is severe, they may have signs of CNS dysfunction such as lethargy, coma, and seizures. Hypertension may be present when calcium concentrations are greater than 15 mg/dL, as a result of either direct hypercalcemic effects on arteriolar tone or renal damage from deposition of calcium phosphate in the renal interstitium. Other tissues that may show signs of calcium deposition are the cornea, skin and subcutaneous tissue, and the falx cerebri.

Laboratory Findings

Serum calcium concentrations are greater than 11 mg/dL (ionized calcium $>$ 5.6 mg/dL). Phosphate may be low (in primary hyperparathyroidism), normal, or high (vitamin D intoxication and hyperparathyroidism secondary to renal failure).

X-ray films of the extremities reveal a zone of increased density at the growing end of the long bones. Metastatic calcifications in subcutaneous tissues, kidney, and the falx cerebri also may be seen.

Differential Diagnosis

The signs and symptoms of hypercalcemia are nonspecific, and diagnosis is usually made after serum calcium concentrations are known. The polyuria exhibited by some patients, even in the presence of dehydration, is thought to result from inhibition of the peripheral action of ADH by excess calcium and can be confused with DI until laboratory reports are back.

Special Tests

Simultaneous measurement of calcium and PTH can be helpful in establishing a diagnosis of hyperparathyroidism if both are elevated. In cases of hypercalcemia resulting from hypervitaminosis D, PTH concentrations will be suppressed. Measurement of serum concentrations of vitamin D metabolites (e.g., 25-hydroxyvitamin D_3 or 1α,25-dihydroxyvitamin D_3) can document the presence of excessive vitamin D.

Treatment

The immediate treatment of hypercalcemia from any cause consists of a calcium diuretic with generous amounts of intravenous fluid containing sodium and potassium. Furosemide can be given at a dose of 1 mg/kg IV every 6 to 8 hours, along with above-maintenance amounts of 5% dextrose/0.45% NaCl, containing 30 mEq of KCl per liter. The rate of fluid administration should produce diuresis of calcium without significant changes in serum sodium and potassium concentrations, but all three electrolytes should be monitored. Furosemide therapy can be discontinued when the serum calcium level is less than 12 mg/dL, but fluid therapy should continue until the concentration equals 10 to 11 mg/dL.

In cases of hypercalcemia from excessive vitamin D intake, cortisone (10 mg/kg/d; maximum, 300 mg) or prednisone (2 mg/kg/d; maximum, 60 mg) can be given orally for a few days to help reduce serum calcium concentrations.

Additional therapy can include oral phosphorus supplements, 1 to 2 g of phosphorus per day, and salmon calcitonin, 5 to 8 MRC* units/kg IV or IM every 6 to 12 hours. In patients with renal disease, peritoneal dialysis plus calcitonin may be the only safe, effective treatment.

Long-term treatment depends on the cause of the hypercalcemia and can include elimination of vitamin D and milk (in hypervitaminosis D) or surgical removal of some of the parathyroid glands (in hyperparathyroidism, primary or secondary).

HYPERTHYROIDISM

The major emergency problems in hyperthyroidism are related to the positive inotropic effects of thyroid hormones on the heart, leading to tachycardia (sometimes severe) and secondary high-output congestive heart failure. The sudden overproduction and/or release of thyroid hormone by the thyroid gland (thyroid storm) occurs only rarely in children.

Pathophysiology

The vast majority of cases of hyperthyroidism in children are caused by Graves' disease, an autoimmune disorder mediated by thyroid-stimulating immunoglobulins. Patients with Hashimoto's thyroiditis can also go through a hyperthyroid stage. Transplacental passage of maternal thyroid-stimulating immunoglobulins can cause serious hyperthyroidism in the neonate, but this is usually a self-limited condition that dissipates in the first 6 months of life as maternal antibodies are metabolized.

* Medical Research Council.

Clinical Features

The major reasons for seeking medical attention are neurologic and cardiovascular problems. The patient may complain of nervousness, agitation, inability to concentrate, or insomnia. Major cardiovascular complaints include palpitations and dyspnea. Other complaints include diarrhea, amenorrhea or dysmenorrhea, hair and skin changes (hair thinning; smooth, dry, warm skin), weight loss (failure to thrive or dehydration), and heat intolerance. In the previously diagnosed hyperthyroid patient, failure to take antithyroid medications can lead to rapid reemergence of symptoms.

Cardiopulmonary examination can reveal tachycardia, systolic flow murmur or the murmur of mitral insufficiency, widened pulse pressure with systolic hypertension, cardiomegaly, and tachypnea. With severe high-output failure, edema, rales, and hepatomegaly are noticeable.

Neurologic findings include agitation, tremor, and hyperactive reflexes.

Almost all patients have a goiter or, rarely, a toxic nodule, and a flow murmur may be audible over the gland. In patients without a goiter, exogenous thyroid hormone intake should be considered. Lid lag and exophthalmos may be present.

Laboratory Findings

With thyroid hormone overproduction, there is elevation of thyroxine (3,3′,5,5′-tetraiodothyronine [T_4]), unbound T_4 (free T_4 [FT_4]), and 3,5,3′-triiodothyronine (T_3). In the severely hyperthyroid patient, T_4 is often greater than 18 to 20 μg/dL; FT_4, greater than 3 ng/dL; and T_3, greater than 250 to 300 ng/dL. Early in the disease the T_3 alone may be elevated (T_3 toxicosis). Except in the rare case of a thyroid-stimulating hormone (TSH)-secreting pituitary tumor, TSH is suppressed to very low or undetectable levels. No clear laboratory distinction can be made between routine hyperthyroidism and thyroid storm. The diagnosis of thyroid storm rests on the presence of severe or accelerating clinical findings such as fever, congestive heart failure, or psychotic changes. Storm can be precipitated by stress (infection, surgery) or radioactive iodine therapy.

Differential Diagnosis

Any condition increasing sympathetic nervous system activity will produce signs and symptoms typical also of hyperthyroidism; such disorders include hysteria, psychiatric disturbances, drug abuse (phencyclidine, amphetamines), and pheochromocytoma. Congestive heart failure can be secondary to rheumatic fever, myocarditis, or congenital heart disease.

Special Tests

If a measurement of FT_4 is not readily available, the FT_4 index can be calculated as the product of the percent T_3 resin uptake times the T_4 level. (Normal index values are 1.25 to 3.50, but laboratories may differ.) If TSH is not suppressed, thyrotropin-releasing hormone (TRH) stimulation test should be done. Autonomous thyroid activity produces a flat TRH test. If the TSH response is not flat, the patient must be evaluated for a pituitary and/or hypothalamic tumor. Autoantibodies to thyroid microsomes and thyroglobulin are frequently found and support the diagnosis of an autoimmune phenomenon.

Treatment

In the patient with severe thyrotoxicosis or storm, β-adrenergic blocking agents should be administered in the emergency department. β-Blockers antagonize the catecholamine-like positive inotropic effects of high levels of thyroid hormones. Propranolol, the β-blocker most widely used, can be used intravenously in the patient with congestive heart failure or severe tachycardia (0.1 mg/kg; maximum dose, 5 mg). The total dose is given as four equal, slow intravenous doses every 10 minutes. Its use requires electrocardiographic monitoring for the development of bradycardia or arrhythmias.

In severe hyperthyroidism and storm, after the administration of propranolol, stress doses of glucocorticoids (e.g., dexamethasone, methylprednisolone) may be administered since they impede the conversion of T_4 to T_3. (For dosages, see "Adrenal Insufficiency.")

Once propranolol and glucocorticoids have been given, thioureas can be begun, even before laboratory results are available if hyperthyroidism is evident clinically. The thiourea drugs, propylthiouracil (PTU) and methimazole (Tapazole), interfere with the synthesis of thyroid hormone. In addition, PTU interferes with the peripheral conversion of T_4 to T_3. The initial dose of PTU is 8 to 12 mg/kg orally (maximum, 600 mg), followed at 8-hour intervals by 6 to 8 mg/kg (maximum, 200 mg). Methimazole can be used in one tenth the dose of PTU. If the patient is unable to swallow, the drug can be given by nasogastric tube. Iodides block the release and production of thyroid hormone while decreasing thyroid gland vascularity. Two to 10 drops of a saturated solution of potassium iodide or of Lugol's solution can be given three times a day, starting several hours after the first dose of PTU.

General support includes cooling by hypothermic blanket (avoid aspirin because it increases metabolic rate) and intravenous fluids as needed to correct dehydration.

Routine initial and chronic therapy involves PTU administration at a dosage of 5 to 7 mg/kg/d or 150 to 175 mg/m^2/d divided into 3 or 4 doses. Methimazole also can be used (one tenth the dose of PTU) and is given two or three times daily, potentially improving compliance. Symptoms of hyperthyroidism usually improve in 1 to 2 weeks; however, laboratory studies take 4 to 6 weeks to demonstrate improvement.

Thioureas can produce significant side effects such as allergic reactions, thrombocytopenia, and leukopenia. With acute infection, patients taking thioureas should have a complete blood count, differential, and platelet count to rule out hematologic abnormalities. The drugs themselves cause a benign leukopenia.

Propranolol (2 to 4 mg/kg/d divided into 4 doses; maximum 160 mg/d) can be used the first several weeks of treatment along with thioureas. Propranolol is stopped once clinical findings have substantially resolved.

HYPOTHYROIDISM

Hypothyroidism is a rare cause of emergencies in children; however, the emergency physician should be familiar with the signs and symptoms of hypothyroidism so that its occasional presence will not be overlooked.

Pathophysiology

Typically, the young child (under 10 years of age) develops hypothyroidism because of an insufficient amount of normal thyroid tissue (anywhere from total absence of the gland to thyroid remnants), often ectopically located, or an enzymatic block in the synthesis of thyroid hormone. In both cases plasma concentrations of TSH are high, but only in the latter does this cause a goiter, since a normal amount of thyroid tissue is present. Hypopituitarism can cause secondary hypothyroidism due to TSH deficiency, but the degree of hypothyroidism is rarely severe.

Autoimmune hypothyroidism due to Hashimoto's thyroiditis or accompanying insulin-dependent diabetes mellitus is not usually seen until at least 10 years of age and is usually accompanied by a goiter.

A transient hypothyroidism may be seen in the postnatal period as a result of maternal ingestion of PTU in the last trimester. A goiter is frequently observed in affected infants, but the hypothyroidism usually resolves by the end of the second week of life.

Clinical Features

In the postnatal period a history of maternal PTU or methimazole ingestion may be obtained. Signs of lethargy, poor feeding, constipation, and difficult, noisy breathing may be reported for infants and young children. Older children may complain of fatigue, constipation, cold intolerance, and dry skin. Adolescent girls may give a history of irregular periods or amenorrhea.

Infants may be floppy and sluggish and have a hoarse cry. The skin may be cyanotic, mottled, or jaundiced, and the abdomen may be distended. The typical "cretin" facies is rarely seen but consists of very coarse features, enlarged fontanelles, flat nasal bridge, eyelid edema, and macroglossia. A goiter may be present in infants with an inborn error in thyroid hormone synthesis or when the hypothyroidism is due to maternal PTU ingestion. There may be respiratory distress from myxedema of the tongue, epiglottis, or larynx. Rarely, a large goiter can compromise breathing or swallowing; the latter situation can be accompanied by vomiting.

Older children may have goiter, dry skin, delayed tooth eruption, delayed secondary sexual characteristics, or short stature with infantile body proportions. Achilles tendon reflexes may show a prolonged relaxation phase.

Laboratory Findings

Specific laboratory tests are not useful in the emergency setting because of the 2- to 4-day delay in obtaining values, even in the best of circumstances. Typically, the serum FT_4 (or total T_4 and T_3 resin uptake) is reduced and TSH is elevated (except in cases of hypopituitarism).

Nonspecifically, normocytic, normochromic anemia can be present, as well as an elevation in serum cholesterol and creatine phosphokinase.

Bone age is of more practical use to the emergency physician in ruling out significant hypothyroidism as the cause of the patient's problem. In the immediate postnatal period, an x-ray film of the infant's knee should demonstrate the distal femoral and proximal tibial epiphyses, since these are universally present at term in normal children. In the older child, an x-ray film of the hand and wrist is obtained and compared with those of normal children at various ages. An atlas for this purpose is usually found in radiology departments. A significant delay in bone age (per radiologist consultation) is compatible with hypothyroidism. Delays also may be suggested by malnutrition, chronic illness, or constitutional delay of adolescence.

Differential Diagnosis

The differential diagnosis is considerable since lethargy, hypotonia, cyanosis, or jaundice in infancy are quite nonspecific, especially in the absence of a goiter. A general laboratory evaluation should be undertaken (see Exhibit 35-2) since the results of thyroid function studies will not be immediately available.

Special Tests

In the older child, serum should be tested for antithyroid antibodies. A thyroid scan can help establish a diagnosis of nongoitrous hypothyroidism, i.e., attributable to thyroid remnants, either ectopic or in their customary location.

Treatment

If a goiter of sufficient size to cause respiratory or swallowing difficulties is present, surgical removal may be indicated. Hypothyroidism in general is treated with replacement thyroid hormone, usually levothyroxine. Although preparations of levothyroxine are slower acting than those of levothyronine, the latter can be more dangerous in their effect on a myxedematous myocardium. It is rarely necessary to use any but levothyroxine preparations. The usual once-a-day oral dose for infants is 0.025 to 0.05 mg/d (tablets are available in both doses) and that for children, 0.05 to 0.15 mg/d.

Serum concentrations of T_4 and TSH can be used to follow patients on replacement therapy; these measurements, in addition to observation for clinical signs of hyperthyroidism, can indicate whether the dose used is excessive. Concentrations of T_4 can increase into the normal range within a week or two, but TSH concentrations may decrease only slowly over the first few months of therapy.

ADRENAL INSUFFICIENCY

Pathophysiology

The zona glomerulosa of the adrenal cortex produces mineralocorticoids (deoxycorticosterone [DOC] and aldosterone) whereas the zona fasciculata produces glucocorticoids (cortisol).

Hypovolemia and elevated serum potassium concentrations stimulate aldosterone release via the renin-angiotensin system. Aldosterone then acts on the distal tubule of the kidney to affect sodium and water retention, with excretion of H^+ and potassium in the urine. In this way aldosterone serves a critical function by maintaining normal levels of total body sodium and water and protecting the body from hyperkalemia, dehydration, and shock. A striking feature of mineralocorticoid deficiency at any age is polyuria, especially in the dehydrated infant.

Corticotropin-releasing factor is released from the hypothalamus during stress or hypoglycemia and stimulates the release of adrenocorticotropic hormone (ACTH) by the pituitary gland. ACTH then acts on the zona fasciculata of the adrenal cortex to stimulate the synthesis and secretion of cortisol. Cortisol is one of the body's major defenses against hypoglycemia and shock and therefore also has a critical function in the body.

Adrenal insufficiency in the newborn period is most commonly caused by congenital adrenal hyperplasia (CAH) resulting from a deficiency in cortisol and aldosterone biosynthesis. In CAH the block in mineralocorticoid and glucocorticoid biosynthesis leads to excessive androgen production. Thus girls usually have ambiguous (virilized) genitalia, but boys appear normal in the first months of life. In CAH decreased aldosterone biosynthesis can lead to salt-losing crises (see "Laboratory Findings"), whereas cortisol deficiency can lead to hypoglycemia.

The most common cause of adrenal insufficiency is adrenal suppression from exogenous glucocorticoids used in the treatment of allergic, inflammatory, or neoplastic diseases. Glucocorticoids administered in pharmacologic doses for more than 4 to 7 days can suppress ACTH release for up to 12 months, with subsequent secondary adrenal insufficiency. Abrupt cessation of replacement in the glucocorticoid-dependent patient can thus precipitate an acute adrenal crisis. Primary adrenal insufficiency (both glucocorticoid and mineralocorticoid insufficiency) is rare in childhood but when present is most often due to an autoimmune process (Addison's disease). Other causes are adrenal hemorrhage, ACTH unresponsiveness, congenital adrenal hypoplasia, or meningococcemia. Addison's disease can be associated with other autoimmune endocrinopathies (e.g., type I diabetes mellitus, hypoparathyroidism).

Clinical Features

Any patient with a history of daily glucocorticoid intake for longer than 3 weeks in the preceding year must be considered to have potential secondary adrenal insufficiency. The patient may have noted weakness, anorexia, vomiting, weight loss, salt craving, and hyperpigmentation prior to coming to the emergency department.

Vital signs may reveal tachycardia and hypotension. Other clinical findings of shock can be present: pallor, poor peripheral perfusion, cool, clammy skin, and disturbed consciousness or coma. With dehydration there may be loss of normal skin turgor, sunken eyes, and dry mucous membranes. Hyperpigmentation of scars, buccal mucosa, skin, pressure points, and exposed and nonexposed skin reflects excessive ACTH secretion and suggests primary adrenal insufficiency.

Laboratory Findings

Glucocorticoid deficiency can cause hypoglycemia as well as acidosis from poor tissue perfusion. Deficient mineralocorticoid activity causes retention of K^+ and H^+ (hyperkalemia and metabolic acidosis) and excessive loss of sodium and water in the urine (hyponatremia, increased BUN and creatinine, and decreased urine output with increased urine specific gravity and osmolality).

Differential Diagnosis

All causes of hypoglycemia, coma, and shock must be considered (e.g., poisoning, hemorrhage, sepsis, anaphylaxis; see Exhibit 35-1).

Special Tests

Whenever adrenal insufficiency is suspected, blood should be drawn for serum cortisol determination. In the nonacute situation a 24-hour urine specimen can be collected for measurement of urinary free cortisol or 17-hydroxycorticosteroids. Dynamic testing includes the metapyrone test and the response to exogenous ACTH. If CAH is a consideration, blood should be sent for 17-hydroxyprogesterone and androstenedione testing.

Initial Therapy

The first priority in the treatment of adrenal crisis is to restore tissue perfusion. After an intravenous line is started, a bolus of normal saline is given at 20 mL/kg or 360 mL/m^2 over 1 hour or less, depending upon the degree of hypotension. Concurrently, 25% dextrose should be given (2 mL/kg) to correct hypoglycemia. Stress doses of a glucocorticoid are then administered: hydrocortisone, 120 to 200 mg/m^2 or 10 mg/kg immediately, and then 120 to 200 mg/m^2/d or 10 mg/kg/d divided every 6 hours. This is accompanied by mineralocorticoid replacement at a dose of 1 mg DOC acetate [DOCA] IM. Methylprednisolone or dexamethasone can be used in doses 1/5 and 1/30 that of hydrocortisone, respectively; however, they provide glucocorticoid effect only, whereas hydrocortisone also has mineralocorticoid activity.

Hyperkalemia greater than 6 mEq/L can produce cardiac arrhythmias and requires aggressive therapy: sodium bicarbonate, 1 to 2 mEq/kg IV over 10 to 15 minutes; calcium gluconate, 50 to 100 mg/kg by slow (5 to 10 minutes) IV drip (maximum single dose = 1 g); or glucose, 500 mg/kg (2 mL of 25% dextrose per kilogram), and insulin, 0.2 U/kg IV, followed by sodium polystyrene sulfonate, 1 g/kg rectally or orally, if tolerated. The plasma glucose concentration should be carefully monitored.

Ongoing Therapy

The full oral replacement dose of hydrocortisone for primary adrenocortical insufficiency is 15 to 25 mg/m^2/d. The appropriate dose for a particular patient must be determined individually, taking into account the patient's growth and development. In infants or patients unable to take oral medications, cortisone acetate can be injected, 30 to 48 mg/m^2 IM every 3 days.

Ongoing mineralocorticoid replacement is also begun after resolution of the acute crisis. If mineralocorticoid deficiency is present, 9α-fluorohydrocortisone is given (0.05 to 0.2 mg/d). In the infant or patient unable to take oral medication, DOCA (1 to 2 mg/d IM), DOC pivulate (25 mg/mo IM), or DOCA pellets (two 250-mg pellets placed SC) can be employed. The pellets' effectiveness can last from 9 to 12 months.

References

1. Bacchus H: *Metabolic and Endocrine Emergencies: Recognition and Management.* Baltimore, University Park Press, 1977.
2. Avery GB: *Neonatology. Pathophysiology and Management of the Newborn,* ed 2. JB Lippincott Co, Philadelphia, 1981.
3. Fulop M, Tannenbaum H, Dreyer N: Ketotic hyperosmolar coma. *Lancet* 1973;2:635–639.
4. Kappy MS, Lightner ES: Low-dose intravenous insulin in the treatment of diabetic ketoacidosis. *Am J Dis Child* 1979;133:523–525.
5. Kappy MS, Morrow G III: A diagnostic approach to metabolic acidosis in children. *Pediatrics* 1980; 65:351–356.
6. Cornblath M, Schwartz R: *Disorders of Carbohydrate Metabolism in Infancy,* ed 2. Philadelphia, WB Saunders Co, 1976.
7. Harrison HE, Harrison HC: *Disorders of Calcium and Phosphate Metabolism in Childhood and Adolescence.* Philadelphia, WB Saunders Co, 1979.

Dennis L. Headings
Robert Ancona
Fred J. Heldrich

36 Infectious Diseases

In terms of true life-threatening emergencies, there are some caused by infections. Meningococcemia, meningitis caused by any agent, staphylococcal pneumonia, peritonitis, epiglottitis, and any infection in the compromised host require emergency evaluation and treatment. Although not always life-threatening, infections and their attendant fevers probably cause more visits to pediatric emergency departments and unscheduled office visits than any other entity. These are emergencies for they require an emergency department visit or an unscheduled visit to the physician to assess this febrile episode. Some of these illnesses are covered in the chapters pertaining to systems involved, others are covered here.

Practically any symptom or sign can be associated with an acute or chronic infection, but fever is, of course, the most universal and general sign of infection. Other symptoms or signs may help to draw attention to a specific organ system. The headache of Rocky Mountain spotted fever (RMSF) or meningitis, the tachypnea of bronchiolitis or pneumonia, the diarrhea with viral or bacterial gastroenteritis, exanthems with common and not so common childhood febrile illnesses, or the immobility of an infected joint are examples of the manner of presentation of specific infectious entities.

Although the ultimate proof of an infectious cause requires growing an organism, this is not always possible. Associated laboratory findings can include an elevated or depressed white blood count, a depressed or elevated platelet count, toxic granulations in granulocytes, metabolic acidosis, or an elevated erythrocyte sedimentation rate. At best these associated laboratory findings are nonspecific. When they are supportive of clinical judgment, they may be considered useful, but when they are contrary to the expected, they certainly do not eliminate the diagnosis.

A few newer, rapid diagnostic laboratory tests have become commercially available, including specific serologic tests to detect the antigens of *Haemophilus influenzae* type B infections, *Neisseria meningitidis* infections, and group B streptococcal infections. The enzyme-linked immunosorbent assay (ELISA) technique has also been adapted for early diagnosis of a number of bacterial and viral diseases. The mononucleosis spot test is, of course, one specific serologic test that can aid in early diagnosis. Most other serologic tests require sera from acute and convalescent stages of illness to demonstrate a rise in the level of serum antibodies against a specific antigen for confirmation of the infectious etiology. Although a fourfold rise in titer is very suggestive of a specific diagnosis, the 2-week delay between samples from acute and convalescent stages does not allow this information to be available when decisions regarding therapy must be made, particularly in emergency situations. Although it is among the oldest of laboratory tests available, the Gram stain of a fluid suspected of being infected remains one of the most useful and easiest means of diagnosing a bacterial infection.

This chapter deals with the common, more severe infectious entities of pediatric practice. The topics concentrate on the signs and symptoms, the differential diagnosis, the evaluation in the first encounter, and the initial treatment of the infection.

SEPTICEMIA

Although used interchangeably with bacteremia, the term "sepsis" can be used with any infection. Bacteremia should apply to a situation in which a positive blood culture is accompanied by mild clinical symptoms, and septicemia should refer to the presence of more severe clinical signs and symptoms accompanying a positive blood culture.

Most septicemias in the pediatric age group are associated with definable sites of infection. Many patients with bacterial meningitis, epiglottitis, osteomyelitis, burn wound sepsis, endocarditis, or infectious arthritis have positive blood cultures, either because of the initial hematogenous spread or because of a continued seeding from the primary site.

Isolated septicemias in the immunologically intact child are unusual and fall into one of three primary syndromes: the late-onset group B streptococcal septicemia, nonlocalized pneumococcal septicemia of infancy, and meningococcal septicemia without meningitis.[1–5]

With any septicemia, whether localized or not, the patient most often appears gravely ill. High fever or hypothermia, abnormal or labored respiration, hypotension, marked irritability or lethargy, and cutaneous signs of disseminated intravascular coagulation, such as petechiae and purpura, are some of the signs and symptoms that may suggest a generalized, severe infection. Specific signs of localized infections with seeding of the blood must also be noted.[6]

The laboratory evaluation of a child suspected of having septicemia should include a complete blood count and differential, a platelet count, blood cultures, and cultures of any other body fluid suspected of harboring infection. Electrolyte studies may demonstrate the metabolic acidosis of severe infections. The complication of an intravascular coagulopathy may be detected by obtaining clotting studies, and the sedimentation rate is an excellent marker of an inflammatory process. Examination of the blood smear may reveal toxic granulations in granulocytes. If pneumonia, osteomyelitis, or arthritis are suspected, x-ray studies also may be valuable. A nuclear scan is of greatest benefit in the early diagnosis of osteomyelitis. In most cases of suspected nonlocalized septicemia, a lumbar puncture also should be performed.

In the case of a severely ill child who is suspected of having septicemia, treatment should not be delayed while extensive laboratory investigations are carried out. With the same intravenous access used to obtain blood for culture, broad-spectrum antibiotics can be pushed before proceeding further.

Given the numerous infections that can be associated with septicemia, almost any bacterial organism is a potential infective agent. Some of the more commonly seen organisms in the pediatric emergency department include *N. meningitidis, Streptococcus pneumoniae, H. influenzae, Escherichia coli, Streptococcus pyogenes* (group A streptococci), and *Streptococcus agalactiae* (group B streptococci).

Meningococcemia

Meningococcemia (meningococcal septicemia) is one of the most serious, rapid and devastating infections seen in the emergency department.[4,5] In addition to the general signs and symptoms of septicemia, cutaneous findings are prominent. Spreading petechiae or purpura in the presence of fever should suggest this diagnosis and necessitate immediate treatment and evaluation. A single petechial lesion should be sufficient to alert the physician to this possible diagnosis. While the typical rash of meningococcemia is petechial, the earliest lesion is a macular, erythematous spot that may blanch on pressure but which will rapidly become petechial. The lesions have no distinct or symmetric pattern of distribution.

The white cell count may be elevated, with an increase in polymorphonuclear cells and band forms. Toxic granules and vacuoles may be seen in the granulocytes. Low serum sodium and elevated blood glucose levels probably reflect a stress reaction secondary to the septicemia. Factors predicting an unfavorable outcome to the disease are a low white blood count, the absence of an associated meningitis, hypotension, purpuric lesions at the time of presentation, thrombocytopenia, petechiae for less than 12 hours, and a low erythrocyte sedimentation rate.

Suspected meningococcemia is a true medical emergency and requires immediate action. In the emergency department blood cultures should be obtained, followed by an initial intravenous dose of both chloramphenicol (25 mg/kg) and ampicillin (100 mg/kg), for although *N. menigitidis* is the organism most commonly associated with this clinical manifestation, a variety of organisms, both Gram-positive and Gram-negative, are potential pathogens. The intravenous line may be maintained with an infusion of 0.2% NaCl in D5W while the patient is transferred to the inpatient ward for further treatment. Support of cardiorespiratory function should be provided as necessary. There must be no delay in initiating treatment. A lumbar puncture should be done to determine the presence of an associated meningitis, but this may be delayed until the patient has been stabilized.

In cases of septicemia and/or meningitis caused by *N. meningitidis*, prophylactic treatment of close contacts and the patient prior to discharge is recommended. Close contacts are those who live in the same house, day-care center contacts, or medical personnel involved in cardiopulmonary resuscitation, intubation, suctioning, or holding for lumbar puncture. Rifampin by mouth in a dose of 10 mg/kg/d up to a total dose of 600 mg twice per day is recommended for 2 days.

Similar recommendations are made when the organism is *H. influenzae*. In this case, however, if the contact is over 5 years of age, only immediate family members and nursery school and day-care center contacts qualify for prophylactic treatment. Therapy should be given for 4 days.

Occult Bacteremia

Bacteremia without localization is an infection most often seen in children less than 3 years of age. Although *S. pneumoniae*[2,3] is the organism most commonly recovered and *H. influenzae* is recovered next in frequency, other organisms may also be found. These patients have high fevers but are without any identifiable site of localized infection. Fever usually occurs precipitously, and the patient may be seen with a febrile seizure. Although studies have been done indicating that the likelihood of bacteremia is directly related to the height of the fever, not infrequently the maximum temperature that the patient may have experienced prior to being examined is unknown, and a relatively low temperature on examination should not reduce the suspicion of bacteremia. Laboratory results that support the probability of bacteremia include a total white blood count greater than 15,000/μL and a shift to the left on differential count with an increase in polymorphonuclear cells and band forms. Unfortunately, none of these tests have the desired sensitivity or specificity, so management of the patient depends in large measure on clinical assessment. The risk of meningitis as a complication is about 5%; thus maximum protection should be provided these patients. Although every child in this age group with high fever and an elevated white blood count is not bacteremic, only a blood culture can provide the diagnosis, and therefore it should be done. Whether to admit each of these patients is debated, but any child who appears ill should be admitted and treated. An important sign of illness is the child's obtunded or inappropriate response to the environment, the examination, or the parents. A lumbar puncture with examination of cerebrospinal fluid should be done if a seizure has occurred. In female children especially, a urine culture should also be obtained.

In those patients for whom blood cultures have been obtained but who are not to be admitted to the hospital, the issue of treatment versus no treatment has not yet been decided; however, there is evidence to suggest a reduction in complications for patients treated prior to the report of the blood culture.[7] Ampicillin or amoxicillin is recommended for those not allergic to penicillin. A trimethoprim-sulfamethoxazole combination is an alternative choice. Following the report of a positive blood culture result, those patients who are well should have the blood culture repeated and therapy continued on an ambulatory basis. Those patients who remain ill should be admitted to the hospital for a full sepsis work-up, including lumbar puncture and intravenous antibiotic therapy, with appropriate medication determined by the culture result.

Hot Babies

One group of patients deserves special comment under this discussion of septicemia. This group, popularized as "hot babies," consists of infants, generally under 6 to 8 weeks of age, who develop fever without any site of infection apparent on physical examination.[8] The following questions must be considered in managing these infants: (1) Should they be evaluated for sepsis? (2) Do they require a lumbar puncture? (3) Should they be treated regardless of laboratory findings until the culture results are known?

As yet, there is no definitive clinical sign or laboratory test to distinguish the septicemic infant from the child who has a febrile upper respiratory tract infection. Infants in this age group do not manifest their infections as typically, or in the same way, as older children and adults, and they do not localize their infections as well. They are, in many ways, compromised hosts and have documented immune deficits. Because of this and because the consequences of sepsis and meningitis in this group of patients are so great, the infant's welfare is better served by being hospitalized, evaluated, and treated until the blood, urine, and cerebrospinal fluid culture results are known.

A major cause of infection in this age group is group B streptococcal sepsis.[1] When occurring after 7 days of age, it is defined as late-onset disease. When infection occurs in the first few days of life, it is considered early onset and is usually encountered while the neonate is still in the hospital, although the trend for early discharge of newborns and mothers after delivery may lead to an increasing emergency department experience with this form of the disease.

Patients with the early-onset form of group B streptococcal sepsis are much more likely to have pneumonia associated with their illness and characteristically have rapid downhill courses, including hypothermia, apnea, hypotension, and disseminated intravascular coagulation. Mortality figures of 25% to 50% are described.

Late-onset group B streptococcal sepsis is defined as occurring any time after 7 days of age up to several months of age. There are no specific signs or symptoms that suggest this particular diagnosis, and these patients have many of the general, nonspecific signs of septicemia. There is a high association with meningitis, and the morbidity figures for this disease are remarkably high.

In the therapy for both forms of the disease, penicillin is the drug of choice.

KAWASAKI SYNDROME

This multisystem disorder of unknown but suspected infectious etiology is also known as mucocutaneous lymph node syndrome. Originally described in Japanese populations, it has now been reported and documented in both endemic and epidemic situations in the United States.[9,10]

There are six major criteria for making a diagnosis of Kawasaki syndrome. Although all may not be present at the same time, five of the six must be noted:

1. fever for more than 5 days that is unresponsive to penicillin
2. conjunctivitis
3. "strawberry" tongue or oropharyngeal erythema
4. swollen, erythematous hands and feet with subsequent desquamation
5. a nonspecific, generalized erythematous rash
6. lymphadenopathy

Lymphadenopathy is the primary criterion most likely to be absent. Additional clinical features can include anemia, elevated white blood cell count, sterile pyuria, increased erythrocyte sedimentation rate, normal antistreptolysin O titer, thrombocytosis, elevated immunoglobulin E levels, and even aseptic meningitis.

In children exhibiting this spectrum of findings, the primary goal is to rule out other diagnoses for which there are more specific therapies. This differential diagnosis includes scarlet fever, toxic shock syndrome, RMSF, Stevens-Johnson syndrome, toxic epidermal necrolysis, serum sickness, and other disseminated bacterial and viral infections. Even collagen vascular diseases such as rheumatic fever, Henoch-Schönlein purpura, and infantile polyarteritis nodosa can be confused with this syndrome.

There are two phases to this illness, each of which can last up to 2 weeks. The first phase is more acute, and the patient is often referred to as looking "toxic" or quite ill, with high fever and rash. The second phase usually includes the arthralgias and desquamation, and it is during this period that the platelet count can be greater than $10^6/\mu L$.

Just as there is no specific diagnostic test, there is no specific treatment for this disorder. Those deaths that have occurred usually have been associated with coronary artery aneurysms and thrombosis, and the risk of this appears greatest during the second phase of the illness when platelet counts are found to be highest (see Chapter 10, "Cardiovascular Disorders"). Because of this, aspirin is usually recommended as supportive treatment both for its antipyretic properties and for its platelet aggregation inhibition properties. Recent studies indicate that intravenous gamma globulin will reduce coronary artery damage.[11] In contrast, corticosteroids appear to be contraindicated because they seem to increase mortality. Complications or areas of involvement that have been reported include hydrops of the gall bladder, iridocyclitis, keratitis, vitreous opacities, and arthritis.

Hospitalization is usually recommended during some part of the illness to rule out other entities, for baseline studies, for symptomatic treatment, and to initiate therapy. The duration of aspirin treatment is an unknown. Most recommendations call for its continuation until clinical signs abate, the sedimentation rate is normal, and thrombocytosis has disappeared. An echocardiographic examination should be done once the acute symptoms subside and again 2 to 3 months later to diagnose coronary artery involvement.

TOXIC SHOCK SYNDROME

Toxic shock syndrome is an illness with fever, a generalized erythematous, macular rash, and hypotension. Although it has been described in boys and younger children, the group most at risk for toxic shock syndrome appears to be menstruating girls and women who use tampons and who have *Staphylococcus aureus* present in the vagina. The etiology is associated with the presence of toxin-producing strains of phage group I *S. aureus*.[12]

The signs and symptoms are typically sudden in onset, with fever, chills, vomiting, diarrhea, myalgia, and abdominal pain. Hypotension develops, usually within 72 hours. Headache and sore throat are frequent complaints. Photophobia and arthralgia may be noted. Physical findings are the maculoerythematous rash, which later peels; hyperemia of the pharynx and conjunctivae; a vaginal discharge; muscle tenderness; tachycardia; and hypotension.[13]

Laboratory features can include positive cultures of *S. aureus* from samples taken from the vagina, cervix, throat, or a localized abscess. Blood cultures are usually negative. The white blood count is significantly elevated; there can be thrombocytopenia and prolonged prothrombin times. The urinalysis and tests of renal function can be markedly abnormal, reflecting ischemic changes or renal failure.

The differential diagnosis includes Kawasaki syndrome, streptococcal infections, RMSF, Stevens-Johnson syndrome, toxic epidermal necrolysis, serum sickness, disseminated bacterial or viral infections, and collagen vascular diseases.[8–10]

This severe multisystem disorder requires rapid, and intensive treatment. These patients must be hospitalized, and the treatment in the emergency department should be aimed at support of vital signs, specifically blood pressure, with fluid therapy and, if necessary, pharmacologic agents. In addition, diagnostic tests should be instituted, and antistaphylococcal treatment with methicillin or nafcillin should be started.

INFECTIOUS MONONUCLEOSIS

Infectious mononucleosis is classically caused by the Epstein-Barr virus, but a similar clinical picture occasionally can be seen with cytomegalovirus, adenovirus, and with viral hepatitis.[14,15] (For a discussion of hepatitis, see Chapter 14, "Gastroenterologic Disorders.")

This infection is a multisystem disease that frequently has hematologic, hepatic, dermatologic, and neurologic symptoms and signs. The onset of illness may be abrupt or insidious, with a prodromal period lasting several weeks. The most common clinical manifestations include fever, generalized malaise, exudative pharyngitis unresponsive to penicillin, cervical adenitis, and splenomegaly. Other less common findings include jaundice, supraorbital edema, and a maculopapular rash. The rash occurs in about 10% of cases but is much more common in the subgroup of patients treated with ampicillin for their pharyngitis; as many as 95% of such patients have a rash. Rare manifestations include urticaria, evidence of myocarditis, pneumonitis, neurologic syndromes such as Guillain-Barré syndrome, seizures, encephalitis, and hemolytic anemias.[13,14]

The laboratory diagnosis depends on the demonstration of atypical lymphocytes in the peripheral blood smear in quantities greater than 10%, a positive mononucleosis spot test, or a positive test for heterophile antibody. Additional laboratory findings may include increases in the levels of Epstein-Barr virus titer, the presence of cold agglutinins, biologic false-positive results from the serologic test for syphilis, and the presence of rheumatoid factor.

Liver function tests in patients with infectious mononucleosis deserve special comment. As previously stated, these patients can be jaundiced, although usually they are not. Almost 100% of the patients do have a viral hepatitis, and almost all have elevated levels of serum transaminases.

Most patients will have had a throat culture at some point in their illness, and this should be encouraged. About 20% will have a concurrent streptococcal pharyngitis accompanying their infectious mononucleosis.

When patients have atypical mononucleosis, the differential diagnosis can be extensive, and the specific diagnosis, elusive. For more typical cases the differential diagnosis includes streptococcal pharyngitis, viral pharyngitis, viral hepatitis, Kawasaki syndrome, and scarlet fever.

Most patients do not need to be hospitalized, and the treatment is primarily symptomatic. Rest, acetaminophen for fever, and counsel regarding precautions for the presence of splenomegaly are the cornerstones of therapy. Corticosteroids should be used only in the presence of upper airway obstruction. Deaths associated with encephalitis, upper airway obstruction, and splenic rupture have occurred, but most patients recover uneventfully in 2 to 4 weeks.

ROCKY MOUNTAIN SPOTTED FEVER

Although named for the Rocky Mountain region of the United States where it was first observed, RMSF is a rickettsial disease that can be seen in any U.S. geographic location. The greatest number of cases reported each year are from the Middle Atlantic states of Maryland, Virginia, and North Carolina.[16]

Rickettsia rickettsii is found in many small woodland rabbits and rodents, who are unaffected by the agent. Its transmission to man is almost always by ticks, who become infected from these small animals, but who can also pass the rickettsiae in vertical transmission from tick mother to tick progeny. The wood tick and the dog tick are most commonly involved, and a history of tick bite or tick exposure is very common and quite helpful in assessing the patient suspected of having RMSF.

The signs and symptoms of RMSF depend on the stage of the disease.[16,17] After an incubation period of 1 to 7 days, the first-stage, nonspecific symptoms appear: fever, malaise, and headache. If there is any specificity at all, it is an unusually severe headache. In some areas where RMSF is common during the spring and summer, the presence of severe headache and a history of tick bite is presumptive evidence of RMSF and treatment is initiated.

The second phase is heralded by the onset of an erythematous macular rash that starts peripherally, especially around the ankles and wrists, and spreads centripetally until most of the body is involved. This rash can involve the palms and soles. After a few days, and especially in the absence of treatment, the rash becomes hemorrhagic with petechiae and purpura.

During the entire course the systemic signs continue and may worsen. In addition, complications may arise, such as disseminated intravascular coagulation, central nervous system involvement, myocarditis, and hypotension.

Depending on the phase of the illness, the differential diagnosis may include Henoch-Schönlein purpura, meningococcemia, leptospirosis, and a variety of viral illnesses with exanthems. The latter include echoviruses, adenoviruses, Epstein-Barr virus of mononucleosis, and atypical rubeola. Although the initial diagnosis is made primarily on the basis of clinical findings, there are a number of helpful laboratory tests. Most patients require a complete blood count and blood culture, and a lumbar puncture may be needed if the clinical appearance suggests meningitis. Serologic evaluation for RMSF previously was based on the Weil-Felix reaction, but specific RMSF complement-fixation or indirect microimmunofluorescent antibody tests are now available. The most specific are the RMSF microimmunofluorescent antibody titer and the fluorescent antibody test applied to a skin biopsy of the rash: these demonstrate the rickettsiae in the tissue.[18,19]

Initial treatment should be started with the clinical diagnosis and may require intense supportive cardiorespiratory measures simultaneously with antibiotic therapy. Rickettsiae are sensitive to both tetracycline and chloramphenicol. Depending on the severity of the illness, both oral and intravenous routes can be used. In both, doses appropriate for septicemia are employed and usually continued for about 7 days.

CELLULITIS

Cellulitis is a bacterial infection of the skin; its severity is determined primarily by the organism involved and the depth of involvement. The most common causative bacteria include *S. pyogenes* and *S. aureus*. *H. influenzae* is a special consideration in the pediatric age group under 6 years, and Gram-negative organisms and anaerobes are also occasionally seen. Gram-negative organisms and anaerobes must be considered, especially in postoperative cases of cellulitis, in diabetic patients, in patients with injuries associated with water, and in those cases of cellulitis following human bites.[20,21]

The signs and symptoms of cellulitis are those of an acute inflammatory reaction: redness, swelling, tenderness, and induration. Crepitance may be elicited where the organisms are gas producers, and *E. coli* and some anaerobes are capable of this, as well as the familiar but unusual *Clostridium perfringens*. Streptococcal cellulitis has sometimes been characterized as having a very explosive course, with the edge of the cellulitis spreading very rapidly. This form of the disease has been termed erysipelas. An even more severe form of cellulitis is necrotizing fasciitis with deep soft tissue involvement, rapid spread, and signs of necrosis.[22] Although characteristically seen with streptococcal infections, it can also be caused by anaerobic organisms and Gram-negative bacteria. Patients with cellulitis are in general more ill than those with the superficial skin infection impetigo. Lymphangitis, positive blood cultures, and systemic signs of toxemia are much more commonly seen.

In *H. influenzae* cellulitis there are several distinguishing features. It is seen almost exclusively in patients under 6 years of age, it most commonly involves the face and periorbital area, and blood cultures are positive in about 70% of cases.[19] *H. influenzae* cellulitis has also been described as having an associated purplish or heliotrope discoloration. Some cases do, but many do not, and cellulitis caused by other organisms, including *S. pneumoniae,* has appeared with identical discoloration.

The evaluation of cellulitis should include a white blood cell count, a blood culture, and culture of an aspirate from the edge of the cellulitis. This can be done using a syringe with a 25-gauge needle, injecting a small amount of sterile saline, and aspirating the fluid. Even if nothing is apparently obtained, culturing should be attempted by flushing the needle and syringe with the blood culture medium. Roentgenograms of the affected area may be helpful in ruling out an underlying osteomyelitis or sinusitis, although bone scans using ^{99m}Tc methylene diphosphonate are more useful than x-ray films in diagnosing early osteomyelitis. In facial cellulitis a careful examination of the teeth may reveal an underlying dental abscess. Additionally, in periorbital disease, the eye must be checked for pupillary reaction and full extraocular muscle mobility. If these are abnormal, an orbital abscess or cavernous sinus thrombosis must be ruled out.

Treatment of uncomplicated cellulitis for patients over 6 years of age should include coverage for streptococci and staphylococci. If the patient is under 6 years of age, consideration of *H. influenzae* infection requires either ampicillin or chloramphenicol: because so many of these patients have positive blood cultures, *H. influenzae* cellulitis can be considered a potentially life-threatening disease requiring chloramphenicol for possible ampicillin-resistant strains. If the patient is diabetic, has a water-associated injury, is recovering from surgery, or has suffered a human bite, initial antibiotic coverage should be considered for Gram-negative and anaerobic organisms. When culture results are known, the treatment can be altered accordingly.

Patients under 6 years of age and all patients with a clinical probability of extension of the infection to the bone should be hospitalized.

PERITONITIS

Peritonitis is an inflammation of the abdominal peritoneal surfaces that can be caused by a number of agents and conditions. The two infectious forms are "primary" peritonitis, seen most frequently in patients with nephrotic syndrome, and "secondary" peritonitis in surgical patients, in whom contamination of the peritoneum has resulted from leakage of a viscus. Meconium peritonitis is a chemical inflammation seen exclusively in the newborn period and is suggestive of bowel atresia or cystic fibrosis.[23,24]

The signs and symptoms of peritonitis include abdominal pain, fever, and vomiting. On physical examination the patient is in obvious pain, with splinting respirations, hypoactive to absent bowel sounds, abdominal guarding, resistance to palpation, and generalized tenderness on percussion. Although rebound tenderness can be elicited, in the patient with peritonitis this can be considered cruel and unusual punishment. The same signs can be elicited by careful percussion. A rectal examination may demonstrate generalized pain.

The list of likely infectious agents should include bacteria such as *S. pneumoniae*, group A streptococci, and Gram-negative organisms. Chemical agents such as meconium and bile and inflammatory responses that are part of a generalized condition such as collagen vascular disease can also produce peritoneal signs. A pneumonia, especially affecting the lower lobes, can mimic peritonitis.

Diagnostic tests include a complete blood count and differential count, a chest film to rule out pneumonia, and abdominal films, which may show ileus, absent properitoneal fat pads, hazy ileopsoas shadows, and even fecaliths in the appendix. In meconium peritonitis, calcifications can be seen. Blood cultures are frequently positive, especially in primary peritonitis. A diagnostic peritoneal aspiration for examination and culture of the fluid may be very helpful.

The treatment of peritonitis depends on whether its cause is primary or secondary. Appendicitis, ruptured viscera, or peritoneal abscesses, causes of secondary peritonitis, require surgery as well as antibiotic therapy. When leakage of gastrointestinal contents has occurred, antibiotic coverage should include an aminoglycoside for Gram-negative organisms and clindamycin for anaerobic bacteria, including the penicillin-resistant *Bacteroides fragilis*.

In primary hematogenous peritonitis the main offending agents include Gram-negative organisms, group A streptococci, and *S. pneumoniae.* Prior to the use of corticosteroids for nephrotic syndrome, *S. pneumoniae* was the most common organism seen, but with the change in therapy, Gram-negative bacteria such as *E. coli* and *Klebsiella pneumoniae* are now found in increasing numbers. Penicillin in combination with an aminoglycoside provides good initial antibiotic coverage. If renal disease is present, however, chloramphenicol may be substituted for the potentially nephrotoxic aminoglycoside.

IMPETIGO

Impetigo is a cutaneous infection usually caused by *S. aureus* and group A streptococci. Any part of the body may be involved, although the face and extremities are the areas most frequently affected. In most cases the symptoms are limited to the typical "honey-crusted" lesions with surrounding erythema. Lymphangitis is rare, although regional lymph nodes may be enlarged. Fever is unusual. When specimens from most lesions are cultured, a mixture of *S. aureus* and *S. pyogenes* is found. However, in the classic form of impetigo, streptococci appear to be responsible for the yellow, thick, crusted lesions, whereas staphylococci cause bullous, vesicular lesions termed "bullous impetigo."[25,26]

Complications of this disorder are rare but include bacteremia, cellulitis, metastatic infection, and acute glomerulonephritis. Culturing specimens for bacteria is not necessary in the majority of cases unless the patient shows signs of more serious infection or fails to respond to traditional therapy. Most cases respond to a combination of either oral penicillin or intramuscular benzathine penicillin and to soaking the lesions to gently debride the crusts. Most cases respond to penicillin treatment even when penicillin-resistant staphylococci are isolated from the lesions. In some cases treatment with a penicillinase-resistant penicillin may be necessary.

STAPHYLOCOCCAL SCALDED SKIN SYNDROME

Staphylococcal scalded skin syndrome (SSSS) usually occurs in young children and has several forms. All variants are caused by *S. aureus* and range from simple bullous impetigo to a generalized erythema and exfoliation. Fever usually accompanies the rash, which classically begins as an erythema involving the face, axillae, and groin, and can progress rapidly to large bullous lesions of the entire body that then exfoliate. The various manifestations are all caused by a toxin (exfoliation) produced by the staphylococci, and cultures of the bullous fluid are sterile.[27]

The differential diagnosis of this disorder includes several acute febrile reactions associated with a generalized erythematous rash. As such, toxic shock syndrome, Kawasaki syndrome, erythema multiforme, and toxic epidermal necrolysis (TEN) must be excluded.

SSSS is most similar to TEN in its clinical appearance; both can be extremely serious and require admission to the hospital. Because TEN is usually associated with a drug reaction, not a staphyloccal infection, a careful history to exclude it is important.[28] Additionally, complete blood counts and cultures of blood and of specimens taken from the lesions should be obtained. In SSSS the staphylococcus is cultured from the skin or nasopharynx and not the exfoliative lesions. SSSS usually spares mucous membranes.

TEN and SSSS have very different treatment regimens, and thus differentation is critical. This may require histopathologic examination of a skin biopsy specimen because the two disorders can be so similar. In SSSS the cleavage plane where bullae form is intraepidermal, whereas in TEN the cleavage plane is deeper, at the epidermal-dermal junction. Because of this, scarring is described in healing TEN but is absent in SSSS.

In SSSS the treatment is based on replacement of fluids and specific antistaphylococcal therapy with either nafcillin or methicillin. Corticosteroids may be contraindicated in SSSS whereas they can be helpful in TEN.

CONJUNCTIVITIS

Inflammation of the conjunctiva of the eye accompanied by an exudate can occur at any age, and infectious agents are frequently implicated. Other causes include allergies and chemicals such as the silver nitrate drops instilled at the time of birth or the chlorine used in swimming pool water.

Among the infectious etiologies, bacterial causes include the gonococcus, pneumococci, group A or B streptococci, staphylococci, and a number of *Haemophilus* species including *H. influenzae*. *Chlamydia trachomatis* is a major cause of conjunctivitis in the neonatal period. The most frequent virus implicated is the adenovirus, which causes epidemic keratoconjunctivitis (adenovirus 8).[29–31]

Purulent discharge from the eye is more commonly seen with bacterial etiologies. The discharge associated with *Chlamydia* or viruses is usually much less purulent and sometimes absent. In addition to the presence and nature of the discharge, the eyes should be checked for corneal involvement and any evidence of iritis. These findings suggest a much more severe problem and require evaluation by an ophthalmologist.

The laboratory evaluation for conjunctivitis is best done by Gram staining and culturing any exudate. Detection of *Chlamydia* requires a Wright or

Giemsa stain of conjunctival scrapings, which are best taken from the upper lid. The inclusion bodies seen within the epithelial cells are characteristic of this disease.

Most patients with conjunctivitis can be treated as outpatients. Exceptions to this are any suggestion of herpes conjunctivitis or a conjunctivitis in a newborn less than a week of age whose laboratory studies show Gram-negative diplococci or a Gram stain suggestive of gonococcal ophthalmitis. In cases of conjunctivitis caused by *Neisseria gonorrhoeae*, treatment requires parenteral penicillin. Herpes infection requires treatment with acyclovir or vidarabine.

LYMPHADENITIS

An inflammation of the lymph nodes may be part of a generalized infection, in which case any or all lymph node groups may be involved; or it may result from a localized infection when drainage by specific lymph nodes produces enlargement and inflammation of the group of lymphatic tissue.[32]

The key characteristics to be noticed in any lymph node enlargement include size, redness of overlying skin, tenderness, and the presence of fluctuation and drainage. Infectious etiologies generally cause swelling, tenderness, and erythema, and they have the potential to fluctuate.

Generalized node involvement is more suggestive of systemic disease such as tuberculosis, syphilis, infectious mononucleosis, cytomegalovirus infections, sarcoidosis, and collagen vascular disease. Although lymphomas and leukemia are a consideration, these disorders do not usually appear with signs of true lymph node inflammation.

Although localized node inflammation can occur anywhere, the most frequent site is the neck, the cervical triangle, and the submandibular nodes. In the presence of typical signs of an inflammatory process, the primary considerations within the differential diagnosis of cervical adenitis are bacterial lymphadenitis, infections caused by atypical mycobacteria, and cat-scratch fever. Those patients with bacterial lymphadenitis typically look more toxemic than patients with the other disorders. They are frequently febrile and may have marked tonsillitis or pharyngitis; their nodes are tender and swollen, with the overlying skin warm and erythematous. In the later stages fluctuation is common. Group A streptococci and *S. aureus* are the bacteria most frequently found to cause this disease.

Mycobacterium tuberculosis can and does cause cervical lymphadenitis (scrofula), but among the numerous disorders that can cause a granulomatous lymphadenitis, the atypical mycobacteria are the most common. Patients with infections caused by atypical mycobacteria are for the most part from 1 to 5 years of age, have normal chest films, and are usually without systemic signs of illness. In addition, over 90% have adenopathy limited to the cervical area, and likewise, in more than 90% it is unilateral.[29] It is also of interest that *M. tuberculosis* usually affects the nodes of the cervical triangle. Atypical mycobacteria are found in soil, and because the submandibular nodes drain the buccal mucosa, ingestion of soil by children in this age group is thought to be the cause of this localized involvement. *M. tuberculosis* lymphadenitis is more likely to show pulmonary involvement on chest films, and the patients usually exhibit systemic signs such as fever, weight loss, and malaise.

Cat-scratch fever is an interesting disorder of suspected but unknown infectious etiology; it generally results in regional lymphadenopathy after a cat scratch and is, like the mycobacterial disorders, a granulomatous reaction. Because scratches are more common on the extremities, the most frequent sites of lymph node involvement are the groin and axilla. Cervical node disease is a pediatric disorder, for about 80% of the cases occur in patients less than 20 years of age.[28] Interestingly, about 80% of the cases also occur in the fall and winter. There are mild to moderate systemic symptoms, and about two thirds of the patients complain of fever and malaise along with the lymph node involvement.

In making a diagnosis among these primary causes of lymphadenitis, a number of clinical and laboratory facts are needed. The nature and location of the lymphadenitis and the presence or absence of systemic signs are important. A search for exposure to cats and actual evidence of cat scratches can be very important. A throat culture to rule out streptococcal pharyngitis or a mononucleosis spot test may be important. A skin test with standard purified protein derivative (PPD-S) is essential. In *M. tuberculosis* infections the PPD-S test is, of course, positive in most cases (greater than 10 mm of induration), and in atypical tuberculosis the PPD-S test is usually positive, demonstrating between 5 and 10 mm of induration. At the present time skin tests for the four groups of atypical mycobacteria (PPD-Y, PPD-G, PPD-B, and PPD-F) are not commercially available. Blood cultures may be indicated, and needle aspiration of the node may offer the only means of bacterial diagnosis by culture.

Treatment depends on the cause of the lymphadenitis. There is no specific therapy for cat-scratch fever but incision and drainage are contraindicated because this may lead to chronic drainage and prolong the usual 1- to 2-month course of the illness. Analgesics, heat, and even repeated needle aspirations may be helpful in this disorder.

In cervical adenitis caused by atypical mycobacteria, surgical excision of the involved lymph nodes is the treatment of choice, and chemotherapy is not required. With *M. tuberculosis* lymphadenitis systemic therapy with at least two primary antituberculosis drugs, usually rifampin and isoniazid, is essential along with a complete evaluation for involvement of other systems by the tuberculous process.

When bacterial lymphadenitis is suspected, unless it is associated with signs of a streptococcal pharyngitis, a penicillinase-resistant penicillin should be used. For intravenous use, either nafcillin or methicillin is appropriate, and in oral use, dicloxacillin is the drug of choice. If fluctuation is present, incision and drainage are usually required to effect a cure.

PREVENTABLE DISEASES

What were once called the "common childhood diseases" are rapidly becoming oddities because medical science has developed relatively safe, effective vaccines that have drastically reduced the incidence of these diseases. The challenge with most of these illnesses is to raise immunization levels to the point that eradication is possible, as has happened with smallpox.

Currently, diphtheria toxoid, tetanus toxoid, and pertussis vaccine are given together as a single injection. The diphtheria-pertussis-tetanus immunization should be given initially as three doses 6 to 8 weeks apart, usually beginning at 6 to 8 weeks of life. Booster immunizations are given approximately 1 year after the third injection, and a second booster, at 4 to 6 years of age. Pertussis immunization is not routinely given after 6 to 7 years of age, but diphtheria and tetanus booster immunizations have been recommended every 10 years. Patients with tetanus-prone wounds should be reimmunized if it has been approximately 5 years since the last tetanus immunization.

Three other formerly common diseases that are currently preventable by a single injection are measles (rubeola), rubella (German measles), and mumps. A single injection, usually given at 15 months of age or later, contains live attenuated virus strains that induce lasting immunity to each of these diseases.

However, despite immunization programs, small numbers of patients still acquire these illnesses, and an awareness of their clinical manifestations is essential.[33–36]

Pertussis

When patients with pertussis have a paroxysmal cough followed by an inspiratory whoop (whooping cough), they can be readily identified. However, in the very young infant and in those in whom only partial immunity exists, the presentation is less characteristic. The illness is caused by *Bordetella pertussis,* although *Bordetella parapertussis, Bordetella bronchiseptica,* and the adenovirus can produce a similar syndrome.

The illness lasts approximately 6 weeks with three stages, each lasting roughly 2 weeks. The first is the catarrhal stage, with progressively worsening upper respiratory tract symptoms of cough, coryza, rhinorrhea, and sneezing. Fever, if present now or during the uncomplicated illness, is only low grade. In the infant, feeding may become poor by the end of this stage. The paroxysmal or spasmodic stage follows when the persistent, irritating cough occurs spasmodically and terminates in an inspiratory whoop frequently associated with vomiting. The face is reddened and suffused; veins are distended. Cyanosis may appear, and the patient seems anxious. In the young infant, apnea is not uncommon. After approximately 2 weeks of such symptoms, the convalescent stage begins, with gradual diminution of symptoms. During this stage intercurrent infections may trigger renewed paroxysms.

Mortality, occurring primarily in infants, is about 1%. Complications include encephalopathy and pneumonia.

The organism may be recovered from the nasopharynx in some cases. An immunofluorescent antibody test permits rapid diagnosis. A striking laboratory finding is a marked lymphocytosis with an elevation in total white blood cell count.

There is no effective treatment, although erythromycin eradicates the organism from the nasopharynx and should be given to the patient as well as to all who are exposed and susceptible. Good nursing care is essential, and hospitalization is advised for the very young.[32–35]

Tetanus

Tetanus is caused by the neurotoxin elaborated by the organism *Clostridium tetani.* This ubiquitous organism is a normal inhabitant in both animal and human intestinal tracts and is found in soil and dust, thus being a potential contaminant following injury. In areas where aseptic technique is not adhered to, even surgical procedures may result in infection from this organism. Tetanus is aptly named "lockjaw" because of the tetanic contraction of skeletal muscles and the early involvement of muscles of the jaw and neck that result in trismus. Involvement of facial muscles results in the sardonic grin or risus sardonicus, and involvement of the muscles of the back and extremities results in truncal hyperextension (opisthotonos), extension of the extremities, and a boardlike abdomen. Urinary retention occurs because of spasm of the sphincter to the bladder.

Tetanic contractions of muscles may be intermittent at first, with progressive shortening of the intervals of relaxation until finally the patient is in a state of continual muscle spasm. At this stage interference with respiration and accumulation of secretions in the tracheobronchial tree may result in asphyxia and death. The sensorium remains clear.

Patients are provoked into episodes of tetanic contractions by external stimuli such as movement, noise, or bright lights. In partially immunized patients, local tetanus has been observed, usually involving muscles in proximity to the wound.

The wound may appear healed and innocent at the time of symptoms, and the organism may not be recovered. Any wound or trauma that favors anaerobic growth is a potential source of infection. The illness is produced by the production of an exotoxin. The incubation period varies from 3 days to 3 weeks. Mortality from this illness is as high as 60%.[33]

Diagnosis is based on the clinical appearance and must be differentiated from bacterial meningitis, encephalitis, strychnine poisoning, rabies, and tetany. Laboratory studies are of value in the differential diagnosis but do not aid in making a specific diagnosis.

Treatment requires the use of human tetanus immune globulin in a dose ranging from 500 to 3,000 U IM, a portion of the dose being given around the wound. Tetanus antitoxin at a single dose of 50,000 to 100,000 U, half IM and half IV, may be used if tetanus immune globulin is not available. If tetanus antitoxin is to be used, testing for sensitivity must be done, and fractionated antitoxin should be used if necessary. The following schedule can be used; each subsequent dose is given at 15-minute intervals if there is no reaction:[33]

0.1 mL of a 1:20 dilution SC
0.1 mL of a 1:10 dilution SC
0.1 mL of undiluted antitoxin SC
0.3 mL of undiluted antitoxin SC
0.5 mL of undiluted antitoxin SC
Remainder intramuscularly

Penicillin should be given for 10 to 14 days.[31] Debridement of a contaminated wound is advisable, and general supportive care is essential. Upon recovery full immunization against tetanus should be provided.[30–33] (See Chapter 30, Table 30-1, for schedule of immunization.)

Diphtheria

Corynebacterium diphtheriae, the infectious agent of diphtheria, produces a membranous nasopharyngitis with involvement of the larynx and trachea. In addition to local pathology, more extensive involvement is caused by dissemination of a toxin elaborated by this organism. Other unusual sites for infection by this organism are conjunctival, aural, dermal, and vulvovaginal.

The incubation period is usually 2 to 5 days, and the early symptoms depend upon the site of infection—usually nasopharyngeal. First, there are signs and symptoms of an upper respiratory tract infection, with low-grade fever followed by a serosanguinous nasal discharge or sore throat with exudate and membrane formation over one or both tonsils. Removal of the membrane leads to bleeding. Cervical lymphadenitis may be striking and creates a bullneck appearance. Laryngeal involvement produces symptoms of croup with cough, hoarseness, and inspiratory stridor. Mechanical obstruction to breathing may be severe. Generalized signs of toxic effects due in large measure to the degree of toxemia, include pallor, weakness, and tachycardia with a weak pulse. Myocarditis may occur early or later in the disease and lead to cardiac failure. Electrocardiographic changes—elevated ST segment, prolongation of the PR interval, and heart block—may be found. A neuritis, resulting in paralyses that usually clear, also may occur. Areas of involvement include the soft palate, extraocular muscles, diaphragm, and extremities.

Diseases to be included in the differential diagnosis are acute streptococcal infections, infectious mononucleosis, peritonsillar abscess, and the croup syndromes of epiglottitis, laryngotracheobronchitis, pharyngeal foreign body, and angioneurotic edema.

Cultures on appropriate media may reveal the organism within 8 hours; however, a clinical decision may be required immediately. A history of no prior immunization is helpful. Antitoxin at doses ranging from 50,000 to 100,000 U IV should be given after testing for sensitivity. If sensitivity exists, the protocol listed in the section on "Tetanus" should be followed. Penicillin, or erythromycin for the penicillin-sensitive patient, should be given for 14 days, and the patient should be hospitalized and isolated until cultures are negative. Active immunization should be provided after recovery.[32–35]

Rubeola

Rubeola, a viral infection also referred to as regular measles or red measles, is characterized by cough, coryza, conjunctivitis, fever, and a rash that occurs on both mucous membranes and skin. There is an incubation period of 8 to 10 days from exposure to onset of symptoms.

Fever and malaise usher in the illness. The fever, mild at first, increases over the next 3 to 4 days and is accompanied by coryza, cough, and conjunctivitis. Eyes are watery, without exudate, and photophobia is marked. The cough is irritating and increases in severity. Twenty-four to forty-eight hours before the onset of the skin rash (usually the third or fourth day of illness), a pathognomonic exanthem, the Koplik spots, appears. The Koplik spots are erythematous macular lesions with a whitish center that are found on the buccal mucosa opposite the molars; they coalesce and cover the entire buccal mucosa, disappearing within 2 to 3 days. The rash begins on the fourth day, first appearing on the neck and behind the ears, then spreading to the face, trunk, and extremities and reaching the feet 3 days after first appearing. At this time the rash begins to fade, first disappearing from the face. At times there is fine peeling of the skin. Temperature returns to normal 4 days after the rash appears. The cough persists, lasting as long as 10 days.

Complications include bacterial infections such as otitis media and pneumonia. A more serious complication is encephalitis.

The laboratory offers no assistance in diagnosis during the acute illness. History of no immunization is helpful.

Treatment of the acute illness is symptomatic. Prophylactic antibiotics should not be used. In the event exposure of the nonimmune patient is recognized, γ-globulin at 0.25 mL/kg can be given to attenuate the disease. If exposure has not been longer than 5 days, measles vaccine can be used.

A variant of rubeola occurring in those patients immunized by the killed vaccine, atypical measles is characterized by fever and an erythematous rash that is usually maculopapular, but may be hemorrhagic, and begins peripherally on the hands and feet. Frequently, there is a localized reaction at the site of the prior inoculation, and pulmonary involvement of viral etiology is not uncommon.

Treatment is supportive, and diseases such as RMSF and meningococcemia must be excluded.

Rubella

Rubella is a mild viral illness also referred to as German measles or 3-day measles. This infection, although usually well tolerated as a childhood disease, carries great risk to the fetus of an infected woman.

The incubation period ranges from 2 to 3 weeks. Symptoms are mild and may consist of only slight malaise and rhinorrhea in the child before the rash appears. The rash is maculopapular and erythematous, more pink than red, with generalized distribution. Postoccipital, postauricular, and cervical nodes may be enlarged and tender. The rash fades within 2 to 3 days, and nodes become nontender but remain enlarged longer. In older children the symptoms may be more pronounced.

When the adenopathy persists, it can be cause for concern, and parents may seek reassurance that it does not represent a malignancy. No treatment is necessary.

Mumps

Epidemic parotiditis is a myxovirus infection primarily involving the parotid glands and other salivary glands; it has the potential also to involve other areas. A large number of infected patients may have subclinical disease.

After an incubation period of 2 to 3 weeks, the illness begins with fever, malaise, anorexia, and headache followed by "ear" pain a day later. Swelling is noted around and behind the ear and gradually increases for 2 or 3 days. Patients may refuse to eat because chewing aggravates the pain. Fever subsides soon after the swelling has attained its peak.

Examination reveals a tender, palpable parotid gland. The ear lobe protrudes secondary to the swelling. Erythema of the underlying skin is not significant. The glands feel tense and firm. Stenson's duct may be erythematous and swollen on the involved side. Frequently, involvement of the second parotid gland follows the first by a day or two.

Submaxillary or sublingual salivary glands also may be affected, and there can be other areas of involvement. Meningoencephalitis may occur in as many as 10% of cases and may occur in the absence of salivary gland involvement. Only in patients beyond puberty is orchitis or oophoritis a manifestation. Pancreatitis may be a cause of abdominal pain and vomiting. Myocarditis, arthritis, and hepatitis also can occur.

There is no specific therapy. Mumps vaccine given after exposure has not been shown effective.

NONPREVENTABLE DISEASES

Although no immunization procedures for protection are available at this time, the following two diseases are included because they conform to the older classification of "common childhood diseases" and are important causes of febrile illness in the pediatric age group.[32–34]

Roseola

Roseola, an illness presumed to be viral and also known as exanthem subitum, usually begins abruptly with high fever, at times producing febrile seizures. It is a disease of infants, occurring in those between the ages of 6 months and 2 years.

Characteristically, there is an abrupt onset with high fever; body temperatures may be 40.0° to 40.5° C (104° to 105° F). The temperature may fluctuate markedly, with daily spikes again going to 40.5° C (105° F). Irritability is an associated finding, being most noticeable when the temperature is highest. After the rash appears, on the third or fourth day, the patient remains afebrile. The rash consists of pink macular or maculopapular lesions that usually remain discrete. It is usually generalized and disappears within a day or two.

During the illness the patient does not appear seriously ill despite the high fever. Physical findings, other than mild lymphadenopathy of occipital, postauricular, and cervical nodes, are lacking. Laboratory studies are useful only for their normal values.

Treatment consists of the use of antipyretics, although febrile seizures may result in hospitalization.

Varicella

Varicella or chickenpox, a herpesvirus infection, is one of the childhood diseases that remains a common entity. A varicella vaccine is presently being tested for use in immunocompromised hosts, but there is no vaccine available for routine immunization.

Following exposure there is an incubation period of 10 to 21 days. The onset is relatively abrupt, with a prodromal period lasting about 24 hours and consisting of malaise, fever, and anorexia. The rash, the characteristic feature of the disease, then occurs in crops, usually more pronounced on the covered portions of the body but appearing in all areas, including mucous membranes and conjunctiva. The more extensive the rash, the higher the fever usually is. These crops of lesions usually appear for 3 successive days. The individual lesions begin as erythematous macules that rapidly become papular and then vesicular with central umbilication. These vesicles are very friable, easily rupturing and then becoming crusted lesions; all this occurs within 12 hours. The lesions are pruritic.

Complications, although unusual, include secondary bacterial infection of the lesions, varicella pneumonia, and encephalitis. Reye's syndrome has been associated with recent varicella infection.

Treatment is entirely symptomatic, but aspirin should not be used because of its association with Reye's syndrome. For immunocompromised patients, varicella-zoster immune globulin or immune plasma should be given within 72 hours of exposure. Patients on corticosteroids should have their dose tapered to physiologic levels and raised again if the disease appears.

References

1. Baker CJ: Group B streptococcal infections in neonates. *Pediatr Rev* 1979;1:5–15.
2. Burke JP, Klein JO, Gezon HM, et al: Pneumococcal bacteremia: Review of 111 cases, 1967–1969, with special reference to cases with undetermined focus. *Am J Dis Child* 1971;121:353–359.
3. Heldrich FJ Jr: *Diplococcus pneumoniae* bacteremia. *Am J Dis Child* 1970;119:12–17.
4. Stiehm ER, Damrosch DS: Factors in the prognosis of meningococcal infection. *J Pediatr* 1966;68:457–467.
5. Koch P, Carson MJ: Meningococcal infections in children. *N Engl J Med* 1958;258:639–643.
6. Owen GM (ed): *Report of the 55th Ross Conference on Pediatric Research.* Columbus, OH, Ross Laboratories, 1966, pp. 10–12.
7. Rosenberg N, Cohen SN: Pneumococcal bacteremia in pediatric patients. *Ann Emerg Med* 1982;11:2–6.
8. Klein JO, Schlesinger PC, Karasic RB: Management of the febrile infant three months of age or younger. *Ped Inf Dis* 1984;3:75–79.
9. Melish ME, Hicks, RV, Larson EJ: Mucocutaneous lymph node syndrome in the United States. *Am J Dis Child* 1976;130:599–607.
10. Melish ME, Hicks RV, Reddy V: Kawasaki syndrome: An update. *Hosp Pract* 1982;17:99–106.
11. Newburger JW, Takahashi M, Burns JC, et al: The treatment of Kawasaki syndrome with intravenous gamma globulin. *N Engl J Med* 1986;315:341–7.

12. Gesler M: Toxic shock syndrome. *Pediatr Clin North Am* 1981;28:433–435.
13. Chesney PJ, Davis JP, Purdy WK, et al: Clinical manifestations of toxic shock syndrome. *JAMA* 1981;246:741–748.
14. Andiman WA: The Epstein-Barr virus and EB virus infections in childhood. *J Pediatr* 1979;95:171–182.
15. Radetsky M: A diagnostic approach to Epstein-Barr virus infections. *Pediatr Infect Dis* 1982;1:425–428.
16. Riley HD: Rickettsial diseases and Rocky Mountain spotted fever—Part I. *Curr Probl Pediatr* 1981;11:1–46.
17. Linnemann CC, Janson PJ: The clinical presentations of Rocky Mountain spotted fever: Comments on recognition and management based on a study of 63 patients. *Clin Pediatr* 1978;17:673–679.
18. Fleisher G, Lennette ET, Honig P: Diagnosis of Rocky Mountain spotted fever by immunofluorescent identification of *Rickettsia rickettsii* in skin biopsy tissue. *J Pediatr* 1979;95:63–65.
19. Hechemy KE, Stevens RW, Sasowski S, et al: Discrepancies in Weil-Felix and microimmunofluorescence test results for Rocky Mountain spotted fever. *J Clin Microbiol* 1979;9:292–293.
20. Fleisher G, Ludwig S, Campos J: Cellulitis: Bacterial etiology, clinical features, and laboratory findings. *J Pediatr* 1980;97:591–593.
21. Phillips JA, Bernhardt HE, Rosenthal SG: *Aeromonas hydrophila* infections. *Pediatrics* 1974;53:110–112.
22. Rea WJ, Wyrick WJ Jr: Necrotizing fasciitis. *Ann Surg* 1970;172:957–964.
23. Fowler R: Primary peritonitis: Changing aspects 1956–1970. *Aust Paediatr J* 1971;7:73–83.
24. Speck WT, Dresdale SS, McMillan RW: Primary peritonitis and the nephrotic syndrome. *Am J Surg* 1974;127:267–269.
25. Peter G, Smith AL: Group A streptococcal infections of the skin and pharynx (Part I). *N Engl J Med* 1977;297:311–317.
26. Burech DL, Koranyi KI, Haynes RE: Serious group A streptococcal diseases in children. *J Pediatr* 1976;88:972–974.
27. Melish ME, Glascow LA: Staphylococcal scalded skin syndrome: The expanded clinical syndrome. *J Pediatr* 1971;78:958–967.
28. Manzella JP, Hall CB, Green JL, et al: Toxic epidermal necrolysis in childhood: Differentiation from staphylococcal skin syndrome. *Pediatrics* 1980;66:291–294.
29. Gigliotti F, Williams WT, Hayden FT, et al: Etiology of acute conjunctivitis in children. *J Pediatr* 1981;98:531–536.
30. Schachter J, Grossman M, Holt J, et al: Infection with *Chlamydia trachomatis:* Involvement of multiple anatomic sites in neonates. *J Infect Dis* 1979;139:232–234.
31. Nichols RL: Infections with *Chlamydia trachomatis:* A commentary. *Pediatrics* 1979;64:269–270.
32. Knight PJ, Mulne AF, Vassy LE: When is lymph node biopsy indicated in children with enlarged peripheral nodes? *Pediatrics* 1982;69:391–396.
33. Feigin RD, Cherry JD: *Textbook of Pediatric Infectious Disease.* Philadelphia, WB Saunders Co, 1981.
34. Krugman S, Katz S: *Infectious Diseases of Children,* ed 7. St. Louis, CV Mosby Co, 1981.
35. Behrman RE, Vaughan VC III: *Nelson Textbook of Pediatrics,* ed 12. Philadelphia, WB Saunders Co, 1983.
36. *Report of the Committee on Infectious Diseases* (1982 Red Book), ed 19. Evanston, IL, American Academy of Pediatrics, 1982.

Jean Jacques Gunning

37 Parasitic Diseases

The inclusion of a chapter on parasitic diseases in this text needs no apology since they are among the most important diseases in the world. There is a pervading misconception among medical students and physicians that in the United States these diseases occur infrequently. That, plus names difficult to pronounce and life cycles impossible to remember, causes these diseases to be largely ignored.

Necessary ingredients for the diagnosis of parasitic or tropical diseases are alertness on the part of the physician and meticulous attention to the details of a good social and geographic history. In general, parasitic diseases can be subdivided into helminthic and protozoal diseases.[1] Commonly, these diseases result in acute or chronic illnesses that may mimic more familiar disease states. For example, a case of acute malaria may well resemble an attack of viral influenza. A different manifestation, and one much easier to recognize, is the asymptomatic patient who has spontaneously expelled a whole or part of a parasitic worm from the intestinal tract.

Alone the signs and symptoms of parasitic diseases are not usually specific enough to be diagnostic. Many serologic tests are done at local hospitals or state health departments. If not, the state will forward the serum to the Centers for Disease Control (CDC) in Atlanta, Georgia. Although some serologic tests can be helpful (e.g., amebic or toxoplasma serology), the diagnosis generally depends on identification or recovery of the parasite from stool, blood, tissue, or cerebrospinal fluid (CSF). Several specimens are frequently required to diagnose malaria in blood. Antacids, barium, antibiotics, and antidiarrheal compounds interfere with the detection of protozoa in the stool. At least three stool specimens may be needed, and these should be collected about 3 days apart.

Quantitation of eggs per gram of feces is helpful to assess the severity of infection and, in some situations, determine if treatment should be administered. This latter consideration depends on the severity of the illness and whether or not the patient will soon return to an endemic zone and become reinfected. In that situation, treatment by removing the parasite and reducing immunity might cause the patient to be more severely reinfected. Another factor is the toxicity of the drug, which must be considered against the deleterious effect of the infection. We are still admonished to "at least cause no harm."

Treatment is with a group of drugs not in general use and largely unfamiliar to most physicians. Close reference should be made to the established pediatric doses listed in this section and in the section on medications. Many drugs listed are unapproved but can be obtained through drug protocols held by the Parasitic Disease Drug Service at the CDC. Telephone consultation can be obtained by calling (404) 633-3311, extension 3496, during working hours and (404) 633-2176 during nights, weekends, and holidays.

HELMINTHIC DISEASES

Worms or helminths are among the most common infections of man throughout the world.[1–3] While the overall incidence in the United States is between 2% and 5%, depending on locality, these organisms infect almost 100% of people in other parts of the globe.[2] Helminthic infections can be separated into two clinical groups: those that cause intestinal tract infections and those that infect other tissues, including the lymphatics, the subcutaneous tissue, and the CSF.

Enterobiasis

Enterobiasis is a lower intestinal tract infection of humans caused by the pinworm *Enterobius vermicularis*. There are virtually no symptoms except perianal pruritus and occasionally vaginal irritation. It is a very common infection of children. The pinworm is acquired by direct fecal-oral transmission. The eggs develop within the upper intestinal tract, and the adults inhabit the lower intestinal tract. There is no tissue migratory phase with this infection.

Manifestations

Worried mothers may bring a child to the emergency department after having seen the small, threadlike worm in the diaper or because the child awakens crying for no apparent reason. The latter is engendered by severe itching caused by the mother pinworm depositing her eggs on the perineum. This can lead to severely disturbed sleep patterns, which in very heavy infestations are thought to interfere with normal growth and development as well as learning ability in school.

Diagnosis

The diagnosis of pinworm infection is made either by seeing the white, 10-mm long, threadlike female worm on the perineum or by identifying the characteristic planiconvex, double-contoured eggs. These eggs contain a motile larva best seen on a cellophane tape-glass slide preparation.

Treatment

A number of excellent drugs are available in single doses: pyrantel pamoate, 11 mg/kg po (maximum, 1 g); mebendazole, 100 mg in children more than 2 years of age. Pyrvinium pamoate, 5 mg/kg po (maximum, 350 mg), also can be given, although it has the disadvantage of staining the diapers bright red. Piperazine citrate, 65 mg/kg/d for 7 days (maximum, 2.5 g/d), can also be used but may cause some giddiness.[4] All of these treatments can be repeated in 2 weeks if necessary. Because pinworm eggs are ubiquitous, reinfection is very common. Stringent hygienic measures probably do not reduce transmission. Treatment of adults and other children in the household only reduces exposure for a brief period and is not recommended.

Trichuriasis

Trichuriasis or whipworm infection is extremely common, especially in the tropics. It is seen most often in the United States as an incidental finding in the stool examination.[2] The patient may be from the southeastern United States or be a recent immigrant or a returning visitor from a tropical country. The colonic mucosa is invaded by the thick end of the whip-shaped worm *Trichuris trichiura*, and the thin end may be seen protruding in the colonic lumen during sigmoidoscopy.

Manifestations

Most often only light infections are seen, and these cause virtually no symptoms. Heavy infections occur usually in children and may cause nausea, abdominal pain, diarrhea, and dysentery. Heavy rectal infections may cause straining during bowel movement, and this, coupled with weight loss in malnourished children, may result in rectal prolapse. The worm causes very slight blood loss, but infections with more than 1000 worms may result in anemia.[2]

Diagnosis

The diagnosis is usually made by finding the characteristic 20- to 50-μm barrel-shaped eggs in the feces. Usually, only egg counts in excess of 3000/g of stool result in symptomatic infections.[2]

Treatment

Mebendazole, 100 mg twice a day for 3 days, should be given. It is only 60% to 70% effective but can be repeated to control heavy infections. It is not recommended in children under the age of 2 years or in pregnant women.[4]

Ascariasis

Ascariasis is an infection of the small intestine and is acquired by ingesting embryonated eggs of the roundworm *Ascaris lumbricoides*. The eggs hatch into larvae in the upper intestine and then penetrate the intestinal wall. The larvae migrate through host tissues and provoke an eosinophilia, especially during pulmonary migration. Infiltrates may be confused with ordinary pneumonia, and wheezing may mimic asthma. The maturing larvae then migrate up the trachea, down the esophagus, and take up lodging in the jejunum. They remain unattached, using their own muscular activity to remain in place.

Manifestations

Most infections are asymptomatic and are diagnosed by routine stool examinations. The adult worm, 15 to 30 cm in length, is occasionally found exiting the host orally or anally during attacks of fever or following antihelminthic medication.[1] Migrating worms can cause intestinal obstruction or obstruct the ampulla of Vater, leading to pancreatitis, jaundice, and ascending cholangitis. Volvulus and intussusception have been reported.

Diagnosis

Examination of the stool reveals the characteristic knobby egg of *Ascaris*. Adult worms have been detected during barium examination of the small intestine.

Treatment

Because certain antihelminthic drugs may not kill or paralyze the *Ascaris* but may cause it to migrate and do mischief, it is important in multiple infection to use a specific anti-ascaris drug. Mebendazole, 100 mg twice a day for 3 days (for children older than 2 years) is very effective. Pyrantel pamoate in a single dose of 10 mg/kg (maximum, 1 g) or piperazine citrate, 75 mg/kg (maximum, 3.5 g) for 2 days, are also excellent.[4] During episodes of intestinal obstruction, intubation with a small-bowel tube and direct instillation of syrup of piperazine may obviate surgery. The worms are tranquilized, generally uncoil, and are passed.

Hookworm Diseases

Infection by *Necator americanus* or *Ancylostoma duodenale* is acquired when skin is penetrated by filariform larvae, which reside in suitable warm, moist earth.

Manifestations

The larvae migrate through tissue and attach finally to the small-intestine mucosa where they suck small amounts of blood for their sustenance. Except for hypersensitivity phenomena during migration and occasional local epigastric symptoms, hookworms generally do not produce symptoms. Iron deficiency anemia is strictly dependent on the nutritional status of the patient and the total numbers of worms present.

Diagnosis

Microscopic examination, including concentration techniques, reveals ova consistent with hookworm species.

Treatment

Mebendazole may be used in children older than 2 years in a dosage of 100 mg po twice a day for 3 days. Pyrantel pamoate in a single dose of 10 mg/kg (maximum, 1 g) is very effective. Thiabendazole, bephenium, or tetrachloroethylene, 0.12 mL/kg (maximum, 5 mL), also may be used in a single dose.[5]

Strongyloidiasis

Strongyloidiasis, like hookworm infections, is acquired when the skin is in contact with suitable soil, thus allowing penetration by the filariform larvae of *Strongyloides stercoralis*. The larvae migrate and come to reside in the jejunal crypts where the female lays eggs. These hatch into rhabditiform larvae upon reaching the intestinal lumen. Some of these larvae may transform into infective filariform larvae within the intestine and autoinfection results. This is one of the few helminths that can multiply within its definitive host. *Strongyloides* has an exceedingly complex life cycle including true parthenogenesis.

Manifestations

During the tissue migratory phase, any hypersensitivity phenomena may occur. Eosinophilia is common. Intestinal symptoms may resemble those of duodenal ulcer. The spectrum may extend from totally symptomless infection to severe malabsorption accompanied by debility, intercurrent infection, and death. In immunosuppressed patients severe hyperinfection may occur because of the autoinfective cycle.

Diagnosis

Since the larvae may be in small numbers, several stool specimens should be examined. Duodenal drainage obtained by tube or string test may also contain larvae. In hyperinfected states larvae may be seen in sputum or CSF. Eggs also may be seen at times in the stool, and these are virtually identical to hookworm eggs.

Treatment
Because of its potential for hyperinfection, this disease should be treated whenever encountered. Thiabendazole, which, unlike mebendazole, is well absorbed, should be given at a dosage of 25 mg/kg po twice a day (maximum, 3 g/d) for 2 days. In disseminated disease, treatment should continue 5 to 7 days.[1] Follow-up examinations are required to assure eradication.

Visceral Larva Migrans

Visceral larva migrans is a manifestation of parasite larvae, usually *Toxocara canis*, migrating through tissues; this provokes an immunologic response of varying intensity, characterized by marked eosinophilia and granulomatous involvement of many tissues and organs. Other parasites, such as *Ascaris*, hookworm, and schistosomes, may produce a similar illness.

The disease is usually acquired by ingesting the eggs of *T. canis*. Frequently, a history of pica is elicited. The eggs hatch into larvae that penetrate the intestinal wall and begin an incomplete tissue migration. Most of them remain in the liver but may reach the brain and the eye.

Manifestations
Mild fever, hepatomegaly, and severe eosinophilia, up to 50% and 60%, are the hallmarks of the illness, and these may persist 1 to 2 years.[2] Pneumonitis can be present. Endophthalmitis and retinal granulomas, which may be confused with retinoblastomas, are infrequent, as are severe central nervous system manifestations. There may be urticaria, pallor, cough, wheezing, and abdominal pain.

Diagnosis
The diagnosis can be confirmed by measuring antibodies against *T. canis*. Liver biopsy may show eosinophilic granulomata and occasionally larvae.

Treatment
Most patients recover completely in about 1 year. Thiabendazole, 25 mg/kg po twice daily (maximum, 3 g) for 5 days, has been helpful but its use is investigational for this disease.[1]

Cutaneous Larva Migrans

Cutaneous larva migrans or creeping eruption is really a subset of visceral larva migrans confined to the skin. It is caused by aberrant wandering, usually of the canine and feline hookworm larvae. Humans are infected when bare skin comes in contact with infected ground.

Ancylostoma brasiliense is the usual parasite. Occasionally, human hookworms, *S. stercoralis*, *Gnathostoma spinigerum*, or the horse botfly *Gasterophilus* may cause the disease.

Manifestations
There is a localized pruritic skin eruption. The migrating larvae cause erythematous, serpiginous tracts. The onset is usually within a few hours of walking barefooted through areas such as beaches or sandboxes or crawling under houses, as is the classic history in the southeastern United States. The lesions are generally on hands, feet, buttocks, shoulders, or back.

Diagnosis
Diagnosis is usually made by inspection of the lesions and by eliciting a history of exposure. Initially, there are itching papules at the point of larval penetration. Within 2 or 3 days, serpiginous tunnels appear in the epidermis. The linear lesions then become elevated and vesicular. Itching and excoriation may lead to secondary infection.

Treatment
Spontaneous resolution is the rule within 2 to 8 weeks. Treatment is with a 10% topical suspension of thiabendazole (500 mg/5 mL) to the advancing edge of the intracutaneous burrow. Oral thiabendazole, 25 mg/kg/d in two doses for 2 days (maximum, 3 g), is also usually effective. Ethylchloride spray is no longer recommended.

Trichinosis

Trichinosis is acquired by ingesting viable, encysted larvae of *Trichinella spiralis* in undercooked or raw meat.[1] Pork or bear meat is the usual vehicle.

Manifestations
The initial intestinal phase is characterized by diarrhea. This occurs during the development of the adults in the small intestine. Larvae are produced, which then migrate through tissues and eventually become encysted. Myositis, fever, periorbital edema, and marked eosinophilia occur. There may be encephalitis and myocarditis.

Diagnosis
The aforementioned symptom complex, severe eosinophilia, and a positive serologic test confirm the diagnosis. The test, however, is not usually positive

until the third week of illness. Muscle biopsy results are positive during the third or fourth week.

Treatment

Thiabendazole, 25 mg/kg/d orally for 2 days, can be given. Severe hypersensitivity reactions can be treated with prednisone.[1]

Helminthic (Eosinophilic) Meningitis

Larval migration through tissues may include the central nervous system and provoke a meningoencephalitis with eosinophilia. Cerebral cysticercosis (from pork tapeworm), trichinosis, toxocariasis (visceral larva migrans), strongyloidiasis, and diseases from other wandering worms have been implicated. Well over a thousand cases of this syndrome have been reported in tropical and subtropical areas, especially in Southeast Asia.[2]

The most common cause has been the rat lungworm *Angiostrongylus cantonensis*. Rats ingest the infective, third-stage larva by eating snails, the intermediate host. Humans acquire the infective larvae in the same manner, although children may pick up the larvae from the slime trail of snails. The larvae penetrate the intestine of the rat and migrate through tissues until finally reaching their definitive home, the pulmonary arteries and veins. There they lay eggs. These hatch into first-stage larvae, which migrate up the trachea and pass out through the rat intestinal tract. Snails ingest these larvae, which develop into infective third-stage forms. Humans or rats eat the snails. The larvae within the raw or poorly cooked snails penetrate the intestinal wall and begin their migration. It is during this migration that the central nervous system may be invaded. Humans are not an ideal host, and the worms seldom reach the pulmonary vasculature but instead are at a dead end in the central nervous system.

Manifestations

Mild fever, acute severe headache, and some meningeal irritation occur. There may be blurring of vision, paresthesias, and palsies of the sixth and seventh cranial nerves. More severe reactions such as coma and convulsions are rare. Spontaneous recovery is the rule. Mortality is less than 0.5%.[2]

Diagnosis

Blood eosinophilia is inconstant. Sampling the CSF reveals an elevated protein and cell count. CSF eosinophilia up to 90% is present.[2] When a needle of sufficient caliber (20 gauge) is used, larvae and young adult worms may be recovered. An antigen made from rat brain larvae has been employed in Thailand to develop a CSF enzyme-linked immunosorbent assay (ELISA) test. This approach looks promising but is not yet available in the United States.

Treatment

Since most cases spontaneously resolve and since therapy might cause worms to die suddenly and potentially accelerate central nervous system reactions, antihelminthic drugs are not generally recommended.[5] Although no evidence of benefit from corticosteroid treatment has been recorded, its use in very severe cases may be considered. No evidence of benefit from the use of any antihelminthic drug exists. If worms are seen in the eye, they should be surgically removed.

Tapeworm Diseases

The tapeworm group of platyhelminths is very diverse. In general, humans may serve as definitive or intermediate hosts. The intermediate or larval forms inhabit various tissues and may cause symptoms by pressure phenomena on vital structures, e.g., cysticercosis of the brain and echinococcosis of the liver or lung. This intermediate form is generally not dealt with at the clinic or emergency department level.

Manifestations

The definitive or intestinal phase of these parasites, despite their awesome length, generally does not cause symptoms, and there are usually no more than three parasites (except with *Hymenolepis nana*). *Diphyllobothrium latum* may compete with the host for vitamin B_{12}. The others, *Taenia solium, Taenia saginata,* and *H. nana* usually do not cause any debility unless the host is marginally nourished. There is no tissue migratory phase in the definitive phase.

Diagnosis

The diagnosis usually is made by seeing the passage of a glistening white proglottid or chain of proglottids in the stool. Eggs may be detected in a routine stool examination.

Treatment

The treatment is niclosamide. The dose varies by body weight: 11 to 34 kg, give 1 g; 34 to 70 kg, give 1.5 g; greater than 70 kg, give 2 g. This single-dose treatment is effective for all intestinal tapeworms except *H. nana,* which must be treated for 1 week.[1] The initial dose is the same, but in young children the dose for the next 6 days is half the initial dose. This drug dissolves the worm, and searching for the scolex (head) is no longer required. If niclosamide is not available, paromomycin, 10 mg/kg po every 15 minutes for four doses, or praziquantel, 15 to 20 mg/kg po in a single dose, can be used.[5]

PROTOZOAL DISEASES

Protozoal diseases of man can be divided clinically into those affecting the intestinal or genitourinary tract, the blood, and the tissues. Asexual reproduction occurs within the human host, and therefore the parasite load may increase. The luminal protozoans are transmitted by direct contact or ingestion. Blood and tissue parasites are generally transmitted by an arthropod vector.

Amebiasis

Amebiasis is primarily an infection of the colon. The disease varies from an asymptomatic carrier state to severe colitis clinically indistinguishable from ulcerative colitis. Abscesses may occur in other organs, most commonly the liver. The protozoan exists as a motile trophozoite that inhabits the surface of the colonic mucosa and in more severe states causes ulcerations and submucosal abscesses. In nondiarrheal states the ameba is passed in the stool as a cyst. These cysts are very resistant, even to chlorination, and are responsible for fecal-oral contamination from fingers, drinking water, or contaminated food. Prevalence rates in the United States vary from 1% to 5%.[3] Venereal transmission among male homosexuals is not uncommon. Strains of ameba acquired in temperate zones are generally avirulent. Invasiveness varies from strain to strain, and amebic liver abscesses are most often encountered in patients who acquired their disease in Mexico, western South America, South Asia, and West and Southwestern Africa.

Manifestations

Amebic dysentery is usually mild, consisting of one to four foul, loose or watery stools daily, containing mucus and blood. There may be mild cecal, right colon, and hepatic tenderness, and chronic mild dysentery may alternate with periods of normalcy. Profuse bloody diarrhea accompanied by cramps, tenesmus, and debility is not unusual but occurs most frequently in immunosuppressed states such as pregnancy, treatment with corticosteroids, and malnutrition.

Hepatic abscesses resulting from amebiasis usually cause chronic, febrile, debilitating illness along with tender hepatomegaly. Occasionally, a fulminant picture of fever in excess of 40° C, severe upper abdominal pain, and leukocytosis with shift to the left may mimic perforated duodenal ulcer, pancreatitis, or acute cholecystitis. Abscesses may be very large, are usually single and in the right lobe, and may cause a "point tenderness" in the right posterolateral area at the lower intercostal spaces. An elevated diaphragm and right shoulder pain may be present.

Diagnosis

Amebic liver abscess is usually diagnosed by a filling defect on a liver scan coupled with a positive amebic serologic test. The latter is positive in well over 90% of cases. The amebae are found in the stool in less than 50% of cases.[6] Needle aspiration of the abscess is required only if there is danger of rupture.

Amebic colitis symptoms may mimic those caused by shigellosis, salmonellosis, and ulcerative colitis. Visualization of the cysts or trophozoites is essential for diagnosis. Material obtained at proctosigmoidoscopy from the region of an ulceration or flecks of bloody mucus have the highest yield for identifying trophozoites. Specimens fixed with polyvinyl alcohol can be stained and are very helpful. Stool samples stained with methylene blue show an overall mononuclear cell background and help to sort out cases of bacterial dysentery and ulcerative colitis. Serologic tests are positive in only about 50% of patients with amebic colitis.

Treatment

For mild or asymptomatic amebiasis confined to the intestinal lumen, diloxanide furoate, 20 mg/kg/d in three doses for 10 days, or diiodohydroxyquin, 30 to 40 mg/kg/d in three doses for 20 days, can be used. In moderate disease metronidazole, 35 to 50 mg/kg/d in three doses for 10 days, should be added to one of the above drug regimens. In severe colitis use the regimen for moderate disease plus emetine, 1 mg/kg/d IM (maximum, 60 mg/kg/d) in 2 doses for 5 days.[4] There is no advantage in using dihydroemetine over emetine at this dosage. Diloxanide and dihydroemetine are only available from the CDC.

Extraintestinal amebiasis (liver abscess) is usually treated initially with metronidazole, 35 to 50 mg/kg/d in three doses for 10 days. Treatment failures happen infrequently, and such patients should be given emetine, 1 mg/kg/d IM (maximum, 60 mg/kg/d) in two doses for 5 days, or chloroquine phosphate, 10 mg base/kg/d po (maximum, 300 mg base) for 3 weeks.[4]

Giardiasis

Giardiasis is a disease of worldwide distribution. Certain areas are notorious for transmission to humans: the Soviet Union and campgrounds and ski resorts in the Sierra and Rocky Mountains. Beavers may serve as a natural reservoir. It is a common disease among populations living under circumstances of poor sanitation and personal hygiene, especially in the tropics. Transmission is by the fecal-oral route or through drinking contaminated water. The cysts survive chlorination. It is the most frequently identified intestinal parasite in the United States.[2]

Manifestations

Typically, a patient seeks medical assistance because of diarrhea that, unlike other traveler's diarrhea, happens later during the course of the trip or upon return home. The infection may be asymptomatic; however, generally there is nausea, flatulence, abdominal cramping, and diarrhea. Stools are usually bulky and foul smelling. Weight loss and malabsorption may occur.

Diagnosis

The diagnosis is made by identifying the characteristic cyst or trophozoite in a stool specimen, or the trophozoite in a duodenal drainage sample, which may be obtained by tube or by a string test (Enterotest). Duodenal biopsy may also yield the diagnosis.

Treatment

Three drugs for treatment of giardiasis are available in the United States: quinacrine, metronidazole, and furazolidone. Quinacrine, at a dose of 6 mg/kg/d po (maximum, 300 mg/d) in three postprandial doses for 5 days, is effective in 80% to 90% of cases. This drug, however, may cause gastrointestinal upsets and occasionally toxic psychoses. Metronidazole, although not licensed for use in this disease, appears better tolerated and is as effective. It is given at 15 mg/kg/d po (maximum, 750 mg/d) in three doses for 5 days. Furazolidone (not to be given to infants under 1 month of age) can also be used, at 6 mg/kg/d in four doses for 7 days.[4] No treatment should be given during pregnancy unless the patient is very symptomatic.

Malaria

Malaria is an acute, remittent, febrile illness characterized by chills, splenomegaly, anemia, and eventually a chronic relapsing course. It is caused by a hemoprotozoan of the genus *Plasmodium. Plasmodium ovale* and *Plasmodium malariae* are much less common than *Plasmodium vivax* or *Plasmodium falciparum.*

Manifestations

Unfortunately, the classic relapsing form of the disease with fevers occurring every 48 to 72 hours is rarely present in an acute case of malaria. Most frequently, the patient appears to have an illness resembling influenza or viral gastroenteritis except that the fever is higher and the chills are more severe. Headache, myalgia, splenomegaly, and anemia are common.

Diagnosis

Thick and thin smears of the peripheral blood are stained with Wright's or Giemsa's stain. The parasites appear as organisms within the red blood cells. The nucleus stains red and cytoplasm blue. Morphologic patterns establish the species causing the infection, which range from ring trophozoites to mature trophozoites. Repetitive ring forms, at times more than one ring per red blood cell, suggest a diagnosis of *P. falciparum* infection. *P. vivax* and the other two species, in addition to ring forms, show further developmental stages in the red corpuscles. This distinction is important because infection by *P. falciparum* is potentially fatal and, if contracted in certain parts of the world, may be highly resistant to chloroquine, and mainstay of treatment.

Treatment

Except for falciparum malaria contracted in South America, Southeast Asia, India, and East Africa, all malarias are treated with chloroquine, 10 mg base/kg (maximum, 600 mg), given immediately and followed by 5 mg base/kg after 6 hours, 24 hours, and 48 hours.[2] Relapses of vivax and ovale malaria are prevented by administering primaquine, 0.3 mg base/kg/d for 14 days. *P. malariae* is thought not to have a relapsing form.

For falciparum malaria resistant to chloroquine and for initial treatment of this malaria when contracted in the aforementioned locales, therapy for an acute attack is with quinine. This drug should be used orally whenever possible, at 25 mg/kg/d in three doses for 3 days. Quinine can be given intravenously, diluted at a proportion of 600 mg to

300 mL saline and infused for at least 1 hour. Quinine controls the acute attack but must be accompanied by pediatric doses of pyrimethamine (body weight ≥ 40 kg: 25 mg twice daily for 3 days; 20 to 40 kg: 25 mg/d for 3 days; 10 to 20 kg: 12.5 mg/d for 3 days; ≤10 kg: 6.25 mg/d for 3 days) and sulfadiazine, 100 to 200 mg/kg/d in four doses for 5 days.[4]

Babesiosis

Babesiosis is caused by the hemoprotozoan *Babesia microti*, which resembles *P. falciparum*. It is contracted by the bite of an infected tick. Generally a disease of animals, it has recently been detected in a small number of humans who were visitors or residents of Long Island or Shelter Island, New York, and Nantucket, Massachusetts.

Manifestations

Babesiosis is an acute febrile illness accompanied by hemolytic anemia, hemoglobinuria, and, at times, jaundice. Chills, sweating, and myalgias are present. Splenomegaly can be detected in the more protracted cases. Most patients have been older than 50 years or immunosuppressed.[1]

Diagnosis

The parasite can be seen in erythrocytes stained with Wright's or preferably Giemsa's stain. They appear similar to malarial parasites. Rings, tetrads produced by budding, basket shapes, and occasionally band forms can be seen. Nuclear material stains red and cytoplasm blue. No pigment or gametocytes are seen. Serodiagnosis, available through the CDC, may be helpful.

Treatment

Chloroquine is not effective. Pentamidine, 2 to 4 mg/kg/d for 15 days, has been used. A combination of quinine and clindamycin has been shown effective.[4] An exchange transfusion may be considered for critically ill patients, especially those who are splenectomized or otherwise immunosuppressed.

Pneumocystosis

Pneumocystis carinii causes severe progressive pneumonitis and severe hypoxemia, generally in immunosuppressed patients. Malnutrition, chemical immunosuppression, and, more recently, the acquired immunodeficiency syndrome (AIDS), recognized in homosexuals, drug abusers, and hemophiliacs, seem to be general prerequisites.

Manifestations

The onset is usually insidious. The patient is hardly febrile, is dyspneic, and has a nonproductive cough. There is tachypnea, air hunger, and cyanosis. There are very few auscultatory findings, in contrast to extensive alveolar infiltrates usually spreading from hilar areas to the periphery. At times, the roentgenogram shows nodular peripheral lesions, which can be confused with other processes. Pleural effusion is rare. Blood gases show severe hypoxemia without hypercarbia.

Diagnosis

The diagnosis is made by identification of the trophozoites or cysts in the sputum, bronchial washings, or lung biopsies. Methenamine-silver or Giemsa's stain are required. Other opportunistic infections are frequent accompaniments of pneumocystosis.

Treatment

Treatment is a combination of trimethoprim, 20 mg/kg/d, and sulfamethoxazole, 100 mg/kg/d, in four doses for 14 days. This may be given orally or intravenously. Pentamidine is strictly a secondary agent and is given at 4 mg/kg/d IM for 14 days.[4]

Toxoplasmosis

Toxoplasma is a genus of ubiquitous, obligate, intracellular protozoans that infect animals and humans; it has a definitive sexual cycle in the intestine of felines. Oocysts of *Toxoplasma gondii* are acquired from excrement of domestic cats. The condition also may be acquired by ingesting cysts in raw or poorly cooked meat. Congenital cases can occur. The infection becomes systemic, and any cells except nonnucleated erythrocytes may be infected with trophozoites (tachyzoites), which may cause death of the cell.

Manifestations

Toxoplasmosis causes severe, often fatal, congenital disease and is part of the "TORCH" syndrome (toxoplasmosis, rubella, cytomegalovirus, herpes, syphilis). Retinitis may be part of acquired or reactivation disease. The usual clinical feature of acquired toxoplasmosis is that of lymphadenopathy. Infection may be asymptomatic, mimicking lymphoma, or may resemble infectious mononucleosis, with lymphocytosis, lymphadenopathy, sore throat, and splenomegaly.

Diagnosis
The aforementioned manifestations, coupled with a negative heterophile or mononucleosis spot test, suggest a diagnosis of toxoplasmosis or cytomegalovirus disease. Diagnosis is established by testing for toxoplasmosis in serum from acute and convalescent stages, and by a specific *Toxoplasma* immunoglobin M test. In some cases biopsy of lymph nodes may suggest the diagnosis. Mouse inoculation with body fluids or infected tissues may also yield the diagnosis. Chorioretinitis may appear as visual loss accompanied by "cotton wool" exudates surrounded by a ring of erythema.

Treatment
Generally, the acquired infectious mononucleosis-like illness requires no treatment. Retinitis should be referred to an ophthalmologist. Treatment, if needed, consists of pyrimethamine, 2 mg/kg/d (maximum, 25 mg) for 3 days followed by 1 mg/kg/d for 4 weeks, and sulfadiazine, 100 to 200 mg/kg/d for 3 or 4 weeks. Spiramycin is not available in the United States.[4]

African Trypanosomiasis

Manifestations
Fever in a recent traveler from Africa, an indolent erythematous nodule occurring 2 or 3 days after the bite of a tsetse fly, and regional lymphadenopathy should cause the examiner to think of trypanosomiasis or sleeping sickness. There is usually severe headache, insomnia, erythema marginatum or a morbilliform rash, peripheral edema, and tender lymph nodes, especially in the posterior cervical chain. All this can occur before central nervous system invasion.

Diagnosis
The trypanosome must be identified in the blood, the CSF, or a lymph node aspirate, using Giemsa's or Wright's stain. It is helpful to centrifuge the blood or CSF and examine the buffy coat of the blood or the sediment of the CSF. Animal inoculation may be needed.

Treatment
During hospitalization, the patient may be treated with appropriate doses of suramin or melarsoprol.

American Trypanosomiasis

American trypanosomiasis or Chagas disease seldom causes acute illness. As in African trypanosomiasis, a traveler from South or Central America with an indolent erythematous nodule or chagoma, usually on an exposed skin surface, can be suspected of having Chagas disease.

Manifestations
The bite of the reduviid bug is generally on the face. Unilateral painless conjunctivitis, eyelid edema, and preauricular node enlargement constitute a complex called Romaña sign. This can persist for several months. The parasite multiplies in tissue and intermittently circulates in the blood. During this period there may be fever, lymphatic involvement, and hepatosplenomegaly. Myocarditis is common in acute disease. Death occurs in 5% to 10% of cases. The remainder lapse into a chronic phase.[1]

Diagnosis
The demonstration of the characteristic *Trypanosoma cruzi* in stained blood films is diagnostic. This is only likely during acute illness. Culture in appropriate media, animal inoculation, or xenodiagnosis using laboratory-reared reduviid bugs, are all helpful.

Treatment
The hospitalized patient can be treated with a nitrofurazone derivative (nifurtimox [Lampit]).

Leishmaniasis

Two manifestations of leishmaniasis are extant: visceral leishmaniasis and cutaneous or mucocutaneous disease. Visceral leishmaniasis (*Leishmania donovani*) can be contracted in India, Russia, China, Middle East, East Africa, the Mediterranean littoral, and certain areas of Central and South America.

Manifestations
The visceral disease causes fever, extreme enlargement of the liver and spleen, lymphadenopathy, weakness, weight loss, and anemia. Mucocutaneous lesions may occur in the African form. The cutaneous disease (*Leishmania tropica* and *Leishmania brasiliensis*) causes chronic ulcerated skin lesions, which may involve the nasal mucosa.

Diagnosis
The leishmania amastigotes may be seen on stained samples from the borders of skin ulcers, liver and spleen biopsies, or bone marrow aspirates. Cultures of these materials may be positive for the promastigotes.

Treatment
The pediatric patient should be hospitalized, and treatment with pentavalent antimony should be initiated.

Amebic Meningitis

Manifestations
Amebic meningitis produces signs and symptoms the same as those for any other form of meningitis. The mononuclear response in the spinal fluid is caused by a free-living ameba of either the genus *Naegleria* or *Acanthamoeba*, which are found in certain freshwater swamps, ponds, hot springs, or brackish water. It is a disease of the summer months and has its onset usually a week or so after swimming. It is thought that the disease is acquired by infection through the nose, and the ameba gains access to the central nervous system through the cribriform plate.

Diagnosis
The diagnosis of this disease can only be made through the astute observations of the person examining the spinal fluid, who might notice the ameboid movements of the organism.

Treatment
Treatment is extremely complicated and survival is unlikely.

References

1. Beaver PC, Jung RC, Cupp EW: *Clinical Parasitology*, ed 9. Philadelphia, Lea & Febiger, 1984.
2. Strickland GT, Hunter GW: *Tropical Medicine*, ed 6. Philadelphia, WB Saunders Co, 1984.
3. Braude AI: *Medical Microbiology and Infectious Diseases*. Philadelphia, WB Saunders Co, 1981.
4. Katzung BG: *Basis and Clinical Pharmacology*. Los Altos, CA, Lange Medical Publications, 1982, chap 54, p 55.
5. Drugs for parasitic infections. *Med Lett Drugs Ther* 1984;26:27–34.
6. Petersdorf RG, Adams RD, Braunwald E, et al (eds): *Harrison's Principles of Internal Medicine*, ed 10. New York, McGraw-Hill Book Co, 1983, pp 1177–1239.

Part X

Psychiatric Disorders and Child Abuse

B. Gregory Fernandopulle

38 Psychiatric Emergencies

Psychiatric emergencies assume grave importance in pediatrics because of both the pathophysiology and psychopathology involved, as well as the dynamics behind the emergency and the consequences of it. The physician is not only faced with a critically ill patient, but very often with an extremely helpless family.[1] Staff members also experience some anxiety, if not anger, particularly if the patient is an adolescent.

The time from birth to the end of adolescence represents from a fifth to a quarter of the life span of an individual.[2] Important developmental changes occur during these years; hence any crisis situation, be it physical or emotional, has great significance during this period.

Table 38-1 gives a brief summary of the relationships between the different developmental norms, as understood from an emotional and cognitive axis.

HISTORY TAKING

Significant facts to be ascertained when taking the history should include details of the following:

1. Developmental history, including history of the mother's pregnancy (e.g., wanted, unwanted). A useful way to ask is, "How easy or difficult was it for you to be pregnant at that time?" Determine also any pathophysiologic insults during the pregnancy (e.g., toxemia, alcohol, smoking, separation).
2. Birth history (birth weight, perinatal problems).
3. Developmental milestones in the four major areas: gross motor control, fine motor control, social response, and language.
4. Personal loss: any parental separations, reactions to death of significant persons or pets, moves in the family, or any other potentially traumatizing experience.
5. School experience, particularly first grade and junior high school. Academic achievement and attitude toward school should be assessed.
6. Family background, including health resources available and stress-producing factors such as the presence of alcoholism, chronic physical disease or emotional illness, multiple separations, substance abuse, degree of flexibility or rigidity in the family, job history.
7. Patient's level of functioning as an individual: outgoing, introverted, reactions to new situations, basic temperament, personality, reaction to stress, a leader or a follower, rigid or flexible person, presence of any chronic illness such as bronchial asthma, diabetes, seizure disorder, attention-deficit disorder.
8. Previous contacts with social services or the law.
9. Determination of who is suffering most. Is it the patient, the family, or the agency that brings the patient in?

TABLE 38-1 Normal Stages of Emotional and Cognitive Development

Age (yr)	Developmental Stages: Emotional	Cognitive
0–2	Attachment, issues of separation, trusting relationship	Thinking is basically egocentric.
3–5	Controlling, independence, issues of being damaged	Thinking is oriented to environment.
6–10	Emotionally less constricted, formation of relationships with family and peers, more industrious	Thinking involves environmental and related factors of time and place; acquisition of knowledge is maximized.
10–17	Formation of identity	Adultlike thinking exists in most areas except when issues are more affect laden; then there is a tendency to regress.

10. Determination of the family's and patient's expectations of each other and of the hospital or physician. An important question that may not have an immediate answer is what, if any, psychologic advantage the crisis brings to the patient and/or the family, e.g., anger, punishment, guilt, depression, or just emotional pain.
11. Inquiry into the resources available for aftercare to bring about needed change as well as to provide some preventive measures in the future.

Because the crisis becomes a great opportunity for change, evaluation of these elements is extremely important in determining the future prognosis of the patient.[1]

COMMONLY ENCOUNTERED SYNDROMES

Suicide

The incidence of suicide increases progressively, starting in the early teens. Most often, it is an impulsive act, subsequent to a loss (strained relationship with parents or boy- or girlfriend, poor school performance, rejection or abandonment, teenage pregnancy).[3] Most of these situations start off with severe anger, which may be denied, followed by feelings of helplessness, hopelessness, and depression.

Common methods for attempting suicide include ingestion of toxic substances or household drugs, with or without alcohol; wrist slashing; hanging or shooting oneself; and automobile accidents, often accompanied by intoxication.[3]

A detailed history, first taken when alone with the adolescent and subsequently alone with the parents, is extremely important. Very often parents want to be in the room during the time the adolescent is interviewed. This may cause complications, including a loss of confidence in the physician by the adolescent. A practical way to start the examination is to tell the parents and the adolescent: "I want to spend some time with Johnny (Jane) alone. I also want to spend some time with the parents alone. What I hear from each will remain between that person and myself. After I have listened to both groups, we will all sit down together, and I will use all the information I have learned, as well as my experience, to tell you what I consider to be in the best interests of all." This usually puts everyone's minds at ease and gives the physician a very good chance of examining each individual closely.

The interview should include a very significant question, especially for the adolescent, which can be as follows: "At what or whom were you angry?" This should be asked in a low-key, gentle, compassionate way. The answer to this question is the key to the problem in most instances, and treatment can be centered around this answer.

An attempt should be made by the physician not only to be fair with the patient and the family, but also to *appear* fair. With adolescents especially, this becomes a significant dynamic in management.

Screening tests for toxic substances and a pregnancy test, when appropriate, should be done in all instances.

Detoxification may be a medical emergency and should be accomplished by admitting either the patient to an intensive care unit or pediatric adolescent ward. Admission for all attempted suicides is appropriate not only for physiologic reasons but also for psychologic reasons. An adolescent requires an enormous degree of emotional support at this stage, as does the family, which is very often confused and frightened by the situation. Hospitalization for a few days provides both the patient and parents time for more rational thinking.

A psychiatric consultation is indicated to evaluate the patient and to plan therapy. Medications during follow-up should be used with care. On discharge, a plan for further care should be clearly defined, e.g., outpatient psychotherapy or counseling for parents.

Acute Psychosis

Patients with an acute psychosis may be seen at any age with symptoms that include loss of reality, hallucinations, delusions, agitated behavior, withdrawal, inappropriate affect, and poor judgment. The cause may be functional or organic; if organic, it may be drug induced and result from the use of street drugs or overuse of prescribed medications. The manifestations from either cause would appear the same, except that in those with an organic cause, there may be either a history of drug ingestion or an underlying organic disease. In the functional group a past history of recurring psychotic episodes may be elicited. In addition to the routine history and physical examination, toxicologic screening is an essential investigation.[3]

Organic Psychosis

Common street drugs that cause psychoses include lysergic acid diethylamide (LSD), phencyclidine hydrochloride (PCP), cocaine, glue (sniffing), large doses of marijuana, jimsonweed (atropine), and other combinations. Some of these can be detected by a toxicology screen.

Medications prescribed by physicians can also produce psychosis when improperly used. Sometimes this is meant as a suicidal gesture. Drugs in this group include antidepressants, antihistamines, muscle relaxants, and antiseizure medication.

A very small group of children and adolescents come to the hospital with acute psychosis-like episodes associated with medical problems: diabetes, seizure disorders (either resulting from the seizure itself and/or a toxic psychosis secondary to antiseizure medications), or acute encephalopathies. These patients should have a comprehensive medical workup, and the medical problem should be addressed accordingly.

Functional Psychosis

Functional psychoses fall into two major categories: pervasive developmental disorders and acute psychoses. Pervasive developmental disorders, including childhood autism, are generally found in younger patients. These patients have a history of withdrawal, agitation, fighting, or acute panic reactions, with the parents or school being unable to handle them. They usually have an ongoing emotional handicap that can be elicited in the history.

Acute psychoses are frequently seen in the teenage child. This may be the beginning of a major psychiatric disorder, e.g., schizophrenia or an affective disorder. A thorough family history of similar problems in previous generations should supplement the normal data base. Both schizophrenia and affective disorders have a strong genetic basis. Some of the early symptoms of acute psychoses may be misinterpreted as variants of normal adolescent behavior until the crisis occurs.

Treatment

Medical or organic causes require specific therapy. The acute psychosis is best treated in a hospital unless a very sophisticated home with a well organized structure is available. A well structured intensive care unit or pediatric ward may be able to handle a patient with a psychotic episode if 24-hour supervision is available. However, if the patient is too destructive, this would not be a prudent course to follow. In this event, admission to a short-term care psychiatric facility is indicated.[1]

Most acute psychotic episodes respond well to aggressive psychopharmacologic management.[1] Agents used include haloperidol or phenothiazine, intramuscularly or orally, every 4 to 6 hours until the acute psychotic episode subsides. All these antipsychotic agents have side effects that should be kept in mind: tremors, muscle twitching, and other parkinsonian symptoms. Side effects can be controlled by using diphenhydramine (Benadryl), 25 to 50 mg IV, or by the use of antiparkinsonian medications.

Hyperkinesis

Hyperkinesis (attention-deficit disorder with or without hyperactivity) is probably the most common disorder seen in a children's psychiatric setting and is recognized with increasing frequency in pediatric practices.[3] These children have problems with short attention span, become easily frustrated, are extremely impulsive, often set fires, wet the bed, and have poor peer relationships. They come into emergency departments for a variety of problems including conduct disorders, drug abuse, and attempted suicide. They are also brought to emergency departments by helpless parents who are on the verge of becoming "burned out" by the constant activity of these children and are unable to deal with them effectively.

As these children reach adolescence, the combination of attention-deficit disorder, low tolerance to frustration, and adolescence itself causes more problems, very often ending in acute crisis, e.g., suicide attempts, problems with the law, and severe depression. Many of these children have a history of stimulant medication (methylphenidate hydrochloride, pemoline, or dextroamphetamine sulfate) for hyperactivity. Some may have also been on phenothiazines or antidepressants.

On clinical examination one can usually verify problems with attention span, frustration with inability to perform tasks, and poor fine motor coordination. Poor school reports and peer relations are very often in the history, as well as ineffective attempts to provide treatment programs in the past.

In acute crisis situations, removing the child from the parent by admitting the child to a ward or placing the child at a relative's home or temporary care facility is useful. Use of a stimulant, such as methylphenidate or amphetamine, should be considered, particularly if it has not been prescribed in the past. This seeming paradox is related apparently to dopamine-serotonin metabolism. Long-term treatment programs should include a family-centered therapy plan in an appropriate clinic setting.

Acute "Medical" Conditions

Examples of acute medical complaints that are symptoms of psychiatric illness include abdominal pain, headaches, vomiting, and wheezing. Patients complaining of these symptoms may have been treated previously in outpatient settings with all investigations having proved negative. However, symptoms continue and increase to crisis proportions. No organic etiology can be found to explain these severe symptoms.[1]

A detailed history and clinical examination is very likely to elicit the sources of stress, e.g., family situation, school, or peer group. The parents often are angry and unable to cope with the problem, although they do not say so directly. It is imperative that the parents and the patient be interviewed separately.

Treatment of these children often necessitates separating the child from the parents for a brief period of time. To attain this end, the child may be admitted to the hospital for a few days. In the hospital the patient can be closely observed and appropriate examinations can be done to exclude organic disease. Medications may be required to reduce anxiety. There should be a review of the resources available at home and in the community to assist these children. Besides psychiatric consultation a social service evaluation may be very useful.

Evaluation of the school program and its appropriateness for the patient is necessary, for this could be the source of the frustration. These children can often be discharged back to the home once a few environmental manipulations have been done and, if necessary, the patient has been temporarily maintained on medication. It is necessary to explain to the parents and the child the chronicity of this handicap and to identify and correct the underlying cause. When medications are effective in alleviating symptoms, the patient and the parents may deny the problem; then the child stops taking the medications and the symptoms recur, very often at a more severe level. Occasionally, it may be necessary to separate these children for a longer period by placing them under foster care or in group homes.

Setting Fires

Setting fires is a dramatic act that frightens parents, school authorities, and any other people around. It is often associated with enuresis and hyperkinetic behavior.[1] Often, it is an expression of an underlying anxiety and depression. A psychiatric consultation should be obtained for every one of these patients. Usually a family-centered treatment program is of help, and a fairly long-term follow-up in these patients is necessary. Most fire setters get over their problems within a relatively short period of time. A few, however, regress, especially when they become anxious or depressed.

Conversion Reactions

Examples of conversion reactions include paraplegia, quadriplegia, blindness, aphonia, weakness of a limb, deafness, and fainting spells. They occur most often in girls, although boys are not an exception; often patients are in the older pediatric age group. A common feature in the background is an overprotective environment that is giving mixed messages to the children. In addition to family members, the school and religious organizations may also be involved. Symptoms usually are very incapacitating and may be acute in onset. Usually, there is a provocation of anxiety. Very often, there is an affective component that is well defined by the symptoms, e.g., anger, guilt, depression, helplessness, and anxiety. The symptoms actually serve the patient's unconscious needs; hence, an acknowledgment of the symptoms in a realistic way is necessary and useful in the resolution of the problem.[3]

Admission to the hospital is warranted. Aside from the detailed history, a complete physical examination and appropriate investigations or specialized consultations may be necessary (e.g., neurology, physical medicine).

A multipronged approach in treatment is useful, e.g., physical therapy, the use of appropriate medications (analgesics, antidepressants, antianxiety drugs), individual psychotherapy, and family counseling. A psychiatrist should be part of the therapy team. Hypnotherapy is a useful adjunct if done by a competent person. On discharge, a family-centered treatment program should be employed for a period of time.

Anorexia Nervosa

Anorexia nervosa has become a fairly common syndrome now with the emphasis in contemporary culture on a slim figure, physical exercise, and health foods.[1] Usually, there is an alternating history of bulimia and vomiting with consequent loss of weight. There is usually the pursuit of thinness as an end in itself and a conflict between eating and losing weight. The weight loss itself can be life threatening. A loss of approximately 25% of normal weight is a strong indication for hospitalization.[1] Failure in outpatient treatment to gain and/or maintain appropriate weight should be considered as an indication for admission. This syndrome is common among young women; however, many young men also are being seen in clinics at present.

A complete medical work-up should be done to rule out organic disease. During hospitalization the most effective way of treating these patients has proved to be one-on-one nursing, 24 hours a day, with oral feedings. The feedings should be progressively increased in terms of calories and kinds of foods. Very often, a sudden addition of a large number of calories and enriched diets causes other symptoms such as diarrhea, further vomiting, and abdominal pain. Medications, nasogastric tube feedings, and intravenous fluids should be used with great caution.

The best results seen now are in those centers following a program of one-on-one nursing, individual therapy, family therapy, group therapy, and attention to other emotional issues (e.g., interpersonal relationships, self image). A behavior-modification type of approach is also useful; for example, gain a certain number of pounds a week, gain "x" number of pounds for discharge, and then maintain that weight during outpatient care. A long-term follow-up is absolutely necessary.

Adoption

Adopted children have a higher incidence of emotional problems.[1] The disorders usually manifest themselves in adolescence. These identity crises are associated with excessive anger, rebellion, and rejection of parents. Patients may run away from home in search of their natural parents. Intense daydreaming with romantic fantasies about one's natural origins is common. If the adoptive parents are middle class, the patient may be sexually acting out with partners of a lower social class. Shoplifting is also a common symptom. Overt psychotic reactions may occur.

Separation of the patient from the parents is usually not necessary. The patient needs help in understanding that rejection of the adoptive parents is, at least in part, a normal quest for identity in adolescence and that guilt, as a consequence of this rejection, is also normal. The parents need emotional support for their feelings of confusion, disappointment, and guilt. Education of the parents and the adolescent about the possible side effects of adoption could help prevent some of these difficulties.

Bereavement

Loss of a parent, sibling, relative, or close friend sometimes becomes an emergency. Symptoms arise within weeks of the event and include suicidal behavior, acute phobias, hysterical conversion, hypochondriasis with reactions of panic to minor injuries, fear of death and dying, regression in toilet training, setting fires, cruelty to pets, and psychotic reactions. In teenagers, delinquency, running away, drug abuse, sexual acting out, teenage pregnancy, and suicidal attempts are not uncommon.

Treatment has to be centered around the child and the parent. In some hospitals there are counselors who specialize in handling such problems. "Compassionate Friends" is a useful referral group. Individual psychotherapy may be necessary for both parent and child.

Fatal Illness

Psychiatric emergencies can arise with the dying child or the parents of a dying child. The child who is suffering a terminal illness may suffer more from guilt, fear of loss of love, and feelings of being abandoned than from the physical disability.

Parents go through different phases of coping, although not necessarily in the order presented: shock and disbelief, denial, anger, depression, and withdrawal. The parents at this time require large amounts of emotional support and understanding of their own feelings and those of the child. Contact with religious personnel or other parents who have had a similar experience is useful.

Indecent Exposure

This is much more common than rape. Studies have shown that these boys and girls by their own behavior, overtly or covertly, often invite this behavior by the perpetrator.[1] A common cause is emotional deprivation on the part of both victim and perpetrator. Aside from examining the perpetrator, who will need psychiatric examination and probably undergo legal proceedings, examination of the victim and the victim's family for possible emotional deprivation and prescription of appropriate treatment are necessary.

References

1. Noshpitz J (ed): *Handbook of Child Psychiatry.* New York, Basic Books Inc, 1979.
2. Lewis M: *Clinical Aspects of Child Development,* ed 2. Philadelphia, Lea & Febiger, 1982.
3. Kaplan HI, Freedman AM (eds): *Comprehensive Textbook of Psychiatry,* ed 3. Baltimore, Williams & Wilkins Co, 1980.

Charles I. Shubin

39 Child Abuse and Neglect

The basic principle in diagnosing suspected abuse or neglect in a child is an incompatibility between the objective findings and the history, either as presented or implied. The number of reports of suspected child abuse seems to be increasing.[1,2] Whether we have reached a peak in reported cases is still unclear, but it is clear that the reported cases represent only the tip of the iceberg.

DEFINITIONS

Definitions are medical, legal, and practical. Child abuse and neglect is medically defined as nonaccidental injury to a minor child (usually under 18 years of age) without adequate explanation and/or failure to provide for needs of the child (medical, environmental, nutritional, educational, and emotional).

Legal definitions vary according to individual state laws.[2] In Maryland, nonsexual abuse is defined as

> physical injury or injuries sustained by a child as a result of cruel or inhumane treatment or as a result of malicious act or acts by any parent, adoptive parent or other person who has the permanent or temporary care or custody or responsibility for supervision of a minor child, or, any sexual abuse of a child, whether physical injuries are sustained or not.[3]

Sexual abuse is defined as

> any act or acts involving sexual molestation or exploitation, including but not limited to incest, rape or sexual offense in any degree, sodomy or unnatural or perverted sexual practices on a child by any parent, adoptive parent or other person who has the permanent or temporary care or custody or responsibility for supervision of a minor child.[4]

A neglected child is defined as

> a child who has suffered or is suffering significant physical or mental harm or injury as a result of conditions created by the absence of his parents, guardian or custodian, or by the failure of that person to give proper care and attention to the child and his problems.[5]

A practical definition to discriminate corporal punishment from abuse is that if the injury requires medical attention, it is child abuse.

CHARACTERISTICS

There are a number of commonly occurring findings that should arouse suspicion of abuse or neglect. A summary of these is given in Exhibit 39-1. (See also Exhibit 31-6 in Chapter 31, "Burns.")

The injured child is usually under 3 years of age. Several studies have suggested that 10% to 20% of

Exhibit 39-1 Indicators of Possible Child Abuse or Neglect

The injured child is under 3 yr of age.
The injuries found are not compatible with the history or are not mentioned in the history.
There is a history of similar episodes or of other suspicious injuries in the past.
There is a prolonged interval between sustaining the injuries and bringing the child in for care.
The activities ascribed to the child and said to be the cause of the injury are not compatible with the child's developmental abilities.
The child has injuries that appear to be in different stages of resolution.
There are soft tissue injuries of an unusual variety or in unexpected locations.
There is evidence of malnutrition, poor hygiene, and inappropriate dress.
The child is brought in by an adult who was not the caretaker at the time of the injury.
There is evidence of sexual abuse.

children under 7 years of age that are seen for emergency care have received nonaccidental injuries; 70% of these children are under 3 years of age.

A history must be obtained from the person caring for the child during the period when the injuries occurred, even if that person did not bring the child in for care. If the injuries found are not compatible with the history or are not mentioned in the history, there are a number of possible explanations. The caretaker could be the abuser and is unwilling to admit guilt, or the caretaker could be shielding the actual abuser or may not know how the child was injured but is unwilling to admit this, as doing so would reflect a lack of responsibility in assuring the child's well-being.

A history of similar episodes or of other suspicious injuries in the past should increase the level of suspicion about the current injury but should *never* be used to decide whether or not to report a suspicious situation. Referral to central registries that have been established in many states may identify a repetitive pattern.

Frequently, there may be a prolonged interval between the time the injuries occur and the time the child is brought in for care. However, extenuating circumstances, such as inability to pay for the visit or lack of transportation, could account for this and may, in themselves, be reasons for referrals to social service agencies.

The examiner must judge the activities ascribed to the child against the child's developmental abilities. The statement that injuries occurred because an infant 4 or 5 months old climbed out of a crib is an example of a history that is incompatible with the child's ability.

TABLE 39-1 Age of Contusions by Appearance

Color of Lesion	Approximate Age
Red, reddish blue, or purple	Initial state
Dark blue, bluish brown, or purple	2–4 d
Green to yellow-green	5–7 d
Yellow to brown	1–2 wk
Return to normal tint	2–4 wk

Source: Reprinted with permission from Wilson EF: Estimation of the age of cutaneous contusions in child abuse. *Pediatrics* 1977; 60:750–752.

Injuries that appear in different stages of resolution must have multiple explanations to account for them. Radiologic findings of fractures in various stages of resolution indicate injuries of different ages. Contusions of soft tissue can be staged according to age, as indicated in Table 39-1.

Soft tissue injuries of unusual variety and in unexpected locations should arouse suspicion. Lesions from direct nonthermal trauma may have the shape of the striking object, such as the loops of an electric cord, the shape of a belt buckle, or the shape of a hand. The question of discriminating child abuse from corporal punishment is most frequently raised in lesions of this type. The circumstances surrounding the striking of the child and the location of the lesion(s) must be considered in answering this question. Most corporal punishment is administered during periods of high emotional stress and relatively low self-control, so the part of the child that is struck and the severity of the injury are usually determined by chance. Even so, children can be and frequently are seriously injured under such circumstances; thus these injuries mandate reporting of suspected abuse.

Thermal injuries, both burns and cold injuries, can also be suspicious because of their shape and location. The injury may take the shape of common hot objects, such as pressing or curling irons, cigarette tips, and heating grills, and an appropriate explanation must be obtained. Burns from hot liquids present special characteristics that permit differen-

TABLE 39-2 Characteristics of Thermal Injuries from Hot Liquids

	Splash	Immersion
Distribution	Irregular, not circumferential	Stocking/glove, sharp line of demarcation
Depth	More superficial, varies from center to edge	Deeper, more even
Typical age and story	Toddler Pulled over container of hot liquid	Infant Put in hot bath water

TABLE 39-3 Behavioral Presentations of Child Sexual Abuse

Precocious sexual interest and/or behavior
Involvement with pornographic materials
Acting-out behaviors, that is, running away
Deteriorating school performance
Poor peer relationship
Seductive behavior
Depression, decreased self-esteem
Aggressive behavior, violent acts
Antisocial behavior such as stealing

tiation of splash from immersion (Table 39-2). (See also Chapter 31, "Burns," and Figure 31-6.)

Concomitant, nonspecific observations, including evidence of malnutrition, poor hygiene (especially in the child too young for self-care), and inappropriate dress for the weather, require care to discriminate, if possible, the effects of poverty from those of neglect. Either case necessitates involvement of social services.

The child may be brought in by an adult who was not the caretaker at the time of the injury(ies) and who is concerned about the child's care when the caretaker appears not to be. Whenever such a question is raised, social service involvement is indicated, usually via a report of suspected child abuse or neglect. Such situations need to be approached cautiously as the adults involved may have competing interests in the child or other motivations for creating the appearance of neglect and/or abuse by the other.

A child who has been sexually abused may present to the physician or other health care providers in a variety of ways (Table 39-3).

Sexually Transmitted Diseases

The finding in a prepubertal child of disease that is transmitted sexually means, until proved otherwise, that child has been sexually abused. Such diseases currently include gonorrhea, syphilis, condyloma acuminata (venereal warts), and Herpes Type II. Some sexually transmitted diseases are also transmitted nonsexually (such as chlamydia, trichomonas, Hepatitis B, and Herpes Type I) and should arouse suspicions of sexual abuse. In such situations, further history should be obtained, additional physical indicators sought, and appropriate laboratory studies performed (cultures for gonorrhea, serology for syphilis, possibly cultures for chlamydia, and Herpes).

Despite the theoretical possibility of transfer of sexually transmitted diseases by fomites or other nonsexual means,[1] the presence of one or more of these infections in a prepubertal child is almost always the result of sexual abuse.

Revelations by the Victim (or Others)

With increasing frequency, child sexual abuse has been presenting as revelations by the victim, either spontaneously or upon questioning. Since there is no way a young child, with the concrete thinking characteristic of this age group, can fabricate or fantasize an experience that represents adult sexual activity unless the child personally experienced the activity, such revelations virtually always are accurate and thus should be believed. Whenever a situation suspicious for child sexual abuse presents, the child must be given an appropriate opportunity to reveal what has been done to him or her and by whom. The number of times the child has to tell his or her story should be kept to the absolute minimum (preferably only once) by coordinating the questioning of the health care provider, the Department of Social Services investigator, the police, and the State Attorney. Where appropriate, anatomically correct drawings and/or dolls should be used to permit the child flexibility in how the story is told.

Sometimes one victim will reveal sexual abuse that is occurring or has occurred to another victim (or victims), such as in a group-care setting. Such revelations should be believed and taken seriously, especially with the younger preschool child.

Occasionally an abuser, spontaneously, under interrogation or while in therapy will reveal that he or she has abused specific children, and such relevations must be followed up.

Behavior Presentations

Virtually any aberrant behavior by a child can be a manifestation of the child having been sexually abused, and a high index of suspicion must be maintained if such children are to be diagnosed correctly. Types of behavior that may be indicative of sexual abuse are listed in Table 39-4. The possibility of the child having been sexually abused must always be kept in mind when evaluating or treating childhood behavior problems.

TABLE 39-4 Presentations of Sexual Abuse

1. Sexually transmitted diseases
   - Gonorrhea, Syphilis, Condyloma Acuminata, Herpes Type II
2. Revelations by victims or others
   - Confessions by abusers
   - Revelations by other victims or witnesses
   - Revelations by child victims, spontaneous or on questioning
3. Behavior presentations
   - Sexual behavior inappropriate for child's developmental level
   - Nonsexual behavior, depression, aggression, school performance

THE REPORTING OBLIGATION

It is only a suspicion that is necessary to mandate a report. Essentially all of the states and territories now have laws that require reporting the suspicion of child abuse and neglect. Reports are made to an investigating agency, usually either the police department or the local department of social services, which is then required to investigate in a timely fashion and to take such actions as needed to protect the child, help the family deal with its problems, and meet the requirements of the law. Failure to report a suspected abuse carries the threat of possible malpractice action against the health care provider when that nonreportage results in further injury or even death to the child. Such malpractice actions have been brought in at least two states, and, at the lower court levels, providers have been held liable for such further injuries. The threat of malpractice should not be the motivating factor in determining the health care provider's willingness to cooperate, but rather concern for the child and the family. It is appropriate for the physician to clearly inform the parent(s) or caretaker of the intention to report. Doing this results in a much greater chance for the relationship between the family and physician to be positive over the long term, even though there is frequently some short-term antagonism.

Exhibit 39-2 Components of History

1. Explanation(s) of the injury(ies) by victim directly, if possible
2. History of previous injuries
3. Past medical history, including illnesses, well-child care, immunizations, parental perceptions as to the health of the child ("He bruises easily.")
4. Family history, including medical history of siblings and other family members
5. Social history, including household composition, usual child care arrangements, socioeconomic circumstances, resources used by family in times of stress (e.g., family, friends, agencies)
6. Behavioral history of child and family, including expectations for the child, perceptions of actual behavior, history of behavior problems
7. History of drug or alcohol abuse and mental illness in child or family
8. Ascertaining if parent/caretaker wants the child placed away from him or her because of fear of harming the child. Direct questioning may be necessary to obtain this information
9. Observation and description of the parent(s)/caretaker's behavior, with as much objectivity as possible. Avoid judgment ("Mother was drunk."); use direct observations ("Mother staggered when she walked and smelled of alcohol on her breath.")
10. Acquisition of information from other sources, documented clearly and nonjudgmentally in the medical record. Use as little medical jargon as possible, as these records are usually read and used by nonmedical persons. Writing records in this manner can frequently result in a reduced need for the provider to be personally involved in the investigative and legal processes that may follow

EVALUATION OF THE CHILD

History

Obtaining a data base about the abused or neglected child and the child's family or caretaker is the single most important component of the evaluation. A history should be elicited from the parent(s)/caretaker about the circumstances surrounding the child's neglect or injury, as well as about the overall socioeconomic and environmental situation. If possible, the examiner should interview directly the person who was caring for the child at the time(s) the neglect or injury could have occurred. This may have to be done by telephone or at a time other than when the child is being seen, since many of these children are not brought for care by this person. It is important to use quotations of what is said by the parent(s)/caretaker. Other sources include the child (even at the earliest verbal age), other members of the household, siblings, relatives, neighbors, and investigators. Care should be taken not to ask leading questions, and, again, quotations should be used liberally. The initial history may be sparse, but further information may become available. Essential to the history is assessment of the potential risk of further harm to the child. Specifics of the history that should be included are shown in Exhibit 39-2.

The Interview of the Sexually Abused Child

The first task in interviewing a sexually abused child is to establish rapport in a situation comfortable to both the child and the interviewer. To prevent the child from having to repeat the events of the abuse, arrangements should be made to have those other professionals who need to hear the child's story present during the history taking. Sometimes this is not possible and/or not appropriate, although Maryland Law currently requires a combined investigation of suspected sexual abuse by the Department of Social Services, the police, and the State Attorney.[2]

The history of the incident(s) should be obtained from the child directly, using terms the child understands. It frequently is helpful to use anatomically correct drawings and/or dolls to get the child to indicate the parts of the anatomy involved, the names of which may be different for the child than for adults. History should be obtained from anyone who has information concerning the situation. This includes other members of the household, social workers, other health professionals, teachers, day care workers, or anyone who may have information that could assist in elucidating what actually happened.

It is important to go through a complete medical history, including a history of past illnesses, especially any history of past similar incidents. Questions concerning the child's allergy to medications are necessary in circumstances where treatment of the child for possible sexually transmitted disease is considered. A complete review of systems is indicated, paying special attention to the genitourinary tract. It is important to ascertain the psychological status of the child. As many incidents are repetitive and occur over extended periods of time, it is important to determine the child's function in school, in his/her family, and with his/her peers.

A critical consideration in taking the history from the child is to remember that once the child has "blown the whistle" on the abuser, he or she may be in immediate danger of further abuse or even death. It is imperative that the examiner and other professionals involved be in a position to protect the child with immediate placement in a safe environment, if this is needed.

Complete documentation of the history (as much as possible in the exact words used by those giving it) should be done in a clear, legible manner as this document frequently is used in the investigation, the legal process for protecting the child, and/or the prosecution of the abuser.

Physical Examination

The two basic principles of physical examination of the suspected abused or neglected child are completeness and documentation. The examination of the child should be as complete as the circumstances permit, including the child's behavior and interaction with the examiner, the family, and others. The examination should be as nontraumatic as possible, especially in cases of suspected sexual abuse. Examination of the genitalia must be part of the total examination and should be gentle. Instruments of any kind are to be used very rarely, if at all. *Never* force an examination. If necessary, use sedation: meperidine hydrochloride (Demerol), 2 mg/kg; promethazine hydrochloride (Phenergan), 1 mg/kg; and chlorpromazine (Thorazine), 1 mg/kg, all in one syringe and given intramuscularly. An evaluation of the child's emotional state and developmental level should be included to permit an assessment of the appropriateness of the parent(s)/caretaker's expectations for the child.

An instant camera can be used to record visible findings. Such photographs should be marked indelibly in the front margins with the child's name, medical record number (if any), the date and time, and name and signature of the person taking the photograph. The photograph is then made a permanent part of the child's medical record by physically attaching it to the medical record, using staples. The plotting of growth curves, when previous data are available, can be helpful.

THE PHYSICAL EXAMINATION OF THE SEXUALLY ABUSED CHILD

As this part of the evaluation of the sexually abused child is frequently necessary for court, careful documentation of the findings, both positive and negative, with legible notes is advisable.

Two basic principles to be followed in the physical examination of the sexually abused child are: first, do a complete physical examination; second, the examination should be as nontraumatic to the child as possible. Because many of these children have been physically abused in addition to having been sexually abused, it is important to do a complete physical examination. Inspection of areas that have been sexually abused is more acceptable to children in the context of a complete examination than as an isolated scrutiny of the abused parts, which could be construed by the child as comparable to the original abuse or worse.

It is important to assure privacy and concern for the child's modesty, and to provide a same-sex chaperone in the situation where the examination is being performed by a professional of the opposite sex. Whenever there is evidence of physical abuse or where the child is less than three years old, an occult trauma x-ray survey is recommended as this may reveal evidence of previous bony injuries that may not be obvious in the physical examination.

It should *never* be necessary to force an examination of the genital area. The vast majority of the time this part of the examination can be done atraumatically by putting it in the context of the complete physical. Having the child relax, not on an examining table but in the lap of a trusted adult, is frequently helpful for a preschool child. The child's willingness to relax and permit examination of the perineum is not a reliable indicator of the child's having been abused, rather the child's resistance to such an examination may suggest the child has been sexually abused.

In those children in whom such an examination is not possible without force, the use of some form of sedation, that is, so-called "lytic cocktail"(meperidine, two milligrams per kilogram; promethazine, one milligram per kilogram; and chlorpromazine, one milligram per kilogram, mixed in one syringe and given intramuscularly) is recommended. In very rare situations, it is necessary to use general anesthesia to adequately examine a sexually abused child.

Recently, new interpretations of findings on examination of the genital and anal areas of sexually abused children have permitted corroboration of histories far more often than previously.[6] In the female, genital sexual injuries can be differentiated from normal anatomy or accidental trauma. This can be done with an understanding of the functional anatomy of this area and a knowledge of the appearance of injured tissue. The external genitalia of the young girl can be divided into anterior and posterior sections by imagining the numbers of a clock face with the 12 anterior (symphysis pubis) and the 6 posterior (toward the anus) so that the introitus is in the center of the clock face. The anterior section would be above the 9 o'clock and 3 o'clock indicators and the posterior section would be below.

Tissue comprising the anterior section is rather tightly attached to the pubic rami and is involved in accidental (straddle-type) injury because of the relative immobility and position of that section of the genitalia relative to the bony pelvis. The posterior section is essentially suspended by the internal muscular supports of the pelvic organs, mostly the levator sling. Because of this suspended structure, this tissue can move considerably and essentially is not injured accidentally. However, during sexual activity, the vagina must be entered with a movement of the penetrating object posteriorly, so sexual molestation would cause injury to the posterior section of the genitalia. As full penetration of the vagina of small girls is very rare, these injuries are of a more subtle nature, comprising stretching and/or tearing of the hymenal or perihymenal tissue, again posteriorly (that is, below the 9 o'clock–3 o'clock line). These injuries, once healed, leave permanent scarring of this tissue which is apparent on close observation (with or without a culdoscope) as white scar tissue, distortion (usually asymmetrical) of the tissue, or both. The finding of such scars in the posterior section of the female genitalia is essentially diagnostic of previous sexual abuse with attempted penetration.

Another useful finding in the examination of the prepubertal girl is the size of the introital opening, which is normally no greater than 1 cm. in diameter and usually much less than that, especially in the younger child. An introital (actually hymenal) opening of greater than 1 cm. would indicate stretching of the introitus, indicating probable sexual abuse.

In both males and females, the anal orifice can demonstrate findings indicative of attempted or actual penetration. These findings are of similar scarring as described above, except there is no anterior/posterior discrimination of accidental versus sexually abusive injury. When the anus is dilated by the passage of a large stool, the stretching occurs from inside, while sexually abusive penetration is from the outside. The injury in passage of a large stool is thus internal (anal fissure or tear) involving the mucosal surface, while penetrating injury is more external, usually at the skin-mucosal border.

The above examinations can be done atraumatically and without invasion of the child (such as use of a speculum) in the vast majority of instances. All that is usually needed is a relaxed patient, a supportive, understanding examiner, and a bright light. Specimens for laboratory studies, as described in the next section, usually can be obtained relatively atraumatically using a flexible swab and sterile saline, if the tissue is dry.

X-ray and Laboratory Studies

All radiologic studies appropriate for the short-term management of the child must be obtained. X-ray films can be invaluable in identifying previously undetected fractures or physical injuries and may indicate the "age" of the trauma. *All* children under 3 years of age with suspected abuse *or* neglect plus any child for whom there is suspicion of injuries detectable radiologically should have survey films taken. Special signs to look for include epiphyseal separations and periosteal thickening, frequently caused by abrupt grasping, shaking, and twisting of the extremities, and transverse or oblique fractures of the midshafts of long bones and fingers as a result of having extremities "rapped." Radiologic findings noted on examinations for intercurrent illnesses may identify previously unsuspected cases. Nuclear medicine scans of bones may indicate injuries before they are evident on x-ray films and thus should be considered in specific cases.

Laboratory tests should be done as individually

indicated. Clotting studies are indicated in children in whom the pattern suggests a possible clotting disorder (such as petechiae, diffuse ecchymoses, or hemarthrosis).

LABORATORY EVALUATION

The laboratory evaluation of the prepubertal child suspected of having been sexually abused would include (*as indicated*): smears and cultures for gonorrhea, serology for syphilis, cell cultures for chlamydia, and/or cultures for Herpes Virus with immuno-identification of Type I or II.

1. UA/UC to rule out UTI or if suspect urinary system trauma
2. Saline prep from vulva, vagina, rectum, mouth to look for sperm (if 72 hr since last assault) or trichomonas (if a discharge or inflammation is present)
3. KOH prep from vulva or vagina if a discharge is present to look for yeast
4. Gram stain of any discharge present for GC or Clue cells. If + for GC, then is diagnostic in child, Rx and save slide in chart in case culture is negative
5. GC cultures (vulvae, vaginal, penile, rectal, pharyngeal) *as indicated* when hx, sx or physical findings suggest likelihood of + result. Remember that vulvovaginal, penile or rectal cultures may be more invasive (and thus more traumatic) than the original molestation. Consider this decision carefully
6. Chlamydial cultures—as for GC above
7. Herpes cultures if suspicious lesion
8. RPR—only if other STD seems likely. Follow up of children examined for molestation reveals they remember the blood drawing more than anything else that was done to them! Likelihood of + very low, especially without other STD
9. Pregnancy test should be done in all post-menarchal females.

Assessment of the Situation

It is the obligation of the physician to reach an impression or assessment of the situation. Only the suspicion of abuse or neglect is necessary to mandate reporting. It is *not* the task of the physician to conclusively prove whether either or both have occurred, but rather to act in the best interests of the child by detecting suspicious circumstances and letting the legally required agencies investigate. Usually, an appropriate impression is "suspected" abuse or neglect, with your perception of the degree of immediate risk to the child for further harm.

MANAGEMENT

Medical or surgical management of the injuries themselves is well covered in other parts of this text; hospitalization is not frequently involved. Management of these cases always results in involvement of other disciplines. The development of multidisciplinary teams to bring together the variety of professionals involved has resulted in better communication and thus better care for these children.

Children whose injuries do not require hospitalization but who require immediate protection may be placed in the home of a relative or in a temporary shelter or foster home. If such placements are not available or the family resists, the only alternative is to admit the child to the hospital, even though there may be no medical indication for admission. When the parent(s)/caretaker will not accept any placement of the child, it becomes necessary for the investigating agency to obtain a court order for emergency guardianship to protect the child.

Investigation of the reported suspicion of abuse or neglect is accomplished by a social service agency or a law enforcement agency. The child must be in a protected environment until the investigation can be completed.

Upon completion of the investigation, a decision will be made concerning further management. This can include legal action, social service support, mental health counseling, attendance at self-help groups (Parents Anonymous), and medical services on a regular basis, or no recommendation other than regular health care with further intervention only as indicated. A plan for long-term follow-up must be devised, with clear allocations of responsibility to specific individuals or agencies to ensure compliance.

LEGAL PROCESSES

Once a report has been made, whether by the practitioner or not, further involvement with the legal system may ensue. Specific rules and regulations differ in various states. A well-documented record with clearly stated conclusions and recommendations may save the practitioner from actually appearing in court as the investigation proceeds. Should the practitioner be required to appear in court, steps should be taken to assure that the appearance is as effective and convenient as possible. This can be done by conferring with the attorney who is calling the practitioner as a witness, so that details of the case and the practitioner's expected testimony are clear to both parties. Court schedules are rarely predictable, so an "on-call" arrangement frequently is the most efficient way for the practitioner to testify.

Criminal prosecution of child abusers is less common than civil petitioning on behalf of the child, but the same guidelines for practitioners' testimony would apply.

PREVENTION

It is clear that even our very best efforts on behalf of abused and neglected children can only partially correct the damage done, and ways to prevent the problem must be sought. Physicians caring for children can help by including extensive anticipatory guidance in the care they provide. When appropriate, parents should be referred to existing programs that teach normal child development and effective parenting skills and principles.

References

1. Bittner S, Newberger E: Pediatric understanding of child abuse and neglect. *Pediatr Rev* 1981;2:197–207.
2. Helfer RG, Kempe CH (eds): *The Battered Child*, ed 3. Chicago, University of Chicago Press, 1980.
3. Annotated Code of Maryland, Family Law Article, Subtitle 9, §5-901,b.
4. Ibid §5-901,j.
5. Ibid Subtitle 7, §5-701,g.
6. Woodling, B.A. "Clinical Signs of Acute and Chronic Sexual Abuse," presentation at Fifth International Congress on Child Abuse and Neglect, Montreal, September 1984.

Bibliography

Goldstein J, Freud A, Solnit AJ: *Beyond the Best Interests of the Child.* New York, The Free Press, 1973.

Goldstein J, Freud A, Solnit AJ: *Before the Best Interests of the Child.* New York, The Free Press, 1979.

Helfer RG, Kempe CH (eds): *Child Abuse and Neglect: The Family and the Community.* Cambridge, MA, Ballinger Publishing Co, 1976.

Shubin CI: Child abuse and neglect: Sexual abuse of prepubertal children. *Maryland Med J* 1985;35:503–508.

Index

F

I

R